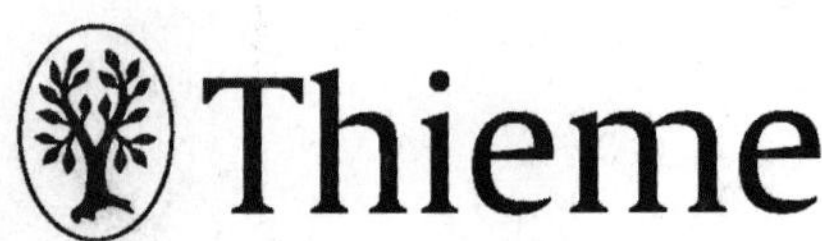
Thieme

Textbook of Plastic, Reconstructive, and Aesthetic Surgery

Volume VI
Aesthetic Surgery

Editor-in-Chief

Karoon Agrawal, MS, MCh
Senior Consultant
Plastic Surgery
National Heart Institute
New Delhi, India

Section Editors

Kuldeep Singh, MS, MCh
Senior Consultant
Department of Plastic, Reconstructive, and Aesthetic Surgery
Indraprastha Apollo Hospitals
New Delhi, India

Lokesh Kumar, MS, MCh, FICS
Senior Director and Head
Department of Plastic and Cosmetic Surgery
BLK Super Specialty Hospital
New Delhi, India

Anil K. Garg, MS, MCh, FISHRS
Plastic Surgeon
Rejuvenate Plastic, Cosmetic, and Hair transplant Centre;
Diplomate of the American Board of Hair Restoration Surgery
Indore, Madhya Pradesh, India

Rakesh Kalra, MS, MCh
Cosmetic and Plastic Surgeon
Ashirwad Hospital
Dehradun, Uttarakhand, India

K. Ramachandran, MS, MCh, MNAMS
Senior Consultant
Apollo Spectra Hospitals
Chennai, Tamil Nadu, India

Thieme
Delhi • Stuttgart • New York • Rio de Janeiro

Publishing Director: Ritu Sharma
Senior Development Editor: Dr Nidhi Srivastava
Director-Editorial Services: Rachna Sinha
Project Manager: Madhumita Dey
Illustrators: Sohaib Alam and Sushil Sardar
Vice President, Sales and Marketing: Arun Kumar Majji
Managing Director & CEO: Ajit Kohli

Thieme Medical and Scientific Publishers Private Limited.
A - 12, Second Floor, Sector - 2, Noida - 201 301,
Uttar Pradesh, India, +911204556600
Email: customerservice@thieme.in
www.thieme.in

Cover design: Thieme Publishing Group
Page make-up by RECTO Graphics, India

Printed in India by Nutech Print Services - India

5 4 3 2 1

ISBN: 978-81-948570-7-5
eISBN: 978-81-948570-3-7

Important note: Medicine is an ever-changing science undergoing continual development. Research and clinical experience are continually expanding our knowledge, in particular, our knowledge of proper treatment and drug therapy. Insofar as this book mentions any dosage or application, readers may rest assured that the authors, editors, and publishers have made every effort to ensure that such references are in accordance with **the state of knowledge at the time of production of the book**.

Nevertheless, this does not involve, imply, or express any guarantee or responsibility on the part of the publishers in respect to any dosage instructions and forms of applications stated in the book. **Every user is requested to examine carefully** the manufacturers' leaflets accompanying each drug and to check, if necessary, in consultation with a physician or specialist, whether the dosage schedules mentioned therein or the contraindications stated by the manufacturers differ from the statements made in the present book. Such examination is particularly important with drugs that are either rarely used or have been newly released in the market. Every dosage schedule or every form of application used is entirely at the user's own risk and responsibility. The authors and publishers request every user to report to the publishers any discrepancies or inaccuracies noticed. If errors in this work are found after publication, errata will be posted at www.thieme.com on the product description page.

Some of the product names, patents, and registered designs referred to in this book are in fact registered trademarks or proprietary names even though specific reference to this fact is not always made in the text. Therefore, the appearance of a name without designation as proprietary is not to be construed as a representation by the publisher that it is in the public domain.

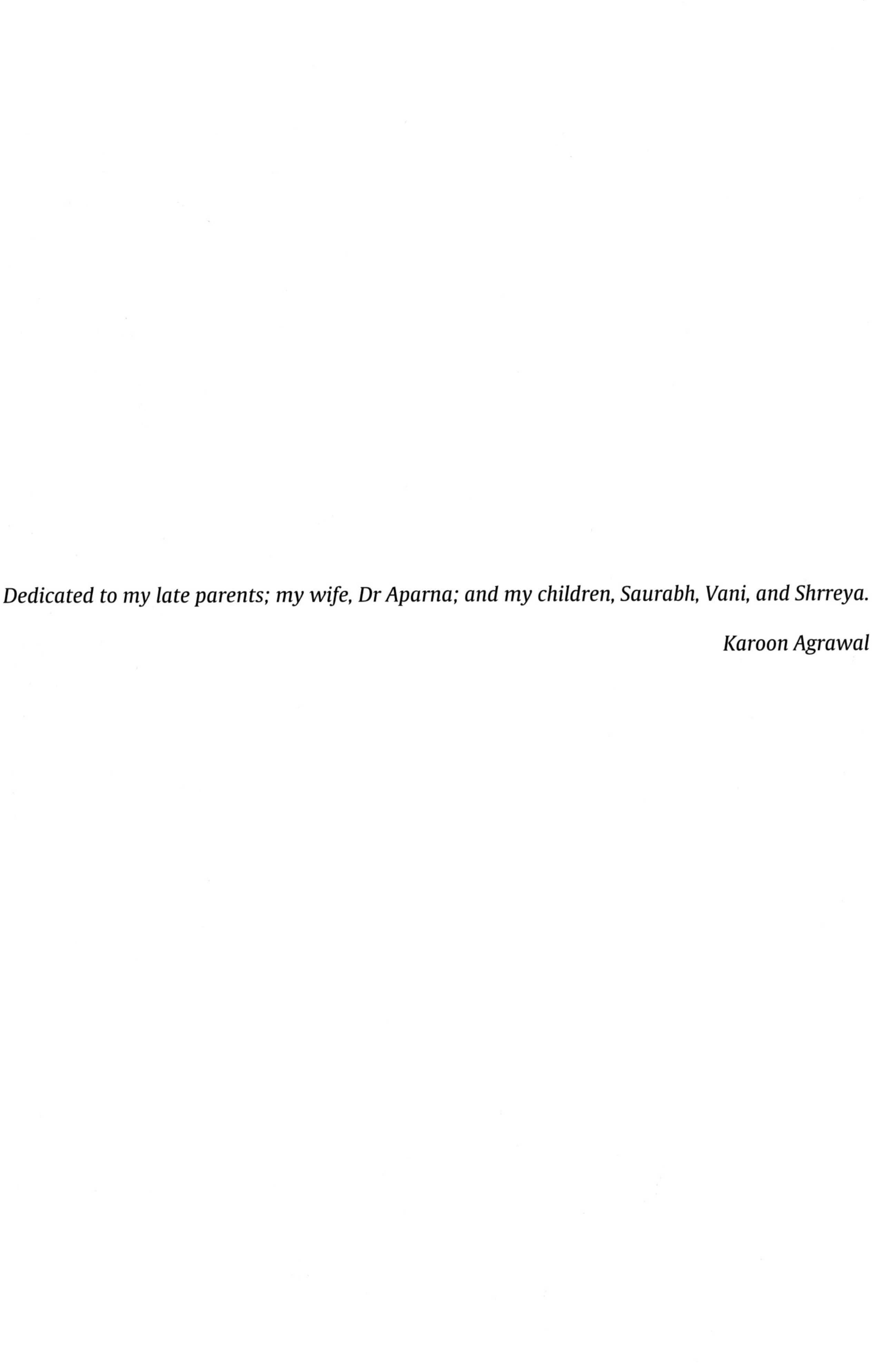

Dedicated to my late parents; my wife, Dr Aparna; and my children, Saurabh, Vani, and Shrreya.

Karoon Agrawal

Contents

Foreword

Do you set down your name in the scroll of youth that are written down old with all the characters of age? Have you not a moist eye, a dry hand, a yellow cheek, a white beard, a decreasing leg, an increasing belly? Is not your voice broken, your wind short, your chin double, your wit single, and every part about you blasted with antiquity? And will you yet call yourself young?

Henry IV, Part 11, Act 1

This is how the bard described middle age. Yellow cheeks, double chins, pendulous abdomen: the despised signs of aging are easily removed by modern aesthetic surgery, simply called by some as Cosmetic Surgery.

Aesthetics are important to Indian lives. Detailed description of arts, music, poetry, and other forms are mentioned in the Vedas. Rhinoplasties and other restorative procedures in the pre-Christian era are well documented and perhaps breathe origins into the present day methodology.

It is doubtful that the term "plastic surgery" was known to many people before the First World War. Wars have always acted as the most potent catalysts for the growth and innovations of surgical skills. Trench warfare of 1914–18 left behind a large number of survivors with gross facial deformities as a result of explosions in confined spaces and shrapnel, and all these people had to be rehabilitated in their civilian roles of peace time. The surgery of the period had no answers to these problems and to meet this challenge a band of Anglo-American surgeons bent their backs to the task. They molded human forms and features and so the term "plastic surgery" was born. The early years of this work extending into the 1920s saw surgeons with extraordinary surgical skills, possessed with creative imagination, inventing ingenious methods, and refinements in established surgical techniques, to make it possible to bridge tissue defects and deficiencies. Transfer of tissues from one part of the body to the other depended on retaining their blood circulation, which required meticulous technique, and therefore precision became a necessity for a plastic surgeon instead of what was a desirable trait. He could now mend large defects in the body without leaving telltale scars. The desirability of the restored part to comply with the beautiful pattern of the normal human body bred in him aesthetic sense. The word art was added to the craft of plastic surgery. Soon this newfound ability was used in the relief of ravages left behind by advancing age. People started flocking to plastic surgeons with sagging faces and other parts of the body, and seeking new leases of active life.

It should therefore become obvious that cosmetic surgery, which is the name by which the layman wishes to call aesthetic surgery, remains a small though demanding branch of plastic surgery—say 10% of the whole. Moreover, it is clear that a good cosmetic surgeon has to be a sound and fully trained plastic surgeon to begin with. The risk of suffering from problems associated with lack of knowledge and insufficient skill will have to be faced by the self-professed specialist.

Plastic surgery is also an attitude of mind. Of the ingredients of such a makeup first must be creative imagination, which would enable the surgeon to visualize the result before commencement of a reconstructive program, i.e., the set goal, and then to back this imagination a technical ability to put in effect what has been revealed. The surgeon must strive to create an effect as near perfect as nature itself. A humane and understanding heart is necessary to guide these efforts.

Short trips abroad, visiting some famous names, and collecting little known diplomas are perhaps the worst ways to get started in this work. I would recommend active apprenticeship with a proficient practitioner of this art as the only reliable mode of learning this demanding and precise branch of surgery. The patients must therefore look for this background in selecting their surgeons, and not get persuaded by writings in the lay press.

Fortunately, however, life's demands are not always of an emergency nature, of life or death, bread or starvation. Our vast social programs and the economic revolution that is taking place in this country aim at putting more and more people beyond the pale of extreme need. The increasing numbers of people who surface from this daily struggle will turn their attention to these requirements. 'The need for beauty is as positive a natural impulsion as the need for food' (L. Burbank). The modern competitive world requires large-scale services of the aesthetic surgeon and so will India.

A doctor's duty lies in making a patient feel better and not necessarily in judging his or her needs. Any surgery, including cosmetic surgery, is connected with pain, with discomfort. The fear of pain is a natural instinct. What are the motives of a person who anticipating pain, discomfort, and knowing the risk of complications willingly enters the hospital, lies down on the operating table to submit to an operation? It must be a chain of psychological reactions,

Note from Section Editors

Being a section editor for the Face section of this volume was an altogether new experience. *Textbook of Plastic, Reconstructive, and Aesthetic Surgery, Volume VI* is intended to be a textbook which would be contemporary as well as remain relevant in the Indian context. The selected authors are people who have extensive experience in this field. The editing, reviewing, and putting together of the chapters in this section required the cooperation of all authors. Working with Dr. Karoon Agarwal is as usual a very active and interactive affair, with him striving to push the envelope, while still remaining within the scope of the book. I feel that this volume will remain relevant to plastic surgeons for a very long time.

Kuldeep Singh, MS, MCh
Senior Consultant
Department of Plastic, Reconstructive, and Aesthetic Surgery
Indraprastha Apollo Hospitals
New Delhi, India

It is my privilege to be associated with *Textbook of Plastic, Reconstructive, and Aesthetic Surgery, Volume VI* as the Section Editor of the general aesthetic section. Aesthetic surgery is an important part of the spectrum of plastic surgery. This is considered to be synonymous with plastic surgery by a layman. Patients undergoing aesthetic surgery have very high expectations. Therefore, one has to provide exceptional outcome in order to satisfy an aesthetic patient. It is quite challenging as one has to maintain a fine balance between achieving sufficient enhancement and yet not giving a surgical look to the final outcome. Our training programs do not empower the young plastic surgeons to take this subspecialty as a career option soon after graduation. Knowledge of ethnic issues is perhaps more important in aesthetic surgery than any other branches of plastic surgery. Lack of reading material is also a major challenge faced by trainees.

An initial proposal by Dr. Karoon Agrawal, our Chief Editor, to bring out a textbook on plastic surgery, which would address these issues, was met with a lot of enthusiasm from all stakeholders. But this initial enthusiasm soon started fading as the magnanimity of the project started sinking in. Frankly speaking, I wanted to give up this responsibility many times but was not allowed to do so by Dr. Agrawal, and his handholding and encouraging words allowed each one of us to complete this mammoth task successfully.

This volume of aesthetic surgery is divided into many sections, each led by a section editor. Because of this shared responsibility, each one of us has been able to do justice to our respective section. Contributors to various chapters were carefully chosen to cover various issues previously lacking in other texts. I am glad that with this last volume, the whole textbook is now available for readers. I am sure this textbook will be of much help to our younger trainees as well as it will serve as a reference text for practitioners.

Lokesh Kumar, MS, MCh, FICS
Senior Director and Head
Department of Plastic and Cosmetic Surgery
BLK Super Specialty Hospital
New Delhi, India

I was excited to have an invitation from Dr. Karoon Agrawal to work on the hair restoration section of *Textbook of Plastic, Reconstructive, and Aesthetic Surgery, Volume VI*. This was a great experience as an editor. Hair restoration is a fusion of art and science. Surgery done by a plastic surgeon who has a sense of aesthetics will undoubtedly be of high quality. The specialty of hair restoration, unfortunately, has remained neglected for a long time, though it is a subspecialty of plastic surgery. Hence, many unqualified persons without an appropriate training perform this surgery, which discredited this procedure in society.

Though hair restoration is a vast field, we have tried to cover almost all parts of this field in order to provide basic knowledge about this process, information about advance techniques, and recent updates in this field.

I extend my sincere gratitude to our chief editor, Dr. Karoon Agrawal, for including hair restoration section in this textbook on aesthetic surgery.

Anil K. Garg, MS, MCh, FISHRS
Plastic Surgeon
Rejuvenate Plastic, Cosmetic, and Hair transplant Centre;
Diplomate of the American Board of Hair Restoration Surgery
Indore, Madhya Pradesh, India

The journey to create an aesthetic surgery section on body and trunk for this textbook has been a passionate labor of love. It is a small section, with very few chapters, but we have tried to cover everything possible. Dr. Karoon Agrawal has been a ring master, keeping an eagle's eye on each activity and guiding not only his section editors but also all contributors.

A lot of importance has been given to understanding the basics, for example, the chapters on obesity and bariatric surgery were developed before the ones on massive weight loss body contouring. The chapter on liposuction has a lot of technical details, so that the reader gains knowledge about the equipment required in this process. Another important factor that was considered was the clinical cross-section of patients from the Indian subcontinent, which is vastly different from the Western patients or even the Far Eastern patients. And lastly, and most importantly, the young plastic surgeons appearing for their qualifying examination as well as the young practitioners settling early in their profession were kept in mind while these chapters were written.

We hope that both clinicians and research-oriented readers shall benefit from this textbook.

Rakesh Kalra, MS, MCh
Cosmetic and Plastic Surgeon
Ashirwad Hospital
Dehradun, Uttarakhand, India

A volume dedicated entirely to aesthetic surgery in the Indian context indicates that we have made significant progress in this direction. When I started aesthetic surgery practice under Dr. S. Arumugam at Apollo Hospitals Chennai, back in 1986, we were trying to start a trend in the field. Little did I realize that we will be writing a volume on aesthetic surgery.

As a section editor of the breast surgery section, I had to formulate the chapters and select the authors who could write on each aspect. The emphasis was on Indian experience. All the authors are plastic surgeons with rich experience and credibility. It was a time-consuming process but at the end of the day it was an exercise worth undertaking. Patients seeking aesthetic breast surgery in the Indian scenario are a little different from those elsewhere. Most of them would not want scars from the surgery, and would want permanent results and long-term solutions. It is extremely important to make them understand not only about the surgery but also about the limitations of its results, scars, longevity of implants, need for revision, etc., thereby clearing up misconceptions. The authors have done a commendable job keeping this in mind, thereby enabling the young postgraduates joining the plastic surgery journey understand its relevance. This textbook will also be a good reference for the experienced plastic surgeons engaged in teaching and practicing aesthetic surgery.

K. Ramachandran, MS, MCh, MNAMS
Senior Consultant
Apollo Spectra Hospitals
Chennai, Tamil Nadu, India

About the Editors

Karoon Agrawal, MS, MCh, is currently a Senior Consultant of Plastic Surgery at National Heart Institute, New Delhi, India. He is also currently the Chairman of Institute Ethical Committee at Institute of Pathology (ICMR), New Delhi, India. He is the founder Editor-in-Chief of the Journal of Cleft Lip Palate and Craniofacial Anomalies and has more than 150 publications in national and international journals and chapters in books of repute.

Kuldeep Singh, MS, MCh, is a Senior Consultant at the Department of Aesthetic, Plastic, and Reconstructive Surgery at Indraprastha Apollo Hospital, New Delhi, India. He has a special interest in nonsurgical rejuvenation of the face, and is an invited faculty in many International and National conferences.

Lokesh Kumar, MS, MCh, FICS, is Senior Director and Head of the Department of Plastic and Cosmetic Surgery at BLK Super Specialty Hospital, New Delhi, India. He was Ethicon visiting Professor in Aesthetic surgery, awarded by Association of Plastic Surgeons of India in 2012 and has been a visiting Professor at various National and International Universities.

Anil K. Garg, MS, MCh, FISHRS, is a Plastic Surgeon at Rejuvenate Plastic, Cosmetic, and Hair transplant Centre and a Diplomate of the American Board of Hair Restoration Surgery (ABHRS). He is currently the president-elect for the Association of Hair Restoration Surgeons of India. He has written numerous chapters in various books pertaining to hair restoration and is also a Co-editor of a book on hair transplant.

Rakesh Kalra, MS, MCh, is a Cosmetic and Plastic Surgeon with concentration of work in Aesthetic Surgery at Ashirwad Hospital, Dehradun, Uttrakhand, India. He is the President of Indian Association of Aesthetic Plastic Surgeons, and Assistant National Secretary of International Society of Aesthetic Plastic Surgery. He is the Founder Member of IMA Blood Bank Society of Dehradun.

K. Ramachandran, MS, MCh, MNAMS, is Senior Consultant, Apollo Spectra Hospitals, Chennai, Tamil Nadu, India. He was the Past President of the Indian Association of Aesthetic Plastic Surgeon and President of Association of Hair Restoration Surgeons of India.

Contributors

Adarsh Chaudhary, MS, FRCS
Chairman
Department of GI Surgery, GI Oncology, and Bariatric Surgery
Medanta-The Medicity
Gurugram, Haryana, India

Aditya Aggarwal, MS, MCh, DNB
Director
Department of Plastic, Aesthetic, and Reconstructive Surgery
Medanta-The Medicity
Gurugram, Haryana, India

Amit R. Peswani, MCh, DNB
Assistant Professor
Department of Plastic Surgery
Topiwala National Medical College
B. Y. L. Nair Charitable Hospital
Mumbai, Maharashtra, India

Aniketh Venkataram, MS, MCh, FDAFPRAS (Belgium), FASAPS (USA)
Consultant Plastic and Hair Transplant Surgeon
Venkat Center for Skin and Plastic Surgery
Bengaluru, Karnataka, India

Anil K. Garg, MS, MCh, FISHRS
Plastic Surgeon
Rejuvenate Plastic, Cosmetic, and Hair transplant Centre;
Diplomate of the American Board of Hair Restoration Surgery
Indore, Madhya Pradesh, India

Anil N. Tibrewala, MS, MCh
Consultant and Plastic and Cosmetic Surgeon
P. D. Hinduja Hospital and Medical Research Center;
Saifee Hospital;
Breach Candy Hospital;
Sir H.N. Reliance Foundation Hospital;
Hinduja Healthcare
Khar, Mumbai, India

Antony Arvind, FRCSI, FRCS (England)
Consultant Plastic, Reconstructive, and Cosmetic Surgeon
Apollo Hospitals
Chennai, Tamil Nadu, India

Arjun Krishnadas, MDS
Assistant Professor
Department of Oral and Maxillofacial Surgery
Amrita School of Dentistry
Ponekkara, Kochi, India

Ashish Davalbhakta, MD, MS, MCh, FRCS (Glasgow)
Consultant and Aesthetic Plastic Surgeon
Advanced Aesthetics and Aesthetics MediSpa;
Professor
Department of Plastic Surgery
Aesthetic Plastic Surgery Maharashtra University of Health Sciences
Pune, Maharashtra, India

Ashok Gupta, MS, MCh, MNAMS, DNB, FRCS (Edinberg), DSc, MPhil, FNAMS
Senior Consultant
Division of Plastic and Reconstructive Surgery
Bombay Hospital Institute of Medical Sciences
Mumbai, Maharashtra, India

Borko Stojanovic, MD
Assistant Professor
Department of Urology and Surgery
School of Medicine
University of Belgrade;
Belgrade Center for Genital Reconstructive Surgery
Belgrade, Serbia

Chiranjiv Chhabra, MD (Dermatology)
Aesthetic Dermatologist and Director
Alive Clinics
New Delhi, India

Deepti Gupta, MS, MCh
Assistant Professor
Department of Burns, Plastic, and Maxillofacial Surgery
Safdarjung Hospital and VMMC
New Delhi, India

Hardeep Singh, MS, MCh
Senior Consultant
Medanta division of Plastic, Aesthetic, and Reconstructive Surgery
Medanta-The Medicity
Gurugram, Haryana, India

Heide Mills, MRCS, ENT
Otolaryngology Specialist Registrar
The Royal London Hospital
Barts Health NHS Trust
Whitechapel, London, United Kingdom

J. Sarah Crowley, MD
Resident
Division of Plastic Surgery
University of California
San Diego, California, USA

James Roy Kanjoor, MS, MCh, FRCS
Senior consultant in Cosmetic Surgery
Roys Cosmetic Surgery Centre
Coimbatore, Tamil Nadu, India

Jijo Joseph, MB, MRCS (Edinberg), DNB
Resident
Department of Plastic Surgery
Apollo First Med Hospital
Chennai, Tamil Nadu, India

K. Ramachandran, MS, MCh, MNAMS
Senior Consultant
Apollo Spectra Hospitals
Chennai, Tamil Nadu, India

Kapil S. Agrawal, MS, MCh
Professor
Department of Plastic Surgery
GSMC and KEM Hospital
Mumbai, Maharashtra, India

Khushbu Mahajan, MD (Dermatology)
Consultant Dermatologist
Kubba Skin Clinic;
Mahajan Skin Centre
New Delhi, India

Klaus Ueberreiter, MD
Chief Plastic Surgeon
Park-KlinikBirkenwerder
Birkenwerder, Germany

Kuldeep Singh, MS, MCh
Senior Consultant
Department of Plastic, Reconstructive, and Aesthetic Surgery
Indraprastha Apollo Hospitals
New Delhi, India

Kulwant S.Bhangoo, MD, FACS, FICS, FIMSA, FAIS, FRCS
Chief of Plastic Surgery
Mercy Hospital;
Clinical Assistant Professor
Department of Plastic Surgery
State University of New York
Buffalo, New York, USA

Lakshyajit Dhami, MS, MCh
Consultant and Aesthetic,Laser, and Plastic Surgeon
Vasudhan Cosmetic Plastic Surgery
Mumbai, Maharashtra, India

Lokesh Kumar, MS, MCh, FICS
Senior Director and Head
Department of Plastic and Cosmetic Surgery
BLK Super Specialty Hospital
New Delhi, India

Manoj Khanna, MS, MCh, DNB
Consultant Plastic and Cosmetic Surgeon
Enhance Clinics
Kolkata, West Bengal, India

Maria Kuriakose, MDS, PhD
Professor
Department of Orthodontics and Dentofacial Orthopedics
Amrita School of Dentistry
Ponekkara, Kochi, India

Marko Bencic, MD
Assistant Professor
Department of Urology and Surgery
Belgrade Centre for Genitourinary Reconstructive Surgery
Belgrade, Serbia

Marta Bizic, MD, PhD
Associate Professor
Department of Urology and Surgery
School of Medicine
University of Belgrade;
Belgrade Center for Genital Reconstructive Surgery
Belgrade, Serbia

Medha Khair Bhave, MS, DNB (General Surgery), MCh, DNB
Plastic Surgeon
Nitin Speciality Clinic
Naupada- Thane West
Maharashtra

Miroslav Djordjevic, MD, PhD
Professor
Department of Urology and Surgery
School of Medicine
University of Belgrade;
Belgrade Center for Genital Reconstructive Surgery
Belgrade, Serbia

Mohan Rangaswamy, MS, DNB, MCh, FRCS
Consultant Plastic Surgeon;
Chief of Surgery
American Academy of Cosmetic Surgery Hospital
Dubai, UAE

Nakul G. Patel, FRCS
Consultant Plastic Surgeon
University Hospitals of Leicester
Leicester, England, United Kingdom

Neeta Patel, MS, MCh
Hon. Plastic and Reconstructive Surgeon
Karuna Hospital;
Navneet Hospital;
HCG hospitals;
Mumbai, Maharashtra, India

Neha Chauhan, MS, MCh
Consultant Plastic Surgeon
Department of Plastic Surgery
La Femme Fortis
Bengaluru, Karnataka, India

Niti Khunger, MD, DDV, DNB
Professor, Consultant Dermatologist, and Head
Department of Dermatology and STD
Safdarjung Hospital and VMMC
New Delhi, India

Peter Scott, MBBCh, FRCS (Edinburgh)
Consultant Plastic and Reconstructive Surgeon
Morningside Mediclinic
Sandton, Johannesburg, South Africa

Pramod Subash, MDS, DNB, MNAMS, MOMSRCPS (Glasgow), FIBCSOMS, Dip. American Board (OMFS)
Professor
Department of Oral and Maxillofacial Surgery
Amrita School of Dentistry
Ponekkara, Kochi, India

Rajat Gupta, MS, DNB
Consultant Plastic Surgeon
RG Aesthetics
New Delhi, India

Rajesh Kumar Watts, MS, MCh
Consultant Plastic Surgeon
Department of Plastic Surgery
Indraprastha Apollo Hospitals
New Delhi, India

Rajesh Rajput, MS, MCh
Aesthetic and Hair Transplant Surgeon
Yavana Aesthetic Clinic
Mumbai, Maharashtra, India

Rakesh K. Khazanchi, MS, MCh
Chairman
Medanta division of Plastic, Aesthetic, and Reconstructive Surgery
Medanta-The Medicity
Gurugram, Haryana, India

Rakesh Kalra, MS, MCh
Cosmetic and Plastic Surgeon
Ashirwad Hospital
Dehradun, Uttarakhand, India

Ranjit Kumar Sahu, MCh
Associate Professor and Head
Department of Plastic Surgery
All India Institute of Medical Sciences (AIIMS)
Jodhpur, Rajasthan, India

Ratchathorn Panchaprateep, MD, PhD, FISHRS
Associate Professor
Division of Dermatology
Department of Medicine
Faculty of Medicine
Chulalongkorn University
Pathumwan, Bangkok, Thailand

Sandeep S. Sattur, MS, MCh
Hair Restorative Surgeon
Hair revive—Centre for Hair Restoration and Skin Rejuvenation;
Wockhardt Hospital
Mumbai, Maharashtra, India

Sandeep Sharma, MS, MCh
Director
AesthetiqueCentre
Alkapuri, Gujarat, India

Sandip Jain, MS, MCh, FRCS
Consultant Plastic and Aesthetic Surgeon
Saifee Hospital;
Breach Candy Hospital;
Wockhardt Hospital;
Bhatia Hospital;
Mumbai, Maharashtra, India

Sanjay Kumar Yadunath Parashar, MS, MCh, DNB, MNAMS, FICS
Plastic Surgeon
Cocoona Centre for Aesthetic Transformation and Day Surgery Hospital;
Dubai London Hospital;
Emirates Hospital
Dubai, UAE

Sanjay Mahendru, MS, MCh
Associate Director
Medanta division of Plastic, Aesthetic, and Reconstructive Surgery
Medanta-The Medicity
Gurugram, Haryana, India

Santdeep Paun, FRCS
Consultant and Facial Plastic Surgeon
The Royal London Hospital
Barts Health NHS Trust
Whitechapel, London, United Kingdom

Satyaswarup Tripathy, MCh
Additional Professor
Department of Plastic Surgery
All India Institute of Medical Sciences (AIIMS)
Jodhpur, Rajasthan, India

Seema Garg, MSc, FISHRS
Hair Transplant Surgeon
Rejuvenate Plastic, Cosmetic, and Hair transplant Centre;
Diplomate of the American Board of Hair Restoration Surgery
Indore, Madhya Pradesh, India

Shivram Bharadwaj, DNB, FRCS (Edinberg), FRCS
Senior Consultant Plastic Surgeon
Apollo Hospitals;
Sundaram Medical Foundation;
Hon. Consultant Plastic Surgeon
Southern Railways Headquarters Hospital
Chennai, Tamil Nadu, India

Shrirang Pandit, MS, MCh
Plastic Surgeon
Poona Hospital and Research Center;
N.M.Wadia Institute of Cardiology
Pune, Maharashtra, India

Slavica Pusica, MD
Assistant Professor
Department of Urology and Surgery
Belgrade Centre for Genitourinary Reconstructive Surgery
Belgrade, Serbia

Soni Nanda, MD (Dermatology)
Consultant Dermatologist and Founder
Shine and Smile Skin Clinic
Max Hospitals
New Delhi, India

Steven R. Cohen, MD
Clinical Professor
Division of Plastic Surgery
University of California;
Medical Director
FACES+Plastic Surgery, Skin and Laser Center
San Diego, California, USA

Subair Mohsina, MS
Senior Resident
Department of Plastic Surgery
Post Graduate Institute of Medical Education and Research (PGIMER)
Chandigarh, India

Sukhdeep Singh, MS, MCh
Consultant
Department of Plastic, Aesthetic, and Reconstructive Surgery
Medanta-The Medicity
Gurugram, Haryana, India

1

Approach to Aesthetic Surgery Patient

K. Ramachandran and Jijo Joseph

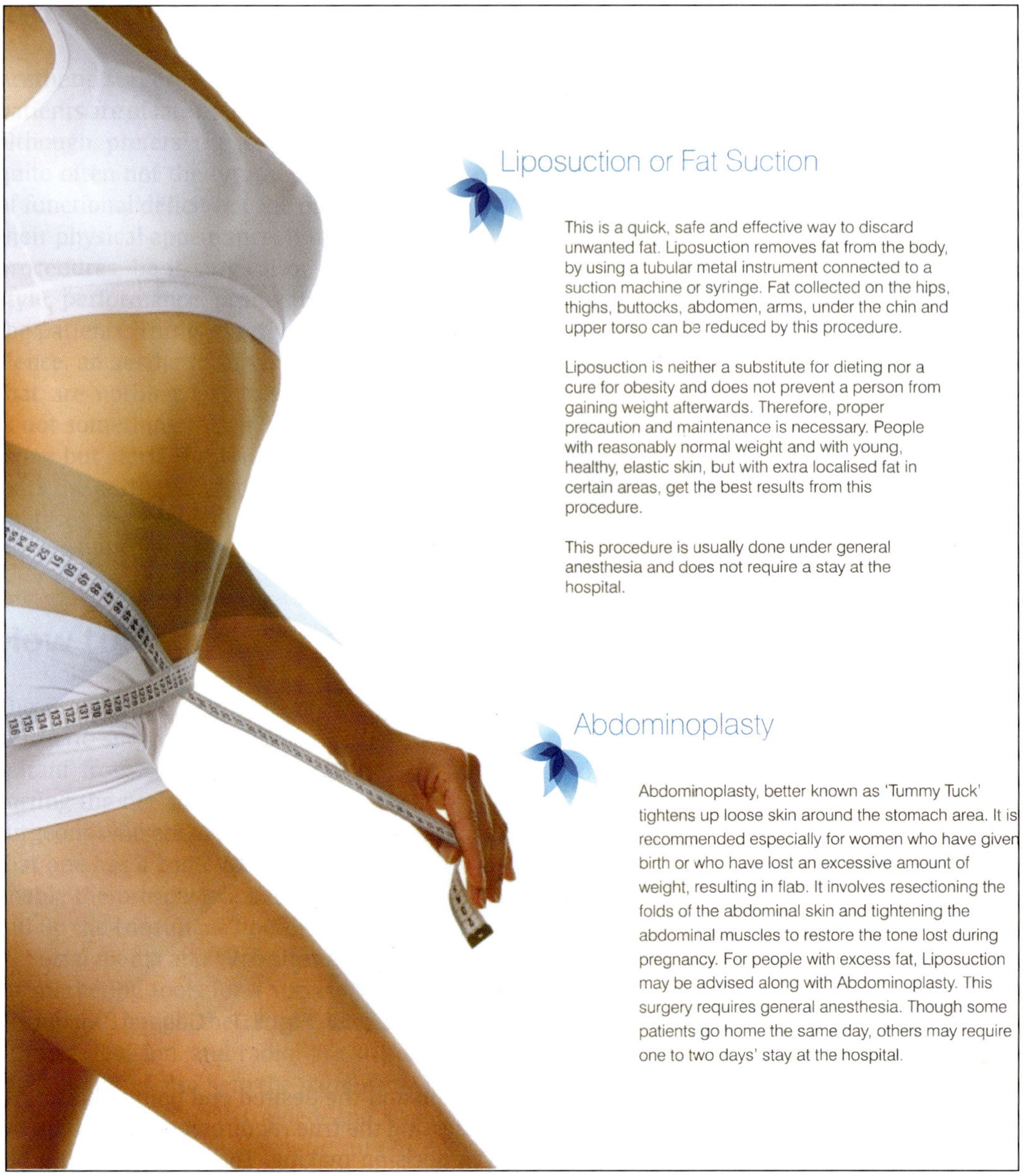

Liposuction or Fat Suction

This is a quick, safe and effective way to discard unwanted fat. Liposuction removes fat from the body, by using a tubular metal instrument connected to a suction machine or syringe. Fat collected on the hips, thighs, buttocks, abdomen, arms, under the chin and upper torso can be reduced by this procedure.

Liposuction is neither a substitute for dieting nor a cure for obesity and does not prevent a person from gaining weight afterwards. Therefore, proper precaution and maintenance is necessary. People with reasonably normal weight and with young, healthy, elastic skin, but with extra localised fat in certain areas, get the best results from this procedure.

This procedure is usually done under general anesthesia and does not require a stay at the hospital.

Abdominoplasty

Abdominoplasty, better known as 'Tummy Tuck' tightens up loose skin around the stomach area. It is recommended especially for women who have given birth or who have lost an excessive amount of weight, resulting in flab. It involves resectioning the folds of the abdominal skin and tightening the abdominal muscles to restore the tone lost during pregnancy. For people with excess fat, Liposuction may be advised along with Abdominoplasty. This surgery requires general anesthesia. Though some patients go home the same day, others may require one to two days' stay at the hospital.

Fig. 1.2 General brochure.

Examination

While doing a physical examination, the privacy of the patient should be respected and utmost gentleness should be observed. The way the patient is dressed at consultation is noted. Is he/she appropriately dressed or rather too casual or flashy or provocative? What does his/her body language indicate? Is he/she shabbily dressed? The consultation suite including the examination area should be done up tastefully.

A proper physical examination is essential in performing the correct surgery. First and foremost step is to "LOOK." This gives a broader picture of the problem. Next step is to "FEEL." This completes the examination. For example, a nasal deformity can be associated with internal nasal valve collapse or absence of nasal bones which cannot be differentiated unless the surgeon performs the "Cottle test" or a proper palpation, examining the bony structure of the nose.

Examining the female patient is always done with a chaperone, preferably a nurse. Also, a lady plastic surgeon when examining a man should always have a nurse with her. Good lighting is necessary. A full size as well as a handheld mirror is essential. One should keep the conversation on during the examination to make the atmosphere informal and comfortable. The body parts to be examined should be adequately exposed while covering the rest of the body. Any irregularity, inequality, asymmetry, etc., should be pointed out. These help in making the patient follow what you are trying to say, and also appreciate certain features of their body/face which they don't seem to have noticed before. Simultaneously, the

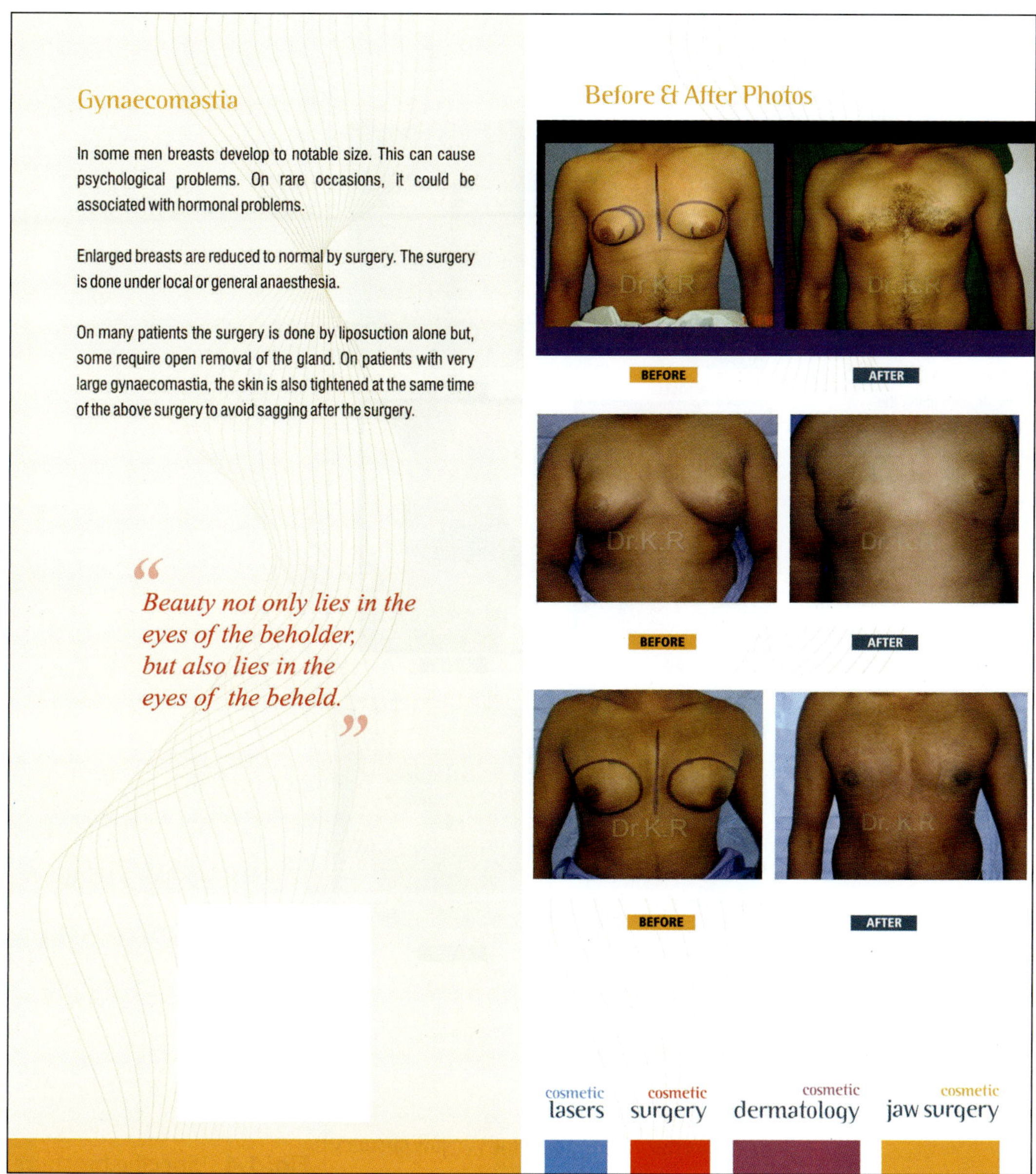

Fig. 1.3 Specific brochure: gynecomastia.

anticipated effects of the procedure can be demonstrated to them. All the features, important points of discussion, and the management plan should be documented, so that they are not missed out.

Problem Analysis

Assessing the Real Problem

This is the most important step in the assessment of a patient who has presented for a cosmetic surgery procedure. It is the sum total of history and physical examination findings. For a particular diagnosis, different treatment strategies are thought of, and from these strategies the best one is chosen based on the patient assessment and their comorbidities, if any. For example, if a patient presents with abdominal skin excess and abdominal wall laxity associated with large ventral hernia, the surgeon might avoid or be cautious about performing liposuction along with abdominoplasty. Similarly if a patient is a chronic smoker, he/she should be put off smoking for at least a period of 3 weeks before the procedure in order to prevent wound-healing problems.[8–10]

Assessing the Patient

This is a very important and sensitive aspect of aesthetic surgery. Not all patients who approach an aesthetic surgeon are candidates for undergoing the procedure. "Effort spent in case selection is time well utilized."[11] The surgeon should

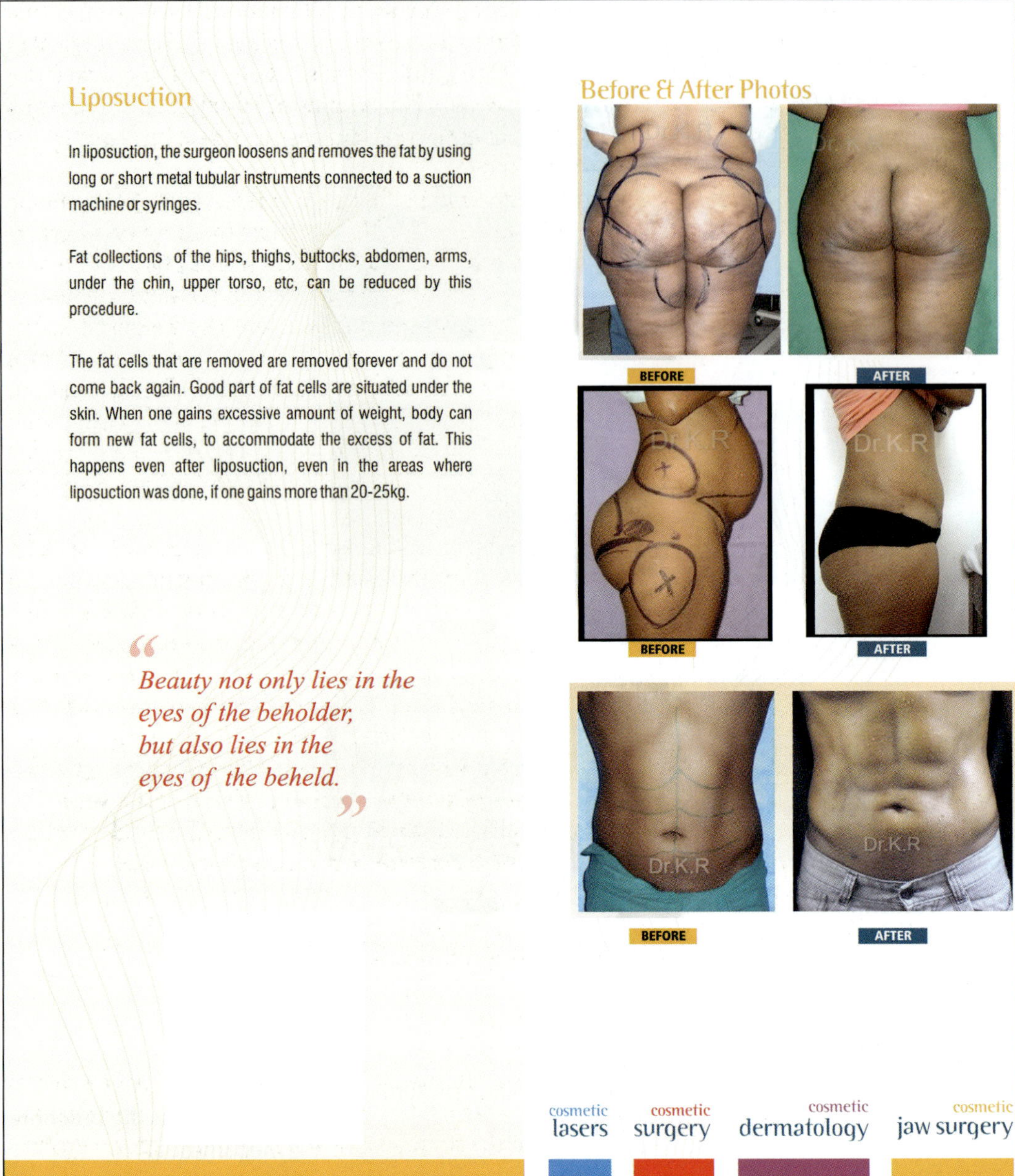

Fig. 1.4 Specific brochure: liposuction.

be very cautious about a patient who is not clear about the problem he/she has. An *ideal patient* who presents for nasal deformity correction should be the one who points out that "my nose is very broad," "I would like to have a sharp nasal tip," etc. This subset of patients is very clear about their objectives and is more realistic about their outcomes.

There is another subset of patients who say "whatever you say, doctor" or "whatever you feel the best, doctor." These patients have only a vague perception of what they want to get corrected and are more likely to be dissatisfied with the outcome.[12] Sometimes, they are testing whether you can find out their problem.

Some patients keep on praising the surgeon. One should be more careful with such patients. The moment they feel that something is not right or some complication has happened, they become hyperanxious and start cursing the surgeon for the unfortunate events that occurred.

There are some patients who repeatedly interrupt the flow of conversation. It is important to talk with the patient rather than just explaining randomly about a procedure. At the same time one should be able to cut off discussions which are irrelevant and continue to concentrate on the areas which are important.

Some prospective patients would have had previous cosmetic surgical procedures elsewhere. They may be unhappy with the results and would have come for a possible revision. One needs to take a close look to see whether the problem being pointed out is really genuine. Is it something that is obvious and needs to be fixed? Be careful of the patient who is bickering and criticizing the previous surgeon while praising you at the time of consultation.

Patients who are on medical treatment for psychological conditions need to be assessed well. An emotional decision to have a surgery on account of a strained relationship or a broken marriage is not a good one. This is called "surgery for secondary gain." Those who are on strong medications/psychotherapy need to get assessed by their physician or psychiatrist.[11,12] Studies have shown that 30 to 70% of patients who sought plastic and cosmetic surgery had some psychiatric problems[13–17] such as body dysmorphic disorder (BDD), depression, etc.[18] A male patient presents with a greater psychological risk than a female.[12] If not evaluated before surgery, it can lead to mental stress if the results are greatly different from patient's expectations or can lead to psychological distress even after successful treatment in those patients who already had psychiatric disorder preoperatively.[4,18]

Diagnosing a patient who has BDD is a challenge as far as aesthetic surgeons are concerned. According to DSM-IV (*Diagnostic and Statistical Manual of Mental Disorders*), BDD is a "psychiatric condition defined as an excessive preoccupation with an imagined or slight defect in appearance, which leads to significant distress or impairment in social, occupational, or other areas of functioning."[19] The hallmark of BDD is the excessive concern or distress over minor or nonexistent flaws in the appearance.[19] Other warning signs include "excessive detailing of the perceived flaw or defect, or contrarily not being able to describe exactly what they are seeking to improve and repetitive behaviors such as mirror checking. Excessive requests for cosmetic surgeries or procedures, dissatisfaction with the results of prior surgery that does not correlate with the objective outcome, camouflaging behavior, unrealistic expectations in terms of cosmetic outcome, expectations that the cosmetic procedure will be the solution to problems in other areas of life are some of the warning signs."[20] To identify these, the surgeon should do a thorough interview at the first consultation and should request for additional records and a psychiatry consultation. Once a patient is identified or suspected of having BDD, an additional checklist should be attached along with the consent form (**Box 1.1**).[20] The low rate of satisfaction in this group of patients,[20] high rate of litigations,[19] and the fact that they may even become more handicapped after a surgical or nonsurgical intervention[20] make them poor candidates for surgery.[19,20] There are even reports of physical threats and even physical harm to the treating aesthetic surgeons by the patients with BDD.[19,20]

Box 1.1 Preoperative checklist for BDD

- I have never been diagnosed with or treated for BDD
- I have undergone plastic surgery procedures in the past, and I have not been unhappy with these procedures
- I consent to contacting my previous plastic surgeon(s)
- I recognize that there is a significant emotional component in choosing an elective plastic surgery procedure
- I understand that the procedure I am seeking may not have the exact outcome that I desire

Abbreviation: BDD, body dysmorphic disorder.

All these factors should be considered and will be of help for the consultant to decide whether to go on or to gracefully decline the procedure.[1] In the initial phase of an aesthetic surgeon's career, it may not be possible for him to make a proper assessment about the psychological status of the patient. Ignoring these factors in a desire to perform more number of surgeries can result in an unhappy patient in spite of the best efforts made to correct the problems he/she presented with. While explaining the pros and cons, one needs to be scientific as well as practical. Explaining against the surgery too is an art.

The end point of aesthetic surgery is "happiness." Unlike any other surgical procedure like an appendectomy or a cholecystectomy where the end point is well defined, aesthetic surgery presents a different situation. Happiness is something which cannot be measured. What would make one person happy may not necessarily satisfy another. It is for this reason that the consultant has to try and analyze the problem faced by the patient and use his interpersonal, clinical skills and judgment to arrive at a decision whether to operate or not,[4] and whether the surgical result can produce the desired happiness which the patient is seeking.

Discussion with the Patient

Explaining Problem

Having listened to the patient about what he or she thinks about the problem, his or her concerns, and what he or she expects from the surgeon, it is the surgeon's turn to explain. The accompanying person should be present during preoperative discussion[21] when the patient talks about the problems and the surgeon explains about the diagnosis and the organic causes of the same. The surgeon should calmly answer all questions, even though they may appear simple and silly and should spend ample time for this.

Sometimes the patient might present alone for consultation. In such case, the surgeon should insist to bring a person with him/her—parent/sibling/spouse/fiancé/close friend[17]—during the second consultation. This is significant because their support may be needed during postoperative recovery period. The discussion in presence of an accompanying person is of immense value in case of an unavoidable problem in the early postoperative period.[17] This has to be discussed with them in the preoperative consultation itself, to ensure their cooperation and favorable response in the postoperative phase.[17]

But this may not be always possible. Some of the patients might not want to disclose that he/she is undergoing a particular surgery. Many patients come from abroad as a part of medical tourism, and hence it won't be cost effective to bring accompanying person(s) with them. In such situations, it is the consultant who should make it very clear to the patient that the procedure will be undertaken with proper formalities and documentation. One should make a final decision whether or not to operate on that patient after proper assessment.

Explaining Solution

Next step is to explain the solution the surgeon can offer. This should be based on the previous steps that have been discussed—history, examination, and problem analysis. The standard in determining how much should be told to the patient is dependent on each patient and is essentially patient centered.[22] Schematic drawings or photographs of previously operated patients can be shown to the patients which will help them obtain a clearer idea about the procedure. Showing representative photographs of the procedures performed can help the patient to understand not only about the surgery but also what to expect from it. Computer simulated imaging (CSI) software that show the "before and after" simulated images work as an adjunctive method of enhancing patient communication.[23] It should not be used as a marketing tool as it is easier to make the patient commit for surgery after showing the simulated images.[23] "It is advisable to demonstrate outcomes that are somewhat less than what the surgeon believes can be achieved" to avoid patient dissatisfaction postoperatively.[23] Remember the adage "promise less deliver more." It is also advisable to provide a copy of CSI containing a disclaimer stating that this is used only for illustration and discussion and does not guarantee the actual surgical results.[21,23]

If there are multiple possible solutions to a particular problem, each one of them should be explained along with the pros and cons of each. Flowcharts might help the patient to understand these solutions better.[21] The financial details of the surgery can be provided at this point. Once the surgeon explains the solutions, the coordinator can take over and explain the cost involved with each type of procedure and explain the reason for the variability in the cost, such as duration, complexity, etc., among different procedures which can help in convincing the patient.

Some of the patients might ask, "Doctor, is this the best solution for me? Isn't the one which I mentioned the better option?" and might quote some procedure or technique which he/she would have seen on the internet, or might have been told by some of his/her friends. At this point in time the surgeon should use his personal experience and knowledge gathered from the literature to explain the pros and cons of each option. Thereafter the onus should be on the patient. One should not be guided by the fear of losing a patient. This can lead to unnecessary bias and suboptimal results.

Explaining Possible Complications

Possible complications, both general and specific, have to be explained in detail, and major ones should be highlighted and preferably be provided in writing.[24] The surgery should not be oversimplified to make it look very trivial and like a parlor procedure. All surgeries carry a certain risk and these should be informed, even though it could be a miniscule risk.[25] Risks from anesthesia and sedation are also discussed. This should be done not only by the surgeon, but also by the anesthesiologist[5] later during preoperative evaluation. It is not right to presume that the patients will refuse surgery if they are warned about the potential risks of surgical treatment.[25]

Even though majority of the patients seeking aesthetic surgery would belong to ASA class 1 category, the fact that they are undergoing an "avoidable surgery" makes it a different situation. Hence the decision of whether or not to take this calculated risk is in the hands of the patient.[25] Reassuring the patient is as important as explaining the complications. He/she should be reassured that "even though there is a possibility that these complications may happen, we are capable of managing that and you may not worry about the same."

If, however, the patient makes repeated visits and is still not able to take a call, he/she may not be a good candidate for the procedure. *Professional Standard for Cosmetic Practise* published by Cosmetic Surgical Practise Working Party (CSWP) of the Royal College of Surgeons (RCS) of England recommended a "cooling off" period of minimum 2 weeks after consultation before invasive surgical procedures could be performed.[2]

Explaining Revision Procedures

Many procedures may require a revision procedure to correct a residual deformity for refining the results. Some of the procedures by themselves require multiple sittings, (e.g., fat grafting, for obtaining optimal results). Explaining these facts preoperatively along with the cost involved in each sitting will help the patients to have a better understanding and help them to be more cooperative.

Preoperative Preparation

Consent Taking

"Every human body of adult years and sound mind has a right to determine what should be done with his own body."[5]

For an aesthetic surgical procedure, obtaining a written informed consent preoperatively is very important, because of the unique doctor–patient relationship in this field.[11] "The most important legal factor for a person giving an informed consent is competency"[5,26] and he/she should consent voluntarily without any coercion, manipulation, or constraint from the surgeon.[5] All the facts discussed with the patient should be reflected in the consent form. This is to be carefully read by the patient and signed. He or she is encouraged to state any doubts they have and appropriate clarification is to be provided. An insufficient informed consent can result in medical litigation.[27] It is ideal to have separate consent form for each procedure which will essentially have two parts: a general part and a specific part (**Fig. 1.5**). The specific part contains those details which are applicable only for that procedure.

It is always better for the surgeon to know few common languages, at least what most of the patient population presenting to him speak. This helps both the surgeon and the patient to understand the physical, psychological, and emotional aspects of the problem better, as well as to build trust. In case the surgeon is not familiar with the patient's language, it is better to get help from an interpreter. Also, the consent should be in a language which they understand, and should be explicitly stated. In case an interpreter is required, the translator should add a written undertaking, stating that he/she has explained everything to the patient in the language they understand. (For further details, refer to Chapter 4 "Ethical and Legal Considerations in Aesthetic Plastic Surgery" in Volume VI.)

Anesthesia

Aesthetic surgical procedures are commonly performed under general anesthesia, or local anesthesia with or without intravenous sedation (MAC—monitored anesthesia care). The choice of anesthesia is dependent on multiple parameters: patient's choice, type (major/minor), complexity of the procedure, comorbid factors, compliance of the patient, etc. The surgeon should explain the pros and cons of different types of anesthesia so that the patient can decide. Studies have shown that administration of local anesthesia can be made pleasing by co-administration of adequate sedation, and infiltration through appropriate needle and in adequate quantity.[28]

Consultation with the anesthesiologist will be helpful in clearing the patient's anxiety about anesthesia.[5] Some surgeons provide an information pamphlet designed by their anesthesia colleague, which contains basic ideas about general anesthesia.

INFORMED CONSENT- REDUCTION MAMMAPLASTY

PART I

1) Breast reduction surgery refers to the reduction of size of the breasts and is usually performed for the relief of the symptoms such as neck pain, bra strap pain, inframammary skin crease infection etc. There are different techniques for performing a reduction mammaplasty each of which is associated with its own advantages and disadvantages. These have been discussed with me.

2) Alternate treatment options include liposuction, wearing special undergarments to support the breasts and also the medicines to reduce the pain.

3) Every effort would be made to reduce the breast to the size discussed; but it may not always be possible to achieve the same. Furthermore, there could be some differences between one side and another.

4) The complications following breast reduction surgery includes altered sensation of nipple-areola and breast skin, irregular contour, asymmetry of both breasts, unfavorable scar, partial or total loss of nipple- areola, unsatisfactory result etc.

5) Breast cancers can occur independent of breast reduction surgery. Hence periodic self-breast examination has to be performed. Breast reduction surgery may interfere with the procedures to stage the breast cancer such as mapping of the lymphatic drainage.

6) Breast reduction surgery can interfere with breast feeding.

PART II

After reading and understanding all these,

1) I hereby give consent to the following procedure_____.

2) I have been advised of the benefits, costs and reason for the procedure as indicated by the clinical observations and/ or diagnostics performed. I acknowledge that no guarantees have been or can be made regarding the likelihood of success or outcomes.

3) I have been advised about the major risks involved in the procedure. Other general complications which can be associated with any surgical procedures such as infection, blood loss, delayed wound healing, wound dehiscence, blood or fluid collection, cardiac or pulmonary complications, blood clot in leg, anesthesia related complications and allergic reactions have also been explained.

4) I have been advised about the existing alternatives in treatment and prognosis of the same and the risk of not having the procedure.

5) I authorize Dr.______________ and such assistants and associates as may be selected by him/ her to perform any part of the above procedures upon myself. I have been advised and I agree that any member of this team may perform any part of my procedures according to his or her stage of training and ability if in the opinion of the above named Surgeon, the experience and the capability of the Assistant Surgeon justifies such a decision.

6) As with any procedure, I am aware of the general and specific complications pertaining to this procedure(s). Therefore, in addition to consenting to the performance of the particular procedure(s), I also consent and authorize the rendering of such other care and treatment as my Surgeon or his designee reasonably believes necessary, should one or more of these and other unforeseen events occur.

7) I give consent to the administration of blood or blood product transfusion during this procedure and immediate post-operative period. I have been informed that despite careful screening in accordance with national and international regulations, there are rare instances of life threatening infections such as AIDS, hepatitis and other viruses or diseases as yet unknown for which screening test do not exist. I also understand that unpredictable reactions may occur which include but are not limited to fever, rash and shortness of breath, shock and in rare occasions death.

8) I consent to the photography or televising of the procedure to be performed for the purpose of advancing medical education; or its publication in scientific journals provided my identity is not revealed by the pictures or descriptions in the accompanying test. In an effort to further medical science and education, I consent to and authorize the presence of and observation of this procedure by qualified observers, as may be authorized by the ____ cosmetic clinics and its regulatory laws and agencies.

9) Having understood the above I give my consent and absolve ____ cosmetic clinics, its doctors and the staff in the event of any complication.

	Signature	Name	Date	Time
Patient				
Witness				
Doctor				
Interpreter				

CONSENT OF THE PATIENT REPRESENTATIVE/ SURROGATE

The patient is unable to consent because ____ and I, _____ (name/relationship to the patient), therefore consent for the patient. I acknowledge that I have had an opportunity to discuss this procedure as stated above with the doctor or doctor's designee and hear by consent to this procedure.

	Signature	Name	Date	Time
Patient representative with relationship				
Witness				
Doctor				
Interpreter				

Fig. 1.5 Consent form for breast reduction. Part I is specific to breast reduction and part II is the general consent form.

Documentation and Photography

Proper documentation of the critical points in history and examination, the solutions offered, the final plan, and appropriately dated preoperative photographs are a must for every case.[4] This should be followed intraoperatively and also through the postoperative period. Detailed documentation helps the surgeon in many ways: (1) to go back in time, see the preoperative and postoperative appearance and to evaluate the results, (2) to provide evidence in case of a litigation,[4] (3) for the purpose of publication and presentations,[29,30] and (4) as a teaching aid.[29,30] Appropriate consent should be obtained before taking the photographs.[30]

Technical details such as contrast, resolution, lighting, magnification, and proper identification[29] should be taken care of during each session for obtaining standard photographs. It is ideal to have a designated photography area in the clinic with standard background, lighting, marked position of camera on a tripod, and marked position of the patient. To make sure that the photographs of each patient taken at each point in time are comparable, four variables have to be looked into: (1) the positioning of the patient, (2) the angle between the patient and the camera, (3) the angle between light and the camera, and (4) the exposure.[29] In all the photographs the shadows should be in the same direction, of approximately same length and similar intensity.[29] The appearance of the patient should also be standardized and "make up" should be avoided so that the true appearance is not camouflaged. (For details, refer to Chapter 24 on "Photography in Plastic Surgery" in Volume I.)

Markings

Appropriate markings are stepping stones for a successful surgery. Adequate time should be spent in marking the operative plan. All the critical points mentioned in the "examination" section should be followed while making the markings. Accompanying persons should not be allowed while the markings are being done, unless the patient is a minor. Areas of deficiency or areas of excess should be marked with appropriate positioning in a well-lit room in front of a full-length mirror in which the patient can see him/herself and participate in the discussion while markings are being done.

Approach to an Unhappy Patient

It is not uncommon to meet a patient who is not happy with the results following a procedure. The causes for unhappiness can be different: either because of a genuinely dissatisfying result or may be the consequence of some psychiatric illness despite achieving an aesthetically acceptable postoperative result.[17]

If the patient presents with below par result and genuinely needs corrective procedure, he/she should be approached with great caution, with a sense of concern and with a pacifying attitude. Handling these patients is tricky and requires experience and expertise. One should be tactful in pointing out the shortcomings and the solutions. One needs to be diplomatic in explaining the situation without blaming the previous surgeon. It is possible to treat these patients, although one may face technical difficulties.

If the patient comes back to the same surgeon, it is a favorable situation. It means that the patient still trusts the surgeon. Hence, the surgeon has the moral responsibility to correct the shortcomings. One should always strive for the result commensurate with the realistic expectations of the patient. If the surgeon finds it difficult or complicated, it is always better to get help from a senior colleague. If the patient presents to a new surgeon and the surgeon is not comfortable with the patient or the procedure, he/she may refer the patient to any other surgeon he/she thinks will be good for the patient.

The patients who are unhappy in spite of achieving a satisfactory result may behave in different ways. Some may take recourse to destructive actions either to themselves or to the surgeon; or they may explore further possibilities of aesthetic surgery or may start litigation.

Different labels have been applied to such "insatiable"[15] aesthetic surgery patients: borderline, ambulatory, latent, incipient, masked, and prepsychotic schizophrenia.[15] A psychiatric-surgical approach should be used to treat such patients. This combined approach along with appropriate timing will help "reduce the intensity of the patients, need for surgery, shorten the course of patient's illness, make the patient's life less chaotic"[15] and will help in attaining a successful surgical result.

The risk of litigation and the chances of becoming "sicker"[15] are higher with those patients who are overtly paranoid or delusional. Hence, these patients are poor candidates for revision surgery and should be discouraged.

Summary

Aesthetic surgery is a field in medicine where the expected end point is perfection and a happy patient. This is not just based on the surgical skills of an aesthetic surgeon, but also on multitude of other parameters. A well-trained and qualified aesthetic surgeon should reach out to the prospective patients/clients through social media, Web sites, and other marketing tools. After adequate evaluation, the biggest challenge is to decide upon whether to go on or to gracefully decline the surgery. If the patient is willing for the surgery after discussing the solutions, realistic outcomes, possible complications, and the cost involved, the surgeon should proceed with the photography and other documentations.

The documentation of the salient points in history, examination, and discussion between the patient and the surgeon, along with appropriate consent and photography, is an integral part of any aesthetic surgery. This will help the surgeon to go back and check the preoperative state of the patient and also use it for research purposes. If a patient returns to the surgeon unhappy, every attempt should be made to rectify the problem. Ultimately, at the end of the day both the surgeon and the patient should be happy.

References

1. Nassab R, Navsaria H, Myers S, Frame J. Online marketing strategies of plastic surgeons and clinics: a comparative study of the United Kingdom and the United States. Aesthet Surg J 2011;31(5):566–571
2. Rufai SR, Davis CR. Aesthetic surgery and Google: ubiquitous, unregulated and enticing websites for patients considering cosmetic surgery. J Plast Reconstr Aesthet Surg 2014;67(5): 640–643
3. Wheeler CK, Said H, Prucz R, Rodrich RJ, Mathes DW. Social media in plastic surgery practices: emerging trends in North America. Aesthet Surg J 2011;31(4):435–441
4. Gorney M. Recognition of the patient unsuitable for aesthetic surgery. Aesthet Surg J 2007;27(6):626–629
5. Ward CM. Consenting and consulting for cosmetic surgery. Br J Plast Surg 1998;51(7):547–550
6. Moore CA, Bokor BR. Anorexia nervosa. In: StatPearls [Internet]. Treasure Island (FL): Stat Pearls Publishing; 2020. https://www.ncbi.nlm.nih.gov/books/NBK459148/
7. Díaz-Marsá M, Alberdi-Páramo I, Niell-Galmés L. Nutritional supplements in eating disorders. Actas Esp Psiquiatr 2017; 45(1, Suppl):26–36
8. Manassa EH, Hertl CH, Olbrisch RR. Wound healing problems in smokers and nonsmokers after 132 abdominoplasties. Plast Reconstr Surg 2003;111(6):2082–2087, discussion 2088–2089
9. Gravante G, Araco A, Sorge R, Araco F, Delogu D, Cervelli V. Wound infections in post-bariatric patients undergoing body contouring abdominoplasty: the role of smoking. Obes Surg 2007;17(10):1325–1331
10. Jabaiti SK. Risk factors for wound complications following abdominoplasty. Am J Appl Sci 2009;6(5):897
11. May JW Jr. Aesthetic surgery 101: resident education in aesthetic surgery, the MGH experience. Ann Plast Surg 2003; 50(6):561–566
12. Wright MR. The male aesthetic patient. Arch Otolaryngol Head Neck Surg 1987;113(7):724–727
13. Connolly FH, Gipson M. Dysmorphophobia: a long-term study. Br J Psychiatr 1978;132:568–570
14. Hay GG. Psychiatric aspects of cosmetic nasal operations. Br J Psychiatr 1970;116(530):85–97
15. Knorr NJ, Edgerton MT, Hoopes JE. The "insatiable" cosmetic surgery patient. Plast Reconstr Surg 1967;40(3):285–289
16. Napoleon A. The presentation of personalities in plastic surgery. Ann Plast Surg 1993;31(3):193–208
17. Reich J. Factors influencing patient satisfaction with the results of esthetic plastic surgery. Plast Reconstr Surg 1975;55(1): 5–13
18. Hayashi K, Miyachi H, Nakakita N, et al. Importance of a psychiatric approach in cosmetic surgery. Aesthet Surg J 2007;27(4):396–401
19. Sarwer DB. Awareness and identification of body dysmorphic disorder by aesthetic surgeons: results of a survey of American Society for Aesthetic Plastic Surgery members. Aesthet Surg J 2002;22(6):531–535
20. Sweis IE, Spitz J, Barry DR Jr, Cohen M. A review of body dysmorphic disorder in aesthetic surgery patients and the legal implications. Aesthetic Plast Surg 2017;41(4):949–954
21. Tebbetts JB, Tebbetts TB, Gorney M. An approach that integrates patient education and informed consent in breast augmentation. Plast Reconstr Surg 2002;110(3):971–978, discussion 979–981
22. Brazier M. Agreeing to treatment: Chapter in medicine, patients and the law. UK: Penguin books; 1992:92
23. Adelson RT. Computer simulated imaging in rhinoplasty. In: Shiffman M, Di Giuseppe A, eds. Advanced aesthetic rhinoplasty. Berlin, Heidelberg: Springer; 2013
24. Armstrong AP, Cole AA, Page RE. Informed consent: are we doing enough? Br J Plast Surg 1997;50(8):637–640
25. Kerrigan DD, Thevasagayam RS, Woods TO, et al. Who's afraid of informed consent? BMJ 1993;306(6873):298–300
26. Nejadsarvari N, Ebrahimi A. Different aspects of informed consent in aesthetic surgeries. World J Plast Surg 2014;3(2): 81–86 Review
27. Park BY, Kwon J, Kang SR, Hong SE. Informed consent as a litigation strategy in the field of aesthetic surgery: an analysis based on court precedents. Arch Plast Surg 2016;43(5): 402–410
28. Maisels DO, Millard DR. Local anaesthesia in cosmetic surgery. Br J Plast Surg 1966;19(2):187–196
29. Jemec BI, Jemec GB. Photographic surgery: standards in clinical photography. Aesthetic Plast Surg 1986;10(3):177–180
30. McG Taylor D, Foster E, Dunkin CS, Fitzgerald AM. A study of the personal use of digital photography within plastic surgery. J Plast Reconstr Aesthet Surg 2008;61(1):37–40

2

Establishing an Aesthetic Surgery Practice

Aditya Aggarwal, Medha Khair Bhave, Vimalendu Brajesh, Sukhdeep Singh, and Rakesh K. Khazanchi

Outpatient Practice Only

This is a small clinic setting with an outpatient department (OPD) and a minor procedure room or operation theater (OT) to collaborate with local hospitals for inpatient work. This option has lesser control over the OT and postsurgical care and the revenue is also shared with the local hospital unit. However, there is lesser administrative work needed and the overhead costs of administration and personnel are also reduced.

Inpatient Practice

This setting includes an OPD with OT and day care/ inpatient facility. To provide patients/clients with a blend of a cosmetic clinic and a relaxing spa experience, creation of a Medspa may be considered. This setting offers greater control over patient care and revenue, yet with it will come additional administrative responsibilities.[4]

The choice between the two options depends upon your vision and aspiration.

Legal Entity of the Practice

This is again dependent on aspirations and could be a proprietorship or a partnership or a company. Please consider legal, financial, and family opinion before the decision is taken. The author suggests creation of a Limited Liability Partnership (LLP) in the early stages of a practice due to its nature of providing a limited liability. An LLP is a business entity in which both partner and corporation exist and a partner is not responsible or liable for another partner's misconduct or negligence. It offers limited liability, offers tax advantages, can accommodate an unlimited number of partners, and is credible. It is registered with the Ministry of Corporate Affairs (MCA). At the same time, it has less compliance than a private limited company and also requires significantly lower cost to start and maintain. There is no requirement of minimal capital and there is no limit to how many partners an LLP can have. The registration cost is low and under Section 40(b), an LLP is not liable to pay any tax. In case of medical negligence or liability, the practice can be safeguarded as the courts cannot attach or auction the partners' movable/immovable assets.

Investment

Funding in an aesthetic practice is needed for:

- Infrastructure: Property purchase or rental and defining the interiors, OT, equipment, LASERs and gadgets like liposuction machines, radiofrequency machine, liposculpture equipment, etc.
- Personnel.
- Overheads.

It may be financially impossible to buy all the expensive technologies being marketed today. Although some new technologies may be mandatory for an upscale practice, look out for rental/leasing opportunities to decrease your financial burden. Choose the correct technology that excites you and incorporate it into your practice to get potentially higher quality patient outcomes. Before spending money on an expensive technology, evaluate the concept carefully in detail before investing in it. Compare it with similar machines and products available from different companies and negotiate a good deal without compromising quality.[5] Always request a demonstration or trial of the technology before using it in your practice. Do not rush to invest into a new product or technology just because it has been well marketed and packaged. It will save a lot of time, unnecessary hassle, and money if the technology/gadget is tried first. It is a good idea to speak to colleagues who have used it earlier, to understand its pros and cons. All new technologies that come into the market are fairly expensive initially with a substantial price drop (depreciate) as soon as these are sold. Subsequent advances in technology over time and more widespread use makes them cheaper (the transition between first generation and second or third generation could be a minor tweak or cosmetic improvement but with a substantial increase in the price of the technology).[6]

Do ensure that these machines are installed well, insured, and covered under warranty with annual maintenance contract (AMC). The company should preferably be able to service it quickly on site and local service engineers should be available. The turnaround time for such repairs should be minimal to minimize financial and patient loss.

Types of Funding Opportunities

1. **Bootstrapped:** This source of funding is your own money, although it may be wise not to use ones' entire savings.
2. **Bank loans:** These can be a source to fund the practice but make sure that the terms and conditions are convenient and the burden of loan repayment should not be like Damocles' sword. The loan amount can always be increased, once the practice is established. The advantage of bank loans is that some of the expenses of the practice can be adjusted against the interest outflow and vital savings can be made.
3. **Investors:** The third source is an investor whose vision overlaps the vision of the clinical team. This should be considered with caution and it is important to judge and manage the expectations as well as to set reasonable time lines about Return on Investment (ROI) for the investor. Due diligence on the legal aspects is a critical pre-requisite if a third-party investor is involved.

Marketing and Patient Outreach

Digital communication has brought about a paradigm shift in the way medical practices are built and sustained.

Earlier, building a practice took years and the name of the doctor spread by word of mouth. With increasing commercialization and competition, patient communication and outreach came into healthcare in a big way. The advent of the digital media further revolutionized the landscape. Now with deft marketing especially on digital platforms aesthetic practice can take off quickly and cater to a wider audience.

National Medical Commission (Medical Council of India) Regulations

The legality of patient communication is governed by the Code of Ethics, 2002 (see Chapter 6) of the Medical Council of India (now the National Medical Commission) but many gray areas remain (**Annexure 2.1**). Therefore, before starting patient communication and outreach in any form it is advisable to consult a medicolegal expert so that one does not fall foul of these regulations.[7,8]

Print Media

This has been the traditional medium for communication, but its use has reduced and undergone a sea change. It now includes the publication of editorials about a medical condition or procedure. Another method is participating in public initiatives around the issue you would like to be related with.

Digital Media

Print medium has been largely superseded by the digital medium as the medium of choice, as it offers a wide choice of methods (Web site, app, Facebook, Instagram, Twitter, blogging, YouTube channels, and many more), greater reach, and can be customized as per your requirements and comfort (**Table 2.2**).

Digital Presence/Identity

The purpose of an identity in the digital domain is to create awareness and provide patients with a point of contact where they can see the facilities, the services offered, and ways to contact you. Having a Web site is a basic way to be present in the digital world. The Web site's landing page should be pleasing and professional. The Web site should be easy to navigate. It is also very important to have a mobile friendly version of the Web site. The patients should find it easy to book appointments and locate the clinic. It is desirable to have a Google profile with the address pinned on Google maps. It is helpful to provide e-brochures about standard procedures as it helps the patients understand the procedures better.

Before and after photographs of your patients, with due consent, generally appeal to the patients checking the Website and the presented results help build credibility. Patient testimonials preferably video testimonials can be added to the Web site to increase the confidence of the prospective patients. Also, it is important to track the visits to your Web site and the pages visited so that those sections can be given more attention. Facebook, Twitter, and Instagram are becoming important channels for connecting with target audiences. They can be used to post information about various medical conditions, procedures, results, or can be a medium to connect on a more human/personal level like anecdotes, interesting facts, personal experiences, etc. Blogging also helps in putting out information about the procedures that you do. It not only provides information to the public but also acts as a way to establish your digital presence. YouTube is a powerful medium which helps you connect to the potential patients and also helps establish your place among your peers. You can have your own channel where you can post edited operative videos, patient information videos, patient testimonials, etc. Operative videos help improve your stature among your peers and also help patients gain greater trust in your abilities (**Table 2.2**).[9]

Table 2.2 Digital presence and marketing

Digital presence	Digital marketing
Mobile friendly Web site	Google advertisements and ratings
Facebook	Search engine optimization
Twitter	Careful use of affiliate channels
Instagram	Social media influencers
YouTube Videos	TV and radio presence

Digital Marketing

Once you have your digital presence then you can market yourself to reach a greater audience. Digital marketing would generally need the services of a professional agency but should have your involvement in creation and vetting of content.

Google advertisements can be customized as per your target audience. Choose the timing depending on the target population. Search engine optimization involves increasing the chances of your Web site or name getting listed higher up on Google search when someone punches in specific key words. It is important to understand about affiliate channels which are sites/apps or entities that get patient queries about different procedures. A practice may choose to be listed on the same sites but remember that some of these systems are easily manipulated. Social media influencers are people/entities that have a significant online following. These may be bloggers talking about beauty, cosmetics, plastic surgery, etc. They may be approached for reviews in case they have undergone a procedure at the clinic. Their word is likely to have greater credibility as it is based on their first-hand experience.

Participating in panel discussions on various platforms including TV and radio helps in creating awareness and highlighting competence.

Digital marketing, despite its multiple advantages, has a flip side. A negative review or comment by an unsatisfied patient also gets spread quickly. It is important that all negative reviews are dealt professionally and with empathy, without divulging any patient details and professional secrets.

Team

Any good practice requires a dedicated, and a professional team of people sharing the same vision working together in a harmonious environment. As the leader of the team, it is the surgeon's responsibility to create a comfortable work environment to nurture the team and ensure commitment and high professional standard. A dress code for the various team members creates a professional environment and the dress can prominently display the logo of your practice.

Front Desk Staff

As they are the first point of contact with the patient, it is very important that the front desk staff are pleasing, well-groomed, and professional in their conduct. They need to be well versed in English and the local language and should be well informed of the services offered in the practice. Among some soft and gentle conducts that make a difference is a personal call on the day of the appointment to confirm the appointment or a cancellation. All phone calls should be answered promptly, preferably within three rings. In telephonic conversations, it is better to have predetermined script. When a patient reaches the clinic, he/she should be made to feel welcome and comfortable—not just in terms of the place but also by the behavior and attitude of the staff. The staff should be facilitators for the patient and should help them with paperwork and insurance issues, etc. While the patient is waiting they could be offered healthy beverage and snacks.

Nursing Staff and Technicians

Nursing staff is needed both for an OPD setting and an inpatient facility. Besides being well trained in nursing, they also need to be well groomed, courteous, and professional in their conduct. As they will also be assisting in procedures, they should be technically well trained about the requirements for various procedures and the working of equipment so that it all feels seamless in front of the patient. In all, patient comfort, safety, and privacy should be paramount. If you have an inpatient facility then trained OT staff and technicians are a requirement. Having well-trained staff reduces stress during surgery, enhances your comfort, and improves results. The staff may need to be trained for some specific procedures that you do, such as hair transplants, LASERS, etc.

Administrative and General Staff

Besides the nursing and front desk staff, the administrative and general staff play an important yet background role in ensuring smooth accounting, salaries, housekeeping, maintenance of the clinic, and many other sundry tasks. The staff can be hired directly or through an agency. The agency may be expensive but provides replacements. The staff should be paid competitive market salaries, and the salary could have an incentive component.

The Art of Consultation

Today, the process of connecting with the surgeon begins much before the first human connect happens; it begins on a tastefully done Web site from which the patient will either mail or call the practice. The response to this mail or phone call is critical and the coordinator who responds must be well versed in the practice and should be able to define the needs of the patient and be able to share appropriate information whether as an e-brochure or a conversation.[10]

The décor of the practice must be elegant and patients should have adequate privacy while the coordinator plans the consultation. The waiting room walls could tastefully display diplomas, degrees, publications, and testimonials in addition to brochures about procedures. The coordinator must ensure that the waiting time for the patient is minimized and they may be offered healthy refreshment at the time.

While ushering the patient in, the coordinator can also alert the physician about the personality of the patient, any previous visits, or any red flags.

It is extremely important for the doctor to dress appropriately. The authors feel a formal apparel and shoes or scrubs with a doctor's apron preferably with the name on it bring a substance to the meeting. The confidentiality and privacy of the meeting must always be ensured. In case students/observers are in attendance, permission for this must be taken from the patient prior to each meeting. The students must have an appropriate demeanor and refrain from making any comments during the consult.

While consulting a female patient it is critical to have another female in attendance. This female is usually a nurse but could also be a female colleague. It is also recommended that the physician not undress a patient, whether male or female, as this may be misconstrued by the patient.

During the consultation, it is important for the doctor to be unhurried and a good listener. Be aware of patients who are very profuse in their praise or very critical, patients whose concern for the deformity is far in excess of the deformity itself, patients who are very demanding and may have unrealistic expectations. It is recommended not to get too involved in the personal and social issues when consulting a patient.

Medical record keeping is a very critical part of the consultation and must be made in detail, including professional photography and surgical plans. It is important to discuss financial issues in a transparent manner and share practical estimates prior to the surgery. This is an important factor and it should be discussed by the doctor or staff who is experienced and skilled in the same. In the beginning of one's career one may choose to conduct each discussion personally, but once the practice is established a reliable staff member may be deputed to perform this critical role.[11]

Informed consent is another important part of the consultation and the doctor should discuss the proposed surgery, alternatives, risks, and benefits, and this discussion should be carefully documented in the patient charts as this is an invaluable medicolegal document.[12]

Use of Technology

Photography and Data Storage

A picture is worth a thousand words. Clinical portrait photographs have become an integral part of an aesthetic practice patient record keeping. DSLR/SLR (digital single lens reflex or single lens reflex) camera with lens in the range of 90 to 105 mm is the preferred choice. A resolution of 3 to 5 megapixel with a fixed, colored background brings uniformity in photographs.[13]

With various available software, a virtual preoperative planning and surgery is also possible if good preoperative photographs are available. It is critical to have the same view with same light exposure in both preop and postop photographs. A designated photography room (with adequate lights and privacy) should be planned for in practice.

With the use of DSLR cameras more surgeries are being video recorded for learning and future reference. This generates very high volume of data, the storage of which is a big challenge. At any aesthetic center with an average three to four surgeries a day the data generated can be as high as 5 to 10 GB per day. Careful storage and an organized filing system helps in quick retrieval of video and photographs.

The commonly used storage devices are hard drives (HDD). They are handy and sturdy but have a low average life span (4–6 yr). Backup data can be stored on DVDs or Blu-ray disks. DVDs have a longer lifespan >25 years. DVD-Rs are not useful as backup storage tools due to inferior lifespan. An average DVD can store data of 4 to 5 GB, which is sufficient for storage of data generated on daily basis at a small aesthetic center. Blu-ray disks are another variant of storage devices with lifespan up to 100 years and storage capacity of 50 to 100 GB. Cloud storage apps provide for unlimited space for data storage which is easily accessible anywhere anytime. Be vigilant that data and patient privacy may not be secure if they are not end-to-end encrypted. Google drive, one drive, and drop box are some examples of nonencrypted cloud storage.

Clinical photographs and digital records mandate utmost safety and confidentiality. Cloud providers that offer local encryption and need passphrase to decrypt them are the safest data storage option but they come at a price.

For Surgical Planning

Aesthetic surgery involves surgery not only of soft tissue but also at the level of skeletal framework. CAD-CAM (computer-assisted designing and computer-assisted manufacture) have now become integral to achieving a good aesthetic result. While professionals are available to help in the planning and printing part, a basic knowledge is essential to understand and achieve good aesthetic results. Horas, Materialize Mimics are few examples.

For Better Communication

Technology can also be used for communication between doctors and staff for smooth functioning of planned aesthetic surgery. Various apps like WhatsApp, Viber, and Facebook Messenger are few examples to communicate the operative list, consumables to be arranged, sequence of surgery, any specific advice, etc.

Quality, Safety, Service

Quality is a perceptual attribute, defined as a measure of a standard of something as against another thing of similar kind. The quality of practice and results should match the peer standards; more importantly, quality is best perceived by the patients, who are at a totally different level of information, understanding, and expectations. Limiting uncontrolled variation in every aspect by setting up protocols and stringently adhering to them is the only way to achieve and maintain quality in practice.

Safety is paramount in surgery but in aesthetic surgery it is indispensable, simply because the patients can live with their problems. Aesthetic desire is considered a requirement above basic health needs by majority. Hence, any mortality or morbidity is looked upon far more harshly than any other specialty.

Service is the core of any practice, more so of aesthetic because of more demanding patients with remarkably high expectations. They want to feel and be treated differently from "unwell" patients. Many even do not want to be referred to as patients but as clients akin to the term used by the nonmedical beauty industry.

These three attributes of practice can be based on one indispensable character—integrity. Ability to look beyond money and acting in the best interest of the patient spells integrity of an aesthetic plastic surgeon. How to incorporate these attributes in practice is an individual prerogative, yet the authors feel the above are critical.

The Aesthetic Surgeon

A qualification in plastic surgery can be augmented with special training, extensive reading, and updating knowledge. Continuing academic and skills updates is essential. Aesthetic norms and demands keep changing. Aesthetic industry includes other beauty businesses like gyms, spas, saloons, fashion, etc. The aesthetic surgeon needs to learn an approach vis-à-vis these businesses where "clients" are wooed routinely with offers. The surgeon must work within legal and ethical boundaries, and developing peer relationships so as to get help when needed is a critical part of that.

Equipment

The cost of aesthetic practice has escalated due to the explosion of technology, which comes at a formidable cost. While some gadgets are more of a gimmick, many others may really make a difference to the quality of results by adding extra dimensions. Moreover, patients are observing the direct marketing by many companies and demand what is trending. For example, radiofrequency tightening of facial skin was in much demand only to fizzle out a few years later due to volume loss and accelerated sagging of skin it led to over a longer period.

It is indeed a demanding task for a plastic surgeon to manage patient demand, finances, and assess the true value of the technology over a period. It is advisable to directly talk to colleagues who are using the technology and seek a realistic opinion. Maintenance of equipment should be regularly done and documented for patient safety as well as legal protection. One must ensure all stipulated safety norms.

Communication and Interaction with the Patient

The patients interact with the aesthetic team at multiple levels.

Before the Consultation

It should be customary to get the patient to fill a form disclosing past illnesses, surgeries, injuries, allergies, and current medication. This document signed by the patient and a witness can serve as legal protection as well as a quick reminder before surgery for safety.

At the Consultation

Adequate time, honest and transparent discussion, writing down patient's expectations, standard clinical photography, and thorough investigations are vital in establishing good doctor–patient relationship. A clear idea about possible complications with incidence should be given. A detailed Informed Consent Process should be followed and consent signed on the day of surgery by both the patient and the surgeon along with a witness identified by the patient. The surgeon should mention particular complications and the expectations that cannot be fulfilled, in his own handwriting, and sign after showing to the patient.

Perioperative Communications

A cordial and empathetic demeanor is a basic essential. Documentation of intraoperative findings and major steps is desired by every patient nowadays. Postoperative instructions should be clear, comprehensive, and customized to patient's needs. It is desirable to have templates for each surgery which can then be modified as per need.

Long-term

One happy patient is a potential advertiser of your services. Taking care of the smallest concerns, availing answering service via staff during critical periods, proactive enquiry about their well-being keeps the patient attached.

Protecting the Practice

Protection should be provided to the surgeon, the team, and the infrastructure and will include various insurances, indemnities, and AMCs. Prevention of sexual harassment at workplace (POSH) policies create confidence in the team and are mandated by the national laws in India (**Table 2.3**). Aesthetic surgeons are frequently called to work as a ghost surgeon by other specialty colleagues. This is a dangerous practice and must be avoided at all costs.[14]

Have a good support team in the form of a lawyer and a chartered accountant (CA). By auditing the accounts well, the CA can help to save more by getting tax breaks and identifying any losses or wasteful practices.

Conclusion

Establishing an aesthetic practice is a fulfilling and rewarding achievement that requires focused efforts (**Table 2.4**). Continuous up-skilling of the team and looking for opportunities such as medical tourism to expand the practice are critical to growing the practice. Continuing with various accreditations such as National Accreditation Board Hospitals (NABH) and Joint Commission International (JCI) helps instill patient confidence. Affiliations with professional organizations such as Indian Association of Aesthetic Plastic Surgeons (IAAPS) as well as International Society of Aesthetic Plastic Surgery (ISAPS) allow the use of their logo in your practice and reaffirms peer standing.

Table 2.3 Protecting the practice

Protection for the surgeon	Protection for the team[a]	Protection of the infrastructure
Professional indemnity	Medical insurance	Insurance of the property (movable and immovable)
Medical insurance	Term life insurance	AMC of expensive machinery
Term life insurance	POSH policies in place	Fire safety and other building norms
Limited liability partnership		Local registration and biowaste disposal process according to national and local laws

Abbreviations: AMC, Annual maintenance contract; POSH, Prevention of sexual harassment at workplace.
[a] Take legal advice for all agreements and read the fine print of insurances.

Table 2.4 Summary

Defining the practice	• Location • Type of practice (individual or group): ➢ Investment type ➢ Legal structure
Patient outreach and connections	• Print and digital media • Legally acceptable patient outreach
Team	• The surgeon, dermatologist, nutritionist, and allied team • Nurses and technicians • Front desk and patient facing teams • Administrative, legal, finance teams
Use of technology	• Photography, documentation of clinical and surgical data, communication with patients and within the team
Quality, safety, and service	• Clear vision and mission and alignment of quality processes to the same
Protecting the practice	• Insurances, indemnity, AMC, HR policies, appropriate licenses and approvals

Abbreviations: AMC, Annual maintenance contract; HR, human resource.

References

1. ISAPS International Survey on Aesthetic/Cosmetic Procedures performed in 2018. https://www.isaps.org/wp-content/uploads/2019/12/ISAPS-Global-Survey-Results-2018-new.pdf. Accessed on June 8, 2020
2. Sachdev M, Britto GR. Essential requirements to setting up an aesthetic practice. J Cutan Aesthet Surg 2014;7(3):167–169
3. D'Amico RA, Saltz R, Rohrich RJ, et al. Risks and opportunities for plastic surgeons in a widening cosmetic medicine market: future demand, consumer preferences, and trends in practitioners' services. Plast Reconstr Surg 2008;121(5):1787–1792
4. Haeck PC. Improving the evaluation and management of the ambulatory and office-based surgical patient. Plast Reconstr Surg 2009; 124(4, Suppl):4S–5S https://pubmed.ncbi.nlm.nih.gov/20827236/. Accessed on June 8, 2020
5. Aurangabadkar SJ, Mysore V, Ahmed ES. Buying a laser: tips and pearls. J Cutan Aesthet Surg 2014;7(2):124–130
6. Ahluwalia J, Gianastano C, Waibel JS. Incorporating aesthetic devices into a dermatologic practice. J Clin Aesthet Dermatol 2020;13(1):18–21
7. Indian Medical Council (Now National Medical Commission). Professional Conduct, Etiquette and Ethics Regulations, 2002, Chapter 6 and 7. https://www.mciindia.org/documents/rulesAndRegulations/Ethics%20Regulations-2002.pdf. Accessed June 8, 2020
8. Nagpal N. Should advertising by aesthetic surgeons be permitted? J Cutan Aesthet Surg 2017;10(1):45–47
9. Venkataram A, Shetty M, Ellur S, Manikavachakan N. Smart apps for the smart plastic surgeon: an update. Indian J Plast Surg 2016;49(1):123–124
10. Bhangoo KS. The art of consultation. Indian J Plast Surg 2014;47(2):167–174
11. Rohrich RJ. The market of plastic surgery: cosmetic surgery for sale: at what price? Plast Reconstr Surg 2001;107(7):1845–1847
12. Cosmetic procedures: Ethical issues; Nuffield Council on Bioethics 2017. https://www.nuffieldbioethics.org/assets/pdfs/Cosmetic-procedures-full-report.pdf. Accessed June 8, 2020.
13. Swamy RS, Most SP. Pre- and postoperative portrait photography: standardized photos for various procedures. Facial Plast Surg Clin North Am 2010;18(2):245–252
14. Piras M, Delbon P, Conti A, et al. Cosmetic surgery: medicolegal considerations. Open Med (Wars) 2016;11(1):327–329

Annexure 2.1

Indian Medical Council (Professional Conduct, Etiquette and Ethics) Regulations, 2002

6.1.1 Soliciting of patients directly or indirectly, by a physician, by a group of physicians, or by institutions or organizations is unethical. A physician shall not make use of him/her (or his/her name) as subject of any form or manner of advertising or publicity through any mode either alone or in conjunction with others which is of such a character as to invite attention to him or to his professional position, skill, qualification, achievements, attainments, specialties, appointments, associations, affiliations, or honors and/or of such character as would ordinarily result in his self-aggrandizement. A physician shall not give to any person, whether for compensation or otherwise, any approval, recommendation, endorsement, certificate, report, or statement with respect of any drug, medicine, nostrum remedy, surgical, or therapeutic article, apparatus or appliance, or any commercial product or article with respect of any property, quality or use thereof or any test, demonstration or trial thereof, for use in connection with his name, signature, or photograph in any form or manner of advertising through any mode nor shall he boast of cases, operations, cures, or remedies or permit the publication of report thereof through any mode. A medical practitioner is however permitted to make a formal announcement in press regarding the following:

- On starting practice.
- On change of type of practice.
- On changing address.
- On temporary absence from duty.
- On resumption of another practice.
- On succeeding to another practice.
- Public declaration of charges.

6.1.2 Printing of self-photograph or any such material of publicity in the letter head or on sign board of the consulting room or any such clinical establishment shall be regarded as acts of self-advertisement and unethical conduct on the part of the physician. However, printing of sketches, diagrams, picture of human system shall not be treated as unethical.

7.11 A physician should not contribute to the lay press articles and give interviews regarding diseases and treatments which may have the effect of advertising himself or soliciting practices; but is open to write to the lay press under his own name on matters of public health, hygienic living or to deliver public lectures, give talks on the radio/TV/internet chat for the same purpose and send announcement of the same to lay press.

7.12 An institution run by a physician for a particular purpose such as a maternity home, nursing home, private hospital, rehabilitation center, or any type of training institution etc., may be advertised in the lay press, but such advertisements should not contain anything more than the name of the institution, type of patients admitted, type of training and other facilities offered, and the fees.

3

Unsatisfactory Results in Aesthetic Surgery: Prevention and Management

Rakesh K. Khazanchi, Hardeep Singh, and Sanjay Mahendru

Introduction

Aesthetic surgery, also known as cosmetic/beauty surgery by lay public, is a branch of plastic surgery that deals with improving the normal. It differs from other surgical procedures in the sense that surgery is done to improve the appearance of the body in the absence of any disease. The aim is to improve the quality of life, body image, and self-esteem and not to treat any disease. This surgery is not need but want based. This aspect adds a different dimension to outcomes after aesthetic surgery. While there may be dissatisfaction due to poor results because of surgery-related complications, the patient may be unhappy because the final outcome does not meet the patient's expectations.

In the past, aesthetic surgery was considered to be the domain of a select group of population mainly the wealthy and those in professions with major emphasis on appearance and beauty. The onset of new millennium has seen a rapid increase in demand for aesthetic surgery with a large number coming from the burgeoning pool of middle-income group. India is among the top five nations in which most aesthetic procedures are performed.[1] With increasing demand, and the supply trying to keep pace with it, a large number of physicians which includes not just plastic surgeons but many from specialties such as Ear, Nose and Throat surgery, Dermatology, Gynecology, Oral and Maxillofacial surgery, and Dentistry are also jumping on to this bandwagon. The resultant increase in competition has led to aggressive marketing with promises made of excellent results. As a result, patients develop unrealistic expectations which are seldom achievable. While known complications of any surgical procedure may compromise the quality of result achieved, it is often the unrealistic expectations that lead to an unsatisfactory outcome. The improvement that is requested is often difficult to measure objectively and there may be gaps in the assessment of results among different observers. Many times the surgeon may have achieved a satisfactory outcome based on clinical and empirical evidence, yet it does not always improve the patient's psychological well-being, self-confidence, or self-esteem.[2] The exact magnitude of problem may be difficult to gauge on account of underreporting and also patients may not come forward with this problem. In one study, 14% of patients undergoing procedures for midface rejuvenation reported unsatisfactory results.[3]

Dealing with unsatisfactory outcomes is therefore an essential learning objective of a surgeon seeking to undertake aesthetic surgery as a career. The first part of this chapter will deal with preventing and avoiding having an unfavorable result. The second part will address dealing with unsatisfactory results.

Prevention

Various causes of unsatisfactory results after aesthetic surgery are listed in **Table 3.1**. Preventive measures start at initial assessment and are continued throughout the management of the patient.

Initial Assessment

First step in avoiding an unsatisfactory result starts at the first consultation. This is done by proper case selection and identifying patients who are more likely to be unhappy with the result regardless of what may be achieved. These patients fall under following categories.

Unclear Objectives

These persons are not clear about the problem and the improvement sought. They are vague and generally unhappy with their body image and expect the surgeon to describe what is wrong with them, describe their flaws, and how they are to be addressed. Aesthetic surgery is about what the patient wants, and not what the surgeon thinks is wrong with the patient. If the patient is unable to describe what is needed or is vague about his/her assessment of the existing deficiency or not clear about the goals, one should tread carefully before operating on such a patient. Multiple consultations may sometimes be required to understand the problem and help the patient develop clarity on what aesthetic surgery can achieve. If there is a mismatch of objectives between the surgeon and the patient, surgery should be avoided.

Very often the surgeon may notice a flaw which the patient may not have noticed, (e.g., a retruded chin in a patient requesting a rhinoplasty). Although not a rule, it is generally unwise to suggest that to the patient. If correction of this flaw is going to significantly enhance the result of

Table 3.1 Causes of unsatisfactory results in aesthetic surgery

Preoperative	Operative	Postoperative
Poor communication	Poor execution	Complications which may cause unexpected morbidity
Unclear objectives		Complications that may compromise the final outcome
Faulty assessment of problem		Poor compliance with postoperative management
Unrealistic expectations		
Doubtful motivation		
Body dysmorphic syndrome		

requested surgery, the surgeon may suggest this additional surgery, but the final choice is left to the patient without any undue pressure from the surgeon. A note of such an offer and patient's response should be made in the medical record.

Unreasonable or Unrealistic Expectations

The second most common patient in this category is the one with unreasonable or unrealistic expectations. This is often seen in patients requesting rhinoplasty and they carry pictures of models from magazines and ask for a nose of a particular type seen in these pictures. There is a general myth among public that plastic surgeons can achieve any desired shape. While it may even be possible to give someone the nose like the one in the picture, the person will never look like the person in the picture and therefore will be dissatisfied. Such patients need to be counseled very carefully and extensively. Surgery should be offered only after the patient has developed an understanding of realistic and achievable goals.

Extraneous Motivation

This is a patient who has questionable self-motivation and is requesting surgery to please someone else. It may be a spouse or a partner, a parent, a sibling, or a friend. It may be a failed relationship, or trying to get a job based on his/her appearance. The extraneous motivation is generally an indication to proceed carefully and the decision will be based on the extent of deficiency sought to be improved and how the patient perceives it. It is not an absolute contraindication but will require careful consideration. The primary indication should be based on patient's perception of the problem rather than how others perceive it. Unfortunately we live in a society where others' perception of appearance may be a necessary requirement for a successful career and this aspect also has to be given some weightage. Many a times the parents prevail upon the patient, for example, a surgery before marriage.

Body Dysmorphic Disorder

One of the keys to avoid an unhappy patient after cosmetic surgery is the ability to identify a patient with body dysmorphic disorder (BDD). Patients with this disorder are preoccupied with an imaginary defect in their physical appearance or have a distorted perception of their body image.[4,5]

This disorder was first introduced by American Psychiatry Association in 1980.[6] Features of this disorder are:

- Preoccupation with one or more perceived defects or flaws in physical appearance that are not observable or appear slight to others. They cause significant distress or impairment in social, occupational, or other important areas of functioning.
- Repetitive behavior like looking at a mirror repeatedly.
- Sometimes accompanied by eating disorders.

There is a high prevalence of BDD in patients seeking aesthetic procedures including aesthetic surgery. Many of these patients take multiple selfies from various angles and point to flaws which are seen in the photos even when they are not so obvious in their actual appearance. They tend to seek unnecessary cosmetic treatments and surgery. They have unrealistic expectations and seek results which are not achievable. They may focus on any part of the body, but the incidence of BDD is highest in patients seeking cosmetic rhinoplasty.[7] Even if a satisfactory result is achieved by a procedure, they may shift their attention to another part of the body.[4]

It is important for the surgeon to make a thorough clinical assessment of patients' concerns and should there be any suspicion of BDD, psychiatric consultation should be sought. This can sometimes be difficult because of the stigma that people may attach to seeing a psychiatrist.

Most surgeons consider BDD to be a clear contraindication to surgery.[8,9] However, others believe that patients with mild-to-moderate BDD with no significant impairment in overall functioning, localized appearance concerns, and realistic expectations may benefit from surgery.[10,11] Choosing these patients is of paramount importance and will require help of a psychiatrist. A frank discussion with the patient may help convince the patient to visit a psychiatrist with the hope that he may recommend surgery.

Besides above, patients with following features should be red flagged and decision to operate or not is made after due consideration:

- Patients appearing to have obsessive compulsive behavior.
- Patients who demand immediate surgery without due consideration.
- Patients who are excessively flattering.
- Patients with past history of litigation.
- Patients with unkempt appearance.
- Patients who seek multiple consultations and criticize other surgeons.

A young aesthetic surgeon at the beginning of his career may be tempted to take on this type of patients but it is wise to seek a second opinion from another more experienced colleague. With experience, identification of such patients comes as a second nature and one would often call this to be a gut feeling of a red flag which must never be ignored.

Preoperative Counseling

Once the decision to undertake a procedure has been made, the next step is presurgical counseling. The purpose of this is to revisit the flaws that are going to be corrected, what can and cannot be corrected, point out any asymmetries that the patient may not have noticed, go over the required preoperative work-up and need for informed consent, alternatives to surgery offered, potential benefits and risks and complications of the procedure, postoperative recovery and care, and the time required for the results to become observable. A meticulous record of this counseling must be maintained.

Preoperative photographs are taken and reviewed jointly by the surgeon and the patient. A checklist of the flaws to

an unhappy patient, good communication, continued access, and resolving queries are the keys to prevent confrontation and litigation. Meticulous record keeping, working knowledge of medical negligence law, and a good malpractice indemnity insurance are essential safeguards against malpractice claims.

References

1. Valikhani A, Goodarzi MA. Contingencies of self-worth and psychological distress in Iranian patients seeking cosmetic surgery: integrative self-knowledge as mediator. Aesthetic Plast Surg 2017;41(4):955–963
2. Honigman RJ, Phillips KA, Castle DJ. A review of psychosocial outcomes for patients seeking cosmetic surgery. Plast Reconstr Surg 2004;113(4):1229–1237
3. Jacono AA, Ransom ER. Anatomic predictors of unsatisfactory outcomes in surgical rejuvenation of the midface. JAMA Facial Plast Surg 2013;15(2):101–109
4. Alavi M, Kalafi Y, Dehbozorgi GR, Javadpour A. Body dysmorphic disorder and other psychiatric morbidity in aesthetic rhinoplasty candidates. J Plast Reconstr Aesthet Surg 2011;64(6):738–741
5. Ribeiro RVE. Prevalence of body dysmorphic disorder in plastic surgery and dermatology patients: a systematic review with meta-analysis. Aesthetic Plast Surg 2017;41(4):964–970
6. França K, Roccia MG, Castillo D, et al. Body dysmorphic disorder: history and curiosities. Wien Med Wochenschr 2017;167(Suppl 1):5–7
7. Veale D, Boocock A, Gournay K, et al. Body dysmorphic disorder: a survey of fifty cases. Br J Psychiatry 1996;169(2):196–201
8. Lee K, Guy A, Dale J, Wolke D. Adolescent desire for cosmetic surgery: association with bullying and psychological functioning. Plast Reconstr Surg 2017;139(5):1109–1118
9. Bouman TK, Mulkens S, van der Lei B. Cosmetic professional's awareness of body dysmorphic disorder. Plast Reconstr Surg 2017;139(2):336–342
10. Bowyer L, Krebs G, Mataix-Cols D, Veale D, Monzani B. A critical review of cosmetic treatment outcomes in body dysmorphic disorder. Body Image 2016;19:1–8
11. de Brito MJ, de Almeida Arruda Felix G, Nahas FX, et al. Body dysmorphic disorder should not be considered an exclusion criterion for cosmetic surgery. J Plast Reconstr Aesthet Surg 2015;68(2):270–272
12. Wang WW, Ford RS, Ford AR, Esq MS, Gupta SC. Medical malpractice risk assessment in plastic surgery. Plast Reconstr Surg 2012;130(5S1):65
13. Mrinmoy Dutta v. Dr AG and Ors. 2016. NCRDC 1524

4

Ethical and Legal Considerations in Aesthetic Plastic Surgery

Ashok Gupta

Preamble

To preserve the credibility, confidence, and reverence bestowed upon physicians since the days of "Lord Dhanvantari," every physician must observe sublime ethical principles even during a crisis; otherwise, one may open floodgates to legal penalties. With the rapidly altering attitude of people toward lifestyle and self-image in the modern competitive society, aesthetic surgery has got tangled in several ethical and legal issues. Conjoined forces of globalization, advertising using mass media, and deviations from old-fashioned beliefs, supplemented with a litigious outlook among people, have clogged the path for a conscious assistance in sound decision making. Hazards associated with aesthetic surgery necessitate thorough deliberation and reasoned evaluation in every patient.

A critical review of the risk and benefit ratio, furthered by a defensive approach, is imperative to safeguard ethical principles in aesthetic surgery. Ethical principles are indispensable while dealing with all the concerns regarding the cognitive and emotional state of a patient. For instance, how does a surgeon respond to a patient who displays evidence of body dysmorphic disorder?

There is a dire need to shield and educate unsuspecting people from the growing lunch-time cosmetic procedure clinics that callously offer unsafe treatments. The author strongly endorses acceptance of aesthetic surgery as a part of the medical reality, implementation of a comprehensive training program, and a postgraduate qualification for aesthetic surgery, which must be suitably conducted at recognized institutions endorsed by a University or a Statutory Authority.

> "A memorandum is written not to inform the reader, but to protect the writer"
>
> "No insurance company ever makes a mistake in your favor"
>
> *Dr Robert M. Goldwyn*[1]

> "Why does the patient want this procedure and does he or she have realistic expectation and understand the limitations of the surgery"
>
> "Trust your judgment; good judgment usually comes from bad experiences. Remember, you can just say no!"
>
> *Dr Rod J. Rohrich*[2]

Historical Aspects

In India, we have been blessed with a code of medical ethics since the days of Charaka and Sushruta. With an unwavering belief in "Altruism" and "Karma; upright actions have solemn values" the foundation for medical ethics and morality was fabricated. The "Hippocratic Oath" (500 BC Greek; first code of medical ethics) is a time-honored doctrine for professional and ethical conduct for medical professionals, highlighting "Do whatever is the best for the patient; patients come first" and "primum non nocere: do no harm."[3]

The term "Medical Ethics" was coined by a British physician Thomas Percival (1794) and the title of his book was *Medical Jurisprudence*. The first "Code of Medical Ethics" implemented by the American Medical Association (1847) was an adaptation of Percival's code.[4] Mercier's verdict (1936) in the French Court pronounced the contractual nature of surgeon–patient relationship. A histrionic shift in medical ethics was witnessed in 1970s consequent to better alertness about "procedural justice." Thereafter, medical ethics slowly reconfigured itself as "bioethics." Currently, aesthetic surgery is passing through an identity crisis as well as an acute ethical dilemma.[5–10]

Bioethical Principles in Aesthetic Plastic Surgery

Conforming to the beliefs of "Biomedical Ethics"[8–12] there are well-defined standards to serve as the ethical basis of a current aesthetic surgery practice.

Autonomy: Each person has a fundamental right to self-determination or self-governance and to accept or refuse any proposed procedure.

Beneficence: Should promote only what is good for the patient. Beneficence is the *only* fundamental principle of medical ethics.

Compassionate care: Patients who are conscious about their appearance and who feel socially disliked are the most probable to benefit from aesthetic surgery.

Dignity: Need to ensure that patients' expectations toward the result are realistic.

Non-maleficence: Primum non nocere.

- Every physician is duty-bound to cause no harm to the patient. It is more important not to harm your patient than to do them good.
- Each of the patients is to be treated ethically on an equal opportunity basis.
- Risk-and-benefit analysis of aesthetic surgery necessitates a protective approach.
- If the procedure is not in the patients' best interests, the surgeon has the right to decline to perform the procedure.
- Aesthetic surgery undertaken by physicians with no recognized qualification or training is a gross violation of the ethical principle of "Non-maleficence."
- A physician has to be equipped with skills to cope up with bad news, treatment failures, patient suffering, medical futility, and death.

Consent and Regulation

History of Surgical Consent

Atrocities committed at Nazi concentration camps during the Second World War (WWII) faced intense criticism from the society. The doctors became targets of public condemnation for conducting nonconsensual trials on patients. "Nuremberg trial" was momentous for the cohorts of informed consent, a term which later formed the "keystone" of policies for human experimentation.[13] The idea that physicians should fully inform patients about medical details in order to aid in their care dates back to the American doctor Hooker (1849), but was not adopted into practice. Consequently, Helsinki Declarations I and II (Modern Version of Hippocratic Oath), adopted first in 1964 at the 18th World Medical Association (WMA) General Assembly, Helsinki (updated last in 2013 at the 64th WMA General Assembly, Brazil), became WMA's best-known ethical doctrines for medical research involving human subjects.[14,15] The Bolam judgment (1957), Bolam v/s Friern Hospital Committee, often referred to as "Bolam criteria," established that standard of care should be judged by an appraisal with the views of an accountable organization of doctors, and adduced revolutions in the law governing the duty of doctors on disclosure of all information to patients regarding risks.[16] It also incorporated a physician's obligation to take rational care to assure that the patient is aware of material risks involved in any recommended treatment and of any equitable alternative or variant. It secured the foundation for the concept of "Informed Consent."

In case of Sidaway v/s Bethlem Royal Hospital and Others (1985), it was observed that "doctor's duty is to exercise rational skill and care with a duty to inform patients during the process of gaining consent" as per the provision of the standard of information agreeing to the "Bolam criteria."[17]

Consent for Surgery

"*Consent*" for any surgery or invasive procedure is defined as "anticipated and firm authorization to acquire an explicit treatment, based on sufficient material information provided towards the expected progress and risks with the possibility of its success and alternate options to it." The word "consent" (an essential obligation) means controlled contract and approval to definite treatment that is free of coercion and deception. "Consent" is perhaps the only principle that runs through all aspects of healthcare provisions today. For any legitimate and effectual consent, three constituents have to be mandatorily included:[18–20]

- **Capacity:** Capability to understand all the information on the forthcoming fears of his or her decision-making ability and aptitude.
- **Disclosure:** Offer all possible information pertinent for taking decision. (Written consent needs to be printed in common man's language in the local vernacular script.)
- **Voluntariness:** Right to exercise his or her decision-making capacity without being exposed to outside force such as intimidation, manipulation, or unjustified influence.

As defined in the Medical Consent Act of 1999 by the General Assembly of Commonwealth of Pennsylvania,[21] a parent or legal guardian of a minor may confer upon an adult person, who is a relative or family friend, the power to consent to medical or surgical treatment on minor under the supervision of a physician, licensed to practice, and to exercise parental rights to obtain records and information. In the Indian setting, the relationship between a surgeon and his or her patient is a contract and thereby covered under the Indian Contract Act (1982) and the Indian Penal Code. The Medical Council of India, Section 7.16 defines: before performing an operation the physician should obtain in writing the consent from the husband or wife, parent or guardian in the case of a minor, or the patient himself as the case may be.[22] Owing to a lack of proper guidelines in Indian consent laws, hospitals and doctors face a dilemma about the best course of action in many gray areas, which needs to be rectified by the concerned professional regulatory bodies.

Modern medical education tends to discourage physician paternalism while emphasizing the importance of patient autonomy and beneficence; however, these two principles are often at odds with each other. It is symbolic of the legal and ethical expression of the basic right to have one's autonomy and self-determination. Any surgeon who performs an operation without a valid consent will be liable under both tort and criminal law and the consequences would be payment of punitive damages, imprisonment, or both.[23]

Consent can be given in the following ways:

- **Advance consent:** Consent given by a patient in advance.
- **Expressed consent:** It may be oral or written. Despite both consents being of equal magnitude, written consent is considered superior due to its evidential value.
- **Implied consent:** It may be implied by a patient's conduct. Anyone coming for consultation on his or her own volition amounts to implied consent for a clinical diagnosis. However, if the assessment involves an examination of the private parts or genitalia, it is suggested to obtain the patient's permission orally.
- **Consent and age:**
  - ➢ Children <12 years: Consent of the parents or guardian only.
  - ➢ Children between 12 and 18 years: Consent of both, the patient and parents or guardian.
  - ➢ Adult patient above 18 years: Consent of the patient only.
- **Proxy consent**: Proxy consent for a minor, incompetent, emergency patient or dead person can be taken from spouse or blood relatives or other relatives,

biological parents or guardian, teacher or warden who brings the child to the doctor, or a stranger who brought such a patient (e.g., in accident cases) or the Medical Superintendent or the person nominated in an Advance Medical Directive.

- **Surrogate consent:** Generally, courts have held that consent by family members with written authorization by two doctors sufficiently protects the patient's interest.
- **Tacit consent:** It means implied consent understood without being stated.

Signature of a witness must also be taken in all the written consents.[18–23]

Condition of Legal Consent

- Surgeon is legally bound to extend truthful information and to ensure the understanding by patient and witness.
- A mentally competent patient has the right to refuse to consent to treatment for any rational or irrational reason or no reason at all, even if he or she could die or suffer from significant harm as a result of this choice.
- It is better to underpromise and overdeliver than to overpromise and underdeliver.
- The patient ought to understand risks, benefits, and cost of the procedure, including the risks of not having the procedure.
- If the patient's expectations are unrealistic and unattainable, it is better to say "NO" and clarify that they cannot be achieved.

Informed Consent

"Informed Consent" was a ceremonial expression used by attorney Paul Gebhard (1957), on behalf of American College of Surgeons in a malpractice suit at US Court.[24,25] It was argued that **(Fig. 4.1)**:

- A patient agrees to a health intervention based on his or her understanding of it.
- The patient has multiple choices and is not compelled to choose a particular one.
- Consent incorporates giving authorization.

Informed consent is included in the doctrines of Article III and IV of the Indian Constitution, which enshrine human rights. Articles 21, 32, and 36 to 51 authorize that personal freedom is sacrosanct and no one can be forced to undergo a particular treatment, unless complied by legal condition. Article 14 guarantees Equality before Law including identical protection of not only any citizen of India, but also all the people within the territory of India.[25] Any procedure performed without effective informed consent amounts to a breach of the rights to self-determination regardless of improvements in the patient's health. Regrettably, most malpractice claims are not results of technical faults, but are due to inadequate communication between the patient and the surgeon.[26–28] "Adequate information" must be furnished by the doctor or a member of the treating team. Informed consent is a keystone of patient-surgeon liaison and respect for autonomy. No one can consent on behalf of a competent adult. "Informed consent is meant to protect people from being coerced into decisions that someone else thought were in their or the state's best interest."[29–31]

Informed consent is the legal obligation of a healthcare provider to educate the patient about the potential benefits and harms of a treatment, while shared decision-making highlights the implication of a scrupulous discussion of all options available to a patient, allowing the patient to direct the treatment decision that is most consistent with his or her values. Consent given for a specific treatment or a procedure will not be legitimate for conducting any other procedure. Any additional procedure may be performed without consent, only if it is necessary to save the life or preserve the health of the patient and it would be unreasonable to delay until the patient regains consciousness and takes a decision. Any consent obtained during the course of surgery is not acceptable.[25–31]

A fresh, written, informed consent must be obtained before every surgical procedure including a re-exploration procedure. Informed consent for anesthesia must be taken by the anesthesiologist as only he or she can impart essential anesthesia-related information and explain the risks involved. Video recording of consent can be done with prior approval.

- Informed consent is mandatory and more than just a signature on a form.
- Potential risks and benefits must be conveyed for all procedures including aesthetic surgery by sharing all evidence the patient may need to comprehend the benefits and risks of the proposed and all possible alternative procedures.
- Patients receiving both oral and written statements retain higher recollection about the risks of various techniques compared to patients getting only verbal communication.
- When a person signs a legal consent for any surgical process but subsequently feels that he or she did not truly consent and can demonstrate misinformation provided to them at the time of signing may annul the said consent's authenticity. Regretfully, a person might challenge the legitimacy of the consent at a future date, claiming that he or she had understood the significance of the consent but had failed to fully apprehend the concerns.

CONSENT TO SURGERY

1. I authorize **DR.-------------------------** to perform ____________________________ by / and under the directions of **DR.______________,** Consultant Surgeon at the _____ Hospital
2. **Dr.____________ / Attending Doctors** have explained to me in details about the medical condition or the problems and the reason why it requires surgery.
3. **Dr.____________ / Attending Doctors** have fully explained to me kind of procedures he will be performing and has explicitly answered all the questions about how these procedures are going to be effective in correcting the medical condition or the problems that I am suffering from.
4. **Dr.____________ / Attending Doctors** have fully explained to me the details of the operative procedure that will be performed on me to my satisfaction.
5. **Dr.____________ / Attending Doctors** have also explained to me in details about the anticipated prognosis of the proposed surgery, the expected side effects of the proposed surgery and also the complications that might arise because of the proposed surgery. It is understood by me that all possible complications cannot be covered and some unexpected / unforeseen events may occur.
6. I am fully satisfied about the information regarding the surgical procedures, risks involved in the procedures, and with a good understanding of those risks, I consent to undergo the procedure on my own free act and will.
7. **Dr.____________ / Attending Doctors** have also explained to me the alternate methods of treatment other than the proposed surgery, along with similar information regarding these; as well as the consequence of no treatment at all.
8. I have been explained all the above-mentioned information **In My Own Language.** I have decided to undergo the surgical procedure, including the administration of blood products, if necessary, as the best means to try to correct the medical condition.
9. I have been explained to my full satisfaction all the salient points of the procedure and risks involved in performing the procedure.
10. I will not hold any of the **Attending Doctors or Dr.__________** and / or the hospital authorities legally responsible in case of any complications post-operatively or thereafter.
11. I understand that during the course of this procedure, **Dr.____________ / Attending Doctors** may find other unhealthy conditions, which may need correction. I therefore, authorize **Dr.____________ / Attending Doctors** to perform any or all such other procedures which he may find necessary to improve or correct my condition.
12. **Dr.____________ / Attending Doctors** have explained to me that this procedure will be performed as a part of a teaching program, and that while performing the procedure, they may invite some of the residents / trainee to attend to the procedure. I have no objections for the same and he has my full consent to do so.
13. I am also willing for documentation of my Clinical Details for Medical Audit / Presentation purpose and give consent to **Dr.____________ / Attending Doctors** to use them for Medical Teaching / Scientific Presentations.
14. I also agree to co-operate fully with the **Dr.____________ / Attending Doctors** and to follow to the best of my ability his / her instructions and recommendations about my care and treatment.
15. I understand that there are risks associated with different type of Anesthesia. I hereby give my consent for any / all types of Anesthesia that may be required for the Operation.
16. I am fully responsible for payment of all my hospital bills for the above mentioned operation / operations and would not hold **Dr.____________ / Attending Doctors** responsible for any discrepancies in the Bills / Accounting at the __________ Hospital, during the course of the treatment.

I confirm that I have not withheld any of my medical conditions and treatment thereupon and have read and fully understood the above CONSENT TO SURGERY before signing it.

I acknowledge that no Guarantee of Success has been given to me as regards the results of the above mentioned procedure.

Witness by:
1)

2)

____
(Signature of Patient, Relative or Legal / Local Guardian for Patient)
Date:

In Presence of:
1)

Fig. 4.1 Sample for informed consent in aesthetic surgeries.

Informed Consent and "Informed Refusal"

An informed consent is the origin of "informed refusal."[25–31] Informed refusal is a newer principle that could be considered the reverse of informed consent, but is less talked about. The law endorses the credence that *refusal* is a patient's right. For instance, a patient who is well-versed with the facts, possible treatment, and risks can refuse to proceed with the treatment for some reason. An informed refusal, in its entirety, demands realistic disclosure of all probable risks linked with not pursuing the suggested treatment.

A critical feature of informed refusal is defense against malpractice litigation; thus, an "informed refusal" must be well documented and be added to the patient's medical record. It is suggested to clarify details in a simple way or use a translator if there is a language barrier between the parties. Informed refusals should ideally be signed in the presence of a witness for verification purposes. A patient can withdraw consent while the procedure is being performed and the doctor is obliged to stop unless stopping the procedure puts the patient's life at risk, in which case the doctor has to stop once that risk no longer exists. The procedure can only continue once the patient's concerns are addressed and resolved and he or she agrees to the same. Professional indemnity will not cover lapses in attaining a valid consent as a lack of it is considered to be intentional error or omission.[25–31]

Informed Consent for Use of Images on Social Media

Casual sharing of images, photographs, and videos divulging intricate anatomy and operative details on social media or live TV shows amounts to violations of the ethical code of professional conduct, etiquette, and ethics regulations of Indian Medical Council.[22] The Social Media Task Force, instituted by American Society of Plastic Surgeons (ASPS), underscores that "no communication with the public be false, fraudulent, misleading or deceptive."[32–34] Images placed online entail the patient's consent, with prior information that once posted online, the images might be perpetually discoverable.[34] Patients have every right to reject utilization of their private images. With additional advancements in digital technology, social media grows to be a crucial component of modern life and thus allows publicity and display tools with caution to observe customary social media rules.[34–37] A recent survey concluded that 59 to 70% of patients planning plastic surgery portrayed the Internet as a useful medium for assessing surgeons and understanding surgical procedures. Almost 60% of plastic surgeons opined that the Internet and social media have proved valuable for the running of surgical practice.[34] Apart from the eternal online presence of photographs, videos, or blog posts, surgeon or patients must also understand the following:[34–37]

- Surgeons have no control over posted content and it can be circulated to unintended viewers.
- Surgeons should offer the opportunity to assess photographs or videos prior to posting online.
- Must obtain consent for the use of photos on social media at the time of operation.
- It also implies a "*quid pro quo*" that could put the patient in a position in which he or she does not want to dissent for fear that they are not living up to their implicit "bargain," wherein precision of the surgery merits a return from the patient by consenting to social media posts.

Even if the Internet provides ample information, it cannot replace the face-to-face consultation which always should remain a detailed process, covering both the risks as well as the limitations of alternative procedures. Patients regularly perusing reality TV reported a larger influence from TV media to pursue surgery, with surgery reality shows seemingly representing reality.[38] Social media plays a big role in our lives today. Remember that even if you have secured your settings for who can view your postings, all of your information is being collected, mined, and stored on the social media platform servers—perhaps is stored forever.

Most social media platforms don't delete user data as at the moment; posts and photos exist in perpetuity. Data are everywhere not just on social media but most of the Cyber Space. Think before you shout. Because the echo is forever.

- All social media platforms lack privacy and that content will exist forever.
- Maintain a professional boundary between you and your patient.
- Protect patient privacy and confidentially at all times.
- Obtain consent for uploading a video or image even if the patient is not directly identifiable.
- Truthfulness and accuracy are simple standards and should be upheld as much as possible.

According to the guidelines of 2011 by American Medical Association (AMA): "physicians must recognize that actions and content posted online may have negative effect on their reputation among patients and colleagues, may have consequences for their medical careers and can harm public trust in the medical profession." Many surgeons are resorting to platforms such as Instagram, Facebook, and Snapchat. This sort of exposure has enlightened a greater number of potential customers to different aesthetic surgeries, allowing people to easily find, observe, and compare procedures to correct perceived body or facial imperfections.[36–38] Privacy of the patient and health condition is non-negotiable. Health information is considered among the most sensitive information.[39] Special permission is necessary for use of an image for any media communications and promotions. Once granted, this permission is extended to all images, including photographs and videos.

Posting about Patients on Social Media Unethical "Medutainment"

Using the patient–physician relationship as a source of entertainment, sensationalizing a procedure for the audience in order to increase notoriety or attract patients is often disguised as efforts to educate the public, to enhance learning and to allay patient fears regarding surgery. This is not responsible marketing, it is unethical and utterly demeans the surgeon's protective duty toward the patient as does objectifying women.[40] However, individuals can modify or withdraw their consent in writing at any time. Social media use is crucial for many surgeons and tremendous openings are created for educating patients, advertising, and interactions. Diligently avoiding The HIPAA violations is an important part of upholding online efficiency. The Privacy Rule strikes a balance that permits important uses of information, while protecting the privacy of people who seek care and healing.[40–42]

Importance of Photographic Records and Documentations[43–45]

- The photographer must ensure that the end product of his photography is treated with the same respect as is accorded to other records of the patient.
- Every patient has a right to refuse to be photographed or to withdraw consent. If a patient decides to withdraw consent, the records must not be used.
- Preoperative photography is obligatory for each and every patient to record any pre-existing asymmetries or defects.
- The patient may notice the asymmetry postoperatively and may attribute it to the surgery.
- In case any intraoperative or postoperative complications develop, it is vital to maintain a full record including photographs of all meetings, detailing the progress of the treatment.
- In case of a legal proceeding in court, these photographic records of complications and treatment are sole admissible defense and will save the surgeon from most liabilities.
- The Medical Council of India (Professional Conduct, Etiquette and Ethics) Regulations, 2002 (4) states that every physician shall maintain the medical records pertaining to his or her indoor patients for 3 years from the date of commencement of the treatment.[22]
- Disposal of any unwanted photographs is another aspect of confidentiality and there is a need for good net security in hospitals.[42–44]

As per the recent Medical Photography Policy towards Best Practice, developed in response to the British Standards Institution (2014) and Institute of Medical Illustrators (2018):[45] All images taken of patients constitute a part of the patient's record irrespective of who has taken the photograph or what device has been used. Clinicians are not permitted to keep personal collections of patient recordings which are not sufficiently consented or recorded in the first instance. Reproduction or copies of recordings may be provided to clinicians for teaching purposes, provided sufficient consent has been sought (Section 7). Reproduction recordings must be transported securely (Section 19) and always stored on secured media devices.

- Any unauthorized photography is a criminal act breaching the General Data Protection Regulation (GDPR)/Current Data Protection and Sections 2 and 8 of the Human Rights Act. The patient has the legal right to expect that their recording(s) is treated in accordance with the Caldicott Principles and that they will be managed appropriately at all times.
- Confidentiality is patient's right under the GDPR and may only be waived by the patient or by someone legally entitled to do so.
- In all cases of clinical recordings, care must be taken to respect the dignity of the patient and to be aware of the religious beliefs and ethnicity of the patient.
- Recordings of the unconscious patient may be taken, provided that informed consent is obtained beforehand or retrospectively.

Legal Concerns on Use of Media in Aesthetic Surgery

Post-PIP Scandal, there has been a mounting demand for execution of strict regulations on cosmetic procedures including Botox and dermal fillers as well. France enacted the "Kouchner law" in 2002 and the UK government published the "Keogh Report" (by NHS medical director Professor Sir Bruce Keogh) in April 2013.[46] The Care Standards Act 2000 introduced autonomous Healthcare National Minimum Standards for aesthetic surgery clinics which was amalgamated by the National Care Standards Commission in England and was replaced by the "Care Quality Commission" under the Health and Social Care Act 2008, sections 62 and 63.[47.]

Aesthetic/Cosmetic surgery tourism is a fast growing market and in a global society the reasons for seeking cosmetic surgery abroad may vary significantly. As Sir Bruce Keogh's review of the industry recently reported, rising demand for cosmetic enhancement has been driven by a number of socio-economic and technological factors, leading to the normalization of serious and potentially harmful cosmetic interventions. In response to the Keogh Review, there have been some developments but not enough to fully protect the cosmetic surgery consumer.

- The General Medical Council also issued new guidance which sets out the standards they expect from doctors who provide cosmetic interventions, including stipulations to market their services responsibly, seek a patient's consent themselves rather than delegate this to somebody else and consider patients' vulnerabilities and psychological needs when making decisions with them about treatment options. While this presumably will not do anything to prevent poorly qualified doctors from offering their services as a cosmetic surgeon, it will, at least, allow prospective consumers of cosmetic surgery services to ascertain whether the surgeon in question is appropriately qualified.

- This could look like the model in France where, following the enactment of the Kouchner law 2002, regulation is much stricter, consent procedures are far more detailed, and additional safeguards regulating advertising and requiring a 'cooling-off' period, to allow the consumer to reflect on the decision, have been brought in.
- The Royal College of Surgeons, UK (2016) incorporated a new regulation to guard patients undergoing aesthetic surgery from "*aggressive marketing.*" It also included the initiative to make a roster of duly certified surgeons, who are suitably qualified to take on definite procedures.
- Issues arising from reality TV shows that project distortion and misinterpretation of surgical results, thus infringing upon the informed consent process and autonomy.
- No communication made with the public should be false, fraudulent, make unjustifiable claims of results, and should not misrepresent one's level of expertise, professional qualification, etc.
- Postings on social network are not to reveal distinctive personal information about patients. Identifying marks or tattoos should be covered or eliminated and all metadata attached to images must be scrubbed to prevent patient identification.
- Body parts not essential for understanding the procedure shown should be deleted.

Importance of "Cooling-off" Period

- The "cooling-off" period is the mandatory minimum time between the consultation where the proposed treatment and its risks are explained and the consultation wherein the decision is taken to proceed with the treatment or otherwise.
- Patients should be examined preoperatively by the surgeon himself or herself and be provided with full and transparent written and verbal information on the procedure and the potential risks.
- The decision to undergo the procedure should be voluntary and the doctors must not pressure patients to make rushed decisions which they may end up regretting, and they must give the patients enough information so they can make an informed choice.
- This two-stage consent with a "cooling-off" period encourages a period of reflection during which the patient has the opportunity to consider the full implications of the proposed procedure and ask additional questions before embarking upon the treatment. This is to avoid hasty decisions and the patients must be told that they can change their minds about whether to proceed with treatment at any point.
- The time frame which depends on the level of invasion and risk of a procedure is specified for each modality and may vary from country to country. The defined "cooling-off" period is mandatory and cannot be decreased, even at the patient's request. In France, a cooling-off period is set even for Botox and dermal fillers.[47]
- In cases where a cosmetic surgery patient is not given a "cooling-off" period, the patient may be entitled to later make a claim for cosmetic surgery compensation.
- Knowing that the procedure may be deficient to honor the targets of a patient with BDD (body dysmorphic disorder), a plastic surgeon "*ought not to perform*" the operation. This is because mutually understood and agreeable expectations cannot be fulfilled within the patient–surgeon relationship.[48–50]

Body Dysmorphic Disorder

BDD is defined as an obsession with an inexplicable or trivial flaw in physical appearance and is a "mental disorder."[48–50] People with BDD consider themselves as to be ugly or deformed, avoid social interactions, and look at surgery as a remedy to improve their self-image. Many patients with BDD repeatedly consult specialists, including plastic surgeons or dermatologists, in pursuit of a panacea to mend their physical appearance. The exact origin of BDD is not known, but is common during the teen years or early adulthood. Most experts agree that many cases of BDD go unrecognized. One red flag to doctors is when patients repeatedly seek plastic surgery for the same or multiple perceived physical defects.

Average onset is 16 years of age (American Psychiatric Association, 2000). While BDD is prevalent in approximately 2% of the general population, the prevalence may be as high as 7 to 15% in the plastic surgery population. According to a major analysis of cosmetic surgery, done by the Medical Defense Union (MDU), an increasing number of patients are suing plastic surgeons over faults during operations designed to improve their appearance.

Common areas of concern for people with BDD[48–50] include skin imperfections including wrinkles, scars, acne, and blemishes, and facial features often involving the nose, but it also might involve the shape and size of any feature, or any visible scar or disfigurement. Patients with such personality disorders will have unrealistic expectations and regardless of the outcome will continue to be irresolute. Thus, proposing aesthetic procedures may not serve the interests of such patients.

Obligation of Results

In case of obligation of results, the surgeon is expected to comply with the commitment to reach a specific result. For the *obligation of results*, the guilt is irrelevant for contractual breach, being enough for the patient to prove that there was no performance that was promised, but not fulfilled by the obligator.[51] The *obligation of means* does not require the concrete result of a purpose, but the commitment to employ all care and techniques available for achieving the desired results. *The patient is responsible for proving that the obligator did not comply with the obligation.* Furthermore, even if a plastic surgeon eventually commits to the achievement of certain results, the nature of the obligation is not defined by it, and there is no change of the *legal category, which is still the same obligation of providing a risky service*, even if it is performed due to force majeure.

Teen Aesthetic Surgery

They think like adults but behave like children.[52–54] When teens and young adults are considering aesthetic surgery, surgeon must consider both the psychological and physical maturity of young patients seeking aesthetic procedures and ensure that the patient possess the intellectual maturity to understand what is involved in the procedure(s), as well as the risks that are inherent in both the surgery and the anesthesia to be administered.[53] Equally important is determining whether the patient's expectations are realistic. According to the American Society for Aesthetic Plastic Surgery, in 2017 more than 229,000 cosmetic procedures, such as nose reshaping, breast lifts, breast augmentation, and liposuction, were performed on patients between 13 and 19 years of age. It is recommended that teenagers discuss potential cosmetic surgery with their parents before consulting a doctor. A significant number of surgeons choose not to perform certain cosmetic procedures on anyone under the age of 18. They feel that young people's bodies are not yet fully developed, and their considerations are still emotionally immature; consequently, teenagers may be contemplating cosmetic surgery for less than valid reasons. Nevertheless, many teenagers benefit from certain cosmetic procedures. It was not until 2004 that the American Society of Plastic Surgeons clarified its position against breast augmentation for patients younger than 18 years. The FDA guidelines suggest waiting until 22 years of age before using gel implants. Only, very essential surgery should be done for teenagers. The consult should be done in the presence of a parent, and even if the teen is above legal consenting age, parental supervision is still needed. A cooling-off period, informed consent under parental supervision, and time to rethink are essential. If a problem is severe enough to cause psychological problems, a psychologist can help in arriving at a decision.[52–54]

Medical Tourism and Aesthetic Surgery: Perils and Profits

Medical tourism in India is growing at a predicted rate of 30% giving it the fourth or fifth position in top global destinations of medical tourism, aesthetic surgery being a part of it. India is experiencing a deluge of medical tourists from the United States, United Kingdom, Canada, Europe, and countries of the Asia Pacific region due to its low cost and high-quality medical services with no or little waiting time. However, a recent survey in Plastic Surgery News raised concerns: "but safety is in question." Scores of hospitals in India are accredited and follow exacting compliance with quality and safety norms as approved by international organizations. The Indian government actively supports medical tourism. It provides "M" multiple entry visa for medical tourists, with validity up to 1 year, and has offered tax breaks to hospitals catering to medical tourists. Globalization has further smoothed the growth of medical tourism. Several challenges including post-treatment care, lack of uniform standards, brain drain, and increased expenses for local people call for immediate attention. While the exact motives for seeking cosmetic surgery abroad may vary, the most common reason is finance.[55,56]

When a person elects to travel abroad to undergo cosmetic surgery, the usual risks of surgery may be magnified on account of various causes. Yet there is little clear evidence to suggest that cosmetic surgery abroad is necessarily dangerous. In a recent study "Sun, Sea, Sand and Silicone," a fruitful attempt was made to track women from different countries, who were undergoing cosmetic surgery in foreign countries. Stark cultural variances were observed in their inclinations and decisions regarding procedures. Sixty-six percent of them were travelling to India or Thailand for breast augmentations and 88% were opting South Korea for eyelid, jawbone, and nose surgery. Those considering traveling to another country to undergo a cosmetic procedure should know the risks associated with the procedure beforehand and ensure that their doctor's facility is licensed in that country. Despite the accreditation strategies, physical safety and legal protection of medical tourists are still uncertain.

Effects of Stress on Economy and Disasters

Plastic surgeons have complained of working harder for the same or lesser income in recent years. A recent survey postulated that incomes of plastic surgeons have remained steady despite plastic surgeons increasing their surgery load by an average of 41% over the last 10 years and that plastic surgeons have adjusted their practice profiles in recent years.[57–59] They have increased their caseloads and shifted their practices toward cosmetic surgery, most likely with the goal of sustaining their income. The strategy appears to have been successful in the short term. Challenges and competition among plastic, cosmetic, reconstructive, and other providers are getting all the more intense. Uncontrolled cosmetic and aesthetic services are an international frontline for surgical, minimally invasive, and nonsurgical options, with several players including Ophthalmology, OBorGYN, ENT, as well as medical spas. Overcoming these undercurrents requires a strategy with a solid foundation: head-and-shoulders above the competition. The analysis reveals that an additional number of surgeons lead to lower fees as most patients are considered to be price-driven. Such a situation is conducive to discounting or EMI and is on a path of even becoming the industry norm. Increasing competition and falling prices for aesthetic surgery may not be a passing barricade for incomes of plastic surgeons unless proactive measures are taken.[58] As per a recent survey by the American Society of Plastic Surgeons (ASPS): The growth was driven largely by increases in minimally invasive procedures, (i.e., Botox, lasers, and soft tissue fillers). It was concluded that a balance of two types of procedures might be the best strategy. "A purely minimally invasive practice seems to be vulnerable to fluctuations in the economic windfalls, while a purely surgical practice would remain unaffected." According to Global Data, a data and analytics company; between 70 and 100% of all the aesthetic procedures performed in the United States are either delayed, postponed, or canceled due to a global pandemic situation like Covid-19. These situations may arise in future as well, and we need to adapt to the regulations, as they are considered to be elective and nonessential.[58]

Physician–Patient Sexual Relationships

A registered practitioner must not only act professionally but also be seen to act professionally (Chapter 7.4 of Ethical Code of Conduct, Etiquette and Ethics Regulations—2002 updated 2016).[22] A physician, being in a position of trust and power, has a duty to act in the interest of his/her patient. She or he must not indulge in any intimate sexual act with patients or exploit them in any manner. The American Medical Association[60] has termed any sexual contact with a concurrent patient or a relative of the said patient as professional misconduct. It states that a physician should terminate the professional relationship before initiating a dating, romantic, or sexual relationship with the concurrent patient. Sexual or romantic relationships with former patients are unethical if the physician uses or exploits trust, emotions, or influence derived from the previous professional relationship. Across the world and practically by all Ethical Boards and Societies: Physicians who enter into sexual relationships with their patients face the threats of deregistration and prosecution. There are many instances wherein physicians have been struck off the register of the General Medical Council (UK) for such violations.[61] In Canada, if a physician engages in sexual activity with a current patient and does not terminate the professional relationship, it is considered sexual misconduct by provincial medical regulatory colleges, even if the relationship is consensual. The Medical Board of Australia, in its guidelines on sexual boundaries in the doctor–patient relationship, calls any sexual relationship with a patient, regardless *of the* patients consent, as unethical and unprofessional.[61–65]

- Sexual misconduct is an abuse of the doctor–patient relationship and can cause significant and lasting harm to patients.
- Patients have a right to feel safe when they are consulting a doctor.
- Sexual relationships between surgeon and patients can conflict with the fiduciary responsibility (legal or ethical relationship of trust with one or more third parties).[61–65]

Sexual Boundary Violation

Any form of sexual relation between physicians and patients is considered sexual abuse.[61–65] A bench of Chief Justice of Delhi High Court in 2018 directed the Medical Council of India to adopt "guidelines on sexual boundaries for doctors" framed by the *Indian Psychiatric Society* (IPS) to be followed by medical practitioners while examining and treating patients: IPS Task Force has well-defined guidelines for *Sexual Boundary Violation (SBV)*: "elephant in the room." It was concluded that sexual relationships between physicians and patients always harm both the patient and the physician. Trust, which is central to an effective physician–patient relationship, is inevitably damaged.[62]

- In view of the power gradient that exists in the doctor–patient relationship, the onus is on the doctor to ensure he or she does not enter into a sexual relationship with a patient.
- The doctor should not touch a patient inappropriately under the guise of a physical examination for his or her own sexual gratification.
- For whatever reason, if a doctor feels it imperative to have a romantic or sexual relationship with a patient (if this does not involve the breaking of any laws), then the doctor should ensure the patient's care is "handed over" properly to another doctor.
- Any nonconsensual sexual activity would amount to sexual abuse or molestation or rape and doctors would be chargeable under Indian Penal Code Section 376-C (d), which relates to sexual abuse, sexual

molestation, adultery, and sexual harassment in the workplace.
- Similar care should be extended to communications with students, colleagues, and other professionals in the multidisciplinary team.

From the above it can be concluded that it would be inappropriate for the physician to get involved in any kind of intimate relationship with their patient whether consensual or not. It would not only attract penal provisions but will lead to professional misconduct resulting in suspension of license. Doctors need to be aware that SBVs can occur in all gender dyads.

Medical Malpractice Insurance: Aesthetic Surgery

Medical malpractice insurance is a critical part of practicing medicine and more so for aesthetic surgery procedures. It has been noted that compared with other specialties, plastic surgery has one of the highest proportions (13%) of physicians facing a malpractice claim. Multiple studies have shown that breast-related surgeries account for 37% of overall claims against plastic surgeons, making it essential for physicians beginning their practices to have an understanding of the types of malpractice policies available.[66]

Two primary categories are occurrence coverage and claims-made coverage.

1. Occurrence policies provide coverage for events insured during the specified policy period. This is the more expansive, since there is no cap on the extent of time that passes before a claim is made. Thus, such policies are riskier for insurers and the most expensive for policyholders.
2. Claims-made policies provide coverage for insured events as long as two conditions are met:
   a. The insured event has occurred.
   b. The policyholder reports the event within the specified coverage period. Premiums for claims-made policies are much more reasonable than the premiums for occurrence policies.

Surgeons can obtain separate and additional coverage to claims-made policies through tail coverage, which provides coverage for claims reported *after* the policy has expired or been canceled. Nose coverage protects physicians for events that took place before a policy took effect.

In India, most of the service providers do not cover aesthetic/cosmetic surgery procedures and it is vital to read the policy document very carefully. Also, almost all indemnity policies do not cover legal defense in criminal cases. The factors that are most important in standard, standalone policy of any professional insurance company are:

- Sum insured.
- Premium payable and often insurance companies refuse to pay for legal defense.
- The minimum deductibles.
- In the professional indemnity policy, you need to be aware of the AOY:AOI ratio (any one year: any one incident). The ratio is generally either 1:1 or 1:2 or 1:4:[66]
  - ➢ If the ratio is 1:1 then you are covered for the entire 100% for any one incident.
  - ➢ If the ratio is 1:2 then for one year you are covered for 50% of the sum insured for one incident.

Important Applicable Legislation and Law

A. IPC section 354B; use of (criminal) force to woman with intent to disrobe: Any man who assaults or uses criminal force on any woman or abets such act with the intention of disrobing or compelling her to be naked shall be punished with imprisonment of either description for a term which shall not be less than 3 years but which may extend to 7 years, and shall also be liable to fine.

B. IPC Section "376C; (d)": Whoever, being on the management of a hospital, abuses such position or fiduciary relationship to induce or seduce any woman either in his custody or under his charge or present in the premises to have sexual relationship with him, such sexual relationship not amounting to the offence of rape, shall be punished with rigorous imprisonment of either description for a term which shall not be less than 5 years, but which may extend to 10 years, and shall also be liable to fine.

C. Sections 80 and 88 of the IPC (Indian Penal Code) contain defenses for doctors accused of criminal liability. Under Section 80 (accident in doing a lawful act) nothing is an offence that is done by accident or misfortune and without any criminal purpose or awareness in the doing of a lawful act in a lawful manner by lawful means and with proper care and attention.

D. In Section 88, a person cannot be accused of an offence if she or he performs an act in good faith for the other's benefit, does not intend to cause harm even if there is a risk, and the patient has explicitly or implicitly given consent.

Landmark Court Judgments

A. The Supreme Court of India in the case AIR 1989 SC 1570 held that if a doctor has adopted a practice that is considered "proper" by a reasonable body of medical professionals, who are skilled in that particular field, he or she will not be held negligent only because something went wrong. It was further laid down that when a doctor is consulted by a patient, the doctor owes to his or her patient certain duties which are:

- Duty of care in deciding whether to undertake the case.

- Duty of care in deciding what treatment to give.
- Duty of care in the administration of that treatment.

Doctors must exercise a conventional degree of skill; however, they cannot give a guarantee of a cure or warranty of the perfection. If the doctor has adopted the right course of treatment, skills, and has worked with a method and manner best suited to the patient, she or he cannot be blamed for negligence, if the patient is not cured. The apex court interalia observed that negligence has many expressions: active, collateral, comparative, concurrent, criminal, gross, hazardous, active and passive negligence, willful or reckless negligence, or negligence per se.

B. The Full bench of Hon'ble Supreme Court of India in a case (AIR 2004, SC 4091: (2004) 6 SCC 42) concluded that extreme care and caution should be exercised while initiating criminal proceedings against medical practitioners for alleged medical negligence. In a well-drafted order, the apex court touched upon the idea that bonafide medical practitioners should not be put through needless harassment. The court said that doctors would not be able to save lives if they were to tremble with the fear of facing criminal prosecution.

"Medical profession is one of the oldest professions of the world and is the most humanitarian one. There is no better service than to serve the suffering, wounded, and the sick. Inherent in the concept of any profession is a code of conduct that underlines the moral values that govern the professional practice and is aimed at upholding its dignity. In the recent times, professionals are developing a tendency to forget that the self-regulation which is at the heart of their profession is a privilege and not a right and the profession obtains this privilege in return for an implicit contract with society to provide good, competent and accountable service to the public. It must always be kept in mind that a doctor's is a noble profession and the aim must be to serve humanity, otherwise this dignified profession will lose its true worth."

References

1. Goldwyn RM. Laws of plastic surgery. Plast Reconstr Surg 2010;126(2):700
2. Rohrich RJ. Streamlining cosmetic surgery patient selection: just say no! Plast Reconstr Surg 1999;104(1):220–221
3. Lakhan SE, Hamlat E, McNamee T, Laird C. Time for a unified approach to medical ethics. Philos Ethics Humanit Med 2009;4:13
4. Pickstone JV. Thomas Percival and the production of medical ethics: the codification of medical morality. Philosophy and Medicine (PHME) Series. R. Baker, ed. 1993;161–178
5. Pandya SK. History of medical ethics in India. Eubios J Asian Int Bioeth 2000;10:40–43
6. Teven CM, Grant SB. Plastic surgery's contributions to surgical ethics. AMA J Ethics 2018;20(4):349–356
7. Sahni AK. Ethical issues, doctor patient relationship & other perspectives. International J Pharm Sci Health Care 2013;6: 34–50
8. Atiyeh BS, Rubeiz MT, Hayek SN. Aesthetic/cosmetic surgery and ethical challenges. Aesthetic Plast Surg 2008;32(6):829–839, discussion 840–841
9. Salehi HR, Mangion AM. Legal aspects of cosmetic and plastic surgery. Int J Adv Stu Hum Soc Sci 2014;3(2):111–115
10. Nejadsarvari N, Ebrahimi A, Ebrahimi A, Hashem-Zade H. Medical ethics in plastic surgery. World J Plast Surg 2016;5(3): 207–212
11. Kumar R, Attri S, Hastir A, Goyal S. Surgical ethics: Indian perspective. Int J Contemp Med Res 2017;4:1096–1099
12. Nandimath OV. Consent and medical treatment: the legal paradigm in India. Indian J Urol 2009;25(3):343–347
13. Shuster E. Fifty years later: the significance of the Nuremberg Code. N Engl J Med 1997;337(20):1436–1440
14. World Medical Association Declaration of Helsinki Ethical Principles for Medical Research Involving Human Subjects. JAMA 2013;2013;310(20):2191–2194
15. Code of Ethics of The American Society of Plastic Surgeons as published by ASPS Ethics Committee, 444 East Algonquin Road, Arlington Heights, IL 60005
16. Lee A. "Bolam" to "Montgomery" is result of evolutionary change of medical practice towards "patient-centered care". Postgrad Med J 2017;93(1095):46–50
17. Sidaway V Board of Governors of Bethlem Royal Hospital and Maudsley Hospital: [1985] 1 All ER 643, [1985] 2 WLR 480, [1985] AC 871, [1985] UKHL
18. Nejadsarvari N, Ebrahimi A. Different aspects of informed consent in aesthetic surgeries. World J Plast Surg 2014;3(2): 81–86
19. Kirby MD. Informed consent: what does it mean? J Med Ethics 1983;9(2):69–75
20. Fenger H. Informed consent in aesthetic plastic surgery. Handchir Mikrochir Plast Chir 2006;38(1):64–67
21. Medical Consent Act General Assembly of Commonwealth of Pennsylvania; Act of Nov. 24, 1999, P.L. 546, No. 52
22. Indian Medical Council Ethical Code of Conduct Professional Conduct, Etiquette and Ethics Regulations—2002
23. Murray AM, Petrone AB, Adcock AK. Utilization of a parental approach to informed consent in intravenous tissue plasminogen activator administration decision-making: patient preference and ethical considerations. Neurol Res Int 2019;2019: 9240603
24. Kristinsson S. The Belmont Report's misleading conception of autonomy. Virtual Mentor 2009;11(8):611–616
25. Kumar A, Mullick P, Prakash S, Bharadwaj A. Consent and the Indian medical practitioner. Indian J Anaesth 2015;59(11): 695–700
26. Wagner RF Jr, Torres A, Proper S. Informed consent and informed refusal. Dermatol Surg 1995;21(6):555–559
27. Sherlock A, Brownie S. Patients' recollection and understanding of informed consent: a literature review. ANZ J Surg 2014;84(4): 207–210
28. Makdessian AS, Ellis DAF, Irish JC. Informed consent in facial plastic surgery: effectiveness of a simple educational intervention. Arch Facial Plast Surg 2004;6(1):26–30
29. Khoo LS, Mazzarone F. Informed consent and failure to disclose: legal perspectives for aesthetic surgeons. PMFA News 2016, 4
30. Murray B. Informed consent: what must a physician disclose to a patient? Virtual Mentor 2012;14(7):563–566
31. Bester J, Cole CM, Kodish E. The limits of informed consent for an overwhelmed patient: clinicians' role in protecting

patients and preventing overwhelm. AMA J Ethics 2016;18(9): 869–886
32. Bennett KG, Berlin NL, MacEachern MP, Buchman SR, Preminger BA, Vercler CJ. The ethical and professional use of social media in surgery: a systematic review of the literature. Plast Reconstr Surg 2018;142(3):388e–398e
33. Spilson SV, Chung KC, Greenfield ML, Walters M. Are plastic surgery advertisements conforming to the ethical codes of the American Society of Plastic Surgeons? Plast Reconstr Surg 2002;109(3):1181–1186
34. Wong WW, Gupta SC. Plastic surgery marketing in a generation of “tweeting”. Aesthet Surg J 2011;31(8):972–976
35. Gutierrez PL, Johnson DJ. Can plastic surgeons maintain professionalism within social media? AMA J Ethics 2018;20(4): 379–383
36. Montemurro P, Porcnik A, Hedén P, Otte M. The influence of social media and easily accessible online information on the aesthetic plastic surgery practice: literature review and our own experience. Aesthetic Plast Surg 2015;39(2):270–277
37. Kisyova R, Rahman SM, Karkhi A. Ethics in aesthetics: social media. J Aesthetic Nurs 2019;8:310–312
38. Crockett RJ, Pruzinsky T, Persing JA. The influence of plastic surgery “reality TV” on cosmetic surgery patient expectations and decision making. Plast Reconstr Surg 2007;120(1):316–324
39. Health Insurance Portability and Accountability Act of 1996 (HIPAA). Public Health Professionals Gateway
40. Mercer C. “Medutainment”: are doctors using patients to gain social media celebrity? CMAJ 2018;190(21):E662–E663
41. Murphy DG, Loeb S, Basto MY, et al. Engaging responsibly with social media: the BJUI guidelines. BJU Int 2014;114(1):9–11
42. Bennett KG, Vercler CJ. When is posting about patients on social media unethical “Medutainment”? AMA J Ethics 2018; 20(4):328–335
43. Bhattacharya S. Clinical photography and our responsibilities. Indian J Plast Surg 2014;47(3):277–280
44. Supe A. Ethical considerations in medical photography. Issues Med Ethics 2003;XI(3):83–84
45. Medical Photography Policy developed by Mid Essex Hospital Services 2018
46. Latham M. “If it ain’t broke, don’t fix it?”: scandals, “risk,” and cosmetic surgery regulation in the UK and France. Med Law Rev 2014;22(3):384–408
47. Griffiths D, Mullock A. Cosmetic surgery: regulatory challenges in a global beauty market. Health Care Anal 2018;26(3): 220–234
48. Hodgkinson DJ. Identifying the body-dysmorphic patient in aesthetic surgery. Aesthetic Plast Surg 2005;29(6):503–509
49. Crerand CE, Franklin ME, Sarwer DB. Patient safety: body dysmorphic disorder and cosmetic surgery. Plast Reconstr Surg 2008;122:1–15
50. Tadisina KK, Chopra K, Singh DP. Body dysmorphic disorder in plastic surgery. Eplasty 2013;13:ic48. body-dysmorphic-disorder-in-plastic-surgery&catid=49. Accessed February 23, 2018
51. de Oliveira Alves RG, de Azambuja LJ. Civil liability of the plastic surgeon in aesthetic procedures. Rev bioét (Impr.) 2012; 20:397–403
52. Singh K. Cosmetic surgery in teenagers: to do or not to do. J Cutan Aesthet Surg 2015;8(1):57–59
53. Wilhite CL. Ethical and legal considerations in teen aesthetic surgery. Plast Surg Nurs 2012;32(1):19–21
54. Paik AM, Mady LJ, Sood A, Eloy JA, Lee ES. A look inside the courtroom: an analysis of 292 cosmetic breast surgery medical malpractice cases. Aesthet Surg J 2014;34(1):79–86
55. Franzblau LE, Chung KC. Impact of medical tourism on cosmetic surgery in the United States. Plast Reconstr Surg Glob Open 2013;1(7):e63
56. Miyagi K, Auberson D, Patel AJ, Malata CM. The unwritten price of cosmetic tourism: an observational study and cost analysis. J Plast Reconstr Aesthet Surg 2012;65(1):22–28
57. Krieger LM, Lee GK. The economics of plastic surgery practices: trends in income, procedure mix, and volume. Plast Reconstr Surg 2004;114(1):192–199
58. Krieger LM. Discount cosmetic surgery: industry trends and strategies for success. Plast Reconstr Surg 2002;110(2): 614–619
59. Liu TS, Miller TA. Economic analysis of the future growth of cosmetic surgery procedures. Plast Reconstr Surg 2008;121(6): 404e–412e
60. The American Medical Association AMA Code of Medical Ethics’ Opinions on Observing Professional Boundaries and Meeting Professional Responsibilities. American Med Assoc J of Ethics 2015;17(5):432-434. http://journalofethics.amaassn.org/2015/05/coet1-1505.html. Accessed 11 September, 2020.
61. Collier R. When the doctor-patient relationship turns sexual. CMAJ 2016;188(4):247–248
62. Kurpad SS, Bhide A. Sexual boundaries in the doctor-patient relationship: guidelines for doctors. Indian J Psychiatry 2017; 59(1):14–16
63. Miller FG, Brody H, Chung KC. Cosmetic surgery and the internal morality of medicine. Camb Q Healthc Ethics 2000;9(3): 353–364
64. Lawrence RE, Brauner DJ. Deciding for others: limitations of advance directives, substituted judgment, and best interest. Virtual Mentor 2009;11(8):571–581
65. The revised Medical Board of Australia guidelines on sexual boundaries. Australian Medical Association. Published: 03 Dec 2018
66. Naik S. Clarification on professional indemnity insurance. GRASP 2020;48:43–45

5

Applications of Regenerative Medicine in Aesthetic Surgery

J. Sarah Crowley, Steven R. Cohen, and Mohan Rangaswamy

Introduction

The concept of regenerative medicine within the scope of aesthetic plastic surgery is the idea of restoring one's youth, and improving beauty and function using or stimulating the body's own cells and tissue. The term "regenerative medicine" was first coined by Dr William Haseltine in 1999 when he used it to describe advancements in tissue engineering to replace human tissue.[1] For facial aging, it has been recognized that volume loss, soft tissue descent, dermal thinning, and sun damage are the main physical signs of aging, and these findings have created a shift toward rejuvenation through serial replacement and regeneration of lost and damaged tissue. Although fillers and implants have been used for this purpose, volume enhancement by fat is ideal as it is natural, easily obtained, autologous, and biocompatible.[2] In addition, fat graft has been shown to improve the quality of skin and improve scars, contractures, and radiation damage.[3] Furthermore, it is an appealing principle of plastic surgery to replace "like with like."[4]

The idea of fat grafting and its reparative and regenerative properties were first described by Neuber in 1893 when he used autologous fat harvested from the arm to fill depressed facial scars.[5] Lexer, a craniofacial surgeon, published on the use of fat grafting for different anomalies including post-traumatic, hemifacial microsomia, knee ankylosis, and in conjunction with tenolysis.[6,7] Fat harvest was done surgically and later by sharp curettes, but true noninvasive liposculpture was first invented by Giorgia Fischer and his father Arpad Fischer in 1974, when they designed the first suction cannula system to harvest fat.[8] Illouz modified it to blunt cannulas and he was one of the first to use lipo-harvested fat as a filling product, calling it "fat cell graft."[9] In 1986, Ellenbogen utilized 4- to 6-mm "pearls" of sharply minced fat as particulate grafts to improve facial atrophy wrinkles, nasolabial folds, and for chin augmentation.[10] However, all the published authors noted the unpredictable success of fat uptake, and it was not until Dr Sydney Coleman described a standardized technique of harvesting, preparing, and injecting fat in 1998 that structural fat grafting became popularized in aesthetic and reconstructive surgery.[11,12] Coleman first described harvesting, processing using centrifugation (separating oil, blood, and fluid), and injecting using 1-mL syringes with small multiple passes.[11] He stated that the key to long-term graft survival lies in the technique of "miniscule amounts," thus increasing the surface area of contact of fat with its surrounding tissues.[2]

Fat Cells

Two different theories have been proposed to explain the mechanism of fat survival, namely "host cell replacement" and "cell survival theory."[13–15] In 1923, Neuhof and Hirshfeld founded the "host cell replacement theory" when they microscopically examined fat and found that the transplanted tissue underwent degeneration initially. These dying cells stimulated phagocytosis and transformation of "wandering cells" into embryonal fat cells with metaplasia into normal mature adipose tissue and sometimes connective tissue.[16] Peer et al stated that the final amount of fat survival depends on the number of viable adipocytes that are grafted and then survive.[17] We now know that aspirated adipose tissue is made up of two constituents, adipocytes with lipid inclusions and the progenitor cells.[13] Studies on adipocyte viability have shown that mature adipocytes are more fragile and are susceptible to trauma and ischemia compared to the more resistant preadipocytes, which have a lower metabolic rate and need for nutrition.[13,14,18,19] Experimental studies on transplanted fat pads in mice clearly showed three zones from the periphery to the center of the graft: the surviving area of 300 microns (adipocytes survived), the regenerating area (adipocytes died, adipose-derived stromal cells survived, and dead adipocytes were replaced with new ones) and the necrotic area (both adipocytes and adipose-derived stromal cells died).[20] This and similar studies form the basis of grafting in small aliquots so that the fat cells are no more than 1 mm from a source of nutrition, i.e., a particle size close to 2 mm in diameter. After grafting, the surviving adipose tissue is long lasting as has been shown in many studies and borne out in personal experiences. Cohen et al showed progressive improvement in facial volume two years after facelifting combined with anatomical and regenerative fat grafting.[21]

Adipocyte-Derived Stem Cells

Adipocyte-derived stem cells (ADSCs) were first described by Zuk et al in 2001. He discovered ADSC from adipose tissue as an alternate source of adult multipotent stem cells.[22] Unlike mesenchymal stem cells (MSC) derived from bone, ADSCs can be obtained relatively painlessly and in large quantities from fatty tissue and are easily processed. Fat tissue contains 500 times more MSCs than bone marrow; the number is mostly independent of host age.[23] The ADSCs belong to the large group of MSCs that are present in several adult and fetal body tissues and share several common features.[24] These cells have the capability of self-renewal and differentiating into other mesodermal derivatives including fat, cartilage, muscle, and bone as well as being induced to form endoderm and ectodermal tissues.[22,25,26] ADSCs have become the most commonly used regenerative cell whether in native form or as culture amplified product.[26] ADSCs secrete factors that promote angiogenesis and antiapoptosis and also have paracrine properties.[27] They are immune modulating, anti-inflammatory, antifibrotic in addition to supporting cell proliferation and maturation when cografted with fat tissue.[28,29]

They may also reverse many of the toxic changes induced by radiation therapy; fat grafts and ADSC are beginning to be used to reverse radiation dermatitis and fibrosis.[30]

Stromal Vascular Fraction

ADSCs are found within the perivascular adipose stroma, and therefore need to be extracted from the surrounding stroma in order to be utilized. Fat tissue can be subjected to collagenase digestion and the resulting infranatant after centrifugation is known as stromal vascular fraction (SVF). It contains multiple different types of cells including ADSCs, pericytes, endothelial progenitor cells, hematopoietic cells, and fibroblasts.[31,32] Mechanical dissociation of fat can also produce SVF, but at lower cell counts than enzymatic digestion.[33] The regenerative properties of SVF are attributed to the many types of growth factors and cytokines that are secreted by the cells within the stroma, particularly when stimulated by ischemia. These growth factors stimulate and promote regeneration through angiogenesis, cell development, and new tissue growth.[34,35] Studies have shown that SVF-enriched fat grafts, also known as cell-assisted lipotransfer (CAL), are retained better than just fat graft alone.[36–39] A unique form of SVF was developed by Yao et al who describes SVF-gel which is a product that has been processed to have high concentrations of ADSCs and other SVF cells without the proinflammatory lipids, and has been shown to produce higher long-term volume retention and rejuvenation effects.[39] Our preferred technique for enzymatic isolation of SVF is the Celution system (Lorem Cytori), mostly used in research studies. For mechanical SVF (not Nanofat), we use Lipocube (Lipocube, Inc.), which creates a cell aggregate SVF that approximates 80 to 85% of the cell counts with similar profiles and viability as enzymatically dissociated SVF.[33]

Nanofat

Tonnard et al first described the concept of "nanofat." Their group mechanically emulsified fat tissue into a liquefied form without connective tissues and called it "nanofat" for facial rejuvenation.[40] Tonnard et al's group was able to isolate $1.975 \times 10^6/100$ mL of SVF cells by enzymatic digestion of their nanofat. Although lower than the cell count of enzymatically obtained SVF, it still contains a significant supply of SVF cells that can be injected through smaller gauge needles (27 gauge). One of the most commonly used mechanical isolation devices for nanofat production is the Tulip Nano Transfer kit (Tulip Medical, Inc.). This method consists of harvesting the fat to obtain 1.5- to 2.5-mm fat parcels using a multihole syringe cannula. These parcels are then made progressively smaller by serial passage through connectors (2.4, 1.4, and 1.2 mm diameters). The emulsified fat is then passed through a device with a two-layered filter of 600 and 400 microns, to reduce the size of the parcels to pass easily through a 27-gauge needle or 25G cannula. However, the overlapping small-sized filters actually trap more extracellular matrix, removing the component where the regenerative SVF cells reside, thus reducing the SVF content.

LipocubeNano was developed as a mechanical isolation device (Lipocube, Inc.) to maximize the amount of matrix and optimize the cell counts of the nanofat.[33] It uses sharp blades inside a closed cubical device to "chop" the fat particles rather than squeeze them through progressively smaller channels and grids. In a comparative study by Cohen et al, LipocubeNano produced a cell count of 2.24×10^6/mL with a cell viability of 96.75%, while the TulipNanoTransfer method produced 1.44×10^6/mL with a cell viability of 96.05%. LipocubeNano produces three different fat products, millifat, microfat, and nanofat, which are used to perform structural grafting in the deep fat compartments, the superficial compartments, and dermis, respectively.[33] This nanofat can pass through 27-gauge needles, penetrate skin when used with microneedling devices, and could be compounded with liposomal and/or exosomal transport vehicles into a unique biocreme for transdermal delivery.[41]

Platelet-Rich Plasma

Platelet-rich plasma (PRP) is another form of autologous tissue product that has been popularized for its regenerative properties. It was first described by Marx et al alongwith its use for growth factor enhancement in bone grafts in the oro-maxillofacial specialty.[42] PRP contains a high concentration of platelets, defined as a platelet count of 1 million/mL. The alpha granules in platelets contain multiple growth factors such as platelet-derived growth factor (PDGF) and vascular endothelial growth factor (VGEF) which are angiogenic, and transforming growth factor-β (TGF-β), epidermal growth factor (EGF), and fibroblast growth factor (FGF) which support cell proliferation.[42] Platelets release these factors upon activation by a process of degranulation. In vitro studies have shown that PRP enhances proliferation of ADSCs in culture while in vivo studies have shown improved volume retention with the addition of PRP to fat grafts in some studies.[43–47] The results have been conflicting in the literature due to inconsistency in the method of PRP preparation, dosing, and lack of objectivity in assessment of end points.[48–50] Platelet-rich fibrin (PRF) is a new form of platelet concentrate and is called second-generation PRP that has been described as easier to utilize in the clinical setting than PRP, with studies showing improved fat graft retention when cotransplanting with PRF compared to PRP.[51]

Facial and Neck Rejuvenation

Facial fat grafting for rejuvenation is perhaps one of the most common applications of regenerative medicine in the field of aesthetic surgery, first popularized by Coleman in the mid-1990s.[11,85] Changes to the aging face include loss of volume, descent of tissues, and facial skeleton losses. Rohrich and Pessa described anatomical fat compartments of the face that are distinctly separated by septal borders.[86] Some are superficial to the muscle and are tightly attached to the skin with numerous fibroseptal bands, and others are deep to the muscles of facial expression and are billowy, cloudlike structures used to cushion and facilitate movement of the muscles that lie above them. It is by observing how these different compartments change over time that one can understand how to perform a precise, anatomic volume enhancement rather than grafting fat randomly to all layers (**Fig. 5.1**).[86]

Our concept is to look at aging as a dynamic process that can be modeled and understood anatomically and eventually physiologically, tissue-by-tissue and cell-by-cell. Almost like viewing a movie and reversing the frames, facial aging is best appreciated by analyzing the patient's own journey by looking at old photographs and understanding how the patient's parents have aged.

Marten and Elyassnia see similar findings and state that the aging face can be categorized into three problems: aging and breakdown at the skin surface, tissue sagging and skin redundancy, and facial hollowing and atrophy. Skin resurfacing procedures can treat most problems at the superficial skin level and the tissue sagging can be addressed with facelift and neck lift. However, facial hollowing and atrophy cannot be corrected with either of these two methods alone and this is where fat grafting is crucial to restoring a youthful and more full appearance. Fat grafting can be used in combination with the facelift to correct facial contour and atrophy.[81] Specifically, for advanced facial rejuvenation, fat grafting alone is not recommended, as facial hollowing rarely occurs without associated sagging tissues. In an attempt to "fill out" the redundant skin, one must then overfill with fat, which often leads to an unnatural look. Instead, fat grafting can be used in conjunction with a lift, typically prior to the start of the facelift, to more precisely correct hollowed areas.[81]

Author's Approach to Facial Rejuvenation with Fat Grafting and Regenerative Cells

The injectable tissue replacement and regeneration (ITR2) is a method of using regenerative cells to reduce and potentially reverse facial aging.[21] This method evaluates the anatomic areas of volume loss topographically, and addresses the anatomic losses of different tissues (skin, fat, and bone) by replacement with different sizes of autogenous fats that are chosen specifically for the area (**Fig. 5.2**). The fat grafts are supplemented with regenerative ingredients including matrix, ADSCs, SVF cells, growth factors, and PRP.[21] Cohen et al describe a systematic approach consisting of syringe aspiration of fat, simple washing, gravity separation and processing to get three types of products. A portion is set aside as millifat (2- to 2.5-mm parcels) and the rest is processed into microfat (1-mm parcels) and nanofat (500 µM) using the Nanocube kit (Lipocube, Inc.). Injection starts in the deep compartments and moves superficially (**Fig. 5.3**). **Millifat** is allocated to the deep temporal region along the preperiosteal lateral supraorbital brow, the upper/lower hemilip at the commissures, glabella, medial supraorbital rims and nasal radix, nasal dorsum, tip and columella (through the domes of the nasal tip), chin mandibular border and gonial angle, and buccal fat compartment. **Microfat** is grafted in a superficial plane for the marionette lines and perioral tissue, superficial temporal fat, medial brows, central/inferior/lateral subcutaneous forehead, and the upper and lower lids,

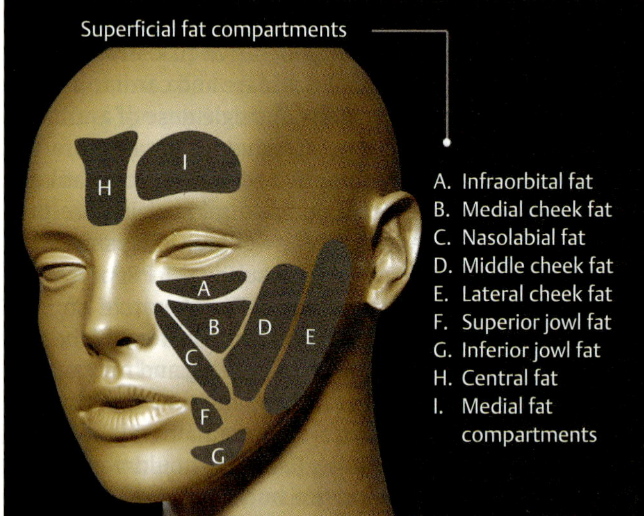

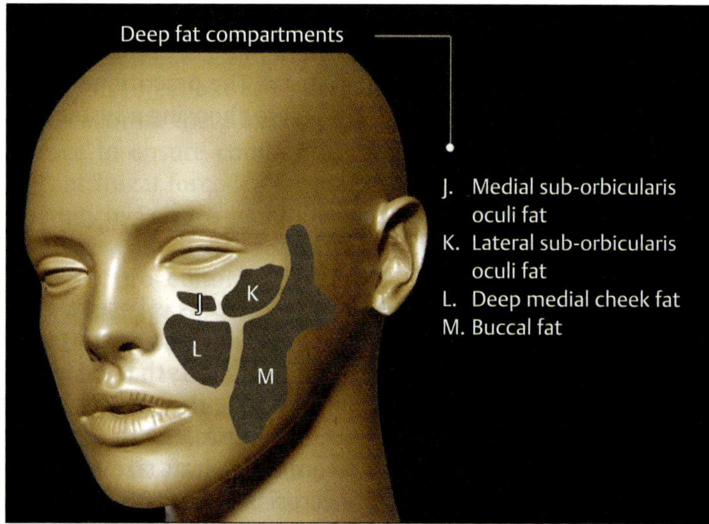

Fig. 5.1 **(a, b)** Superficial and deep fat compartments of the face.

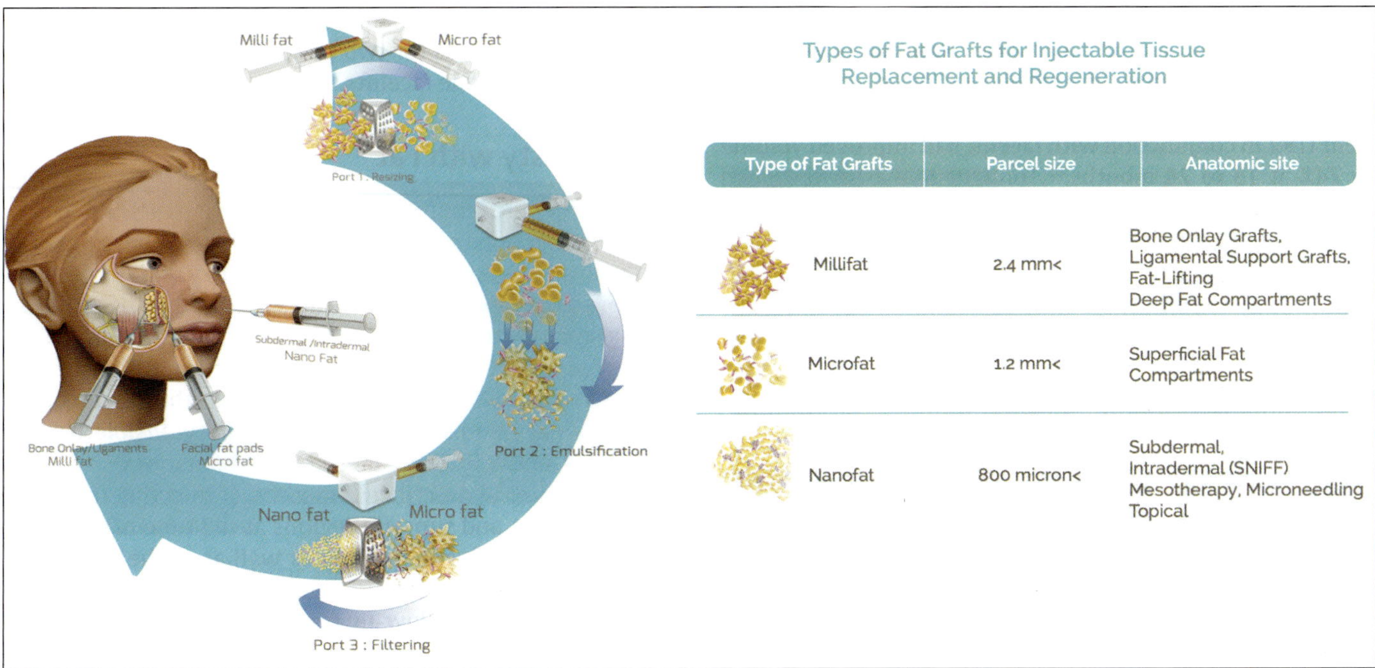

Type of Fat Grafts	Parcel size	Anatomic site
Millifat	2.4 mm<	Bone Onlay Grafts, Ligamental Support Grafts, Fat-Lifting Deep Fat Compartments
Microfat	1.2 mm<	Superficial Fat Compartments
Nanofat	800 micron<	Subdermal, Intradermal (SNIFF) Mesotherapy, Microneedling Topical

Fig. 5.2 Description of millifat/microfat/nanofat.

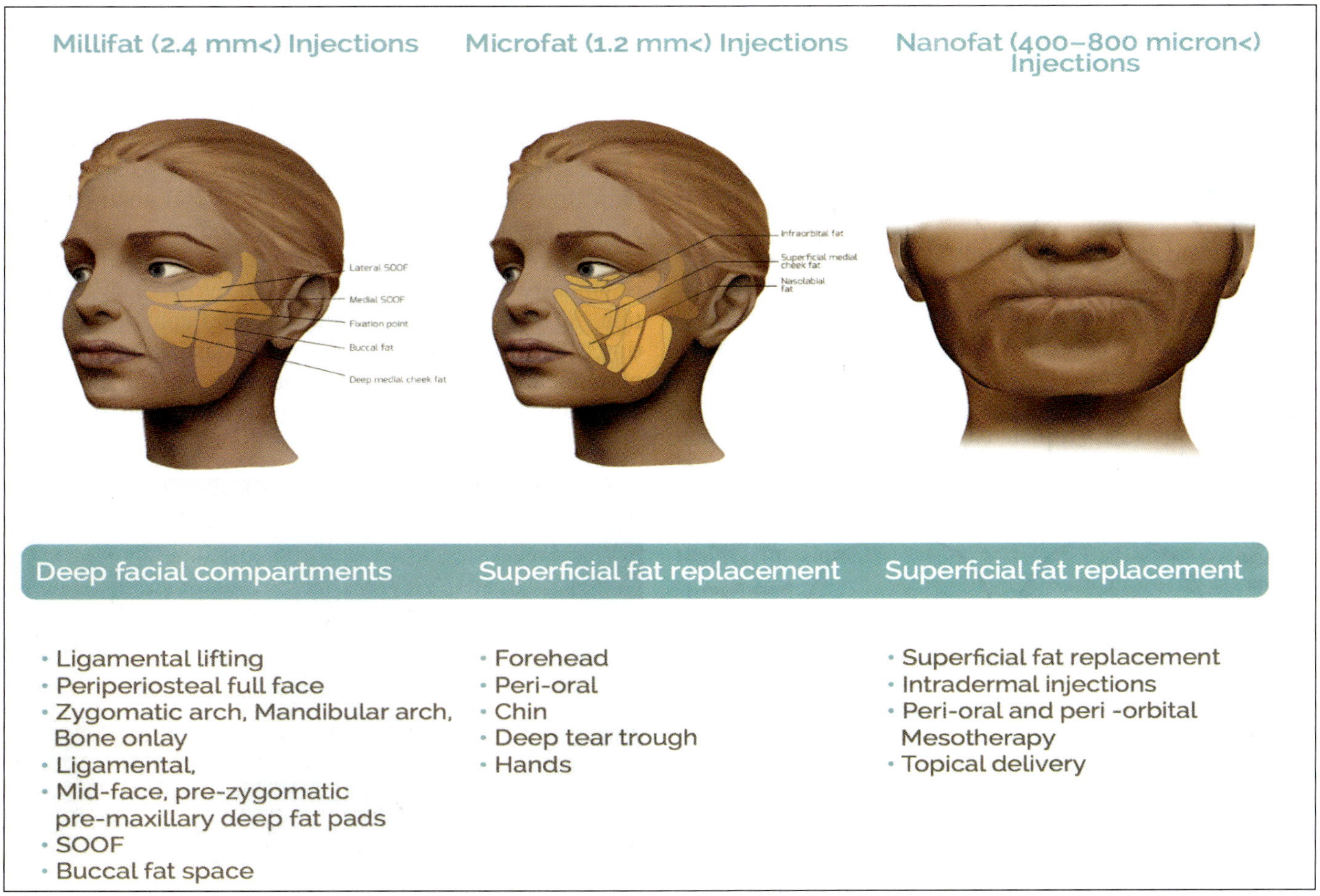

Fig. 5.3 Millifat/microfat for superficial and deep fat compartments, areas of bone loss, and tissue regeneration of the face, and nanofat for superficial fat replacement.

of fat from the sacral region is particularly important to exaggerate lumbar lordosis and enhance perceived gluteal projection. The fat is collected in a sterile container, and is decanted and rinsed with Ringer's lactate or Normal Saline. Clindamycin 300 mg may be added to the solution. The fat is transferred either using 60-mL syringes for injection or autoinjected using power-assisted vibration with the roller pump reversed.

Technique of fat injection is incredibly important here and must be done in small aliquots with a 3.7-mm cannula in an antegrade and retrograde fashion, fanning motion. No more than 5 to 10 mL of fat should be injected with each pass and in multiple planes for even homogenous distribution. The planes should always be in the superficial or deep subcutaneous space. No fat is placed below the muscular fascia or into the muscle as described by Del Vecchio's safe gluteal augmentation technique.[110,111] Avoidance of deep muscular layers is critical to avoid accidental intravenous injection. The correct angling of the cannula parallel to the injection plane is important and ultrasound guidance is a valuable safety adjunct in order to help avoid the danger zone[110] (**Fig. 5.14**). Overcorrection can cause compression and death of transplanted fat.[84] **Figs. 5.15 and 5.16** show our preop and 6-month postop images of liposculpture with gluteal augmentation.

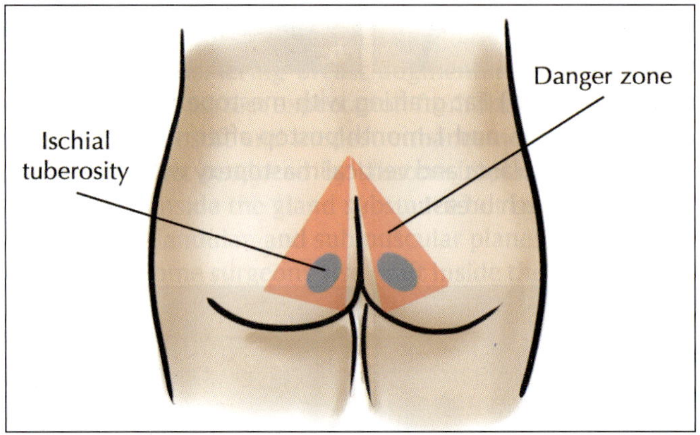

Fig. 5.14 Danger zone of the buttock and area with greatest risk of gluteal vessel injury and fat embolism.

Genital Rejuvenation

Vaginal rejuvenation was first introduced into the medical literature in 2007 and has increased in interest in the past several years, along with the introduction of scrotal rejuvenation in 2018.[112] Genital rejuvenation can be considered

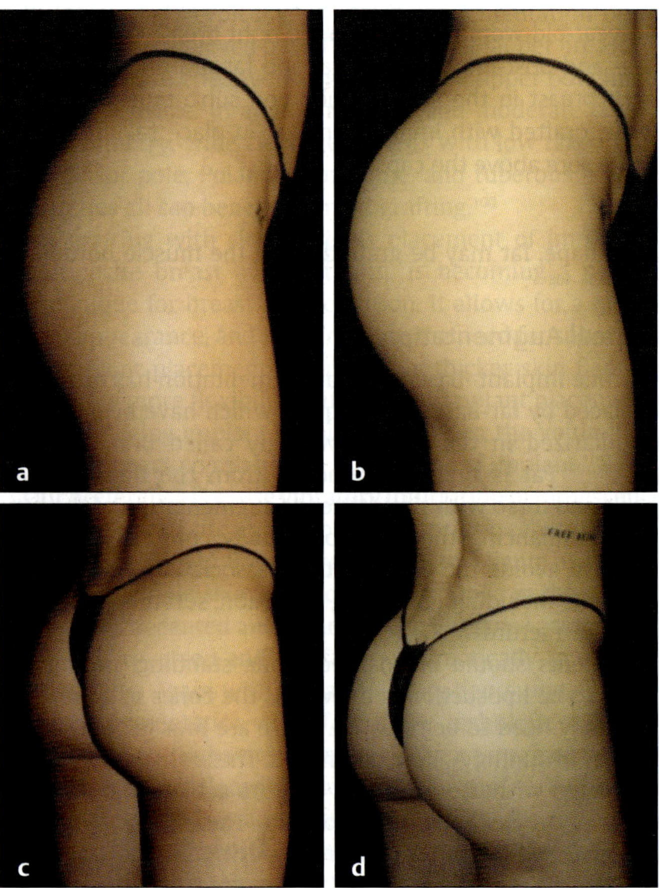

Fig. 5.15 (a–d) Gluteal augmentation with fat in a 29 year-old-woman: pre- and post 6-months follow-up with liposculpture of the flanks and abdomen with bilateral subcutaneous gluteal augmentation with 400 mL per buttock.

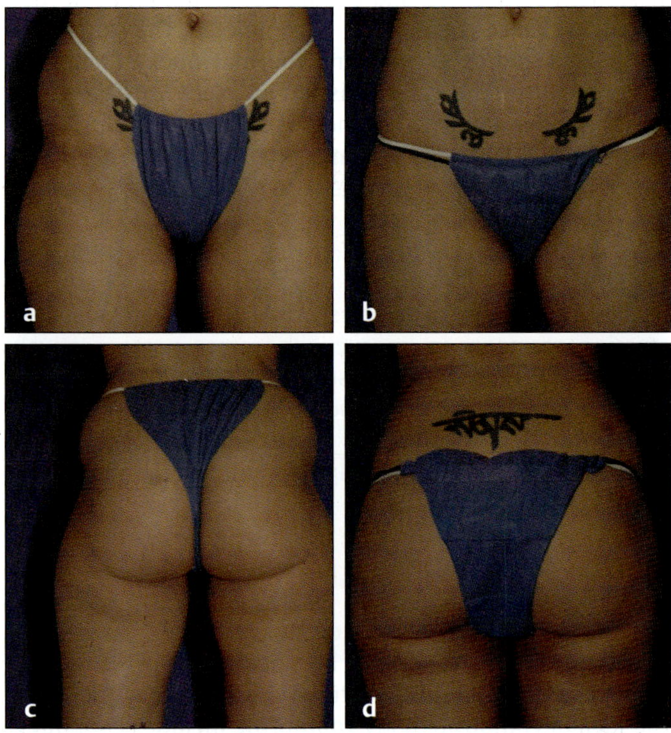

Fig. 5.16 (a–d) Gluteal augmentation with fat in a 28-year-old-woman: pre- and post 6-months follow-up with liposculpture of flanks and abdomen with bilateral subcutaneous gluteal augmentation with 300 mL per buttock.

for local hair loss, atrophy, excess tissue, and skin laxity. Regenerative cells are an integral part of genital rejuvenation in combination with resections, Mons liposuction, muscle tightening, and laser.[113] Fat is harvested and processed as described previously. Fat grafting is done using blunt 1.5- to 2-mm cannula by retrograde technique, depositing small aliquots to each labia major starting by superior entry. The Mons pubis may also require fat grafts. Micro and nanofat are used in vaginal mucosa, introitus, and at the G spot enhancement of sexual sensation.[114] PRP has also been used alone or in combination to rejuvenate the exterior and interior with further improvement of lichen sclerosus as well.[113,115] A recent study by Menkes et al studied 50 women with genitourinary syndrome of menopause.[116] Women received microfat in the labia majora and nanofat in the vagina. The women's vagina health index and female sexual distress scale-revised showed significant improvement following treatments and with 80% of patients normalized at 6-month follow-up.[116]

Hand Rejuvenation

Throughout history, how worn and aged one's hand appears has been a way to distinguish social class, so it is no wonder that many patients have had interest in improving the aesthetic appearance of their hands. The elderly or aged hand has poor skin quality with pigmentations, skin laxity, visible veins and tendons, and loss of subcutaneous fat emphasizing arthritic appearance.[111,117] There have been qualitative measures to grade the soft tissue atrophy of the hand including Zhou's Grading system and the Merz Hand Grading Scale to evaluate the improvement following hand rejuvenation. Fat grafting is the most superior way to achieve younger looking hands due to its ease of technique and ability to truly rejuvenate the skin changes from the inside.[118] The Coleman technique has been used to prepare the fat for grafting. The point of entrance is the dorsal wrist fanning out toward the dorsum of the hand.[117] Using small syringes, the fat is injected while withdrawing the cannulas in small aliquots of 0.3 mL or less. Many small tunnels should be formed to maximize surface area. At the end, the hand should have a puffy slightly overfilled appearance. An additional small volume of fat should be injected at the base of each finger.[118] Microfat is used for subcutaneous replacement and nanofat microneedling and biocreme for dermal and skin regeneration (**Fig. 5.17**). The patients are given a pump container with the Nanofat Biocreme, which they keep refrigerated and use until it is gone.

Hair Restoration

Androgenic alopecia occurs due to androgens (dihydrotestosterone) causing "miniaturization of hair follicles" or the depletion of the anagen stage, with increase in the resting hair follicles and telogen.[119] Current ways to treat androgenic alopecia include drugs such as finasteride, minoxidil (which have systemic effects) and surgical procedures including hair transplantation, which is considered the gold standard in hair restoration. Male pattern loss in females is not so easily managed by hair transplantation. The use of stem cells for treatment of alopecia has seen a growing interest as multipotent stem cells can regenerate hair follicles with sebaceous organs in the skin.[119] Cohen was the first to transplant enzymatically obtained SVF into a woman with androgenic alopecia in 2009, which led to a number of clinicians and researchers to utilize cell therapy methods to address this distressing condition. Adipose tissue has been found to have an antiadrenergic effect through conversion of the DHT into weak 3-alpha diol through a 3-alpha reductase activity.[120] Fukuoka et al injected ADSCs medium intradermally into 22 patients with alopecia for a total of six sessions, and hair numbers were found to be significantly increased after treatment in both men and women.[121] The most promising published study to date is the STYLE trial by Kuka et al, a randomized, blinded controlled multicenter trial of 71 patients. The patients were randomized into four groups: Puregraft fat with high-dose adipose-derived regenerative cells (ADRCs), Puregraft fat enriched with low dose of ADRCs, Puregraft fat alone, and saline injections in the fourth group. At week 24, there was a statistically significant difference in hair count between the low-dose ADRC group and no fat saline control group.[122]

Correction of Permanent Filler Complications

Several permanent nonreversible fillers have been used for aesthetic purpose on the face, breasts, body, and buttocks in the past three decades by qualified and unqualified practitioners. Chief among them are polyacrylamide, polymethyl methacrylate (PMMA), Bio-alcamid, and silicone oils. Initially touted as safe, it soon became apparent that they may cause terrible complications even after several years out in the future. One of the authors is seeing increasing numbers of patients with almost incorrigible problems resulting

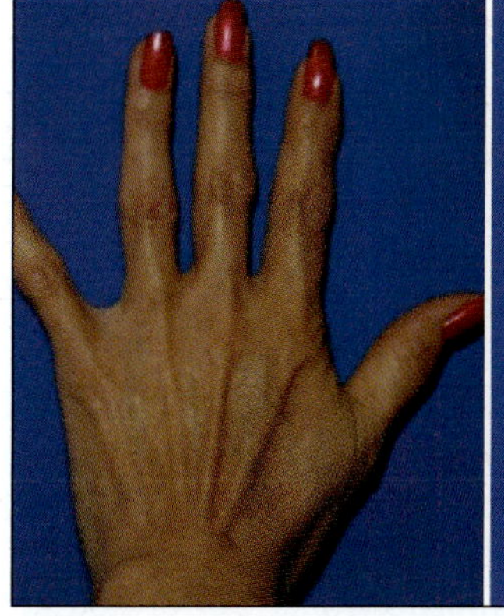

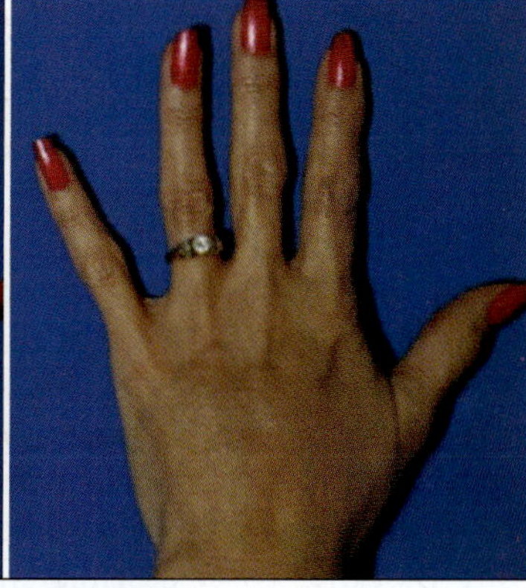

Fig. 5.17 Fat grafting for hand rejuvenation in 61-year-old-woman with microfat injected to dorsum of hand through single incision at hand/wrist junction and nanofat microneedling. A total of 12 mL injected per hand.

several years after permanent filler injections. The problems are mainly in the face and buttocks but have also been seen in breasts, hands, genitals, nose, and feet. The presentations include cold abscesses, hot abscesses, Peau d' orange skin, inflammatory masses, nodules, repeated inflammations, chronic sinuses, contour problems, hardness of tissues, pain, paralysis, migration, and tissue atrophy. The patients continue to suffer without reliable treatment; attempts at removal often result in deformity, nerve damage, or persistent sinuses.

The fillers cause chronic low-grade inflammation, space effects, pressure, and fibrosis leading to atrophy of all tissue layers, dermal thinning, and loss of anatomical layers. Chronic/recurrent sinuses and nonhealing ulcers, chronic ill health, and deformity often lead to reactive depression. Ultrasound scans show "snow storm" appearance with total loss of tissue layers. On magnetic resonance imaging (MRI) they appear hyper intense on T2-weighted and short tau inversion recovery (STIR) images with peripheral rim enhancement in case inflamed. MR images reveal the distribution and pattern of fillers. Unfortunately, in most cases, it is distributed diffusely in several layers and is nearly impossible to remove without oncological types of resections.

There is no consensus or guidelines on how to treat them. Mere injections of corticosteroids, especially in superficial tissues, do not address the problem at all and leads to further atrophy and deformities. Internal laser "melting' of fillers is promoted by some but is not logical and leads to nonselective destruction, further compounding the problem. Since this is a problem of tissue destruction, chronic inflammation, and intense fibrosis, a regenerative approach is more logical.

Regenerative fat cells, nanofat, SVF, and culture amplified ADSC-enriched fat have been found to be very useful. Over the last 6 years, an algorithmic protocol has been developed as follows. Briefly, the patient is examined clinically and by MRI. The problem is then classified as abscess like, localized large fillers deposits, diffuse inflammatory mass, or a combination. When possible (lakes, abscess, and large pools of fillers) filler is evacuated through mini-incisions or by facelift approach for face. This helps to reduce filler load. Transmucosal incisions are forbidden, although patients request them; this is to prevent introduction of infection and to avoid nerve damage. In inflammatory masses with acute exacerbation, systemic high-dose pulse steroids (we use prednisolone as 30-, 30-, 20-, 20-, 10-, 10-mg tapering pulse) along with antibiotics are used first. Deep injections of diluted corticosteroid (triamcinolone 5 mg/mL) also help to provide rapid improvement. This is followed by injection of autologous ADSCs or nanofat at several points at different depths at 2-cm intervals. Softening is observed after 3 to 4 months. Vaser-assisted liposuction is performed to soften the mass, remove fat plus filler, and create channels in which more fat with or without ADSC (or SVF) is grafted. Vaser is safe when used in superficial planes and with adequate hydration of tissues and lower powers (typically 50%). This step is repeated once or twice more after a minimum gap of 4 months. One can usually observe progressive decrease of fibrosis and resistance to cannula with each session. Dermal scars, ulcers, and sinuses usually heal and good improvement in tissue texture and vitality is observed (**Fig. 5.18**). Tissue restoration after necrosis has also been reported in such cases with injections of SVF.[123,124]

Once the tissue vitality has been restored, procedures like scar revisions, facelifts, body lifts, and larger volume fat grafts (for gluteal area) may be performed safely to achieve specific goals (**Fig. 5.19**). Particularly in the gluteal area, the loose floppy skin flaps may be overlapped after deep de-epithelization of one flap (**Fig. 5.20**). Fat grafting is done conservatively and in multiple sessions for gradual corrections, mindful of the fact that the host tissues are far from normal and we do not want fat necrosis to add to the problems. Migration of fillers from buttocks into the tissue planes of the thighs is seen sometimes; this is treated by open drainage, negative pressure dressings, and delayed fat grafting. Regenerative cells have enabled treatment of such previously incorrigible problems in a safe and fairly predictable way, adding yet another application of fat and stem cells.

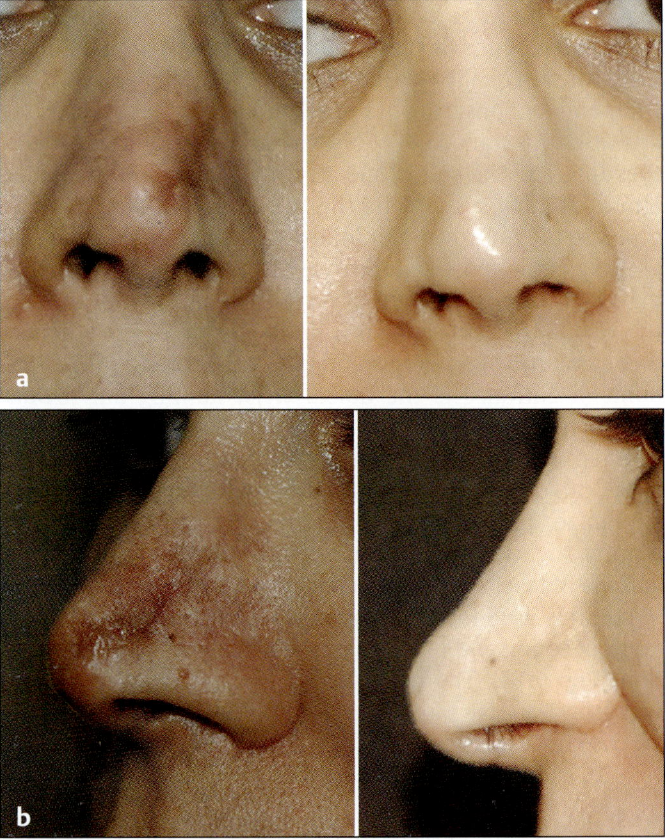

Fig. 5.18 Chronic ulceration and granuloma following injection of permanent fillers post rhinoplasty. She underwent two sessions of nanofat grafting by **sharp needle intradermal fat** (SNIF) grafting technique 5 months apart. Result 10 months after the second session.

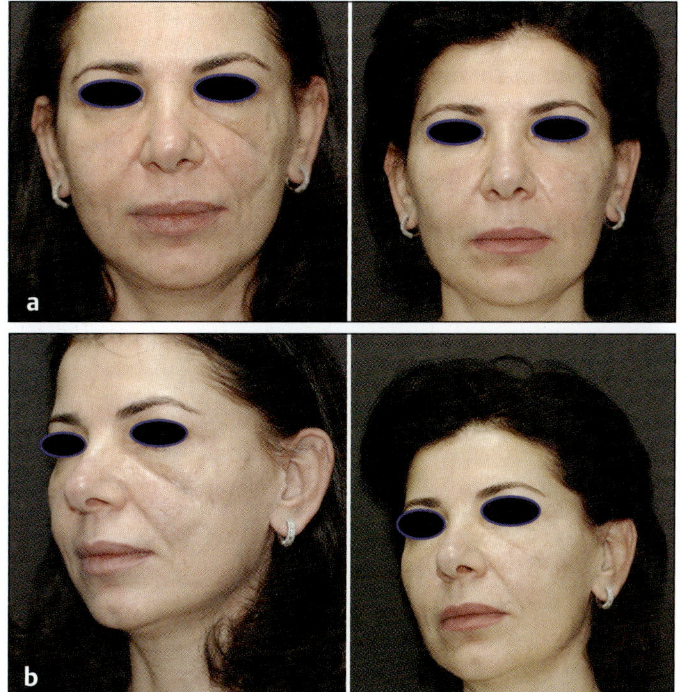

Fig. 5.19 (a, b) Scarring, soft tissue destruction, and deformity of left side following multiple procedures to deal with filler complications: incisional drainage, resections, laser destruction, and steroid injections. She also had deep fibrotic nodules in the right cheek. Result after one session of micro and nanofat grafting followed by two sessions of ADSC-enriched fat grafting and scar revision.

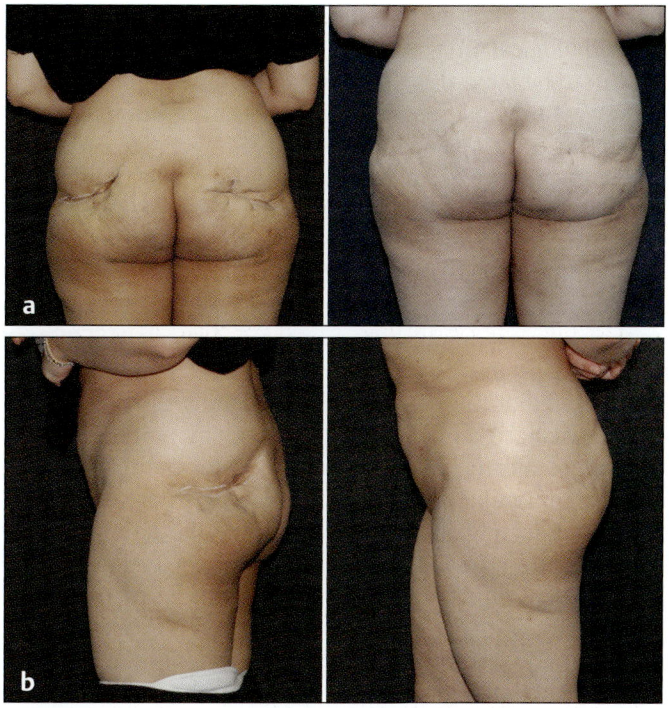

Fig. 5.20 (a, b) Destruction of buttocks after radical debridement done for life-threatening invasive sepsis following permanent filler injections. Reconstruction by scar excision, removal of filler residues, double breasting of de-epithelized flaps, and ADSC-assisted fat grafting (450 mL of fat and 85 million cells per side) at a second stage. Result 8 months after fat grafting.

Complications and Safety Profile of the Use of Regenerative Cells

Use of regenerative cells as described in this chapter has been associated with very few complications especially when correct techniques were used.[125–127] Complications may be subdivided into mild or serious, early or late, aesthetic or potentially medical issues. Swelling and bruising are common early side effects and need not be considered as complications unless excessive or prolonged. Bruises may leave behind hemosiderin deposits in the skin, resulting in prolonged grayish discoloration difficult to treat. Lactoferrin (an iron chelator)-based creams have been found useful.[128]

Excessive volumes or large boluses can result in fat necrosis; the dead fat can produce prolonged edema, induration, and mild inflammatory signs. Ultrasonic therapy sessions twice weekly have been found to be useful to reduce problems, although it will not influence the fat survival. Both fat necrosis and hematoma can get secondarily infected. Infection after fat grafting is rare; however, fat grafting is to be treated as a proper surgical procedure with rigorous aseptic technique. It is desirable to reduce the time spent by the fat ex vivo and ensure prompt grafting both to enhance survival and reduce infection. Irregularities and asymmetries may be prevented by technical accuracy but cannot be eliminated altogether; this may require touch-up procedures.

In the medium time frame from 1 to 6 months, the major concern is the retention of volume. With correct technique, stable results may be noted at 4 months, prior to this fat may decrease in volume up to 49% but may recover volume due to regeneration from the precursor cells. It is best therefore to delay any touch-up corrections for at least 6 months. Excessive growth of the fat is seen rarely, especially if the patient gains weight. This can be addressed by Vaser-assisted gentle liposuction.

The initial concerns about stimulating malignancies in the breast or of masking underlying malignancy have been laid to rest and breast fat grafting is now a standard procedure.[98] Wrong technique, specifically injecting large boluses using bigger syringes can lead to failure of vascularization. Dead fat in breasts can degenerate into oil cysts and calcific nodules (dystrophic calcification).[129] This complication can be reduced drastically by paying attention to graft particulate size and proper distribution in the host bed. Small oil cysts and small calcifications visible only on radiological imaging are more common. Calcification produced by fat grafting is however mammographically different from the microcalcifications of cancer; but it is best to avoid this by using good technique.

Fat grafting of buttocks has seen a huge rise in numbers since 2011 but several fatal and non-fatal pulmonary fat embolisms reported in the past decade led ASPS to declare fat grafting of the buttock region as the most dangerous aesthetic procedure.[130] Fat entering the rich venous plexus deep to the gluteus maximus was suspected. A special ASERF task force was established to investigate these fatalities which concluded that this complication is entirely associated with intramuscular grafting of fat in gluteus maximus.[131] Safety guidelines include using larger bore blunt cannulas, avoiding intramuscular entry, keeping cannulas pointed toward the skin, injecting while moving the cannula, patient in jack-knife position, and constant awareness of cannula tip.[132] Grafting by vibratory devices is a useful tool that expands the spaces, distributes the fat better, and has been shown to be safe.[133] Performing the surgery using local anesthesia with sedation offers another layer of protection since the muscle tone is intact and the patient will react if muscle is breached.

Even nonfatal fat emboli may lead to long-term pulmonary insufficiencies in survivors as the fat does not break down unlike blood clots.[134] Fat emboli may migrate to the arterial side via a patent foramen ovale (PFO) and result in strokes. Up to 2 to 10% of the population may have PFO, which explains strokes in survivors and fat emboli in the cerebral circulation in the fatalities.[135]

The Future Direction of Regenerative Cells

The results of clinical applications in diverse fields of aesthetic and reconstructive plastic surgery are very exciting and promising. This field is also an area where clinical applications have gone far ahead of basic science, although the latter is playing catch-up. There is a need for better standardization of techniques and quantitative prognostication of cell counts, survival percentages, and volumes. This requires well-controlled animal and clinical studies. Studies directed at customization of the regenerative cells toward specific applications, cellular subtypes, synergy with growth factors, use of cell-free growth factors, exosomes, and cell-free matrix could result in greater precision and new applications.[136,137]

The role of scaffolds is almost in its infancy, although in the laboratory, scaffolds have been shown to enhance and control the growth of the stem cells. Another future direction is the seeding of biosynthetic constructs with autologous stem cells to prefabricate implants that will integrate with host tissue. What we know so far is a tantalizing preview of vast future possibilities in the field of regenerative medicine to maintain and enhance human quality of life and longevity.

References

1. Haseltine WA. Interview: commercial translation of cell-based therapies and regenerative medicine: learning by experience. Interview by Emily Culme-Seymour. Regen Med 2011;6(4): 431–435
2. Coleman SR. Structural fat grafts: the ideal filler? Clin Plast Surg 2001;28(1):111–119
3. Coleman SR. Structural fat grafting: more than a permanent filler. Plast Reconstr Surg 2006; 118(3, Suppl):108S–120S
4. Moseley TA, Zhu M, Hedrick MH. Adipose-derived stem and progenitor cells as fillers in plastic and reconstructive surgery. Plast Reconstr Surg 2006; 118(3, Suppl)121S–128S
5. Neuber, F. Fettransplantation Bericht uber die Verhandlungen der Deutscht Gesellsch Chir. Zentralblatt fur Chirurgie 1893; 22:66.
6. Lexer E. Die freien transplantationen. Stuttgart 1919–1924
7. Egro FM, Coleman SR. Facial fat grafting: the past, present, and future. Clin Plast Surg 2020;47(1):1–6
8. Fischer G. Liposculpture: the "correct" history of liposuction. Part I. J Dermatol Surg Oncol 1990;16(12):1087–1089
9. Illouz YG. Body contouring by lipolysis: a 5-year experience with over 3000 cases. Plast Reconstr Surg 1983;72(5):591–597
10. Ellenbogen R. Free autogenous pearl fat grafts in the face: a preliminary report of a rediscovered technique. Ann Plast Surg 1986;16(3):179–194
11. Coleman SR. Structural fat grafting. Aesthet Surg J 1998;18(5): 386, 388
12. James IB, Coleman SR, Rubin JP. Fat, stem cells, and platelet-rich plasma. Clin Plast Surg 2016;43(3):473–488
13. Tremolada C, Palmieri G, Ricordi C. Adipocyte transplantation and stem cells: plastic surgery meets regenerative medicine. Cell Transplant 2010;19(10):1217–1223
14. Bellini E, Grieco MP, Raposio E. The science behind autologous fat grafting. Ann Med Surg (Lond) 2017;24:65–73
15. Leong DT, Hutmacher DW, Chew FT, Lim TC. Viability and adipogenic potential of human adipose tissue processed cell population obtained from pump-assisted and syringe-assisted liposuction. J Dermatol Sci 2005;37(3):169–176
16. Neuhof H, Samuel H. The transplantation of tissues. Appleton; 1923:1–297
17. Peer LA. Cell survival theory versus replacement theory. Plast Reconstr Surg 1955; (16):161–168
18. von Heimburg D, Hemmrich K, Haydarlioglu S, Staiger H, Pallua N. Comparison of viable cell yield from excised versus aspirated adipose tissue. Cells Tissues Organs 2004;178(2):87–92
19. Wolter TP, von Heimburg D, Stoffels I, Groeger A, Pallua N. Cryopreservation of mature human adipocytes: in vitro measurement of viability. Ann Plast Surg 2005;55(4):408–413
20. Eto H, Kato H, Suga H, et al. The fate of adipocytes after nonvascularized fat grafting: evidence of early death and replacement of adipocytes. Plast Reconstr Surg 2012;129(5): 1081–1092
21. Cohen SR, Womack H, Ghanem A. Fat grafting for facial rejuvenation through injectable tissue replacement and regeneration: a differential, standardized, anatomic approach. Clin Plast Surg 2020;47(1):31–41

22. Zuk PA, Zhu M, Mizuno H, et al. Multilineage cells from human adipose tissue: implications for cell-based therapies. Tissue Eng 2001;7(2):211–228
23. Strioga M, Viswanathan S, Darinskas A, Slaby O, Michalek J. Same or not the same? Comparison of adipose tissue-derived versus bone marrow-derived mesenchymal stem and stromal cells. Stem Cells Dev 2012;21(14):2724–2752
24. Klingemann H, Matzilevich D, Marchand J. Mesenchymal stem cells: sources and clinical applications. Transfus Med Hemother 2008;35(4):272–277
25. Zuk PA, Zhu M, Ashjian P, et al. Human adipose tissue is a source of multipotent stem cells. Mol Biol Cell 2002;13(12):4279–4295
26. Zuk PA. The adipose-derived stem cell: looking back and looking ahead. Mol Biol Cell 2010;21(11):1783–1787
27. Rehman J, Traktuev D, Li J, et al. Secretion of angiogenic and antiapoptotic factors by human adipose stromal cells. Circulation 2004;109(10):1292–1298
28. Hong KY, Kim IK, Park SO, Jin US, Chang H. Systemic administration of adipose-derived stromal cells concurrent with fat grafting. Plast Reconstr Surg 2019;143(5):973e–982e
29. Bashir MM, Sohail M, Bashir A, et al. Outcome of conventional adipose tissue grafting for contour deformities of face and role of ex vivo expanded adipose tissue-derived stem cells in treatment of such deformities. J Craniofac Surg 2018;29(5): 1143–1147
30. Yasemin Benderli Cihan HB. Role of autologous fat graft in the treatment of radiotherapy toxicity. Nursing and Palliative Care. 2008
31. Rohrich RJ, Wan D. Making sense of stem cells and fat grafting in plastic surgery: the hype, evidence, and evolving U.S. Food and Drug Administration Regulations. Plast Reconstr Surg 2019;143(2):417e–424e
32. Simonacci F, Bertozzi N, Grieco MP, Grignaffini E, Raposio E. Autologous fat transplantation for breast reconstruction: a literature review. Ann Med Surg (Lond) 2016;12:94–100
33. Cohen SR, Tiryaki T, Womack HA, Canikyan S, Schlaudraff KU, Scheflan M. Cellular optimization of nanofat: comparison of two nanofat processing devices in terms of cell count and viability. Aesthet Surg J Open Forum 2019;1(4):1–11
34. Salgado AJ, Reis RL, Sousa NJ, Gimble JM. Adipose tissue derived stem cells secretome: soluble factors and their roles in regenerative medicine. Curr Stem Cell Res Ther 2010;5(2): 103–110
35. Salibian AA, Widgerow AD, Abrouk M, Evans GR. Stem cells in plastic surgery: a review of current clinical and translational applications. Arch Plast Surg 2013;40(6):666–675
36. Gentile P, De Angelis B, Pasin M, et al. Adipose-derived stromal vascular fraction cells and platelet-rich plasma: basic and clinical evaluation for cell-based therapies in patients with scars on the face. J Craniofac Surg 2014;25(1):267–272
37. Li J, Gao J, Cha P, et al. Supplementing fat grafts with adipose stromal cells for cosmetic facial contouring. Dermatol Surg 2013;39(3 Pt 1):449–456
38. Chang Q, Li J, Dong Z, Liu L, Lu F. Quantitative volumetric analysis of progressive hemifacial atrophy corrected using stromal vascular fraction-supplemented autologous fat grafts. Dermatol Surg 2013;39(10):1465–1473
39. Yao Y, Cai J, Zhang P, et al. Adipose stromal vascular fraction gel grafting: a new method for tissue volumization and rejuvenation. Dermatol Surg 2018;44(10):1278–1286
40. Tonnard P, Verpaele A, Peeters G, Hamdi M, Cornelissen M, Declercq H. Nanofat grafting: basic research and clinical applications. Plast Reconstr Surg 2013;132(4):1017–1026
41. Cohen SR, Goodacre AK, Womack H, et al. Topical Nanofat Biocrème improves aesthetic outcomes of nonablative fractionated laser treatment: a preliminary report. Aesthet Surg J 2020;40(8):892–899
42. Marx RE, Carlson ER, Eichstaedt RM, Schimmele SR, Strauss JE, Georgeff KR. Platelet-rich plasma: growth factor enhancement for bone grafts. Oral Surg Oral Med Oral Pathol Oral Radiol Endod 1998;85(6):638–646
43. Li F, Guo W, Li K, et al. Improved fat graft survival by different volume fractions of platelet-rich plasma and adipose-derived stem cells. Aesthet Surg J 2015;35(3):319–333
44. Modarressi A. Platelet rich plasma (PRP) improves fat grafting outcomes. World J Plast Surg 2013;2(1):6–13
45. Seyhan N, Alhan D, Ural AU, Gunal A, Avunduk MC, Savaci N. The effect of combined use of platelet-rich plasma and adipose-derived stem cells on fat graft survival. Ann Plast Surg 2015;74(5):615–620
46. Atashi F, Jaconi ME, Pittet-Cuénod B, Modarressi A. Autologous platelet-rich plasma: a biological supplement to enhance adipose-derived mesenchymal stem cell expansion. Tissue Eng Part C Methods 2015;21(3):253–262
47. Cervelli V, Bocchini I, Di Pasquali C, et al. Platelet rich lipotransfer: our experience and current state of art in the combined use of fat and PRP. BioMed Res Int 2013;2013:434191
48. Rigotti G, Charles-de-Sá L, Gontijo-de-Amorim NF, et al. Expanded stem cells, stromal-vascular fraction, and platelet-rich plasma enriched fat: comparing results of different facial rejuvenation approaches in a clinical trial. Aesthet Surg J 2016;36(3):261–270
49. Frautschi RS, Hashem AM, Halasa B, Cakmakoglu C, Zins JE. Current evidence for clinical efficacy of platelet rich plasma in aesthetic surgery: a systematic review. Aesthet Surg J 2017;37(3):353–362
50. Sclafani AP, Azzi J. Platelet preparations for use in facial rejuvenation and wound healing: a critical review of current literature. Aesthetic Plast Surg 2015;39(4):495–505
51. Liao HT, Marra KG, Rubin JP. Application of platelet-rich plasma and platelet-rich fibrin in fat grafting: basic science and literature review. Tissue Eng Part B Rev 2014;20(4):267–276
52. Xiong S, Yi C, Pu LLQ. An overview of principles and new techniques for facial fat grafting. Clin Plast Surg 2020;47(1):7–17
53. Padoin AV, Braga-Silva J, Martins P, et al. Sources of processed lipoaspirate cells: influence of donor site on cell concentration. Plast Reconstr Surg 2008;122(2):614–618
54. Ullmann Y, Shoshani O, Fodor A, et al. Searching for the favorable donor site for fat injection: in vivo study using the nude mice model. Dermatol Surg 2005;31(10):1304–1307
55. Rohrich RJ, Sorokin ES, Brown SA. In search of improved fat transfer viability: a quantitative analysis of the role of centrifugation and harvest site. Plast Reconstr Surg 2004;113(1): 391–395, discussion 396–397
56. Klein JA. Tumescent technique for local anesthesia improves safety in large-volume liposuction. Plast Reconstr Surg 1993; 92(6):1085–1098, discussion 1099–1100
57. Klein JA. The tumescent technique: anesthesia and modified liposuction technique. Dermatol Clin 1990;8(3):425–437
58. Lewis CM. Comparison of the syringe and pump aspiration methods of lipoplasty. Aesthetic Plast Surg 1991;15(3): 203–208
59. Keck M, Kober J, Riedl O, et al. Power assisted liposuction to obtain adipose-derived stem cells: impact on viability and differentiation to adipocytes in comparison to manual aspiration. J Plast Reconstr Aesthet Surg 2014;67(1):e1–e8

60. Smith P, Adams WP Jr, Lipschitz AH, et al. Autologous human fat grafting: effect of harvesting and preparation techniques on adipocyte graft survival. Plast Reconstr Surg 2006;117(6): 1836–1844
61. Lee JH, Kirkham JC, McCormack MC, Nicholls AM, Randolph MA, Austen WG Jr. The effect of pressure and shear on autologous fat grafting. Plast Reconstr Surg 2013;131(5):1125–1136
62. Erdim M, Tezel E, Numanoglu A, Sav A. The effects of the size of liposuction cannula on adipocyte survival and the optimum temperature for fat graft storage: an experimental study. J Plast Reconstr Aesthet Surg 2009;62(9):1210–1214
63. Meyer J, Salamon A, Herzmann N, et al. Isolation and differentiation potential of human mesenchymal stem cells from adipose tissue harvested by water jet-assisted liposuction. Aesthet Surg J 2015;35(8):1030–1039
64. Cohen SR, Hewett S, Ross L, et al. Regenerative cells for facial surgery: biofilling and biocontouring. Aesthet Surg J 2017; 37(suppl_3):S16–S32
65. Strong AL, Cederna PS, Rubin JP, Coleman SR, Levi B. The current state of fat grafting: a review of harvesting, processing, and injection techniques. Plast Reconstr Surg 2015;136(4): 897–912
66. Condé-Green A, de Amorim NF, Pitanguy I. Influence of decantation, washing and centrifugation on adipocyte and mesenchymal stem cell content of aspirated adipose tissue: a comparative study. J Plast Reconstr Aesthet Surg 2010;63(8): 1375–1381
67. Ramon Y, Shoshani O, Peled IJ, et al. Enhancing the take of injected adipose tissue by a simple method for concentrating fat cells. Plast Reconstr Surg 2005;115(1):197–201, 202–203
68. Ferraro GA, De Francesco F, Tirino V, et al. Effects of a new centrifugation method on adipose cell viability for autologous fat grafting. Aesthetic Plast Surg 2011;35(3):341–348
69. Kurita M, Matsumoto D, Shigeura T, et al. Influences of centrifugation on cells and tissues in liposuction aspirates: optimized centrifugation for lipotransfer and cell isolation. Plast Reconstr Surg 2008;121(3):1033–1041, discussion 1042–1043
70. Aronowitz JA, Ellenhorn JD. Adipose stromal vascular fraction isolation: a head-to-head comparison of four commercial cell separation systems. Plast Reconstr Surg 2013;132(6): 932e–939e
71. Sesé B, Sanmartín JM, Ortega B, Matas-Palau A, Llull R. Nanofat cell aggregates: a nearly constitutive stromal cell inoculum for regenerative site-specific therapies. Plast Reconstr Surg 2019;144(5):1079–1088
72. Dohan Ehrenfest DM, Rasmusson L, Albrektsson T. Classification of platelet concentrates: from pure platelet-rich plasma (P-PRP) to leucocyte- and platelet-rich fibrin (L-PRF). Trends Biotechnol 2009;27(3):158–167
73. Dohan Ehrenfest DM, Bielecki T, Del Corso M, Inchingolo F, Sammartino G. Shedding light in the controversial terminology for platelet-rich products: platelet-rich plasma (PRP), platelet-rich fibrin (PRF), platelet-leukocyte gel (PLG), preparation rich in growth factors (PRGF), classification and commercialism. J Biomed Mater Res A 2010;95(4):1280–1282
74. Dhurat R, Sukesh M. Principles and methods of preparation of platelet-rich plasma: a review and author's perspective. J Cutan Aesthet Surg 2014;7(4):189–197
75. Kakagia D, Pallua N. Autologous fat grafting: in search of the optimal technique. Surg Innov 2014;21(3):327–336
76. Khouri RK Jr, Khouri RK. Current clinical applications of fat grafting. Plast Reconstr Surg 2017;140(3):466e–486e
77. Pu LL, Coleman SR, Cui X, Ferguson RE Jr, Vasconez HC. Autologous fat grafts harvested and refined by the Coleman technique: a comparative study. Plast Reconstr Surg 2008; 122(3):932–937
78. Lin TMLS, Lai CS. The treatment of nasolabial fold with free fat graft: preliminary concept of micro-autologous fat transplantation (MAFT). 2nd Academic Congress of Taiwan Cosmetic Society 2007
79. Kao WP, Lin YN, Lin TY, et al. Microautologous fat transplantation for primary augmentation rhinoplasty: long-term monitoring of 198 Asian patients. Aesthet Surg J 2016;36(6):648–656
80. Zeltzer AA, Tonnard PL, Verpaele AM. Sharp-needle intradermal fat grafting (SNIF). Aesthet Surg J 2012;32(5):554–561
81. Marten TJ, Elyassnia D. Fat grafting in facial rejuvenation. Clin Plast Surg 2015;42(2):219–252
82. Sadati KS, Corrado AC, Alexander RW. Platelet-rich plasma (PRP) utilized to promote greater graft volume retention in autologous fat grafting. Am J Cosmet Surg 2006;23:203–211
83. Cohen SR, Womack H. Injectable tissue replacement and regeneration: anatomic fat grafting to restore decayed facial tissues. Plast Reconstr Surg Glob Open 2019;7(8):e2293
84. Ghavami A, Villanueva NL. Gluteal augmentation and contouring with autologous fat transfer: part I. Clin Plast Surg 2018;45(2):249–259
85. Coleman SR. Facial augmentation with structural fat grafting. Clin Plast Surg 2006;33(4):567–577
86. Rohrich RJ, Pessa JE. The fat compartments of the face: anatomy and clinical implications for cosmetic surgery. Plast Reconstr Surg 2007;119(7):2219–2227, discussion 2228–2231
87. Tonnard P, Verpaele A, Carvas M. Fat grafting for facial rejuvenation with nanofat grafts. Clin Plast Surg 2020;47(1):53–62
88. Thomas WW, Bucky L, Friedman O. Injectables in the nose: facts and controversies. Facial Plast Surg Clin North Am 2016;24(3):379–389
89. Nguyen PS, Baptista C, Casanova D, Bardot J, Magalon G. Autologous fat grafting and rhinoplasty. Ann Chir Plast Esthet 2014;59(6):548–554
90. Cárdenas JC, Carvajal J. Refinement of rhinoplasty with lipoinjection. Aesthetic Plast Surg 2007;31(5):501–505
91. Cohen SR, Womack HA, Hauch AT, Delaunay F, Trivisonno A. Treatment of nasal aging and possible long-term nasal enhancement with fat using injectable tissue replacement. Plast Reconstr Surg Glob Open 2019;7(5):e2242
92. Trivisonno A, Cohen SR, Magalon G, et al. Fluid cartilage as new autologous biomaterial in the treatment of minor nose defects: clinical and microscopic difference amongst diced, crushed, and fluid cartilage. Materials (Basel) 2019;12(7):1062
93. Czerny V. Drei plastische Operationen. III. Plastischer Ersatz der Brustdrüse durch ein Lipom. Arch F Klin Chir 1895;50:544–550
94. Alvarez R, Ridelman E, Rizk N, et al. Assessment of mammographic breast density after sleeve gastrectomy. Surg Obes Relat Dis 2018;14(11):1643–1651
95. Cohen O, Lam G, Karp N, Choi M. Determining the oncologic safety of autologous fat grafting as a reconstructive modality: an institutional review of breast cancer recurrence rates and surgical outcomes. Plast Reconstr Surg 2017;140(3):382e–392e
96. Veber M, Tourasse C, Toussoun G, Moutran M, Mojallal A, Delay E. Radiographic findings after breast augmentation by autologous fat transfer. Plast Reconstr Surg 2011;127(3): 1289–1299
97. Coleman SR, Saboeiro AP. Primary breast augmentation with fat grafting. Clin Plast Surg 2015;42(3):301–306, vii

98. Fraser JK, Hedrick MH, Cohen SR. Oncologic risks of autologous fat grafting to the breast. Aesthet Surg J 2011;31(1):68–75
99. Del Vecchio DA, Bucky LP. Breast augmentation using pre-expansion and autologous fat transplantation: a clinical radiographic study. Plast Reconstr Surg 2011;127(6):2441–2450
100. Bravo FG. Parasternal infiltration composite breast augmentation. Plast Reconstr Surg 2015;135(4):1010–1018
101. Auclair E, Anavekar N. Combined use of implant and fat grafting for breast augmentation. Clin Plast Surg 2015;42(3): 307–314, vii
102. Del Vecchio D, Wall S Jr. Expansion vibration lipofilling: a new technique in large-volume fat transplantation. Plast Reconstr Surg 2018;141(5):639e–649e
103. Del Vecchio DA. "SIEF" (simultaneous implant exchange with fat): a new option in revision breast implant surgery. Plast Reconstr Surg 2012;130(6):1187–1196
104. Pereira LH, Sterodimas A. Composite body contouring. Aesthetic Plast Surg 2009;33(4):616–624
105. Hoyos AE, Millard JA. VASER-assisted high-definition liposculpture. Aesthet Surg J 2007;27(6):594–604
106. Danilla S. Rectus abdominis fat transfer (RAFT) in lipoabdominoplasty: a new technique to achieve fitness body contour in patients that require tummy tuck. Aesthetic Plast Surg 2017;41(6):1389–1399
107. Saad AN, Pablo Arbelaez J, De Benito J. High definition liposculpture in male patients using reciprocating power-assisted liposuction technology: techniques and results in a prospective study. Aesthet Surg J 2020;40(3):299–307
108. Saad A, Combina LN, Altamirano-Arcos C. Abdominal etching. Clin Plast Surg 2020;47(3):397–408
109. Condé-Green A, Kotamarti V, Nini KT, et al. Fat grafting for gluteal augmentation: a systematic review of the literature and meta-analysis. Plast Reconstr Surg 2016;138(3):437e–446e
110. Villanueva NL, Del Vecchio DA, Afrooz PN, Carboy JA, Rohrich RJ. Staying safe during gluteal fat transplantation. Plast Reconstr Surg 2018;141(1):79–86
111. Conlon CJ, Abu-Ghname A, Davis MJ, et al. Fat grafting for hand rejuvenation. Semin Plast Surg 2020;34(1):47–52
112. Cohen PR. Genital rejuvenation: the next frontier in medical and cosmetic dermatology. Dermatol Online J 2018;24(9): 13030/qt27v774t5
113. Cihantimur B, Herold C. Genital beautification: a concept that offers more than reduction of the labia minora. Aesthetic Plast Surg 2013;37(6):1128–1133
114. Herold C, Motamedi M, Hartmann U, Allert S. G-spot augmentation with autologous fat transplantation. J Turk Ger Gynecol Assoc 2015;16(3):187–188
115. Cohen PR, Riahi RR. Platelet-rich plasma and genital rejuvenation. Skinmed 2019;17(4):272–274
116. Menkes S, SidAhmed-Mezi M, Meningaud JP, Benadiba L, Magalon G, Hersant B. Microfat and nanofat grafting in genital rejuvenation. Aesthet Surg J 2020;sjaa118
117. Fantozzi F. Hand rejuvenation with fat grafting: a 12-year single-surgeon experience. Eur J Plast Surg 2017;40(5): 457–464
118. Hoang D, Orgel MI, Kulber DA. Hand rejuvenation: a comprehensive review of fat grafting. J Hand Surg Am 2016; 41(5):639–644
119. Gentile P, Garcovich S. Advances in regenerative stem cell therapy in androgenic alopecia and hair loss: Wnt pathway, growth-factor, and mesenchymal stem cell signaling impact analysis on cell growth and hair follicle development. Cells 2019;8(5):E466
120. Epstein GK, Epstein JS. Mesenchymal stem cells and stromal vascular fraction for hair loss: current status. Facial Plast Surg Clin North Am 2018;26(4):503–511
121. Fukuoka H, Suga H. Hair regeneration treatment using adipose-derived stem cell conditioned medium: follow-up with trichograms. Eplasty 2015;15:e10
122. Kuka G, Epstein J, Aronowitz J, et al. Cell enriched autologous fat grafts to follicular niche improves hair regrowth in early androgenetic alopecia. Aesthet Surg J 2020;40(6):NP328–NP339
123. Kim JH, Ahn DK, Jeong HS, Suh IS. Treatment algorithm of complications after filler injection: based on wound healing process. J Korean Med Sci 2014;29(Suppl 3):S176–S182
124. Kim JH, Park SH, Lee BH, Jeong HS, Yang HJ, Suh IS. Early intervention with highly condensed adipose-derived stem cells for complicated wounds following filler injections. Aesthetic Plast Surg 2016;40(3):428–434
125. Kim IA, Keller G, Groth MJ, Nabili V. The downside of fat: avoiding and treating complications. Facial Plast Surg 2016;32(5):556–559
126. Yoshimura K, Coleman SR. Complications of fat grafting: how they occur and how to find, avoid, and treat them. Clin Plast Surg 2015;42(3):383–388, ix
127. Toyserkani NM, Jørgensen MG, Tabatabaeifar S, Jensen CH, Sheikh SP, Sørensen JA. Concise review: a safety assessment of adipose-derived cell therapy in clinical trials: a systematic review of reported adverse events. Stem Cells Transl Med 2017;6(9):1786–1794
128. Brizzio E, Castro M, Narbaitz M, et al. Ulcerated hemosiderinic dyschromia and iron deposits within lower limbs treated with a topical application of biological chelator. Veins Lymphatics 2012;1:18–26
129. Mineda K, Kuno S, Kato H, et al. Chronic inflammation and progressive calcification as a result of fat necrosis: the worst outcome in fat grafting. Plast Reconstr Surg 2014;133(5): 1064–1072
130. Cárdenas-Camarena L, Bayter JE, Aguirre-Serrano H, Cuenca-Pardo J. Deaths caused by gluteal lipoinjection: what are we doing wrong? Plast Reconstr Surg 2015;136(1):58–66
131. Mofid MM, Teitelbaum S, Suissa D, et al. Report on mortality from gluteal fat grafting: recommendations from the ASERF task force. Aesthet Surg J 2017;37(7):796–806
132. Whitfield RM, Rios LM Jr, DiBernardo BE. Making fat transfer to buttocks safer. Aesthet Surg J 2017;37(10):1199–1200
133. Abboud MH, Dibo SA, Abboud NM. Power-assisted gluteal augmentation: a new technique for sculpting, harvesting, and transferring fat. Aesthet Surg J 2015;35(8):987–994
134. Ajemba O, Zia H, Lankachandra K, et al. Pulmonary histopathology of a case of fat embolism (FE) in a patient and its similarity to an animal model of FE. FASEB J 2014; 28(S1)
135. Fisher DC, Fisher EA, Budd JH, Rosen SE, Goldman ME. The incidence of patent foramen ovale in 1,000 consecutive patients. A contrast transesophageal echocardiography study. Chest 1995;107(6):1504–1509
136. Wang L, Hu L, Zhou X, et al. Exosomes secreted by human adipose mesenchymal stem cells promote scarless cutaneous repair by regulating extracellular matrix remodelling. Sci Rep 2017;7(1):13321
137. Young DA, Ibrahim DO, Hu D, Christman KL. Injectable hydrogel scaffold from decellularized human lipoaspirate. Acta Biomater 2011;7(3):1040–1049

Face

6

Anatomy of Aging Face and Its Assessment

Sanjay Kumar Yadunath Parashar

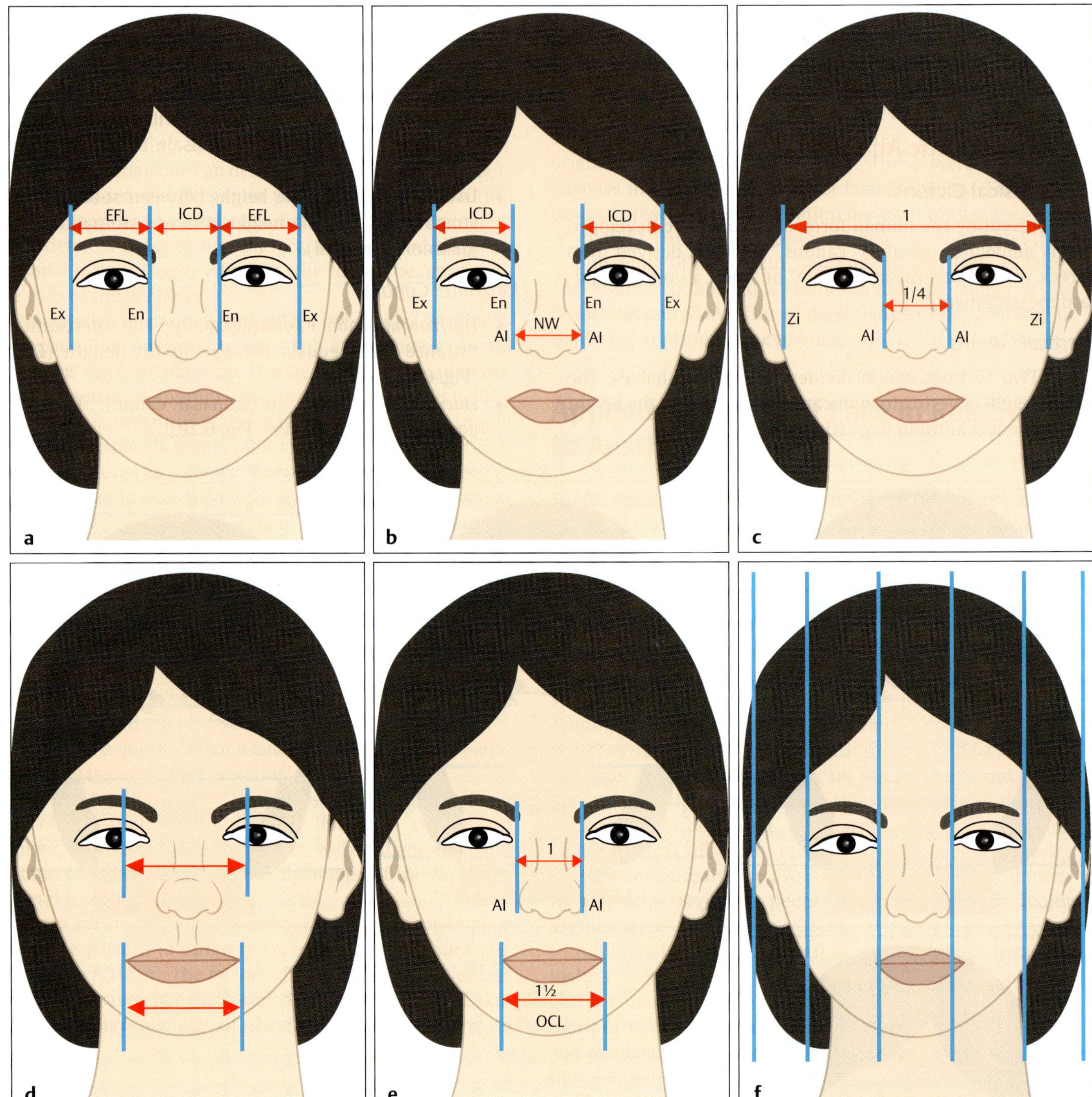

Fig. 6.2 (a–f) The horizontal canons. **(a)** Horizontal canon 1 (orbital canon): the intercanthal distance (ICD) equals the eye fissure length (EFL). **(b)** Horizontal canon 2 (orbitonasal canon): the ICD equals the nasal width (NW). **(c)** Nasofacial canon: the width of the ala equals one-fourth the distance between the zygions. **(d)** Orofacial canon: oral commissure length is equal to the distance between medial corneal limbi. **(e)** Orofacial canon: oral commissure length is equal to one-and-a-half times of interalar distance. **(f)** Face is also divided vertically into fifths with the distance equal to the ICD. Al, alare; EFL, eye fissure length; En, endocanthion; Ex, exocanthion; NW, nasal width; OCD, intercanthal distance; OCL, oral commissure length; Zi, zigion.

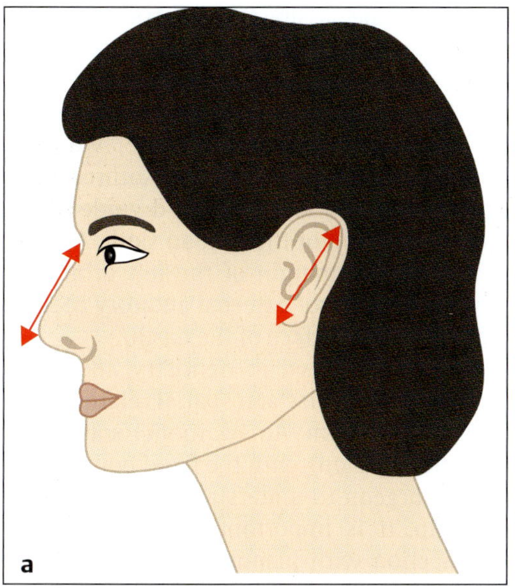

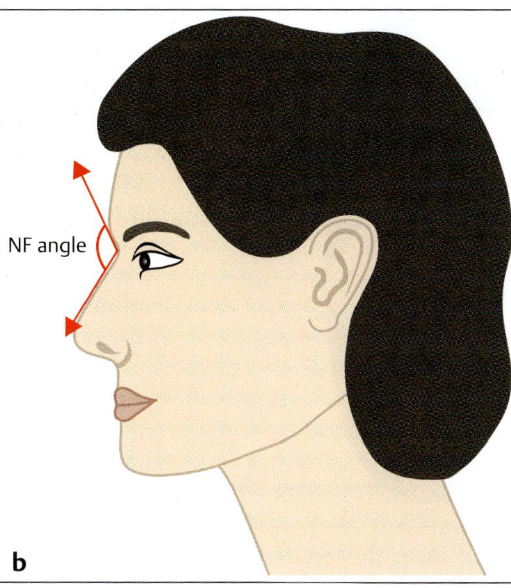

Fig. 6.3 Inclined canons. **(a)** Nasoaural canon: the inclination and proportion of the nasal dorsum is equal to that of ears. **(b)** Nasofrontal angle: forehead makes an angle with the nose of 130+/–7 degrees in males and 134+/–7 degrees in females. NF angle, nasofrontal angle.

- Nasofacial canon: The width of the ala equals one-fourth the distance between the right and left zygion (**Fig. 6.2**c).
- Orofacial canon: Oral commissure length is equal to distance between medial corneal limbi (**Fig. 6.2d**).
- Orofacial canon: Oral commissure length is equal to one and a half times of interalar distance (**Fig. 6.2e**).
- Face is also divided vertically into fifths with the distance equal to the ICD (**Fig. 6.2f**).

Inclined Canons

- Nasoaural canon: The inclination and proportion of the nasal dorsum is equal to that of ears (**Fig. 6.3a**).
- Nasofrontal angle: Forehead makes an angle with the nose of 130+/–7 degrees in males and 134+/–7 degrees in females (**Fig. 6.3b**).

However, studies using direct anthropometry and photogrammetric analyses in white and Asian subjects found variations in these proportions, with the width of the eyes and nasal widths often being either less than or greater than the ICD.[13] Other studies of Indian, African American, Turkish, Chinese, and Korean subjects have reported that some of the neoclassical canons may fit a few subjects and they do not represent the average facial proportions.[14–16]

In the past, human forms and canons were depicted in a way the artist preferred, but for reconstructive and cosmetic surgery, realistic sizes and proportions are assessed using anthropometric techniques.[17]

Angles and Proportions of Aesthetic Nose

Twentieth century saw the development of objective measurements and proportions. Jacques Joseph (1865–1934) strongly emphasized the importance of nasal profile for cosmesis of face. He defined the angles and proportions of an aesthetic nose. There are 16 nasal proportion indices that determine length, width, slope, and angle of nose. There are three main angles: nasofrontal, nasolabial, and nasal tip angle and two main inclinations dorsum and columella. Nasal index is the width divided by length times 100 (NI = width/length × 100). This index classifies nose into Leptorrhine, Mesorrhine, and Platyrrhine. Mario González-Ulloa (1913–1995) introduced the concept of profile-plasty. He believed that the glabela, subnasale point, and pogonion should be in line and should be perpendicular to Frankfurt horizontal.[18]

Concept of Golden Proportion

R.M. Ricketts popularized the concept of “golden proportion” in facial surgery. Egyptians originally defined the golden proportion. The Greek Letter phi (ϕ) is used to indicate the number 1.618 and the aesthetically attractive ratio is 1:1.618 (**Fig. 6.4**).[19] Ricketts advocated the use of golden proportion for planning orthognathic surgery. Generally, these canons in themselves do not have great practical value for soft tissue procedures because there are individual variations and desires. Measuring the face cannot replace the surgeon’s judgment.

Cephalometric Analysis

It is the study and measurement of human head, with the help of radiography. It comprises of fixed hard and soft tissue landmarks (**Fig. 6.5**). It helps to analyze the facial planes and angles. Horizontal planes are Frankfurt, Sella-Nasion, Basion-Nasion, Palatal, occlusion, and mandibular planes. The vertical planes are facial, A-Pog line, facial axis, and esthetic planes. These planes allow us to measure angles. Down’s analysis provides diagnostic information for orthognathic surgery. On the other hand, Steiner separately analyzed skeletal, dental, and soft tissue for treatment planning.[20]

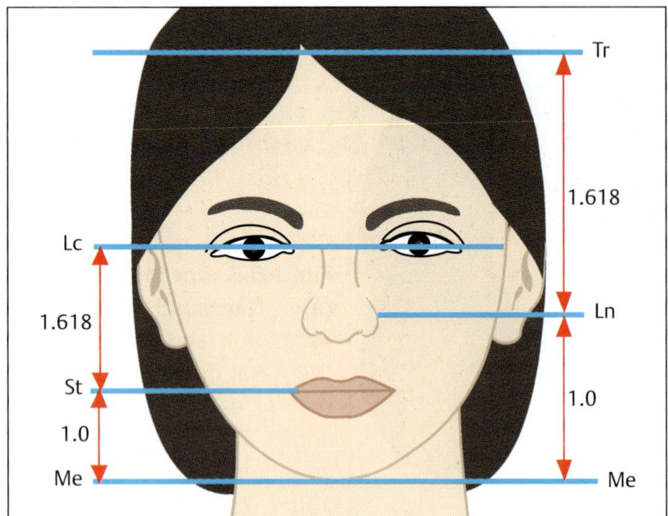

Fig. 6.4 The golden proportion of face: the aesthetically attractive ratio of the face is 1:1.618. Lc, the point at the lateral canthus of the eyes; Ln, the point at the lateral rim of the nose; Me, soft-tissue menton; St, Stoma; Tr, trichion.

A Frankfurt horizontal line passing through trichion, glabela, subnasale, menton will give us horizontal proportions of the face. Assessment of vertical proportions helps in identifying asymmetries that may be missed in gross examination.

The *Frankfurt plane* (auriculo-orbital plane) was the term established at the World Congress on Anthropology in Frankfurt, Germany in 1884 for a standard guideline to determine anatomical position of the human skull. A plane passing through the inferior margin of the left orbit (left orbitale) and the upper margin of external auditory meatus (the porion) is parallel to the surface of the earth.[21]

Cephalometric analysis is used in dentistry and facial plastic surgery, to measure the size and spatial relationships of the teeth, jaws, and cranium. An additional soft tissue imposition in the radiology along with the fixed bony points helps a facial plastic surgeon to understand the soft tissue and bony relationship. It is important when diagnosing facial forms in connection with planning for orthodontics and skeletal surgery (**Fig. 6.6**).

For further details, refer to Chapter 7 on "Principles and Techniques of Nonsurgical Facial Rejuvenation" in Volume VI.

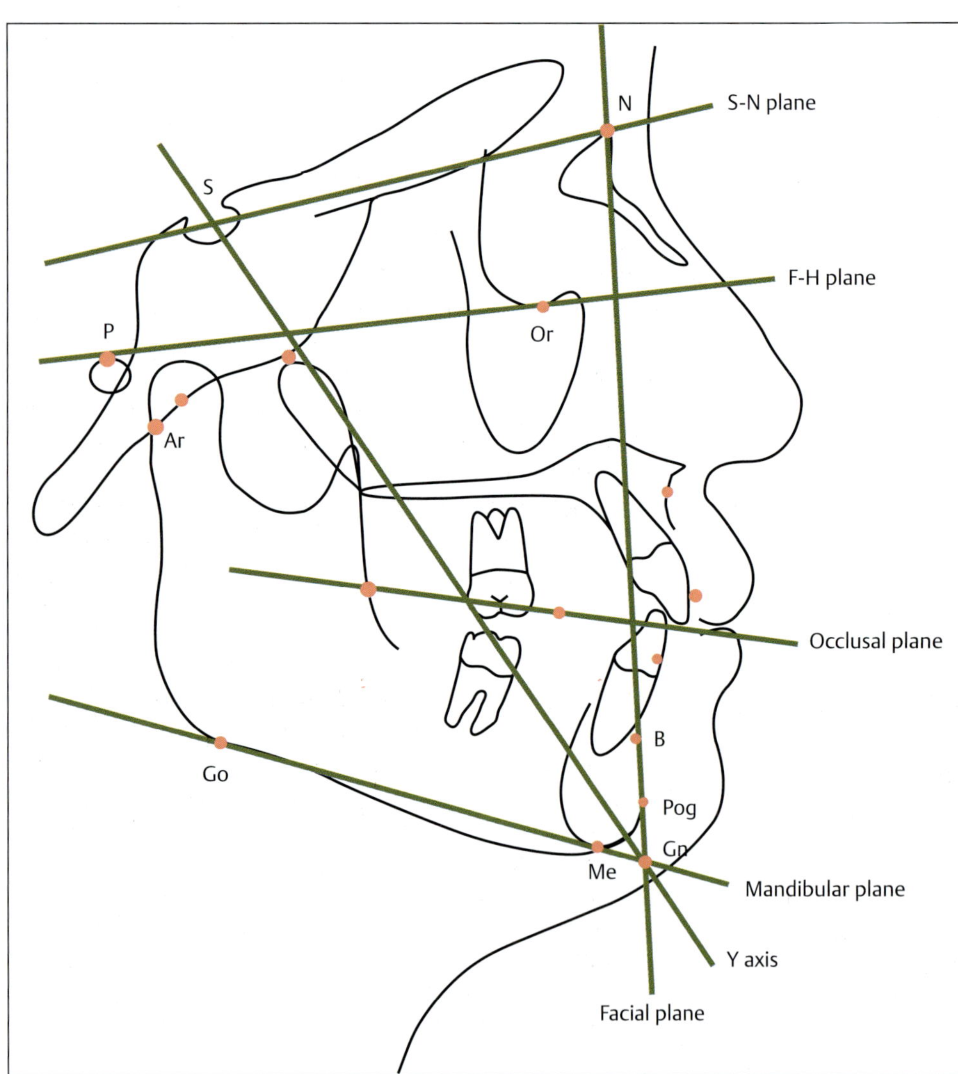

Fig. 6.5 Cephalometry with facial planes and angles. Horizontal planes: Frankfurt horizontal plane, Sella-Nasion, Basion-Nasion, Palatal occlusion, Mandibular planes. Vertical planes: facial axis, A-Pog line, esthetic planes. S, sella; N, nasion; P, porion; Or, orbitale; Ar, articulare; A, subnasale; B, supramentale; Pog, pogonion; Gn, gnathion; Me, menton; Go, gonion.

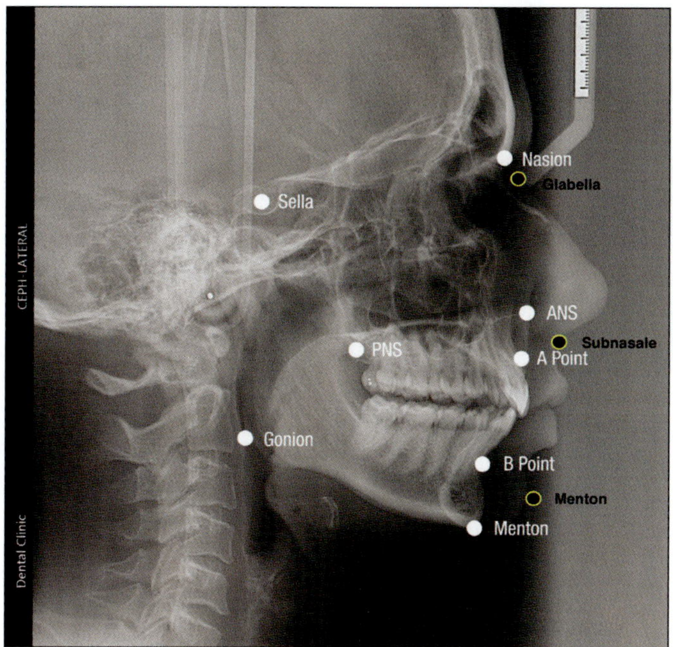

Fig. 6.6 Cephalometric soft tissue and bony points. ANS, anterior nasal spine; PNS, posterior nasal spine. gonion.

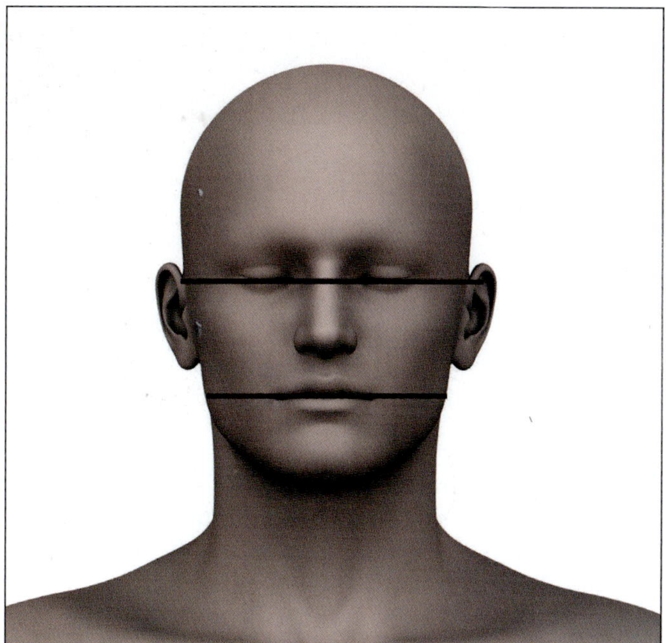

Fig. 6.7 Segments of the face: upper face segment between the trichion and palpebral fissure, midface segment from palpebral fissure to oral commissure, and lower face segment from oral commissure to the lower part of neck.

Mendelson and Wong's Division of Face

Bryan Mendelson and Chin-Ho Wong[22] have beautifully described the anatomy of aging skin. They have divided the face into medial and lateral parts. The lateral face is more fixed than the medial face and the retaining ligaments approximately divide it. According to Mendelson and Wong the medial part is more functional and mobile; it is further divided into superolateral part that overlies the zygomatic bone and inferomedial part overlying the vestibule of the oral cavity. This is described in greater detail while describing the anatomy of midcheek.

Facial Segments

The conventional method of dividing the face into upper, middle, and lower face allows us to understand the anatomy and its clinical and aesthetic implications (**Fig. 6.7**).

Upper Face Segment

Extent

Upper face extends from the hairline to the palpebral fissure (line passing through the medial and lateral canthi). It includes the forehead, eyebrow, and upper eyelid. The medial forehead overlies the frontal muscle and lateral forehead overlies the temporalis muscle.

Applied Anatomy

Skin

Skin of face undergoes significant aging changes. Understanding the details of skin in each anatomic subunit of face will help understand the aging process.

Dermis is the key component of the skin that changes with aging. It consists of collagen, elastic fibers and ground substance, (i.e., mucopolysaccharides, hyaluronic acid, and chondroitin sulfate.[1]

- *Eyelid skin:* Eyelid skin is thinnest in the face and it contains hair follicles, sweat glands, and sebaceous glands. However, the hair grows in the lash only, sebaceous glands secrete in between the conjunctiva and cornea (Gland of Zeis) and into the eyelashes (Meibomian glands). The sweat glands (Glands of Moll) open near the base of the eyelashes. Rest of the upper eyelid skin is devoid of dermal appendages that prevent it from re-epithelizing following an injury to the eyelid skin.

It does not have subcutaneous fat layer and is firmly adherent to the orbicularis oculi muscle.

- *Forehead skin:* The skin is more sebaceous in the central part than in periphery of the forehead and is very closely approximated to the frontalis muscle with minimal fatty tissue. Therefore the muscle contraction causes accordion-like effect on the skin, increasing the risk of wrinkling. The skin of forehead has a larger

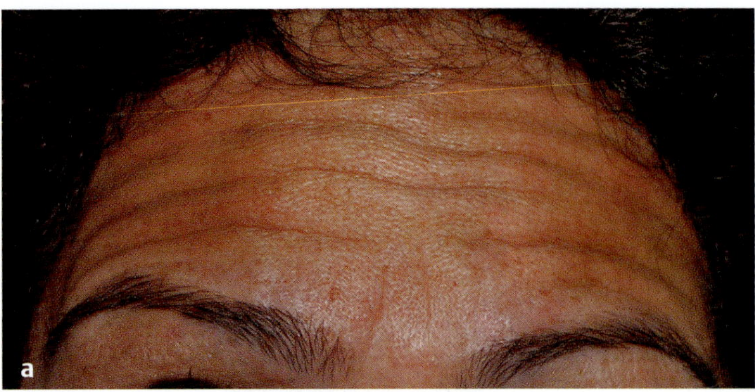

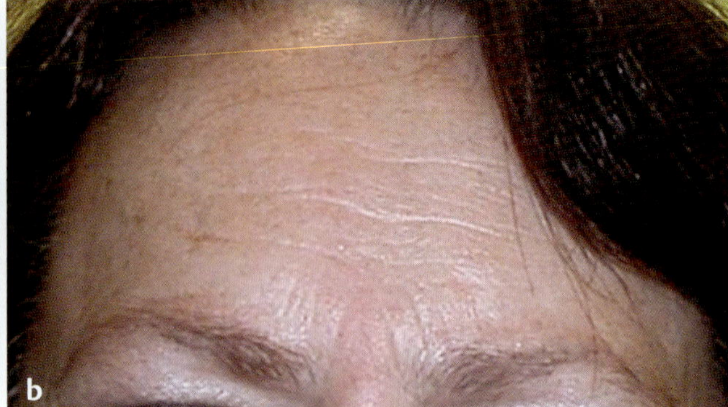

Fig. 6.8 **(a)** Deep furrows on dynamic movement in thick skin. **(b)** Fine wrinkles on dynamic movement in thin skin patient.

number of dermal appendages and sebaceous glands, allowing the skin to regenerate rapidly. People with thick skin form deep furrows and on the contrary thin skin forms fine lines or wrinkles (**Fig. 6.8a, b**).

Forehead Muscles

- *Frontalis muscle:* It originates in the galea aponeurotica on both sides of the frontal region and inserts in the dermis of the eyebrow region and works as brow elevators. The muscle glides on the periosteum because of loose areolar tissue under the deep galeal fascia. The deep galeal fascia is more firmly adhered to the periosteum medially than laterally. Hence the lateral brow is more mobile. There is an intermediate zone on the temporal line where the superficial temporal fascia and galea are firmly adhered to the periosteum and it is called as "line-of-fusion." This zone requires release during temporal or endoscopic browlift for adequate elevation of the brow (**Fig. 6.9**).

The temporal branch of the facial nerve is the motor innervations to the muscle.

- *Corrugator supercilii:* These are paired muscles that originate medially from the frontal bone near the superomedial part of orbital rim and are inserted laterally in the dermis of eyebrows. These have two heads, with one being transverse and the other oblique. Therefore, these become bulky muscles causing significant contraction and skin bunching in the glabellar region.

The motor innervation is via the temporal branch of the facial nerve that enters the muscle belly laterally.[23]

- *Procerus muscle:* It originates in the nasal bones in the midline and is inserted into the dermis of glabellar skin. It causes horizontal lines and oblique lines on the nasal dorsum called as "Bunny lines."

Buccal branches of the facial nerve, which enters the muscle infraorbitally medial to the medial canthus, supply the muscle.[24]

- *Temporalis muscle:* Temporalis muscle is a masticatory muscle. It is located laterally in the forehead region and occupies the temporal fossa. It originates

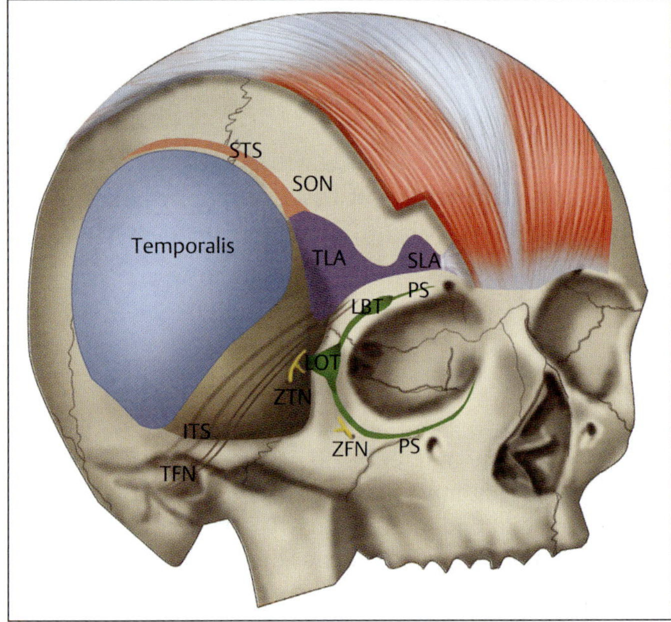

Fig. 6.9 The upper temporal space and the retaining ligaments of the temple. The boundaries of the space are the superior temporal septum (STS) and the inferior temporal septum (ITS), which are extensions of the temporal ligament adhesion (TLA). No structures cross the temporal space. The TLA continues medially as the supraorbital ligamentous adhesion (SLA). Inferior to the temporal space is the triangular-shaped area of important anatomy (stippled). Crossing level 4 in this area are the medial and lateral branches of the zygomatic temporal nerve (ZTN) and the sentinel vein. The temporal branches of the facial nerve (TFN) course on the underside of the temporal-parietal fascia over the area immediately inferior to the ITS. The periorbital septum (PS, *green*) is on the orbital rim at the boundary of the orbital cavity. The lateral orbital thickening (LOT) and the lateral brow thickening (LBT) are parts of the periorbital septum. SON, supraorbital nerve; ZFN, zygomaticofacial nerve. (Source: Dr. Levent Efe, CMI. With permission from Mendelson B, Wong C-H. Anatomy of the aging face, section 1: aesthetic surgery of face. Plastic Surgery, Vol. 6. 3rd ed., 83.)

from squamous part of the temporal bone and is inserted into the coronoid process of mandible. It is a very active muscle and is often a cause of "tension headache." There are many surgical options oriented around temporalis muscle-induced headaches.[25] The motor innervations are from mandibular branch of the trigeminal nerve.

There are fat pads located above and below the muscle and together they provide volume to the temporal fossa (**Fig. 6.10**).

Temporal Fascia

Temporoparietal fascia (TPF) is the extension of superficial musculoaponeurotic system (SMAS) superiorly in the forehead.[26]

TPF is divided into two layers in the upper part of temporal region, deep inner and superficial outer part. Superficial part is continuous with SMAS. Just deep to this layer lies the frontal branch of the facial nerve and frontal branch of the superficial temporal vessels. The deep part of fascia is flimsy and is loosely attached to the deep temporal fascia. The DTF splits just above the zygomatic arch enveloping a fat pad; inferiorly it fuses and attaches with the periosteum of zygomatic bone. The deep layer of temporal fascia envelops the temporalis muscle (**Fig. 6.11**). However in the middle thirds

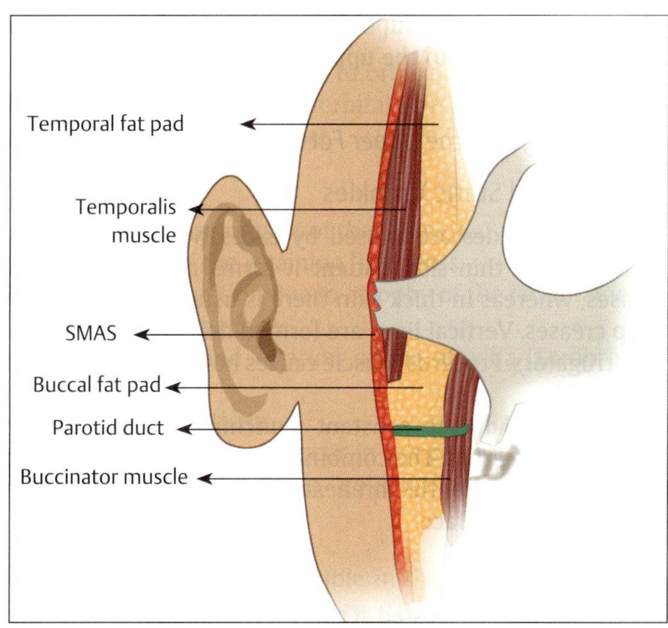

Fig. 6.10 Buccal pad of fat is located in the cheek between buccinator and masseter muscle and the temporal extension is located deep to the temporalis muscle. Atrophy of this deep fat causes temporal hollowing. SMAS, superficial musculoaponeurotic system.

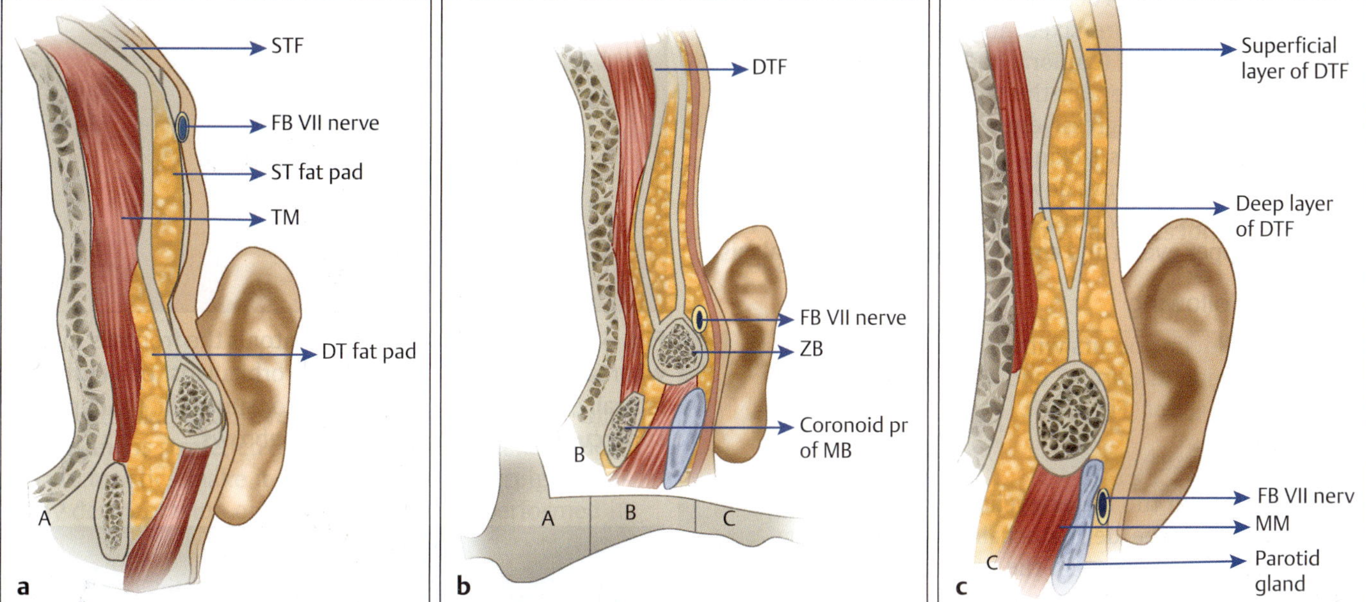

Fig. 6.11 Diagrammatic representations of anatomical structures around temporal fascia at different levels. **(a–c)** Temporoparietal fascia (TPF) is divided into deep inner and superficial outer layers. Superficial part is continuous with superficial musculoaponeurotic system (SMAS). The deep part of fascia is loosely attached to the deep temporal fascia. And, it splits just above the zygomatic arch enveloping a fat pad. Inferiorly it fuses and attaches with the periosteum of zygomatic bone in the proximal **(c)** and distal third region **(a)** of zygomatic arch. In the middle third part **(b)** the superficial and deep part of fascia attaches separately and directly to the periosteum of the zygoma. The frontal branch of the facial nerve below the zygomatic arch lies under the masseteric fascia. At the middle third level of zygoma it is under the SMAS layer. At the anterior third of zygoma it is located deep to the deep layer of fascia. So, the risk of frontal nerve injury is less if the dissection is in the subcutaneous plane. DT, deep temporal; DTF, deep temporal fascia; FB, frontal branch; MM, masseter muscle; pr of MB, process of mandible; ST, superficial temporal; STF, superficial temporal fascia; TM, Temporalis muscle; ZB, zygomatic bone.

bulge due to weakening of the orbicularis muscle and orbital septum. Subsequent changes in the lower eyelids are thinning of the skin and displacement of lid cheek junction with apparent increase in the vertical length of the lower eyelid. Further changes occur in the lateral canthus with changes in the shape and size of the palpebral aperture.

Tear Trough Deformity

The change in the lid-cheek junction is the cause of tear trough deformity or "nasojugal groove." The combination of displacement of fat from the inferior orbital rim, attenuation of the orbital ligaments, and underlying bony resorption aggravates the tear trough deformity. The depression continues laterally along the lateral part of the inferior orbital rim forming "palpebromalar groove." This is the beginning of the "V" deformity that eventually becomes a "Y" deformity.

The furrows or grooves that divide the midcheek are palpebromalar groove, nasojugal groove, and midcheek groove. The nasojugal and midcheek groove forms the "true tear trough" deformity (**Fig. 6.15**).

Malar Bags

Malar segment that overlies the zygomatic bone consists of thick pad of fat. Attenuation of the malar cutaneous ligament causes the fat to bulge out causing "malar fat bags." The proximal pulling effect of the malar cutaneous ligament forms the "midcheek groove" and completes the "Y" deformity. This breaks the youthful convex contour of the midcheek into three parts as aging progresses. The "malar bag" may atrophy in some people as age advances, causing sagging of skin and folding over the underlying malar ligaments. This is called as "festoons" (**Fig. 6.17**).

Prominent Nasolabial

The nasolabial segment of the midcheek undergoes significant aging changes. The firm layer of fat is held by the orbitomalar ligaments superolaterally in a young patient and the nasolabial fold appears only on smiling. With aging changes and volumetric changes in the face, the fold deepens as the nasolabial segment descends inferomedially. Barton[30] classified the severity of nasolabial fold: 0 , no visible fold; 1, minimal fold; 2, moderately deep fold; and 3, very deep fold (**Fig. 6.18**).

Lower Face Segment

Extent

The lower face extends from the oral commissure to the clavicle bones inferiorly.

Anatomy

Skin

The skin over the chin is thick with compact subcutaneous fat, in the lateral part over the mandibular area it is relatively thin, and has increased risk of pigmentation in type IV and type V skin types.

Neck skin is thin and superficial fascia of neck is composed of fatty tissue of variable thickness. The inner layer of the superficial fascia is elastic layer closely integrated to the platysma muscle. The deep fascia of the neck invests the deeper structures of the neck. The skin-superficial fascia, platysma unit, glides freely over the deep fascia. The only anchorage points are superiorly along the mandibular border and premasseteric area.

Platysma Muscle

Platysma originates from the deep fascia of deltoid and pectoral muscles. It courses over the clavicle and extends superomedially. The anterior fibers interlace under the symphysis menti and posterior fibers cross the mandible. Some fibers are inserted into the mandible in the oblique line, rest of the fibers merge with the SMAS layer of the face.

Raul Gonzalez[31] described that the anterior edges of the platysma are attached to the deep cervical fascia near the hyoid bone, whereas the posterior edge is attached

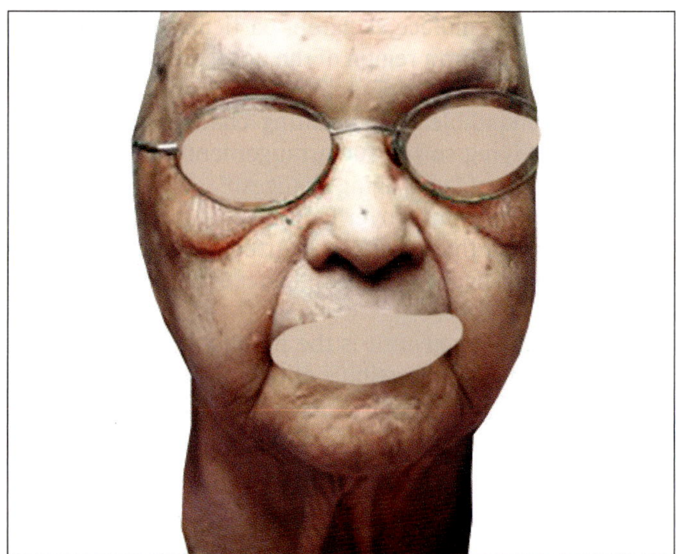

Fig. 6.17 The "malar bag" may atrophy in some people as age advances, causing sagging of skin and folding over the underlying malar ligaments. This is called as "festoons."

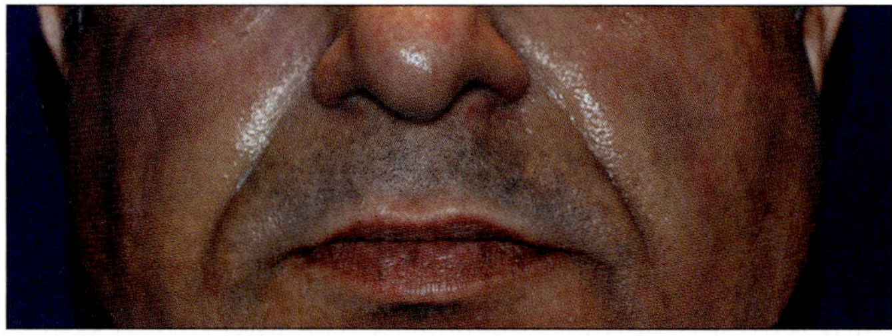

Fig. 6.18 Prominent nasolabial fold, Barton type 3.

to the same fascia at the angle of mandible. In between the edges, muscle is loosely adhered to the fascia. He showed that the loss of tone of the cervical skin and platysma muscle is more evident at the lateral part. Excessive skin in the central part of the neck is mostly related to excessive weight loss. Skin and platysma muscle are very closely associated and therefore loss of skin tone is associated with a loss of platysma tone.

Aging Changes

Wrinkles and Creases

Perioral lines form around the lower lip. Initially, they are dynamic and later creases appear at rest. Smokers have higher risks of deep perioral lines. They are also called as "lip bleeds" as the lip stick applied on the lip drips into these creases. They are uncommon in Fitzpatrick skin type V and VI.

Down-Turned Oral Angles

The oral commissure is horizontal in young people but with aging it drops down as the modiolus displaces inferiorly.

Marionette Lines or Labiomandibular Folds

It forms at the corner of the mouth due to combination of skin laxity and muscle overlap.

Medially in between the SMAS and buccinator muscle lies the buccal pad of fat. The inferior part of the buccal fat descends with aging and forms the typical fullness of labiomandibular fold.

Jowls are fatty deposits that accumulate along the inferior border of the mandible. The combination of fat deposit, skin sagging, attenuation of masseteric cutaneous ligament and descent of the buccal pad of fat all can aggravate the jowls. The mandibular cutaneous ligament anteriorly limits the jowl.

Platysmal Bands

With aging, the platysmal support in the midline and superolaterally is attenuated. The anterior edge of platysma descends inferiorly causing neck folds. The skin muscle complex forms folds; the platysma muscle causes bands that bow strings as the face is animated.

Fat Accumulation

Excessive fat accumulates in the submental and submandibular region of the skin obliterating the angle of the mandible. The fat is also accumulated around the angle of the mandible making the face appear wider with age. The appearance of "double chin" makes the neck appear shallower (**Fig. 6.19**).

Layers of the Face

The face has five layers similar to the scalp. These layers are skin, subcutaneous layer, musculoaponeurotic layer, loose areolar tissues, and deep fascia/periosteum (**Fig. 6.20**). Scalp layers are skin, subcutaneous tissue, galea aponeurotica, loose areolar tissue, and periosteum.

Layer 1

Skin comprising of the epidermis and dermis.

Layer 2

Subcutaneous tissue is composed of fatty tissue that are arranged in layers and tightly bound by fibrous septa. The thickness of fatty layer varies in the face, with it being most in the midface region. Retinacular cutis fibers encapsulating the fat tissue are more compact superficially, tightly binding the fat cells and are more diffuse in the deeper plane loosely enclosing the fat cells. The vertical fibers of the retinacular system firmly hold the cutis of the skin and some of the ligaments run as deep as the periosteum. This forms the "retaining ligaments" of the face. The horizontal fibers separate the fatty tissue into layers and it becomes less dense as you go deeper.[29]

Facial Fat Units

The author described the facial fat units based on cadaveric studies and clinical analysis of 164 patients who underwent liposuction of face and neck to improve the contour and rejuvenate the face (**Fig. 6.21a, b**).

Subcutaneous fat deposits in the face with age change the shape of the face. A smooth oval face in females and sharp square face in men are signs of youthful and healthy face. Deposition of fat in some parts of the face can change the

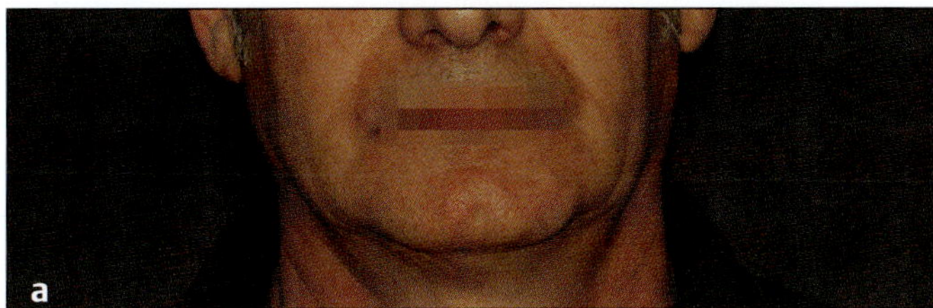

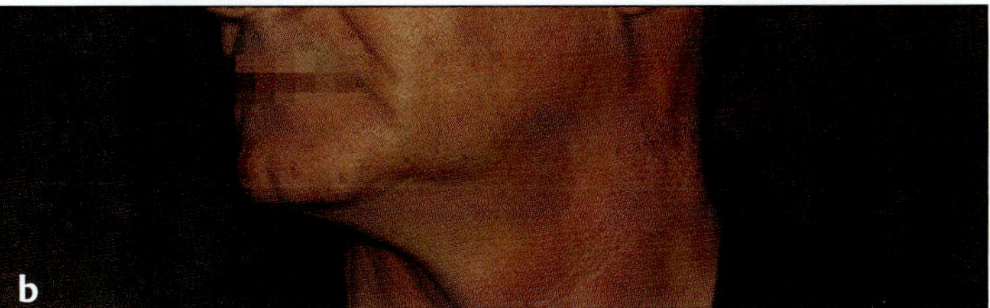

Fig. 6.19 **(a, b)** Aging changes in lower face: down-turned oral angles, labiomandibular folds, jowls, and platysmal bands. **(a)** Frontal view. **(b)** Lateral view.

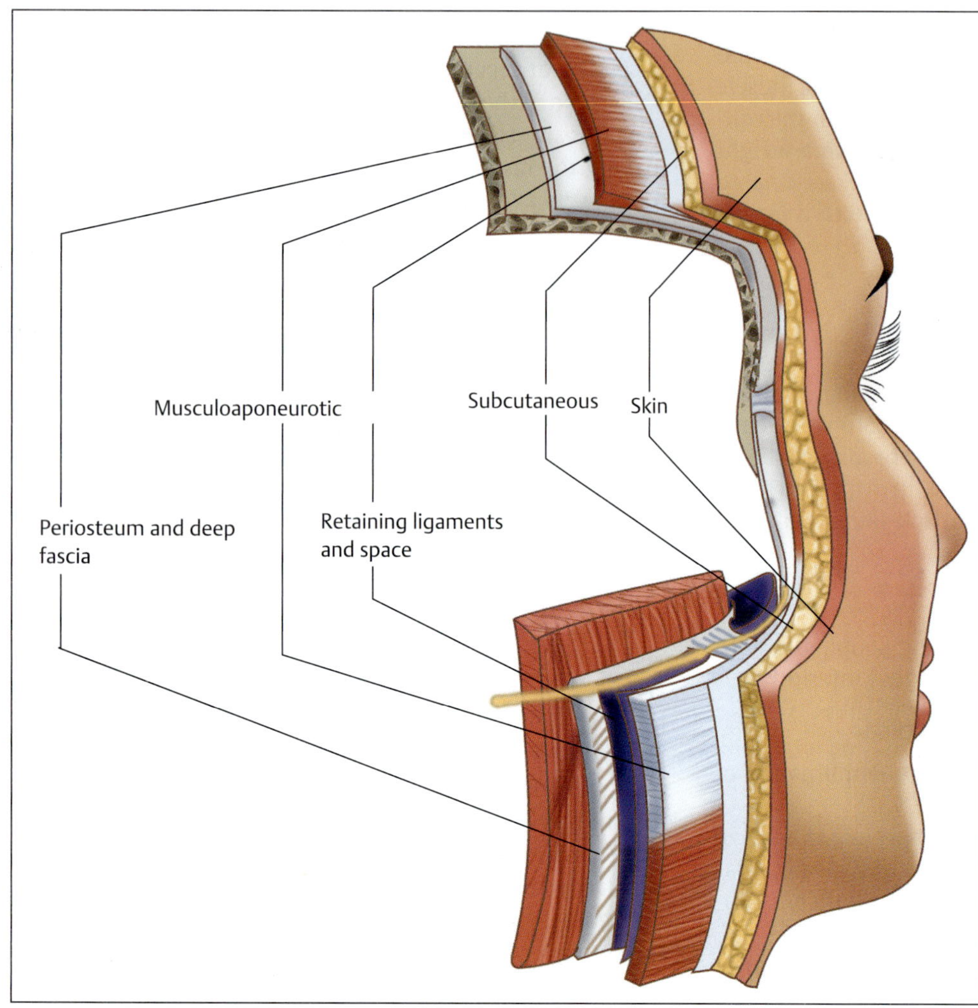

Fig. 6.20 The face is constructed of five basic layers. This five-layered construct is most evident in the scalp but exists in the rest of the face also, with significant modification and compaction for functional adaptation. Layer 4 is the most significantly modified layer, with alternating facial soft tissue spaces and retaining ligaments. Facial nerve branches also transition from deep to superficial in association with the retaining ligaments through layer 4. (Source: Mendelson B, Wong C-H. Anatomy of the aging face, section 1: aesthetic surgery of face. Plastic surgery, Vol. 6. 3rd ed., page 79.)

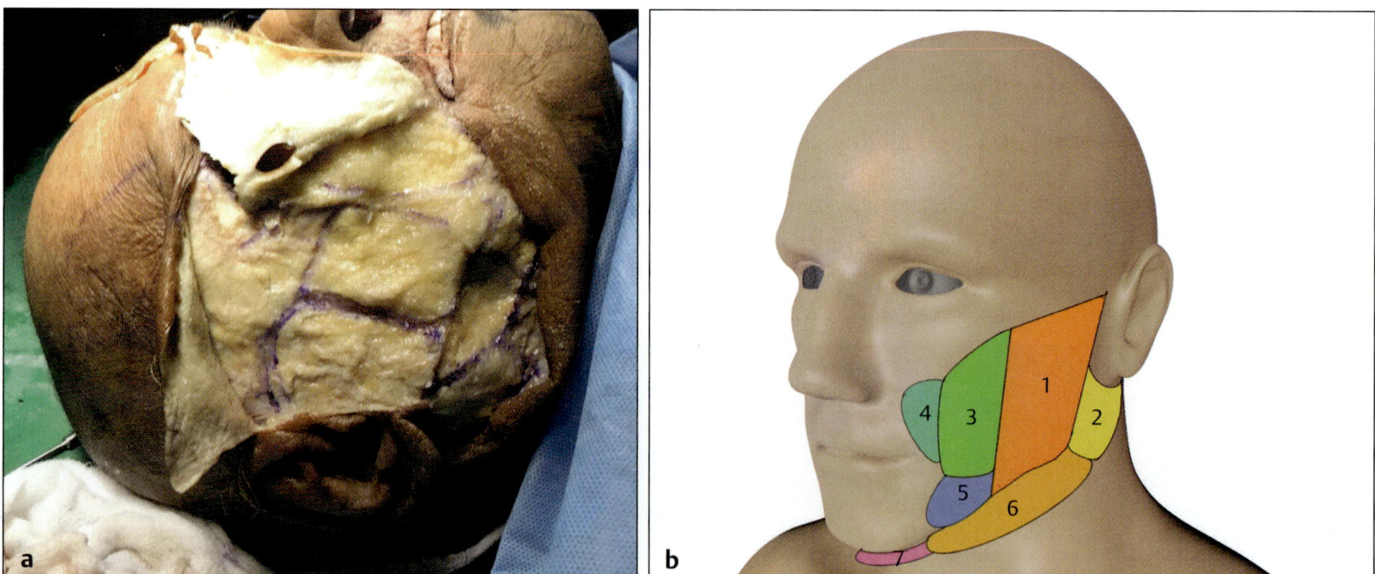

Fig. 6.21 **(a, b)** Facial fat units. There are seven areas in the face where fat can alter the shape of the face. **(a)** Cadaver showing the superficial fat layer with zones marked. **(b)** (1) Preauricular zone, (2) mastoid zone, (3) buccal zone, (4) nasolabial zone, (5) jowls, (6) submandibular zone, (7) submental zone.

shape to irregular oval, round, or wide. Some of these zones can be treated by liposuction to restore the shape of the face.

Author proposes that there are seven areas in the face where fat can alter the shape of the face.

- Preauricular zone: Fat deposits in subcutaneous tissue and SMAS of preauricular region increase the size of the face, making it round. The primary reason is weight gain. This fat can be removed by careful liposuction using fine cannulas.
- Mastoid zone: A youthful face has a nice contour at the angle of the jaw with sternocleidomastoid muscle imparting a youthful and healthy appearance to the face and neck region. Excess accumulation of fat occurs in this region both in men and women, obliterating the contours. Combination of fat deposits in preauricular and mastoid areas gives a wide look to the face. Performing liposuction, focusing on this zone, improves the contour of the face.
- Buccal zone: Buccal fat is composed of subcutaneous fat, SMAS fat, and buccal pad of fat. Excess fat accumulates in all the three layers of the fat and combined with fat displacement the face contour changes to round. The subcutaneous fat is amenable to liposuction but the buccal pad of fat needs surgical removal intraorally.
- Nasolabial zone: This is a small zone lateral to the nasolabial fold. It can be due to midface descent and/or fat accumulation with weight gain. Liposuction of this zone has risk of sagging skin and wrinkling.
- Jowls zone: This is a zone of displaced fat from midface in addition to subcutaneous deposits. Even a small pocket of fat takes away the youthful look of the face. Liposuction can reduce the jowls but surgical correction is more definitive solution to this problem.
- Submandibular zone: Fat deposits in the submandibular zone obliterate the jaw line and contour of the neck. But submandibular gland ptosis can accentuate the defect and has to be carefully assessed.
- Submental zone: Fat deposits in this zone occur very early in the age. Fat deposits in submental zone causes "double chin" deformity.

The clinical implications are discussed later in the chapter.

Layer 3

Musculoaponeurotic layer: This layer is similar to galea aponeurotica of scalp with its occipitofrontalis muscle unit. This layer continues in the face with the superficial group of facial muscles. These muscles are orbicularis oculi, orbicularis oris, and platysma, and they do not directly originate from the bone. However, facial muscles also have a deep layer of muscles that originate from underlying bones, e.g., zygomaticus major and minor, levator labii superioris, levator angulii oris, depressor labii inferioris, and depressor anguli oris.

In scalp there is a free gliding space between the upper three layers which act as a composite layer, i.e., skin, subcutaneous tissue, and galea musculoaponeurotica that move over the periosteum. There are no cutaneous ligaments in the scalp.

Superficial Musculoaponeurotic System (SMAS)

SMAS constitutes the third layer of face (**Fig. 6.22**). It is a thick fascial layer that extends from superficial temporal fascia superiorly to superficial cervical fascia inferiorly. In the lower face it tends to be muscular being the cranial extension of platysma. In midface and upper face it is aponeurotic with fibrofatty components and continues across the zygomatic arch as superficial temporal fascia which blends

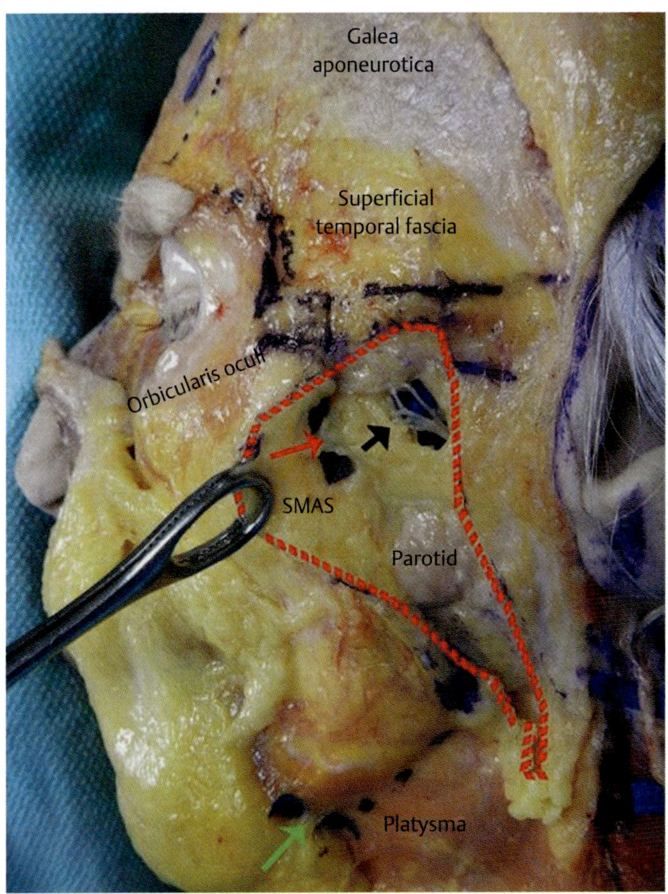

Fig. 6.22 Superficial musculoaponeurotic system (SMAS): cadaver dissection of the left face. Skin and subcutaneous tissue have been reflected medially. The SMAS is incised and undermined for a short distance (red dots delineate the incised edges of the SMAS). A small SMAS flap is held in ovum forceps. Underneath the SMAS the parotid gland can be seen, and the frontal rami of the facial nerve travelling to cross the zygomatic arch can be appreciated (*black arrow*). The outline of the zygomatic arch and the lower mandibular border are marked in *blue*. A *red arrow* points to a sub-SMAS retaining filament with a *blue* background. A *green arrow* points to a fibrous filament retaining the skin to the lower mandibular border with a *blue* background. Age and gender of the cadaver are unknown.

with frontalis muscle, galea aponeurotica, and orbicularis oculi.[32] The SMAS consists of three-dimensional architecture of collagen fibers, elastic fibers, fat cells, and muscle fibers. Alireza Ghassemi published an anatomical study of SMAS in cadavers at multiple levels: forehead, parotid, zygomatic and infraorbital (IO) region, nasolabial fold, and lips. He described two architectural models of SMAS. Type 1 is a meshwork of fibrous septa which envelops lobules of fat and has viscoelastic properties. The interconnecting fibrous network is connected to periosteum via retaining ligaments. This morphology is found in parotid, zygomatic and IO region, and lateral part of nasolabial folds. Type 2 is a meshwork of intermingled collagen, elastic, and muscle fibers without distinct fat lobules and is located in medial part of nasolabial region, upper and lower lips. SMAS is closely related to facial nerve as it progresses from lateral to medial aspect, where it branches and becomes more superficial. In addition, SMAS constitutes a compartment through which blood vessels penetrate to supply overlying skin.[33,34]

These two architectures have distinct clinical significance. Type 1 is more viscoelastic so it is susceptible to aging process but at the same time is useful in elevation, mobilization, and repositioning of soft tissue during rhytidectomy. Type 2 has firm connection to muscles of the lips and it directly influences lip movements.

Layer 4

Layer 4 comprises of retaining ligaments, soft tissue spaces, deep layers of fascial muscles, and branches of facial nerve. In the face, the top three layers act as composite segment but it does not freely glide all over the face because of retaining ligaments. These ligaments that run from periosteum to the dermis compartmentalize the face. In between the ligaments, the tissues move adequately with contraction of muscles.

The retaining ligaments are more abundant in the periphery than in the medial part of the midface. There is less support to the medial cheek, causing more sagging and formation of nasolabial folds.[35]

Layer 5

The deepest and the last layer is the deep fascia overlying the masseter (masseteric fascia) and temporalis (deep temporal fascia) and formed by periosteum in medial part of the face. In the neck it continues as investing layer of the deep fascia.

Fat Pads of Face

Suborbicularis Oculi Fat (SOOF)

SOOF described by May et al[36] and later by Aiache and Ramirez[37] is a specialized layer of fat that lies deep to the lower lid orbicularis muscle. This fat allows gliding movement of the orbicularis muscle. It has two parts, medial and lateral as described by Rohrich et al[38] (**Fig. 6.23**).

The lateral SOOF is located at the lateral orbital rim and it extends from lateral canthus to the lateral orbital thickening. The medial part of SOOF extends from lateral canthus to the medial limbus of the cornea. The deep medial cheek fat is inferior to medial SOOF. The inferior boundary of SOOF is the tear trough.

Retroorbicularis Oculi Fat (ROOF)

M. Charpy in 1909 described a layer of fat underneath the eyebrow extending from midpart of eyebrow to lateral part of eyebrow. ROOF can contribute to upper eyelid heaviness and resection of this fat can help decrease heaviness of the upper lid and lateral brow[39] (**Fig. 6.23**).

There are some fatty layers that have special characteristics. Malar pad of fat overlies the zygomatic bone and it is firmly adhered to the periosteum. Malar pad of fat has extensive fibrous septa that are adhered to the skin.

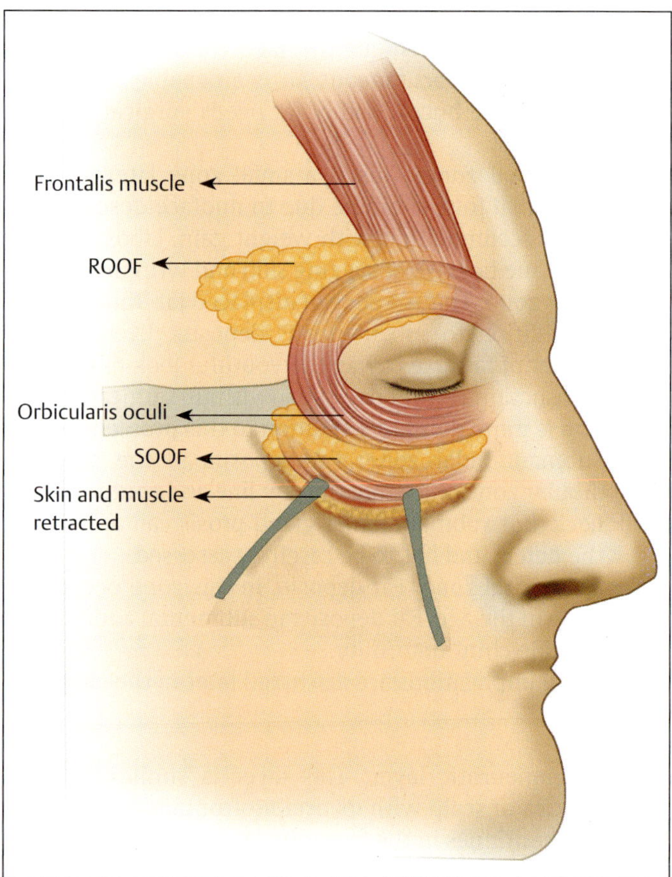

Fig. 6.23 Three morphological forms of retaining ligaments of the face. ROOF, Retroortbicularis oculi fat; SOOF, suborbicularis oculi fat. (Source: Mendelson B, Wong C-H. Anatomy of the aging face, section 1: aesthetic surgery of face. Plastic surgery, Vol. 6. 3rd ed., page 80.)

Buccal Fat Pad

Heister first described buccal fat in 1732 as "Glandular Morlares"; Bichat later in 1802 described it as fatty in nature with special characteristic to allow mastication. It is also called "masticatory fat" and it separates the muscles of mastication. The average weight ranges from 8 to 11.5 g as demonstrated in cadaveric studies.[40]

Parts of Buccal Fat

Main body of fat constitutes 20 to 30% of the total volume of fat. It has four extensions:

1. Buccal fat proper constitutes 30 to 40% of the total buccal fat volume. Part of the buccal fat is buttressed between buccinators and SMAS anterior to the masseter muscle. Posteriorly it is sandwiched between masseter and buccinators. Buccal part is divided in to upper one-third and lowers two-third by parotid duct. Below the parotid duct lies a large buccal branch of facial nerve. Part of this fat is fairly superficial and it descends with aging causing bulge below the oral commissure (**Fig. 6.24a–c**).
2. Pterygoid extension: This is posterior extension of buccal fat that lies between the pterygoid muscles.
3. Deep temporal fat is extension behind the temporal muscle overlying the squamous part of temporal bone.
4. Superficial temporal extension lies between the temporalis muscle and deep temporalis fascia.

Retaining Ligaments of Face

Retaining ligaments are tiny fibrous structures that support the facial soft tissue in a youthful position and were first described by McGregor and later by Furnas and Stuzin et al.[8,41]

Stuzin and Mendelson[41,42] described that the ligament is in inverted "L" shape where the horizontal limb is formed by zygomatic cutaneous ligaments and vertical limb is along the anterior border of masseteric muscle formed by masseteric cutaneous ligaments (**Fig. 6.25**).

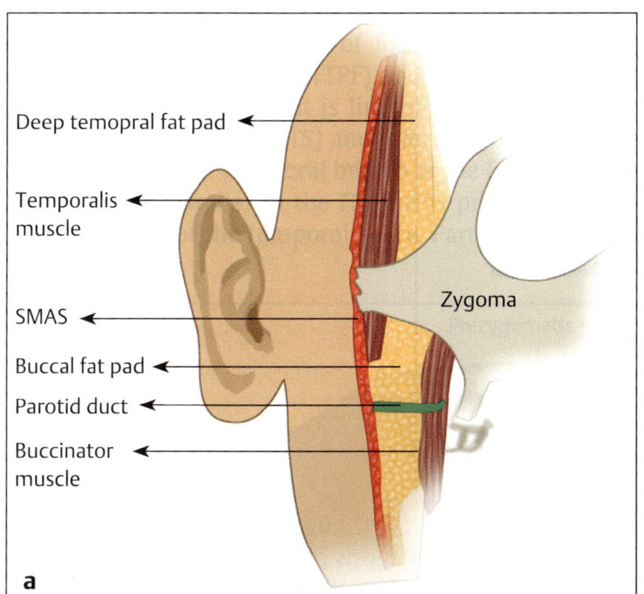

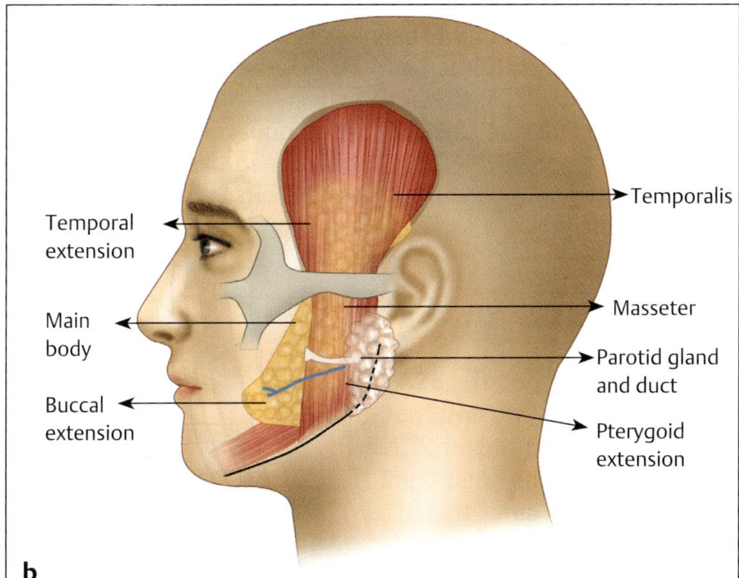

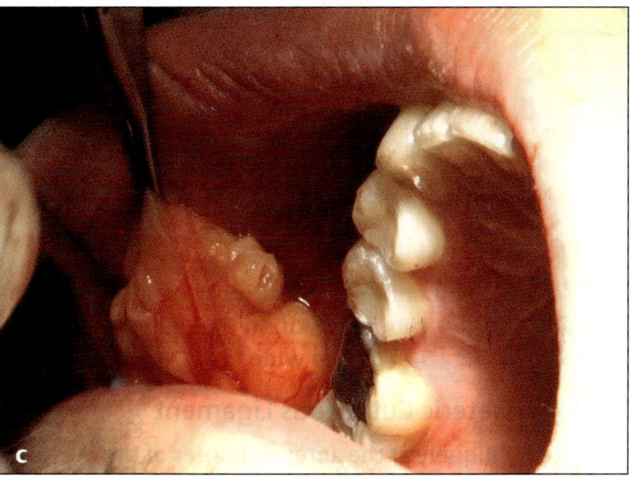

Fig. 6.24 Buccal pad of fat. **(a)** Sagittal anatomy. **(b)** Surface marking. **(c)** Intraoperative fat appearance. SMAS, superficial musculoaponeurotic system.

at the inferior part and runs below and parallel to mandible. It enters the platysma from underneath and forms a plexus.

Blood Supply

Key to avoiding complications in any facial treatment includes having an in-depth knowledge of vascular anatomy. Vascular supply of face-lift flap, location of vessels to prevent inadvertent vascular damage while performing injectable fillers and risks of excessive bleeding can be avoided if you keep in mind the anatomy during the procedure[9] (**Fig. 6.29**).

Transverse facial artery (TFA) is the main artery that nourishes the skin of the face. It is a branch of superficial temporal artery and it arises deep to the parotid gland. It accompanies the buccal branch of the facial nerve in the same plane lying under the parotidomasseteric fascia. A large perforator arising from TFA is located near the zygomatic ligament below the bone. The TFA anastomoses extensively with lacrimal, IO, and facial arteries.

Facial Artery

Lee et al[50] presented an extensive cadaveric work on the course and pattern of branching of facial artery.

They classified three patterns of facial artery branches:

1. Type I nasolabial pattern (51.8%).
2. Type II nasolabial pattern with IO trunk (29.6%).
3. Type III forehead pattern (18.6%).

The level of the facial artery and its branches also varies significantly. In 85.2% cases they run on the surface of facial muscles.

Superficial Temporal Artery

Superficial temporal artery bifurcates in front of the auricle into frontal and parietal branches. The frontal branch runs parallel to eyebrow toward the forehead and parietal branch runs vertically up in the parietal region.

Supraorbital Artery

Supraorbital artery, a branch of ophthalmic artery, runs along with the supraorbital nerve and exits the supraorbital notch. It divides into superficial and deep branch supplying the forehead muscles, skin, and frontal bone.

Supratrochlear Artery

It is also a branch of the ophthalmic artery and exits the orbital bone in the medial part along with the nerve counterpart.

Skin Types

The Fitzpatrick skin type (**Table 6.1**) is a skin classification first developed in 1975 by Thomas Fitzpatrick,[2] a dermatologist from Harvard Medical School. The aging pattern in the skin types varies and is a useful guide to analyze an aging face.

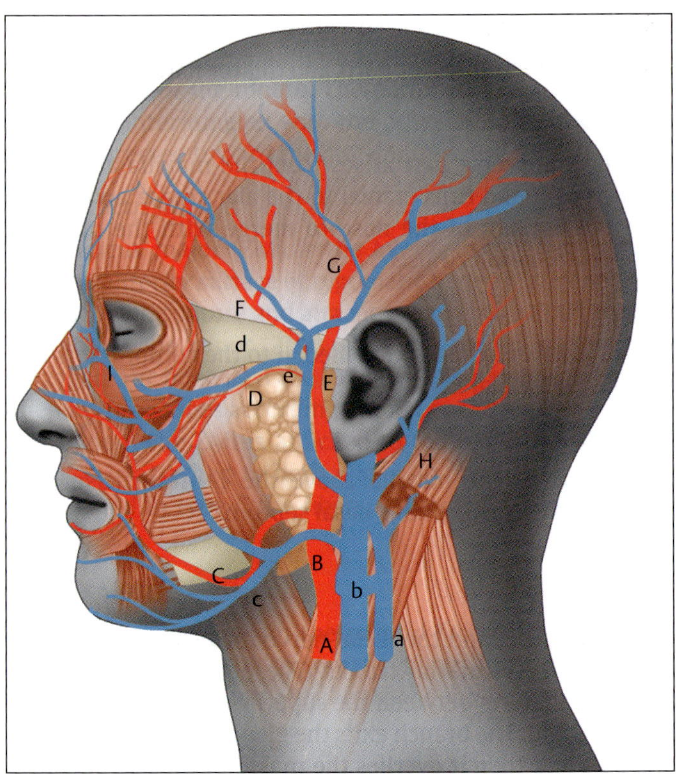

Fig. 6.29 Facial blood circulation: (A) common carotid artery, (B) external carotid artery (ECA), (C) facial artery, (D) transverse facial artery, (E) superficial temporal artery, (F) frontal branch of superficial temporal artery (STA), (G) parietal branch of STA, (H) posterior auricular artery, (I) angular artery. (a) Jugular vein, (b) external Jugular vein (EJV), (c) facial vein, (d) transverse facial vein, (e) superficial temporal vein.

Type I, II, and III tend to have more skin wrinkling, sagging, sunspots, and photo damage due to low melanin content and thinner dermis. On the other hand, type IV, V, and VI tend to have more pigmentation changes than wrinkling due to thicker and compact dermis. In addition, darker skin types have more cornified cell layers and greater lipid content.

There is a large variation of skin type among people of Indian subcontinent due to diversity of genes and cultural traits. India predominantly comprises two population groups, the lighter-skinned Aryans and the darker-skinned Dravidians, hence the aging pattern also varies. Variations are found in people who live in different geographical areas of India: north Indians with more Aryan descent and south Indians with more Dravidian descent and then there are interracial mixes.[51] On the other hand, eastern part of India has oriental descent; hence, in India, we see a range of skin types from type III to VI. There is also a striking variation in the facial morphology across India. The facial index (ratio of facial length to facial width) varies among Indians from different geographical regions. This is described later in the chapter.

Table 6.1 Fitzpatrick skin type classification

Type	Color	Reaction to UVA	Reaction to sun
I	Caucasian; blonde or red hair, freckles, fair skin, blue eyes	Very sensitive	Always burns easily, never tans; very fair skin tone
II	Caucasian; blonde or red hair, freckles, fair skin, blue eyes or green eyes	Very sensitive	Usually burns easily, tans with difficulty; fair skin tone
III	Darker Caucasian, light Asian	Sensitive	Burns moderately, tans gradually; fair to medium skin tone
IV	Mediterranean, Asian, Hispanic	Moderately sensitive	Rarely burns, always tans well; medium skin tone
V	Middle Eastern, Latin, light-skinned, black, Indian	Minimally sensitive	Very rarely burns, tans very easily; light or dark skin tone
VI	Dark-skinned black	Least sensitive	Never burns, deeply pigmented; very dark skin tone

Abbreviation: UVA, ultraviolet A.

Skin Texture Changes

The textural changes in face also add to the aging process. These changes are uneven pigmentation, which may be due to combination of hormonal changes, sun exposure, and postinflammatory changes. Freckles are light brown spots that develop with aging and are directly related to sun exposure. "Skin tags' or polyps are small excess of skin hanging with a pedicle and they are prevalent in face, neck, axilla, and groin (**Fig. 6.30**).

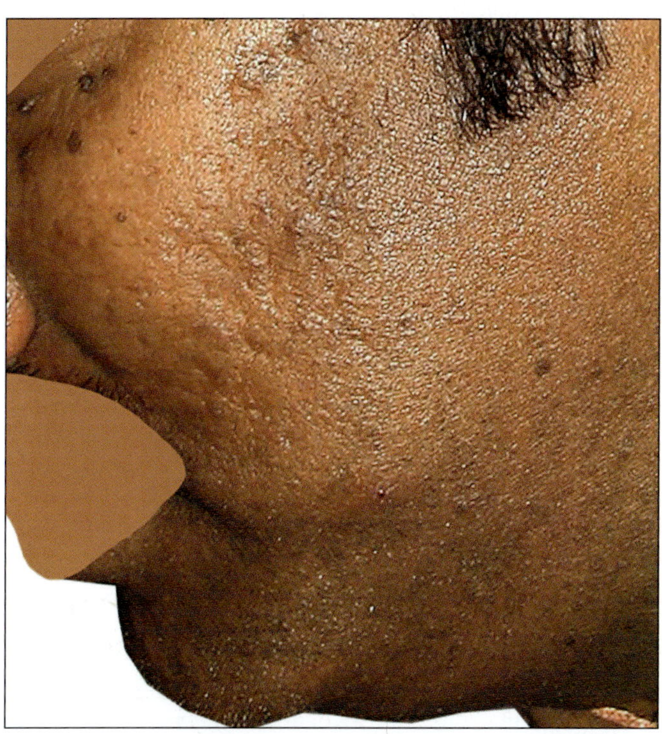

Fig. 6.30 Skin texture changes: uneven pigmentation, freckles, skin tags, etc.

Aesthetic Units of Face

Aesthetic units of face were first described by González-Ulloa in the context of facial reconstruction and placement of scars.[52] Cadaver dissections were performed and finally 40 regions of body and 14 of face were described based on skin thickness and histology.

Menick incorporated visual perception of people looking at their faces and further described the facial aesthetic units based on the ridges, valleys, and convex and concave shapes visible with light reflexes of different parts of the face.[53] This led to establishments of subunits like nasal and lip subunits.

There are three important reasons the aesthetic subunits of face are important for antiaging management of the patient:

1. *Volumetric changes* of aging are different in each aesthetic subunit of the face. Lateral forehead, orbital units, and medial cheek units undergo volume loss as compared with other subunits of the face. Lateral cheek units and neck units gain volume with aging.
2. *Textural changes*: Generally, the skin is more sebaceous in the medial part of the face than the periphery. Lateral forehead, zygomatic unit, and lateral cheek unit have higher risk of pigmentation. Any ablative procedures such as peeling or CO_2 laser are done with caution in these subunits of the face.
3. *Healing process*: The healing process of skin varies in facial subunits. Scars appear better if they are located at the borders of the subunit. Scars in the sebaceous skin do not heal very well.

Fattahi[54] (**Fig. 6.31**) further described the facial subunits (**Table 6.2**) that allow us to individually assess the zones and compare it to the other side for symmetry. Although each subunit has its own proportion but what is fairly standard is that the more symmetric face a person has, the more attractive the person appears.

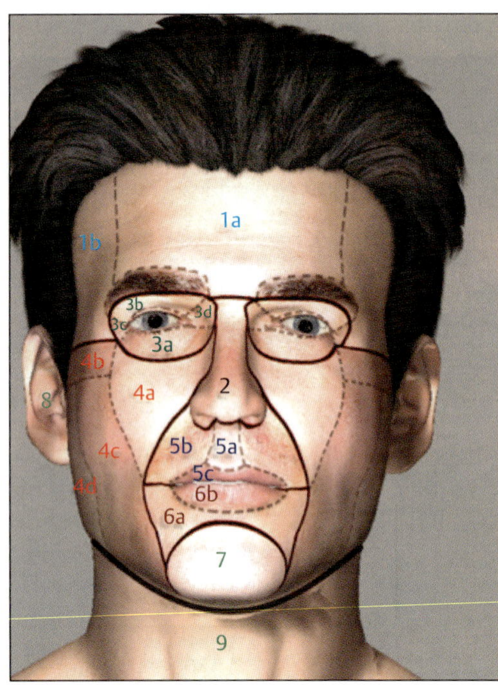

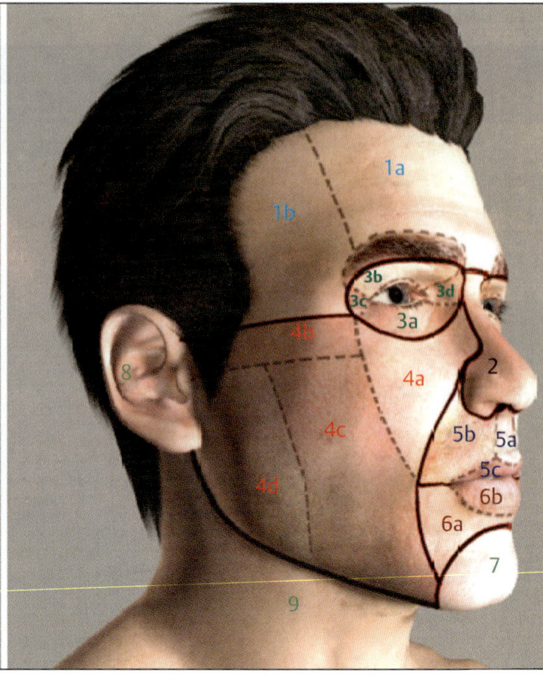

Fig. 6.31 Aesthetic units of face. (Used by permission of author Davide Brunel, http://www.med-ars.it/.)

Table 6.2 Facial aesthetic units (Fattahi)

Forehead unit	• Central subunit • Lateral subunit • Eyebrow subunit
Nasal unit	
Eyelid units	• Lower lid unit • Upper lid unit • Lateral canthal subunit • Medial canthal subunit
Cheek unit	• Medial subunit • Zygomatic subunit • Lateral subunit • Buccal subunit
Upper lip unit	• Philtrum subunit • Lateral subunit • Mucosal subunit
Lower lip unit	• Central subunit • Mucosal subunit
Mental unit	
Auricular unit	
Neck unit	

Skeletal Anatomy of Face

The facial bones are the structural foundations of face. The facial skeleton consists of 14 stationary bones and a mobile lower jawbone. These bones form the basic shape of face apart from providing muscle attachment for function and expressions. The facial skeleton is believed to grow continuously and differentially throughout life. The vertical height of facial bones increases continuously with age unless supervening factors such as tooth loss intervene. Males have more prominent brow ridges, differently shaped orbits, larger pyriform aperture, and larger jaw than females. In addition, they differ in rate and extent of bony changes with aging.[55,56]

Bony Changes with Age

It is a well-established fact that facial changes with aging are a result of structural changes in the soft and bony tissue.[54]

The changes in the bones are predominantly in the periorbital bones, maxillary bones, and prejowl area of mandible. This results in change of position of overlying muscle and suspension structures. The areas most affected by these changes and resulting changes include lateral brow ptosis, prominent medial orbital pad of fat, tear trough deformity, malar mounds, deep nasolabial folds, and deepening of prejowl sulcus.

It is important to understand the bony changes to accomplish a complete and harmonious rejuvenation.

Periorbital Region

The orbital aperture increases with age in both area and width due to resorption of superomedial and inferolateral aspects of the rim.

Midface

It comprises of maxilla in medial and middle thirds and zygoma in the lateral third. It has been demonstrated that midface retrusion occurs with aging irrespective of dentulous status. The maxilla undergoes more changes than zygoma.

Perinasal Changes

The noses lengthen and tip droops because of changes in the bony foundation. The pyriform aperture enlarges with aging and the posterior displacement of the bony rim is greatest at the lower part of aperture causing retrusion of columella, posterior displacement of alar base, and deepening of nasolabial folds.

Lower Face

The most recent study showed that the mandiblular angle increases, whereas the ramus height and mandibular body height and length decrease. Yet another observation was reduced skeletal projection in prejowl area that leads to exaggeration of jowls.

Aging Changes among Indians

India is a diverse country with more than 2,000 ethnic groups.[57] Merely referring the Indian skin as "Asian skin" or Fitzpatrick type V is inadequate.

There are few publications describing the skin color differences across India, but literature is deplete of varying facial morphology and aging pattern in India. It is time that we organize a study to classify the Indian faces to deal with the aging changes. Indian skin color classified as fair, wheatish brown, medium brown, dark brown, and intense dark is described[56] in dermatological journals. It is explained in the context of pigmentary changes in the skin. The morphology of face in Indian subcontinent varies from north to south and east to west. Broadly it can be classified using facial indices into the following types (the facial framework is expressed as the facial index, which is the ratio of facial length to facial width) (**Fig. 6.32a–e**):

- Hypereuryprosopic: Short broad face with facial index less than 80.
- Euryprosopic: Short or broad face or both with a facial index of 80 to 85.
- Mesoprosopic: Face of average width with a facial index of 84.0 to 87.9.
- Leptoprosopic: Long, narrow, or a long narrow face with a facial index of 88.0 to 92.9.
- Hyperleptoprosopic: Very long narrow face with a facial index of 93.

Generally, north Indians are tall, fair, and thin, while south Indians are short, stout, and broad. The climates of these two regions are different, and hence, according to the environment, facial features also differ.[51,57]

The common aging concerns among north Indians are dynamic and static wrinkles, sagging skin, jowls, and neck laxity. On the contrary, south Indians are concerned about deep forehead furrows, tear trough deformity, deep nasolabial folds, and fat bulges in the jaw lines and neck.

In authors' experience there are two main concerns in Indian patients' aging changes and soft tissue disproportion. Generally, north Indians have leptoprosopic and hyperleptoprosopic morphology with skin types III to IV. The common aging concerns in them are:

- Dynamic and static wrinkles.
- Brow ptosis.
- Excess eyelid with deep nasolabial folds, marionette, perioral lines.
- Jowls and neck aging.
- Skin texture changes such as freckles, pigmentations, and skin tags.
- On the other hand, south Indians have hypereuryprosopic and euryprosopic morphology with type V skin.

The common aging concerns are:

- Lower eyelid excess and bags.
- Pigmentary changes.
- Dark circle and IO depressions.
- Midface aging with nasolabial fold, cheek waviness, marionette folds.
- Lower face aging such as jowls and double chin.

Authors also recognized that soft tissue disproportion is a significant concern in Indian population. Lipoadiposity with fat deposits in various face zones, as described earlier in this chapter, changes the shape of the face (**Fig. 6.33a–e**).

- Irregular oval: The fat displaces in the lower part of the face including jowls and jaw line.
- Round shape: The fat deposit is in the cheek and neck areas.
- Pear shape: The face appears trapezoid with excess fat deposits in the jaw line and mastoid region and often occurs in men.
- Square shape: This is a common change that occurs in eastern Indian patients with wide bone structure aggravated by fat deposits, skin laxity, and masseter hypertrophy.

Assessment of Aging Face

Patients seeking treatments for aging are of diverse skin types and age groups. Some patients are able to identify the problem or concern they have, whereas others may simply complain of tired looks. There is a changing trend in the age group of the patients seeking antiaging treatment. Younger patients are seeking treatment for minimal early signs of aging or simply prevention.

A thorough understanding of the aging changes and a systematic approach to assessment will allow better outcome for the treatment. The initial consultation is important to understand their needs. Handing the patient with a mirror in a well-lighted room and asking them to elaborate on their concerns is necessary to make a plan.

Melvin Shiffman[58] proposed a clinical classification for facial aging (**Table 6.3**). The four different areas of face that are affected by aging are tear trough, cheek fat loss, nasolabial fold, and jowl prominence. He further states that the first change of aging is the stage 1 with appearance of tear

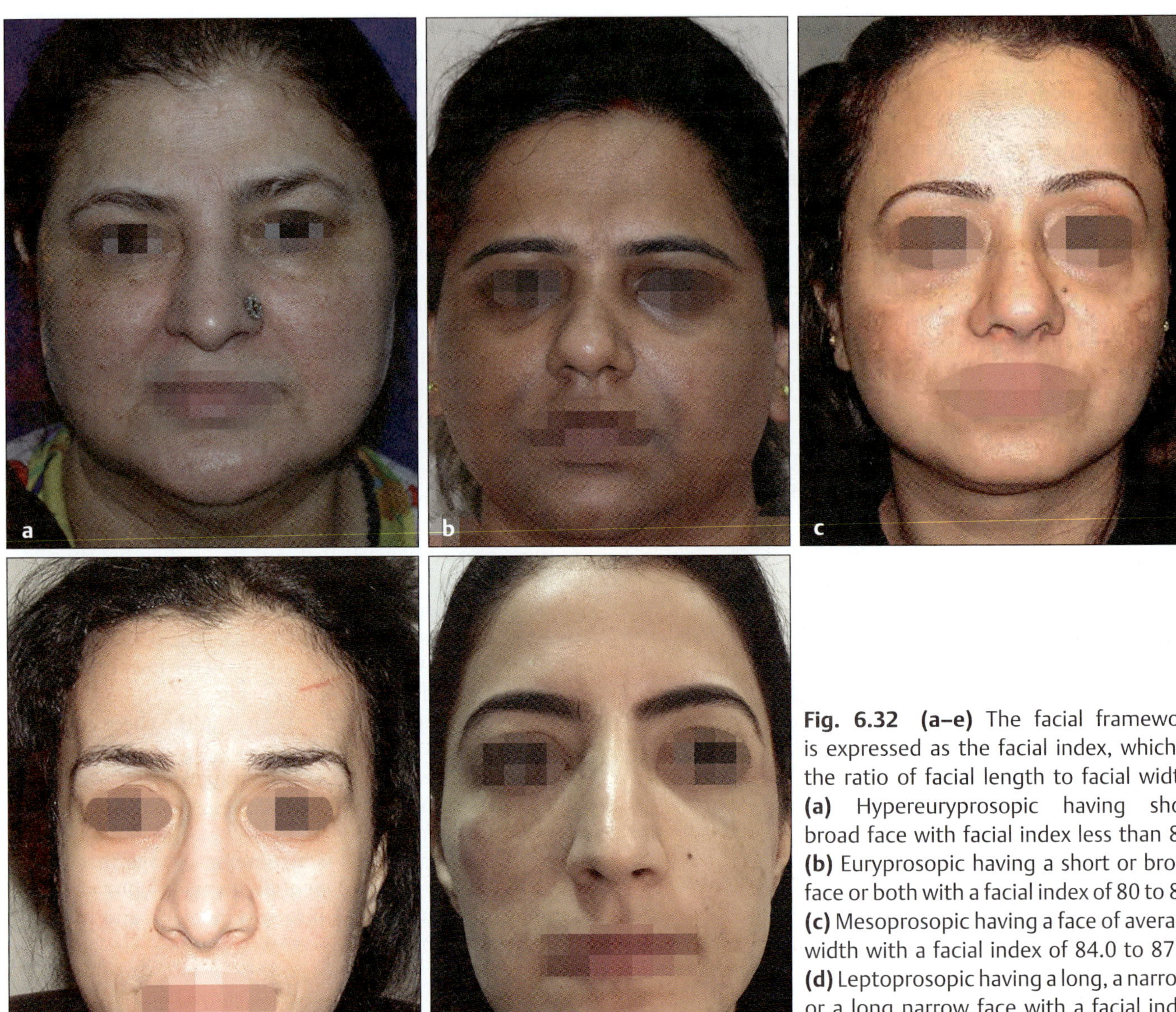

Fig. 6.32 **(a–e)** The facial framework is expressed as the facial index, which is the ratio of facial length to facial width. **(a)** Hypereuryprosopic having short broad face with facial index less than 80. **(b)** Euryprosopic having a short or broad face or both with a facial index of 80 to 85. **(c)** Mesoprosopic having a face of average width with a facial index of 84.0 to 87.9. **(d)** Leptoprosopic having a long, a narrow, or a long narrow face with a facial index of 88.0 to 92.9. **(e)** Hyperleptoprosopic having a very long narrow face with a facial index of 93.

trough deformity and slight nasolabial fold depth. It progresses to stage 4 with severe changes in all areas.

Patient Concerns

It is similar to eliciting "history of primary illness" where the patients enumerate their concerns. After they have listed their concerns, ask them leading questions regarding each part of the face. The method will be clear later in the chapter.

Medical History

A detailed evaluation of health is a prerequisite with enquiry on hypertension, diabetes mellitus, bleeding disorders, allergies, smoking, etc. These patients are more prone to excessive bleeding and bruising even after minimal invasive procedures. Smokers have high incidence of complications after face lift or blepharoplasty. A patient undergoing major surgery needs complete evaluation of respiratory, cardiac, renal, and hepatic system. A complete drug history is essential to prevent bleeding disorders, drug interactions, deep vein thrombosis, etc. In elderly and high-risk patients, a complete preanesthetic evaluation is mandatory.

Weight fluctuation causes volume changes in the face and can exaggerate the signs of facial aging. Is patient educated to maintain healthy lifestyle to prevent its effect on the face? Chronic sun exposure is the commonest cause of pigmentation. The pigmentation is more prominent in IO, malar, and temporal regions, reducing the glow of the face and giving more tired appearance.

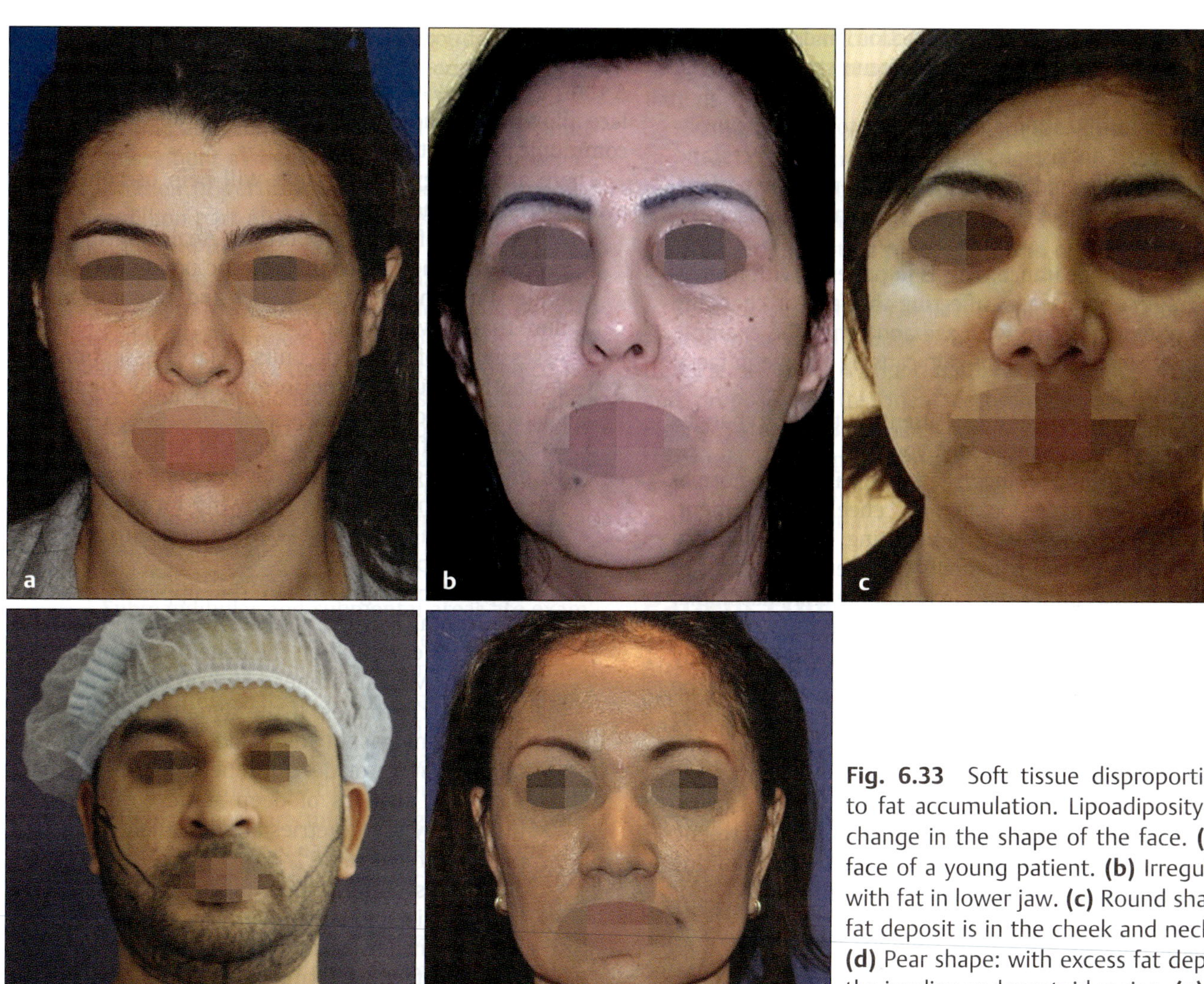

Fig. 6.33 Soft tissue disproportion due to fat accumulation. Lipoadiposity causes change in the shape of the face. **(a)** Oval face of a young patient. **(b)** Irregular oval with fat in lower jaw. **(c)** Round shape: the fat deposit is in the cheek and neck areas. **(d)** Pear shape: with excess fat deposits in the jaw line and mastoid region. **(e)** Square shape: in patients with wide bone structure aggravated by fat deposits and skin laxity.

Table 6.3 Shiffman classification of facial aging

Stage	Tear trough depth	Cheek fat loss	Nasolabial fold depth	Jowl prominence
Stage 0	None	No Loss	None	None
Stage 1	Slight	No loss	Slight	None
Stage 2	Mild	Slight loss medially	Mild	Slight
Stage 3	Moderate	Moderate	Moderate	Moderate
Stage 4	Severe	Severe	Severe	Severe

Past Procedures

A detail history of previous procedures on the face is recorded. Any history of facial resurfacing by peeling or laser is important to understand the skin healing. History of permanent fillers such as polyacrylamide may cause problem if any invasive procedure is performed. Past history of any procedures that may cause internal scarring such as thread lift is important for any further treatment.

Psychological Assessment

The challenging part of any aesthetic procedure is the psychological response of the patient. It can vary from

Table 6.6 Treatment options

Options	Advantages	Disadvantages	Risks vs. benefits	Patient choice
Nonsurgical skin tightening Radiofrequency based Ultrasonic based	• Minimal risk • No downtime • Natural outcome if any	• Unpredictable outcome • Repetitive procedures • Nondramatic outcome • Expensive	• Economic risks with unpredictable outcome	
Fillers/fat grafting	• Mild improvement in NL, LM, PZ areas • Minimal risks • Minimal downtime	• Large volume required • May look unnatural • May require more sessions • No benefit to Neck	• Moderate risks, moderate outcome	
Thread lifts	• Dramatic improvement • Minimal downtime • Minimal risks • Minimal discomfort • No scars	• Multiple threads required • Long-term outcome unpredictable • Threads may break causing asymmetry • Risks of extrusions, etc. • Expensive	• Good outcome, moderate risks but longevity unpredictable	
Facelift and neck lift	• Dramatic improvement • Long-term outcome • Multiple problems addressed	• Risks • Discomfort • Scar • Downtime	• Good outcome, moderate-to-high risks, long term, cost effective	

Abbreviations: LM, labiomental; NL, nasolabial; PM, palpebromalar region.

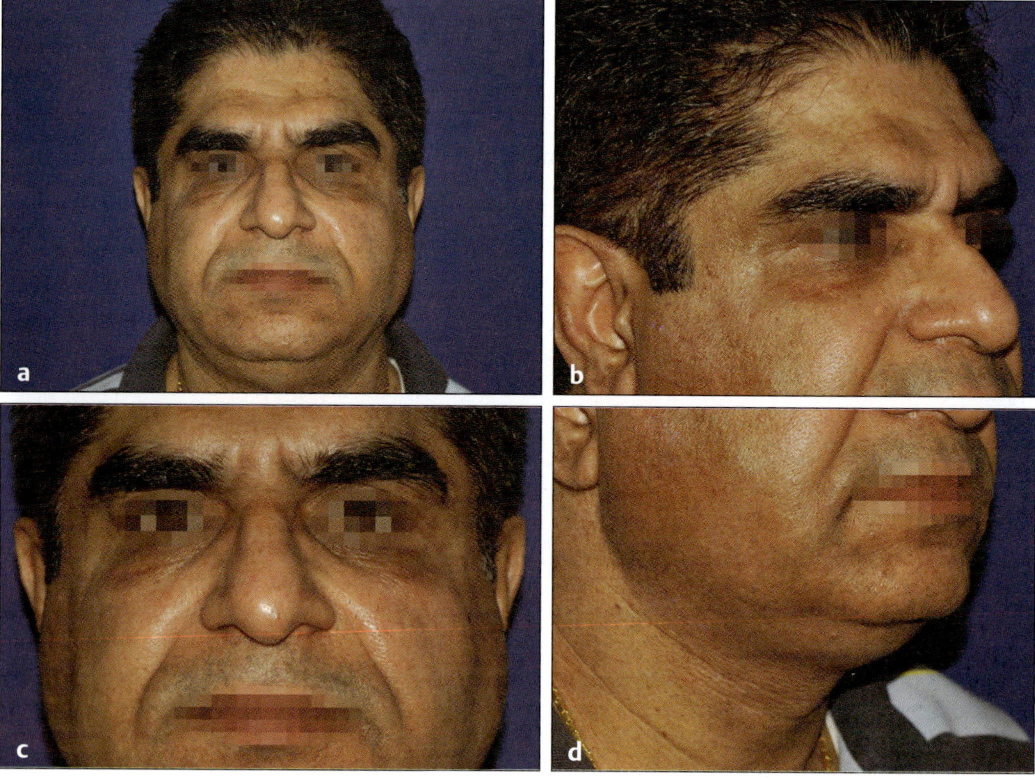

Fig. 6.34 Refer to **Table 6.4** for assessment proforma and analysis of face with proposed treatment in this male patient of 52 years age seeking facial rejuvenation. **(a)** Full face and neck. **(b)** Upper face. **(c)** Midface. **(d)** Lower face.

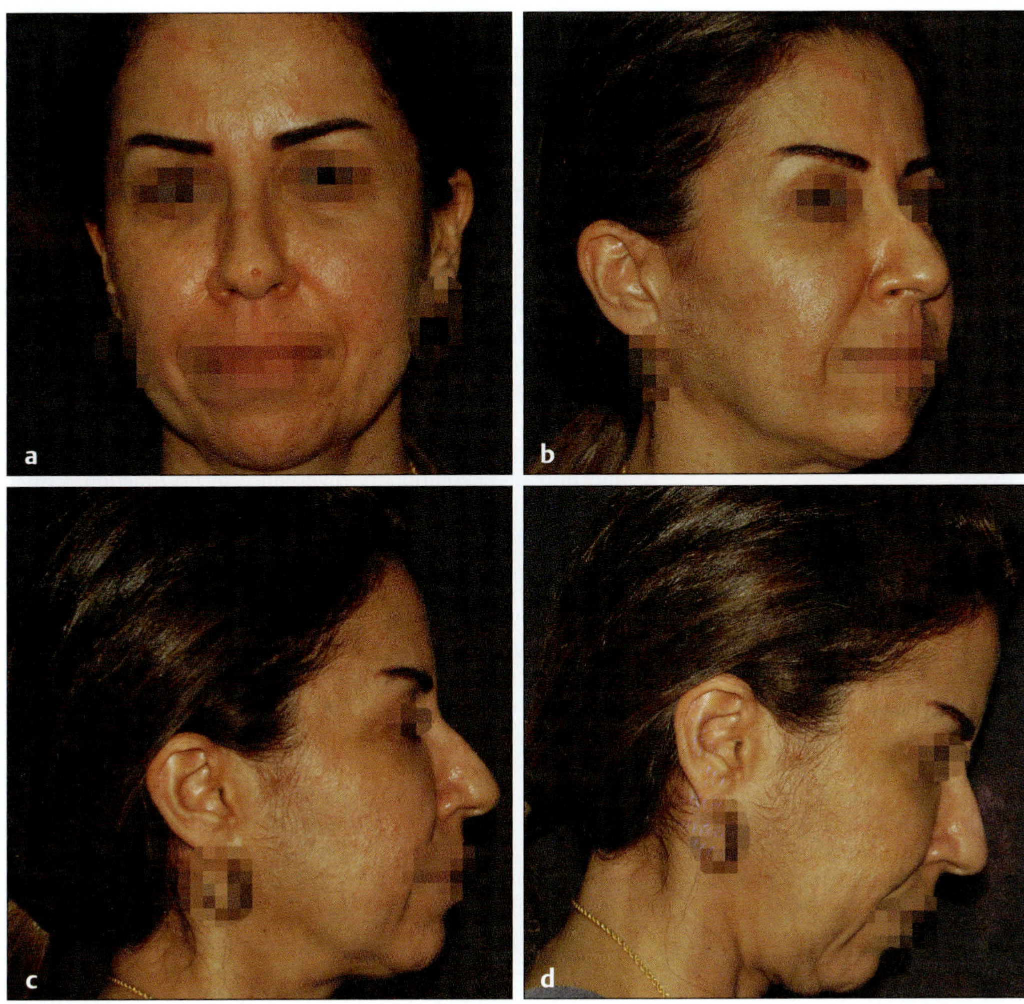

Fig. 6.35 Refer to **Tables 6.5 and 6.6** for assessment proforma and analysis of face with proposed treatment in this female patient of 48 years age seeking facial rejuvenation. **(a)** Frontal view. **(b)** Oblique view. **(c)** Profile. **(d)** Neck flexed position.

References

1. Khazanchi R, Agarwal A, Johar M. CME: anatomy of aging face. Indian J Plast Surg 2007;40(2):223–229
2. Odunze M, Cohn A, Few JW. Restylane and people of color. Plast Reconstr Surg 2007;120(7):2011–2016
3. Ogeng'o J. The changing face of human anatomy practice: learning from history and benefiting from technology. Anat J Afr 2014;3(2):308–312
4. Bhattacharya S. Sushrutha: our proud heritage. Indian J Plast Surg 2009;42(2):223–225
5. Deeper B, Pushpalatha K. A glimpse of our past: contributions of Sushruta to anatomy. Anat J Afr 2014;3(2):362–365
6. Paul MD, Calvert JW, Evans GRD. The evolution of the midface lift in aesthetic plastic surgery. Plast Reconstr Surg 2006;117(6):1809–1827
7. Mitz V, Peyronie M. The superficial musculo-aponeurotic system (SMAS) in the parotid and cheek area. Plast Reconstr Surg 1976;58(1):80–88
8. Furnas DW. The retaining ligaments of the cheek. Plast Reconstr Surg 1989;83(1):11–16
9. Whetzel TP, Mathes SJ. The arterial supply of the face lift flap. Plast Reconstr Surg 1997;100(2):480–486, 1657, discussion 487–488
10. Little JW. Volumetric perceptions in midfacial aging with altered priorities for rejuvenation. Plast Reconstr Surg 2000;105(1):252–266, discussion 286–289
11. Ramirez OM. Three-dimensional endoscopic midface enhancement: a personal quest for the ideal cheek rejuvenation. Plast Reconstr Surg 2002;109(1):329–340, discussion 341–349
12. Naini FB. Facial aesthetics: concepts and clinical diagnosis. Wiley-Blackwell; 2011:18–44
13. Farkas LG, Hreczko TA, Kolar JC, Munro IR. Vertical and horizontal proportions of the face in young adult North American Caucasians: revision of neoclassical canons. Plast Reconstr Surg 1985;75(3):328–338
14. Karaca Saygili O, Cinar S, Gulcen B, Ozcan E, Kus I. The validity of eight neoclassical facial canons in the Turkish adults. Folia Morphol (Warsz) 2016;75(4):512–517
15. Husein OF, Sepehr A, Garg R, et al. Anthropometric and aesthetic analysis of the Indian American woman's face. J Plast Reconstr Aesthet Surg 2010;63(11):1825–1831
16. Porter JP, Olson KL. Anthropometric facial analysis of the African American woman. Arch Facial Plast Surg 2001;3(3):191–197
17. Fang F, Clapham PJ, Chung KC. A systematic review of interethnic variability in facial dimensions. Plast Reconstr Surg 2011;127(2):874–881

18. Vegter F, Hage JJ. Clinical anthropometry and canons of the face in historical perspective. Plast Reconstr Surg 2000;106(5): 1090–1096
19. Ricketts RM. Divine proportion in facial esthetics. Clin Plast Surg 1982;9:401–22
20. Bashour M. History and current concepts in the analysis of facial attractiveness. Plast Reconstr Surg 2006;118(3):741–756
21. Gosman SD. Anthropometric method of facial analysis in orthodontics. Am J Orthod 1950;36(10):749–762
22. Mendelson BC, Wong CHS. Surgical anatomy of the middle premasseter space and its application in sub-SMAS face lift surgery. Plast Reconstr Surg 2013;132(1):57–64
23. Hwang K, Kim YJ, Chung IH. Innervation of the corrugator supercilii muscle. Ann Plast Surg 2004;52(2):140–143
24. Hwang K, Jin S, Park JH, Chung IH. Innervation of the procerus muscle. J Craniofac Surg 2006;17(3):484–486
25. Kurlander DE, Punjabi A, Liu MT, Sattar A, Guyuron B. In-depth review of symptoms, triggers, and treatment of temporal migraine headaches (Site II). Plast Reconstr Surg 2014;133(4):897–903
26. Abul-Hassan HS, von Drasek Ascher G, Acland RD. Surgical anatomy and blood supply of the fascial layers of the temporal region. Plast Reconstr Surg 1986;77(1):17–28
27. Wong CH, Mendelson B. Facial soft-tissue spaces and retaining ligaments of the midcheek: defining the premaxillary space. Plast Reconstr Surg 2013;132(1):49–56
28. Mendelson BC, Jacobson SR. Surgical anatomy of the midcheek: facial layers, spaces, and the midcheek segments. Clin Plast Surg 2008;35(3):395–404, discussion 393
29. Lambros V. Observations on periorbital and midface aging. Plast Reconstr Surg 2007;120(5):1367–1376, discussion 1377
30. Barton FE Jr. Rhytidectomy and the nasolabial fold. Plast Reconstr Surg 1992;90(4):601–607
31. Gonzalez R. Composite platysmaplasty and closed percutaneous platysma myotomy: a simple way to treat deformities of the neck caused by aging. Aesthet Surg J 2009;29(5):344–354
32. Rohrich RJ, Pessa JE. The fat compartments of the face: anatomy and clinical implications for cosmetic surgery. Plast Reconstr Surg 2007;119(7):2219–2227, discussion 2228–2231
33. Hashem AM, Couto RA, Duraes EFR, et al. Facelift part I: history, anatomy, and clinical assessment. Aesthet Surg J 2020;40(1): 1–18
34. Ghassemi A, Prescher A, Riediger D, Axer H. Anatomy of the SMAS revisited. Aesthetic Plast Surg 2003;27(4):258–264
35. Accioli de Vasconcellos JJ, Britto JA, Henin D, Vacher C. The fascial planes of the temple and face: an en-bloc anatomical study and a plea for consistency. Br J Plast Surg 2003;56(7):623–629
36. May JW Jr, Fearon J, Zingarelli P. Retro-orbicularis oculus fat (ROOF) resection in aesthetic blepharoplasty: a 6-year study in 63 patients. Plast Reconstr Surg 1990;86(4):682–689
37. Aiache AE, Ramirez OH. The suborbicularis oculi fat pads: an anatomic and clinical study. Plast Reconstr Surg 1995;95(1): 37–42
38. Rohrich RJ, Arbique GM, Wong C, Brown S, Pessa JE. The anatomy of suborbicularis fat: implications for periorbital rejuvenation. Plast Reconstr Surg 2009;124(3):946–951
39. Naik MN, Honavar SG, Das S, Desai S, Dhepe N. Blepharoplasty: an overview. J Cutan Aesthet Surg 2009;2(1):6–11
40. Lang J. Clinical anatomy of the masticatory apparatus and peripharyngeal spaces 100,101. 1st ed. ; 1995:99–107
41. Stuzin JM, Baker TJ, Gordon HL. The relationship of the superficial and deep facial fascias: relevance to rhytidectomy and aging. Plast Reconstr Surg 1992;89(3):441–449, discussion 450–451
42. Mendelson BC. Surgery of the superficial musculoaponeurotic system: principles of release, vectors, and fixation. Plast Reconstr Surg 2001;107(6):1545–1552, discussion 1553–1555, 1556–1557, 1558–1561
43. Ozdemir R, Kilinç H, Unlü RE, Uysal AC, Sensöz O, Baran CN. Anatomicohistologic study of the retaining ligaments of the face and use in face lift: retaining ligament correction and SMAS plication. Plast Reconstr Surg 2002;110(4):1134–1147, discussion 1148–1149
44. DiFrancesco LM, Anjema CM, Codner MA, McCord CD, English J. Evaluation of conventional subciliary incision used in blepharoplasty: preoperative and postoperative videography and electromyography findings. Plast Reconstr Surg 2005; 116(2):632–639
45. Rogers CR, Mooney MP, Smith TD, et al. Comparative micro-anatomy of the orbicularis oris muscle between chimpanzees and humans: evolutionary divergence of lip function. J Anat 2009;214(1):36–44
46. Choi DY, Hur MS, Youn KH, Kim J, Kim HJ, Kim SS. Clinical anatomic considerations of the zygomaticus minor muscle based on the morphology and insertion pattern. Dermatol Surg 2014;40(8):858–863
47. Furnas DW. Landmarks for the trunks and the temporofacial division of the facial nerve. Br J Surg 1965;52:694–696
48. Freilinger G, Gruber H, Happak W, Pechmann U. Surgical anatomy of the mimic muscle system and the facial nerve: importance for reconstructive and aesthetic surgery. Plast Reconstr Surg 1987;80(5):686–690
49. Salinas NL, Jackson O, Dunham B, Bartlett SP. Anatomical dissection and modified Sihler stain of the lower branches of the facial nerve. Plast Reconstr Surg 2009;124(6):1905–1915
50. Lee JG, Yang HM, Choi YJ, et al. Facial arterial depth and relationship with the facial musculature layer. Plast Reconstr Surg 2015;135(2):437–444
51. Prasanna LC, Bhosale S, D'Souza AS, et al. Facial indices of north and south Indian adults: reliability in stature estimation and sexual dimorphism. J Clin Diagn Res 2013;7(8):1540–1542
52. González-Ulloa M. Regional aesthetic units of the face. Plast Reconstr Surg 1987;79(3):489–490
53. Menick FJ. Artistry in aesthetic surgery: aesthetic perception and the subunit principle. Clin Plast Surg 1987;14(4):723–735
54. Fattahi TT. An overview of facial aesthetic units. J Oral Maxillofac Surg 2003;61(10):1207–1211
55. Mendelson B, Wong CH. Changes in the facial skeleton with aging: implications and clinical applications in facial rejuvenation. Aesthetic Plast Surg 2012;36(4):753–760
56. Pessa JE. An algorithm of facial aging: verification of Lambros's theory by three-dimensional stereolithography, with reference to the pathogenesis of midfacial aging, scleral show, and the lateral suborbital trough deformity. Plast Reconstr Surg 2000;106(2):479–488, discussion 489–490
57. Hourblin V, Nouveau S, Roy N, de Lacharrière O. Skin complexion and pigmentary disorders in facial skin of 1204 women in 4 Indian cities. Indian J Dermatol Venereol Leprol 2014;80(5):395–401
58. Shiffman M. Facial aging: a clinical classification. Indian J Plast Surg 2007;40(2):178–181
59. Gorney M. Recognition of the patient unsuitable for aesthetic surgery. Aesthet Surg J 2007;27(6):626–629
60. Parashar S. How can a plastic surgeon avoid getting into trouble or litigation? Medicolegal aspects of dermatology & plastic surgery. 1st ed. Jaypee Publication; 2019:400–409

7

Principles and Techniques of Nonsurgical Facial Rejuvenation

Niti Khunger, Soni Nanda, and Khushbu Mahajan

Table 7.3 Glogau photoaging and wrinkle scale

Group	Classification	Average age in years	Type of wrinkles	Skin characteristics
I	Mild	25–35	No or minimal wrinkles	Early photoaging Mild pigmentary changes No keratosis Does not require makeup
II	Moderate	35–50	Wrinkles in motion	Early-to-moderate photoaging: Few brown spots visible (lentigos) Seborrheic keratosis and DPN palpable, few visible Parallel smile lines begin to appear Needs makeup to conceal
III	Advanced	50–65	Wrinkles at rest	Moderate-to-advanced photoaging Multiple brown spots (senile lentigos) Multiple seborrheic keratosis and DPN Visible capillaries (telangiectasias) in fair skin Needs heavy makeup to conceal
IV	Severe	60–75	Full of wrinkles	Severe photoaging Favre-Racouchot syndrome may be seen Senile comedones Multiple brown spots Multiple seborrheic keratosis and DPN Yellowish and sallow complexion in fair skin Cannot wear makeup because it cakes and cracks

Abbreviation: DPN, dermatosis papulosa nigra.
Source: Modified from Glogau 1996.[8]
Note: Ages are representative as it depends on degree of sun exposure.

The second step is a detailed counseling and discussion to have a rejuvenation plan, a timeline and expectation alignment. The expected outcomes of treatment, cost and likely complications should be discussed. An informed consent should be taken including all details and possible adverse effects. The patient must be given an opportunity to take an active part in decision making.

The third step is standardized photographic documentation (**Fig. 7.1**). Patients often forget what they initially looked like and comparative before and after photographs help in convincing patients. Pre-existing asymmetry and other issues must be demonstrated and documented.

Skin rejuvenation has two components: patient directed and physician directed **(Table 7.4)**. Proper knowledge and application of both these components is an integral part of a successful aesthetic practice, and combining both modalities leads to a complete facial regimen, maximizing results and patient satisfaction.

Patient-Directed Techniques for Rejuvenation

These include the use of products on the skin such as sunscreens, moisturizers, retinoids, α-hydroxy acids, and various antioxidants present in cosmeceuticals to both maintain youthful skin and rejuvenate damaged skin.[9] Since the use of these products is in control of the patient, they are patient directed. There is a wide variety of products available to prevent, reduce, and repair the aging skin. Though several factors such as smoking, hormones, and obesity contribute to the appearance of the aging skin, photoaging or UV light in sunlight plays a major role.

Sunscreens

Photoprotection and sunscreens form an integral part of any facial rejuvenation regimen and also help to reduce the risk of PIH following procedures. Sunscreens alter the effects of UV radiation on the skin by absorption and/or reflection. Protection from sunlight through the use of sunscreens can significantly reduce the risk of photoaging, provided they are correctly applied. An ideal sunscreen should provide broad-spectrum photoprotection (290–760 nm), be photostable, nontoxic, and aesthetically acceptable and affordable. Both UVA and UVB blockers are required. Sunscreens can be broadly divided into chemical (organic), physical (nonorganic), or a combination of both (**Table 7.5**).[10] Chemical sunscreens can further be classified into UVA protectors, UVB protectors, or broad-spectrum filters offering both UVA and UVB protection. Salicylates are good UVB absorbers, TDSA (terephthalylidene dicamphor sulfonic acid, ecamsule,

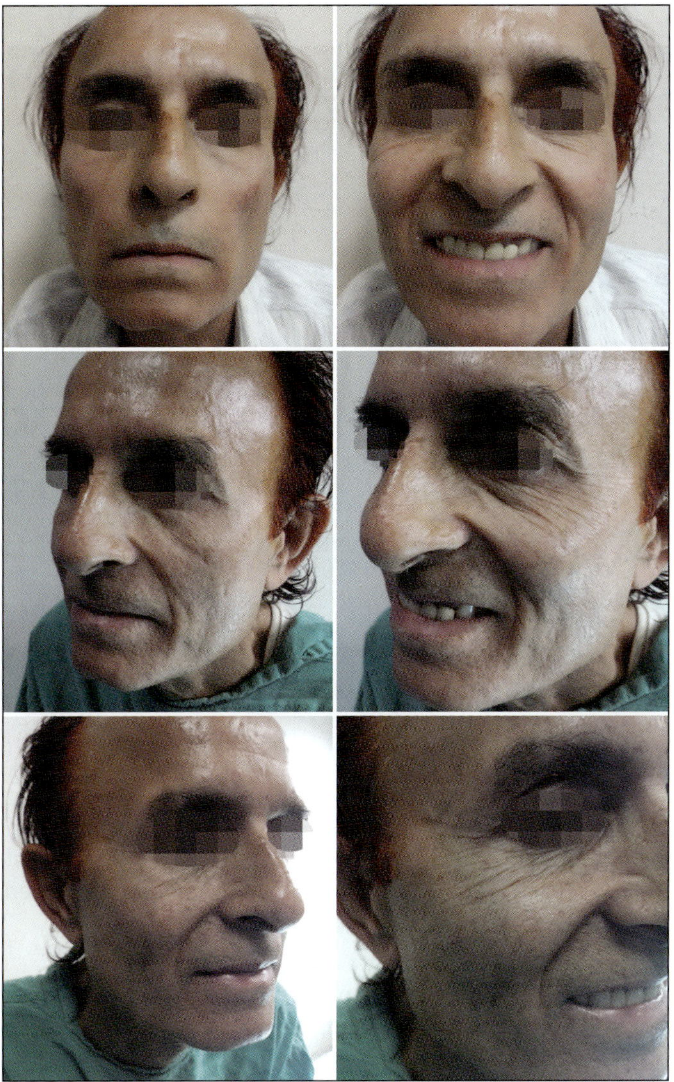

Fig. 7.1 Standardized photographs static and dynamic.

Mexoryl SX), DPDT (disodium phenyl dibenzimidazole tetrasulfonate), DHHB (diethylamino hydroxybenzoyl hexyl benzoate) are good UVA sunscreens. Zinc oxide and titanium oxide are used as physical blockers and are especially useful in children and sunscreen allergic individuals.

There are sunscreen-related indices which are commonly misunderstood, e.g., sun protection factor (SPF). It is actually UVB sunburn protection factor, defined as the ratio of the least amount of ultraviolet energy (UVB) required to produce minimal erythema on sunscreen-protected skin to the amount of energy required to produce the same erythema on unprotected skin. Internationally agreed procedures define protected skin as that to which a 2 mg/cm^2 layer of sunscreen has been applied.[11] It is important to know that a sunscreen with an SPF of 15 blocks about 93% of UVB radiation, while one with an SPF of 30 blocks about 97% of UVB radiation. This 4% difference in SPF may not make a lot of difference in aesthetic appeal as a higher SPF sunscreen is generally more uncomfortable because of higher concentration of active ingredient. Sometimes patients complain of worsening of skin color despite use of sunscreen with high SPF. This is because a good SPF value will not protect the skin from the entire UV spectrum and is just a measure of protection against UVB rays.

Another important point of consideration is the amount of sunscreen applied. Sunscreen should be applied properly to all sun-exposed areas (in a concentration of 2 mg/cm^2), and allowed to dry completely before sun exposure. It should be reapplied every 2 hours, and also after swimming, vigorous activity, excessive perspiration, or toweling. We can use the concept of fingertip unit (FTU) to establish the amount of sunscreen to be applied. One FTU is the amount of topical preparation that is squeezed out from a standard tube (with 5-mm nozzle) along an adult's fingertip. A fingertip is from the end of the finger to the first crease in the finger (**Fig. 7.2**).

Table 7.4 Nonsurgical skin rejuvenation techniques

Patient directed	Action	Physician directed	Action
Photoprotection and sunscreens	Prevents photoaging, reduces pigmentation	Chemical peels	Smoothens the skin, even tone, reduces pigmentation, reduces wrinkles, improves texture
Moisturizers	Reduces dry skin, barrier repair, reduces fine lines	Microdermabrasion	Smoothens the skin, even tone
Topical retinoids	Reduces fine wrinkles, even skin tone, skin lightening	Microneedling	Reduces wrinkles, improves texture
Alpha-hydroxy acids	Reduces wrinkles, smoothens the skin, even skin tone, skin lightening	Botulinum toxin	Reduces dynamic wrinkles
Topical antioxidants and cosmeceutical	Repair creams, reduces wrinkles, skin lightening	Fillers	Plumps the skin and underlying atrophy, reduces hollows, reduces static wrinkles
		Platelet-rich plasma	Improves texture, hastens recovery
		Photorejuvenation by energy-based devices	Improves skin laxity, tightens the skin Ablative devices improve texture and fine lines

Table 7.5 Classification of topical sunscreens

Organic (chemical)			Inorganic (physical)
UVA filters	UVB filters	Broad-spectrum filters	
Benzophenones	PABA derivatives—Padimate O	Ecamsule (Mexoryl SX)	Zinc oxide
Avobenzone	Cinnamates	Silatriazole (Mexoryl SL)	Titanium dioxide
Ecamsule	Salicylates	Bemotrizinol (Tinosorb S)	Calamine
Meradimate	Ensulizole	Bisoctrizole (Tinosorb M)	Iron oxide

Abbreviations: PABA, *p*-aminobenzoic acid; UV, ultraviolet.

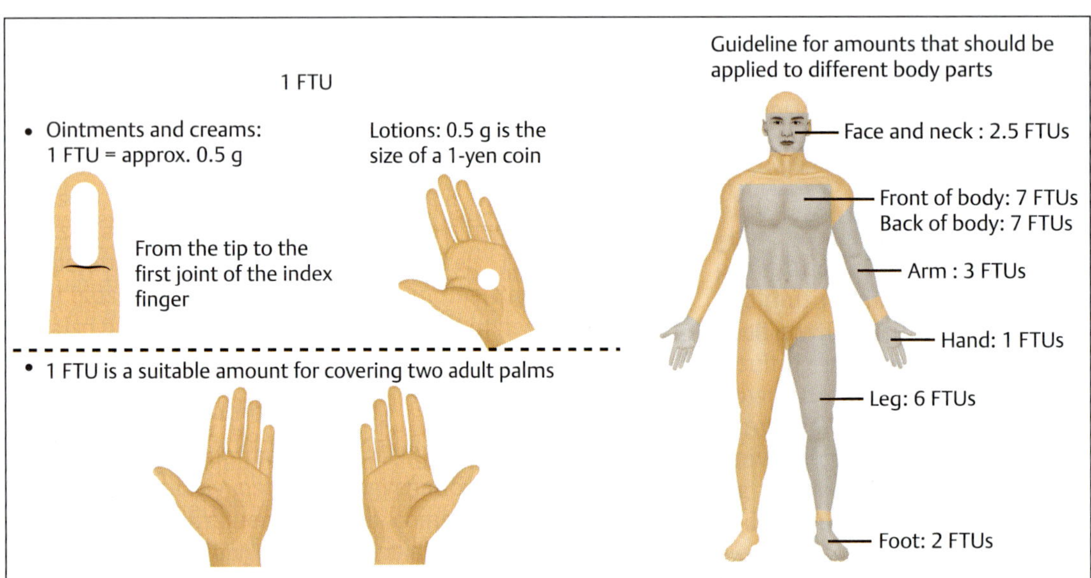

Fig. 7.2 Fingertip unit and amount of sunscreen required.

One FTU is enough to treat an area of skin twice the size of the flat of an adult's hand with the fingers together. Based on the area to be treated, FTUs are as follows: face and neck: 2.5 FTU; a full hand (front and back): 1 FTU; an entire arm and hand: 4 FTU; front of chest and abdomen: 7 FTU.

Schneider[12] suggested the teaspoon rule to ease the calculation of amount. He suggested 3 mL each (slightly more than half a teaspoon) for each arm and for the face and neck, and 6 mL (slightly more than a teaspoon) for each leg, chest, and back. Sometimes sunscreens are associated with adverse effects like stinging, burning sensation, redness, and aggravation of acne. Few ingredients like *p*-aminobenzoic acid (PABA), PABA esters, benzophenones, and avobenzone are known to cause contact allergic dermatitis and photosensitivity. To overcome these either we change the formulation or shift to a purely physical blocker. It must be emphasized that chemical sunscreens which absorb UV light and physical sunscreens which reflect UV light can both prevent photoaging, but cannot reverse changes that have already occurred, unless they contain additional antiaging products.[13]

Moisturizers

Moisturizers prevent water loss from the skin, reduce the dryness which comes with aging, reduce fine wrinkles, and also act as vehicles to transport active ingredients. They are an active part in the antiaging regimen as they decrease transepidermal water loss and some also have wound healing, antipruritic, and anti-inflammatory actions.

Moisturizers are of four main types.[14,15] *Emollients* are mainly lipids and oils such as squalene, cholesterol fatty acids, and hyaluronic acid which help in hydrating and softening the skin. They are useful in sensitive skins and may also act as barrier creams, depending on the oil content. *Humectants* are hygroscopic compounds which attract water from two sources, from the dermis into the epidermis and in humid conditions from the environment. They include glycerin, urea, sorbitol, and alpha-hydroxy acids. Ammonium lactate is a humectant which reduces dryness and scaling of the skin by reducing abnormal thickening of the stratum corneum and increasing cohesion between corneocytes. However high concentrations of humectants can be irritating and should be avoided in sensitive skins. *Occlusives* physically block transepidermal water loss and maintain the water content and include lanolin, petrolatum, mineral oil, and silicones like dimethicone and zinc oxide. *Protein rejuvenators* like collagen, elastin, and keratin help in skin rejuvenation by replenishing essential proteins.[14,15] Petrolatum, dimethicone, and glycerin are common products in moisturizers.

Moisturizers should be noncomedogenic, hydrating, cosmetically elegant, and hypoallergenic. Maximum benefits of moisturizers can be derived by applying at the right time and the right way. They should ideally be lightly applied on moist skin along the direction of the hair follicles. Application can be repeated one to three times daily, depending on the skin. Additives such as sunscreens, antioxidants, vitamins, botanicals, and cosmeceuticals are frequently incorporated to enhance the effects. Irritant reactions, contact dermatitis, and acneiform eruptions are adverse effects that can occur with moisturizers.

Topical Retinoids

Topical retinoids are the major products that have proven antiaging effects. They are effective exfoliators and increase epithelial cell turnover.[16] They increase collagen in the papillary dermis by inhibiting matrix metalloproteinases and collagenases. They also decrease wrinkles by inducing epidermal hyperplasia, glycosaminoglycan deposition, thickening stratum corneum, and also decrease keratinocyte and melanocyte atypia.[16] Topical tretinoin is recommended as the first-line therapy for photoaging, and its benefits usually take at least 4 months. However, patients can develop retinoid dermatitis in the first 2 to 4 weeks of therapy that manifests as skin irritation, redness, stinging, dryness, and peeling. Hence they should be applied for short duration only in the initial phase.

Alpha-Hydroxy Acids and Topical Antioxidants

Alpha-hydroxy acids such as glycolic acid, pyruvic acid, lactic acid also have antiaging properties. Topical antioxidants such as topical vitamin C, vitamin E, and botanical cosmeceuticals such as polyphenols are part of topical rejuvenating creams that play a role in maintenance of skin rejuvenation programs.[17]

Physician-Directed Techniques for Rejuvenation

These are techniques which are performed by trained physicians. The advantage is that since they are minimally invasive they can be performed in an office setting and do not require elaborate operation theatre (OT) setups. They have minimal downtime and less risk of adverse effects. However they may require multiple sessions to be effective. There is a plethora of nonsurgical rejuvenating techniques and devices available today, such as botulinum toxin, fillers, chemical peels, microdermabrasion (MDA), microneedling, and energy-based devices such as lasers, radiofrequency, and high intensity microfocussed ultrasound, and regenerative therapies such as platelet-rich plasma (PRP) **(Table 7.4).** Since they act by different mechanisms and target different depths, an aesthetic surgeon can successfully combine techniques to give optimal results. Botulinum toxin, fillers, and threads have been discussed in Chapters 8 and 9, on "Nonsurgical Rejuvenation of the Face using Botulinum Toxin and Fillers" and "Threads in Aesthetic Surgery" in Volume VI.

Chemical Peels

Despite the advent of many technologies, chemical peels remain a popular method of rejuvenating aging and sun-damaged skin. Chemical peeling is a technique of application of an exfoliating chemical agent or combination of agents that leads to a controlled destruction of the layers of the skin. This is followed by regeneration leading to an improved appearance in texture and tone.[18] Based on the level of exfoliation, chemical peels can be very superficial (up to stratum corneum only), superficial (entire epidermis up to basal layer), medium depth (epidermis and papillary dermis), and deep peels (epidermis and dermis up to midreticular dermis). They may be used singly or in combination, simultaneously or sequentially, with other procedures to enhance results.

Value of Chemical Peels in Aesthetic Practice

There has been a resurgence in the use of chemical peels because they offer many advantages. According to statistics by the American Society of Plastic Surgery, 1.38 million chemical procedures were performed in 2018, up 1% from 2017 and up 20% as compared to 2000.[2] It was the third most common nonsurgical procedure after botulinum toxin injection and soft tissue fillers.

History of Chemical Peels and Resurfacing[19]

Skin resurfacing for beauty has been practiced since prehistoric times, where women would use rocks and shells to abrade the surface of their skin. In Babylonia and India, women used pumice stones to exfoliate the top layers of the skin for beautification. The Egyptians, Greeks, and Romans are also documented to have used acids and balms for chemical peeling. Gypsies were reportedly the first group to use phenol for deep chemical peels, and they passed secret chemical peel recipes between generations. During mid-1800s, Ferdinand Hebra, a Viennese dermatologist, heralded the use of chemical peels, and in 1834, Friedlieb Runge, a chemist, used them as a part of a professional treatment. In 1927, H.P. Bame, an American plastic surgeon, helped push phenol peeling as a part of plastic surgery. In 1946, an American plastic surgeon, Joseph Urkov, reported on the success of chemical peeling, claiming to have treated 2,000 patients for various skin problems with croton oil peeling. These were further made popular by dermatologists like MacKee, who reported on their use in acne scars. The Baker-Gordon formula with croton oil became popular. The alpha-hydroxy acids were studied by Van Scott and Yu. During 1970s, the use of phenol and trichloroacetic acid (TCA) peels became more common among dermatologists and plastic surgeons, and chemical peels evolved into what they are today. Since then various agents have been used for chemical peeling, with newer agents being added day to day.

Mechanism of Action[19]

Chemical peels act by causing wounding of the skin that is followed by remodeling and regeneration. The results depend on the depth of wounding. Very superficial peels exfoliate the stratum corneum only, whereas superficial peels exfoliate the entire epidermis from the stratum corneum down to the papillary dermis at a depth of about 60 micron. They act by causing epidermolysis due to decreased corneocyte adhesion and increased collagen deposition in the dermis. This causes thinning of the stratum corneum, increase in epidermal thickness, and uniform distribution of melanin, which leads to improvement in skin texture and skin tone. Medium-depth peels cause exfoliation of the epidermis and the papillary dermis to reach the upper reticular dermis at a depth of 450 micron. They cause coagulative necrosis of cells by precipitation of proteins followed by regeneration and neocollagenosis. Deep peels reach up to the mid-reticular dermis, leading to extensive cell necrosis up to a depth of about 600 micron (**Fig. 7.3**).

The stages of wound healing after a chemical peel and the time taken to complete repair depend on the depth of skin necrosis. Superficial peels cause coagulation, inflammation, and then re-epithelialization, whereas the medium-depth peel and deep peels, apart from coagulation and inflammation, also cause granulation tissue formation, angiogenesis, and remodeling of collagen and matrix in the dermis. The stages of wound healing are a continuous process.

Coagulation with inflammation is the first stage of wound healing which occurs after chemical peeling.[20] Coagulation and precipitation of proteins lead to necrosis and degeneration of stratum corneum and keratinocytes. Neutrophils act as scavengers and decontaminate the wound. Platelets release platelet-derived growth factor (PDGF), epidermal growth factor (EGF), fibronectin, fibrinogen, and histamine. The macrophages also secrete collagenase which debride the wound, cytokines, interleukins, and tumor necrosis factors which stimulate fibroblast to promote collagen and promote angiogenesis. They also secrete transforming growth factor (TGF) which stimulates keratinocytes.

The phase of coagulation and inflammation is followed by tissue proliferation. In superficial peels where the basement membrane is intact, epithelial cells migrate from basement membrane and the normal epidermis is restored in 2 to 3 days. In deep peels keratinocytes start to migrate from appendages and surrounding normal skin. Superficial peels which cause epidermal injury primarily cause epidermal regeneration. The interfollicular epithelial stem cells in the skin fuel re-epithelialization process by stimulating the proliferation of the basal cells. The appendages, particularly the stem cells in the bulge area of the pilosebaceous follicles, contribute to the regeneration; hence, re-epithelialization of the facial skin is faster as compared to nonfacial skin, because of a greater number of pilosebaceous follicles on the face. The basal cells proliferate, differentiate, and move upwards, restoring cell-to-cell adhesion and construction of a smooth semipermeable horny layer with intact barrier function.

During medium depth and deep peels, the mechanisms of dermal wound healing are stimulated. The erythema that develops following a chemical peel is due to new capillary formation in that area caused by angiogenesis that begins with endothelial cell migration. Granulation tissue formation

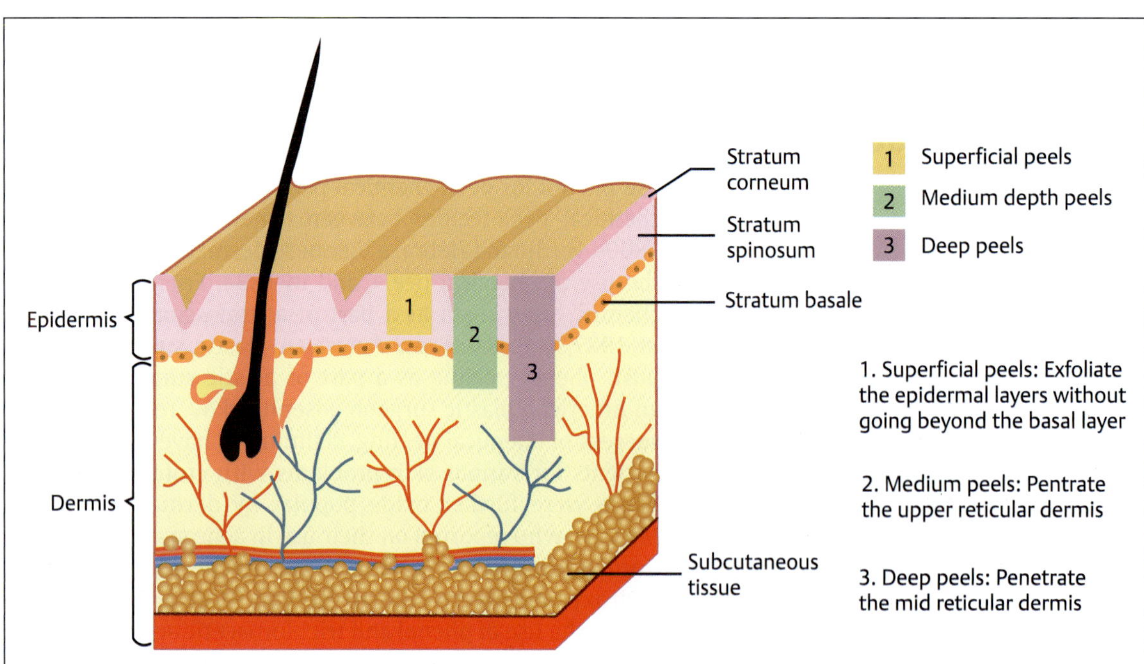

Fig. 7.3 Depth of chemical peels.

begins on the second day of chemical peel. Fibroblasts differentiate to produce collagen and other ground substance. Growth factors, fibronectin, and glycosaminoglycans are also involved.

The phase of tissue remodeling involves reorientation of collagen in a parallel fashion. It plateaus after 21 days. Collagen remodeling is the reason for rejuvenation and reduction in wrinkles that takes place after deep peels. Re-epithelialization in deep peels begins on day 3 and continues until day 10 to 14. Occlusive ointments prevent dehydration and promote faster re-epithelialization, with less tendency for delayed healing, which may occur with dry crusting.

The final stage of wound healing, fibroplasia, continues well beyond the initial closure of the peeled wound and continues with neoangiogenesis and new collagen formation for 3 or 4 months. Prolonged erythema lasting 2 to 4 months can occur in unusual cases of sensitive skin or in those with contact dermatitis. New collagen formation can continue to improve texture and rhytides for a period of up to 4 to 6 months.

Indications

Chemical peels are cutaneous resurfacing procedures used for a wide variety of cosmetic conditions such as pigmentation, photodamage, acne, mild facial scarring, dilated pores, and skin rejuvenation. The common pigmentary disorders for which peels are used include melasma, freckles, and lentigenes, and PIH. Patient alignment is very important before starting peels for any pigmentary disorder as the response may not be complete and recurrences may occur. The choice of peeling agent depends on the desired depth of the peel, which is dependent on the depth of the treating pathology, indication, and the patient's skin type **(Table 7.6)**. Using the correct depth of the peel is critical for a successful outcome.[21]

Superficial Peels

These are indicated for the treatment of pigmentation such as melasma, PIH, mild photoaging, Glogau scale I, skin rejuvenation, improvement of skin texture, and even skin tone **(Fig. 7.4)**. The common peeling agents used include glycolic acid 20, 35, 70%, salicylic acid 20, 30%, TCA 15, 25%, retinol 5, 10%, tretinoin 1%, and combination peels containing mandelic, pyruvic, kojic, citric, or lactic acid. They are safe in all skin types.

Medium-Depth Peels

They are indicated for deeper pathologies such as fine wrinkles, Glogau photoaging scale type II, superficial scars, deeper pigmentary abnormalities like lentigines, actinic and seborrheic keratosis, and textural changes (**Fig. 7.5**). The common medium-depth peeling agents include glycolic acid 70%,

Table 7.6 Classification of chemical peels and their indications

Depth of peel	Histological level	Peeling agents	Indications	Expected outcomes
Very superficial	Exfoliation of the stratum corneum, without any epidermal necrosis	SA 20% GA 30–50% (1–5mins) TCA 15% Retinoic acid 3–5% Jessners peels 1–3 coats MA 30%	Skin glow, comedonal acne	Good
Superficial	Destruction of the full epidermis, up to the basal layer	GA 50–70%, till erythema TCA 25–35% Jessners peel >4 coats Pyruvic 40–50% SA 30% +TCA 20% Jessners + TCA 20%	Dyschromia Melasma PIH Dilated pores Fine wrinkles Photoageing I	Good Recurrence can occur in melasma
Medium depth	Destruction of the epidermis, papillary dermis up to the upper one third of the reticular dermis	GA 70% + TCA 35% Jessners + TCA 35% Solid CO2 + TCA 35% Rarely used TCA 50% Phenol 88% Pyruvic >60%	Fine wrinkles Photoageing II	Fair to good
Deep peel	Necrosis of the entire epidermis and papillary dermis, with inflammation extending to the mid-reticular dermis	Baker-Gordon 2.1% croton oil in 50%phenol Hetter –0.4–1.6% croton oil in 35% phenol	Deep wrinkles Skin laxity	Fair to good Increased risk of complications

Abbreviation: GA, glycolic acid; MA, mandelic acid; SA, salicylic acid; TCA, trichloroacetic acid.

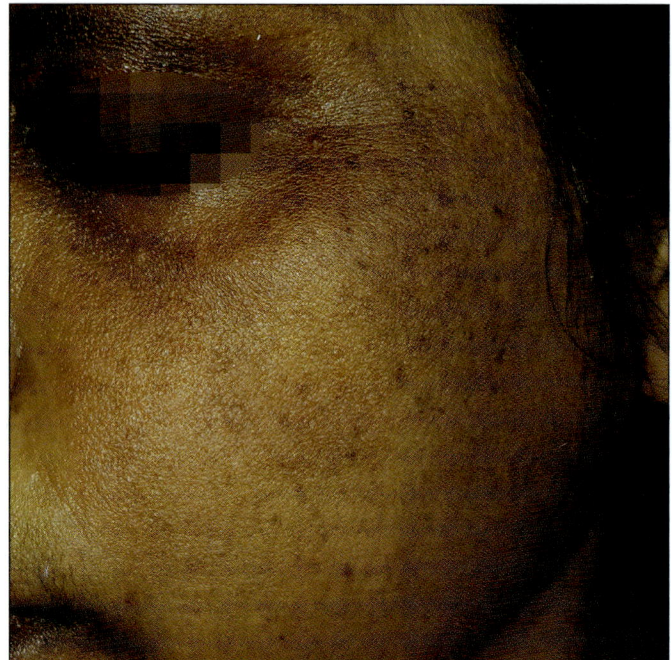

Fig. 7.4 Photoaging Glogau Type II in a 38-year-old female showing patchy irregular pigmentation and brown spots—indication for superficial chemical peels.

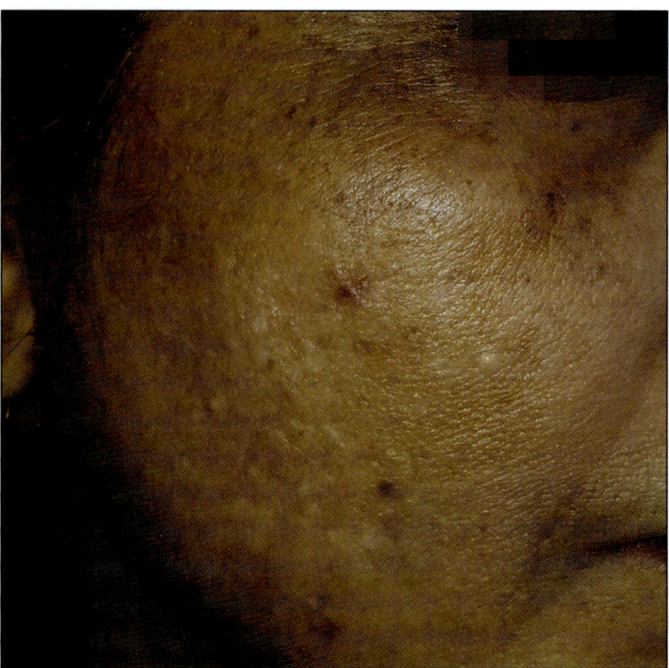

Fig. 7.5 Photoaging Glogau Type III showing senile lentigines, melasma, dermatosis papulosa nigra, and superficial wrinkles—indication for medium-depth chemical peels.

TCA 35 to 50% and combination peels, Jessner peel with 35% TCA (Monheit), 70% glycolic acid with 35% TCA (Coleman).[22] Pyruvic acid 50% is also useful as a medium-depth peel for photoaging.[23] However, medium-depth peels should be used with great caution in dark skin patients, Fitzpatrick skin type 4 and 5, due to the risk of PIH and scarring.

Deep peels were used for severe photoaging, Glogau type III and IV, and deep wrinkles and acne scars. Phenol in the Baker-Gordon formula (88% phenol, croton oil 8 drops, septisol) was the most popular. The advantage was that they were one-time procedures, leading to dramatic results. But there are many disadvantages as they require an OT setup, cardiac and renal monitoring, and have a prolonged downtime and a high risk of pigmentary changes and scarring. They have now largely been replaced by lasers.

Contraindications

Chemical peels are contraindicated in the presence of open wounds and active infections such as folliculitis, warts, herpes simplex, etc. These should first be treated before beginning chemical peels. Prophylactic acyclovir should be given to patients with a history of herpes simplex. They should be done cautiously in patients with history of photosensitivity and patients with unrealistic expectations. Deep peels are relatively contraindicated in dark skins as they can cause permanent depigmentation and scarring.

Peeling Agents

A wide variety of peeling agents are available and the choice and strength of the agent depends on the depth required and the condition to be treated. The current trend is to use combination peels, which have a wide safety margin (**Table 7.7**).

Peels for Pigmentation

In pigmentary disorders, peels should not be used as the first line of treatment. These are used as adjunct to medical therapy. Superficial peels like glycolic acid (<35%), salicylic acid (20–30%), lactic acid, phytic acid, and ferulic acid done at 2- to 4-week intervals are preferred (**Fig. 7.6**). Addition of topical vitamin C and pigmentation booster (citric acid, kojic acid, arbutin) can improve the results without making the skin sensitive. Combination peels like glycolic/salicylic peels followed by yellow peel (retinoic acid, kojic acid, azelaic) have also been found to be useful. Spot peels have been found to be useful in cases of localized pigmentation.

Medium-depth peels have been found to be useful in conditions like macular amyloidosis and lichen planus pigmentosus (**Fig. 7.7**). In cases of melasma, peels should be used as adjunct to topical treatment.[24] Both superficial and medium-depth peels have been found to be useful (**Fig. 7.8**). Enough gap should be given between two sessions of peels for the skin to recover completely from the inflammatory effect of previous session. For freckles and lentigenes, TCA peel 25% spot applications have been found to be useful. Post acne pigmentation responds well to monthly sessions of combination superficial peels containing salicylic (20%) and mandelic acid (10%).[25]

Overzealous use of peels can lead to increased sensitivity of skin and worsening of pigmentation in some cases. Also in acne-prone skin medium-depth peels can lead to flare-up of

Table 7.7 Peeling agents and complications

Depth of peel and indications	Superficial peels for mild photoaging type 1	Medium-depth peels for moderate photoaging type 2	Deep peels for severe photoaging types 3 and 4	Peels for pigmentation	Peels for skin glow
Peeling agents	Glycolic acid 35–50% for 1–2 minutes Lactic acid Salicylic acid 30% TCA 10–25% Jessner peel 1–3 coats Pyruvic acid Retinoic acid Ferulic acid Mandelic acid Phytic peel Combination peels	Glycolic acid 50–70% TCA 25–35% Pyruvic 40–70% Jessner peel + 35% TCA	Phenol peels—Baker-Gordon formula	Salicylic acid 20% Mandelic acid 30–40% Kojic acid Lactic acid Citric acid Hydroquinone Ferulic acid Azelaic acid Retinol peel—yellow peel Combination peels	Glycolic acid 20% Lactic acid Ferulic acid Mandelic acid Combination peels
Safety	Safe for all skin types	Cautious use in darker skins	Avoid in darker skins	Safe for all skin types	Safe for all skin types
Frequency	Every 2 wk	Once in 6 mo	One-time procedure	Every 2–4 wk	Every 2 wk
Complications	Erythema, burning, irritation, pruritis, infection, pigmentation	Prolonged erythema, edema, burning, irritation, pruritis, infection, pigmentation, scarring	Delayed healing, depigmentation, scarring, systemic cardiotoxicity	Erythema, burning, irritation, pruritis, infection, pigmentation	Dryness, irritation

Abbreviation: TCA, trichloroacetic acid.

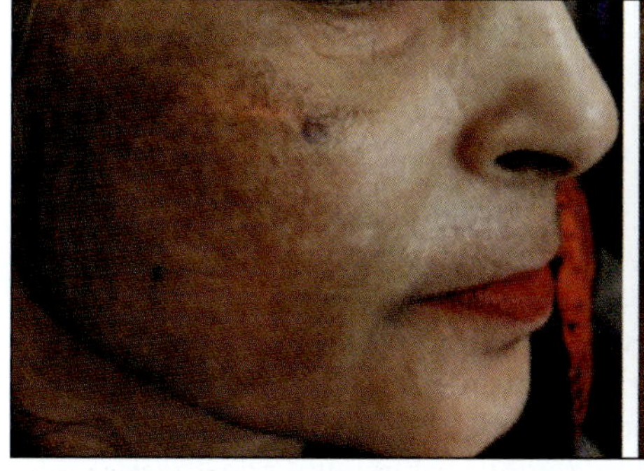
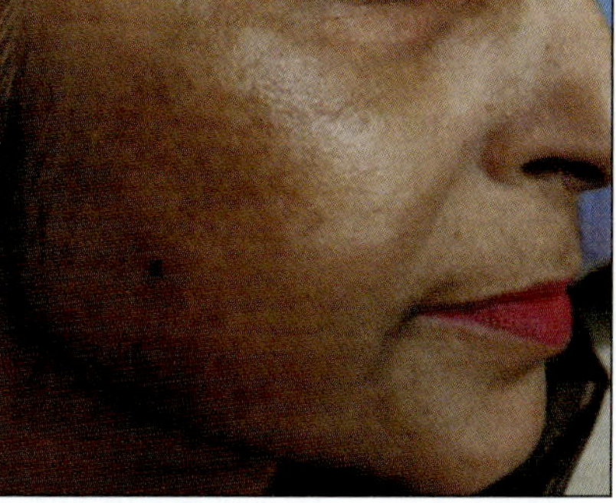

Fig. 7.6 Improvement of hyperpigmentation and skin texture following topical sunscreens, skin lightening agents, and sequential chemical peels with salicylic acid 20% and 15% Trichloroacetic acid at 2 weekly intervals for four peels.

acne. Hence judicious use of appropriate peels is advocated in pigmentary conditions after proper priming of the skin.

Peels for Skin Rejuvenation

Peels done for skin rejuvenation, also referred to as "glow peels" or "party peels" are peels done for instant glow with zero downtime. A party peel may contain a single peeling agent or a combination of peeling agents with skin-brightening substances. The commonly used peeling agents like glycolic acid, salicylic acid, kojic acid, mandelic acid, and lactic acid are used in very low concentration (**Fig. 7.9**). Lipohydroxy acid 5 or 10%, a newer lipophilic derivative of salicylic acid, is a useful peel for acne and skin rejuvenation.[22] Azelaic acid and mandelic acid superficial peels are also useful in aging.[26] Also a variety of skin-brightening agents like pentapeptide-13, oligopeptide-34, arbutin, 3-O-ethyl ascorbic acid, and licorice are used. Some of the preparations also contain fruits (protease), polypeptides, and hyaluronic acid.

Glow peels are usually gel-based peels which are rubbed into the skin, kept for a longer time and followed by a mask/serum application. These peels usually do not have any do's and don'ts unlike the conventional peels. Also these can be performed by a trained practitioner. These peels are safe for

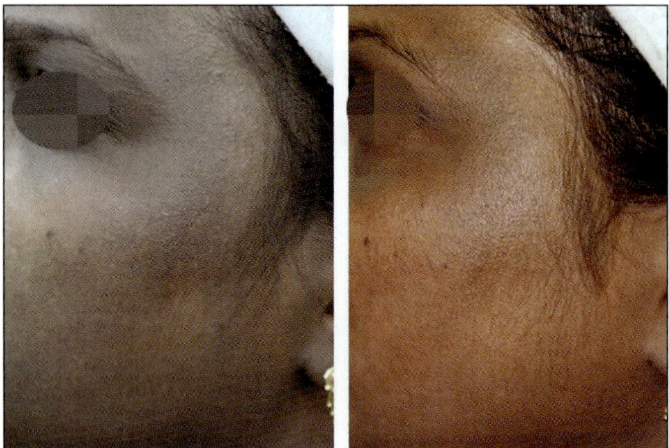

Fig. 7.7 A case of lichen planus pigmentosus. Result after four sessions of medium-depth peels 25% trichloroacetic acid (TCA) at 6 weekly intervals.

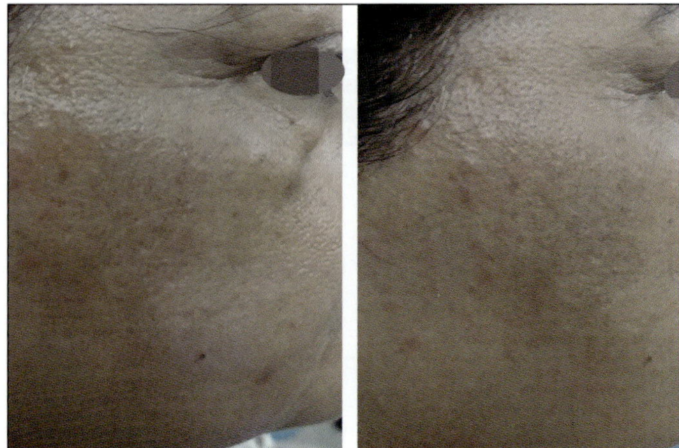

Fig. 7.8 Mixed melasma. Results after six sessions of superficial peels with a combination peel containing salicylic acid 20% and mandelic acid 10% at 4 weekly intervals.

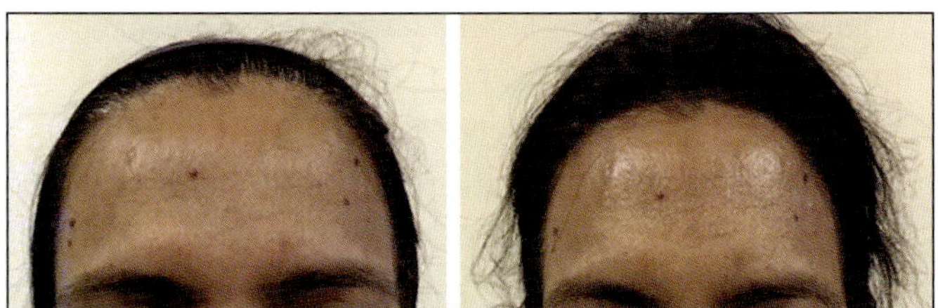

Fig. 7.9 Glow peel with 90% lactic acid after a single session. (The images are provided courtesy of Dr Atula Gupta, Gurgaon, Haryana, India.)

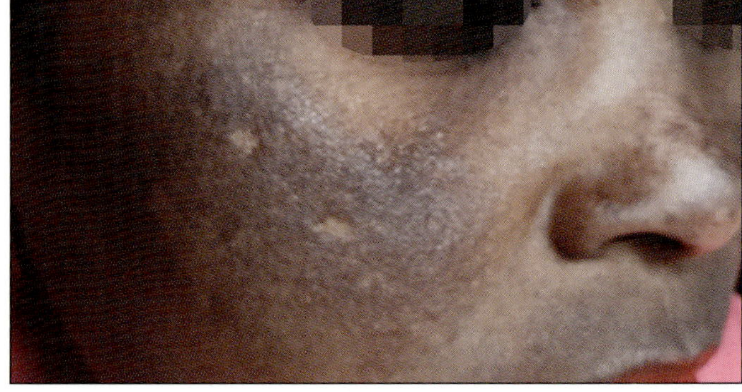

Fig. 7.10 Exogenous ochronosis due to prolonged use of hydroquinone.

all skin types and can be repeated frequently. These peels improve the skin texture if done at monthly intervals of 6 to 8 months. These are also useful for decreasing post-peel inflammation caused by clinical strength peels. However, the results are temporary and do not last for a long time.

Procedure

The procedures for chemical peels include pre-peel priming, peel application, and post-peel care.[27,28] Priming before a peel is essential to ensure a uniform peel, reduce the risk of complications, detect intolerance to agents, and ensure compliance of the patient. Priming should begin at least 2 to 4 weeks before a peel. Sunscreens, skin-lightening agents like hydroquinone, and topical retinoids like tretinoin or adapalene are the chief topical products for priming the skin before a peel. Hydroquinone (2–5%) is a phenolic compound that reduces risk of PIH. Prolonged use can lead to exogenous ochronosis which appears as a bluish gray pigmentation, with change in texture of the skin and is very resistant to treatment **(Fig. 7.10)**.[29] It should be suspected in all patients complaining of worsening of pigmentation following application of hydroquinone and other phenolic compounds. In cases of intolerance, alternative skin-lightening agents such as kojic acid (2–5%), salicylic acid (5–10%), azelaic acid (10–20%), citric acid, arbutin, glycolic acid (6–12%), or topical corticosteroids can be used. Topical corticosteroids should be applied for short duration; not exceeding 6 to 8 weeks as it can lead to complications such as skin atrophy, telangiectasia, acne, and hypertrichosis (**Fig. 7.11**).[30]

Superficial peels do not require anesthesia, but medium-depth peels may require pain control in anxious patients with a cooling fan or ice pack. Deep phenol peels require an OT setup and sedation, regional or general anesthesia.

Prior to peeling, the patient washes the face and removes all makeup. The skin is cleaned with alcohol or pre-peel cleanser and oily skin is degreased with acetone. The hair is pulled back with a band or cap, and the head should be up at least 45 degrees. All practices of infection control must be followed. The neutralizing agent must be kept ready. The sensitive areas such as medial and inner canthi, and nasal and oral commissures, may be protected with petrolatum. The peeling agent is poured in a small glass cup and applied with firm even strokes using a brush or cotton bud. Application is along cosmetic units of the face, beginning with the forehead, followed by cheeks, nose, chin, and lastly perioral and periocular areas (**Fig. 7.12**). A feathering technique should

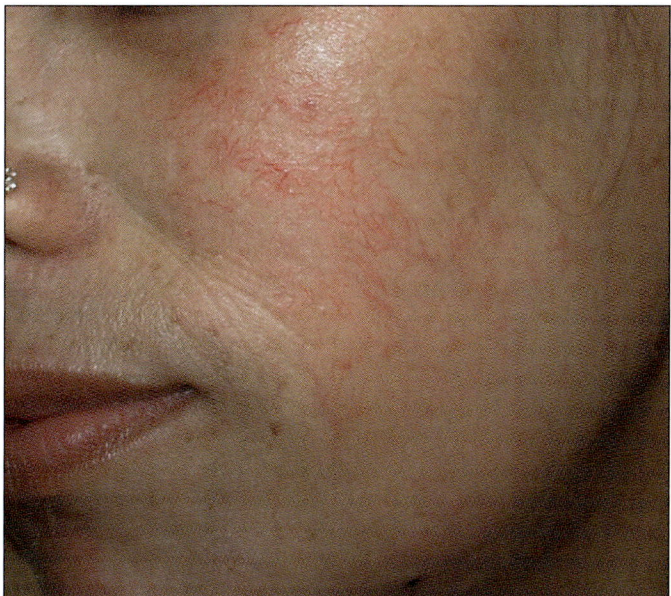

Fig. 7.11 Persistent telangiectasia due to steroid misuse.

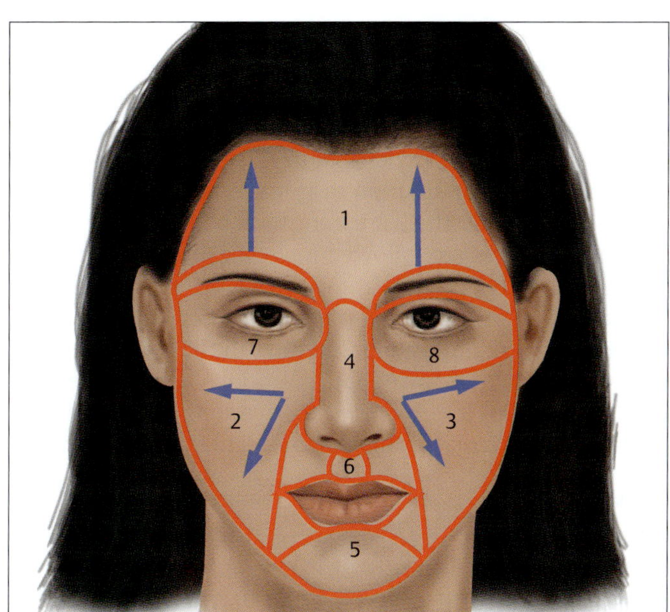

Fig. 7.12 Cosmetic units of the face and direction of strokes of application of the chemical peel.

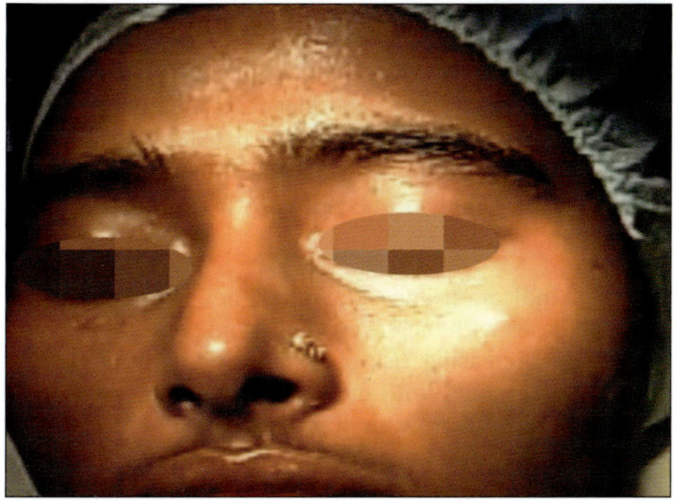

Fig. 7.13 End point of chemical peel—erythema following application of 70% glycolic acid.

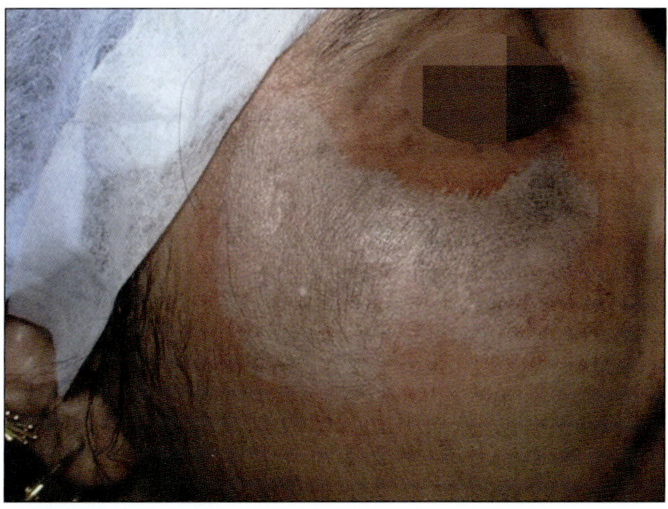

Fig. 7.14 End point of medium depth chemical peel—frosting following application of 25% trichloroacetic acid (TCA).

be applied at the edges. In areas of wrinkling and the periocular areas, the skin should be stretched before applying the peel to prevent pooling of the peeling agent. The peel should be neutralized with cold saline or neutralizing agent, once the end point is reached.[27] The end point of glycolic acid peel is erythema (**Fig. 7.13**), whereas the end point of TCA peel is frosting (**Fig. 7.14**). Frosting occurs due to coagulation of proteins. The degree of frosting depends on the concentration of TCA. A sunscreen should be applied before patient leaves the clinic.

Good postprocedure care enhances outcomes and reduces complications. The patient must be given written instructions regarding sun protection and topical applications. Mild peeling or flaking of the skin can occur and patients should be instructed not to forcibly peel off the skin and should apply a noncomedogenic moisturizer. In a superficial peel, the skin returns to normal in 3 to 5 days, whereas re-epithelialization may take 5 to 7 days in a medium-depth peel.

Deep Phenol Peels[5,28]

The deep Baker-Gordon peel requires a surgical setting, IV sedation, IV hydration with cardiac and renal monitoring, due to the risk of arrhythmia. It can be applied with or without occlusion. Occlusion is accomplished using a petrolatum dressing or tape. Following the application of the peel, skin necrosis occurs with exudation, inflammation, and facial edema. Pain management and nonsteroidal anti-inflammatory agents are crucial in this phase. Gentle soaks with dilute vinegar solution to remove necrotic epidermal debris and prevent thick crust formation from the serosanguinous exudates are followed in the healing phase, which takes about 2 to 3 weeks. Croton oil peeling with lower concentrations of phenol is reported to be safer by varying the concentration of croton oil according to the cosmetic units of the face, such as lower concentrations around the eyes than the cheeks. It is reported to give long-lasting results, but still carries a risk for hypopigmentation and scarring.

Results

Kubiak et al[31] compared a sequential peel of 70% glycolic acid with 15% TCA versus 35% TCA alone in 40 patients with photoaging, Glogau type II and III. They found significant improvement in all skin parameters such as elasticity, hydration, melanin index, and erythema index in both groups. The sequential GA/TCA group fared better in hydration and melanin index, while the 35% TCA peel was more effective in reducing wrinkles, but with lower tolerability. In another split face study in 50 patients, lipohydroxy acid 5 to 10%, a derivative of salicylic acid, was as effective as glycolic acid 20 to 50% in reducing facial hyperpigmentation and fine lines/wrinkles.[32] Prestes et al compared 85% lactic acid versus 70% glycolic acid versus sunscreen alone and reported that both peels were effective in reducing wrinkles around the eyes as compared to no effect with sunscreen alone.[33] Superficial peels have shown efficacy in periorbital rejuvenation and pigmentation.[34,35] Tretinoin peels 1% and retinol peels are useful peeling agents for melasma, PIH, and improvement of photoaging.[36–38] Medium-depth and deep peels are effective for wrinkles and aging skin, but have a low margin of safety.[5]

Combination Techniques

Chemical peels are often combined with other rejuvenation techniques such as botulinum toxin and fillers as they fill the gap to provide improved surface texture, and with microdermabrasion (MDA) and microneedling to enhance results. Superficial peels can be combined at the same time, but medium-depth and deep peels should precede the injectables at least 2 weeks before.[21] Temporary fillers like hyaluronic acid may be safely combined, but semipermanent fillers should be avoided as there is a theoretical risk of biofilm formation.[21] They can also be cautiously combined with resurfacing lasers and microneedling radiofrequency to enhance effects (**Figs. 7.15 and 7.16**).

Complications[21,39,40]

Chemical peels are relatively safe procedures if they are performed under supervision, choosing the right peel for

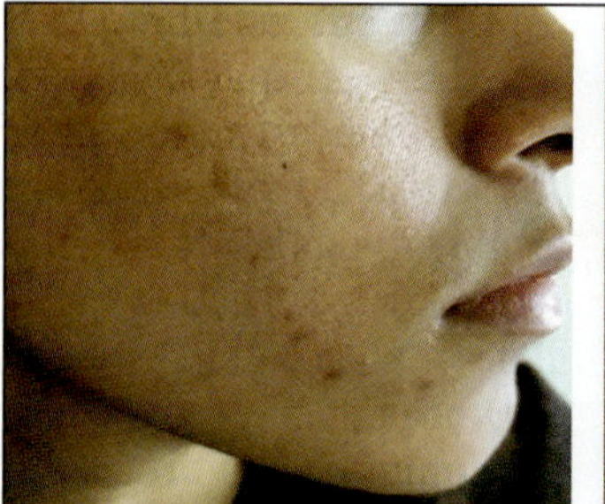
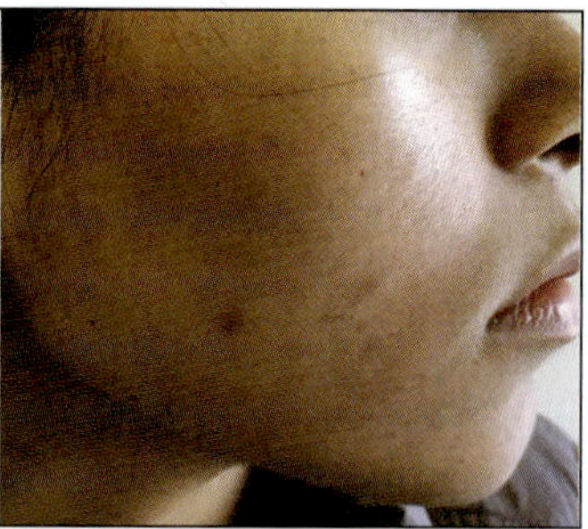

Fig. 7.15 Open pores in a young female: Chemical peels with salicylic acid 30%, two sessions and microneedling radiofrequency (MNRF) two sessions. (The images are provided courtesy of Dr Atula Gupta, Gurgaon, Haryana, India.)

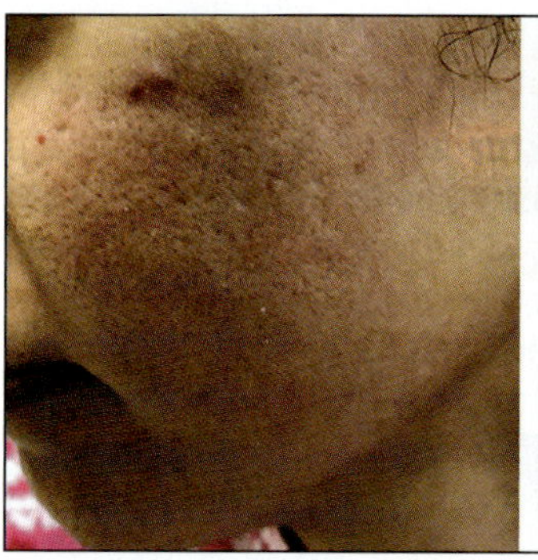
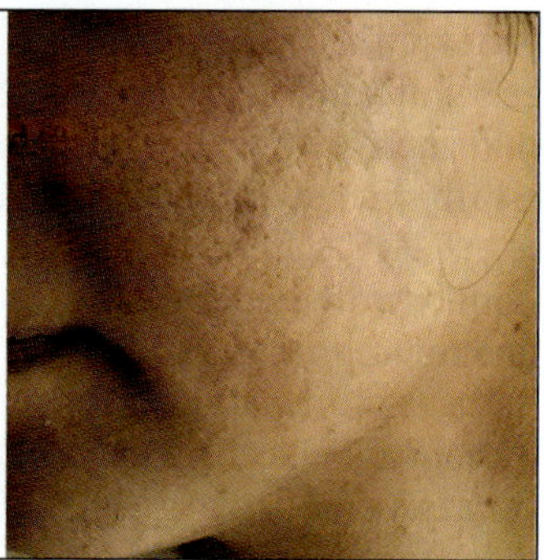

Fig. 7.16 Open pores in an older female with skin laxity. Chemical peels with modified Jessner peel four sessions and microneedling radiofrequency (MNRF) four sessions. (The images are provided courtesy of Dr Atula Gupta, Gurgaon, Haryana, India.)

the right indication and skin type. The risk of complications increases with increasing depth and darker skin types. Patients at increasing risk of complications include those with sensitive skins, with outdoor occupations, and poorly compliant patients.[40] Complications with superficial peels are rare and unmet expectations is the commonest complication.[39] Prolonged erythema, sensitive skin, and PIH are common complications that can occur with overzealous peeling (**Fig. 7.17**).

Conclusion

Chemical peels are effective techniques for skin rejuvenation and play a major role in improvement of skin texture, skin tone, and other signs of photoaging. Alpha-hydroxy acids including glycolic acid, mandelic acid and lactic acid, pyruvic acid (alpha ketoacid), salicylic acid and its derivatives (betahydroxy acid), trichloroacetic acid, and the retinoids, tretinoin and retinol, are safe and effective superficial peels for skin rejuvenation in all skin types, with proper precautions. Medium-depth peels using higher strength of TCA alone or in combination with high-strength glycolic acid are to be used judiciously in darker skin types. Deep peels with phenol and croton oil are risky in darker skins.

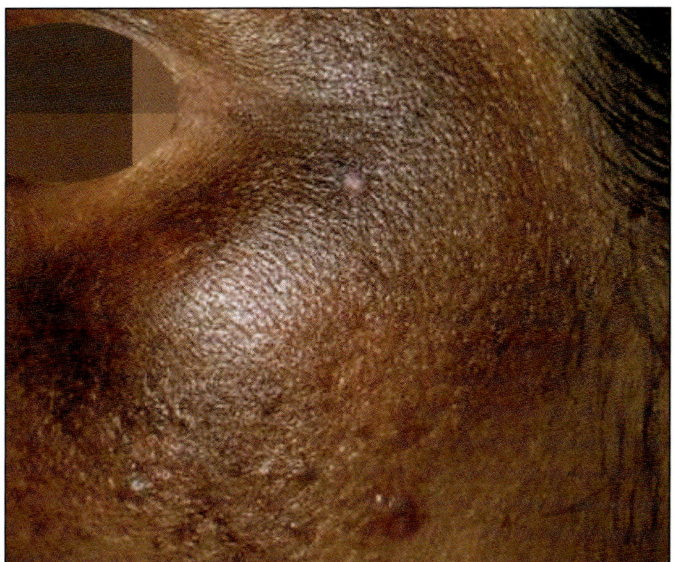

Fig. 7.17 Postinflammatory hyperpigmentation occurring as a complication of chemical peel.

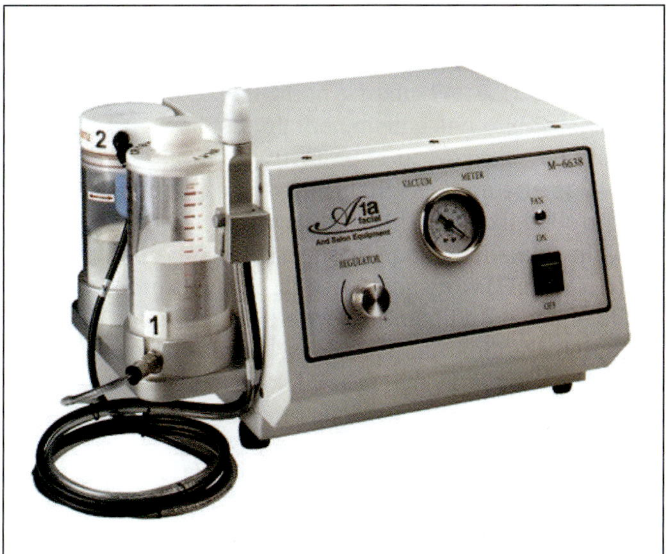

Fig. 7.18 Equipment for microdermabrasion using crystals.

Microdermabrasion

Microdermabrasion (MDA) is a commonly performed office-based procedure, being done since 1985. It can be done by a trained clinician, aesthetician, medical assistant, or nurse without the use of anesthesia. It was introduced by Marini and Lo Brutto as a milder treatment modality than the routinely performed chemical peels and dermabrasion procedures and reported to be clinically effective by Monteleone in 1988.[41] Over the past few decades, it has become one of the most commonly done noninvasive cosmetic procedure.

Devices

There are two types of MDA equipment: crystal MDA and diamond MDA. In crystal MDA, mildly abrasive crystals are propelled against the skin at a predetermined flow rate, under the control of a handheld vacuum system. The most common crystal used is aluminum oxide. Sodium chloride, magnesium oxide, and sodium bicarbonate crystals are less commonly employed (**Fig. 7.18**). Diamond MDA is a crystal-free system, in which diamonds embedded in the handpiece provide the abrasive stimulus (**Fig. 7.19**). While crystal MDA leads to superficial exfoliation, diamond MDA can be useful for deeper scars. Also, diamond MDA can be used in patients having allergy to crystal and is not associated with any possible ocular side effects.

Mechanism of Action

The crystals cause gentle mechanical abrasion of the skin which leads to the removal of the stratum corneum or dead cell layer. MDA has also been shown to affect deeper layers of the epidermis and dermis. It causes a rearrangement of melanosomes in the basal layer of the epidermis, flattening of rete ridges at the dermal-epidermal junction, increased collagen fiber density at the dermal-epidermal junction, and vascular ectasia in the reticular dermis.[42] MDA also causes an upregulation of wound-healing transcription factors and matrix metalloproteinases in the dermis.[43] In addition to the cosmetic benefits of MDA, studies have shown improved skin permeability and enhanced delivery of transdermal medications dosed on an area of the skin treated with MDA. Hence, crystal MDA is combined with superficial peels to enhance the penetration without increasing the side effects. Diamond MDA acts as a similar abrasive modality and the penetration can be increased by increasing the number of passes.

Indications

It is used mainly to improve uneven skin tone and texture, photoaging, enlarged pores, fine wrinkles, and scars, including acne scars.[42,44] Tan et al[42] conducted a study on 10 patients with skin type 1 to 3 and found that there was an immediate increase in the roughness of skin, skin temperature, and a decrease in the sebum content which was not maintained in between the sessions. They reported a good improvement in seven patients with respect to photoaging and skin elasticity and flattening of wrinkles after five to six treatments at weekly interval.[42] Shim et al also reported significant improvement in skin roughness/textural irregularities, mottled pigmentation, and overall skin complexion in photodamaged skin.[44] It may also be used for striae and melasma. Diamond MDA is useful for acne scars.

Contraindication

MDA is contraindicated in the presence of any viral or bacterial infection.[45] In individuals with contact allergies to

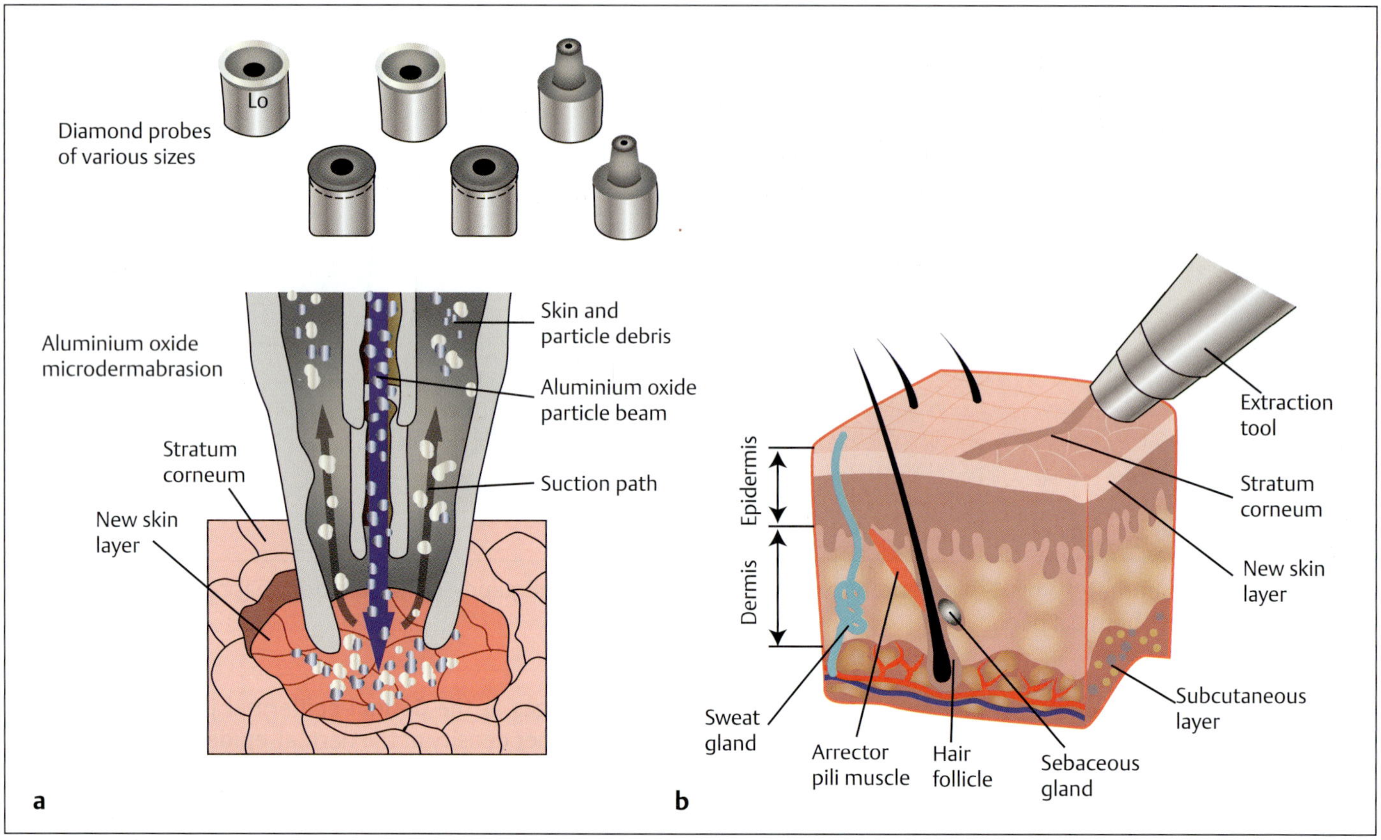

Fig. 7.19 (a) Crystal microdermabrasion. **(b)** Diamond microdermabrasion.

the aluminum crystals, a different crystal or a crystal-free system should be used.[46] Hypertrophic scarring, keloidal tendency, rosacea, and telangiectasias are considered relative contraindications.

Procedure

After cleaning the area to be treated with a mild cleanser, adequate eye protection is ensured for both the patient and the operator. The skin is stretched with the nondominant hand. The device tip is put over stretched skin at an angle of around 45 degrees such that microcrystals strike the skin surface at an angle and produce microtrauma to the skin. The device tip usually has a 4- to 6-mm opening. The used crystals and the dead skin are simultaneously aspirated by negative pressure into a container which is thus discarded. The entire area is covered with small passes, maintaining a gentle pressure throughout the treatment (**Fig. 7.20**). The second pass is perpendicular to the first pass to avoid streaks in the skin.In between two passes the crystal on the skin is cleaned with a soft brush. Number of passes to be given need to be individualized depending on the skin type and the condition to be treated. Patients often require four to six treatments at 1 to 4 weeks interval to achieve the desired results. Patients are advised proper skin care routine, cleansing the skin with a mild cleanser and to avoid other parlor services during the period of MDA treatment.

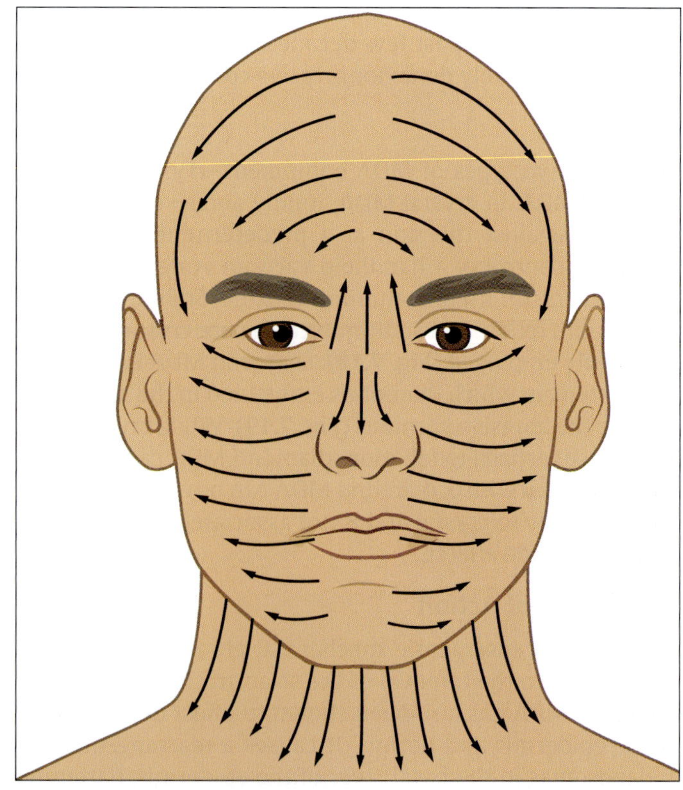

Fig. 7.20 Direction of strokes in microdermabrasion.

Limitations

MDA has not been found to be useful for deep wrinkles, scars, ice-pick acne scars, and PIH.[44] Efficacy of MDA in melasma is controversial. A combination of MDA with peels might be useful in some cases.[47] Extreme caution should be exercised while combining these modalities in darker skin types due to the risk of PIH.

Complications

The technique is considered safe for all Fitzpatrick skin types and complications are minimal. Vigorous MDA may cause tenderness, swelling, redness, petechiae, and bruising specially on sensitive skin. Eye irritation can occur if the crystals come in contact with the conjunctiva.[42] The eyes should be protected during the procedure by placing a moist gauze over the eyes of the patient. The operator should wear protective goggles and mask. There is an increased risk of autoinoculation of viral cutaneous lesions (e.g., molluscum contagiosum) and reactivation of latent herpes simplex virus in an affected dermatome.[48] In few cases skin may become more sensitive to photodamage for a few days after the procedure. In case of any complication, appropriate medical treatment and hand holding of the patient needs to be done.

Conclusion

MDA is a simple, safe, and easy to perform superficial skin resurfacing procedure done by both doctors and aestheticians. This procedure is considered safe for all skin types and ages and is used to improve a variety of cosmetic skin conditions.

Microneedling

Microneedling, also called as percutaneous collagen induction (PCI), is a simple, safe, effective, and minimally invasive office-based procedure which requires minimal training. As a principle it was introduced by Orentreich and Orentreich in 1995.[49] They demonstrated that introducing a needle beneath retracted scars and wrinkles stimulates collagen. Fernandes used a similar technique and followed it by the development of the dermal roller.[50] Microneedling is a procedure involving superficial and controlled puncturing of the skin by rolling with miniature fine needles, which is done using either a dermaroller, a dermapen, or a dermastamp. Microneedling helps in collagen induction and dermal remodeling without causing any damage to the epidermis. Its role as a transdermal delivery system for therapeutic drugs and vaccines is being extensively evaluated; the detail is given in the later part of the chapter.

Mechanism of Action

Microneedling leads to multiple microscopic wounds with minimal superficial bleeding in the dermis and sets up a wound-healing cascade with release of various growth factors.[51] Neovascularization or neocollagenesis is initiated by migration and proliferation of fibroblasts and laying down of intercellular matrix.[52] Liebl et al[53] have proposed another hypothesis to explain how microneedling works. According to them a rapid change in the inner electrical potential triggers increased cell activity and the release of various proteins, potassium, and growth factors from the cells into the exterior, leading to the migration of fibroblasts to the site of injury, and hence, collagen induction (**Fig. 7.21**). PCI treatment preserves the epidermis while stimulating collagen deposition, thereby reducing the risk of post-treatment complications and patient downtime.

Indications

It is being used for a wide variety of aesthetic conditions like skin rejuvenation, acne scars, posttraumatic and burn scars, alopecia, hyperhidrosis, and stretch marks (**Fig. 7.22**). Moreover, new indications are being added and the instrument used is being improved on a regular basis.[54] The use of microneedling as a technique for transdermal drug delivery is also being extensively explored.[55]

Contraindications

Contraindications include active acne, any local viral/bacterial infection like warts or herpes labialis, and presence of eczema or psoriasis lesions. Keloidal tendency, blood dyscrasias, and patients on chemotherapy/radiotherapy are relative contraindications.

Devices

The standard medical dermaroller has a 12-cm long handle with a 2 × 2 cm wide drum-shaped cylinder at one end studded with 8 rows and 24 circular arrays of 192 fine microneedles, usually 0.5 to 3 mm in length and 0.1 to 0.25 mm in diameter (**Fig. 7.23**).[56] The instrument is presterilized by gamma irradiation. Dermarollers with narrow width of drum are useful for smaller area like nose, eyes, and scalp treatments. Home dermarollers usually have a 0.5-mm needle depth. These are useful for skin rejuvenation and do not cause any pain or side effects. Clinically 0.5- to 1-mm dermarollers are used for fine wrinkles and skin rejuvenation and 1.5- and 2-mm-sized needles are commonly used for scars.

Modern automated microneedling devices have increasingly replaced the manual dermaroller. A single-use, sterile needle cartridge with a range of needle configurations is fitted on the device. The depth can be adjusted according to the site and the needles move back-and-forth rapidly penetrating the skin.

Procedure

The patient should be explained about the procedure in detail and aligned regarding the results, downtime, and the need for multiple sessions. The skin should be primed for at least 2 weeks with regular use of sunscreen and mild retinoid preparations at night. The procedure is done under local anesthetic. The skin should be cleaned with spirit, and

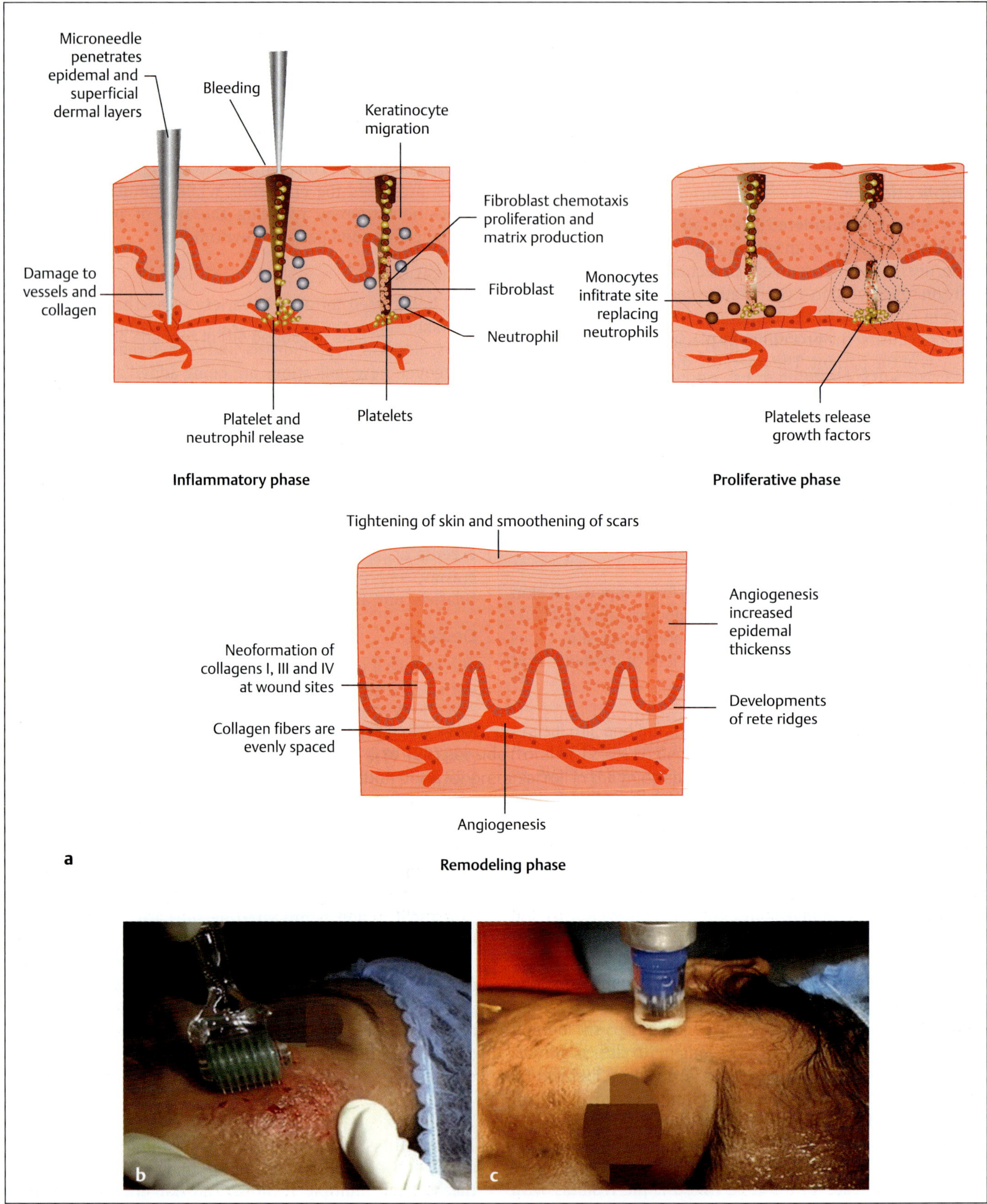

Fig. 7.21 **(a)** Mechanism of action of microneedling. **(b)** Microneedling with the dermaroller till the endpoint of pinpoint bleeding. **(c)** Microneedling with the Dermapen (R).

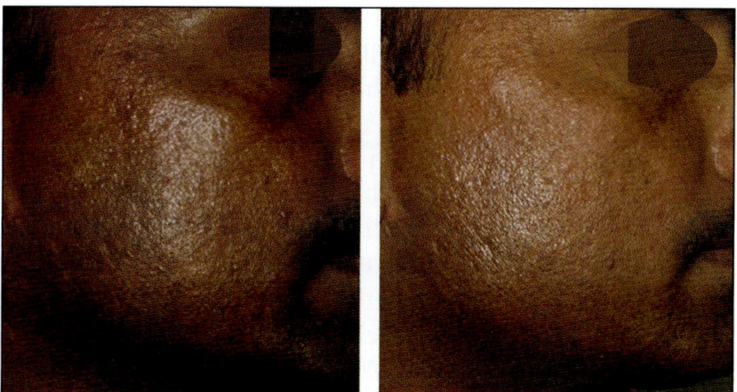

Fig. 7.22 Skin rejuvenation following four sessions of microneedling and topical vitamin C application immediately after the procedure.

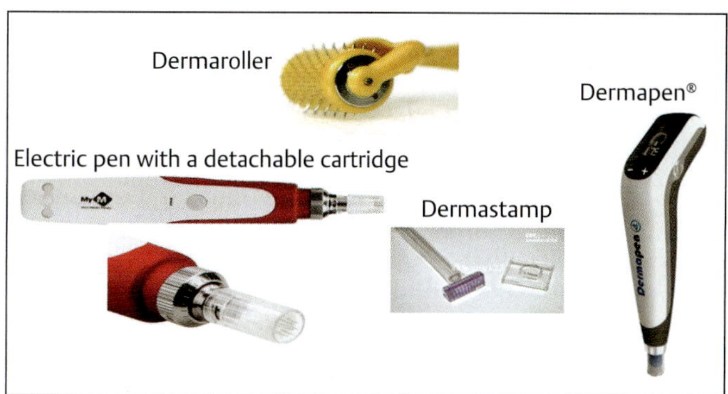

Fig. 7.23 Microneedling devices.

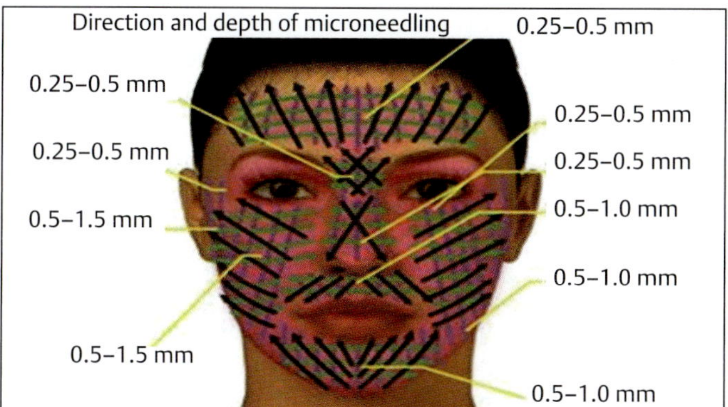

Fig. 7.24 Depth and directions of microneedling for facial rejuvenation.

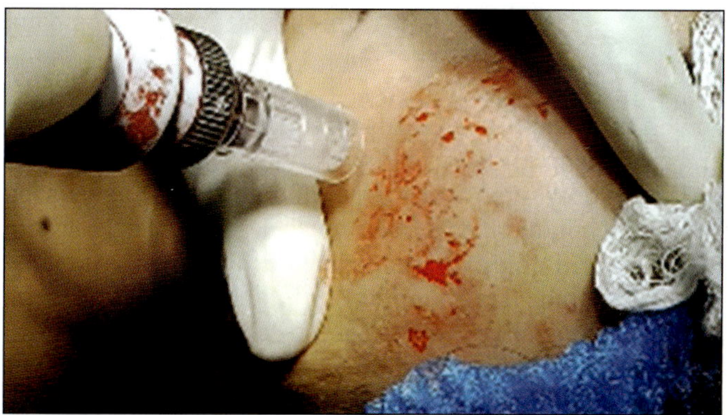

Fig. 7.25 End point of microneedling—erythema or pinpoint bleeding points.

a thick coat of eutectic mixture of lignocaine and prilocaine/tetracaine is applied for 45 minutes to 1 hour. Maintaining full aseptic precautions, skin is stretched with one hand and the dermaroller is held in the other. Dermaroller is held at an angle and with firm pressure four to five passes are given each in vertical, horizontal, and oblique directions on the affected area (**Fig. 7.24**). End point is pin-point bleeding points which can be easily controlled by applying pressure (**Fig. 7.25**). The area is cleaned with wet saline gauze and ice packs can be used for patient comfort. Antiseptic cream is applied and the patient is advised to avoid excessive sun exposure and chemical use for the next 1 week. Slight erythema and edema can be present for 2 to 3 days depending on the depth of needles used, skin type, and the indication for which the procedure was done. The patient should be instructed to wash the face with plain water for 24 hours. No makeup is allowed. After 24 hours a cleanser and physical sunscreen may be used. Swimming, strenuous activity, sweating, direct sunlight should be avoided for 1 to 2 days following treatment.

There is no downtime and the patient can resume daily work the very next day. Treatments are performed at 3- to 8-week intervals and multiple sittings are needed to achieve the desired effect on the skin. Since new collagen maturation takes time, the final results should be assessed only after 3 to 6 months.

Results

In a study by Domyati et al[57] 10 patients with Fitzpatrick skin type III and IV and Glogau class II to III wrinkles were subjected to six skin microneedling sessions at 2-week intervals. A statistically significant increase in collagen types I, III, and VII, and tropoelastin was observed. In another study of 10 patients treated with microneedling for upper lip rhytides demonstrated a mean 2.3-fold reduction in wrinkle severity using the Wrinkle Severity Rating Scale (WSRS) 30 weeks after the completion of two treatment sessions.[58] It also improved neck aging as reported by Fabbrocini et al.[59] Among various techniques available for skin rejuvenation, microneedling is a safe and effective technique.[60,61] It can be combined with other regenerative therapies such as PRP and enriched stem cell therapy to enhance results.[62]

Complications

This is a safe technique; however, there are few complications. Transient erythema, edema, bruising may be noted. Folliculitis, aggravation of acne, tram track scarring, and PIH are rare complications.[54]

Conclusion

A review of microneedling highlights that results are encouraging for a variety of conditions including scars, acne, melasma, photodamage, skin rejuvenation, hyperhidrosis, and alopecia. The main advantage is that the epidermis is preserved while promoting production of dermal collagen and elastin. Overall, it is a safe, simple, and efficacious technique for facial rejuvenation of all skin types.

Platelet-Rich Plasma

Platelet-rich plasma (PRP) is an autologous serum therapy that is processed to deliver high concentrations of platelets and growth factors. It is being increasingly used in hair and skin rejuvenation, either alone or synergistically in combination with lasers, microneedling, fillers, and fat graft due to its effect on wound healing.[63]

Mechanism of Action

Alpha granules within the platelets contain various growth factors such as PDGF, vascular endothelial growth factor (VEGF), EGF, TGF-β, and insulin-like growth factor (IGF). These are responsible for promoting stem cell regeneration, soft tissue remodeling, angiogenesis, and cell proliferation. PRP causes skin rejuvenation through angiogenesis, neocollagenesis, and adipogenesis. PRP has also shown to increase collagen density and dermal elastic fibers leading to skin rejuvenation.[64] PRP with autologous fat also improves fat survival.

Indications

PRP therapy is indicated for the treatment of wrinkles, especially periorbital and neck rhytides, improvement of skin texture and skin tone. It can reduce healing time if combined with fractional ablative CO_2 laser.[65]

Contraindications

Absolute contraindications to the procedure are platelet dysfunction syndrome, chronic liver disease, local infection, septicemia, hypofibrinogenemia, and anticoagulant use. Patients on corticosteroids and immunosuppressive drugs, thrombocytopenia, and autoimmune conditions are relative contraindications.[63]

Procedure

There is a lack of standardization on the preparation of PRP, though a platelet count of 1 million/mL has become the working definition for therapeutic PRP.[66] PRP can be prepared by single-spin or double-spin method. In the double-spin method, a sample of venous blood is drawn in a sterile tube containing an anticoagulant acid, citrate dextrose. The sample is centrifuged at 1,200 rpm for 10 minutes for sedimentation of the RBC. The supernatant plasma-containing platelets are transferred into another sterile tube without an anticoagulant and centrifuged at a higher speed in a hard spin 3,500 rpm for 5 minutes to obtain a platelet concentrate. The platelet pellet is at the bottom and the lower one-third is the PRP. The upper two-third is platelet-poor plasma (PPP), which is removed. The platelet pellets are suspended in a minimum quantity of plasma (2–4 mL) by gently shaking the tube. Thirty mL of whole blood yields about 3 to 5 mL of PRP. In the single-spin method whole blood with anticoagulant is centrifuged at high speed. This results in separation of three layers: the bottom layer consisting of RBCs, the middle layer consisting of platelets, which is the buffy coat and WBCs, and the top layer which is the PPP layer. The supernatant PPP is removed and the buffy-coat layer is transferred to another sterile tube. It is centrifuged at low speed to separate WBCs or a leucocyte filtration filter is used.

The PRP can also be prepared by using commercial kits. There is no consensus on whether the PRP should be with or without activation with calcium.[67] The PRP can either be injected after topical anesthesia at intervals of 4 to 6 weeks or applied topically following microneedling or CO_2 fractional laser therapy. If the PPP is heated up to 100°C, it turns opaque with a gel-like consistency. It can thus be used as an inert biofiller.[68]

Results

PRP combined with fractional laser therapies and microneedling improves wound healing, reduces erythema, and shortens recovery time.[69] Combining PRP with hyaluronic acid-based fillers has become very popular as the "Vampire facelift" promoted by celebrities world over via social media. The fillers act as a scaffold and growth factors from PRP enhance skin rejuvenation and soft tissue augmentation.[56] Long-term improvement has been reported with skin texture, nasolabial folds, horizontal neck bands, and facial rhytids. Significant improvements have also been reported in the periorbital region with improvement in rhytids and skin tone.[64] PRP and platelet-rich fibrin matrix (PRFM) combined with autologous fat has been reported to enhance treatment outcomes and increase fat survival.[70]

Complications

Though it is safe, bruising can occur following PRP injection. A single report of skin necrosis and blindness in one eye has been reported following PRP for bilateral cosmetic PRP injections to rhytids in the glabellar region.[71]

Conclusion

Autologous PRP has shown significant benefit either alone or in combination with other techniques for facial rejuvenation. However, the methods still require standardization and effects may be variable.

Photorejuvenation

Photorejuvenation (photofacial) is a commonly performed cosmetic procedure, to give patients a clear, firm, and youthful skin with no downtime. Various light-based devices are used, hence the term "photorejuvenation."

Mechanism of Action

During photorejuvenation, light stimulates the underlying cells to enhance the body's natural process of cell regeneration, leading to improvement in skin texture. It promotes significant collagen production by targeting the dermal fibroblasts. The laser or intense pulsed light (IPL) also targets melanin and breaks it down to improve and lighten complexion. Mid-infrared lasers have been found to stimulate the production of collagen I, III, and VIII, and trophoelastin production.[72] Similarly light waves are absorbed by the hemoglobin in the red blood cells which damages the blood vessel walls, making red colorations on the skin less visible.[73] In photodamaged skin, photofacials lead to increased collagen deposition in upper papillary and reticular dermis and better arrangement of elastin fibers. In such cases dermal dendritic cell is considered to be the biological target leading to activation of heat shock protein 70 and procollagen 1.[74]

Indications

Photorejuvenation helps in improving skin texture, reducing hyperpigmentation, decreasing superficial wrinkles and fine lines, improving acne especially inflammatory lesions, and increasing the blood circulation.[75] In author's experience, this procedure has been found to be especially useful in patients having dry, damaged skin due to excess steroid use or excess use of resurfacing lasers or deep peels **(Fig. 7.26)**. Patients with rosacea and abnormal flushing also show good results after four to six sessions. It is an excellent modality for treatment of photoaging.

Contraindications

Contraindications include history of photosensitivity and seizures, especially those induced by strong light when IPL is used.

Devices

Photorejuvenation can be done using a number of nonablative lasers. These include pulsed dye lasers (PDL) targeting microvessels and IPL targeting both melanin and microvessels. Cutoff filters 570- to 645-nm wavelengths also show epidermal thickening, new rete ridge, and dermal collagen formation, and a decrease in degenerated elastic fibers.[74]

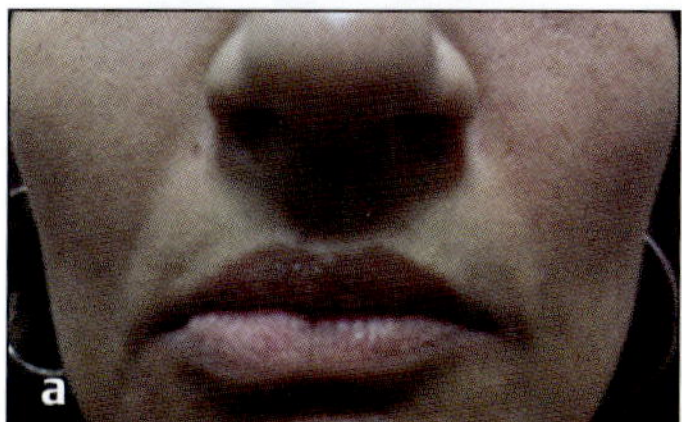

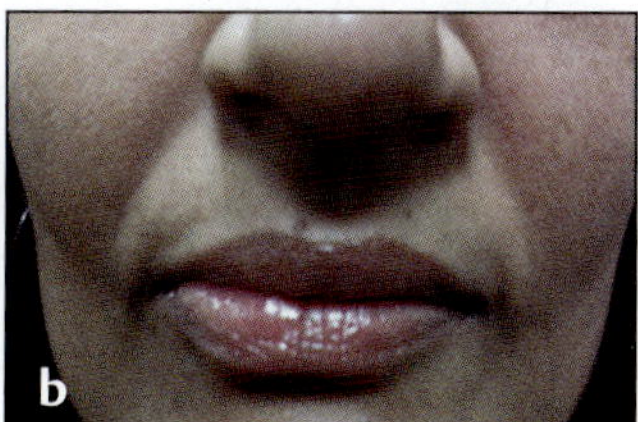

Fig. 7.26 Photorejuvenation. **(a)** Dry lusterless skin before treatment. **(b)** After 4-monthly sessions of photofacials with intense-pulsed light.

Mid-infrared lasers targeting dermal water and collagen like 1,320-nm Nd:YAG and low-intensity diode (wavelength) are also used and have been found to be very good for antiaging but do not improve pigmentary or vascular abnormalities.[75]

Procedure

In photofacial treatments first the area to be treated is cleaned with a mild cleanser following which laser/IPL light is given over the entire area. This is either done by contact devices in which the handpiece is held in contact with the skin or in certain devices light is delivered from a distance. The end point for rejuvenation is slight warmth and redness over the treated area. The energy given and the number of passes depend on the laser being used, skin type, and the indication.

Adequate eye protection for the operator and the patient needs to be ensured. These treatments are usually performed at a gap of 4 weeks. Multiple sessions are required to get the optimum results. IPL photorejuvenation targets deeper layers of the skin, so they are usually combined with more superficial treatments such as MDA and chemical peels. Usually a gap of 2 weeks is recommended between a session of photorejuvenation and peel/MDA.

Results

There is level 1 evidence for treatment of melasma, acne vulgaris, and telangiectasias and level 2 evidence for treatment of lentigenes, acne rosacea, capillary malformations, actinic keratosis, and sebaceous gland hyperplasia with photofacials.[56] A study by Negishi et al has shown excellent improvement in more than 90% cases of pigmentation, more than 83% of telangiectasias, and 65% of skin texture in Asian skin with IPL photofacials.[76]

Limitations

Photofacials are not useful for severe photoaging, deep wrinkles, excessive skin laxity, PIH. Its usefulness in melasma is still debatable.

Complications

Photofacial is considered a very safe procedure for all skin types, with practically no downtime. Erythema and minor blisters which heal without scarring have been reported.[76]

Conclusion

Photofacial as a skin rejuvenation procedure has been gaining popularity in the recent past due to excellent safety profile and a wide range of aesthetic issues that can be improved.

Energy-Based Devices

Radiofrequency-Based Devices

Radiofrequency (RF) is emerging as a gentler, nonablative skin-tightening device that delivers uniform heat to the dermis at a controlled depth.

Mechanism of Action

It utilizes energy to generate heat in tissues through rapid movement of charged particles, which leads to collagen denaturation and tissue contraction when a critical temperature is reached (65–75°C).[77] At a lower temperature there are higher chances of epidermal damage because the threshold for epidermal burn is 44°C. Depth of penetration is inversely proportional to frequency used.[78] Following treatment, coagulated columns in the dermis are followed by cellular infiltration, neovascularization, granulation tissue formation, leading to thickening and contraction of collagen fibers. This is followed by remodeling, leading to neocollagenization[79] (**Fig. 7.27**).

RF uses electrothermal energy which is not chromophore/skin type dependent causing nonselective tissue heating and thus theoretically is suitable for all skin types.[80] In contrast to lasers, where temperature gradient is maximum on the skin surface, here the thermal gradient is reversed, with the temperatures highest in the deeper levels. Thus, RF treatment is associated with minimal downtime. Radiofrequency has also proven to be useful and effective in neck treatment without significant downtime or risks.

Microneedling Radiofrequency

Microneedling radiofrequency (MNRF) combines two procedures commonly used in rejuvenation, (i.e., microneedling and radiofrequency which complement each other by synergistic action). The concept of using needles as the electrodes allowing the RF energy to be delivered directly into the dermis was proposed in a pilot study by Hantash and colleagues in 2009.[81] Since the RF energy was fractionated among several delivery and return needles, it was also termed as "microneedling fractional radiofrequency (RF)." RF microneedling can deliver heat at greater depths than laser, 3 mm or more with certain devices.[80]

Indications

RF energy devices are used for tightening and treatment of rhytides, acne, acne scars, cellulite, and stretch marks. They are particularly useful for face and neck tightening (**Fig. 7.28**).

Contraindications

Active infection at treatment site, patients with pacemaker, keloidal tendency, patient on anticoagulants and immunosuppressives, pregnancy, lactation, and systemic illness like epilepsy or cardiovascular ailments are contraindications to treatment.

Devices

Those with insulated needles offer the advantage of deeper penetration of electrothermal energy sparing the epidermis and thus minimizing the risk of PIH, whereas noninsulated needle will dissipate heat throughout the length of needle resulting in larger coagulation zones, more downtime and slower healing and increased chances of nonspecific epidermal injury. In monopolar devices, energy flows from an active electrode within the operator's handpiece to a grounding pad (passive electrode) placed distally on the patient's body. Its advantage is that the energy can be deposited deep into dermis and fibroseptal network (**Fig. 7.27**).

In bipolar RF the energy flows between two adjacent electrodes, both contained within the operator's handpiece. Compared with monopolar RF, bipolar RF provides higher energies but less depth penetration. Variable needle length

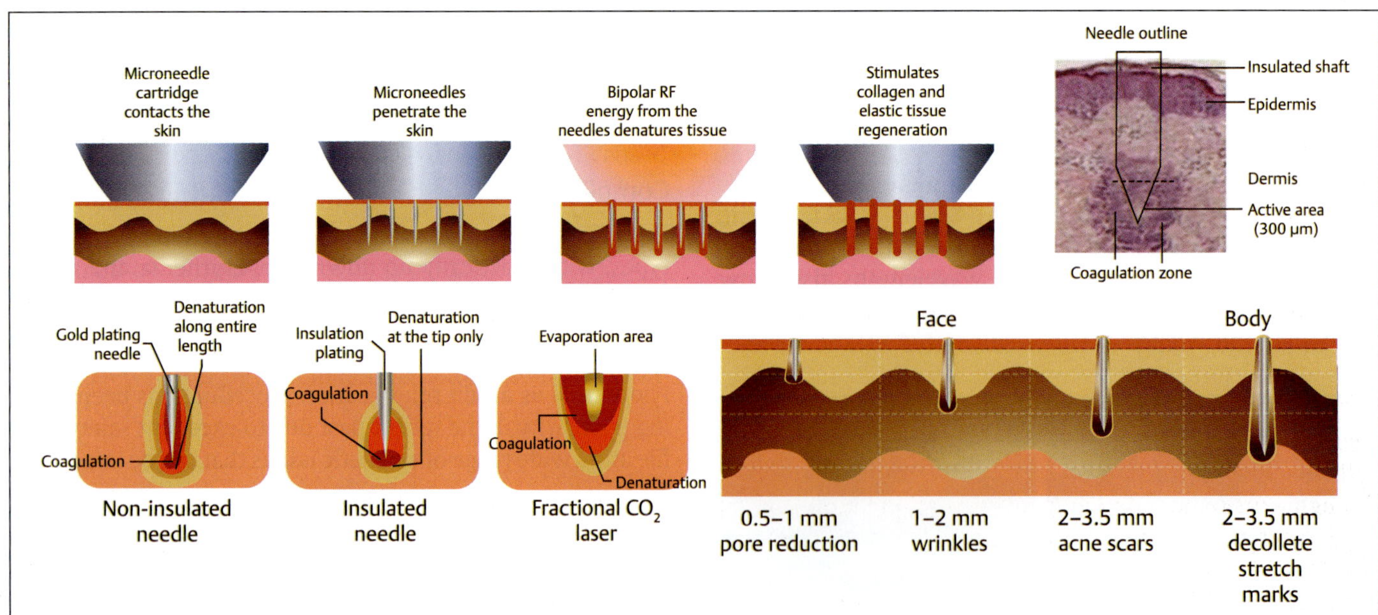

Fig. 7.27 Mechanism of action of microneedling radiofrequency (MNRF) and differences between insulated and noninsulated needles.

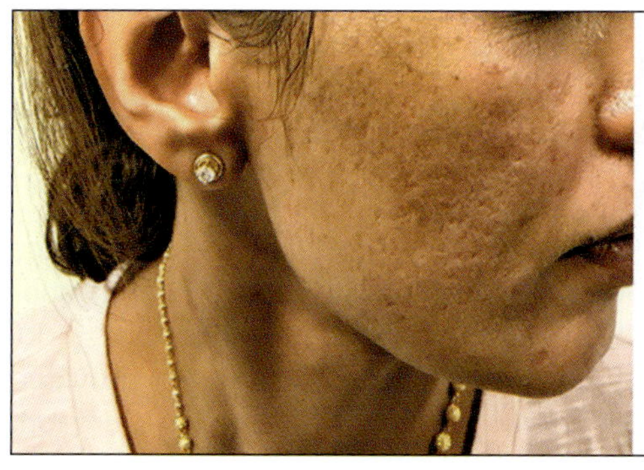
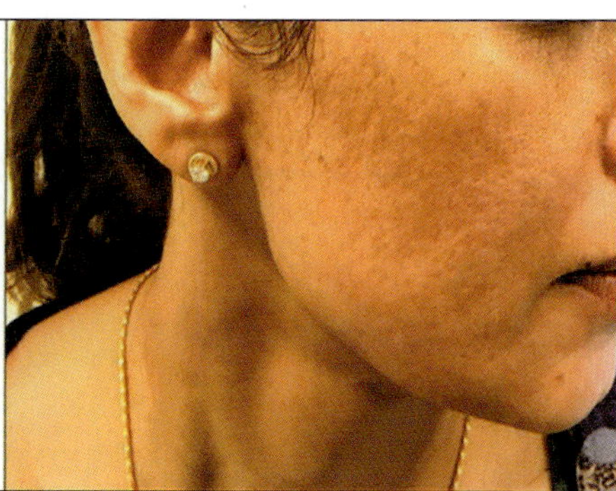

Fig. 7.28 Freckles with scars treated with combination of Q-switched Nd: YAG laser 1,064nm five sessions with chemical peel glycolic acid, Kojic peels (Sesglicopeel K—Sesderma) three sessions and microneedling radiofrequency (MNRF) four sessions. (The images are provided courtesy of Dr Atula Gupta, Gurgaon, Haryana, India.)

gives more flexibility to treat different conditions at different sites. Fixed length devices offer multiple tips to work at different levels. However, the thermal zone will vary with the angle of action on the skin (perpendicular being ideal), skin resistance, quality of needle, and number of needles (more needles means more resistance). With manual insertion, the procedure is operator dependent and so the speed and direction of performing the procedure may bring about variability in results. Mechanical insertion devices avoid these operator variabilities. Few devices monitor temperature and impedance, which gives instantaneous feedback to the handpiece to maintain the temperature at 67°C during each pulse.

Procedure

The treatment area is cleansed and topical anesthetic cream is applied for 45 minutes to 1 hour followed by recleansing of face. Sterility during and immediately after procedure is important, as there is disruption of skin barrier, following micropuncture wounds. Studies have shown that the amount of collagen produced is directly dependent on the intensity of heating;[82] however, there may be a plateau effect and thus increasing energies beyond a point may increase downtime and complications without any reasonable increase in results.[83] Larger radiothermal zones (RTZ) means more downtime. Minimal bleeding is expected and should be wiped with sterile gauze, which is not there with noninsulated needles. Postprocedure pain and discomfort may be there along with some redness, edema, and skin flaking for 2 to 3 days. Postprocedure precautions include sun protection, moisturization, maintaining sterility of treatment site, and keeping the head up while sleeping for 2 days.

Results

There have been quite a few studies using MNRF as an antiaging tool in the improvement of skin laxity and texture through skin remodeling and collagen stimulation. One of the largest multicenter studies conducted by Calderhead et al[84] on 499 patients with wrinkles from five study centers using fractional RF system reported 80 to 88% satisfaction with minimal downtime and adverse effects. Another study on 100 patients reported 100% response rate for rhytides and 95% for laxity.[85] Clementoni et al[86] performed a pilot study using fractional high-intensity-focused radiofrequency in 33 patients with neck laxity and found histological as well as clinically significant difference with decrease in cervicomental and gnathion angles. MNRF can also be combined with other resurfacing procedures like lasers and injectables especially when dealing with both epidermal and dermal pathologies.

Complications

Procedural complications include petechiae, bruising, flare up of acne, redness, swelling, superficial burns, and PIH. Long-term complications include scarring and altered skin texture; however, they are extremely rare. Complications are more likely procedural rather than due to device. To minimize complications[80] firm and equal pressure should be maintained on handpiece, keeping it perpendicular to skin surface. One should choose appropriate power settings, avoiding high energy and pulse stacking, and should allow skin cooling between pulses.

Conclusion

MNRF is a safe and effective antiaging procedure with minimal downtime and precise action on the dermis.

Monopolar Radiofrequency Device

Thermage is a noninvasive, nonablative device that uses monopolar radiofrequency energy to bulk heat underlying skin while protecting the epidermis to produce skin tightening. It is used for the treatment of facial wrinkles including the periorbital region. It received FDA approval for the treatment of periorbital wrinkles in 2002, facial rhytids in 2004, and all rhytids in 2005. The Thermage CPT (Solta Medical, USA) system consists of three components: a generator, a cryogen unit, and a handpiece connected to a disposable treatment tip.[87,88] Cryogen spray cools the inner side of the membrane of the tip to cool the epidermis. Sensors are placed at all corners of the tip to ensure uniform contact and distribution of RF energy. The Thermage FLX system (AccuREP technology, Solta Medical, USA) is the most recent device. It was released in 2017.

It is mainly useful for patients between 35 and 60 years with mild-to-moderate facial and neck laxity and rhytids with realistic expectations (**Fig. 7.29**). Patients with severe

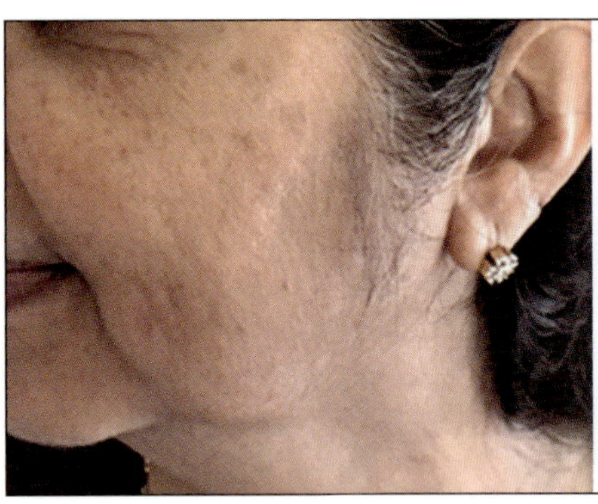
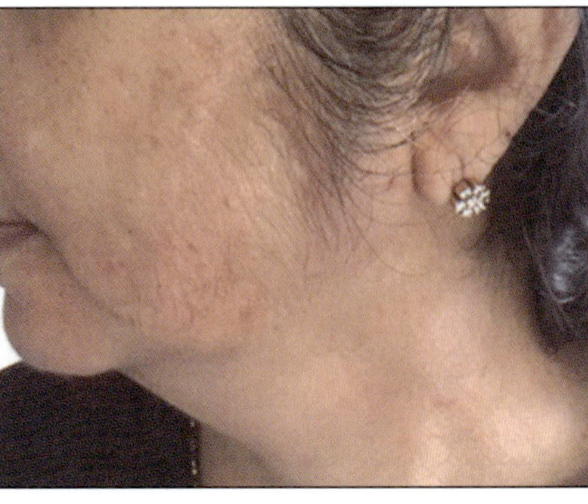

Fig. 7.29 Skin laxity of the lower face treated with polydioxanone (PDO) monofilament threads and monopolar RF four sessions. (The images are provided courtesy of Dr Atula Gupta, Gurgaon, Haryana, India.)

laxity and deep rhytids, obese patients with extremely loose redundant skin are poor candidates for this procedure. It is contraindicated in patients with a pacemaker or any implanted electronic device, presence of active skin infection, or pathology at the treatment site. Smoking, pregnancy, autoimmune conditions, prior radiation therapy, and other conditions that impair wound healing are also relative contraindications.

Procedure

All metal jewelry, makeup, and lotions should be removed. A temporary grid system is placed on the clean treatment area, which guides the provider on pulse placement with the treatment tip. Coupling fluid is placed generously on the treatment area. There are three tips available for face, body, and eye, with different repetitions or pulses (face tip: 600 and 900 REPs; eye tip: 450 REPs), and these are chosen based on site and area to be treated. Pressure is evenly applied to the skin and pulses are laid down in an adjacent, but not overlapping, fashion. Two passes are performed over the entire treatment area. Then, additional three to five vector passes are performed in the direction in which the skin tightening/lift is desired. When treating over bony prominences, tissue is moved such that more skin and subcutaneous fat is centered over the bony area, which decreases pain and sensitivity. While treating eyelids, sterile plastic eye shields must be placed to prevent ocular injury. Full contact with the treatment tip membrane is essential for proper dispersion of energy; otherwise the machine refuses to fire. Intensity of RF energy is increased to a level which the patient perceives as hot but tolerable. No topical anesthesia cream is used. The grid is removed after treatment with isopropyl alcohol and the skin is gently cleansed. Immediately postprocedure redness, edema, and some skin tightening is expected.

Fitzpatrick et al[87] reported at least 1 point improvement in Fitzpatrick wrinkle score in 83.2% of treated areas and eyebrows lifted by at least 0.5 mm in 61.5% in 86 patients who received a single treatment with the ThermaCool (TC) System for periorbital tightening and were evaluated for 6 months after treatment. Alster and Tanzi found that single treatment with Thermacool is effective in significantly improving cheek and neck laxity. Nasolabial and melolabial folds were more responsive to treatment than the jowls, and mandibular ridge.[89]

Complications are very few especially after adoption of multiple-pass, low-fluence treatment algorithm by most physicians, with persistent erythema and edema being the most common complications.

Ultrasound-Based Devices

High-intensity-focused ultrasound (HIFU) treatment has recently been introduced as an effective antiaging tool. When ultrasound waves are microfocused to a point in living tissue, molecular vibration results and heat is generated at 60°C, creating microthermal zones at predetermined depths in the mid-to-deep dermis up to the superficial musculoaponeurotic system (SMAS). This causes contraction of collagen and tissue coagulation with subsequent formation of new collagen without affecting the epidermis.[90,91] Focused ultrasound is superior because of its capability to reach deeper tissues without affecting superficial tissues. Unlike RF energy, HIFU can heat deeper tissue to between 60°C and 70°C without damaging the skin and does not require surface cooling.[92] Suh et al reported that HIFU treatment increased the elastin and collagen fiber concentration in the dermis and led to dermal thickening.[93]

The Ulthera system (Ultherapy), a device working on this principle, was approved by the US FDA in 2009 for noninvasive eyebrow elevation, but is commonly used for panfacial and submental treatments. Depending on the device settings, the target tissue can be set to variable depths: 1.5 mm, 3.0 mm (targets deep dermis) or 4.5 mm (targets the SMAS and platysma).[92] The Ulthera system delivers transcutaneous microfocused ultrasonic energy from an operator-controlled handpiece and a monitor which allows direct visualization of the delivered energy so that specific structures such as bone can be avoided. The focal energy delivered in predetermined "lines" results in discrete intervals between coagulation zones that promote healing.

Indications

Candidates between 20 and 50 years of age with facial or periorbital rhytides with realistic expectations are suitable. Unlike RF devices, HIFU can be performed in patients with pacemakers and devices in situ.

Contraindications

Patients on anticoagulant therapy, infection at the treatment site, and those with unrealistic expectations should not be taken up. Caution in cases of pre-existing hyaluronic acid (HA) filler in the face, as the filler can be disrupted or disintegrated. The imaging handpiece permits the operator to see the underlying filler and avoid it.

Procedure

Topical anesthetic cream is applied 1 hour before the treatment. Ultrasound gel is then applied to the skin. The operator moves the probe parallel to the first exposure line and places the second row of ultrasound exposures 3 to 5 mm from the first line. The probes come in various depths and are used according to the depth of target area, which can be deep dermis or the superficial muscle layer.

Results

Several studies have demonstrated the efficacy and safety of HIFU in facial skin tightening. Serdar et al[94] performed HIFU on face and neck of 75 patients by using two different probes with focal depth of 3 and 4.5 mm. Three months after treatment the patient satisfaction was 78% and physician assessment showed 80% improvement in nasolabial, jawline, submental, and neck areas, each evaluated separately. Nineteen patients (25.3%) reported pain, five patients (6.7%) had transient erythema, and two patients (2.7%) had both transient erythema and pain; all adverse effects were resolved after the procedure. Park et al[95] also reported HIFU as an effective and safe method in the treatment of facial wrinkles and suggested that HIFU has its effects on multiple aspects such as skin tone, facial contour, tightness of the skin, facial lifting, and the improvement of wrinkles. Shome et al in a recent Indian study reported that 85% patients showed improvement which was maintained at 1 year.[96]

Complications

The most common complications related to HIFU include erythema, edema, and pain, all of which subside within days without treatment. Bruising, PIH, paresthesia, and less commonly fat atrophy and neurologic complications have been described.[97]

Conclusion

HIFU is a noninvasive, skin-tightening tool with the advantage of actions at deeper level with no effect on epidermis. It is a relatively new technique but the clinical data favors it as an emerging effective antiaging tool.

Future Prospects

Scientific advances in nanotechnology and regenerative medicine along with technology are rapidly changing. Innovations in drug delivery, nonsurgical techniques, cosmeceuticals, and personalized medicine are some of the future prospects that are going to change the way we approach aging medicine. Molecular-level interventions to prevent telomeres shortening, genomic interventions, noninvasive tissue contouring, skin-tightening techniques, nutritional medicine, and microrobotic tissue-rebuilding techniques are some of the innovations expected in the future.[98] The plastic surgeon practicing cosmetic surgery must be familiar with these aspects of aesthetic surgery and medicine.

Conclusion

The demand for noninvasive or minimally invasive skin rejuvenation techniques has increased exponentially in the past few decades. The advent of botulinum toxin, fillers, chemical peels, microneedling, microdermabrasion (MDA), lasers, and other energy-based devices have catapulted the nonsurgical procedures to the top over surgical aesthetic procedures. Regenerative therapies like platelet rich plasma (PRP), biofillers, stem cell therapy, nanofat transfer, etc., are emerging as exciting techniques that act synergistically with other interventions. Newer technologies such as photorejuvenation, radiofrequency and laser-based devices, and ultrasound-based therapies are contouring the aging population as never before. The spotlight is also on patient-directed topical products such as sunscreens, moisturizers, retinoids, alpha-hydroxy acids, and topical antioxidants which form the cornerstone of maintenance programs following interventions. In general, minimally invasive nonsurgical techniques offer great benefit with low risk of complications and reduced costs and downtime as compared to conventional surgical methods. The future lies in personalized medicine that can prevent, reverse, and repair the effects of aging. A thorough knowledge of the nonsurgical methods of facial rejuvenation is essential for a practicing aesthetic surgeon. It is in the greater interest of the plastic surgeon to provide a comprehensive approach to a patient-seeking facial rejuvenation. A successful integration of various modalities can optimize results and lead to greater patient satisfaction.

References

1. Fisher GJ, Kang S, Varani J, et al. Mechanisms of photoaging and chronological skin aging. Arch Dermatol 2002;138(11): 1462–1470
2. The American Society of Plastic Surgeons. 2018 National plastic surgery statistics: cosmetic and reconstructive procedure trends. https://www.plasticsurgery.org/documents/News/Statistics/2018/plastic-surgery-statistics-full-report-2018.pdf Accessed March 2020
3. ISAPS International Survey on Aesthetic/Cosmetic Procedures. 2018. https://www.isaps.org/wp-content/uploads/2019/12/ISAPS-Global-Survey-Results-2018-new.pdf. Accessed March 2020

4. Durai PC, Thappa DM, Kumari R, Malathi M. Aging in elderly: chronological versus photoaging. Indian J Dermatol 2012;57(5): 343–352
5. Starkman SJ, Mangat DS. Chemical peel (deep, medium, light). Facial Plast Surg Clin North Am 2020;28(1):45–57
6. Sachdeva S. Fitzpatrick skin typing: applications in dermatology. Indian J Dermatol Venereol Leprol 2009;75(1):93–96
7. Vashi NA, de Castro Maymone MB, Kundu RV. Aging differences in ethnic skin. J Clin Aesthet Dermatol 2016;9(1):31–38
8. Glogau RG. Aesthetic and anatomic analysis of the aging skin. Semin Cutan Med Surg 1996;15(3):134–138
9. Commander SJ, Chang D, Fakhro A, Nigro MG, Lee EI. Noninvasive facial rejuvenation. Part 1: patient-directed. Semin Plast Surg 2016;30(3):129–133
10. Latha MS, Martis J, Shobha V, et al. Sunscreening agents: a review. J Clin Aesthet Dermatol 2013;6(1):16–26
11. Griffin ME, Bourget TD, Lowe NJ. Sun protection factor determination in the United States. In: Lowe NJ, Pathak M, Shaath N, eds. Sunscreens, development, evaluation and regulatory aspects. 2nd ed. New York: Marcel Dekker; 1997:499–512
12. Schneider J. The teaspoon rule of applying sunscreen. Arch Dermatol 2002;138(6):838–839
13. Shanbhag S, Nayak A, Narayan R, Nayak UY. Anti-aging and sunscreens: paradigm shift in cosmetics. Adv Pharm Bull 2019;9(3):348–359
14. Sethi A, Kaur T, Malhotra SK, Gambhir ML. Moisturizers: the slippery road. Indian J Dermatol 2016;61(3):279–287
15. Wan DC, Wong VW, Longaker MT, Yang GP, Wei FC. Moisturizing different racial skin types. J Clin Aesthet Dermatol 2014;7(6):25–32
16. Griffiths CE, Russman AN, Majmudar G, Singer RS, Hamilton TA, Voorhees JJ. Restoration of collagen formation in photodamaged human skin by tretinoin (retinoic acid). N Engl J Med 1993;329(8):530–535
17. Helal NA, Eassa HA, Amer AM, Eltokhy MA, Edafiogho I, Nounou MI. Nutraceuticals' novel formulations: the good, the bad, the unknown and patents involved. Recent Pat Drug Deliv Formul 2019;13(2):105–156
18. Khunger N; IADVL Task Force. Standard guidelines of care for chemical peels. Indian J Dermatol Venereol Leprol 2008; 74(74, Suppl):S5–S12
19. Brody HJ, Monheit GD, Resnik SS, Alt TH. A history of chemical peeling. Dermatol Surg 2000;26(5):405–409
20. Stegman SJ. A comparative histologic study of the effects of three peeling agents and dermabrasion on normal and sundamaged skin. Aesthetic Plast Surg 1982;6(3):123–135
21. O'Connor AA, Lowe PM, Shumack S, Lim AC. Chemical peels: a review of current practice. Australas J Dermatol 2018;59(3): 171–181
22. Rendon MI, Berson DS, Cohen JL, Roberts WE, Starker I, Wang B. Evidence and considerations in the application of chemical peels in skin disorders and aesthetic resurfacing. J Clin Aesthet Dermatol 2010;3(7):32–43
23. Ghersetich I, Brazzini B, Peris K, Cotellessa C, Manunta T, Lotti T. Pyruvic acid peels for the treatment of photoaging. Dermatol Surg 2004;30(1):32–36, discussion 36
24. Sarkar R, Arsiwala S, Dubey N, et al. Chemical peels in melasma: a review with consensus recommendation by Indian Pigmentary Expert Group. Indian J Dermatol 2017;62(6): 578–584
25. Garg VK, Sinha S, Sarkar R. Glycolic acid peels versus salicylic-mandelic acid peels in active acne vulgaris and post-acne scarring and hyperpigmentation: a comparative study. Dermatol Surg 2009;35(1):59–65
26. Wójcik A, Kubiak M, Rotsztejn H. Influence of azelaic and mandelic acid peels on sebum secretion in ageing women. Postepy Dermatol Alergol 2013;30(3):140–145
27. Khunger N. Getting started: step by step chemical peels. 2nd ed. New Delhi, India: Jaypee Medical Publishers; 2014:7–15
28. Soleymani T, Lanoue J, Rahman Z. A practical approach to chemical peels: a review of fundamentals and step-by-step algorithmic protocol for treatment. J Clin Aesthet Dermatol 2018;11(8):21–28
29. Khunger N, Kandhari R. Dermoscopic criteria for differentiating exogenous ochronosis from melasma. Indian J Dermatol Venereol Leprol 2013;79(6):819–821
30. Coondoo A, Phiske M, Verma S, Lahiri K. Side-effects of topical steroids: a long overdue revisit. Indian Dermatol Online J 2014;5(4):416–425
31. Kubiak M, Mucha P, Rotsztejn H. Comparative study of 15% trichloroacetic acid peel combined with 70% glycolic acid and 35% trichloroacetic acid peel for the treatment of photodamaged facial skin in aging women. J Cosmet Dermatol 2020;19(1):137–146
32. Oresajo C, Yatskayer M, Hansenne I. Clinical tolerance and efficacy of capryloyl salicylic acid peel compared to a glycolic acid peel in subjects with fine lines/wrinkles and hyperpigmented skin. J Cosmet Dermatol 2008;7(4):259–262
33. Prestes PS, Oliveira MM, Leonardi GR. Randomized clinical efficacy of superficial peeling with 85% lactic acid versus 70% glycolic acid. An Bras Dermatol 2013;88(6):900–905
34. Vavouli C, Katsambas A, Gregoriou S, et al. Chemical peeling with trichloroacetic acid and lactic acid for infraorbital dark circles. J Cosmet Dermatol 2013;12(3):204–209
35. Dayal S, Sahu P, Jain VK, Khetri S. Clinical efficacy and safety of 20% glycolic peel, 15% lactic peel, and topical 20% vitamin C in constitutional type of periorbital melanosis: a comparative study. J Cosmet Dermatol 2016;15(4):367–373
36. Khunger N, Sarkar R, Jain RK. Tretinoin peels versus glycolic acid peels in the treatment of Melasma in dark-skinned patients. Dermatol Surg 2004;30(5):756–760, discussion 760
37. Sadick N, Edison BL, John G, Bohnert KL, Green B. An advanced, physician-strength retinol peel improves signs of aging and acne across a range of skin types including melasma and skin of color. J Drugs Dermatol 2019;18(9):918–923
38. Kligman DE, Draelos ZD. Combination superficial peels with salicylic acid and post-peel retinoids. J Drugs Dermatol 2016; 15(4):442–450
39. Khunger N. Step by step: chemical peels. 2nd ed. New Delhi, India: Jaypee Medical Publishers; 2014:283–301
40. Nikalji N, Godse K, Sakhiya J, Patil S, Nadkarni N. Complications of medium depth and deep chemical peels. J Cutan Aesthet Surg 2012;5(4):254–260
41. Shpall R, Beddingfield FC III, Watson D, Lask GP. Microdermabrasion: a review. Facial Plast Surg 2004;20(1):47–50
42. Tan MH, Spencer JM, Pires LM, Ajmeri J, Skover G. The evaluation of aluminum oxide crystal microdermabrasion for photodamage. Dermatol Surg 2001;27(11):943–949
43. Karimipour DJ, Kang S, Johnson TM, et al. Microdermabrasion: a molecular analysis following a single treatment. J Am Acad Dermatol 2005;52(2):215–223
44. Shim EK, Barnette D, Hughes K, Greenway HT. Microdermabrasion: a clinical and histopathologic study. Dermatol Surg 2001;27(6):524–530
45. Grimes PE. Microdermabrasion. Dermatol Surg 2005;31(9 Pt 2): 1160–1165, discussion 1165

46. Salik E, Løvik I, Andersen KE, Bygum A. Persistent skin reactions and aluminium hypersensitivity induced by childhood vaccines. Acta Derm Venereol 2016;96(7):967–971
47. Cotelessa C, Persis K, Fargnoli MC, Mordenti C, Giacomello RS, Chimenti S. Microabrasion versus microabrasion followed by 15% trichloroacetic acid for treatment of cutaneous hyperpigmentation in adult females. Dermatol Surg 2003;29(4): 352–356
48. Karimipour DJ, Karimipour G, Orringer JS. Microdermabrasion: an evidence-based review. Plast Reconstr Surg 2010;125(1): 372–377
49. Orentreich DS, Orentreich N. Subcutaneous incisionless (subcision) surgery for the correction of depressed scars and wrinkles. Dermatol Surg 1995;21(6):543–549
50. Fernandes D, Signorini M. Combating photoaging with percutaneous collagen induction. Clin Dermatol 2008;26(2): 192–199
51. Ablon G. Safety and effectiveness of an automated microneedling device in improving the signs of aging skin. J Clin Aesthet Dermatol 2018;11(8):29–34
52. Fabbrocini G, Fardella N, Monfrecola A, Proietti I, Innocenzi D. Acne scarring treatment using skin needling. Clin Exp Dermatol 2009;34(8):874–879
53. Liebl H, Kloth LC. Skin cell proliferation stimulated by microneedles. J Am Coll Clin Wound Spec 2012;4(1):2–6
54. Hou A, Cohen B, Haimovic A, Elbuluk N. Microneedling: a comprehensive review. Dermatol Surg 2017;43(3):321–339
55. Waghule T, Singhvi G, Dubey SK, et al. Microneedles: a smart approach and increasing potential for transdermal drug delivery system. Biomed Pharmacother 2019;109:1249–1258
56. Bahuguna A. Micro needling: facts and fictions. Asian J Med Sci 2013;4:1–4
57. El-Domyati M, Barakat M, Awad S, Medhat W, El-Fakahany H, Farag H. Multiple microneedling sessions for minimally invasive facial rejuvenation: an objective assessment. Int J Dermatol 2015;54(12):1361–1369
58. Fabbrocini G, De Vita V, Pastore F, et al. Collagen induction therapy for the treatment of upper lip wrinkles. J Dermatolog Treat 2012;23(2):144–152
59. Fabbrocini G, De Vita V, Di Costanzo L, et al. Skin needling in the treatment of the aging neck. Skinmed 2011;9(6):347–351
60. Ramaut L, Hoeksema H, Pirayesh A, Stillaert F, Monstrey S. Microneedling: where do we stand now? A systematic review of the literature. J Plast Reconstr Aesthet Surg 2018;71(1):1–14
61. Bonati LM, Epstein GK, Strugar TL. Microneedling in all skin types: a review. J Drugs Dermatol 2017;16(4):308–313
62. Lee HJ, Lee EG, Kang S, Sung JH, Chung HM, Kim DH. Efficacy of microneedling plus human stem cell conditioned medium for skin rejuvenation: a randomized, controlled, blinded split-face study. Ann Dermatol 2014;26(5):584–591
63. Peng GL. Platelet-rich plasma for skin rejuvenation: facts, fiction, and pearls for practice. Facial Plast Surg Clin North Am 2019;27(3):405–411
64. Sand JP, Nabili V, Kochhar A, Rawnsley J, Keller G. Platelet-rich plasma for the aesthetic surgeon. Facial Plast Surg 2017;33(4): 437–443
65. Na JI, Choi JW, Choi HR, et al. Rapid healing and reduced erythema after ablative fractional carbon dioxide laser resurfacing combined with the application of autologous platelet-rich plasma. Dermatol Surg 2011;37(4):463–468
66. Rughetti A, Giusti I, D'Ascenzo S, et al. Platelet gel-released supernatant modulates the angiogenic capability of human endothelial cells. Blood Transfus 2008;6(1):12–17
67. Dhurat R, Sukesh M. Principles and methods of preparation of platelet-rich plasma: a review and author's perspective. J Cutan Aesthet Surg 2014;7(4):189–197
68. Dashore S, Dashore A. Platelet-poor plasma-based biofiller: an innovative alternative to expensive hyaluronic acid-based fillers for treatment of chicken pox scars. J Am Acad Dermatol 2019; S0190–9622(19)32493–4
69. Shin MK, Lee JH, Lee SJ, Kim NI. Platelet-rich plasma combined with fractional laser therapy for skin rejuvenation. Dermatol Surg 2012;38(4):623–630
70. Sclafani AP. Safety, efficacy, and utility of platelet-rich fibrin matrix in facial plastic surgery. Arch Facial Plast Surg 2011; 13(4):247–251
71. Kalyam K, Kavoussi SC, Ehrlich M, et al. Irreversible blindness following periocular autologous platelet-rich plasma skin rejuvenation treatment. Ophthal Plast Reconstr Surg 2017; 33(3S, Suppl 1):S12–S16
72. Preissig J, Hamilton K, Markus R. Current laser resurfacing technologies: a review that delves beneath the surface. Semin Plast Surg 2012;26(3):109–116
73. Purschke M, Laubach HJ, Anderson RR, Manstein D. Thermal injury causes DNA damage and lethality in unheated surrounding cells: active thermal bystander effect. J Invest Dermatol 2010;130(1):86–92
74. Goldberg DJ. Current trends in intense pulsed light. J Clin Aesthet Dermatol 2012;5(6):45–53
75. Waibel JS. Photorejuvenation. Dermatol Clin 2009;27(4):445–457, vi
76. Negishi K, Tezuka Y, Kushikata N, Wakamatsu S. Photorejuvenation for Asian skin by intense pulsed light. Dermatol Surg 2001;27(7):627–631, discussion 632
77. Arnoczky SP, Aksan A. Thermal modification of connective tissues: basic science considerations and clinical implications. J Am Acad Orthop Surg 2000;8(5):305–313
78. Beasley KL, Weiss RA. Radiofrequency in cosmetic dermatology. Dermatol Clin 2014;32(1):79–90
79. Zheng Z, Goo B, Kim DY, Kang JS, Cho SB. Histometric analysis of skin-radiofrequency interaction using a fractionated microneedle delivery system. Dermatol Surg 2014;40(2):134–141
80. Weiner SF. Radiofrequency microneedling: overview of technology, advantages, differences in devices, studies, and indications. Facial Plast Surg Clin North Am 2019;27(3):291–303
81. Hantash BM, Ubeid AA, Chang H, Kafi R, Renton B. Bipolar fractional radiofrequency treatment induces neoelastogenesis and neocollagenesis. Lasers Surg Med 2009;41(1):1–9
82. Hruza G, Taub AF, Collier SL, Mulholland SR. Skin rejuvenation and wrinkle reduction using a fractional radiofrequency system. J Drugs Dermatol 2009;8(3):259–265
83. Phothong W, Wanitphakdeedecha R, Sathaworawong A, Manuskiatti W. High versus moderate energy use of bipolar fractional radiofrequency in the treatment of acne scars: a split-face double-blinded randomized control trial pilot study. Lasers Med Sci 2016;31(2):229–234
84. Calderhead RG, Goo BL, Lauro FAA, Gursoy D, Savant SS, Wronski A. The clinical efficacy and safety of microneedling fractional radiofrequency in the treatment of facial wrinkles: a multicenter study with the INFINI system in 499 patients. 2013. www. lutronic.com
85. Alexiades-Armenakas M, Newman J, Willey A, et al. Prospective multicenter clinical trial of a minimally invasive temperature-controlled bipolar fractional radiofrequency system for rhytid and laxity treatment. Dermatol Surg 2013;39(2):263–273
86. Clementoni MT, Munavalli GS. Fractional high intensity focused radiofrequency in the treatment of mild to moderate laxity of

the lower face and neck: a pilot study. Lasers Surg Med 2016; 48(5):461–470

87. Fitzpatrick R, Geronemus R, Goldberg D, Kaminer M, Kilmer S, Ruiz-Esparza J. Multicenter study of noninvasive radiofrequency for periorbital tissue tightening. Lasers Surg Med 2003; 33(4):232–242
88. Ruiz-Esparza J, Gomez JB. The medical face lift: a noninvasive, nonsurgical approach to tissue tightening in facial skin using nonablative radiofrequency. Dermatol Surg 2003;29(4):325–332, discussion 332
89. Alster TS, Tanzi E. Improvement of neck and cheek laxity with a nonablative radiofrequency device: a lifting experience. Dermatol Surg 2004;30(4 Pt 1):503–507, discussion 507
90. White WM, Makin IR, Barthe PG, Slayton MH, Gliklich RE. Selective creation of thermal injury zones in the superficial musculoaponeurotic system using intense ultrasound therapy: a new target for noninvasive facial rejuvenation. Arch Facial Plast Surg 2007;9(1):22–29
91. Chan NP, Shek SY, Yu CS, Ho SG, Yeung CK, Chan HH. Safety study of transcutaneous focused ultrasound for non-invasive skin tightening in Asians. Lasers Surg Med 2011;43(5):366–375
92. Gutowski KA. Microfocused ultrasound for skin tightening. Clin Plast Surg 2016;43(3):577–582
93. Suh DH, Shin MK, Lee SJ, et al. Intense focused ultrasound tightening in Asian skin: clinical and pathologic results. Dermatol Surg 2011;37(11):1595–1602
94. Aşiran Serdar Z, Aktaş Karabay E, Tatlıparmak A, Aksoy B. Efficacy of high-intensity focused ultrasound in facial and neck rejuvenation. J Cosmet Dermatol 2020;19(2):353–358
95. Park H, Kim E, Kim J, Ro Y, Ko J. High-intensity focused ultrasound for the treatment of wrinkles and skin laxity in seven different facial areas. Ann Dermatol 2015;27(6):688–693
96. Shome D, Vadera S, Ram MS, Khare S, Kapoor R. Use of microfocused ultrasound for skin tightening of mid and lower face. Plast Reconstr Surg Glob Open 2019;7(12):e2498
97. Alam M, White LE, Martin N, Witherspoon J, Yoo S, West DP. Ultrasound tightening of facial and neck skin: a rater-blinded prospective cohort study. J Am Acad Dermatol 2010;62(2): 262–269
98. Dobke M, Hauch A. Targeting facial aging with nano and regenerative technologies and procedures. Plast Aesthet Res 2020;7:1

8

Nonsurgical Rejuvenation of the Face using Botulinum Toxin and Fillers

Kuldeep Singh and Chiranjiv Chhabra

- **Introduction**
- **Botulinum Toxin**
  - Upper Face
    - Glabellar Lines and Eyebrows
    - Browlift and Reshaping
    - Forehead Lines
    - Periorbital Area
    - Adverse Effects
  - Midface
    - Scrunch Lines
    - Nasal Tip Ptosis
    - Gummy Smile
    - Adverse Effects
  - Lower Face
    - Perioral Lines
    - Marionette Lines
    - Puckered or "Popply" Chin
    - Adverse Effects
- **Injectable Fillers**
  - Upper Third of Face
    - Forehead and Suprabrow
    - Periorbital (Periocular) Area
  - Midface
    - Tear Trough
    - Lateral SOOF
    - Nasolabial Fold
    - Nose
  - Lower Face
    - Perioral Rejuvenation
    - Marionette Folds/Lines
    - Chin
    - Jawline
  - Adverse Effects of Fillers
    - Pain
    - Edema and Bruising
    - Erythema
    - Infections
    - Nodules and Lumps
    - Tyndall Effect
    - Hypersensitivity Reactions
    - Malar Edema
    - Vascular Compromise
- **Full-Face Rejuvenation**
  - Assessment
  - Planning and Execution
- **Conclusion**

Introduction

Aging is a natural physiological phenomenon characterized by both intrinsic and extrinsic changes in the body. Age-related skin changes are visible and come into focus early. The pain of visible aging leads a person to seek a solution to his/her aesthetic problem. Many of the age-related changes are inevitable but can be slowed down by adopting wiser lifestyles, an appropriate skin care routine, and timely medical intervention in the form of procedures like dermal filler injections, neurotoxins, energy-based devices, chemical peels, regenerative medical solutions, and many more options. The Gold standard for antiaging is a combination approach.

In this chapter we will be concentrating on the use of hyaluronic acid (HA) fillers and neurotoxins to address aging issues. We are well aware that aging can be categorized into photoaging and chronological aging. Facial aging is a sum total of changes occurring in four layers: skin, fat, muscle, and bone. Bone—resorption; soft tissue—atrophy; fat—resorption and migration; skin atrophy. Four Rs of facial rejuvenation were earlier described by Woffles Wu,[1] but in today's context there are actually 6 Rs which are needed. Therefore as clinicians we should adopt the 6R technique of what can be called the comprehensive age management (CAM) plan (**Box 8.1**).

The concept of aging and beauty has been evolving rapidly over the past decade. In our practice of injectables spread over 20 years, we have observed the following:

- Patients are seeking aesthetic intervention at an earlier age. In a study of patients coming for facelifts, 32% reported having received injectables for facial rejuvenation starting at an average age of 37 years.[2,3] Now, even in India the patients are coming in their 30s for antiaging, as well as seeking enhancement of facial features as early as the 20s.[4]
- Earlier mostly women were seeking aesthetic improvement, now men are also seeking solutions in ever increasing numbers, though women still form the majority of patients in an aesthetic clinic.
- Earlier the focus was on looking younger. Now the focus is on (enhancement) beautification as well as looking more youthful.

Box 8.1 Comprehensive age management (CAM) plan

R1 Relax—The hyperdynamic muscles of the face
R2 Restore—The depleted soft tissue volume
R3 Rejuvenate—Improve skin laxity
R4 Resurface—Improve skin quality, texture, and pigmentation
R5 Reshape—Give support to the bony profile of the face and enhance landmarks
R6 Rehabilitate—Constant upkeep by follow-ups and touch-ups

The mindset of the treating physician is also changing from antiaging alone toward enhancement along with antiaging, contributing to better outcomes.

Botulinum Toxin

BontA is one of the serotypes produced from fermentation of clostridium botulinum in an anaerobic environment. In a nutshell, intramuscular injection of BontA inhibits the release of acetylcholine from motor nerve terminals, from autonomous nerve terminals, as well as secretomotor terminals having acetylcholine as neurotransmitter.

Botulinum toxin A (specifically OnabotulinumA) has been approved for more than 25 indications worldwide for indications involving bigger muscles including cervical dystonia, lower and upper limb spasticity, and for smaller muscles like glabellar frown lines, strabismus and blepharospasm. It is also approved for use in migraine, axillary hyperhidrosis and neurogenic overactive bladder.

In 2002, FDA approved Botox for treating frown lines, crow's feet, and forehead lines for aesthetic improvement. Double-blind, placebo-controlled trials by Carruthers et al[5] have established safety and efficacy of the toxin, supported also by many studies across Asia. The response rate was uniformly >80%, with a median duration of 120 days. Its onset of action appears in 3 days in most of the patients, with almost half of them reporting the effect in 24 hours.[6] Adverse effects were reported in a large series of 537 patients (treating glabellar lines and crow's feet), where authors[7] observed that overall incidence was not different in BontA versus placebo. Eyelid ptosis (3.2%) occurred in a significantly higher number in the BontA than in the placebo group, and interestingly, occurred only when the glabellar lines were injected. As the number of treatment cycles increased, the incidence of this adverse effect decreased to 0.8%.

From among various serotypes, viz., A, B, C1, D, E, F, and G, serotype A (Onabotulinum A—Botox, Incobotulinum A—Xeomin, Abobotulinum A—Dysport) is commonly used.

The only serotype B used is Rimabotulinum B toxin (Myobloc). The new kid on the block is Jeuveau (Prabotulinum toxin A),[8] which has already undergone Phase III studies for safety and efficacy in the treatment of glabellar lines. There are other newer toxins which are undergoing Phase IIa trials, like the RT002, also known as Daxibotulinum toxin A.[9]

Most of the BontA preparations are complex, with a protective protein shell called NAP (neurotoxin-associated protein), except Xeomin where all the proteins have been removed during the purification process. Onabotulinum A (Botox) preparation comes as a vacuum dried powder, while the rest come as lyophilized powders. Rimabotulinum B comes as a reconstituted solution.

Unpreserved saline was used to reconstitute Onabotulinum A earlier, but use of even preserved saline shows no decrease in efficacy, and is also less painful.

Sterile water does not decrease efficacy, but the injection is extremely painful. Agitation/foaming of the solution is known to produce no reduction in efficacy. Storage after reconstitution in normal saline has been found to have no reduction in efficacy for 2 to 6 weeks in various studies.[10,11]

Dilution has also been a subject of controversy, with current recommendations for Onabotulinum A ranging from 1 to 3 mL, 2.5 mL being the current standard recommended dilution. It was observed in a study by Hsu et al in 2004[12] that BontA showed greater diffusion with greater dilution, and Carruthers et al in 2007[13] showed more ptosis in the higher dilution group while treating the glabella, although the difference was not statistically significant. We personally prefer a dilution of 2 mL for a vial of 100 U (50 U/mL) for most indications.

Upper Face

Glabellar Lines and Eyebrows

Onabotulinum A was approved by the FDA for use in glabellar lines only in 2002, although it has been used for the same indication for over two decades as an off-label indication.

It is the first effective and noninvasive technique for browlift and improvement in glabellar lines described by Carruthers et al in 2003.[14] They showed that both dynamic and resting glabellar lines improved with botulinum toxin. Subsequently, it was also used for treating forehead lines, lines in the periocular area and other lines.

It has been seen that injection of Onabotulinum A into the procerus and corrugator supercilii not only relaxes the glabella, but also the medial frontalis due to deeper diffusion. This also causes lowering of the medial end of the eyebrows and elevation of the middle and lateral brow, mostly to our advantage in improving the shape of the eyebrows. Twenty to twenty-four units when injected in women, and 20 to 40 units in men will give an adequate response in the glabellar region (**Fig. 8.1**). Indian consensus guidelines suggest 16 to 20 units over three to five points[7] with the lateral points staying medial to the midpupillary line, at least 1 cm above the eyebrow.

Browlift and Reshaping

A detailed knowledge of muscle anatomy is necessary to perform this advanced indication of toxin (**Fig. 8.2**). Carruthers[15] in a study showed lateral, then medial and middle eyebrow elevation by injecting 20 to 40 U of toxin in the glabella alone. Injection into the orbicularis oculi muscle at various points in the brow can give a browlift by relaxing the orbicularis oculi muscle at those specific points, thereby allowing the frontalis to elevate that part of the brow (**Fig. 8.3a, b**). By manipulating these points we can modify the shape of the eyebrows to our advantage. Horne and Rohrer[16] described central eyebrow elevation by selectively treating the inferomedial and lateral frontalis, allowing the central part to arch up. Ahn et al[17] injected at three points in the lateral brow and produced an average of 4-mm elevation of lateral brow. While attempting the eyebrow lift in men, if at all needed, care should be taken to keep the shape horizontal, or it will appear feminized.

Forehead Lines

Injection of Botulinum toxin can alleviate dynamic lines, but also mild resting lines, improving with each successive injection.[18] When injecting the forehead for horizontal lines, all injection points must be at least 2 cm above the orbital rim (**Fig. 8.4a–d**) to prevent brow ptosis. Injection of 10 to 20 U in women and 20 to 30 in men had been originally recommended. However, in a consensus meeting[18] recommendations were made to reduce dose to almost half of that being used earlier, to get a more natural look. However, it was also recommended to follow up at 2 weeks to determine the need for further treatment. A Global Aesthetics consensus meeting in 2016[19] recommended a combination of toxin and fillers as the optimal treatment of forehead lines. Indian Consensus guidelines[7] however recommend a dose of 6 to 8 U in women and 10 to 12 U in men, with addition of fillers for static lines.

Relaxing of the medial frontalis muscle can lead to a hyperactive lateral edge of the muscle, causing the eyebrows to "spock", which is easily treated by injecting 2 U of BontA in the hyperactive area 2 cm above the brow (**Fig. 8.5a, b**).

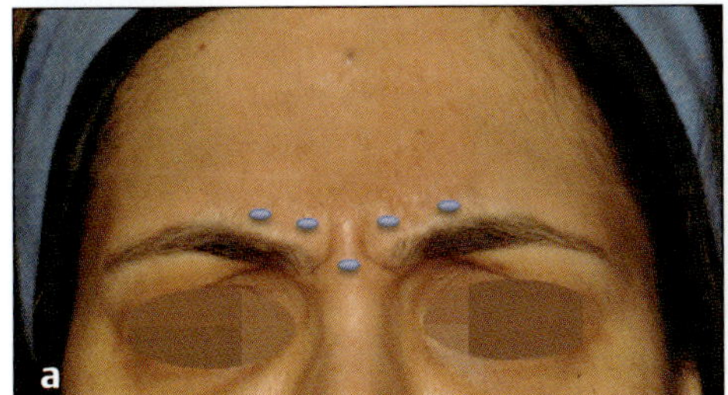

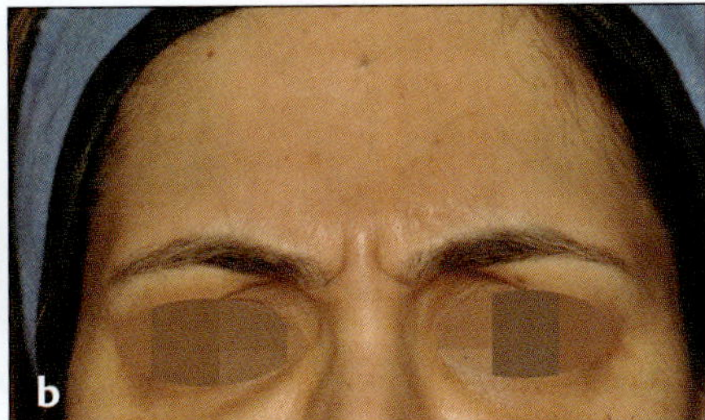

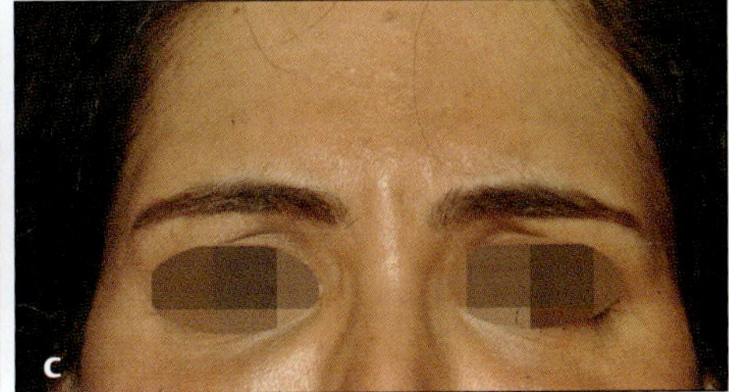

Fig. 8.1 Patient desired improvement in glabellar complex but did not want a frozen expression. **(a)** Twenty units of Onabotulinum A injected into the procerus and corrugator muscles distributed over five points, 4 U per point. **(b)** Before injection, and **(c)** effect at 2 weeks showing a relaxed procerus and corrugator muscles with consequent improvement in the appearance.

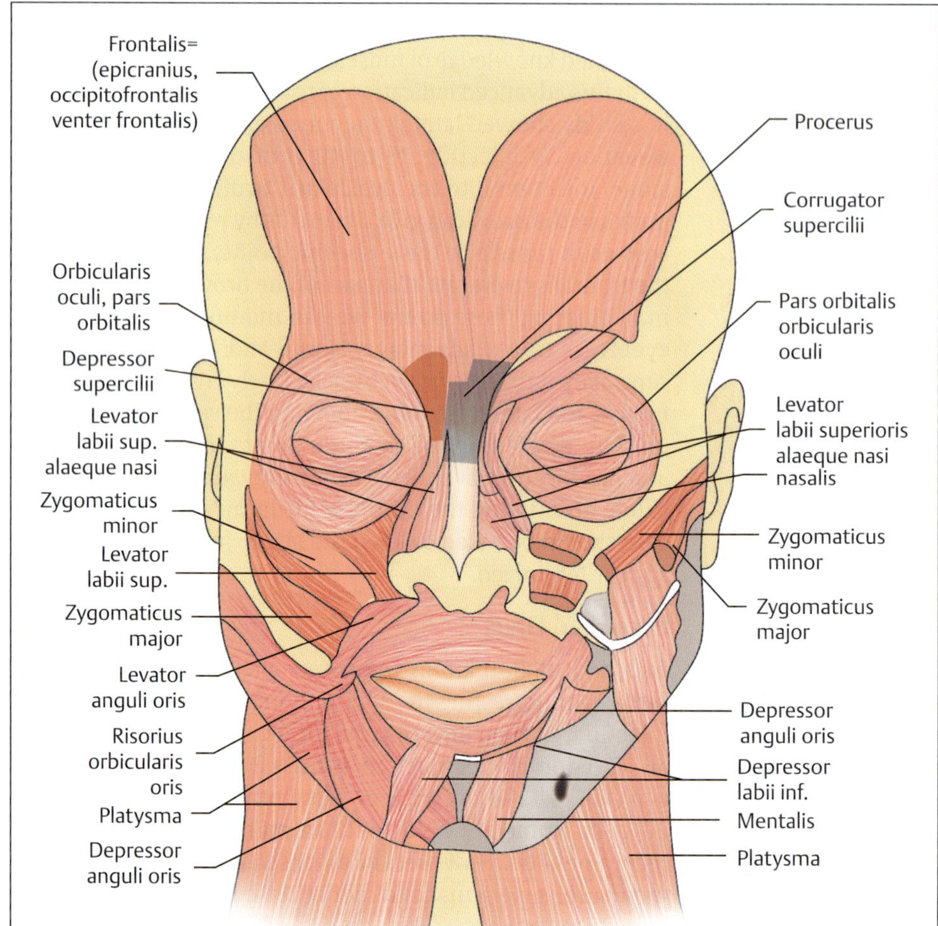

Fig. 8.2 Muscles of the face, highlighting the upper face target muscles for Botulinum toxin. inf, inferioris; sup, superioris.

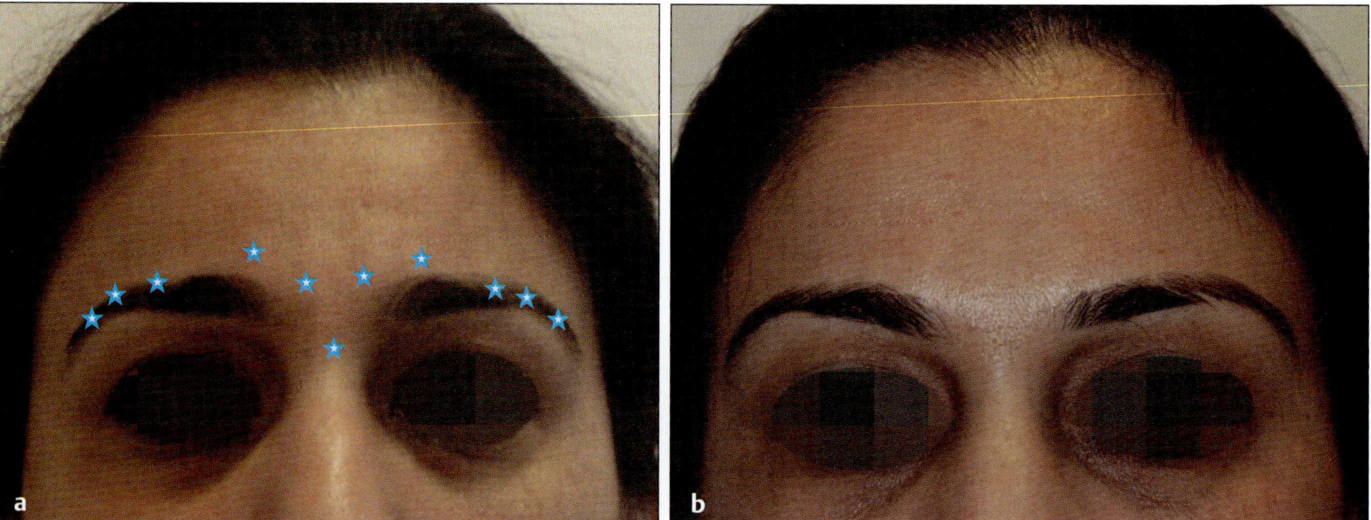

Fig. 8.3 Eyebrow lift and reshaping. **(a)** Injection is done in the glabellar region as well as the points where the eyebrow needs to be lifted. Five points in the glabella (as described in **Fig. 8.1**), and three points in the eyebrow, 2 U each 1 cm apart as shown, placed subdermally to block the orbicularis oculi brow depressor action at specifically those points, allowing the frontalis to lift. **(b)** Postinjection after 14 days showing lowering of medial eyebrow and elevation of mid and lateral brow.

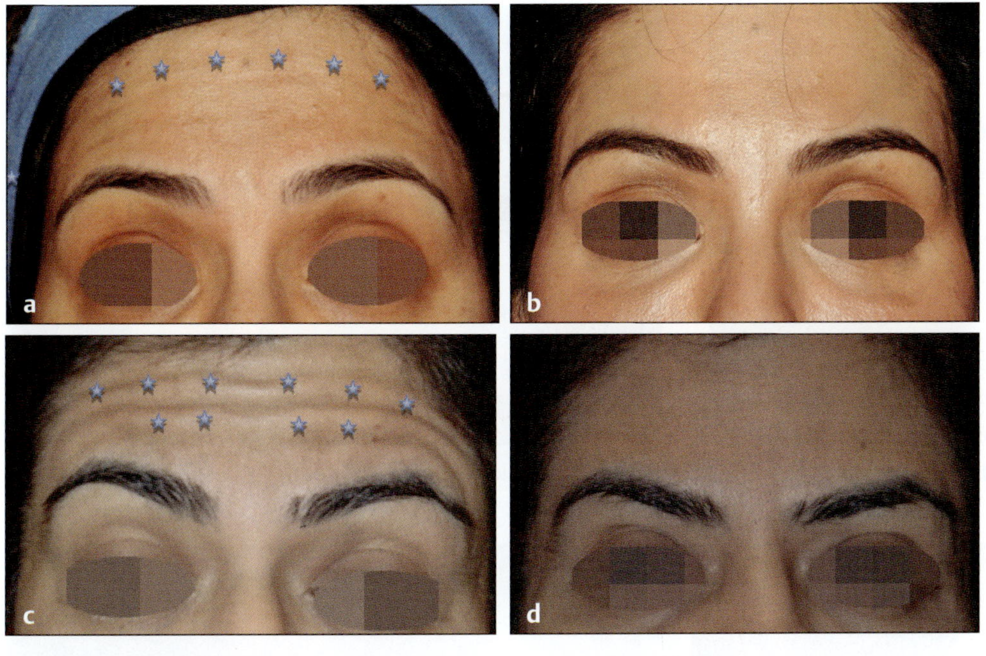

Fig. 8.4 Treatment of forehead horizontal rhytides. **(a, c)** Inject 8 to 12 U of botulinum toxin A into the frontalis at multiple points (usually 6–10). These patients have also had glabellar lines injected. **(b, d)** Post-treatment with botulinum toxin A.

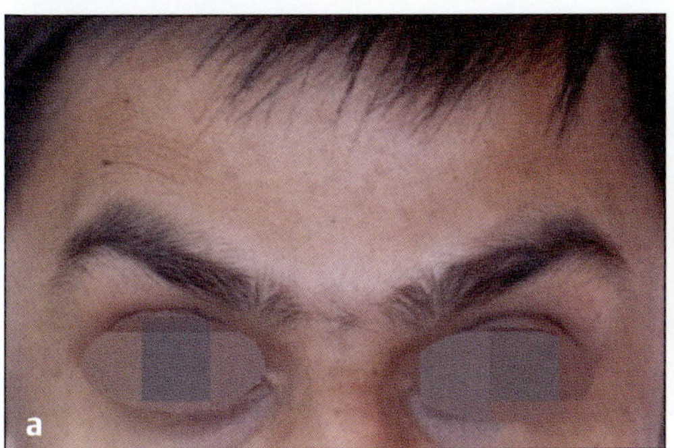

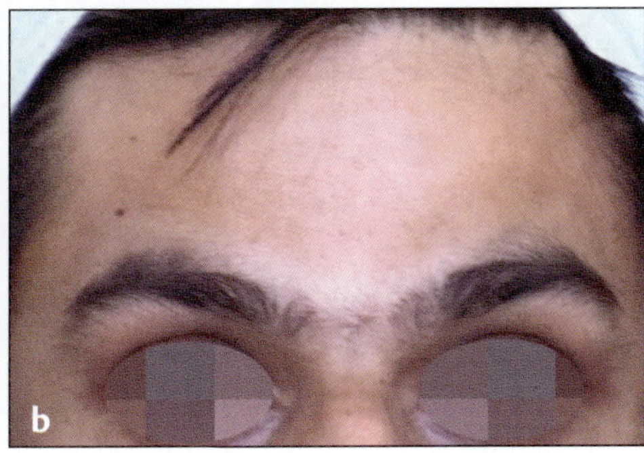

Fig. 8.5 Spocking of the eyebrows caused by a hyperactive lateral frontalis. **(a)** Spocked eyebrows, **(b)** treated by 2 U of BontA 2 cm above the spock in the lateral frontalis.

Caution: In older patients, preexisting conditions like dry eyes or post-Lasik surgery status may precipitate/worsen dry eyes after BontA treatment.

Periorbital Area

The periocular region shows signs of aging in the form of under eye dark circles, compounded by volume loss with eyes appearing sunken, or visible tear troughs. In addition, there may be brow ptosis, hooding of the eyelid as well as presence of lateral hyperdynamic lines called crow's feet **(Fig. 8.6)**. Commonly in younger people, the last one may be the only problem present. Some people have hypertrophic pretarsal orbicularis (eyelid roll), which may cause eyes to narrow or shut completely during smiling **(Fig. 8.7)**. Also, there may be lines in the infraorbital region extending from the medial limbus to crow's feet, known as infraorbital rhytides.

Crow's Feet

It is advisable always to seat the patient upright with head supported and hair safely out of the way with a hairband. In the periocular region we inject subdermally (as the orbicularis is adherent to the undersurface of the skin in this area with very little s/c fat) raising a bleb, at least 1 to 1.5 cm away from the lateral orbital rim. Usually three such injections are made in the upper, middle, and lower crow's feet lines. Visible veins in the area should be avoided to prevent/minimize bruising. A second row may be injected 1 cm lateral to the three points, if crow's feet are marked and extend laterally (**Fig. 8.8a**, with red dots indicating an optional second row). Six to twelve units of Onabotulinum A are recommended on either side[7] (**Fig. 8.8a**).

A word of caution against chasing crow's feet into the cheek. Considering that the inferolateral part of the orbicularis oculi is the only cheek elevator, it can cause problems with smiling. Also, if we go beyond the zygomatic bone into the cheek, we may inject inadvertently into the main elevator of the angle of mouth, the zygomaticus major muscle, causing a drop in the level of the angle of mouth, with resultant asymmetry if it is unilateral.

Hypertrophic Pretarsal Orbicularis

This causes eyes to close while smiling, can be treated with 1 to 2 U of Botox in the midpupillary line 3 mm below lash

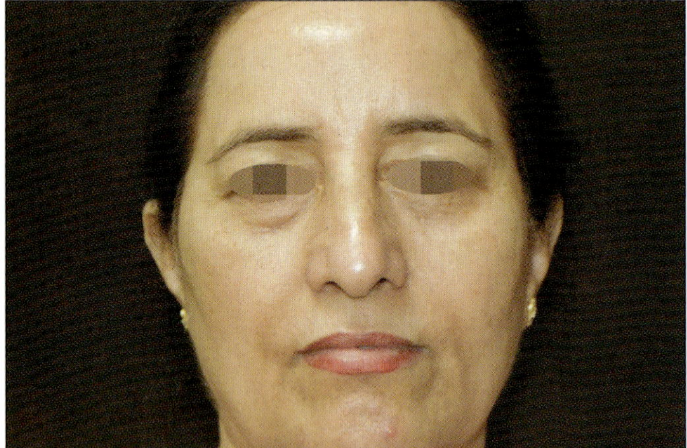

Fig. 8.6 Aging changes in the periocular area.

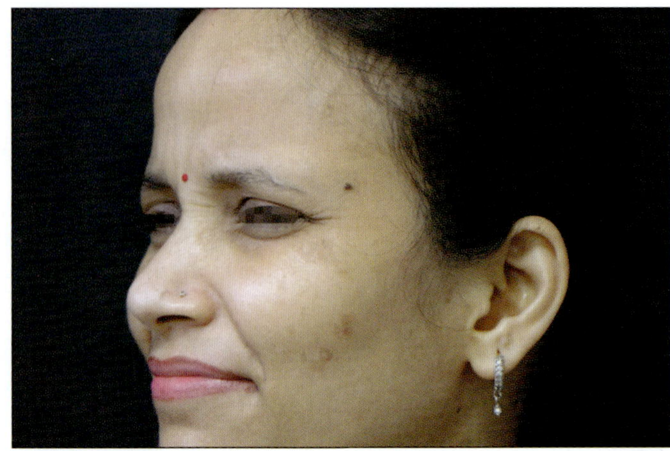

Fig. 8.7 Eyelid roll in a younger person.

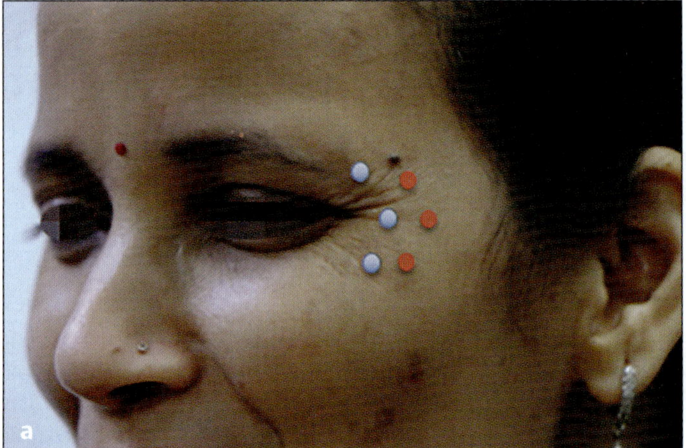

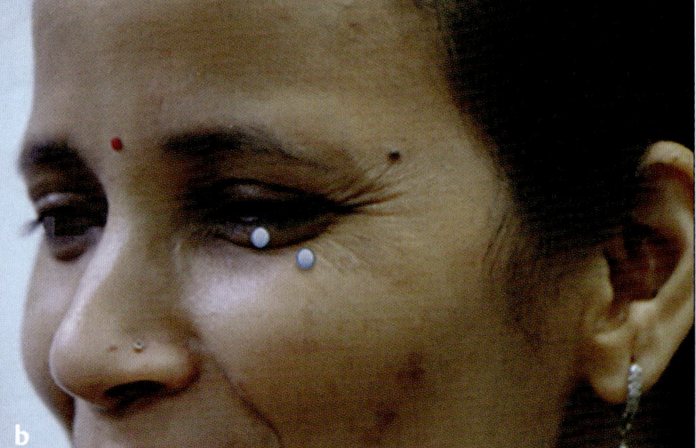

Fig. 8.8 Injection points for periocular rhytides (crow's feet), pretarsal roll, and infraorbital lines. **(a)** Three points (*blue dots*) BontA into the lateral orbicularis oculi muscle, 6 to 12 U per side (total of 12–24 U) depending on the severity of wrinkles; red dots indicate an optional second row. **(b)** Injection point for pretarsal roll in the midpupillary line 3 mm below lash margin, and infraorbital crow's feet point 7 mm from lash margin, between midpupil and lateral canthus.

margin[20] (**Fig. 8.8b**). Likewise, hyperactive infraorbital orbicularis can be treated with an additional 2 U about 7 mm below lid margin midway between the midpupil and the lateral canthus (**Fig. 8.8b**). Flynn et al in 2001 compared 2 U in the lower eyelid midpupillary line alone, with 2 U in midpupillary line plus 3 points in the crow's feet. Both resulted in widening of the eye, but the latter was more effective.[21] It is not advisable to treat orbicularis near the medial canthus, to avoid inhibiting the action of the lacrimal pump leading to epiphora.

Adverse Effects

Bruising is a common adverse effect, which can be prevented by avoiding visible veins. If there is bleeding from the injection point, give gentle pressure for 5 minutes, with instructions not to exercise, or bend head forward and downward for 24 hours. An ice pack will help minimize the bruising.

Other common adverse effects in the glabella, forehead, and brow regions possibly are edema, headache, brow ptosis, and upper eyelid ptosis. A 5.4% incidence of blepharoptosis (upper eyelid ptosis) has been reported in a multicenter study by Carruthers in 264 patients, declining to 1% in a subsequent study.[5,7,22] It is important that while injecting the glabellar region, one should inject the lateralmost point of the corrugator very superficial (just subdermal), and staying at least 1 cm above the orbital rim for prevention of lid ptosis (**Fig. 8.3a**). It is presumed to occur because of diffusion of toxin along the supraorbital notch (following the superior ophthalmic vein) to the levator palpebrae superioris, or in the preperiosteal plane.[23] Ptosis appears at about 7 days after injection. Usually treatment is conservative as it resolves spontaneously in 2 to 3 weeks. Apraclonidine 0.5%,[24] phenylephrine 2.5%, naphazoline 0.05%, and brimonidine 0.2%[25] eye drops have been used with varying degrees of success. The risk of using these eye drops in older people, especially those with a narrow gonial angle, is of precipitating acute narrow angle glaucoma.

Brow ptosis has been seen following injection of forehead lines within 2 cm of the eyebrows, blocking the action of the lower frontalis. Treatment is to inject the 3 points described earlier to elevate lateral brow.

Injections in the periocular region should be done very cautiously in the elderly, as they have dry eyes, a lax lower eyelid, and a lax orbital septum. A lower eyelid snap test will give an idea of preexisting laxity of the lower eyelid. Performance of a snap test and testing for a dry eye are mandatory requirements before planning injections in this region. In patients with lower eyelid eye bags, injection into the preseptal orbicularis would result in aggravating the eye bags[26] and even appearance of festoons[27] due to relaxation of the preseptal orbicularis, whereas in patients with a positive snap test, injection of toxin would cause paralytic ectropion and epiphora, if the lower eyelid pretarsal orbicularis is treated **(Fig. 8.9a, b)**.

Lip ptosis[28] or sometimes even cheek ptosis (the lateral orbicularis oculi functions as an accessory cheek elevator)[29] can occur in less than 1% of patients, and could be due to diffusion/injection into the inferolateral orbicularis oris fibers,[29] or the zygomatic muscles. This usually resolves in 2 to 3 weeks, but can also be helped by weakening the angle depressor (2 U into the DAO) on that side, thereby allowing a weakened elevator to lift the angle of mouth and the cheek.

Midface

Anatomy of the midface is different in many ways from the upper face. The skin is tighter, muscles are more densely adherent, and wrinkles are often static than dynamic. The muscles of the midface are closely interdependent on the muscles of the lower face. Much lower doses of botulinum toxin are used in the midface and lower face than in the upper face. Adverse effects easily occur in the midface due to disturbance in the interbalance of muscles, rather than just by diffusion which is mostly the case in the upper face. In many areas of the midface, better results are obtained by fillers, use of energy-based devices, and invasive procedures like rhytidectomy. The commonly injected areas in the midface are the scrunch or "bunny" lines, a dynamic drooping nose tip, and correction of a gummy smile.

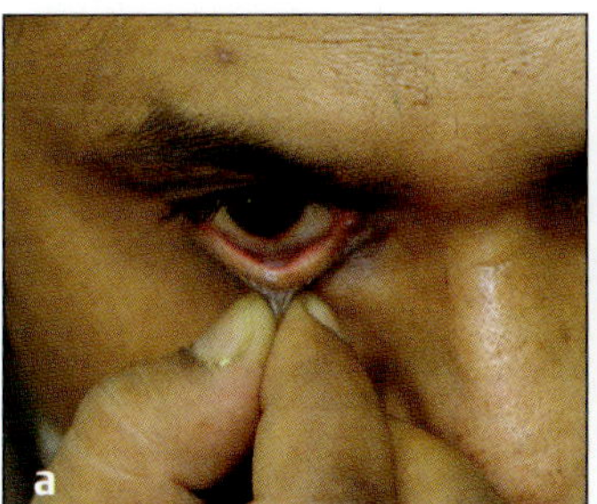

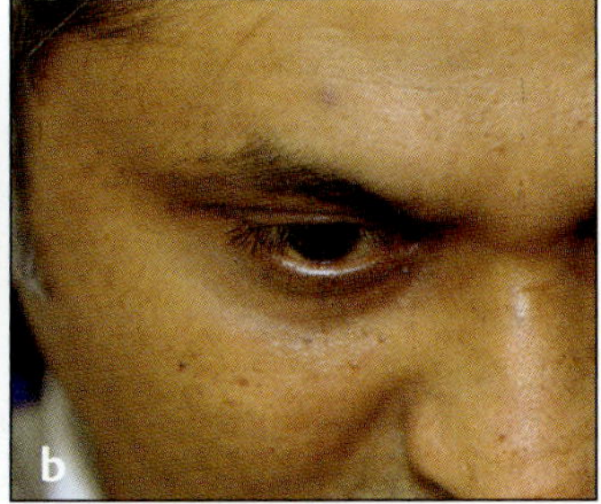

Fig. 8.9 **(a)** Snap test to determine laxity of the lower eyelid. **(b)** Quick return to normal position indicates a negative test.

Scrunch Lines

These are oblique lines in the upper part of the sides of the nose caused by contraction of the nasalis muscle. They may be present de novo when they are called bunny or scrunch lines, or appear after correction of glabellar lines as a compensatory mechanism (called "Botox sign"). Scrunch lines are treated at the same time as the glabella.[30] The lines are produced by the contraction of the transverse fibers of the nasalis muscle. If hyperactive, and not treated initially with the glabella, then will need to do so in the follow-up visit at 2 weeks. Injection is done at a point on the nasal bones on their side away from the angular vessels and the levator labii superioris alaeque nasii (LLSAN). Two to four units are injected on either side[19] **(Fig. 8.10)**.

Nasal Tip Ptosis

Dynamic nasal tip ptosis is when the nasal tip rotates downward while talking, depressing the upper lip or smiling. It is because of the action of a hyperactive depressor septi (DS) muscle. It can be associated with a short upper lip, transverse crease across the upper lip, or a gummy smile. DS arises from the region of the anterior nasal spine (ANS) and inserts into the caudal border of the cartilaginous septum, some orbicularis fibers, and along the nasal mucosa under the ala. In some people the LLSAN fires simultaneously to pull the alar base upward and backward, facilitating the rotation, and causing a gummy smile **(Fig. 8.11)**.

The treatment of this dynamic nasal ptosis is to inject 2 to 4 U of Botulinum toxin A just above the labiocollumellar junction. Two additional units may be injected in the columella, with supplemental doses of 2 U in each dilator naris (into each alar rim in its middle), a total of 3 to 10 U.[19] And if the LLSAN is hyperactive, pulling the ala backward and upward as well as causing a gummy smile, it is advisable to simultaneously inject toxin 2 U in the LLSAN on either side as for a gummy smile[31] **(Fig. 8.12a, b)**.

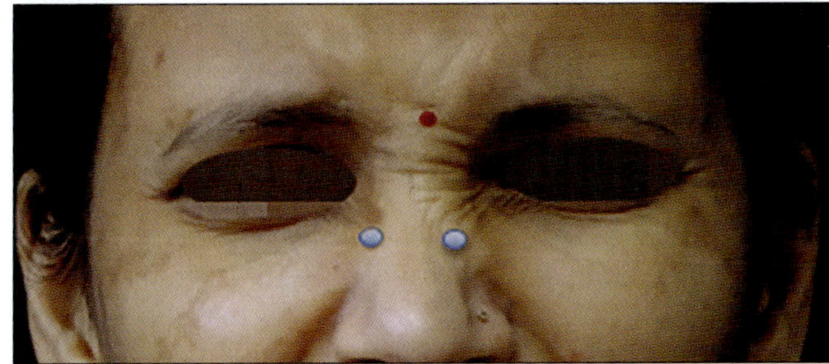

Fig. 8.10 Scrunch (bunny) lines (more prominent on the left side) and the points to be injected for correction with BontA toxin. Also, we can clearly observe the contracted glabella, transverse facial lines caused by contraction of the procerus, and pretarsal hypertrophic orbicularis (lower lid rolls).

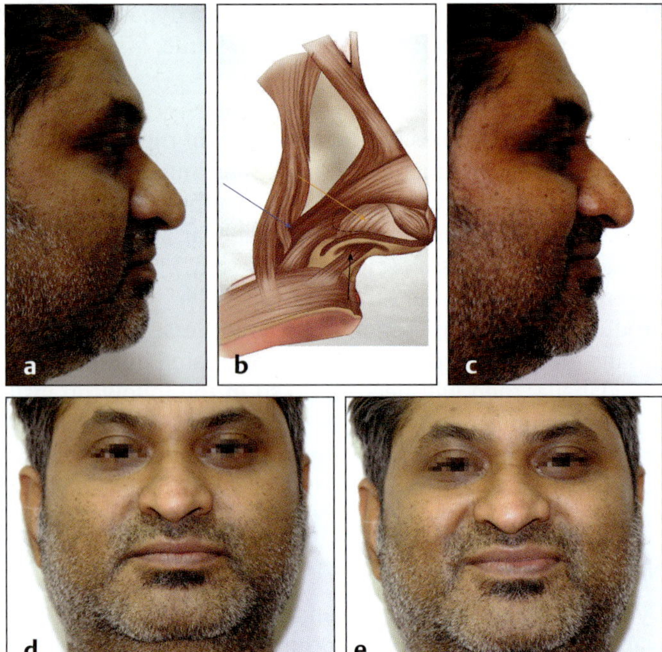

Fig. 8.11 The dynamic drooping nose tip **(a)** in repose, **(b)** showing muscles responsible: levator labii superioris alaeque nasii (LLSAN) (*blue arrow*), dilator naris (*yellow arrow*), and **(c)** Smile firing up all three muscles. **(d)** Frontal view in repose. **(e)** Frontal view smiling with drooping tip, dilated nostrils, and pulled-up alae.

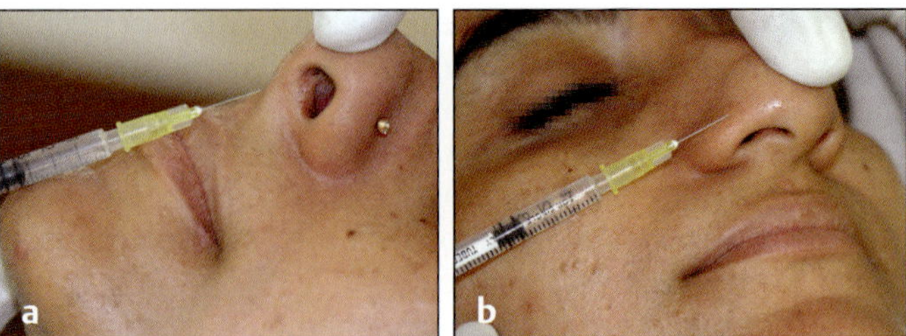

Fig. 8.12 Injection technique for dynamic drooping nose tip. **(a)** Depressor septi muscle being injected after lifting the tip of the nose away from the orbicularis. **(b)** Additional units being injected midway on the alar rim into the dilator nares.

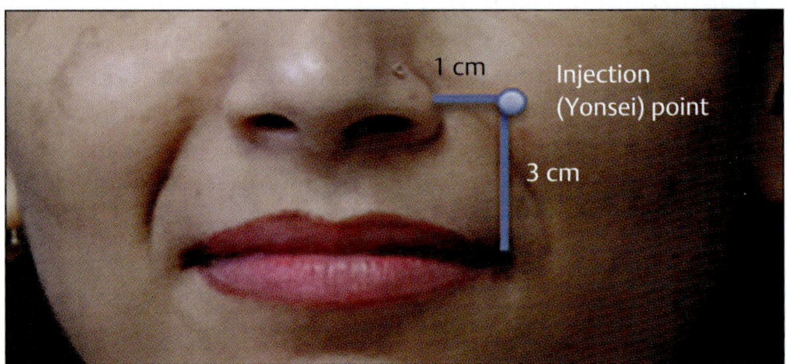

Fig. 8.13 Injection point described as the Yonsei point by Hwang et al in 2009 as the confluence of three muscles: levator labii superioris alaeque nasii (LLSAN), levator labii superioris (LLS), and zygomaticus minor.

Gummy Smile

Excessive show of gums during smile or laugh is called a "gummy smile." It is frequently associated with a short furrowed upper lip, and in some people a dynamic drooping tip of nose, occasionally all three features at the same time. Optimum tooth exposure has been assessed to be full crown height of the central incisors and 2 mm of upper gingiva.[32] Women generally show more gum than men who prefer a half-incisal show. Reasons for a gummy smile include an increased interlabial space, excessive contraction of upper lip elevators, often in combination with a genetically short upper lip, decreased upper incisor crown height, and increased vertical height of the maxilla. Four types of gummy smile have been described: anterior, posterior, mixed, and asymmetric, and different injection techniques recommended for each type.[33]

Those with gummy smile caused by hyperactive elevators of the upper lip are ideal candidates for Botulinum toxin A treatment. If cephalometry reveals normal dimensions, and 2 mm of upper incisor is seen in repose, then it is presumed that exposure of excess gingiva is due to hyperfunctional muscles.

Hwang et al in 2009 described the "Yonsei point" where all three muscles meet (LLSAN, LLS, and zygomaticus minor), which is about 10 mm lateral to the alar base and 30 mm above the horizontal lip line. Here the muscles are subdermal and dose of Botox required is less.[34]

Benedetto[30] recommends 2 U of toxin in the alar-facial groove into the palpable LLSAN just over periosteum. If the central gingiva is exposed more, then 1 U is injected in the DS. Another method described by Polo[35] is to inject 1 to 2 U in the central lip elevators given transmucosally. Polo[35] injected 2.5 U each at 2 points per side, first at the Yonsei point, and the second 2 cm lateral to it, only if the gummy smile extended laterally[33] (**Fig. 8.13**). He achieved a mean lowering of lip by 5.1 mm at 2 weeks. Effect lasts for 3 to 6 months.[35] **Fig. 8.14a, b** shows a young lady with a gummy smile with no malocclusion, only hyperactive elevators, which is the right indication for Botulinum toxin A.

Adverse Effects

While injecting "scrunch lines," if the injection is too lateral or low, we can get asymmetry and ptosis of the upper lip, or even epiphora from diffusing into medial orbicularis fibers.[30] Hematoma can result from puncturing of the angular vessels.

In case of injections for the "drooping tip of the nose," only dynamic drooping tip will respond to injection. Diffusion from injecting the DS can affect the upper lip elevators and the sphincteric action of the orbicularis causing upper lip

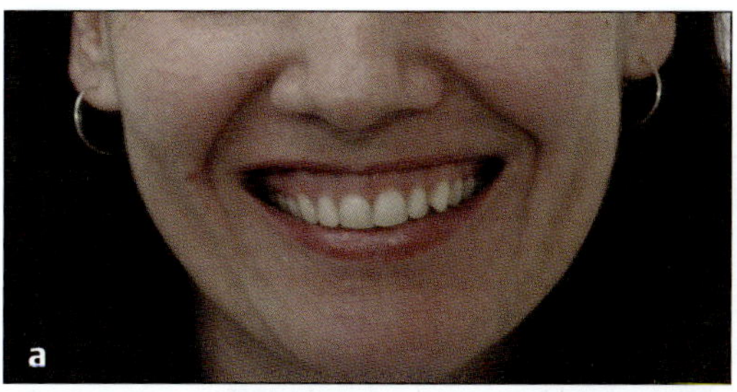
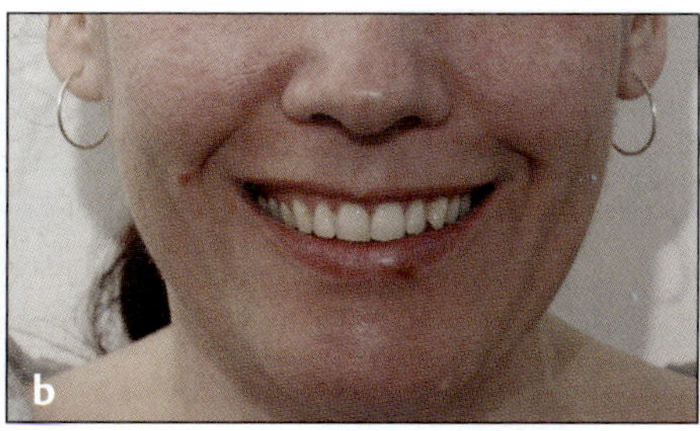

Fig. 8.14 Gummy smile and its treatment. **(a)** Lady with gummy smile from hyperactive lip elevators. **(b)** After 2 U of botox at the Y point.

lengthening, thinning, effacing of the philtrum, asymmetry, and difficulty with eating, swallowing, and speaking.[36]

On the other hand, treating the gummy smile, the risk of producing asymmetry is high, and high doses here are likely to produce upper lip ptosis and incompetence of the oral sphincter with its attendant problems.

The key is that in the midface, only experienced injectors of toxin can safely venture, as due to extensive interdependence of muscles, risk of diffusion into adjacent muscles is high.

Therefore, the doses need to remain small, and no massage should be done post injection.

Lower Face

The orbicularis oris muscle, the depressor anguli oris (DAO), depressor labii inferioris (DLI), mentalis, and the platysma muscles are responsible for the complex movements in the lower face. Aging affects them by increased resting tone and repetitive movements causing a crease/creases, and also by underlying bony resorption. Marionette lines are thought to result from DAO hyperactivity, assisted partly by bone and fat resorption, plus gravity pulling down lax tissues. The hyperactive mentalis muscle accompanied by bony absorption in the chin region also leads to an upwardly displaced chin eminence and a popply chin **(Fig. 8.10)**.

Excessive blocking of perioral muscles will cause issues with speaking, whistling, and expression. Therefore, mild, functional blocks are needed. It is preferable to have a lesser dilution of the reconstituted BontA solution to minimize diffusion in this area.

Perioral Lines

They form as a result of repetitive actions of the orbicularis oris muscle such as in smoking, habitually pursing lips, playing particular wind instruments, and these usually occur in women. Men develop them less due to presence of beard hair preventing inward turning of skin. Also, women have problems of lipstick bleeding into these grooves all the time. Perioral lines are also worsened by aging and prolonged sun exposure causing thinning of the skin. Dynamic perioral lines will respond better to botulinum toxin, whereas static lines will benefit from a combination approach with fillers as well as using a fractionated laser like CO_2 as adjunctive therapy.

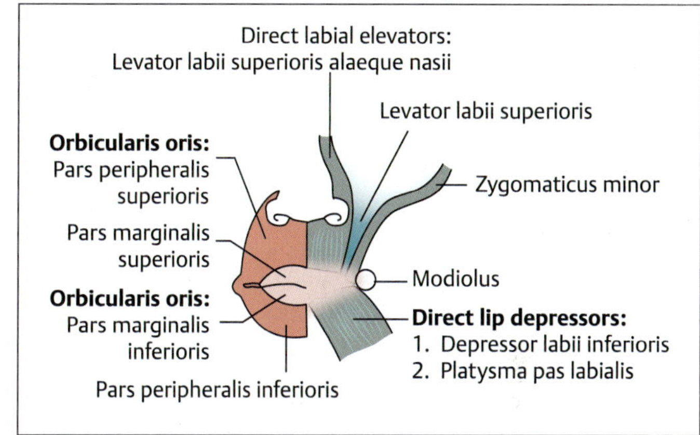

Fig. 8.15 Anatomical parts of Orbicularis oris muscle and its relationship with various muscles of the face.

The orbicularis oris is a complex muscle with intrinsic (deep) and extrinsic (superficial) fibers. There is also criss-crossing of fibers from above down and vice versa. The superficial fibers are divided into pars marginalis (in the vermilion) and pars peripheralis (in the skin part). Each is divided into four parts: right and left, upper and lower. The peripheralis arises mostly from the modiolus where the elevators and depressors contribute (**Fig. 8.15**).

Technique

Perioral lines need 1 to 2 U of toxin to be injected very superficially raising a bleb, just above the white roll at 2 points on either side of the midline in the upper lip, and 1 point on either side in the lower lip.[36] The objective being only to inject the superficial fibers, and maintaining symmetry to prevent any resultant functional asymmetry. Addition of HA fillers in the lines will help smoothen out the rhytides **(Fig. 8.16a, b)**. Lipstick running out into the skin is best corrected by injecting fillers (not BontA) in a linear manner along the white roll.

Marionette Lines

Marionette lines extend from below the angles of the mouth downward and outward till the lower border of the mandible ending in the prejowl sulcus. They are also called the labiomandibular groove and give the impression of sadness and disapproval. They are usually caused by a hyperactive DAO muscle which is a triangular muscle originating from

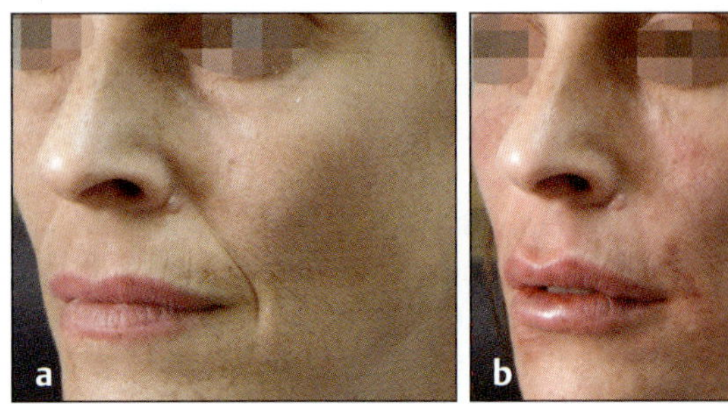

Fig. 8.16 Combination treatment of perioral lines. **(a)** Static perioral lines in the upper as well as lower lip running across the vermillion border causing lipstick bleed. **(b)** After 4 U of toxin followed by hyaluronic acid (HA) filler after 2 weeks in the lines as well as vermillion border and volume increase of the lip.

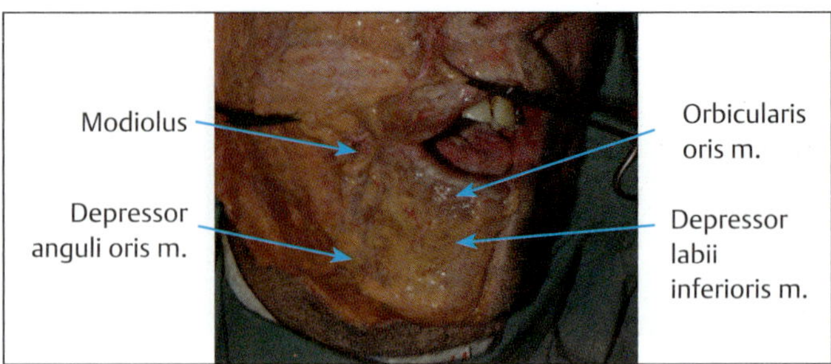

Fig. 8.17 Cadaver dissection showing muscles of the lower thirds of the face and the modiolus.m, muscle.

the posterior part of the oblique line of the mandible superficial to the DLI muscle. It converges and inserts into the modiolus, with some fibers decussating with the orbicularis oris, risorius, levator anguli oris, and inferiorly posterior fibers with the platysma (**Fig. 8.17**).

Injection of BontA is safely done by keeping closer to the mandibular border on a line dropped from a point 1 cm lateral to the angle of mouth, thus injecting into the lower third of the muscle near its posterior border (**Fig. 8.18**). One can start with 2 U the first time, and then increase in subsequent injections up to 4 U/side. This helps improve the smile in people having excessive downturning of the angle of mouth, as well as partly smoothen out marionette lines. In addition, an extra point can be injected at the lower border of the mandible where its posteriormost fibers meet the platysma. Injection should be kept superficial as it overlies the DLI muscle.

Most older patients will require volume support with filler under the angles of the mouth, often extending all the way to the prejowl sulcus to simultaneously correct loss of soft tissue support in the area. Poor dental support caused by loss of teeth also contributes to this, and should be kept in mind (refer to the section on fillers).

Puckered or "Popply" Chin

In a lot of people both men and women, mostly the latter, contractions of a hyperactive mentalis cause a puckering of the chin—localized or generalized across the front of the chin. Many people involuntarily keep puckering their chin, but in the elderly where there is resorption of the bone in the chin area, a hyperactive mentalis causes the chin to ride upward in the front of the mandible. This can be well brought out by making the surprised look action with eversion of the lower lip.

The paired mentalis muscles arise from either side of the midline from the incisive fossa and insert into the skin of the front of the chin over a wide area. In a cleft chin the fibers do not meet in the midline. Some fibers also decussate with the

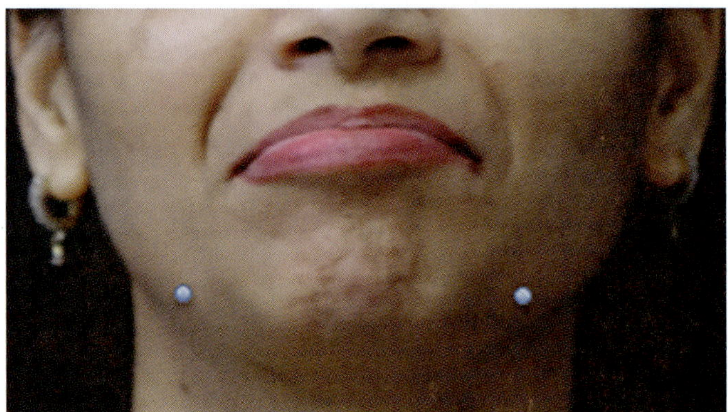

Fig. 8.18 Injection points for the depressor anguli oris.

orbicularis in the upper part and with the DAO laterally. It elevates the chin, causes chin of the front of chin to pucker, and helps in eversion of the lower lip.

Toxin injection into the mentalis is used to treat chin dimpling, as well as helping the chin not ride upward while speaking, which gives an impression of decreased vertical height of the lower third of face, as well as increasing depth of the labiomental crease. Usually 2 to 4 U of botulinum toxin is injected in 2 points deep into the muscle in front of the mental protuberance.[36] This is adequate if the chin is cleft, or wide and square. However, in a narrow and pointed chin, this may lead to diffusion laterally into the DLI muscle, and therefore many people prefer to inject 4 U in a single point in the midline in the lower half of the muscle **(Fig. 8.19a–c)**.

A popply chin might require diluted toxin to be injected very superficially at multiple points. Fillers may be required after 2 weeks to improve chin position and contour, as well as to efface the labiomental groove. BontA injection is preferably made in the chin prominence at one point in the midline or at 2 points very close to the midline to avoid lateral diffusion into the DLI (**Fig. 8.19a–c**). A popply chin may require a more superficial injection with very diluted BontA strength.

Adverse Effects

Injection of toxin into the perioral lines can cause difficulty in speaking, whistling, pouting, or blowing which usually lasts for a few days in almost every patient. However, if higher

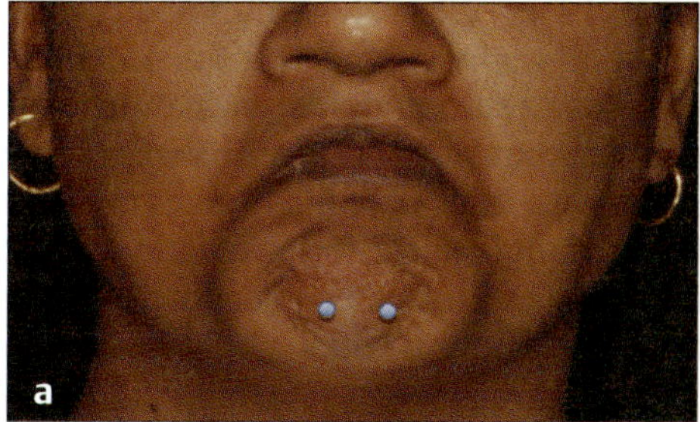

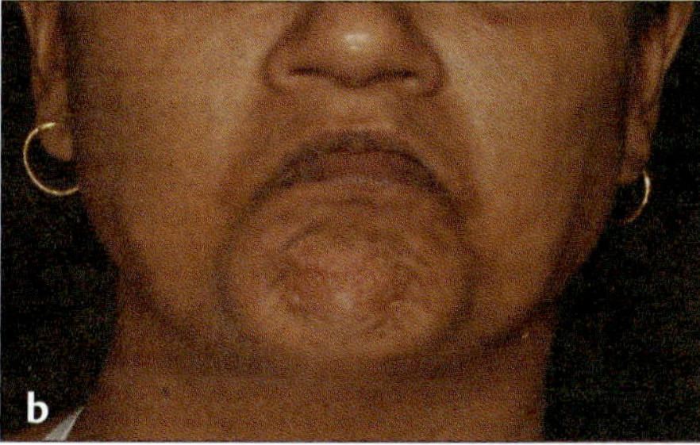

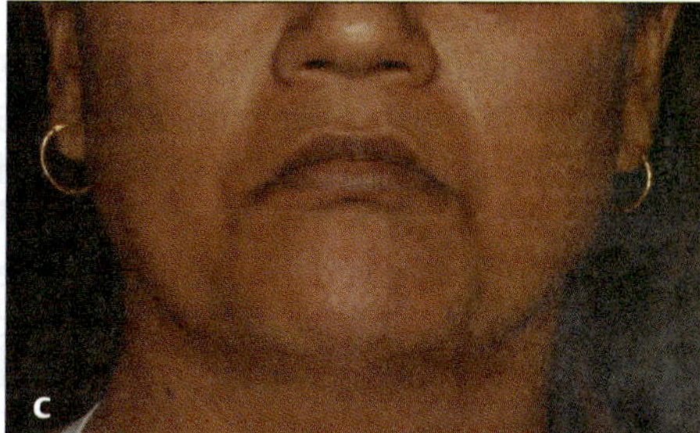

Fig. 8.19 **(a)** Hyperactive mentalis causing severe puckering of the chin in a wide square chin. Three to four units of toxin is injected at each of the two points deep into the muscle. **(b)** Pretreatment picture showing the puckering caused by an active pair of mentalis muscles. **(c)** Posttoxin and hyaluronic acid (HA) filler to chin. Four units of botulinum toxin A were injected into the mentalis muscle in the midline followed 2 weeks later by HA filler injection in the chin area.

doses are injected, all these symptoms become more severe and persist till the effect goes away. Also, drooling can occur in some cases. Injection into the philtrum is avoided as it results in flattening of the same. The points to be injected should be symmetrical and equal in dose, otherwise asymmetry can result. Orbicularis oris is the only inverter of the lips, and paralysis can lead to loss of sphincter control as well as difficulty in pronouncing bilabial sounds, making public speaking difficult.

The DAO is another muscle where one can easily get into trouble by injecting close to the DLI especially in the area where fibers of muscles overlap as they both originate from the oblique line of the mandible. Since the DLI lies deeper and partially anterior to the DAO, the injections should be kept superficial and in the posterior and inferior parts of the DAO. If toxin diffuses into the DLI, it produces a classic deformity caused by inability to pull the affected half of the lip downward while speaking (**Fig. 8.20**).

When the mentalis is injected at two points, one should be careful about diffusion into the DLI laterally, or the orbicularis upwards. Massage of the chin should especially be avoided, to avoid dispersal of toxin. Too high a dose can lead to dribbling of liquid while drinking.

The DAO, DLI, and the mentalis are all evertors of the lower lip.[37] If we manage to block all three, the DAO and mentalis by design, and the DLI by accidental diffusion, it can cause severe inversion of the lip along with involuntary biting of the lower lip and buccal mucosa.

While injecting the lower face we should take note that the lower face muscles are small, thin, of lower mass, and so need less toxin to show response. They are not forgiving when overdosed and can easily result in complications.

Injectable Fillers

Fat was one of the earliest fillers used in the face, which has gradually evolved into microfat and nanofat transfer, refueling interest with the current body of work in stem cells. Collagen as a filler was widely used in the 1980s and 1990s but its limitation was the short duration of effect (3–4 mo),

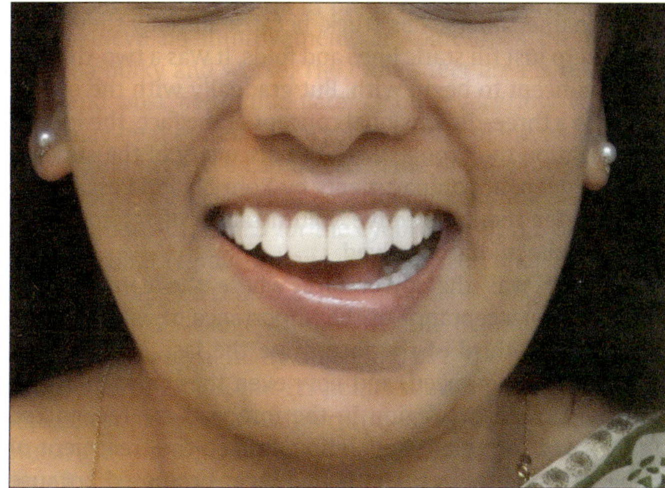

Fig. 8.20 Botulinum toxin A injection into the depressor anguli oris (DAO) on the right side has diffused into the right depressor labii inferioris (DLI) causing lower lip to remain up while smiling. (The image is provided courtesy of Dr Chytra Anand, Bengaluru, Karnataka, India.)

and its delayed hypersensitivity. Collagen as a filler occupied pride of place till the Hylan (hyaluronic acid) gels came in.

In 2003, Restylane was the first HA product to get FDA approval. HA was discovered at Columbia University by Karl Meyer and John Palmer.[38] They isolated it in bovine vitreous humor in 1943. HA is a polymer of disaccharides composed of D-glucuronic acid and DN-acetyl glucosamine, which has widely been used as a filler to treat rhytides, folds, and volume loss in recent times. HA acts as a scaffold for elastin and collagen, is hydrophilic, and can hydrate the skin. As we age, the naturally existing HA in our skin decreases, thereby leading to loss of volume, elasticity, and turgor of the skin.

Initially, extracted HA was from animal sources, but the current source of production is bacterial (NASHA—nonanimal stabilized hyaluronic acid). Hyaluronic gel can be found as biphasic or monophasic types, latter being a homogenous solution. Medical-grade silicone (Silikon 1000) was introduced in 1997 for ophthalmic use, although off-label use was permitted by FDA.[39]

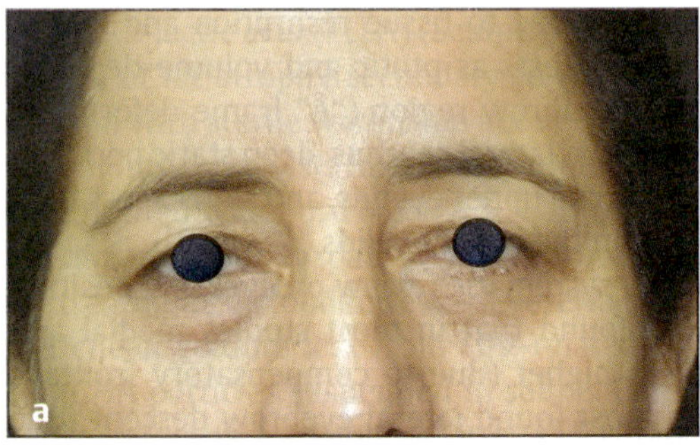

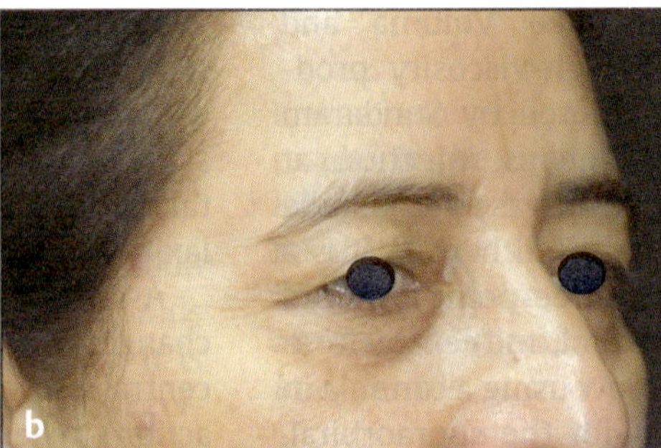

Fig. 8.24 (a, b) Sixty-year-old female showing signs of periorbital aging: ptotic lateral brow, dermatochalasis upper lid, infraorbital skin excess with eye bags, and infraorbital hollowing. Temple hollowing and eyebrow volume depletion contributing to eyebrow descent.

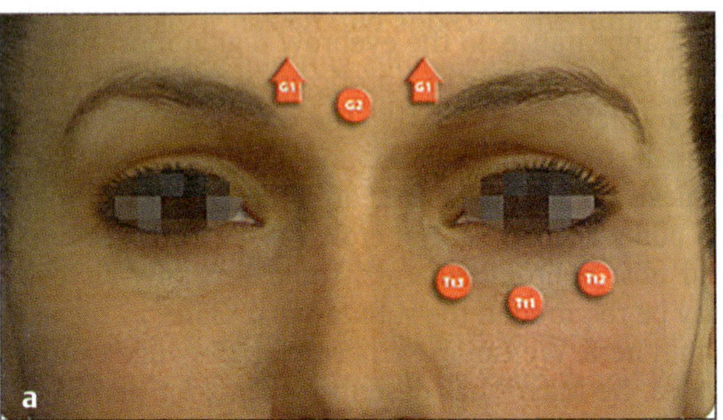

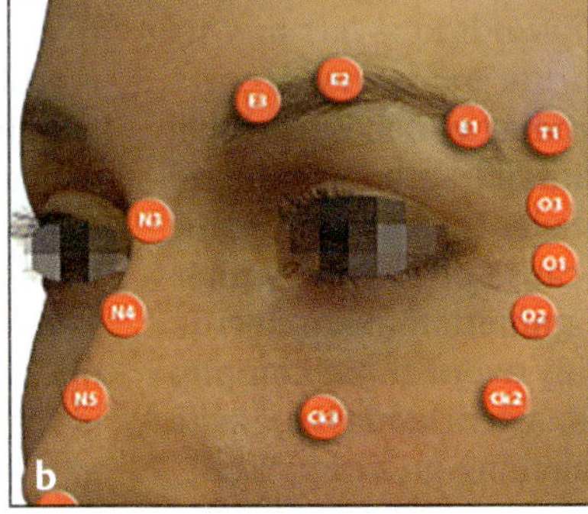

Fig. 8.25 (a, b) MD Codes points described by de Maio for periorbital rejuvenation. These are guidance points. (Adapted from de Maio 2020.[49])

Midface

Treating the midface primarily involves treating the zygomaticomalar area (lateral cheek), the infraorbital region (medial cheek), and the tear trough. For the purpose of treatment, we can use as reference Hinderer lines on the face as shown in **Fig 8.26**.

In youth, the middle third of face has a convexity which progressively flattens with age. The convexity in the mid face is maintained by the malar fat pads supported by the zygomatic bones. According to Rohrich and Pessa[43] the **malar fat pad** is divided into three compartments–medial fat compartment of the cheek (superolateral to the nasolabial fat pad), and middle and the lateral temporal-cheek fat. The zygomaticomalar region contributes to the lateral projection on the face due to the projection of the zygomatic bone. In childhood, this part is not projected but it reaches maximum development in the second decade.

The lateral suborbicularis oculi fat (SOOF) and the malar fat pad are responsible for the projection of the most anterior part of the cheek. The aging of the adipose compartments have a central role in facial aging. Aging is happening because of both ptosis of soft tissues (fat and skin) and the hypotrophy of the deep fat compartment. The reduction of volume in the deep fat compartments leaves the overlying superficial fat compartments and skin unsupported. Loss of deep midfacial fat leads to loss of support for both the medial cheek fat and the lower eyelid, with unmasking of the infraorbital rim and the orbital fat. This also contributes to the exaggerated nasolabial folds (NLFs) **(Fig. 8.27)**.

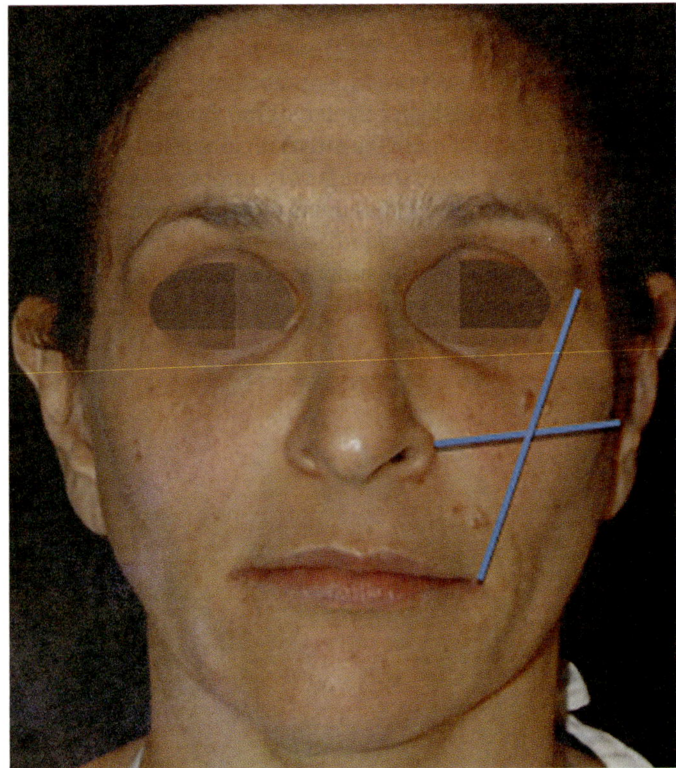

Fig. 8.26 Hinderer lines divide the midface into four compartments: medial malar, lateral malar, submalar, and area superolateral to the nasolabial fold (one line is drawn from the tragus to the alar groove and another one from the lateral end of the eyebrow to the oral commissure).

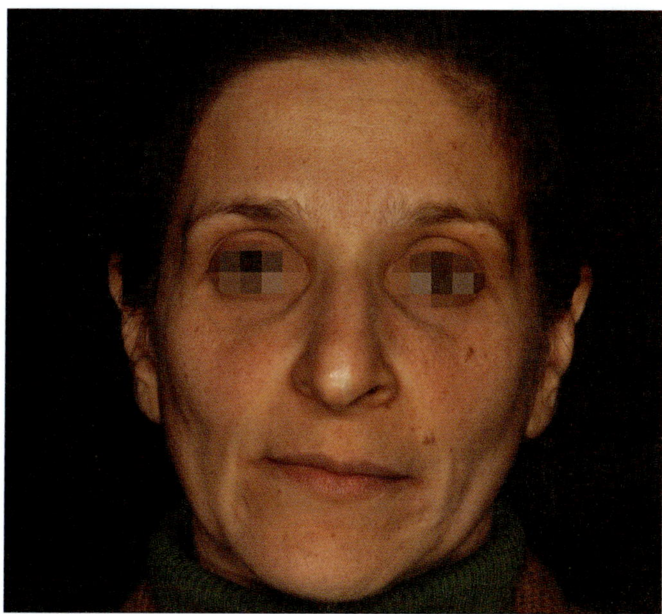

Fig. 8.27 The aging midface in a 47-year-old Indian lady. There is aging in four layers: bone, muscle, fat pads, and skin.

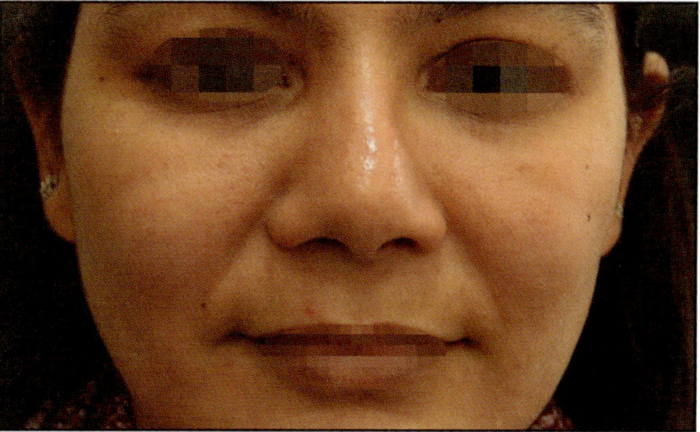

Fig. 8.28 "Midcheek groove" seen in a young lady. It corresponds to the site of the zygomatic ligament, and is a continuation of the nasojugal groove laterally. "Tear trough" extends from medial canthus to midpupil, "nasojugal groove" from midpupil to lateral canthus, and "midcheek groove" beyond that.

There are numerous retaining ligaments in the midface and attenuation of these ligaments with age also is known to contribute to ptosis of soft tissues. The zygomatic ligament is formed at the confluence of septa where all three compartments meet, and corresponds to the midcheek groove (**Fig. 8.28**).

The hollows appear where the ligaments are attached, and the bulges where the ptotic fat pads descend (**Fig. 8.28**). Pessa[53] has shown that with age there is a posterior inferior rotation of the skeleton toward the base of the skull. This reduces the bony support to the soft tissues, and happens much later in life.

Skin laxity, ligamentous laxity, atrophy of deep fat compartments with simultaneous hypertrophy of superficial fat compartments, and later in life bony remodeling all contribute to aging of the face (**Fig. 8.27**).

Tear Trough

The tear trough is a commonly seen facial feature in the Indian face, appearing sometimes in the teens, and which worsens as we age. It is an infraorbital depression starting at the medial canthus, and extending inferolaterally along the lower orbital rim and from the midpupillary point may continue into the nasojugal fold and more laterally into the midcheek groove. The tear trough is a significant area of concern in the Indian face. Majority of Indians suffer from varying degrees of tear trough because of anatomical considerations such as deep set eyes, recessed infraorbital rim, and deficient soft tissue support in relation to the lower eyelids.

Technique

It is widely believed that the deep compartment of the midface should be volumized first, thereby lifting the cheeks to a varying extent, spontaneously improving the NLFs and bringing down the filler volume requirement of the tear trough and the nasojugal fold, as well as that of the NLF.

When volumizing with fillers, we can inject with needle or microcannulas. We can use the linear fan technique or give supraperiosteal bolus injections. Selection of the appropriate technique depends on various factors—the age of the patient, the degree of volume loss, quality of overlying skin, degree of skin laxity, area to be injected, vascular pattern in the area, possible risk of arterial complications associated with that region, and largely also depends on the skill sets of the injector.

In younger subjects, an eight-point lift has been described by Mauricio de Maio,[54] which provides boluses of filler in the zygomatic arch area, lateral malar and medial malar area, the nasolabial groove (upper one-fourth), below the angles of mouth for support, prejowl sulcus, angle of mandible, and the hollow buccal region (**Fig. 8.29**).

Patients who have very little skin laxity and mild degree of volume loss will benefit greatly from this technique, also at the same time economizing on the amount of filler used. However, this approach may not work in older patients with more volume loss and significant degree of skin laxity. In the latter, volume has to be primarily replaced in the deep fat compartments, and also borrow in addition, some of the points of the 8 point lift. Midface filling is easier with a single point in the lateral malar area entering the prezygomatic space, going up to the tear trough and the nasojugal fold (**Fig. 8.30**).

Pain relief is good with Xylocaine 2% with adrenaline at the point of entry of the cannula and a zygomaticofacial nerve block (placed on the summit of the zygoma), aided by lidocaine combined fillers. The tear trough can also be filled separately using a 25-gauge cannula entering from the midcheek area (**Fig. 8.31**).

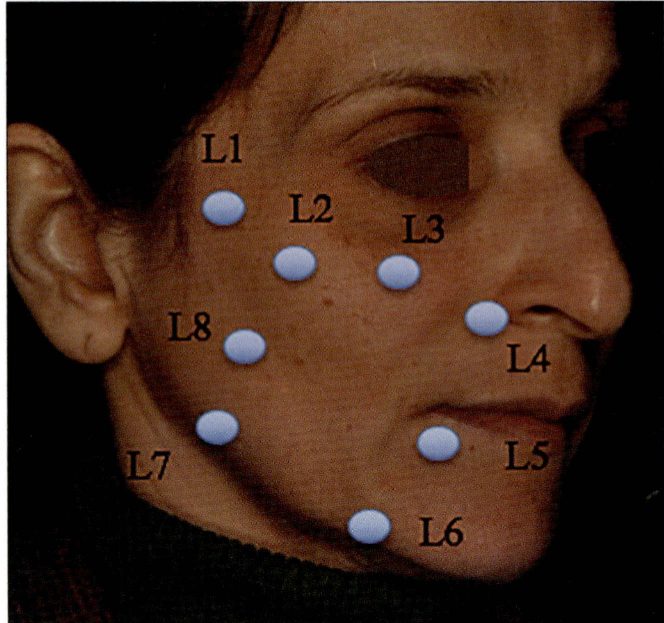

Fig. 8.29 Eight-point lift as described by de Maio. L1: zygomatic arch, L2: body of zygoma, L3: medial malar, L4: piriform fossa, L5: below oral commissure, L6: prejowl sulcus, L7: angle of mandible, L8: preauricular/buccal hollow.

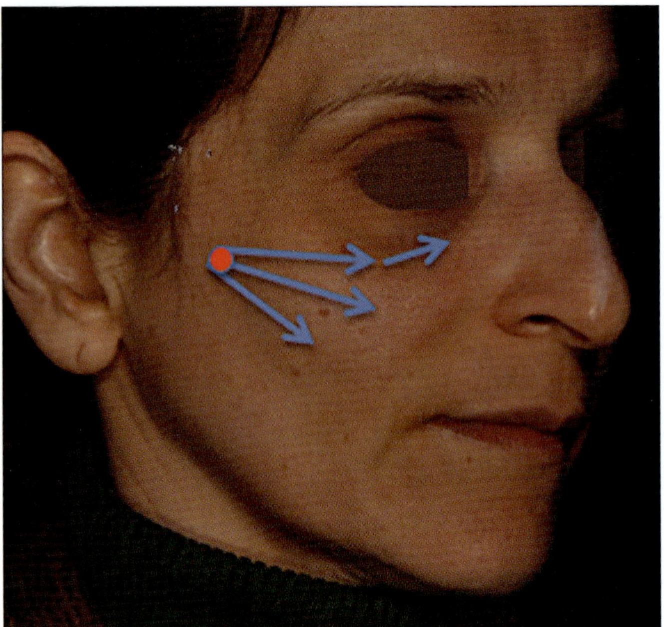

Fig. 8.30 Midface volumization via an access point (*red dot*) above the zygomatic ligament into the prezygomatic space, suborbicularis oculi fat (SOOF), tear trough, and deep medial cheek fat compartment. Same access point can then be used to fill superficially bilayered approach. Usually a 25-gauge blunt flexible cannula is used.

It is preferable to treat the tear trough with a low- or medium-density filler placed supraperiosteally, deep to the orbicularis oculi muscle in the area of the SOOF. The most medial part of the tear trough is challenging to correct as the orbicularis muscle is attached to the bone with the medial-most part of the orbicularis-retaining ligament (ORL) called the tear-trough ligament and it is not possible to inject beneath it. Also, there is practically no fat support under the skin and skin quality is often compromised. In the tear-trough region there is a risk of overcorrection with fillers making the product visible and palpable. If the product is placed superficially it becomes visible as a bluish discoloration (Tyndall effect).

If there are preexisting malar bags, then while correcting the tear trough, one may aggravate the malar edema. In such cases, one should avoid injecting into the medial SOOF. A low G′ filler placed supraperiosteally in small amounts is the key to a good result, and also avoids what is called the FOS (facial overfilled syndrome) described by Cotofana et al.[55]

Lateral SOOF

This is injected using a needle in boluses with a high G′ filler supraperiosteally, or with a cannula as part of a lifting and volumizing combination. Casabona et al in 2019[56] demonstrated that filler injection in the lateral SOOF (i.e., lateral to the line of ligaments separating the medial from lateral face) will have a significant lifting effect, and therefore will reposition displaced tissues, making volumization easier and resulting in less volume of filler needed for volumizing the medial part. In another study Casabona et al[57] using a cannula showed that injecting the G point (corresponding to the lateral SOOF) alone shows a significant lift of the lower lid, inferior aspect of ala of nose, angle of mouth, and dermal location of the mandibular ligament.

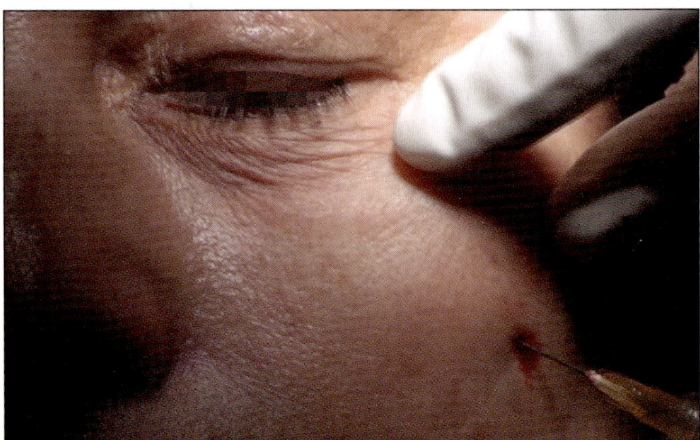

Fig. 8.31 Access to tear trough from the midcheek area with a 25-gauge cannula.

So, lateral injection leads to a lift, whereas medial injection leads to volumization. Also, the lateral SOOF injection is the most efficient in terms of a lift as SVC (surface volume coefficient—volume injected to lift obtained) with 0.5 mL value being 93%, and for 1 mL to be 95%.

Nasolabial Fold

This is part of the perioral area, and once the midface is done, some filler can be deposited in the upper third of the fold, deep close to the periosteum (**Figs. 8.32 and 8.33**). The facial vessels changing to angular vessels are close to the alar base, and avoiding intravascular injection is central to safety. Note is to be made that in post-facelift patients, the anatomy may be disturbed, and one has to be extra careful in avoiding adverse reactions. So, stay on the bone, aspirate before injecting, use small aliquots, and inject slowly, intermittently. The rest of the NLF is dynamic, affected by all the volumization which has been done before coming to the NLF, viz., the temple, zygomatic arch, and body, and the deep medial cheek compartment. De Maio[49] has described three points for the NLF: NL1, NL2, NL3. NL1 is at the piriform fossa (described earlier as the upper one-third). The remaining two are injected in the subdermal plane in very small amounts by linear threading to just efface the sharpness.

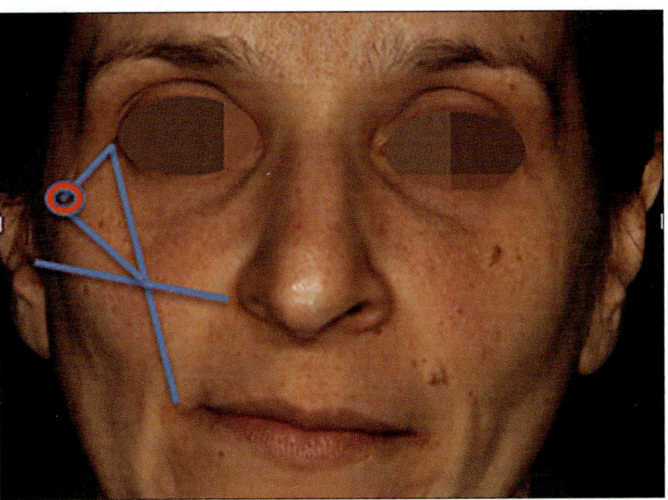

Fig. 8.32 "G" point described by Casabona[57] presenting lateral suborbicularis oculi fat (SOOF) to achieve optimum lift, so that tissues are lifted to more optimum position so that volume required in the medial face is reduced.

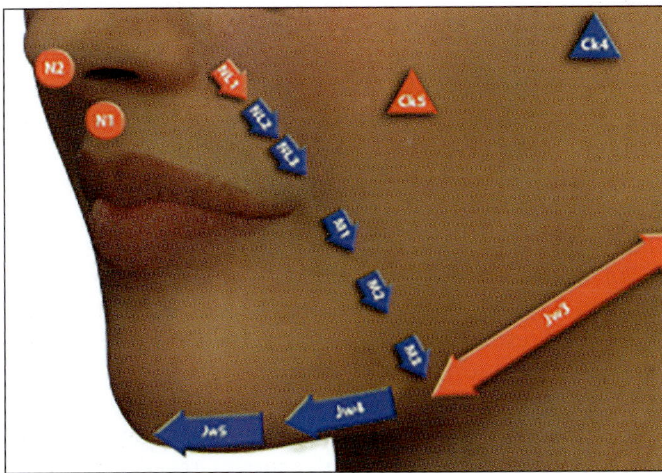

Fig. 8.33 MD Codes for nasolabial folds: NL1, NL2, NL3. These are guidance points. (Adapted from de Maio 2020.[49])

Nose

The nose is an area which will be of special interest to plastic surgeons, as many patients are not willing to undergo surgery for minor imperfections of the nose. Also, many with low-profile noses are not sure of whether they will like the augmented look. So they get nasal augmentation done using filler as a trial, and progress to a surgical rhinoplasty later.

Technique

A complete nerve block is given to the nose, like that given for a rhinoplasty under local anesthesia. The point of entry is planned in the infratip area. Using a 23- or 25-gauge, 50-mm cannula, the dorsum, supratip, nasolabial angle, and the columella can be augmented. In cases who have premaxillary hypoplasia, subalar injection and injection lateral to the alar base are also done, which helps in narrowing of the nostrils to a certain extent (**Figs. 8.34 and 8.35**). A secondary benefit arising from augmentation of the low-profile dorsum in an oriental-featured person is that it reduces/eliminates epicanthal folds (**Fig. 8.36**).

A needle is preferred over a cannula by many injectors for nasal augmentation, using a direct approach in the midline. The preperiosteal plane is injected proximally and the distal half preperichondrially.[58,59] Postrhinoplasty minor aberrations like mild residual deviation of the dorsum or a depression can be corrected easily using a filler. Caution has to be observed to avoid vascular complications in this area.[59]

Lower Face

Lower face is a very interesting area for rejuvenation as it is very important for the pleasant appearance of the face. A well-contoured jawline is desirable in men and women,

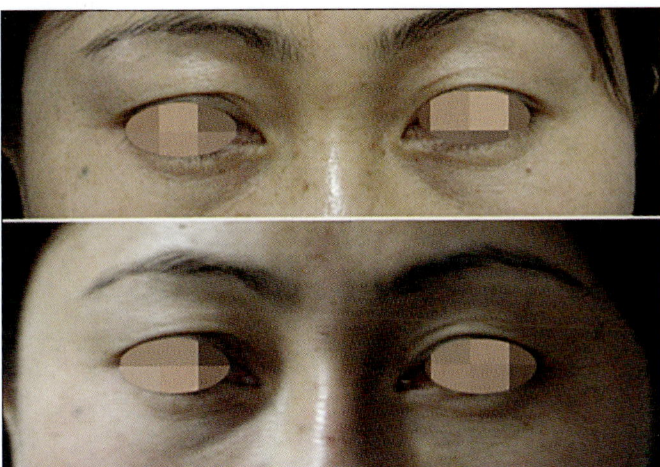

Fig. 8.34 Raising the bridge in oriental noses has the additional benefit of effacing in the epicanthal folds.

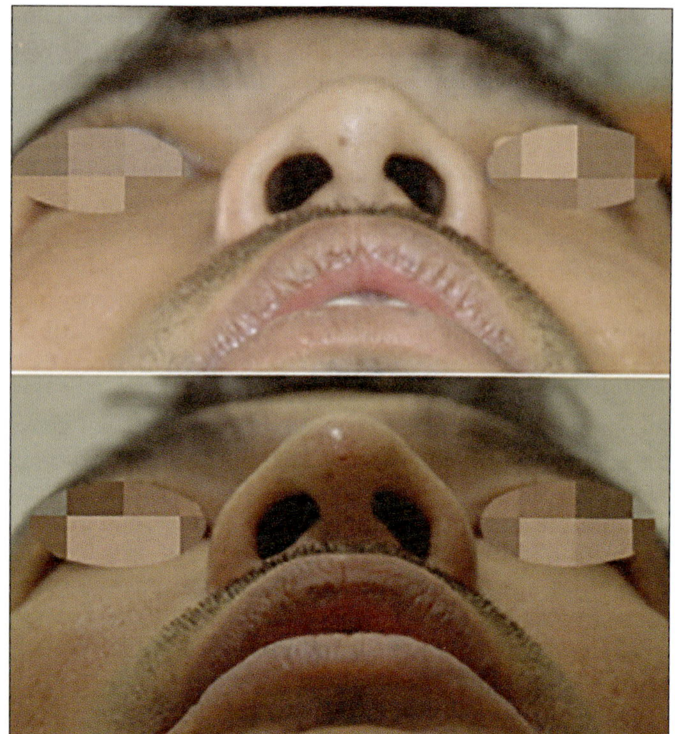

Fig. 8.35 Nasal tip can be reshaped to make it sharper and more projecting.

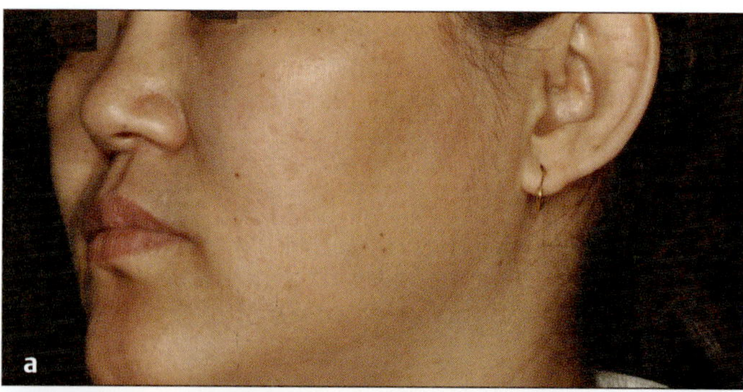

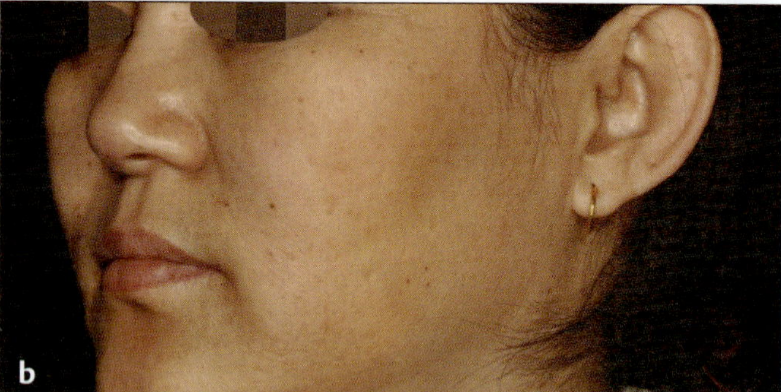

Fig. 8.36 Nonsurgical rhinoplasty in an oriental nose elevating the whole dorsum from the radix to the tip, also correcting the maxillary retrusion and improving the profile (inclination and length) of the upper lip to enable a comfortable lip closure at rest.

giving a perception of beauty and youth. It is also key to sexual dimorphism, defining male and female characteristics. The nonsurgical rejuvenation and beautification of the lower third of the face is becoming more frequent. Injectable fillers can reshape the jawline, lift soft tissues, and improve facial proportions, effectively improving the appearance of the area. This area is amenable to surgical rejuvenation procedures and many a times combined approach gives highly satisfactory result.

Perioral Rejuvenation

Aging shows early on in the perioral region. This would include the lips, areas above and below, smokers' lines (bar code), marionette lines, and chin. The aging lips show progressive loss of volume and structure. They lose definition as the philtral columns and cupids bow fade, the upper lip becoming thin and elongated and convex, while the lower lip becomes thin and inverted.[60] The elongated upper lip falls over the lip angles and becomes continuous with the marionette line worsening its appearance **(Fig. 8.37)**. Better results are achieved by combining fillers with neuromodulators. It is always advisable to have a conservative approach by using lesser product. Permanent fillers should be avoided in the lips, and BontA dose used in the lips should be very small as the perioral muscles are very small and there is atrophy with age.

Technique

When treating lips with filler we have to restore definition, add volume to lip bulk, correct asymmetry, lift lip angles, and support the lower lip at the commissures by filling the marionette triangle **(Fig. 8.38)**.

Fillers offer good support to the hollow under the angles of mouth which was causing them to downturn, and injection of supporting bars of filler right along the marionette line to the prejowl sulcus will support the angle of mouth even better (**Fig. 8.37**). One should always assess dental alignment and labial/buccal support before planning filler in this area.

The lips can be enhanced by defining the white rolls with subdermal filler placement, augmenting the flattened philtral ridges, and restoring volume to the vermillion if needed (**Fig. 8.38a, b**). Medium-to-thin viscosity fillers serve our purpose. The injections are mostly made by needle, and not by cannula. It is good to keep filler in separate compartments in the lip. Safe injection area is the dry part of vermillion and in the subcutaneous plane.

For smokers' lines, BontA injections as mentioned in the segment on toxin, and streaks of filler in the smokers' lines give a good result **(Fig. 8.17)**. Perioral rejuvenation with fillers is combined usually with neuromodulators for the DAO and the mentalis, as these two muscles, if hyperactive, pull the angles of mouth down and the lower lip down, respectively. Always try to slightly under correct, review at 2 weeks and add any more filler if that is needed.

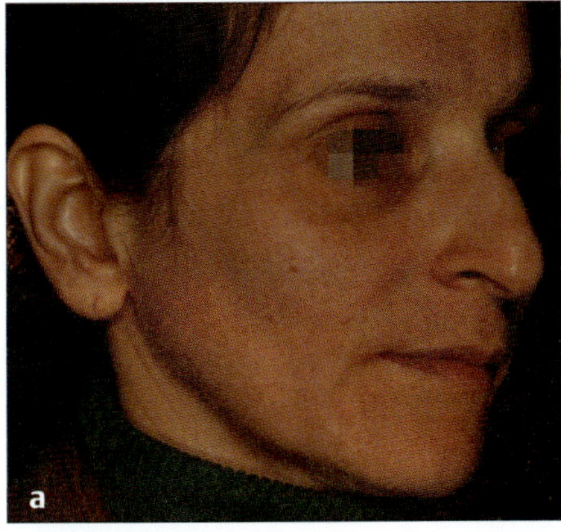

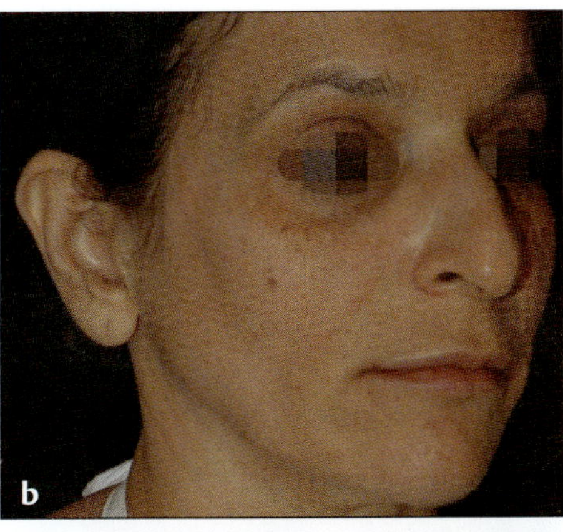

Fig. 8.37 Perioral rejuvenation with hyaluronic acid (HA) fillers. HA fillers were injected in the nasolabial fold, marionette lines, marionette triangle, lips, mental crease, and chin.

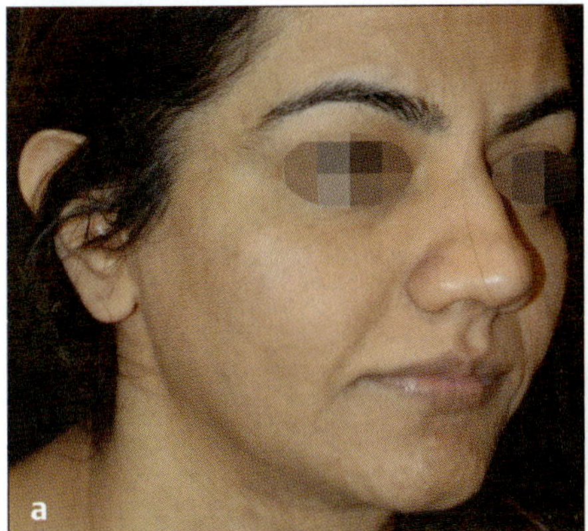

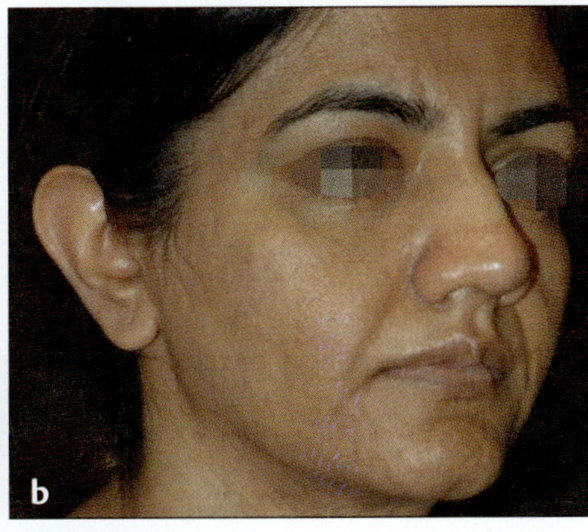

Fig. 8.38 **(a)** A 45-year-old lady with loss of lip volume and definition of lip margin. **(b)** One mL hyaluronic acid (HA) filler was used to improve the angle of the lips, white roll, philtral creases, and lip volume.

Marionette Folds/Lines

These lines are responsible for droopy lips and the sad and aging look. Initially, aging starts as the marionette line appears, and with progressive underlying soft tissue loss, it develops into the marionette triangle. Then, aided by a hyperactive DAO, the fold extends vertically downward from the commissure to the prejowl sulcus at the site of the mandibular ligament.

Technique

In an aging face, it is prudent to start by lifting and repositioning the midface before treating the perioral region. Having dealt with the midface, using a needle we can start by placing an HA filler of medium viscosity under the oral commissure in a triangle medial to the marionette line to support the lateral lower lip from below (M1) (**Fig. 8.39**). In case the marionette triangle is wider, then we can use a 25-gauge cannula to evenly fill and support it. The remainder of the fold has to be filled for two reasons: one is to construct a continuous pillar of filler to support the commissure, and second to efface the marionette fold, injecting in the subdermal plane. The lowest point (M3) coincides with the prejowl sulcus where the injection is done at the preperiosteal level. In younger people a hyperactive DAO is usually the reason, but associated poor dental canine and premolar support may need fillers in addition to the toxin (**Fig. 8.40**).

Chin

This is one of the least understood features of the face in the process of aesthetic facial improvement. A person with a well-formed and projected chin is perceived to have a strong personality, with a recessed chin implying weakness and an indecisive nature. This may be totally untrue but appearances do matter. We often notice that people with chin deficiency tend to grow beards to make themselves look aesthetically appealing. Some of the chins where implants are done can be suitably managed by filler injections, though the injections will have to be repeated every year. However, mandibular dimorphism with coexistent malocclusion (Class II) needs to be ruled out because that should be treated surgically.[61] The aging chin loses underlying soft and bony tissue, with the overlying skin becoming lax and irregular, and coupled with a hyperactive mentalis, the chin rides upward.

Technique

We place HA fillers with high viscosity and high G′ supraperiosteally to add anterior projection and elongation of the chin. This can be done precisely with a needle though many clinicians prefer to combine it with a cannula. In women, the effort is to keep the chin narrow, whereas in men it is kept more square. Additional filler may be required in the superficial planes also, as the deep fat compartment is small and cannot accommodate much filler. Often if there

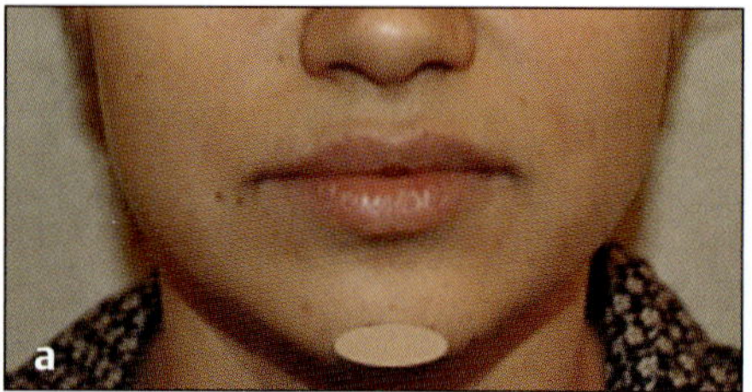

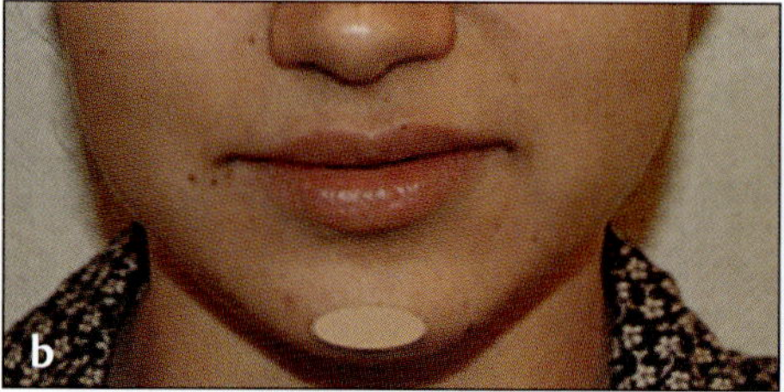

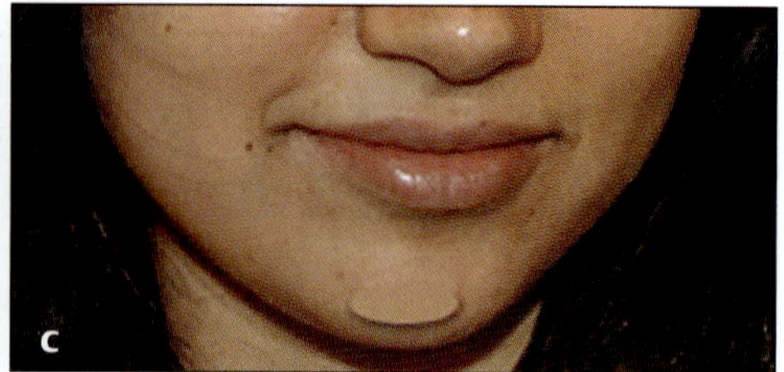

Fig. 8.39 **(a)** A 26-year-old lady with a sad expression due to downturned angles because of a hyperactive depressor anguli oris (DAO) and poor support behind the angles of mouth. **(b)** After Botulinum toxin in the DAO. **(c)** Two weeks later filler under the commissures and the M1, M2, and M3 points of MD Codes were needed because of poor soft tissue support.

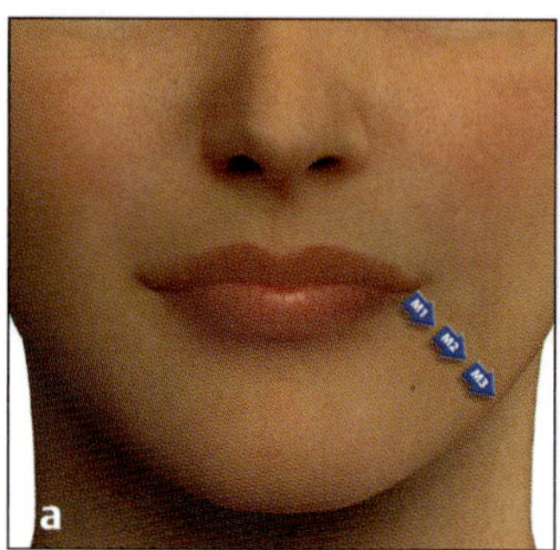

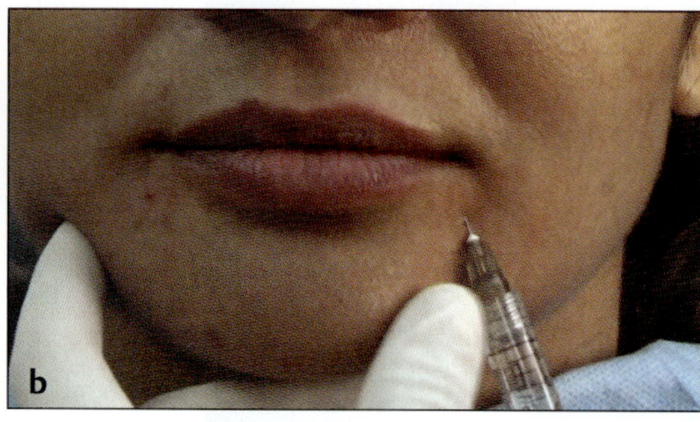

Fig. 8.40 (**a**) MD Codes for marionette lines.[49] **(b)** Injecting under the commissure (M1) with needle.

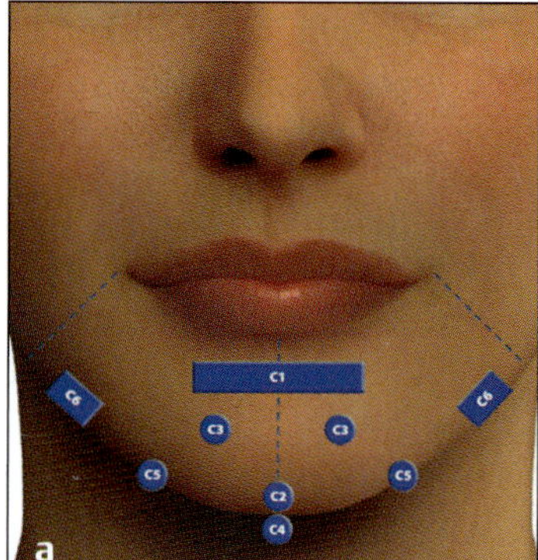

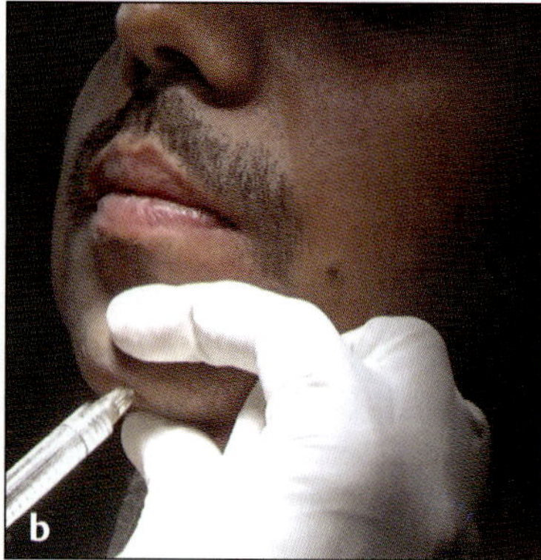

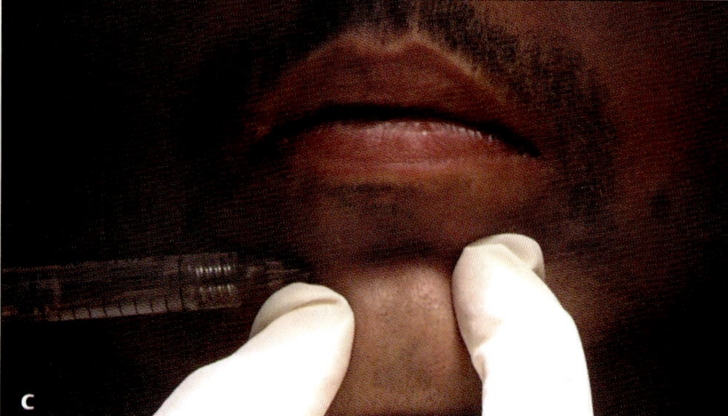

Fig. 8.41 **(a)** Chin MD Codes.[49] **(b)** Injecting the deep fat compartment of the chin at C2. **(c)** Injecting the labiomandibular groove: C1. Caution: Injecting too deep may end up piercing the lip mucosa.

is a coexisting hyperactive mentalis, Botulinum toxin A is injected in the midline, with 2 to 4 U helping to relax the chin. It also prevents migration of filler, as well as increases longevity of filler. Filler alone also creates a mechanical block to the hyperactivity of the mentalis muscle and thereby smoothens the chin. MD Codes for the chin as described by de Maio[49] gives one a good guide to assessing, injecting, and documenting chin filler injection (**Fig. 8.41**).

Jawline

The lower face is very significant as far as perception of aging is concerned. Many women seek aesthetic medical intervention when they notice appearance of jowls and a sagging jawline. The reasons for an aging jawline are multiple, ranging from skin laxity, relative decrease in fat compartments, and absorption of bone on the mandible, resulting in a jowl, prejowl sulcus, and a poorly defined jawline. The jawline should be straight and smooth from the chin to the gonial angle. The gonial angle measured by Upadhyay et al in 2012[62] was 129 degrees with no difference in men and women, and horizontally lies at the level of the oral commissure. The jawline is more horizontal in men, with the angle prominent and everted.

Technique

To improve the jawline we need a more comprehensive approach than just treating the jawline itself. For best results we need to address the middle face first, followed by the lower face. We treat from superiorly to inferiorly. The filler (HA fillers commonly) can be injected either by needle, or a combination of needle and cannulas. Once the midface filler injections help reposition the tissues by lifting them, the jawline can be defined and enhanced from the chin to the angle of mandible.

Given below are the points and the sequence of injecting to get optimal results.[49] Also mentioned is the depth (plane) of injection, with approximately 0.05 to 0.1 mL per injection in case of a needle being used (**Figs. 8.42 and 8.43**):

- Lateral cheek lift by injecting at the zygomatic arch—supraperiosteal.
- Lateral cheek lift by injecting at the zygomatic eminence—supraperiosteal.
- Anterior projection of the cheek, (i.e., the medial malar area)—supraperiosteal.
- Upper preauricular region—subcutaneous.
- Lower preauricular region inferior to the tragus—subcutaneous.
- Mandibular angle—supraperiosteal.[63]
- Postjowl sulcus—supraperiosteal and subcutaneous both.
- Prejowl sulcus—supraperiosteal and subcutaneous both.
- Marionette triangle—subcutaneous.
- Chin—supraperiosteal and subcutaneous both.

For a subcutaneous injection on the jaw line into the superficial fat compartment, it is advisable to pinch the skin to avoid the facial vessels at the anteroinferior angle of the masseter.[63] It is important not to inject into the jowl bulge as it will exaggerate it. The jowl is the no go zone while improving the definition of the jawline.

Adverse Effects of Fillers

Soft tissue augmentation is among the most popular aesthetic procedures in the world today. With proper training of anatomy, injection technique, and asepsis, results are pleasing and well tolerated. Still, in the best of hands, complications can occur. An in-depth knowledge of side effects is essential for early detection and treatment of these complications.

Though generally safe, complications can occur with temporary fillers. Compared to temporary fillers, permanent filler complications are difficult to treat since the product does not dissipate and remains in the body. The products available for augmentation can be divided into biodegradable, semibiodegradable, and nonbiodegradable. This classification correlates with the longevity of the results—as being temporary (results last 6–12 mo), semipermanent (duration up to 18 mo), or permanent (up to a lifetime). The complications may be injector related, patient related, or product related.

The most frequent, early onset complications with fillers are related to the injection site, such as pain, erythema, edema, ecchymosis, and bruising. These mostly resolve in 4 to 7 days and patient should be made aware prior to the procedure. Other complications are inappropriately placed filler,[64] vascular occlusion, hypersensitivity, malar edema, and paresthesias. Delayed onset complications include delayed onset edema, inflammatory and noninflammatory nodules, biofilms, and delayed hypersensitivity.

Pain

This is due to hydrostatic separation of the tissue during the injection as well as due to multiple needle punctures. Pain can be minimized by topical anesthetic creams, icing, distraction techniques, and inclusion of lidocaine in the filler material which now comes in prepackaged syringes.

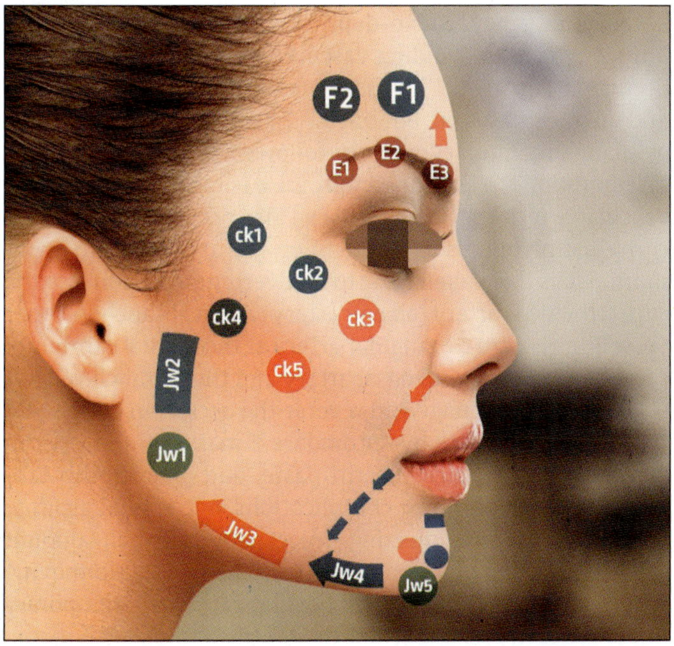

Fig. 8.42 Jawline rejuvenation schema. (Adapted from de Maio 2020[49].)

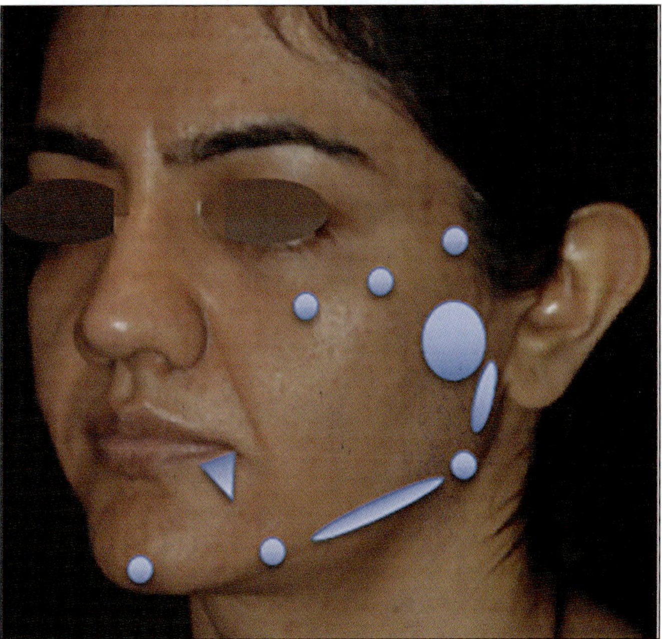

Fig. 8.43 Comprehensive 10-point jawline rejuvenation will get optimal results.

Edema and Bruising

HA fillers are known to cause injection site–related edema and bruising. Bruising is due to extravasation of blood due to puncturing a vein inadvertently, or due to preexistent coagulopathies. Chances of bruising can be minimized by avoiding highly vascular areas, using smaller gauge needles (27–31 gauge), slower injections, injecting smaller volumes in one prick, minimizing the number of pricks, or using blunt cannulas.

It is advisable to discontinue blood thinning medications in case it is safe to do so about 7 days prior to injection. To reduce bruising during the procedure it is advisable to apply firm pressure on the site of bleeding, apply cold compresses, and topical vitamin K cream postprocedure.[65]

Erythema

It is caused by hyperemia of superficial capillaries, can also occur postmassage, and is usually temporary. Mostly nothing is needed for erythema, but if it persists then antihistamines, medium potency topical steroid, and Vitamin K creams can be prescribed. If redness persists for several days it may be indicative of hypersensitivity.

Infections

As with any procedure that breaches the skin, acute skin infections can occur after fillers injections and could be bacterial, fungal, or viral. Acute infections can be minimized by more stringent aseptic cleaning techniques utilizing alcohol or chlorhexidine. Acute bacterial infections which are most likely seen are due to staphylococcus and streptococcus, and may present as single or multiple tender erythematous and/or fluctuant nodules. These may be accompanied by fever and fatigue. Infections should not be confused with hypersensitivity reactions which is accompanied by itching and absence of fever.[66]

Early onset skin infections should be treated immediately with oral antibiotics against *Staphylococcus aureus*. In more serious cases IV antibiotics should be administered. When a lesion that appears infectious in nature appears more than 2 weeks after the filler injection, it may be suggestive of an atypical mycobacterial infection. An infection may rarely manifest as an abscess from one week to several years after the treatment.

Rarely (in <1.5%), there may be reactivation of herpes that may occur 24 to 48 hours postinjection. Postfiller if herpes is activated, it should be treated with antiviral therapy and appropriate antibiotics.

Nodules and Lumps

Sometimes inadequate assessment, improper injection technique, and incorrect placement of product may result in placement of too much volume in a small area, resulting in visible lumps. These are very evident in the periorbital and perioral areas. Persistent nodules and lumps are normally resistant to the normal HA degradation process and may not resolve spontaneously. They can be reversed by hyaluronidase injections intralesionally.[67]

Tyndall Effect

In the tear-trough region, a bluish discoloration is observed over the injected area. This is due to injecting excessive product of a high G′ in too superficial a plane. This is due to a Tyndall effect, (i.e., scattering of light by particles in a suspension). High-frequency blue light is scattered more easily than red light by a thick layer of a high concentration filler placed superficially and becomes the predominantly visible light.

Hypersensitivity Reactions

Though rare, the reaction can manifest as acute, excessive, persistent swelling following filler injection. The reaction can last for >6 weeks. Fillers are essentially foreign bodies and some people may develop a hypersensitivity to the product as a result of IgE-mediated immune response (type 1 hypersensitivity reaction or a delayed type IV hypersensitivity).

Malar Edema

This can develop, or existing malar edema can get exaggerated, while injecting the tear troughs and periorbital hollowing in patients prone to preexisting malar edema (those with malar bags). This happens because the fillers further compromise the already compromised lymphatic circulation.[68]

Vascular Compromise

It is a rare but critical complication and should be managed as an emergency. An in-depth knowledge of facial anatomy is crucial to avoiding vascular complications. Vascular occlusion can result in tissue necrosis and disfigurement and in rare cases in blindness. Tissue necrosis manifests as blanching and severe pain followed later by violaceous discoloration.[69] Vascular compromise is mostly due to intravascular arterial occlusion and can also occur due to external compression of vessels by the filler. The area prone to maximum risk is the glabella due to inadvertent injection into the supratrochlear artery (an end artery) and its branches. Other vessels at risk are the angular artery at the medial canthus of the eye and the lateral nasal artery and their branches.

To limit the damage and reverse the occlusion one should perfuse the area with hyaluronidase,[70] massage, apply warm compresses and nitroglycerin paste, and give aspirin tablets. To prevent vascular complications, one should aspirate every time before injecting, inject slowly, small amount (<0.1 mL) in one place and also keep the needle tip moving while injecting. Though complication rates with temporary fillers are low, it is important to identify and manage them.

Full-Face Rejuvenation

Patients many times come with specific issues related to some areas of the face, like the glabellar frown lines, or tear troughs, or NLFs, or just the jowls.[71] But sometimes, they come with global issues like looking older, tired, or just not looking good. Other times, they may come with emotional issues like "I look angry, or sad, or tired." The tendency to only treat specific issues does not always bring about a happy patient or a favorable outcome.[72] This happens because the features of aging are global, and we did not assess/ appreciate the overall shape, proportions, symmetry, or sexual dimorphism in the face.

Assessment

A detailed full-face assessment should be done, which takes into account, the shape of the face, the proportions (or averageness) of different thirds of the face, symmetry, features of sexual dimorphism. Faces age differently depending on their structural framework; faces with prominent structural features like high cheekbones offer less of sag and more of deflation or volume deficiency. Contrast this with those with poor structural support to the midface, having heavy chubby faces and small lower third of faces, causing mostly descent with tissue excess in the midface making lower third deficiency even more prominent.

Planning and Execution

Note should be made as to what features are contributing to deterioration of that face, and also how that face is going to age in future. This will finally decide the general direction of our global rejuvenation plan as suggested earlier. We always start treating from the top—temples, forehead, brows—to midface lifting and volumizing, and go onto lower third which is primarily correcting proportion and restoring features (**Fig. 8.44**). Then individual features are restored and enhanced, if not already dealt with.

Faces with mild-to-moderate issues can be dealt best by combination treatments consisting not only of injectables but preceded many times by energy-based treatments which lay the groundwork for a tighter skin envelope to optimize nonsurgical treatment. A definite line should be drawn as to whether a surgical option would achieve a better outcome, entirely on its own, or with adjunctive injectable treatment in most of the cases. Unpleasant and unfavorable outcomes usually arise from trying to solve all problems with only one modality—nonsurgical or surgical.

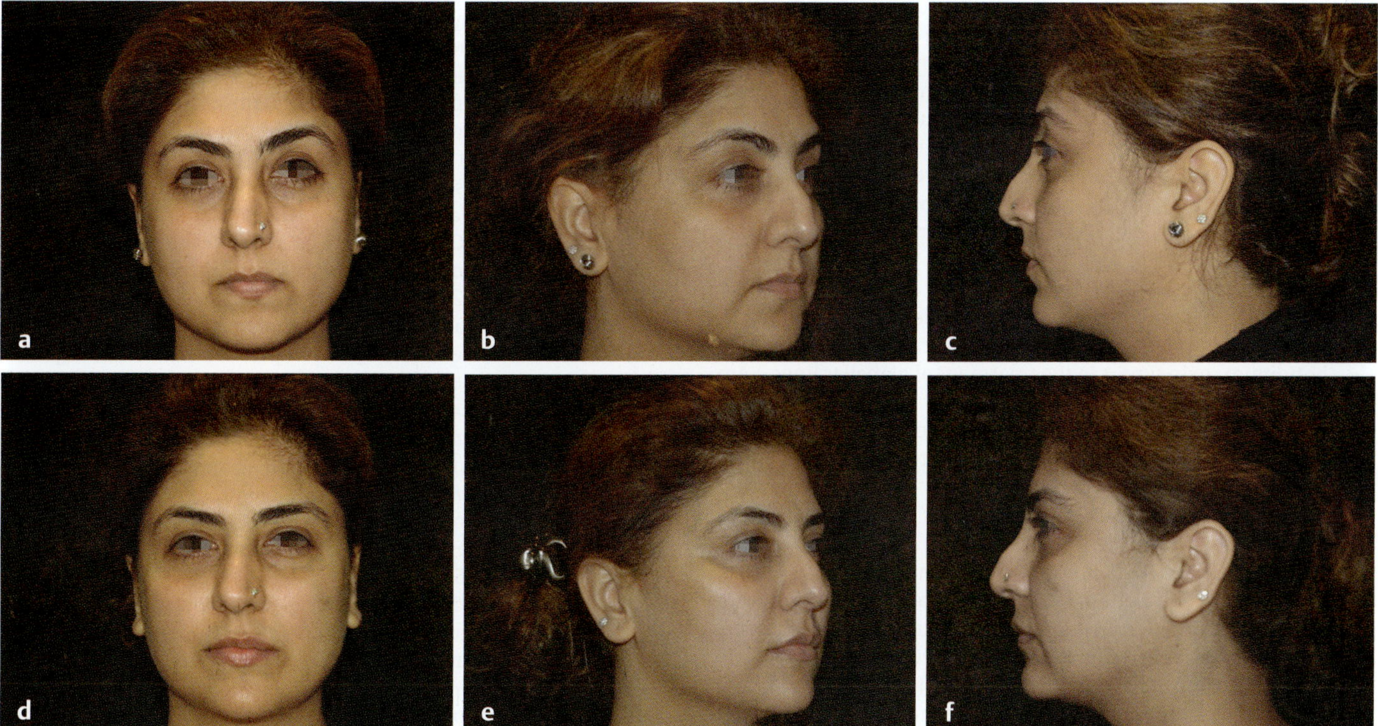

Fig. 8.44 **(a)** Frontal view: pretreatment. **(b)** Right oblique view: pretreatment. **(c)** Left profile view pretreatment. **(d)** Frontal view: post treatment—note improved chin height and proportion of lower ⅓rd of the face to middle and upper ⅓rd and raised lid cheek junction. **(e)** Right oblique view: post treatment—better positioned cheek eminence, lip profile, and chin contour. **(f)** Left profile view: post treatment—note increased chin height and improved lip profile.

Conclusion

A combination of neurotoxins and filler injections is the Gold Standard for treating the aging face by nonsurgical means. Neurotoxins work to reduce or ameliorate rhytides as well as alter facial expressions. To deliver optimal results we need to understand the functional interplay between the facial muscles. Temporary fillers are preferred to the permanent fillers. The cornerstone of a good treatment is a proper facial assessment. Satisfactory results cannot be achieved if the clinician underassesses the face or does not understand what the patient wants. Therefore, it is wise to plan a full-face treatment with fillers over multiple sessions. It is important to understand that we should inject the right product, in the right plane, in the right amount, and in the right patient. A good understanding of the facial anatomy is important to perform safe and effective treatment.

References

1. Wu W. Non-surgical facial rejuvenation with the 4R principle: innovative uses of BOTOX and facelifting with the Woffles Lift, a barbed suture sling. In: Aesthetic surgery of the facial mosaic. Berlin, Heidelberg: Springer; 2006
2. Jacono AA, Malone MH, Lavin TJ. Nonsurgical facial rejuvenation procedures in patients under 50 prior to undergoing facelift: habits, costs, and results. Aesthet Surg J 2017;37(4):448–453
3. Wollina U, Goldman A. Minimally invasive aesthetic procedures in young adults. Clin Cosmet Investig Dermatol 2011;4:19–26
4. Kapoor KM, Chatrath V, Anand C, et al On behalf of the Indian Facial Aesthetics Expert Group Consensus Recommendations for Treatment Strategies in Indians Using Botulinum Toxin and Hyaluronic Acid Fillers. Consensus recommendations for treatment strategies in Indians using botulinum toxin and hyaluronic acid fillers. Plast Reconstr Surg Glob Open 2017; 5(12):e1574
5. Carruthers JA, Lowe NJ, Menter MA, et al; BOTOX Glabellar Lines I Study Group. A multicenter, double-blind, randomized, placebo-controlled study of the efficacy and safety of botulinum toxin type A in the treatment of glabellar lines. J Am Acad Dermatol 2002;46(6):840–849
6. Beer KR, Boyd C, Patel RK, Bowen B, James SP, Brin MF. Rapid onset of response and patient-reported outcomes after onabotulinum toxin A treatment of moderate-to-severe glabellar lines. J Drugs Dermatol 2011;10(1):39–44
7. Carruthers A, Carruthers J, Lowe NJ, et al. For the BOTOX® Glabellar Lines I & II Study Groups. One-year, randomised, multicenter, two-period study of the safety and efficacy of repeated treatments with botulinum toxin type A in patients with glabellar lines. J Clin Res 2004;7:1–20
8. Beer KR, Shamban AT, Avelar RL, Gross JE, Jonker A. Efficacy and safety of prabotulinum toxin A for the treatment of glabellar lines in adult subjects: results from 2 identical phase III studies. Dermatol Surg 2019;45(11):1381–1393
9. Carruthers J, Solish N, Humphrey S, et al. Injectable daxibotulinum toxin A for the treatment of glabellar lines: a phase 2, randomized, dose-ranging, double-blind, multicenter comparison with onabotulinum toxin A and placebo. Dermatol Surg 2017;43(11):1321–1331
10. Sloop RR, Cole BA, Escutin RO. Reconstituted botulinum toxin type A does not lose potency in humans if it is refrozen or refrigerated for 2 weeks before use. Neurology 1997;48(1): 249–253
11. Hexsel DM, De Almeida AT, Rutowitsch M, et al. Multicenter, double-blind study of the efficacy of injections with botulinum toxin type A reconstituted up to six consecutive weeks before application. Dermatol Surg 2003;29(5):523–529, discussion 529
12. Hsu TS, Dover JS, Arndt KA. Effect of volume and concentration on the diffusion of botulinum exotoxin A. Arch Dermatol 2004;140(11):1351–1354
13. Carruthers A, Carruthers J, Cohen J. Dilution volume of botulinum toxin type A for the treatment of glabellar rhytides: does it matter? Dermatol Surg 2007;33(1 Spec No.):S97–S104
14. Carruthers J, Lowe NJ, Menter MA, Gibson J, Eadie N, For the Botox Glabellar Lines II Study Group. Double-blind, placebo-controlled study of the safety and efficacy of botulinum toxin type A for patients with glabellar lines. Plast Reconstr Surg 2003;112(5):21S–30S
15. Carruthers A, Carruthers J. Eyebrow height after botulinum toxin type A to the glabella. Dermatol Surg 2007;33:S26–S31
16. Horne DF, Rohrer TE. Shaping of the eyebrows with botox. In: Hartstein ME, Holds JB, Massry GG, eds. Pearls and pitfalls in cosmetic oculoplastic surgery. New York, NY: Springer; 2008
17. Ahn MS, Catten M, Maas CS. Temporal brow lift using botulinum toxin A. Plast Reconstr Surg 2000;105(3):1129–1135, discussion 1136–1139
18. Carruthers A, Carruthers J, Fagien S, Lei X, Kolodziejczyk J, Brin MF. Repeated onabotulinum toxin A treatment of glabellar lines at rest over three treatment cycles. Dermatol Surg 2016;42(9): 1094–1101
19. Sundaram H, Liew S, Signorini M, et al; Global Aesthetics Consensus Group. Global aesthetics consensus: hyaluronic acid fillers and botulinum toxin type A-recommendations for combined treatment and optimizing outcomes in diverse patient populations. Plast Reconstr Surg 2016;137(5):1410–1423
20. Carruthers JD, Faris SE. Neurotoxin injection for lower eyelid roll. In: Kontis TC, ed. Cosmetic injection techniques: a text and video guide to neurotoxins and fillers. Lacombe VG: Thieme Verlagsgruppe; 2013: Ch. 10, p. 32
21. Flynn TC, Carruthers JA, Carruthers JA. Botulinum-A toxin treatment of the lower eyelid improves infraorbital rhytides and widens the eye. Dermatol Surg 2001;27(8):703–708
22. Carruthers A, Carruthers J, Cohen J. A prospective, double-blind, randomized, parallel- group, dose-ranging study of botulinum toxin type A in female subjects with horizontal forehead rhytides. Dermatol Surg 2003;29(5):461–467
23. Ramey NA, Woodward JA. Mechanisms of blepharoptosis following cosmetic glabellar chemodenervation. Plast Reconstr Surg 2010;126(5):248e–249e
24. Wijemanne S, Vijayakumar D, Jankovic J. Apraclonidine in the treatment of ptosis. J Neurol Sci 2017;376:129–132
25. Mendonça TB, Lummertz AP, Bocaccio FJ, Procianoy F. Effect of low-concentration, nonmydriatic selective alpha-adrenergic agonist eyedrops on upper eyelid position. Dermatol Surg 2017;43(2):270–274
26. Paloma V, Samper A. A complication with the aesthetic use of Botox: herniation of the orbital fat. Plast Reconstr Surg 2001;107(5):1315
27. Goldman MP. Festoon formation after infraorbital botulinum A toxin: a case report. Dermatol Surg 2003;29(5):560–561, discussion 561

28. Frankel AS. Botox for rejuvenation of the periorbital region. Facial Plast Surg 1999;15(3):255–262
29. Kane MA. Classification of crow's feet patterns among Caucasian women: the key to individualizing treatment. Plast Reconstr Surg 2003; 112(5, Suppl):33S–39S
30. Benedetto A. Cosmetic uses of botulinum toxin A in the midface. In: Benedetto A, ed. Botulinum toxins in clinical aesthetic practice. Essex, UK: Informa Healthcare; 2011:104–139
31. Dayan SH, Kempiners JJ. Treatment of the lower third of the nose and dynamic nasal tip ptosis with Botox. Plast Reconstr Surg 2005;115(6):1784–1785
32. Bilal R. The gum and tooth show preference during smile by the patients visiting Qassim university dental hospital. Int J Applied Dent Sci 2016;2(1):24–27
33. Mazzuco R, Hexsel D. Gummy smile and botulinum toxin: a new approach based on the gingival exposure area. J Am Acad Dermatol 2010;63(6):1042–1051
34. Hwang WS, Hur MS, Hu KS, et al. Surface anatomy of the lip elevator muscles for the treatment of gummy smile using botulinum toxin. Angle Orthod 2009;79(1):70–77
35. Polo M. Botulinum toxin type A in the treatment of excessive gingival display. Am J Orthod Dentofacial Orthop 2005;127(2): 214–218, quiz 261
36. Carruthers J, Fagien S, Matarasso SL; Botox Consensus Group. Consensus recommendations on the use of botulinum toxin type a in facial aesthetics. Plast Reconstr Surg 2004; 114(6, Suppl):1S–22S
37. Benedetto AV. Cosmetic uses of botulinum toxin A in the lower face and upper chest. In: Botulinum toxin in clinical dermatology. UK: CRC Press, Informa Group; 2006: Ch 5, pp. 205–206
38. Simoni RD, Hill RL, Vaughan M, et al. JBC Centennial. The discovery of hyaluronan by Karl Meyer. J Biol Chem 2002;277:61–62
39. Coleman SR. Injectable silicone returns to the United States. Aesthet Surg J 2001;21(6):576–578
40. Mest DR, Humble G. Safety and efficacy of poly-L-lactic acid injections in persons with HIV-associated lipoatrophy: the US experience. Dermatol Surg 2006;32(11):1336–1345
41. Summary of safety and effectiveness data. https://www.accessdata.fda.gov/cdrh_docs/pdf5/P050052B.pdf. Accessed August 20, 2020
42. Eça LP, Pinto DG, de Pinho AM, Mazzetti MP, Odo ME. Autologous fibroblast culture in the repair of aging skin. Dermatol Surg 2012;38(2):180–184
43. Rohrich RJ, Pessa JE. The fat compartments of the face: anatomy and clinical implications for cosmetic surgery. Plast Reconstr Surg 2007;119(7):2219–2227, discussion 2228–2231
44. Vedamurthy M. Beware what you inject: complications of injectables—dermal fillers. J Cutan Aesthet Surg 2018;11(2): 60–66. http://www.jcasonline.com/text.asp?2018/11/2/60/240031. Accessed August 9, 2020
45. de Maio M. Myomodulation with injectable fillers: an innovative approach to addressing facial muscle movement. Aesthetic Plast Surg 2018;42(3):798–814
46. Rho NK, Chang YY, Chao YY, et al. Consensus recommendations for optimal augmentation of the Asian face with hyaluronic acid and calcium hydroxylapatite fillers. Plast Reconstr Surg 2015;136(5):940–956
47. Kim J. Novel forehead augmentation strategy: forehead depression categorization and calcium-hydroxyapatite filler delivery after tumescent injection. Plast Reconstr Surg Glob Open 2018;6(9):e1858
48. Sundaram H, Carruthers J. The glabella and central brow. In: Carruthers J, Carruthers A, eds. Procedures in cosmetic dermatol: soft tissue augmentation. 3rd ed. London: Elsevier Saunders; 2013:88–99
49. de Maio M. MD Codes™: a methodological approach to facial aesthetic treatment with injectable hyaluronic acid fillers. Aesthetic Plast Surg 2020. https://doi.org/10.1007/s00266-020-01762-7
50. Rzany B, DeLorenzi C. Understanding, avoiding, and managing severe filler complications. Plast Reconstr Surg 2015; 136(5, Suppl):196S–203S
51. Papageorgiu K, Mancini R, Garneau HC, Chang S-H, Jarullazada I, King A. A Three-Dimensional Construct of the Aging Eyebrow: The Illusion of Volume Loss. Aesth Surg J 2012;32(1):46-57
52. Papageorgiou KI, Mancini R, Garneau HC, et al. A three-dimensional construct of the aging eyebrow: the illusion of volume loss. Aesthet Surg J 2012;32(1):46–57
53. Pessa JE. An algorithm of facial aging: verification of Lambros's theory by three-dimensional stereolithography, with reference to the pathogenesis of midfacial aging, scleral show, and the lateral suborbital trough deformity. Plast Reconstr Surg 2000;106(2):479–488, discussion 489–490
54. De Maio M. Treatment planning. In: de Maio M, Rzany B, eds. Chapter 4: Injectable fillers in aesthetic medicine. Berlin, Heidelberg: Springer Link Verlag; 2014:52–55
55. Cotofana S, Gotkin RH, Frank K, Lachman N, Schenck TL. Anatomy behind the facial overfilled syndrome: the transverse facial septum. Dermatol Surg 2020;46(8):e16–e22
56. Casabona G, Frank K, Koban KC, et al. Lifting vs volumizing: the difference in facial minimally invasive procedures when respecting the line of ligaments. J Cosmet Dermatol 2019;10.1111/jocd.13089 (Online ahead of print)
57. Casabona G, Bernardini FP, Skippen B, et al. How to best utilize the line of ligaments and the surface volume coefficient in facial soft tissue filler injections. J Cosmet Dermatol 2020;19(2): 303–311
58. Harb A, Brewster CT. The nonsurgical rhinoplasty: a retrospective review of 5000 treatments. Plast Reconstr Surg 2020; 145(3):661–667
59. Scheuer JF III, Sieber DA, Pezeshk RA, Campbell CF, Gassman AA, Rohrich RJ. Anatomy of the facial danger zones: maximizing safety during soft-tissue filler injections. Plast Reconstr Surg 2017;139(1):50e–58e
60. Lévêque JL, Goubanova E. Influence of age on the lips and perioral skin. Dermatology 2004;208(4):307–313
61. Arroyo HH, Olivetti IP, Lima LF, Jurado JR. Clinical evaluation for chin augmentation: literature review and algorithm proposal. Rev Bras Otorrinolaringol (Engl Ed) 2016;82(5):596–601
62. Upadhyay RB, Upadhyay J, Agrawal P, Rao NN. Analysis of gonial angle in relation to age, gender, and dentition status by radiological and anthropometric methods. J Forensic Dent Sci 2012;4(1):29–33
63. de Maio M, Wu WTL, Goodman GJ, Monnheit G. Facial assessment and injection guide for Botulinum toxin and injectable hyaluronic acid fillers: focus on the lower face. Plast Reconstr J 2017;140(3):393e–404e
64. Cohen JL. Understanding, avoiding, and managing dermal filler complications. Dermatol Surg 2008;34(Suppl 1):S92–S99
65. King M. The management of bruising following nonsurgical cosmetic treatment. J Clin Aesthet Dermatol 2017;10(2):E1–E4

66. Funt D, Pavicic T. Dermal fillers in aesthetics: an overview of adverse events and treatment approaches. Clin Cosmet Investig Dermatol 2013;6:295–316
67. Daines SM, Williams EF. Complications associated with injectable soft-tissue fillers: a 5-year retrospective review. JAMA Facial Plast Surg 2013;15(3):226–231
68. Funt DK. Avoiding malar edema during midface/cheek augmentation with dermal fillers. J Clin Aesthet Dermatol 2011; 4(12):32–36
69. Beleznay K, Humphrey S, Carruthers JD, Carruthers A. Vascular compromise from soft tissue augmentation: experience with 12 cases and recommendations for optimal outcomes. J Clin Aesthet Dermatol 2014;7(9):37–43
70. DeLorenzi C. New high dose pulsed hyaluronidase protocol for hyaluronic acid filler vascular adverse events. Aesthet Surg J 2017;37(7):814–825
71. Sobanko JF, Taglienti AJ, Wilson AJ, et al. Motivations for seeking minimally invasive cosmetic procedures in an academic outpatient setting. Aesthet Surg J 2015;35(8):1014–1020
72. Michaud T, Gassia V, Belhaouari L. Facial dynamics and emotional expressions in facial aging treatments. J Cosmet Dermatol 2015;14(1):9–21

9

Threads in Aesthetic Surgery

Neeta Patel

Age and the Face

Aging is an inevitable natural consequence of sustained cellular metabolism. Nowhere are its effects on the body more visible than on the skin, which is exposed and continually subjected to external insults along with internal factors that drive senescence.[1] With its beauty, uniqueness, and complexity of the tissues it comprises, the face, which is a window to one's personality, becomes the most important unit for aesthetic concern. A combination of factors including gravity, loss of soft tissue elasticity, bone resorption, and subcutaneous fat redistribution are all seen to contribute to the visible changes of facial aging. The resorption of dental bones, in particular, effaces the scaffolding under the soft tissue, causing loss of skeletal projection, while a decrease in ligament elasticity leads to sagging of the overlying soft tissue.[2,3] Therefore, any corrective measures involving the face are contingent upon a thorough understanding of these specific changes occurring during aging.

Traditionally, standard surgical facelifts involve indelible stigmas comprising long incisions, undermining, superficial musculoaponeurotic system (SMAS) plication and tightening to lift, reposition, and fix tissues at appropriate positions. However, fallouts include telltale scars, morbidity, and downtime, resulting in overall patient intimidation. Besides, several patients who show early signs of aging and seek rejuvenation may not be good candidates for such radical intervention. The incessant search for solutions that are less invasive yet productive in giving results that would satisfy our patients has seen a rapid rise in many nonsurgical methods that could be done in the office without the associated trade-offs that surgery entails. Each patient is a unique individual and while it is important to try and meet their demands, it is equally important to customize treatments and lessen the collateral consequences that surgery entails. Among the number of modalities globally available today, plastic surgeons should be adept in choosing the right treatment for the patient. This chapter will focus on the use of threads as rejuvenation tools, either alone or in conjunction with other modalities, for both aesthetic and closely related aesthetic procedures.

"THREADING" Through History

The use of threads dates back to the ancient Egyptians who implanted gold sutures under the skin, to enhance the beauty of Cleopatra.[4] While the Eastern world used gold needles and threads along with acupuncture to improve "aura," the Russians used gold threads in grids under the skin to tighten facial tissues.[5] In fact, building upon these early pioneers, Andamyan from Moscow blended gold threads with absorbable polyglycol sutures and patented them in 2000.[6] However, smooth sutures "cheese-wired" the holding tissue, which led to experimentation with roughened/barbed sutures as improvisation in as early as the 1950s. In this regard, the general surgeon J. H. Alcamo was first granted a patent for barbed sutures in 1964,[7] though no evidence exists of their usage at that time. The 1970s saw popularization of the "curl-lift" (Guillemain) technique[8] using simple surgical sutures (absorbable or nonabsorbable) placed subcutaneously and anchored to fixed tissues to provide lift. Following Ruff, H. J. Buncke, internationally renowned as the father of modern microsurgery, patented his unidirectional barbed sutures as "Surgical methods using one-way sutures" in 1999,[9] which was thereafter acquired by the Quill corporation. Simultaneously, G. L. Ruff used unidirectional barbed threads to lift the face, buttocks, and breast, which he patented in 2001 as the Contour ThreadLift.[10]

Since 1975, M. A. Sulamanidze (Moscow) had started working on the concept of procedures that would "reduce skin space, causing retraction and adaptation through minimally invasive surgery." After a series of improvements, he created threads of multipoint anchorage,[11,12] where cannulas were used instead of needles and skin punctures instead of incisions, making the process even less invasive. He named this the "Aptos Thread lift" (anti-ptosis). Classically, it was a short, bidirectional, barbed thread made of 2–0 polypropylene for positioning along the lines and contours of the face. In 2003, he developed the "Dynamic Aptoslift" using smooth, coiled polypropylene springs (Aptos Springs), which allowed for lifting and fixing soft tissues even when in motion. Woffles Wu incorporated Aptos sutures in his practice, but found them too fragile and short in length. Subsequently, by combining the techniques of Des Fernandes (Cape Town, South Africa) and Sulamanidze's concept, he developed the "Woptos Lift" and a longer version of threads. The name was later altered to the "Woffles lift."[13] This version also compensated for possible cheese wiring of the bend in the suture, by using X-interlinked sutures.

Threads started gaining popularity in different forms and textures to achieve the same effect the world over. In this regard, Nikolay Serdev used semielastic, antimicrobial, braided long-term absorbable polycaproamide threads made in Bulgaria, which he called Serdev sutures,[14,15] not just for the face but also for various other areas of the body such as breast, buttocks, and thighs which are in use even today.

Anatomical Considerations and Methodology

Thread lifting is a minimally invasive procedure with the objective to maximize the possibility of a favorable lift and repositioning of tissues without any collateral damage to the surrounding structures. To this effect, accurate anatomical knowledge of the face is mandatory. For simplicity, the face can be divided into three sections, *viz.* the upper third (forehead and brows), the middle third, and the lower third (chin, jawline, and neck) to simplify facial assessment and treatment. In the midface, the central facial triangle made up of the eyes, nose, mouth, and malar bones is a key determinant of perceived beauty. Hence the goal of any youthful rejuvenation procedure should be the restoration of harmony between these features.[16]

Important Anatomical Observations

- Mendelson and Wong[2,3,17] observed that the anterior part of the face is more susceptible to aging than the lateral. By drawing a vertical line from the lateral canthus downward the medial (frontal) mobile part of the face is demarcated. This area is more amenable to floating threads, because of its dynamic nature and lack of anchoring points.[18]
- The lateral part, which shows lesser signs of aging than the frontal, does however contain anchoring points (temporal fascia) which therefore allows anchored lifts in this area. The posterior half of the face (mastoid area) has skin intimately connected to the deeper fascia and muscle and hence less amenable to any pulling force.
- Regardless of broad facial demarcations, soft tissue sagging is also dependent on strength of attachment to the skeleton. Areas resistant to ptosis are generally supported by connective tissues, vessels, and nerves. It follows, therefore, that areas of least resistance are easiest to lift.[19]

Pinch Anatomy

In order to avoid damage to underlying important anatomical structures such as blood vessels and nerves, when inserting the thread, Kim and coworkers[20] developed the concept of "pinch anatomy." This involves gently pinching the skin above the proposed point of insertion, to assess the depth and course of main blood vessels and nerves underlying the dermis. The knowledge of the extent of inclusion of these structures in the pinched skin will determine the plane of insertion of the thread so as to prevent damaging them. For instance, as the facial nerve traverses the zygomatic arch, it snakes below the superficial musculoaponeurotic system (SMAS) and moves close to the bone. A gentle pinch of the skin above the zygomatic area was shown to exclude this nerve and blood vessels from the pinch, thus facilitating a safe procedure. Fig. 9.1 depicts important anatomical structures susceptible to injury during thread lift (**Fig. 9.1**). **Fig. 9.2** depicts the method used to prevent damage to underlying structures.

Types of Threads

Threads can be divided into three main categories (**Figs. 9.3–9.7**).

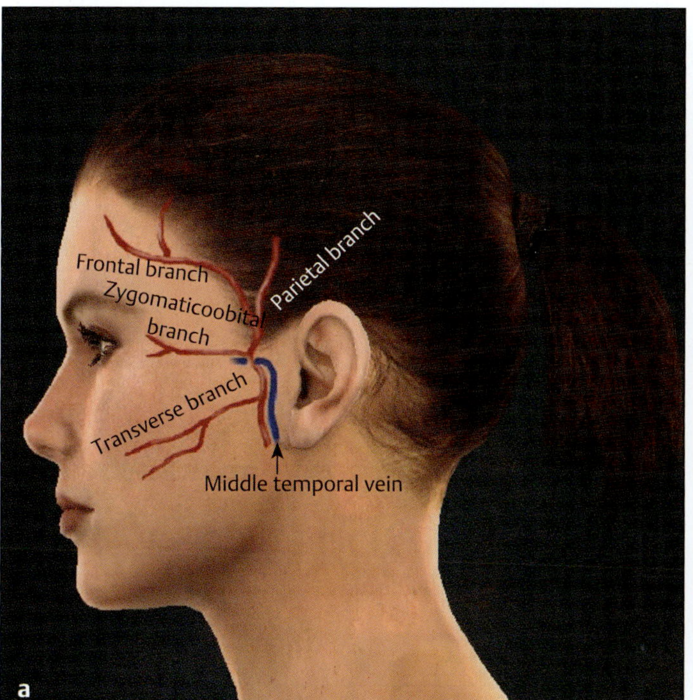

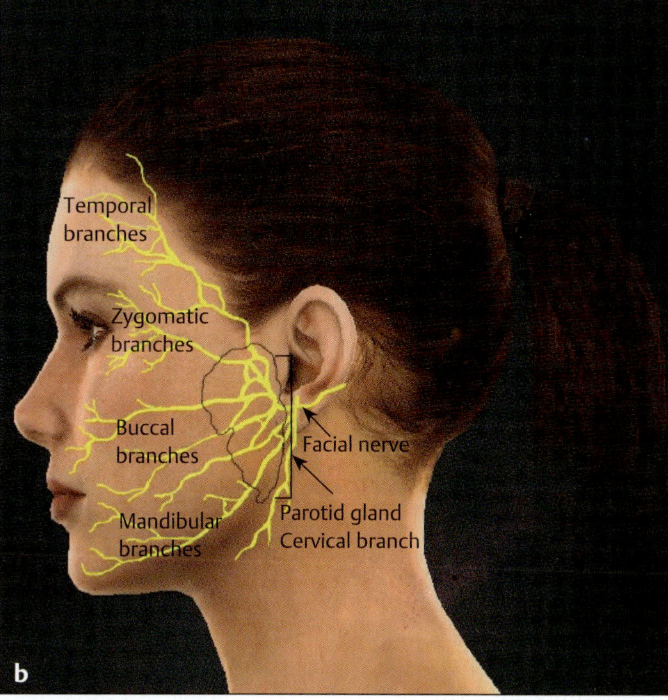

Fig. 9.1 Anatomical structures vulnerable to damage during thread lifting. **(a)** Superficial temporal artery with the branches: frontoparietal, zygomatico-orbital, and transverse, as well as the middle temporal vein. **(b)** Facial nerve with its five main branches (frontotemporal, zygomatic, buccal, mandibular, and cervical) as well as the parotid gland. (The images are provided courtesy of Dr Prashanti Patel, Mumbai, Maharashtra, India.)

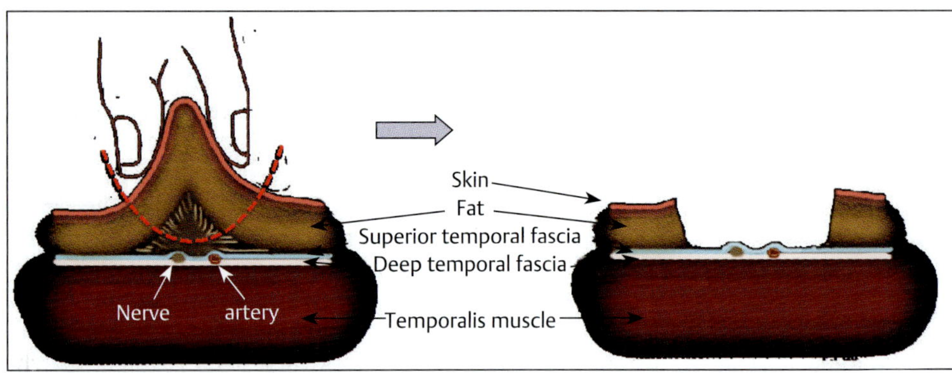

Fig. 9.2 Pinch anatomy. (Adapted from Kim et al 2019.[20]) (The image is provided courtesy of Dr Prashanti Patel, Mumbai, Maharashtra, India.)

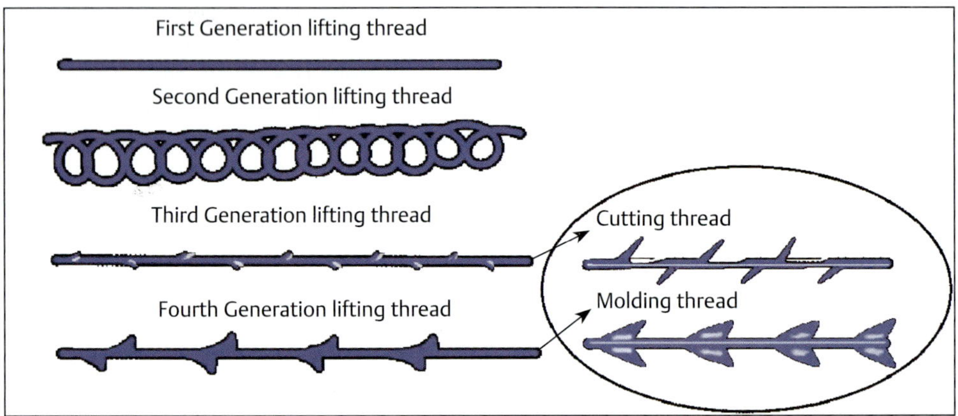

Fig. 9.3 Various types of polydioxanone (PDO) threads. With each generation of threads, the lifting effect gets better due to more surface area in contact with the surrounding tissue. (Diagram adapted from Kim et al 2019.[20]) (The image is provided courtesy of Dr Prashanti Patel, Mumbai, Maharashtra, India.)

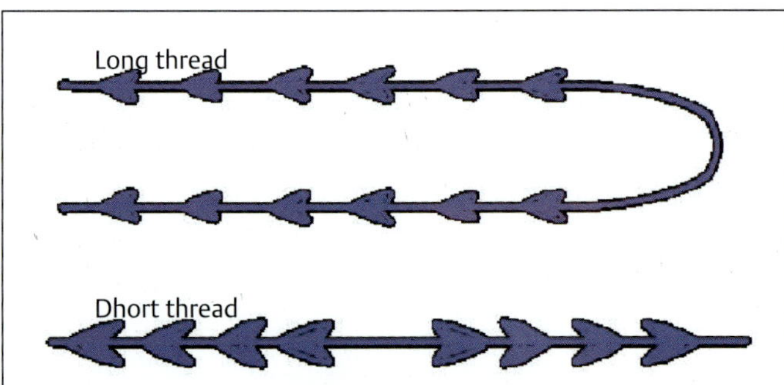

Fig. 9.4 Long and short threads. Bidirectional cogs with zigzag threads are good at fixing the lift effect made by the cogs. Twister threads are mono threads but having more surface area, thus giving more volumization (filler effect). (The image is provided courtesy of Dr Prashanti Patel, Mumbai, Maharashtra, India.)

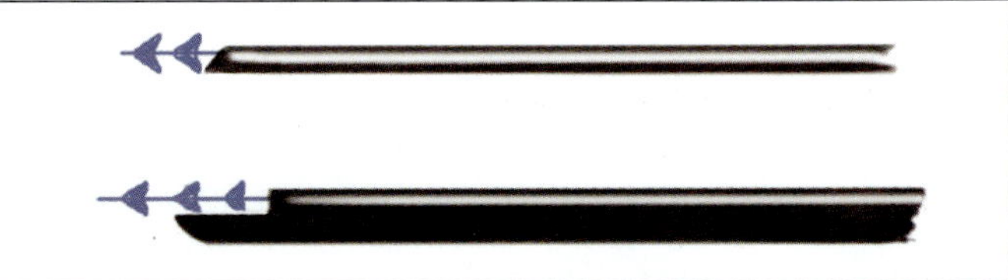

Fig. 9.5 Thread with needle and cannula. (The image is provided courtesy of Dr Prashanti Patel, Mumbai, Maharashtra, India.)

Mode of Absorption

Absorbable Threads

These include threads made of polydioxanone (PDO): smooth monothreads, those with uni- or bidirectional barbs or cog,[21] and poly-L-lactic acid (PLLA): (Silhouette Soft, Sculptra in solid form).

Nonabsorbable Threads

These include the APTOS thread, Contour Thread, and Woffles thread made of polypropylene.

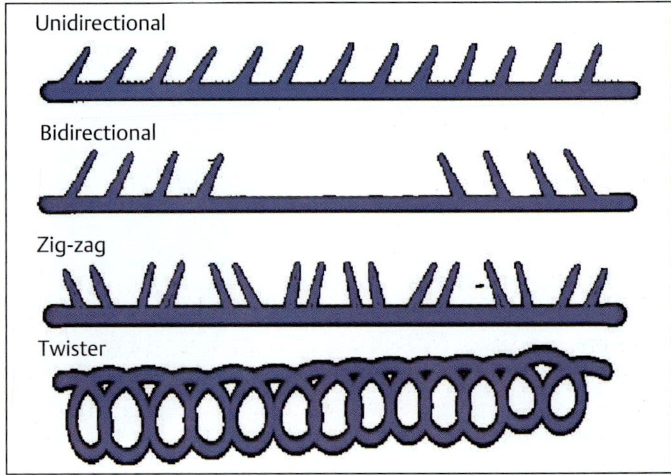

Fig. 9.6 Different types of cog threads. (The image is provided courtesy of Dr Prashanti Patel, Mumbai, Maharashtra, India.)

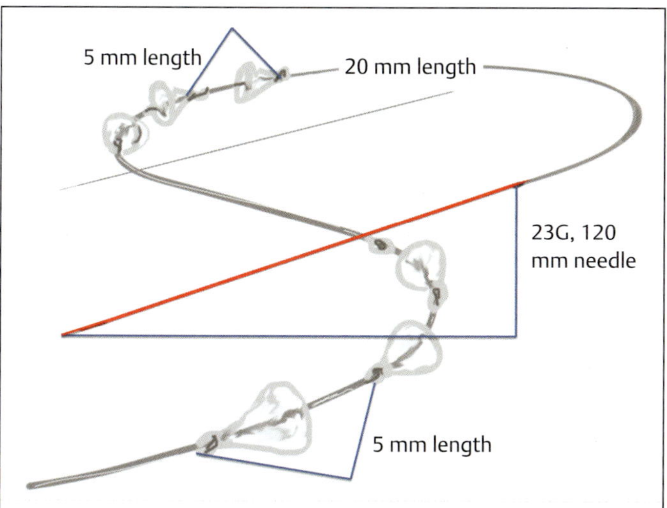

Fig. 9.7 Design of the silhouette soft thread (PLLA—poly-L-lactic acid). (The image is provided courtesy of Dr Prashanti Patel, Mumbai, Maharashtra, India.)

Surface Characteristics

Smooth Threads

- **Absorbable:** These are basically floating threads made of PDO. They can be used alone or along with other cogs. They can also be used as spirally twisted monofilaments. They are mainly used as volumizers with little effect on lift.
- **Nonabsorbable** smooth threads are not very popular as they "cheese wire" (cut through) and cause early relapses.

Barbed (Corrugated) Threads[22]

- **Unidirectional** threads, which function by anchoring to surrounding structures in one plane with the other end anchored to the deep temporal fascia. These are not very effective.
- **Bidirectional** threads are inserted using cannulas and give two-way anchorage provided by the barbs engaging the tissue.
- **Cog** threads are absorbable PDO unidirectional, bidirectional, and multidirectional threads.[23]
- **Cones** (made of PLLA) absorbable threads inserted with needles attached at both ends.

Length of Threads

Different lengths of threads are chosen as per the procedure selected for thread lifting.[24] Short sutures of less than 90 mm in length are used as floating threads in patients with mild laxity of tissues and are of plain, screw, spiral, or cog variety.

In contrast, patients with moderate-to-severe aging manifesting as jowls, or requiring use in other body areas need lengths greater than 90 mm. These are typified by the APTOS 2/0, 4/0 threads, Silhouette Soft, and Contour Thread.

Mechanics of Thread Lifting

Threads conceptually achieve a lift by shifting the skin and subcutaneous tissue to a more favorable position (higher position) without cutting the skin or surgically undermining it. The advantages are minimal instrumentation, less pain, and almost no morbidity compared to conventional surgery. The different types of threads described in the preceding section cause tissue lift in two ways: purely mechanical and with tissue reaction. With regard to the former, Kim and coworkers[20] have simplified the concept with the following terminology. *The fixing point* of the thread is generally immobile such as the deep temporal fascia and experiences maximum tension. *The hanging point* (the other end of the thread) is situated directly in the tissues to be lifted, or to a tissue above it (to which it is well connected) to be lifted. Finally, *the direction* refers to the vector of pull from the hanging point to the fixed point.

Of the *barbed* threads, the **nonabsorbable** polypropylene threads sized 2–0/3–0 with 20 prominences every 0.5 mm along their length allow physical engagement of tissues at every barb along the thread. However, since they are nondegradable, reversals are difficult. On the other hand, *barbed bioabsorbable* PDO threads are made by cutting or molding method and chosen in accordance to the pulling force needed. They initially provide mechanical lift by physical engagement; however, with time, as a reaction with adjacent tissues and biodegradation of the thread, there is additional neocollagenesis, angiogenesis, and dermal thickening which result in tightening and volumization, thus complementing the lift.

Unidirectional cogs provide suspension of the tissue only in one direction and the thread needs to be anchored to a fixed point. These are not as effective as bidirectional ones, wherein the forward and reverse facing cogged segments simultaneously fix lifted tissues and prevent them from slipping. However, a good result can be obtained when a large number of threads are used.

The mechanism of action of **floating monofilament absorbable** threads is tissue reaction following injury, followed by angiogenesis and neocollagenesis along the path of the thread. This also results in tightening along with volumization over time. When used in a grid-shaped design or along the vector, it maximizes benefits. Often, monothreads are used along with barbs/cogs to give a volumized effect along with superficial skin tightening which enhances the results of the latter.

The **absorbable poly-L-lactic acid** (PLLA) threads induce type I, II, III collagen deposition but elicit lesser inflammatory stimulation than the PDO threads and are longer lasting with 2-year duration. They also achieve volumizing effect when used as cones (Silhouette Soft sutures);[25] though unlike hyaluronic acid the volumization occurs along with the degradation of the thread over time (2 years). The cones (8/12/16 in number) on each half of the bidirectional thread are mobile between knots at uniform intervals along the thread. This arrangement allows immediate lifting of the soft tissues due to subcutaneous tissue binding and repositioning by gathering at a point, along with neocollagenesis. They are particularly useful for lifting in difficult areas such as the periorbital, malar, as well as the nose (tip) and neck, because of the IR unique mechanism of lift. In addition, these threads come equipped at both ends, with two 23-gauge, 12-cm needles, which are flexible and allow for treatment on curved surfaces, thus reducing pain and bleeding compared with PDO sutures. However, PLLA do have certain drawbacks when compared with PDO threads, in that they are less elastic and easily breakable, expensive, and may result in severe bleeding if inappropriately inserted. This technique requires experience, knowledge, and skill, and therefore, is not recommended for the beginner.

Treatment Planning, Simulation, and Marking

Thread lift, though a unique and versatile rejuvenation tool, is not suitable for all patients seeking facial rejuvenation. It is imperative to thoroughly counsel patients regarding their specific needs and expectations versus what can be realistically achieved. Candidates should be selected by evaluating the extent and location of skin ptosis, and assess whether thread lift alone would suffice or combination with other modalities would be more beneficial to achieve the best result.

Simulation

Following selection of the thread, the surgeon should simulate the procedure by using one/both hands and fingers to manually lift the desired facial area to predict the result of the procedure. This manipulation is done with the patient sitting upright preferably in front of a mirror.

Marking

After simulation the vectoral path corresponding to the desired lift effect should be marked with a temporary marker. The entry (starting) and exit (ending) points on the main vector line are marked to confirm the thread length (**Fig. 9.8**).[20] Prophylactic antibiotics may be prescribed depending on the surgeon's preference. The skin around the area of thread lift including the hairline area should be thoroughly cleaned and well prepped.[24]

Anesthesia

- **Monothreads:** Topical anesthesia such as a 7 to 15% mixture of EMLA (eutectic mixture of local anesthetics) is applied 45 minutes before the procedure, in case of superficial monothreads.
- **Barbs/cogs/long threads:** Local anesthesia in the form of a 1 to 2% lidocaine solution with epinephrine (1:200,000) is injected at entry and exit points.[20]

Method

The needle is inserted perpendicular to the skin and subcutaneous layer. It is then gently angled horizontally and pushed in the direction of the marked vector toward the point of exit on the skin; the other hand supports the skin firmly to allow passage.

The needle is gently pulled out and the thread with the cones follows into the tract. Once the thread is fully inserted, the needle is cut and kept aside .With the nondominant hand, the skin is pushed upwards in the direction of the vector as its cones engage, keeping the dominant hand holding the thread end. Some skin wrinkling (temporary) may be seen at the point of needle insertion.

Note: These guidelines remain the same for any type of thread (cog/barb) in the lateral part of the face. Refer to **Fig. 9.9** for general tips and guidelines in inserting threads.

Cutting of the Thread

After insertion, the thread is not pulled before cutting. Rather the skin is pushed upward over it and then cut and buried. Any resultant skin folds are temporary and resolve in a short time (**Fig. 9.8e**). Postoperatively cold compression is applied to minimize swelling and bruising.

Thread Lifts in Specific Areas of the Face

Brow Lift

Anatomical Considerations

Anatomically the tissues above the brow are more firmly attached as compared to the tissues below the eyebrow in the periorbital area; hence, the force used by the thread inserted here may not be enough to give an appreciable lift.

In performing an absorbable thread-lifting procedure to elevate the brow area, it is advisable to insert the thread into the supraperiosteal plane in the frontalis muscle area and into the subcutaneous fat layer in the temporalis muscle area.

By pinching the skin before insertion, vessels and nerves underlying can be protected.

Brow lifting is a procedure that lifts both the lateral part of forehead and temple and is done in two different anatomical areas simultaneously (**Fig. 9.10**).

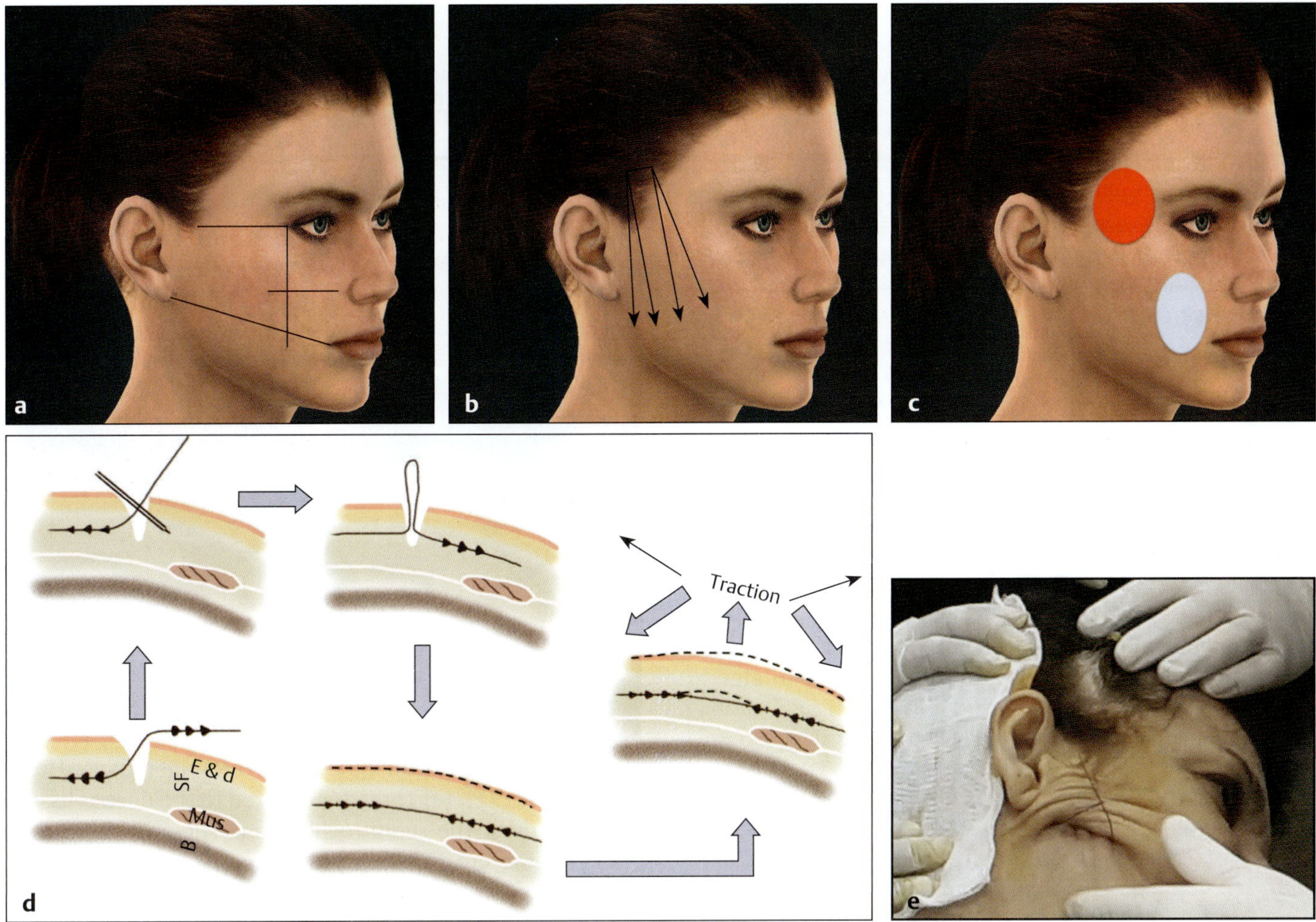

Fig. 9.8 **(a)** Depiction of reference lines (to aid vector planning) marked before the procedure. **(b)** Thread trajectories in the face: A blunt tool (awl) or disposable needle is used to make the entry point (one or more threads per hole) to be anchored in the temporal region. **(c)** "Special" areas of the face: The orange round area shows the temporal site of possible (temporary) skin wrinkling or folding after insertion of thread. The oval white area below shows the area of possible resistance to thread passage due to underlying ligaments. **(d)** Thread insertion (diagrams adapted from Kim et al 2019[20]): The lifting process follows the direction of the arrows. Here, the procedure shown is with Silhouette Soft cones with attached needle but it also applies to barbed threads. **(e)** Cutting of the thread.Abbreviations: B, bone; Mus, muscle; SF, subcutaneous fat; E&d, epidermis and dermis. The dotted lines in the tissue depict curvature of skin due to traction by the inserted thread. (The image is provided courtesy of Dr Prashanti Patel, Mumbai, Maharashtra, India.)

Points of caution in the forehead and brow area:

- Bleeding is more likely to occur here than the lower face.
- Knowledge of vascular anatomy is very important.
- Cannula is better than a needle.
- Local anesthetic with adrenaline helps minimize bleeding.
- Surgically, tissues and fat excised during a blepharoplasty often decreases this bulk and gives a more visible lift.
- Headaches up to a week are common. Botulinum toxin given to the upper face a week before the procedure can help to a great extent, along with enhancing results.

Midface and Jowls (Figs. 9.11–9.13)

Points of caution in the midface and jowl:

- Preoperatively, malar prominence should be noted, which can get exaggerated if already full.
- Simulation must be performed to test which pulling vector is effective. The most effective vectors are determined and treatment planned accordingly.
- Thread lifting and volumizing effects are considered simultaneously here.
- A good lift is obtained when the angle subtended by the mandibular line on the horizontal is greater than or equal to 30 degrees.[20]

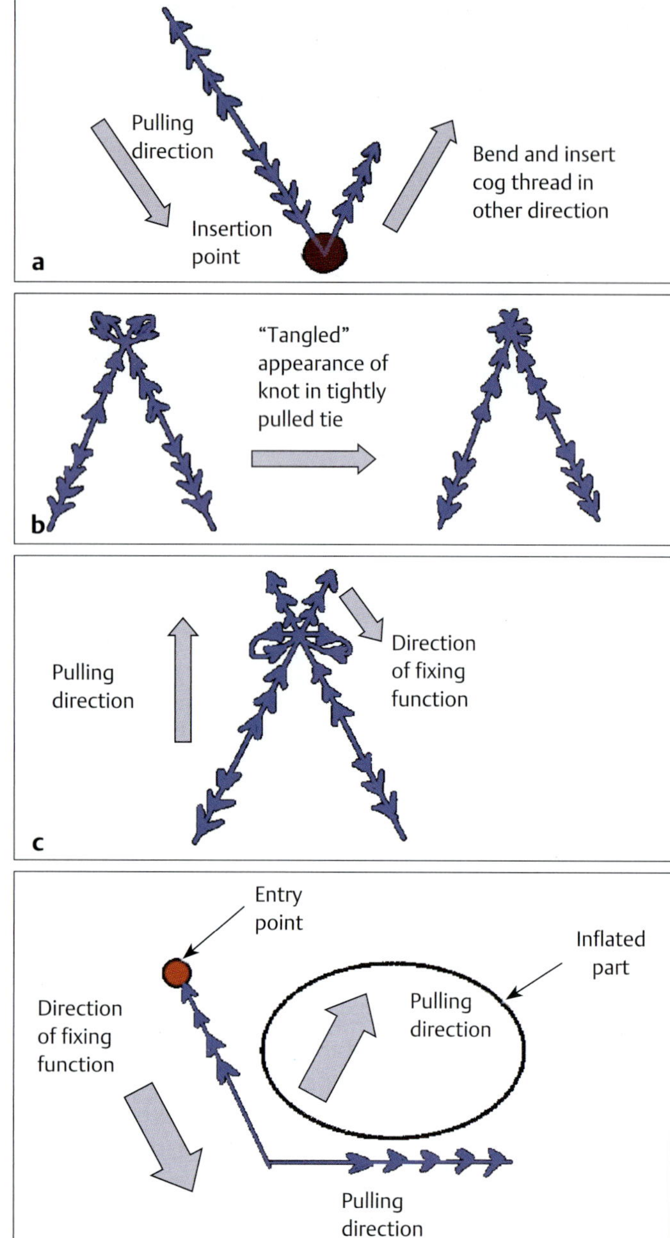

Fig. 9.9 **(a–c)** General tips and guidelines in the techniques of insertion and fixation of cogs (adapted from Kim et al 2019[20]). **(d)** The technique used in the face to improve the jawline. (The images are provided courtesy of Dr Prashanti Patel, Mumbai, Maharashtra, India.)

Neck

Neck lifts are useful in people with mild skin sagging and a good amount of subcutaneous fat (1.5 cm or more), but not recommended for older patients with heavier skin sagging and very little fat. It is contraindicated in severe cases (can worsen an existing "turkey gobbler" effect).

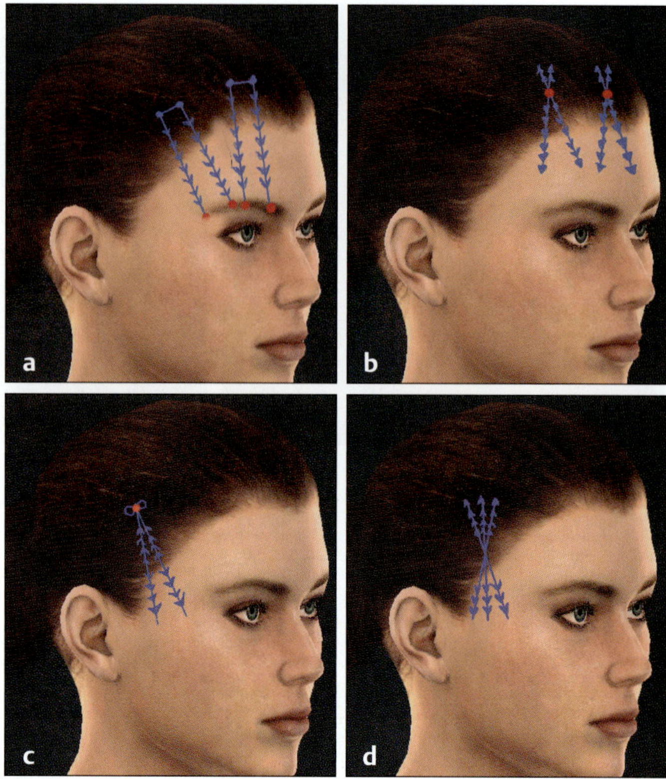

Fig. 9.10 Various techniques used in brow lift (adapted from Kim et al 2019[20]). **(a)** Threads anchored to the deeper tissues in the hairline. The supratrochlear and supraorbital arteries (which come out in the subcut tissue) should be avoided. Set entry point where it is relatively flat than curved. The exit point is on the corrugator muscle fibers. More the ptosis, more the number of threads will be needed. **(b)** X-method: cog threads are crossed and fixed to the hairline. Force of pull is more than using parallel threads as the subcut tissue here is very thick. May exaggerate existing horizontal forehead lines. **(c, d)** Threads used to lift the lateral orbital and brow area. They can be knotted or an X-method can also be used for a more effective pull. (This image is provided courtesy of Dr Prashanti Patel, Mumbai, Maharashtra, India.)

Method

The procedure is shown in **Fig. 9.14**. Thread is inserted from the two medial points and taken out laterally. Pulling the thread simultaneously after engaging the cogs in the soft tissue along the thread trajectory from its lateral exit points makes the central area (submental) taut and thus flattening it (taking in the sag). Insertion trajectory of the thread is as shown in **Fig. 9.15**.

Monothreads can be added in the submental area under the skin to fortify the tightening effect. They can also be added to fill out the horizontal fine wrinkles as volumizers. Points of caution in the neck:

- The patient should be supine with neck slightly extended.

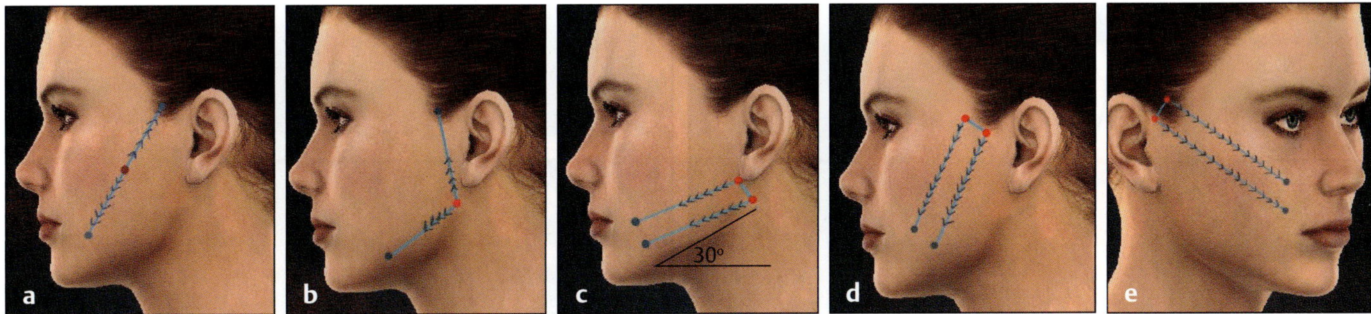

Fig. 9.11 **(a–e)** Different thread trajectories in the face for mild cases of a ptotic jowl (adapted from Kim et al 2019[20]). **(a, b)** A bidirectional thread inserted through the middle of two exit points. The lowest cone/barb/cog are fixed in the jowl and the topmost in the temporal hairline. Point of needle insertion is in the middle of the two exit points. **(b)** The same concept as **(a)**, but at an angle and specifically improves the jawline and not the marionette line. Entry point is approximately 1 fingerbreadth inside from the mandibular angle or right behind. When the angle between each half of the thread is greater than the angle between the mandibular body and ramus, the results are much better. **(c)** For prominent or moderately sagging jowl with marionette lines: One thread is used, but it has an effect similar to that of using two cog threads; two vector lines are marked. One in the upward direction toward the temporal area and the other, more horizontal, going backwards from the chin to the angle of the jaw. **(d, e)** Two ways to lift the marionette lines and jowl area using one or more cogged threads inserted in parallel. The nasolabial fold **(e)** can be lifted well if the end point of the lower thread is directed toward it. By lifting the skin above the nasolabial folds, the malar area can be volumized with the gathering tendency of the bidirectional cogs. (This image is provided courtesy of Dr Prashanti Patel, Mumbai, Maharashtra, India.)

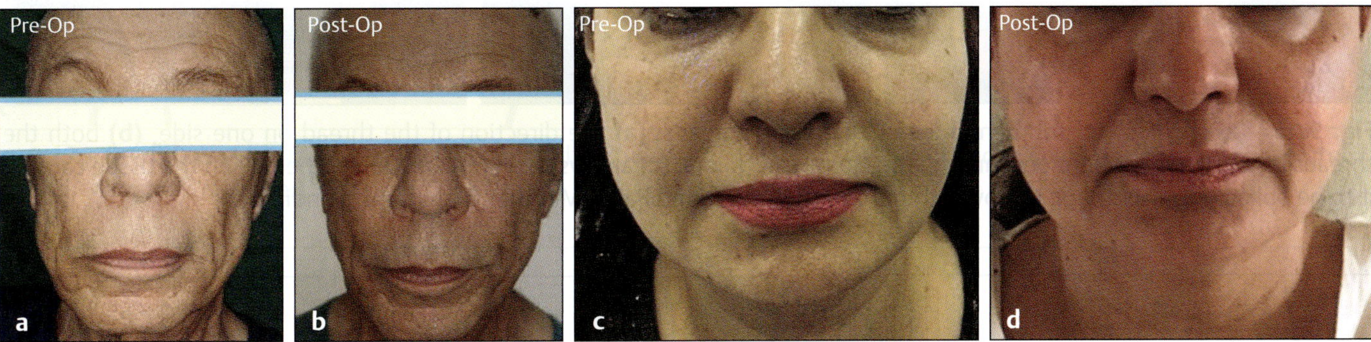

Fig. 9.12 **(a)** Thread lift using bidirectional polydioxanone (PDO) threads. **(b)** Thread lift using bidirectional polydioxanone (PDO) threads.

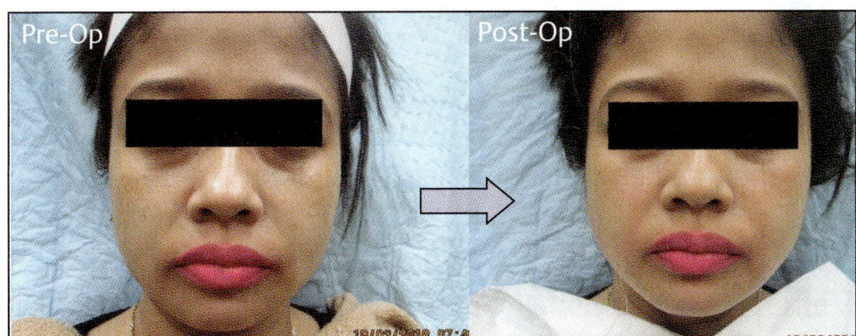

Fig. 9.13 Thread lift using Silhouette Soft poly-L-lactic acid (PLLA) threads.

- The skin pinch by the nondominant hand should be the guiding tunnel to insert the thread.
- The needle is continuously "guided and guarded" by the two fingers of the nondominant hand from the point of insertion till exit.

Threads Used to Lift Other Body Parts

Apart from the face, threads also have been used to lift mild-to-moderate sag of the arms, thighs, buttocks, and breasts with reasonable results. Insertion of four or more 12-cm-long MULTIFIX threads, comprising 2–0 nonabsorbable, polypropylene with multidirectional cogs, have been shown to lift flaccid arms following liposuction. Similar usage of threads was reported for the inner thigh,[26] and in buttock lifts.[15] Here subdermal fat tissue is pulled, repositioned, and volumized, using a suture connecting the deep fibrous tissue with the gluteus maximus fascia to achieve increased anteroposterior diameter (**Fig. 9.16**).[15,26,27]

With respect to breast lift, Sulamanidze et al[28] have reported the insertion of hypodermic underbreast Aptos threads followed by suspension of the breast on the clavicle (**Fig. 9.17**). This was referred to as a "hypodermic bodice" and utilized a cellulocutaneous flap generated through

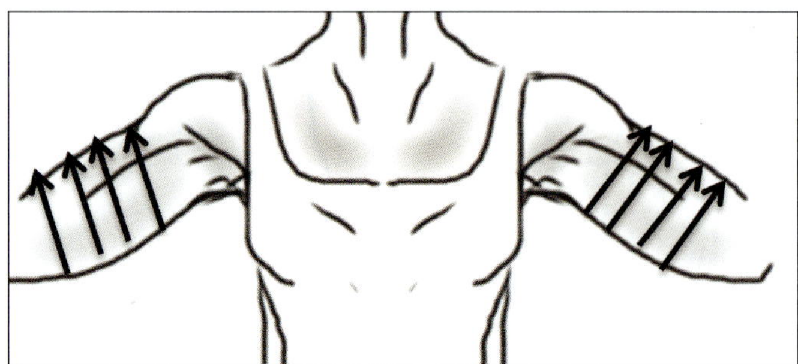

Fig. 9.19 Vectors for inserting threads in arm lift. (The image is provided courtesy of Dr Prashanti Patel, Mumbai, Maharashtra, India.)

oris muscle to erase marionette lines[26] a week before insertion of threads.

Threads in Facial Palsy

Several reports attest to the efficacy of threads in correcting asymmetry of the face affected by facial palsy. Recently, Dua and Bhardwaj[31] used subdermal suspension absorbable PDO sutures together with dermal fillers and neurotoxin to treat ptosis occurring due to facial muscular dystrophy. To treat asymmetry arising from facial palsy, Alam percutaneously applied nonabsorbable Gore-Tex-based implants in the nasolabial fold suspended with Prolene sutures in the deep temporal fascia.[32] This procedure allowed restoration of the nasolabial fold while also repositioning the mouth aesthetically and showed long-lasting results, testifying to their effectiveness. Bidirectional barbed polypropylene sutures (triple convergence thread) have also been used in other instances of the palsied hemiface correction, due to their excellent biocompatibility, low surgical complexity, low cost, and their ease of adaptability with other surgical procedures.[33,34] However, when comparing the materials used in threads, braided polyester (Ethibond Excel) and braided polyester blended with polytetrafluoroethylene (PTFE) showed better loadbearing ability and resistance to stretch than did polypropylene.[35]

Factors Affecting Thread Lift Procedures

On an untreated and well-selected patient, thread lift can give a very satisfying result; however, special conditions can adversely influence thread-lift results. Most have to do with prior procedures done or pathologies affecting the face. Scars resulting from zygomatic or orthognathic surgeries, previous facelifts, or acne scars which have fibrotic connections to the underlying subcutaneous tissues do not allow easy passage of a cannula or needle. Facial liposuction also increases the proportion of fibrotic fatty tissue compared with an untreated face. Similarly, one should wait for at least a year between ultrasound procedures for the face (HIFU) and a subsequent thread lift, to resolve fibrotic connections that can hamper needle movement.[20]

Complications and Troubleshooting

Thread lifting is not a surgery and its success is highly dependent on the right selection of patient (best for one with mild skin laxity) choosing the appropriate thread, as well as detailed counseling regarding realistic expectations. Some patients may not show desired results with only thread lifting and may need combination treatments. For patients with severely sagging skin, and high expectations, a surgical facelift may be the only option. Besides the patient and the treatment plan, it is important that the threads used are proven safe for use. Certain materials used in threads have been shown to have cytotoxic characteristics even though they are licensed for use.[36]

Overall, thread lift is an extremely safe and easy procedure which can be carried out in the outpatient clinic with minimum to no morbidity. The complications mentioned below occur rarely and when adequate precautions are not taken.[20]

Bleeding, Bruising, and Hematomas

Bleeding occurring at the thread entry point, but stopping within a minute, is due to small blood vessel injury and can be ignored. However, if it continues over a minute, a medium-sized vessel (superior temporal vein/artery) may have been damaged; in which case, the needle should be inserted through a new entry point, preferably medial to the hairline which is relatively safer. Bleeding is seldom seen when a cannula is used instead of a needle. Late-onset bleeding (hematoma) is extremely rare and occurs due to cogs repeatedly irritating capillaries. The area should be iced and compressed. Knowledge of underlying anatomy is imperative.

Pain and Stiffness

If the underlying cause is infection, oral antibiotics should be prescribed. Hematoma-induced pain can be treated with ice compression. Cogs may disengage from tissue and hang, causing pain, which is treated by massaging/molding for several days up to a month. If there is persistent skin irritation by thread ends, they have to be removed.

Skin Folds

Usually temporary and seen if the skin is too thin or too many thick threads have been inserted into one hole, or the force used during the procedure is excessive. The skin overlying the thread may look palpably raised, especially while smiling (animation). This usually resolves with time.

Thread Protrusion and Migration

If threads emerge out of the skin or through the oral mucosa, they can be cut and removed, usually without repercussions. Thread migrations occur due to incorrect cutting of bidirectional cog threads or breakage of PDO threads, which therefore do not remain anchored and move with facial expressions (**Fig. 9.20**).

Dimpling of Skin

Skin may appear dented when cog threads are not positioned evenly in the subcutaneous fat and overlying dermis, resulting in imbalanced pull and sunken skin, especially aggravated by animation. This can occur immediately after the procedure or within a month and can be improved by physically molding the skin using finger, still the cogs get untangled and snap back to their original position.

Sunken Cheeks

Most often a feature of older patients, as such they are not good candidates for thread lift to start with, as the procedure may exaggerate (worsen) the effect.

Unsatisfactory Lift

Heavier jowls can be resolved by inserting longer threads or many short ones to exert stronger pull. However, in severely hypertrophic/heavy faces, options other than thread lift should be considered.

Temporary Paralysis of Facial Nerve Branches

Sometimes loss of facial sensation is also accompanied by temporary paralysis due to the local anesthetic rather than actual damage by a cannula. The patient, therefore, needs only to be reassured.

Elevation of the Lateral Canthus

This may occur if the distance between the thread and the lateral orbital rim is less than an inch or two fingerbreadths, or when the thread is forcibly pulled. It generally resolves spontaneously.

Infection

Prevention of infection by observing good asepsis is better than treating it later on. The entry points and the concerned area of the face should be cleaned well and hairline suitably prepared. The surgeon should particularly prevent hair from being entangled in the entry points while inserting the needle.

Difficulty in Doing the Procedure due to Underlying Scarring and Fibrosis

It is important to note the past history of such cases, and an adequate cooling-off period before doing a thread lift is necessary.

Conclusion

Thread lifting cannot replace surgery, but has its unique place in the armamentarium of the surgeon. Judicious use of this tool for the right patient can give a very favorable result or buy time until the candidate is ready for surgery. It is important to realize though that where only threads do not suffice, multimodal combinations with threads often serve the purpose and allow for greater flexibility in approach.

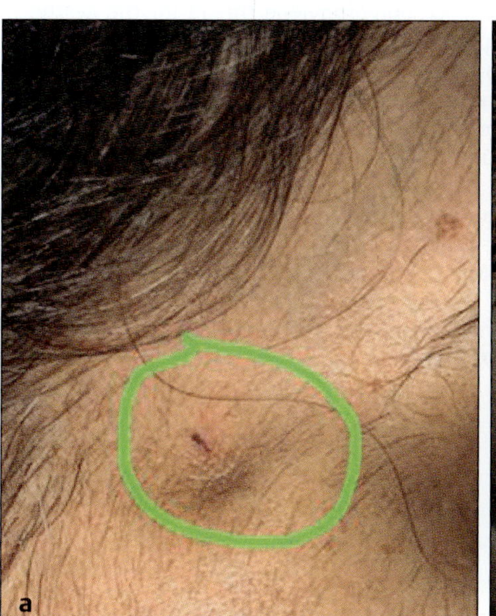

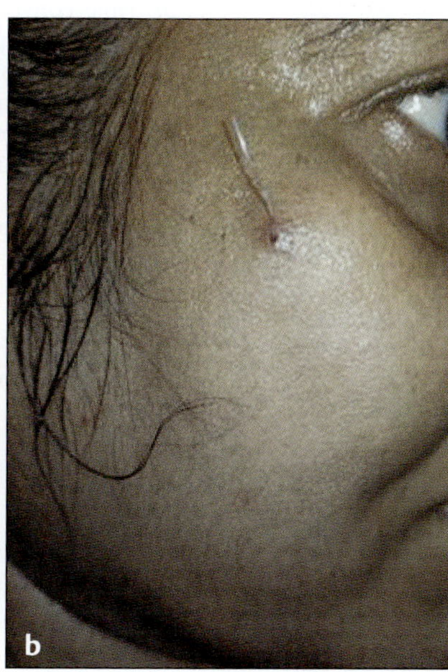

Fig. 9.20 Possible complications of thread lift. **(a)** Thread visible on skin surface. **(b)** Thread protruding from skin surface.

In author's opinion the last word on threads is yet to be written as it is still evolving and holds great promise in the aesthetic and functional plastic surgery horizon.

References

1. Gruber F, Kremslehner C, Eckhart L, Tschachler E. Cell aging and cellular senescence in skin aging: recent advances in fibroblast and keratinocyte biology. Exp Gerontol 2020;130:110780
2. Mendelson B, Wong CH. Anatomy of the aging face. Ch. 6. In: Warren RJ, Neligan PC, eds. Plastic surgery, Vol. 2. Aesthetic surgery of the face; 2013:78–92
3. Mendelson B, Wong CH. Changes in the facial skeleton with aging: implications and clinical applications in facial rejuvenation. Aesthetic Plast Surg 2012;36(4):753–760
4. Connell R. A golden stitch in time saves nine years of aging. Mainchi Newspapers; 2005. http//mdn.mainichimsn.co.jp/Waiwai/archive/news/2005/07/20050706p2g00mOdm01900 0chtml
5. Kress D. The history of barbed suture suspension: applications, and visions for the future. In: Cueteaux CG, ed. Simplified facial rejuvenation. Berlin: Springer; 2008:247–256
6. Andamyan AA. Method for skin rejuvenation. US Patent 6,086,578; 2000
7. Alcamo JH. Surgical suture. US Patent 3,123,077; 1964
8. Guillemain R. Le "Curl lift," la profession médicale. Chir Plast Estét March 1970
9. Buncke HJ. Surgical methods using one-way suture. US Patent 5,931,855; 1999
10. Ruff GL. Barbed bodily tissue connector. US Patent 6,241,747B1; 2001
11. Sulamanidze MA, Fournier PF, Paikidze TG, Sulamanidze GM. Removal of facial soft tissue ptosis with special threads. Dermatol Surg 2002;28(5):367–371
12. Sulamanidze MA, Paikidze TG, Sulamanidze GM, Neigel JM. Facial lifting with "APTOS" threads: feather lift. Otolaryngol Clin North Am 2005;38(5):1109–1117
13. Wu WT. Barbed sutures in facial rejuvenation. Aesthet Surg J 2004;24(6):582–587
14. Serdev N. Scarless Serdev suture methods in brow and face lifts. Int J Cosmet Med Surg 2001;1:9–15
15. Serdev N. Serdev suture for scarless buttock and ultrasonic liposculpture of the buttocks. Int J Cosmet Med Surg 2003;5(1): 27–34
16. Coleman SR, Grover R. The anatomy of the aging face: volume loss and changes in 3-dimensional topography. Aesthet Surg J 2006;26(1S):S4–S9
17. Wong CH, Mendelson B. Newer understanding of specific anatomic targets in the aging face as applied to injectables: aging changes in the craniofacial skeleton and facial ligaments. Plast Reconstr Surg 2015; 136(5, Suppl):44S–48S
18. Han HH, Kim JM, Kim NH, Park RH, Park JB, Ahn TJ. Combined, minimally invasive, thread-based facelift. Arch Aesthetic Plast Surg 2014;20(3):160–164
19. Sulamanidze M, Sulamanidze G. Facial lifting with APTOS methods. J Cutan Aesthet Surg 2008;1(1):7–11
20. Kim B, Kim B, Oh S, Jung W. The art and science of thread lifting. Singapore: Springer; 2019
21. Gamboa GM, Vasconez LO. Suture suspension technique for midface and neck rejuvenation. Ann Plast Surg 2009;62(5):478–481
22. Kalra R. Use of barbed threads in facial rejuvenation. Indian J Plast Surg 2008; 41(1, Suppl):S93–S100
23. Suh DH, Jang HW, Lee SJ, Lee WS, Ryu HJ. Outcomes of polydioxanone knotless thread lifting for facial rejuvenation. Dermatol Surg 2015;41(6):720–725
24. Yongtrakul P, Sirithanabadeekul P, Siriphan P. Thread lift: classification, technique, and how to approach to the patient. World Acad Sci Eng Technol 2016;10(12):558–566
25. Goldberg DJ. Stimulation of collagenesis by poly-L-lactic acid (PLLA) and -glycolide polymer (PLGA)-containing absorbable suspension suture and parallel sustained clinical benefit. J Cosmet Dermatol 2020;19(5):1172–1178
26. Padín VL. Experience in the use of barbed threads and non-barbed Serdev sutures in face and body lift: comparison and combination. In: Serdev N ed. Miniinvasive Face and Body Lifts: Closed Suture Lifts or Barbed Thread Lifts. Rijeka: InTech;2013:333
27. In: Serdev N ed. Miniinvasive Face and Body Lifts: Closed Suture Lifts or Barbed Thread Lifts. Rijeka: InTech; 2013.
28. Sulamanidze M, Sulamanidze G, Sulamanidze K. Mastopexy: how to reach consistent results: new methods. In: Serdev N, ed. Miniinvasive face and body lifts: closed suture lifts or barbed thread lifts. 2013:231
29. Des Fernandes MB. Percutaneous suspension sutures to change the nasal tip. In: Serdev N ed. Miniinvasive Face and Body Lifts: Closed Suture Lifts or Barbed Thread Lifts. Rijeka: InTech; 2013
30. Atiyeh BS, Dibo SA, Costagliola M, Hayek SN. Barbed sutures "lunch time" lifting: evidence-based efficacy. J Cosmet Dermatol 2010;9(2):132–141
31. Dua A, Bhardwaj B. A case report on use of cog threads and dermal fillers for facial-lifting in facioscapulohumeral muscular dystrophy. J Cutan Aesthet Surg 2019;12(1):52–55
32. Alam D. Rehabilitation of long-standing facial nerve paralysis with percutaneous suture-based slings. Arch Facial Plast Surg 2007;9(3):205–209
33. Citarella ER, Sterodimas A, Green AC, Sinder R, Pitanguy I. Use of triple-convergence polypropylene thread for the aesthetic correction of partial facial paralysis. Aesthetic Plast Surg 2008;32(4):688–691
34. Perrone M. Use of triple-convergence polypropylene thread for the aesthetic correction of partial facial paralysis caused by the facial nerve injury. Rev Col Bras Cir 2012;39(5):368–372
35. Humphrey CD, McIff TE, Sykes KJ, Tsue TT, Kriet JD. Suture biomechanics and static facial suspension. Arch Facial Plast Surg 2007;9(3):188–193
36. Aitzetmueller MM, Centeno Cerdas C, Nessbach P, et al. Polydioxanone threads for facial rejuvenation: analysis of quality variation in the market. Plast Reconstr Surg 2019;144(6):1002e–1009e

10

Surgical Rejuvenation of Upper Face

Kulwant S. Bhangoo

Introduction

Much attention has been focused on the midface and the lower face and neck with regard to rejuvenation of the aging face. In contrast, the upper part of the face has been relatively ignored. This might be because the signs of aging usually affect the midface and lower face much before affecting the upper third of the face.[1]

The upper third of the face comprises the forehead, glabella, temples, eyebrows, and the upper eyelids. Here again, redundancy of the upper eyelid skin usually forestalls the changes in the brow and forehead. Blepharochalasia of the upper eyelids is followed by ptosis of the eyebrows and rhytides of the glabella and forehead. Rejuvenation of the midface and lower face without addressing the upper third will result in a disassociated and disharmonious overall appearance.

Rejuvenation of the Upper Third of the Face

The upper third of the face consists of the forehead, glabella, temples, eyebrows, and upper eyelids anatomic subunits (**Fig. 10.1**).

Before considering any treatment options, it is important to evaluate the various anatomic factors contributing to the aging process (**Box 10.1**). Surgical methods for rejuvenating each one of these anatomic units are listed in **Box 10.2**.

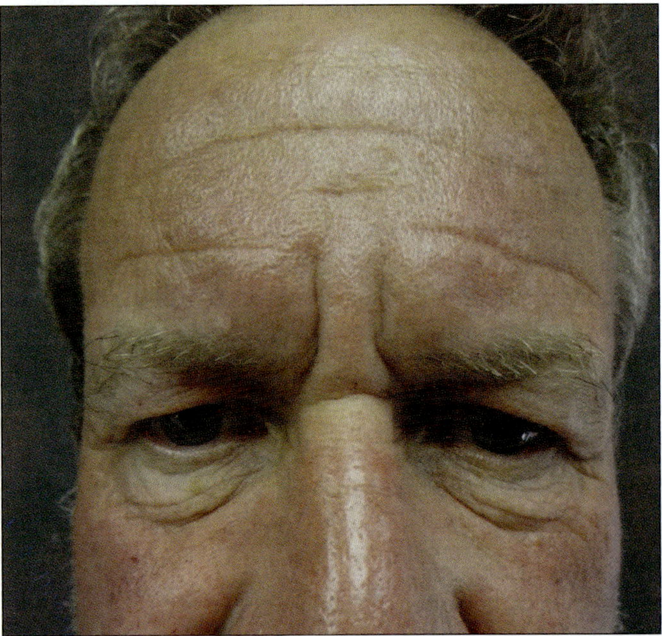

Fig. 10.1 Aging of upper third of face—Receding hairline, transverse forehead creases, glabellar rhytides, brow ptosis, skin redundancy of upper eyelids.

Box 10.1 Evaluation of upper third aging: Patient evaluation—Anatomic factors

- Forehead height
- Frontal and temporal hairline
- Frontal and brow hair abundance
- Skin quality, texture, thichkness, mobility and elasticity
- Mobility of scalp (galeal)
- Forehead wrinkling, degree and depth
- Temporal rhytides
- Eyebrow position, mobility and symmetry
- Glabellar rhytides
- Upper eyelids
- Degree of dermatochalasia
- Upper eyelid skin redundancy
- Lateral canthal hooding
- Lacrimal glands
- Sub Brow fat ptosis
- Preaponeurotic fat
- Preseptal fat pads
- Floppy lid
- Browptosis coexistence
- LID crease
- LID ptosis

Box 10.2 Procedures for rejuvenation of upper third of the face

- Fat grafting and fillers
- Midforehead lift
- Dermal fat grafts for forehead rhytides
- Coronal browlift
- Pretrichal browlift
- Endoscopic browlift
- Temporal lift
- Direct brow lift
- Dermal fat grafts for glabellar rhytides
- Transpalpebral resection of corrugator and procerus
- Transpalpebral browpexy with suture
- Endotine browpexy
- Upper blepharoplasty

Evaluation of Upper Third Facial Aging

In assessing the upper third of the face, attention is paid to the forehead in rest and animation to evaluate the rhytides. Brow position is evaluated by assessing the position of medial, middle, and lateral brow. There are gender variations with regard to the brow position. In the female, the distance between the brow and the upper lid margin is much more than in the male patient. Furthermore, in the female the lateral brow is usually higher than in the male (**Fig. 10.2a, b**).

Redundancy of skin and rhytides in the temporal region should be assessed and addressed if need be.

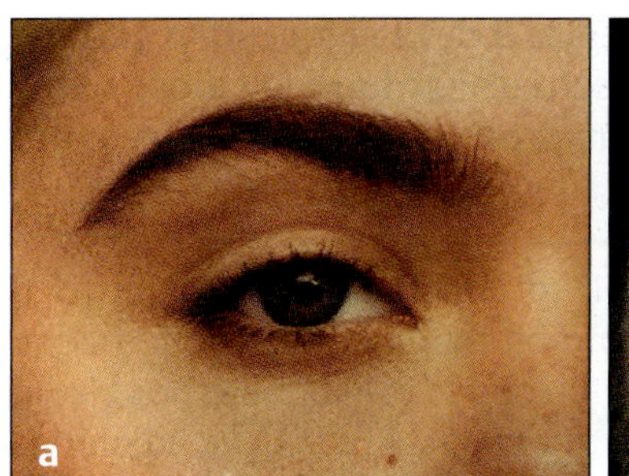
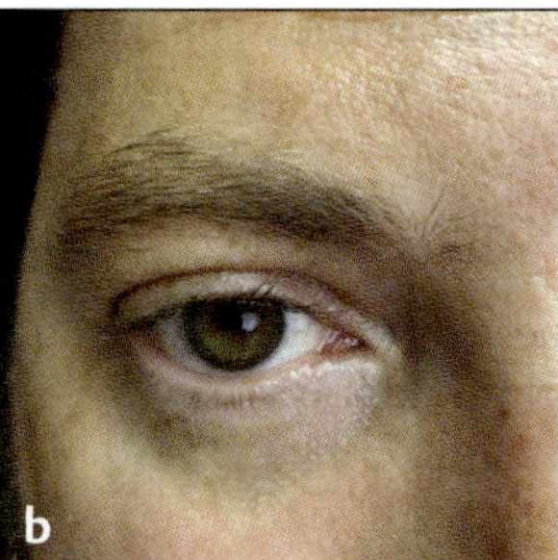

Fig. 10.2 **(a)** Female eyebrow. **(b)** Male eyebrow.

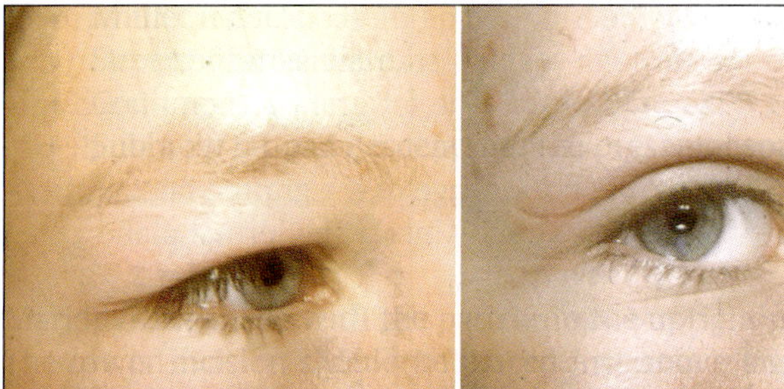

Fig. 10.3 Absent lid crease pre- and postop.

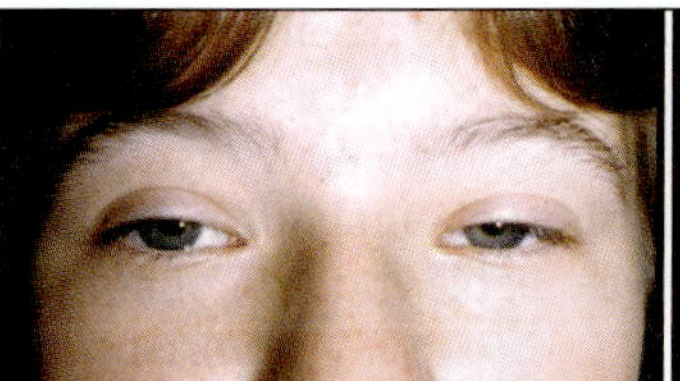
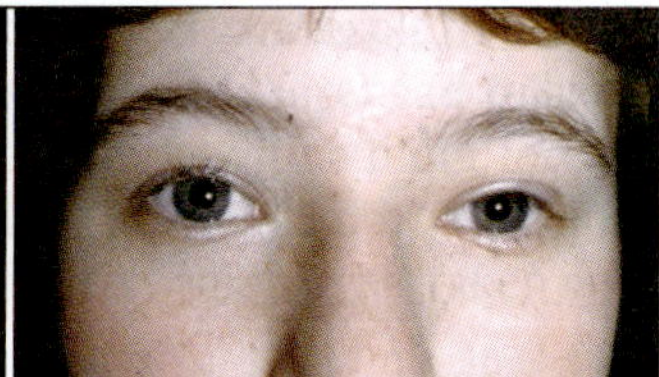

Fig. 10.4 Lid ptosis pre- and postop.

Assessment of the distance between the lid margin and the brow is also important in evaluating brow ptosis. Aging of the upper eyelids is the result of not only excess skin, but also other factors. The upper eyelid redundancy frequently results in the inability of the patient to elevate the lid above the 180-degree horizontal meridian. There may also be herniation of the fat pads in the medial, middle, and lateral compartments, which should be carefully evaluated. The descent of subbrow fat into the upper eyelid will result in a heavy upper eyelid. Redundancy of orbicularis oculi muscle can result in the so-called "floppy" upper lid which usually occurs in older and overweight patients.[2] Excess skin laterally can result in hooding which should be evaluated and addressed by modifying the skin incision during blepharoplasty.

Careful evaluation should be made as to the co-existence of brow ptosis which should be addressed, if present, when dealing with upper blepharoplasty. The presence of lid ptosis should be recognized and addressed if present. Removal of excess skin only when there is co-existence of brow ptosis will result in a sub-optimal outcome.

Brow ptosis and redundancy of the upper eyelid skin will make an individual wrinkle the forehead by contracting the frontalis muscle to raise the eyebrows as a compensatory maneuver. This, in turn, leads to creation and aggravation of forehead rhytides. Furthermore, it gives the individual a constantly "surprised" expression. Brow position is important, as a low eyebrow gives a sad and unhappy look, whereas a high brow gives a surprised and frightened look.

There are ethnic variations in the appearance of the upper eyelid.[3] Most notably, in the South Asian and oriental patients there may be absence of the upper lid fold or crease which can be created during upper blepharoplasty (**Fig. 10.3**).[4] If there is ptosis of the eyelid, then it will warrant correction (**Fig. 10.4**).

Pertinent Anatomy

Skin	-	Texture. Rhytides rest and animation.
Ligaments	-	Periorbital septa and adhesions, temporal crest transition from supraorbital to temporal parietal fascia.
Muscles	-	Frontalis, corrugator supercilii, procerus, orbicularis oculi.
Nerves	-	Supraorbital nerve, supratrochlear nerve, zygomaticofrontal nerve, zygomaticotemporal nerve.
Vessels	-	Supraorbital vessels and supratrochlear vessels, sentinel vein.

Surgical Rejuvenation of Upper Third of Face

Fat Grafting and Fillers for Facial Rejuvenation

Autologous fat grafting has grown in popularity in recent years. Autologous fat is the most biocompatible filler material which is freely available from the patient. It is long lasting and less expensive than other synthetic fillers. Autologous fat graft and dermal fillers have many applications in rejuvenation of the mid and lower face. It is used for volumizing and correcting depressions resulting from tissue atrophy due to advancing age. Both fat grafts and fillers can also be used to correct folds, such as nasolabial folds and marionette lines and perioral rhytides. As far as the upper third of the face is concerned, it has rather limited applications. Its applications are limited to correcting forehead and glabellar rhytides. It is also used in enhancing upper eyelid fullness and for correcting postsurgical upper lid hollowness resulting from overresection of fat during blepharoplasty.

When using fat to correct forehead and glabellar wrinkles, it is important not to inject it directly into the rhytides like the synthetic fillers. The forehead skin is taut and not distensible. Direct injection will require a lot of pressure which will damage the delicate fat cells. A tunnel should be created in the subdermal plane directly under the wrinkle. This is done through a small stab incision in the skin and by using a lacrimal probe. The fat graft is then placed into this tunnel, and the small incision is closed with a single 6–0 catgut suture to prevent leakage of the grafted fat. Synthetic fillers can be injected directly into a subdermal plane under the wrinkles.

Fat grafts and fillers can also be used for correcting temple hollowness resulting from subcutaneous fat atrophy with advancing age (**Fig. 10.5**). Fat grafts are also in vogue for enhancing upper eyelid fullness due to atrophy because of advancing age or to correct iatrogenic hollowness resulting from excessive resection of fat during blepharoplasty (**Fig. 10.6**).

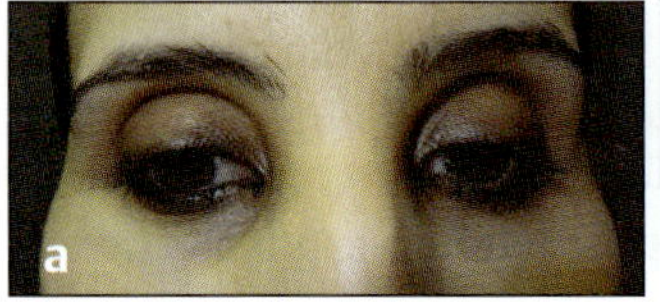

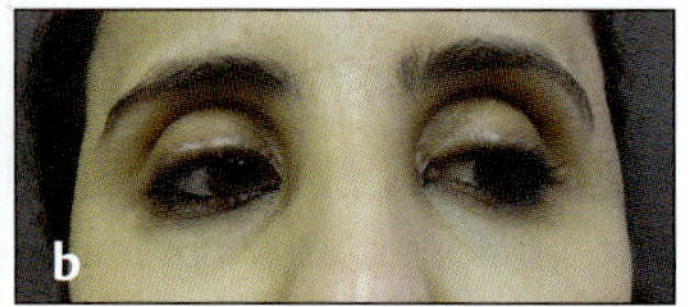

Fig. 10.5 Temporal hollow. **(a)** Preoperative picture. **(b)** Post fat grafting picture.

Fat grafts in the upper eyelids can also be used to correct the A-frame deformity resulting from excessive fat resection during upper blepharoplasty (**Fig. 10.7**). Platelet-rich plasma (PRP) can improve fat grafting outcomes.[5]

Rejuvenation of the Aging Forehead

Forehead Plasty—Direct Excision

The prominent feature of forehead aging is the development of deep transverse creases. There are several ways of dealing with this. In the past, direct excision was made using an incision, as shown in the diagram in **Fig. 10.8a, b**. This works well in older patients with fair skin. Although mid-forehead incision allows direct access to the underlying structures such as the procerus muscle and the corrugator supercilii muscle, the procedure is seldom recommended. This is because direct excision in the mid-forehead area can result in unsightly scars in individuals with dark skin. This can also result in prolonged hyperesthesia and numbness of the scar and beyond due to injury to the supraorbital and supratrochlear neurovascular bundles.[6]

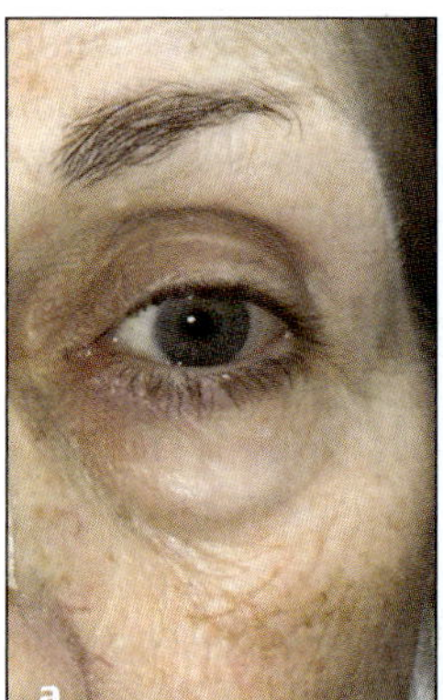

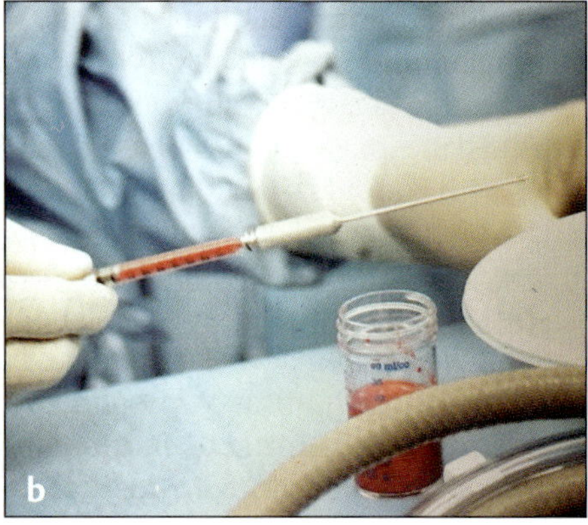

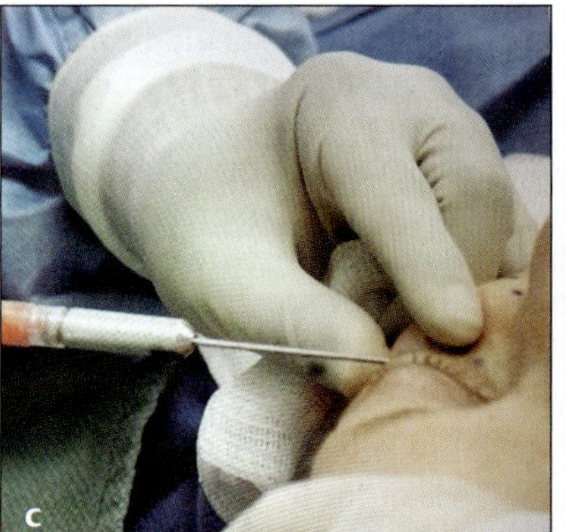

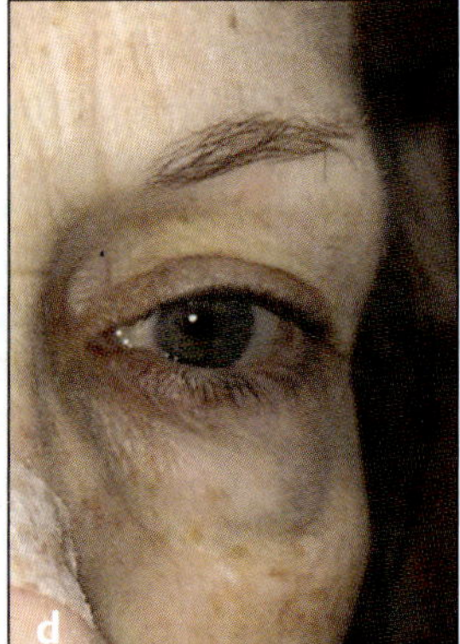

Fig. 10.6 **(a)** Hollow lid due to overresection of fat during blepharoplasty. **(b, c)** Fat grafting. **(d)** Hollowness corrected by fat grafting.

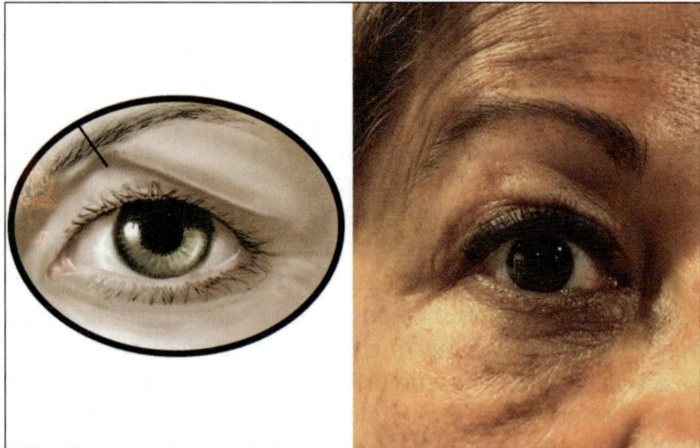

Fig. 10.7 A frame deformity.

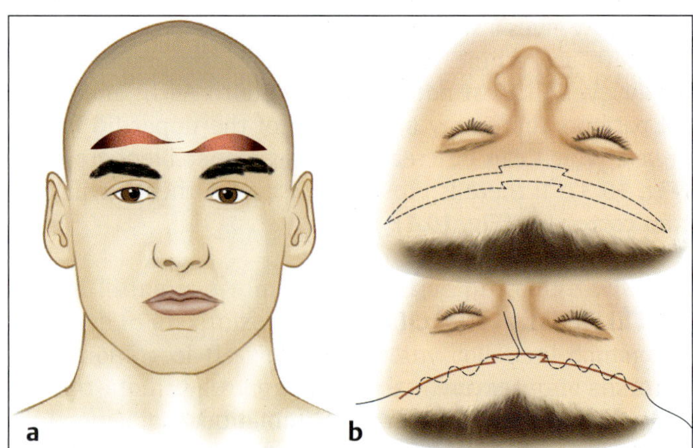

Fig. 10.8 **(a)** Direct excision for forehead rhytides. **(b)** Mid-forehead incision.

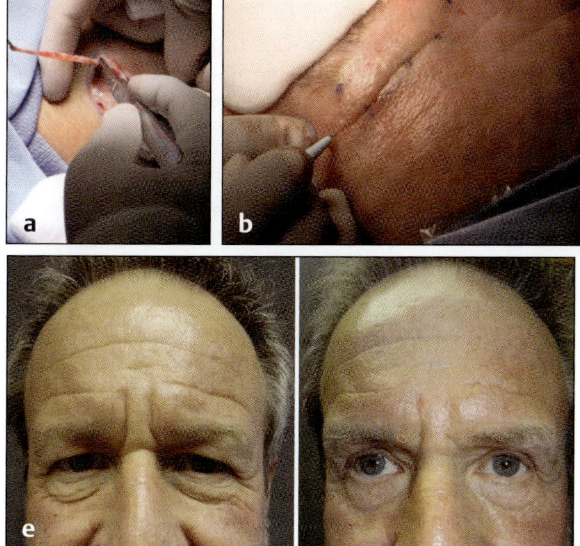

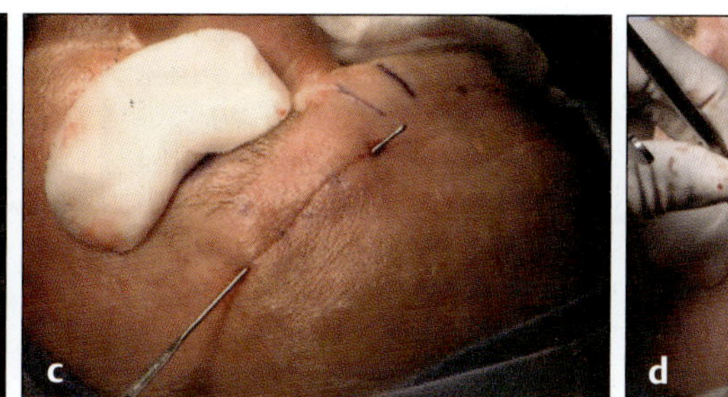

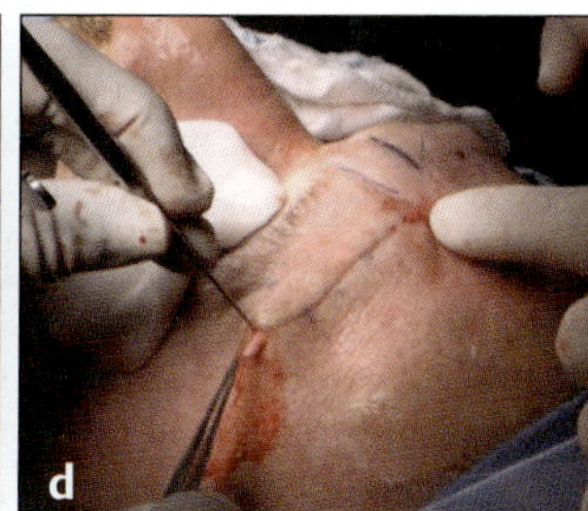

Fig. 10.9 **(a)** Harvesting of dermal fat graft from groin. **(b)** Forehead crease marked and small incision made at both extremities of the crease. **(c)** Subdermal tunnel made with blunt lacrimal probe. **(d)** Dermal fat graft milked into forehead crease—initial placement with traction suture with straight Keith needle with blunt-end leading. **(e)** Dermal fat graft for forehead creases pre- and postop.

Forehead Plasty—Dermal Fat Grafts

The author prefers to correct deep forehead creases by insertion of dermal fat grafts. These grafts can be harvested from a preexisting scar. If there are no scars then the groin crease can be used. An elliptical incision is outlined in the groin crease. The dermal fat grafts are harvested by making an incision through the epidermis only. The marked area is then de-epithelialized. An incision is then deepened on either side and the dermal fat graft is harvested and cut into thin strips measuring 2 mm in width (**Fig. 10.9a**). Some amount of fat is left attached under the dermis depending on the depth of the skin creases.

The forehead creases are marked. A small incision is made at either extremity of the crease (**Fig. 10.9b**). Undermining is then performed with a blunt-tipped lacrimal probe. This undermining should be done in a subdermal plane (**Fig. 10.9c**). The grafts are then inserted into these tunnels. Placement of the grafts is facilitated by tying a suture to the graft and inserting it into the tunnel with a straight Keith needle. The needle is then inserted into the tunnel with the blunt end leading and retrieved from the opposite side. The dermal fat graft is then carefully milked into the forehead crease (**Fig. 10.9d**). The incisions are closed with a single 6–0 catgut suture. This is the least aggressive way of dealing with forehead creases with long-lasting permanent results (**Fig. 10.9e**).

Coronal Forehead Lift

Coronal forehead lift is among the oldest methods of treating the aging forehead.[7] The scar is located a few centimeters behind the hairline. It treats all aspects of the aging forehead and brow. It allows access to the procerus and the corrugator supercilii muscles to correct the frown lines. It also eliminates the forehead creases in many cases. Coronal forehead lift has many disadvantages. The scar can be unsightly in dark-haired individuals (**Fig. 10.10**). It elevates the hairline and makes the forehead taller. It vertically lengthens the upper third of the face. There is prolonged hyperesthesia and numbness of the scalp which can be bothersome. This procedure does not allow fine-tuning of the brow position. Contraindications include a high forehead and receding hairline.

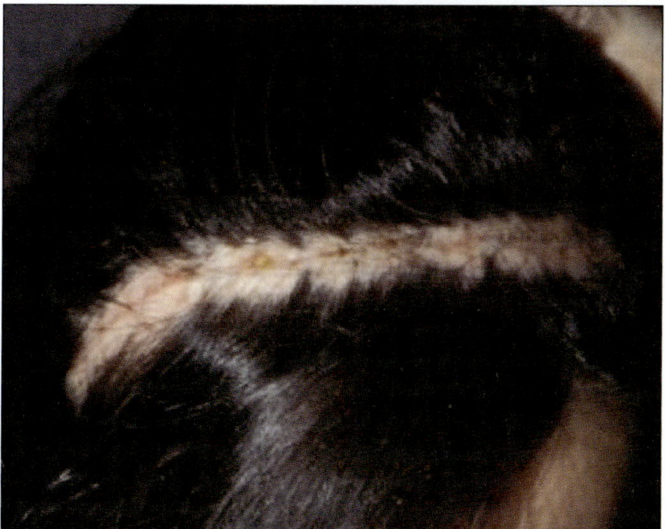

Fig. 10.10 Unsightly coronal forehead lift scar.

Technique

The procedure can be done under local anesthesia but preferably under general anesthesia, especially when it is combined with other facial rejuvenation procedures. A small strip of hair can be shaved (**Fig. 10.11a**). This is done in a calculated way so that the shaved area is the extent of the scalp, anterior to the incision, that will be resected at the

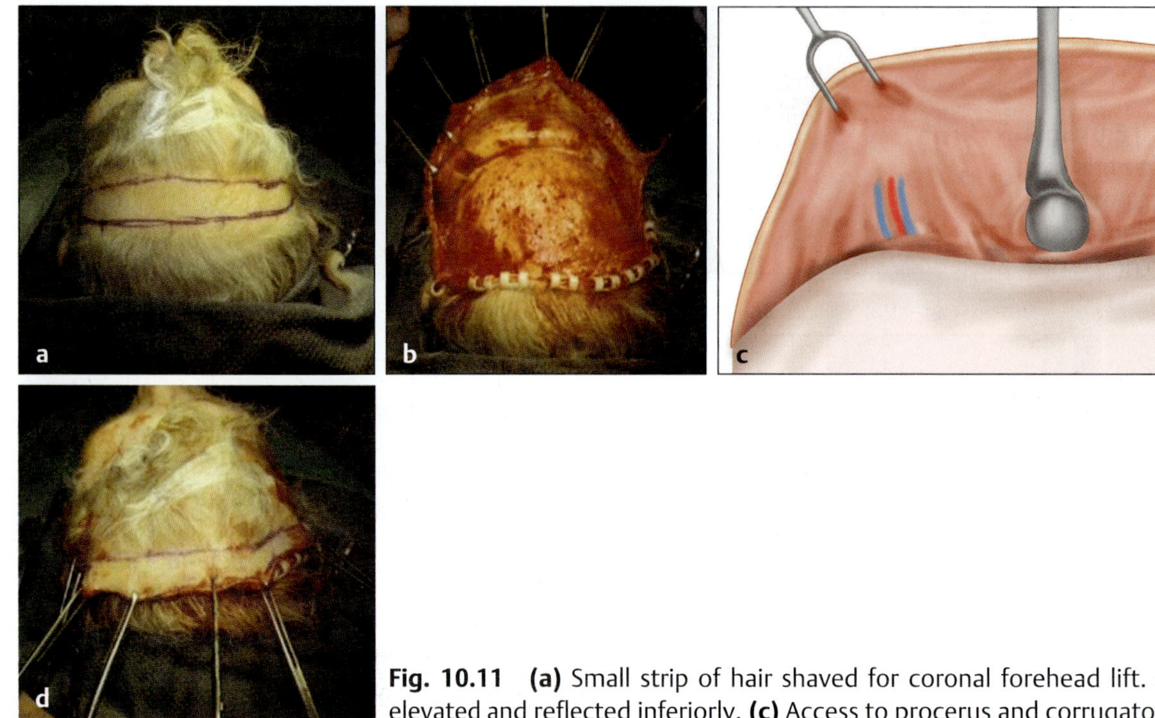

Fig. 10.11 **(a)** Small strip of hair shaved for coronal forehead lift. **(b)** Frontal scalp flap elevated and reflected inferiorly. **(c)** Access to procerus and corrugators. **(d)** Skin resection.

end of the procedure, thus leaving no non-hair-bearing area along the incision site. A coronal incision is then made from just above the ear from one side to the other. Using blunt and sharp dissection, undermining is performed in the loose subgaleal plane above the periosteum. The frontal scalp flap is elevated and reflected inferiorly (**Fig. 10.11b**). Bleeding in this plane is minimal and effectively controlled by electrocautery. After the tissues surrounding the neurovascular bundles of the supraorbital complex are encountered, blunt dissection is performed with a fine hemostat for identifying, isolating, and preserving the important supraorbital and supratrochlear neurovascular bundle. The procerus muscle and the corrugator supercilii muscles are identified and transected if required (**Fig. 10.11c**). After establishing hemostasis the flap is pulled superiorly and the amount of redundant scalp tissue is gauged by manually pushing the two skin flaps toward each other (**Fig. 10.11d**). The excessive tissue from the frontal flap is then excised in small segments. The excision at all times parallels the direction of the hair follicles. Closure is done with multiple subcuticular 3–0 polydioxin sutures in the galea and the dermis. All tension should be eliminated at the margin in order to prevent alopecia. Alopecia along the scar can be disturbing. It can be particularly noticeable in dark-haired individuals (**Fig. 10.10**). Final closure of the incision can be done with skin staples. Drains are not usually necessary, and pressure dressing applied for 48 hours will prevent postoperative hematoma.

Pretrichial Forehead Lift

In patients who have a high forehead or a receding hairline, a coronal browlift will further elongate the forehead. In these individuals, a forehead lift can be performed using the pretrichial forehead lift. In this procedure there is no vertical forehead lengthening. It preserves the hairline. This procedure also treats all aspects of aging forehead and brows. There is immediate scar camouflage within the hairline if the incision is placed correctly and if the wound is closed meticulously. The disadvantages include the possible visible scar in the event of impaired healing. There is also prolonged hyperesthesia and dysesthesia of the scalp due to injury to the supraorbital neurovascular bundle.

Technique

An incision is made along the hairline. The incision should be angled and made parallel to the direction of the hair follicles so as to minimize damage to the hair bulbs along the incision line. The rest of the procedure is similar to that as described for the coronal browlift (**Fig. 10.12a**). A reverse beveling of the incision to partially transect several hairline hair follicles allows some eventual hair growth through the resulting scar, thus facilitating camouflage of the scar (**Fig. 10.12b**). This is accomplished by growth of the partially transected hair follicles that will eventually grow through the scar (**Fig. 10.12c**).

Endoscopic Browlift

Since the advent of endoscopic browlift by Isse and Vasconez in 1992,[8] the procedure and instrumentation have significantly evolved to its present state.[9] The procedure has actually replaced the previously done, more aggressive, procedures such as coronal browlift.[7] Furthermore, it has gained tremendous patient acceptance compared to the previous procedures.

The procedure is now readily accepted by patients because of small incisions and small resultant scars, ability to expose and release periorbital adhesions, allow excision of corrugator and procerus muscles, allow preservation of sensory nerves due to endoscopic magnification. The scars are short and risk of alopecia is less, and, more importantly, there is no sensory loss or dysesthesia.

Scalp elevation is established by fixation devices as opposed to scalp skin excision as with other methods shortening the operative time and minimizing blood loss. Advantages and disadvantages of the endoscopic browlift are listed in **Table 10.1**.

Indications

Patients with short forehead, flat forehead, and nonreceding hairline are the good candidates, while persons with high and convex forehead, receding hairline, deep rhytides, and thick skin are the unfavorable candidates.

Patient Evaluation for Endoscopic Browlift

It is important to select the right patient for this procedure. Evaluation of the patient for endoscopic browlift should be performed with the patient sitting upright (**Fig. 10.13a–c**). When the patient has blepharochalasia of the upper eyelids and brow ptosis, they have a tendency to artificially elevate their brows by contracting their frontalis muscles. This results in deep forehead rhytides. More importantly,

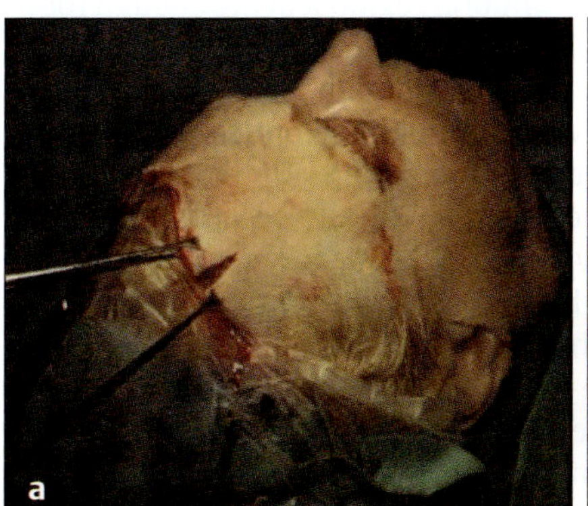
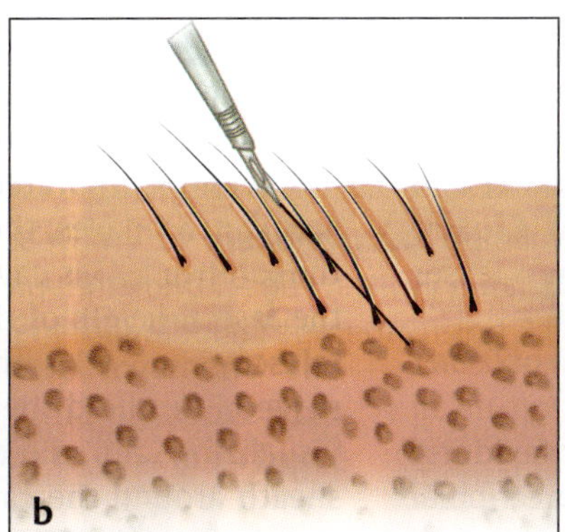
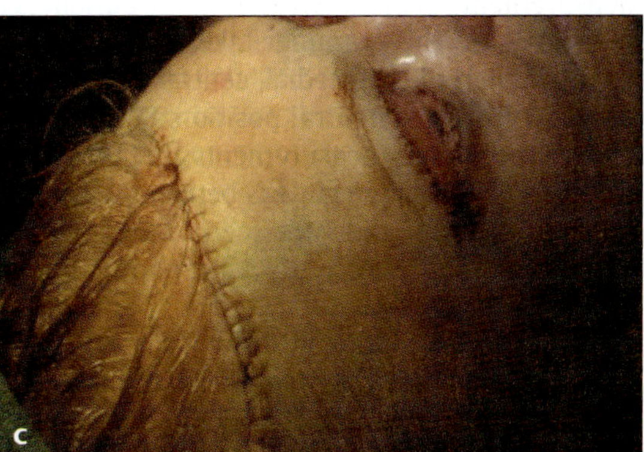

Fig. 10.12 **(a)** Segmental excision of skin. **(b)** Pretrichial incision—oblique to avoid injury to hair follicles. **(c)** Closure of pretrichial forehead lift.

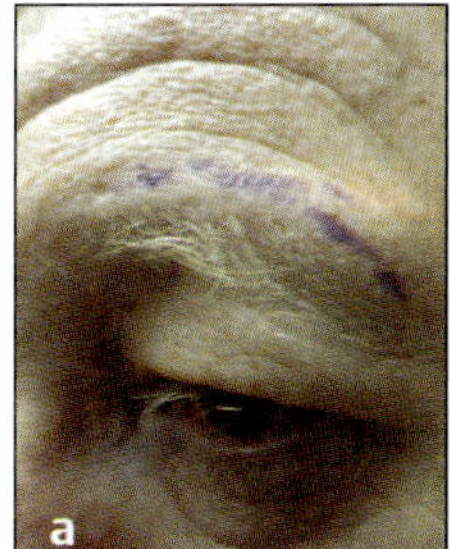
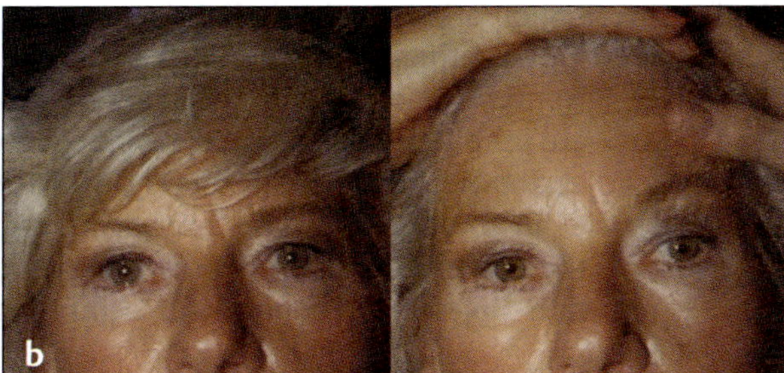
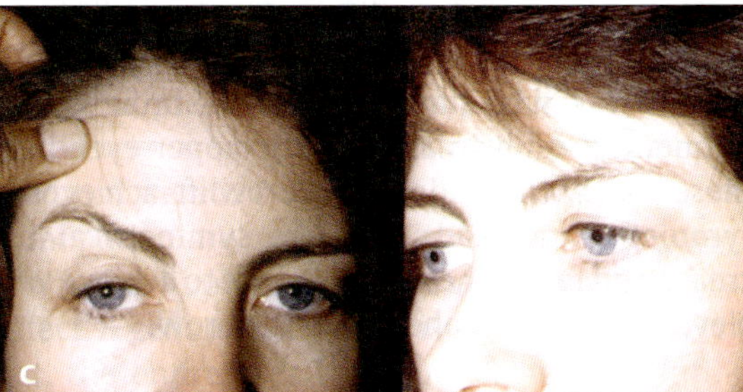

Fig. 10.13 **(a)** Assessment of brow ptosis—markings show the brow is below the orbital rim. **(b, c)** Evaluation for endoscopic browlift.

Table 10.1 Advantages and disadvantages of endoscopic browlift

Advantages	Disadvantages
• It can be performed through small incisions • Surgery is less invasive than other traditional methods • It allows for release of periorbital adhesions and ligaments and accurate elevation of brows • It is useful in correcting brow asymmetry • Allows for excision of procerus and corrugator muscles • Allows endoscopic magnification during corrugator and procerus myomectomies • There are no sensory disturbances as with other procedures • No alteration of hairline • No alopecia	• Requires expensive instrumentation • There is a long learning curve • Requires general anesthesia • Expensive fixation devices • Technology dependent

of the temporal region and a temporal lift is also required, another incision can be made in the temporal region. These incisions can be made with a #15 blade. Some surgeons recommend deepening these incisions with electrocautery in order to prevent bleeding from the skin edges to prevent clouding of the optic instruments. However, this can result in alopecia around the resultant scars due to destruction of hair follicle because of the heat from cautery. For this reason, the author has abandoned using electrocautery to deepen the incisions.

The endoscope and the sheath are introduced through one incision and the instruments, such as the elevators, dissectors, suction, and cautery, are inserted through the other incision (**Fig. 10.17a**).

Creation of Optical Cavity

There is no naturally occurring cavity in the forehead. An optical cavity is created by placing an endoscope in a sheath that has a 30-degree shelf at its end. This elevates the skin flap and creates the optical cavity. If there is fraying of tissues that obscures the visual field, a suture placed on the overlying skin and applying traction on it will elevate the flap and allow visualization.

Undermining

Blind dissection is performed over the frontal and parietal regions.[11] This dissection is performed in a subgaleal plane using a sharp periosteal elevator. It is important to perform the undermining posteriorly in the parietal region from one side to the other in order to allow for posterior glide of the undermined forehead flap. After completing the dissection of the parietal scalp, attention is directed toward the frontal region. Through the three incisions and using a sharp-curved elevator, subperiosteal dissection is performed in a blind manner down to the orbital rim. This dissection can be performed very expeditiously and is usually bloodless if the dissection is performed in the proper plane. If a temporal lift is required, the dissection is performed separately through a temporal incision, taking care to protect the frontal branch of the facial nerve. The frontal and temporal

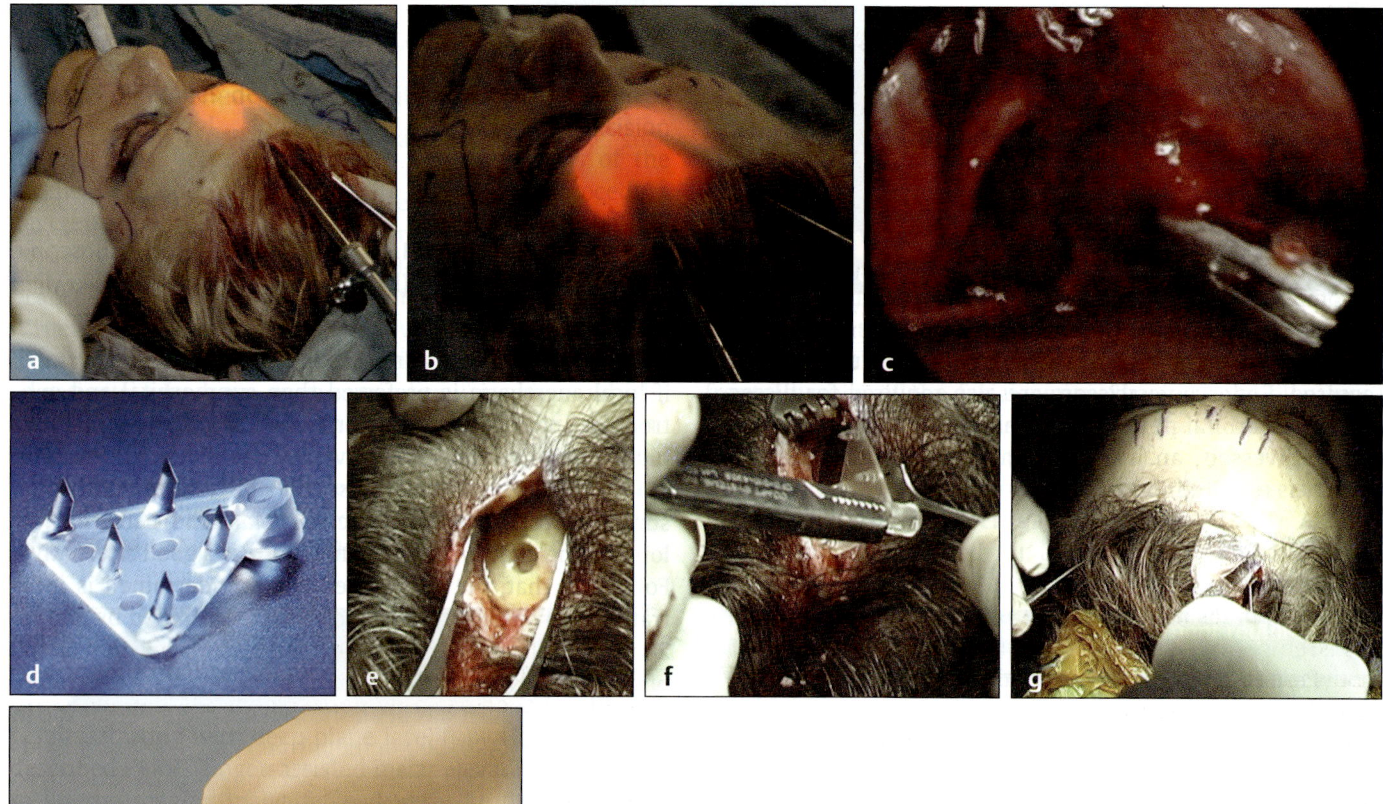

Fig. 10.17 **(a)** Endoscope and sheath inserted into one incision; instruments inserted through the other incisions. **(b)** Endoscopic browlift—releasing the brow. **(c)** Corrugator supercilii muscles removed by grasping forceps, supraorbital and supratrochlear neurovascular bundles on either side. **(d)** Forehead endotine. **(e)** Drill hole for endotine. **(f)** Endotine inserted into drill hole. **(g)** Scalp pulled posteriorly. **(h)** Digital pressure to engage endotine.

dissections are then joined to each other. The fusion of the galeal and the temporal parietal fascia is termed a conjoined fascia. This conjoined fascia is pushed upward and the elevator is inserted onto the bone at a point approximately 7 cm above the brow. Joining these two dissections at 7 cm above the brow will ensure protection of the frontal branch of the facial nerve. It is frequently necessary to incise the conjoined tendon between the temporal and frontal planes with a sharp elevator or an endoscopic scissors.

Release of Periosteum

The release of periosteum along the supraorbital rim is a key aspect of endoscopic browlift procedure. Releasing the attachment of the periosteum from the supraorbital rim allows the undermined frontal flap to be displaced posteriorly. Under direct vision, the periosteum is incised laterally with the sharp edge of the periosteal elevator (**Fig. 10.17b**). It is then continued medially. In so doing, the supraorbital nerve and the adjacent vessels are visualized under direct vision and protected. There is usually a large vein in close proximity to the supraorbital neurovascular bundle which should be protected. Medially, supratrochlear nerves are identified and protected.

Procerus and Corrugator Myomectomy

Under direct vision, the procerus muscle is identified in the middle. Using grasping forceps this muscle can be removed in small pieces. Bleeding is controlled with electrocautery.

The corrugator supercilii muscles are similarly removed by using the grasping forceps and removing the muscle piecemeal (**Fig. 10.17c**). It is important to protect the supraorbital and supratrochlear neurovascular bundles and the blood vessels around these nerves during this procedure. Bleeding can be controlled using electrocautery. Excision of the procerus muscle will result in correction of the deep transverse line in the radix area and the corrugator resection will correct the vertical rhytides or frown lines in the glabella.[12]

Fixation

Several methods of fixation of the elevated brow following endoscopic browlift have been used in the past (**Box 10.4**).[13] These have included sutures to attach the forehead flap to periosteum, insertion of a K-pin into the outer table and through the staples in the incision.[14] These are left in place for a few days and then removed. Cortical tunneling of the outer table of the skull has been used and is an economic way of fixation. This entails making a tunnel between the outer and inner layers of the skull using a motorized sharp drill. Other fixation devices that have been used in the past include the use of metal screws. These have been abandoned because they will interfere with magnetic resonance imaging (MRI) should the patient need one in the future. The screw heads are also palpable and can be bothersome. Mitek screws frequently used by orthopedic surgeons are buried into the bone, have also been used in the past. These also are objectionable because of the fact that they are retained metal foreign body. Most recently, forehead endotine has been used (**Fig. 10.17d**).The endotine has the advantage that it provides three-point fixation which is more effective than the one-point fixation as offered by other methods. Furthermore, the endotines are absorbable.[15] The newer generation of endotines are absorbed in 6 weeks. This allows for fixation without a retained metallic foreign body. The placement of the endotines is achieved by first making a marking in the bone after pulling the forehead flap posteriorly. A drill hole is made (**Fig. 10.17e**). The bone debris is irrigated from the drill hole. The endotine is then inserted into the hole (**Fig. 10.17f**). The scalp is then pulled posteriorly (**Fig. 10.17h**) and engaged into the tines with digital pressure (**Fig. 10.17h**). This allows for elevation of the forehead and the brow. The incisions are closed with 3–0 Vicryl for the deeper layer and skin staples for surface closure. A drain is not normally required as the dissection is pretty much avascular. A pressure dressing may be applied for 48 hours (**Figs. 10.18–10.20**).

Box 10.4 Fixation devices for the elevated brow following endoscopic browlift

- Periosteal suture
- Cotical tunnel
- K-pin
- Screws
- Mitex screws
- Absorbable screws
- Endotine forehead

Temporal Lift

In some patients there is laxity of tissue in the temporal region, resulting in ptosis of the lateral aspect of the eyebrow. The temporal lift can be performed through a coronal or a pretrichial forehead lift;[16] however, it can also be done as an independent procedure. The temporal lift is ideal for elevating the lateral aspect of the brow (**Fig. 10.21**). The scar is camouflaged in the temporal hairline. It improves the brow position and corrects temporal tissue laxity.

Fig. 10.22 shows a patient who has undergone upper blepharoplasty with unsatisfactory correction of the lateral aspect of the brow. She subsequently underwent a browpexy.

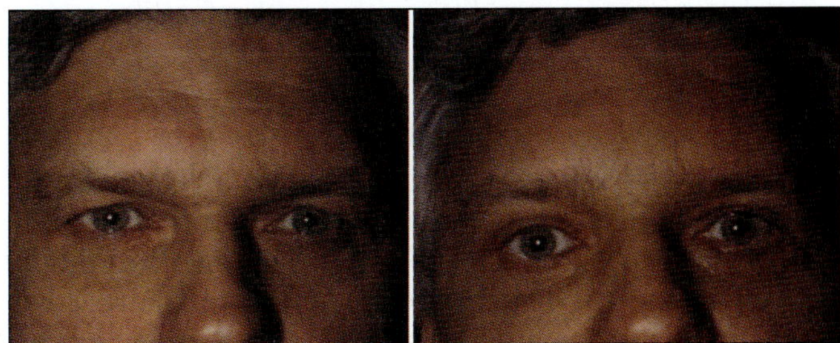

Fig. 10.18 Endoscopic browlift pre- and postop.

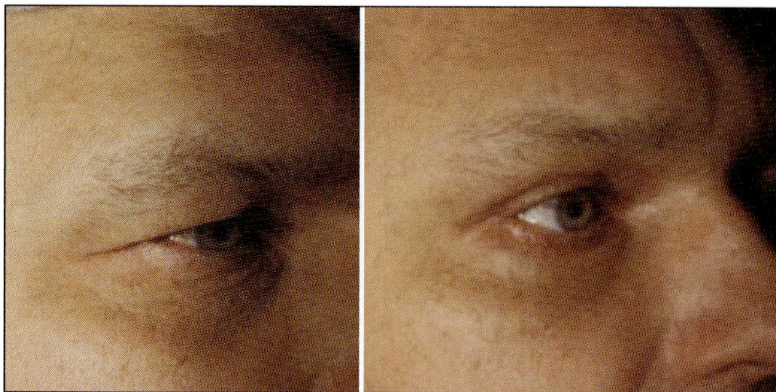

Fig. 10.19 Endoscopic browlift in a male patient—pre- and postop.

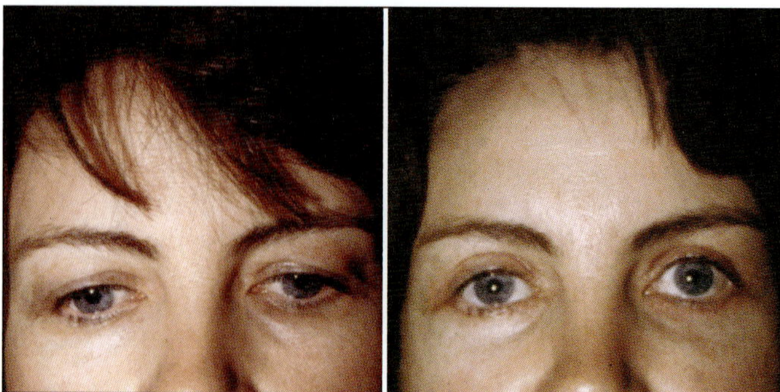

Fig. 10.20 Endoscopic browlift in a female patient—pre- and postop.

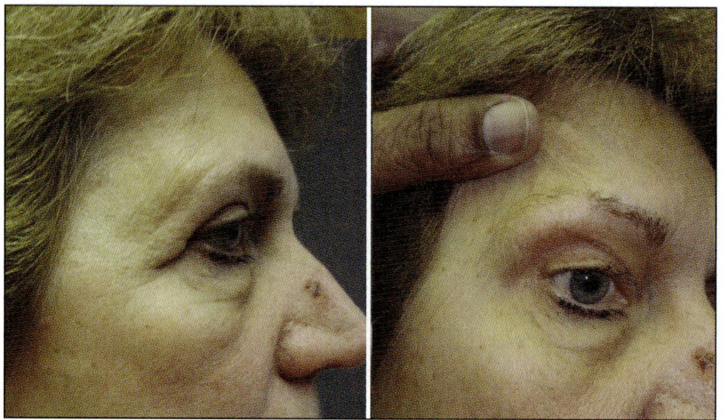

Fig. 10.21 Temporal lift assessment—Correction of lateral hooding by elevation of the temple.

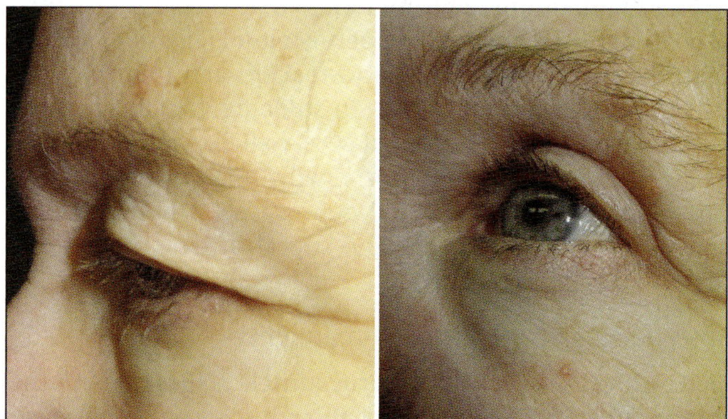

Fig. 10.22 Patient has undergone upper blepharoplasty with unsatisfactory correction of lateral aspect of brow due to temporal laxity.

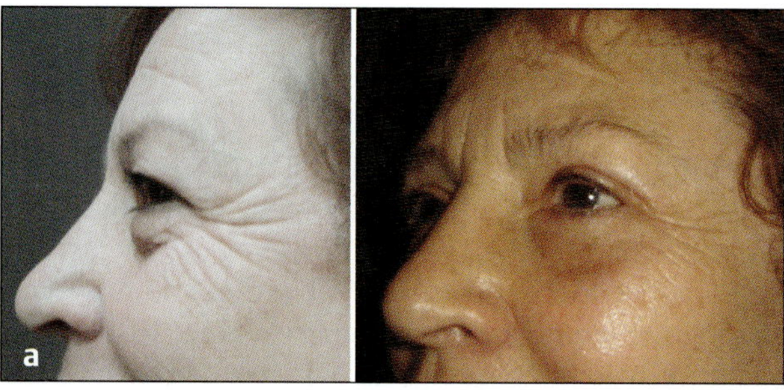

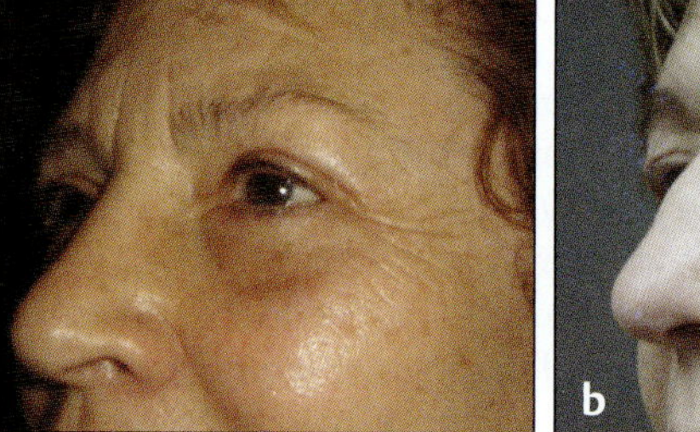

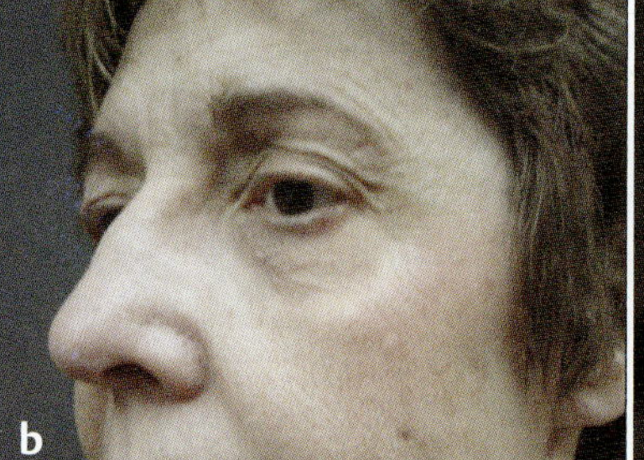

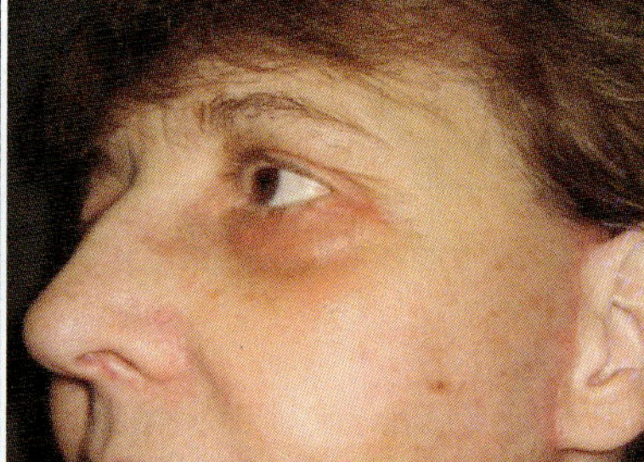

Fig. 10.23 **(a, b)** Temporal lift with facelift.

There was still laxity of the brow laterally which required a temporal lift for its correction. **Fig. 10.23a, b** shows a patient who underwent temporal lift together with a facelift.

Technique

Incision is marked as shown in **Fig. 10.24a** in the temporal region with the patient sitting up. A zigzag incision is preferred. This incision is placed about 3 cm posterior to the temporal hairline. The procedure can be performed under local anesthesia or under general anesthesia when it is being done in conjunction with other procedures. The incision is carried up to the level just above the thick, shiny, deep temporalis fascia. In a predominantly blunt dissection, the temporal flap is undermined in this avascular plane to just above the level of the brow and the redundant lateral canthal skin (**Fig. 10.24b**).

The frontal branch of the facial nerve should be marked preoperatively and protected during this procedure. It is, therefore, recommended that blunt dissection be performed under direct vision aided by a good fiberoptic light. The frontal branch is probably more at risk from stretching or injury from cautery than from the actual transection. Therefore, electrocautery should be used with caution and away from the location of the frontal branch of the facial

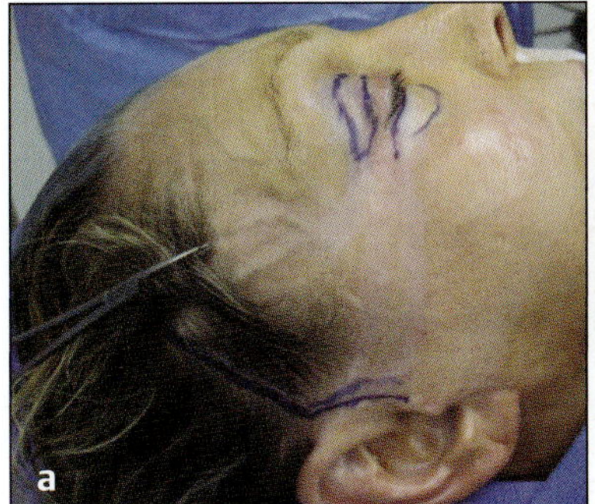

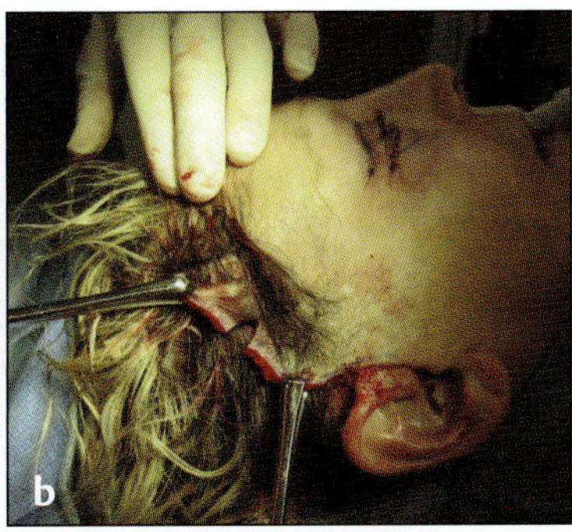

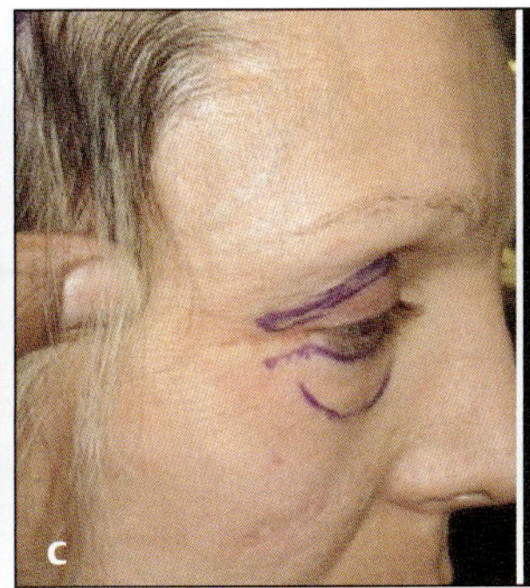

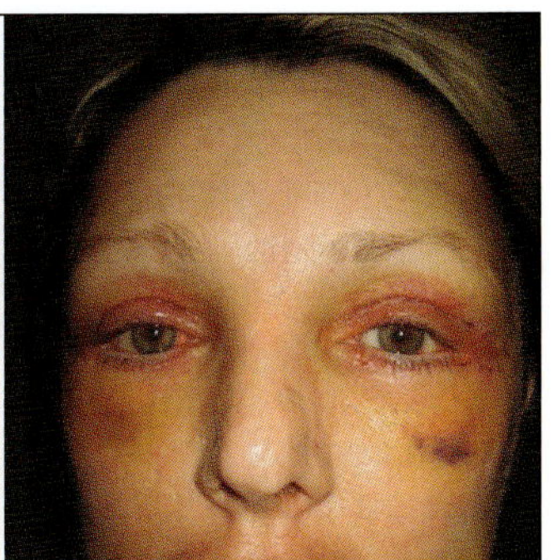

Fig. 10.24 **(a)** Incision markings for temporal lift. **(b)** Incision placed for temporal lift. **(c)** Temporal lift pre- and postop.

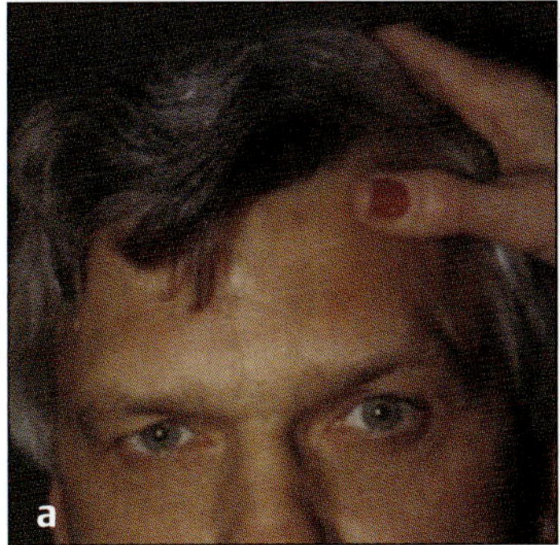

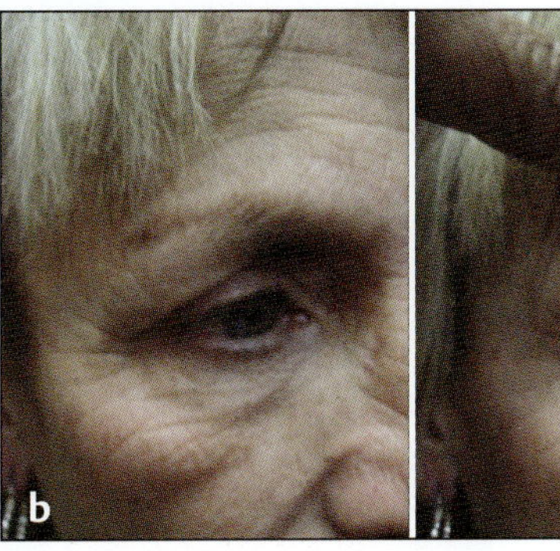

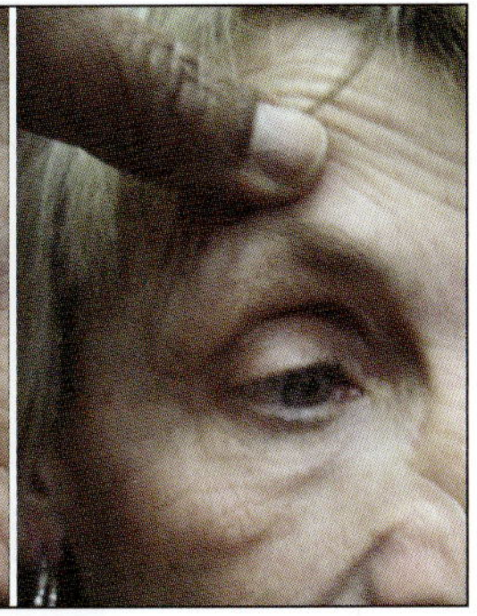

Fig. 10.25 **(a)** Assessment of brow ptosis—digital elevation. **(b)** Brow is digitally raised to determine desired elevation.

nerve. The skin flap is then advanced upward and laterally. A few key sutures of 3–0 polydioxin or PDS are inserted through the dermis. The redundant flap is then segmentally excised. Care is taken to ensure that all tension is taken by the dermal tissues away from the wound margins to prevent alopecia. Surface closure can be performed using skin staples. **Fig. 10.24c** shows the immediate postoperative result.

Brow Ptosis

Ptosis of eyebrows is a prominent feature of aging of the upper third of the face. It is evaluated by assessing the position of the brow relative to the supraorbital rim (**Fig. 10.25a, b**). Normally the eyebrow is at or slightly above the orbital rim. Descent of the eyebrow below the orbital rim gives the patient a sleepy look and can also have a functional implication in accentuating the patient's blepharochalasia with resultant decrease in visual field. Ptosis of the eyebrow can involve the entire brow or can be most pronounced medially in the mid-forehead area or laterally.

Direct Browlift

In certain cases, particularly in older, fair-skinned patients, direct excision of the skin above the brow can result in elevation of the brow. The elliptical excision can be performed over the entire brow if the ptosis involves the whole extent of the brow. Alternatively, it can be performed in the medial, mid, or lateral part depending on the location of the brow ptosis (**Fig. 10.26**).

This procedure can be done under local anesthesia. An elliptical skin incision is made just above the brow taking care to preserve the brow hair follicles. Through this incision the orbital component of the orbicularis muscle can be identified. Through this approach, the subbrow fat pad can be addressed. If the subbrow fat pad is very prominent it can be excised. In some cases, there is ptosis of the subbrow fat in the upper eyelid. Through this approach, a subbrow fat pad ptosis can also be corrected. The skin flap is then elevated superiorly and excised segmentally (**Fig. 10.27**). Meticulous closure is required to prevent an unsightly scar. This procedure works well in older patients as indicated in **Fig. 10.28**. In younger patients, it can result in unsightly scars (**Fig. 10.29a, b**). The advantage of this procedure is that it allows for accurate brow elevation and preserves the forehead and scalp sensation. Patients should be carefully selected and should have abundant brow hair. This procedure is also very effective in correcting brow asymmetry. This procedure does not alter the forehead height.

Glabellar Rhytides—Frown Lines

Correction of frown lines is one of the most frequently requested cosmetic procedures. Correction of glabellar frown lines can be accomplished by nonsurgical and surgical methods. Nonsurgical methods usually result in temporary correction of the glabella frown lines. These

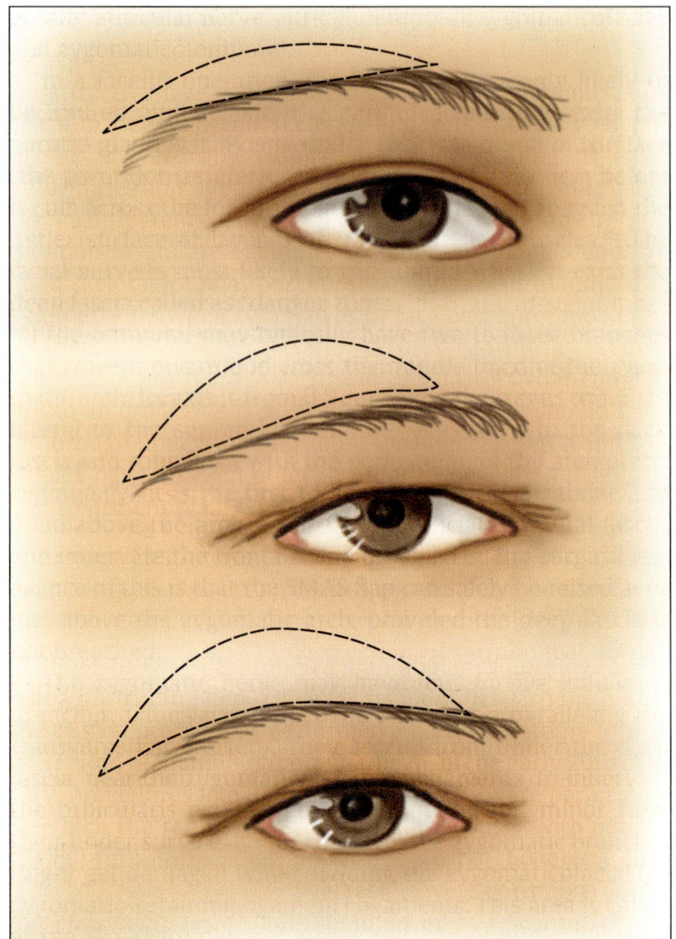

Fig. 10.26 Direct skin excision for lateral, mid, and total brow ptosis.

can be accomplished by using neurotoxins or fillers. For further detail, refer to Chapters 7 and 8 on "Principles and Techniques of Nonsurgical Facial Rejuvenation" and "Nonsurgical Rejuvenation of the Face using Botulinum Toxin and Fillers" in Volume VI.

Surgical correction of glabellar frown lines can be achieved in two ways:

- Placement of fat or dermal fat grafts.
- Resection of corrugator and procerus supercilii muscle.

Placement of Fat and Dermal Fat Grafts for Glabellar Rhytides

Deep forehead and glabellar frown lines can be corrected surgically by doing fat grafts. Fat harvested from another source can be injected into the frown lines. Some surgeons prefer to pretreat the fat with platelet-rich plasma (PRP) platelets. It is difficult to directly inject the fat into the forehead rhytides which will require great force due to nondistensibility of tissues. This will result in destruction of the fat cells resulting in a poor take. It is preferable to make a very tiny incision with a microblade and then make a tunnel using a lacrimal probe just under the dermis. The fat can then be injected into this pocket. A suture is placed in order to prevent leakage of the injected fat. This is usually done with a single 6–0 nylon suture.

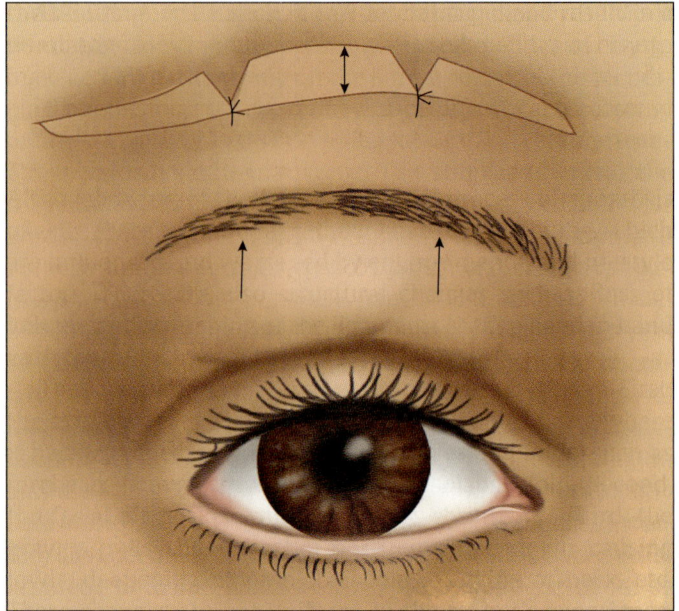

Fig. 10.27 Direct excision of subbrow fat and segmental excision of skin above.

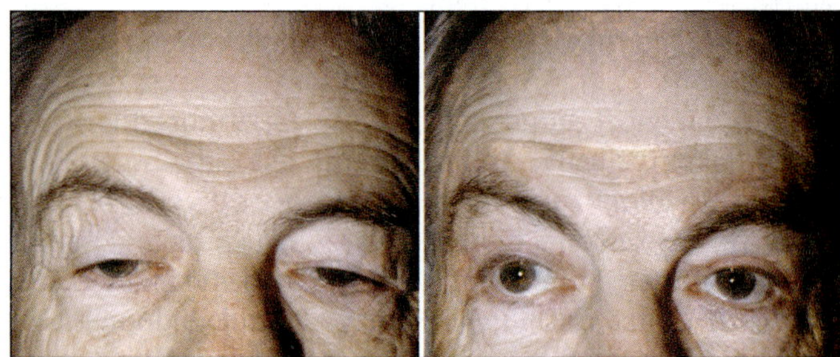

Fig. 10.28 Direct browlift in older patient pre- and postop.

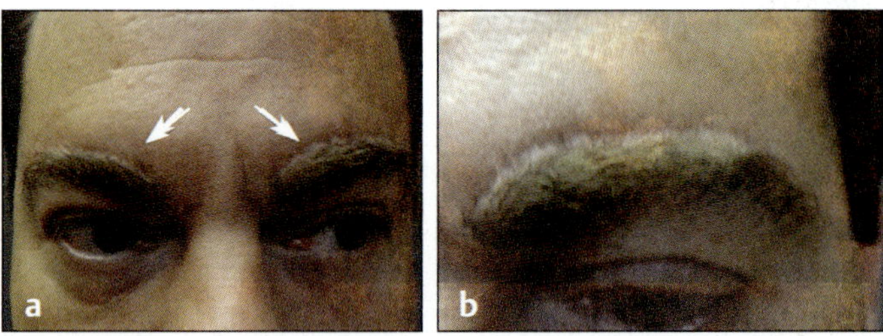

Fig. 10.29 (a, b) Unacceptable scar from direct excision.

The author prefers correction with dermal fat grafts. Fat is frequently resected during upper blepharoplasty. This can be saved and then inserted into the grooves as described above. If the grooves are deep and very prominent, then a dermal fat graft is preferred. A dermal fat graft can be harvested during concurrent surgical procedures such as a facelift; if not, a strip of dermis and fat can be harvested from any scar that the patient may have. If there are no scars, the author prefers to use the inguinal crease. A strip of dermis and underlying fat is then harvested. For placement of the dermal fat graft, a tiny incision is made at the upper and lower extremity of the frown line. A subdermal tunnel is then created by using a lacrimal probe. A suture is then placed at one end of the dermal fat graft. If available, a straight Keith needle should be used. The needle is then inserted through the lower incision with the blunt end leading the insertion. The blunt end is then retrieved from the upper incision and the dermal fat graft is then squeezed into the tunnel to correct the frown line (**Fig. 10.30**). The small incisions can usually be closed with single fast absorbing 6–0 catgut sutures. **Fig. 10.31** shows the result of glabellar dermal fat grafts.

Corrugator and Procerus Resection for Glabellar Rhytides

Correction of frown lines is one of the most frequently sought-after cosmetic procedures. It is usually treated by injecting a neurotoxin, such as Botox or Dysport. Such injections give only a temporary correction—lasting between 3 and 4 months.

Permanent correction of frown lines is accomplished by transecting a segment of corrugator supercilii and procerus muscles during endoscopic browlift and during transpalpebral blepharoplasty.[17]

Excision of a segment of corrugator supercilii muscle can be performed at the time of the upper blepharoplasty procedure. Dissection is performed through the medial part of the upper eyelid incision. After making the skin incision, the upper lid margin is retracted superiorly. Under direct vision and using loupe magnification, dissection is continued toward the supraorbital rim. Supratrochlear nerves should be identified and preserved. By spreading the scissors, the corrugator supercilii muscle is identified. The muscle is freed from its attachment to the bone in its midportion.[18] A segment of muscle measuring approximately one centimeter in length is then resected (**Fig. 10.32**). In patients who have hypertrophic muscles this segment can then be replaced. It will result in fibrosis and prevent a recurrence and also prevent a depression at the site of the resection. In thinner patients, it is not necessary to replace this piece of resected muscle. This will result in elimination of the glabellar frown lines. It will take some time for the results to become noticeable. Fat or dermal fat grafts can also be used to further augment the result and achieve immediate results.

The procerus muscle can also be excised through the same transpalpebral approach as described for corrugator resection, taking care to protect the supratrochlear neurovascular bundle.

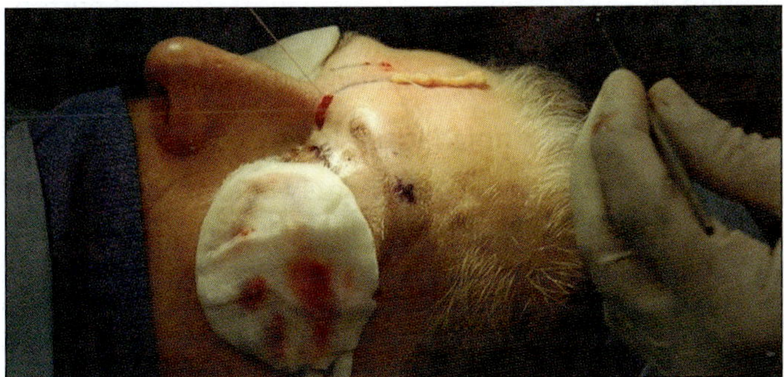

Fig. 10.30 Glabellar dermal fat graft.

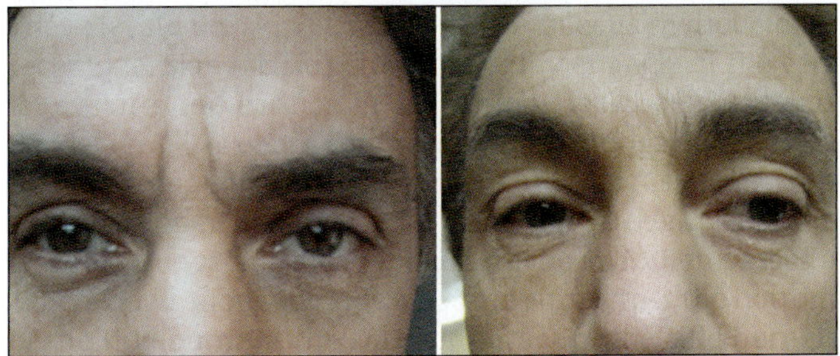

Fig. 10.31 Glabellar dermal fat graft pre- and postop.

Transpalpebral Browpexy—Sutures or Endotine

Effective elevation of the brow can also be performed through the transpalpebral approach, frequently combined with upper blepharoplasty. Accurate evaluation is extremely important. This should be performed with the patient sitting upright. The brow is digitally raised to determine the extent of the desired elevation. At that point, redundancy of upper eyelid skin is also appraised in the event that an upper blepharoplasty is concomitantly planned. It is frequently asked whether one should do the browpexy first or the upper blepharoplasty first in order to prevent excessive excision of the skin. In the author's experience, it is preferable to do the upper blepharoplasty first by evaluating the extent of redundant skin in the manner described above. Having done the blepharoplasty, the browpexy can then be performed. This is done by making the incision along the supratarsal crease laterally or through the lateral aspect of the upper blepharoplasty incision. The eyebrow is elevated digitally. The dissection is then performed with electrocautery through the

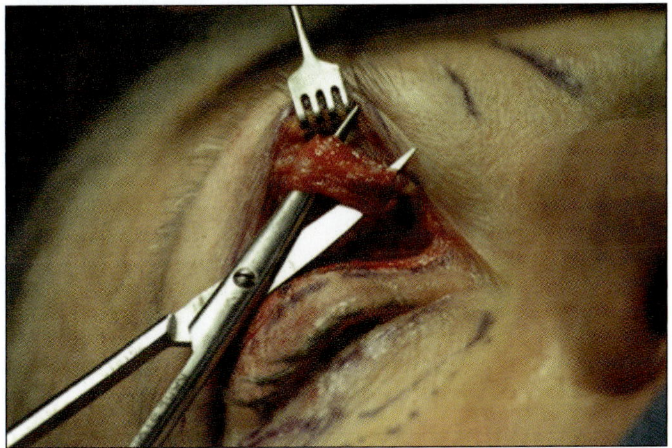

Fig. 10.32 Corrugator resection to correct glabellar rhytides.

orbital component of the orbicularis oculi muscle laterally down to the orbital rim. Frequently there is prominence of subbrow fat pad. If required, this can be excised under direct vision. If there is ptosis of the brow fat pad into the upper eyelids then this can also be addressed at the same time. The periosteum over the supraorbital rim should be preserved in order to get a good bite for fixation with the suture. A non-absorbable suture such as 4–0 Ethibond or Mersilene is then inserted through the periosteum 1 cm above the orbital rim and then a bite is taken through the undersurface of the brow (**Fig. 10.33a, b**). The suture is then tied with multiple knots. By digital palpation, fixation is confirmed. **Fig. 10.34** shows upper blepharoplasty and browpexy with suture fixture.

Alternatively, the fixation of the brow to the supraorbital rim can be performed with an absorbable endotine device. The endotine is made of an absorbable material. It has three tines as shown in the diagram. After performing the dissection down to the supraorbital periosteum as described above, the location of the placement of the endotine is marked (**Fig. 10.35a**). The periosteum is then scraped from that area. A drill hole is then made with a special drill provided with the endotine (**Fig. 10.35b, c**). A suture is then placed through the periosteum and through the two holes at each extremity of the endotine to prevent the endotine from being displaced postoperatively in case it gets dislodged. It is important to remove all bone debris from the drill hole by irrigating prior to insertion of the endotine. The endotine is then pressed snugly into the drill hole (**Fig. 10.35d**). The sutures along the extremities of the endotine described above are then tied with 4–0 Vicryl sutures. This provides additional security as far as the possibility of displacement of the endotine postoperatively is concerned. The eyebrow is then carefully positioned and digitally pressed to engage into the tines (**Fig. 10.35e**). The incision in the orbital orbicularis oculi muscle is repaired with 6–0 Vicryl sutures. The skin is closed with 6–0 running and interrupted nylon

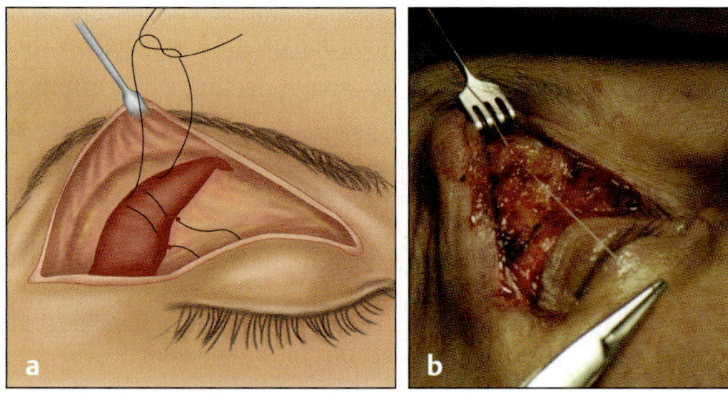

Fig. 10.33 (a, b) Transpapebral browpexy suture.

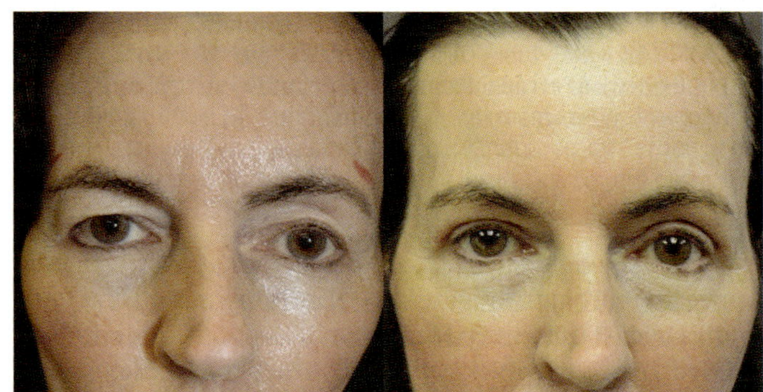

Fig. 10.34 Upper blepharoplasty and browpexy with suture fixation.

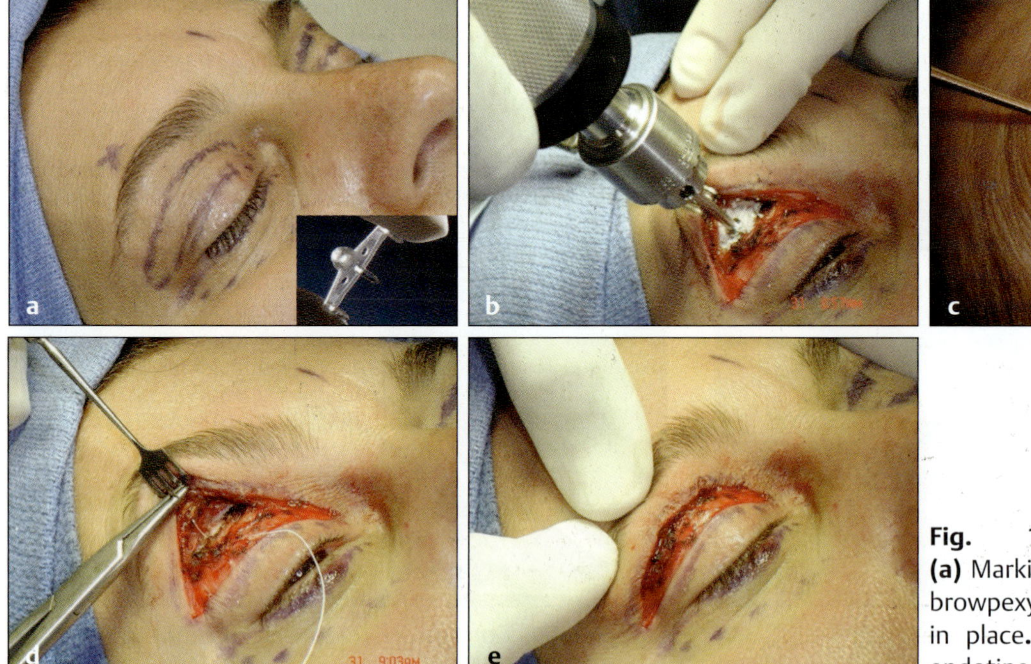

Fig. 10.35 Endotine browpexy. **(a)** Markings. **(b)** Drill used for endotine browpexy. **(c)** Hole created. **(d)** Endotine in place. **(e)** Engaging brow into the endotine with digital pressure.

sutures. Gauze pads are then placed over the brow and maintained in place with steri-strips in order to exert pressure postoperatively to prevent hematoma. This dressing is left on for 5 days.

If the endotine is used, the patient will sometimes feel a bulge in that area. This may also be tender. The bulge usually disappears after 6 weeks as the material is absorbable. During that time, the brow is fixated in its new position due to fibrosis. The patient should be appraised about this preoperatively. **Figs. 10.36–10.39** show the result of endotine browpexy.

Complications of Forehead Plasty and Browlift

Possible complications of forehead and browlifting procedures include hematoma, flap necrosis, infection, alopecia, injury to the seventh nerve, scalp hypesthesia, scalp paresthesia, neuralgia, incision pruritus, widening of the scar, depigmentation of scar, brow asymmetry, elevated hairline, and abnormal hairline. Most of these complications are avoidable by using a meticulous technique. A hematoma should be promptly addressed and evacuated; otherwise, it can result in necrosis of the overlying skin.

Upper Blepharoplasty

Upper blepharoplasty is one of the most commonly performed aesthetic facial surgical procedures. It is performed for both functional and cosmetic reasons. Redundancy of upper eyelid skin can result in compromise of peripheral visual field, particularly on upward and outward gaze (**Fig. 10.40**). Upper blepharoplasty can result in improvement of peripheral visual field. When there is redundancy of upper eyelid skin, the patients tend to raise their eyebrows to compensate for the redundancy and this results in a constantly surprised look. Furthermore, it results in transverse wrinkling of the forehead.

Evaluation for Upper Blepharoplasty

A thorough medical history is taken to rule out any systemic disease that could affect the upper eyelids, such as thyroid dysfunction and myasthenia gravis, dry eye syndrome, and blepharospasm. The coexistence of brow ptosis should be ruled out and, if present, it will also need to be addressed. The integrity of levator muscles and aponeurosis should be assessed and treated at the time of excess skin resection if indicated. Skin redundancy should be carefully assessed to avoid under- or overresection. If there is coexistent brow ptosis, the brow should be digitally elevated to its normal position and the excess skin is then evaluated.

If browpexy or brow elevation is planned, it should be performed first to avoid a lagophthalmos which can occur if the lid skin is first excised and the brow secondarily elevated. The herniation of fat pads is assessed in each of the three compartments. It is frequently most pronounced in the medial compartment. Descent of subbrow fat into the lid is assessed and may need to be addressed. Hyperplasia of orbicularis oculi can result in floppy lids and may require resection.

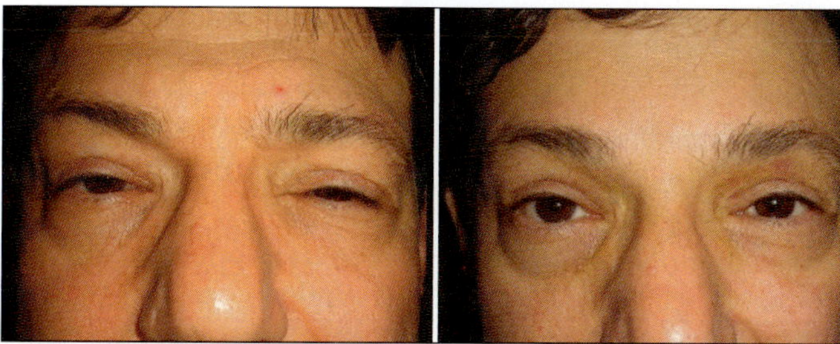

Fig. 10.36 Endotine browpexy in a male patient—pre and postoperative pictures front views.

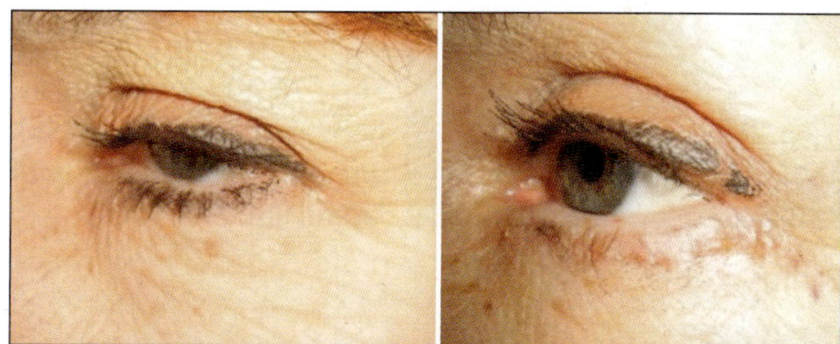

Fig. 10.37 Endotine browpexy pre- and postop—lateral views.

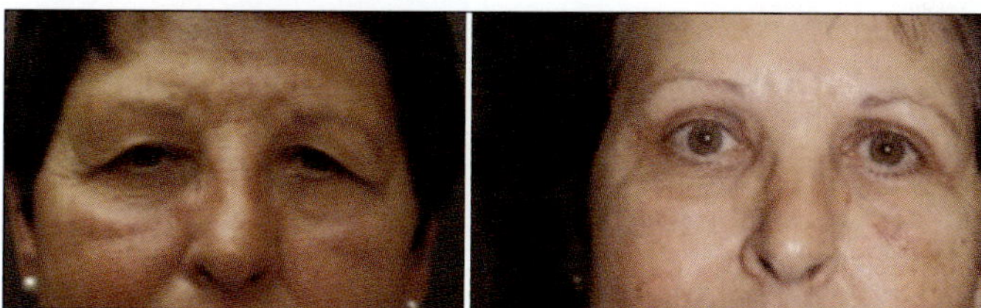

Fig. 10.38 Endotine browpexy in a female patient—pre- and postop.

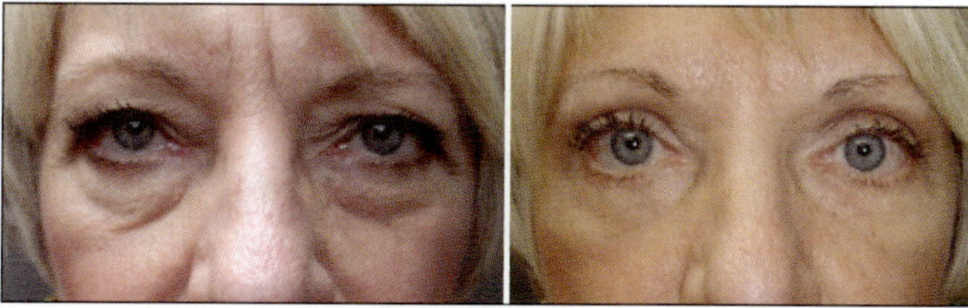

Fig. 10.39 Preop and Postop of a 56-year old female who had many of the procedures discussed in this chapter, namely dermal fat grafts to glabellar frown lines, corrugator resection, endotine browpexy and upper blepharoplasty.

It is important to evaluate the patient properly for upper blepharoplasty. The patient should be sat upright. Gross vision should be checked in both eyes as many patients have impaired vision in one eye without being aware of it. The patient is asked to relax the forehead. When that is done, the exact amount of redundant skin can be evaluated and marked. Furthermore, it is important to note the presence of herniated fat pads. These are most prominent in the medial compartment.

Lateral fullness of the eyelid could be due to herniation of fat pads but is more frequently due to either prolapse of subbrow fat pad into the upper eyelid or ptosis of the lacrimal gland (**Fig. 10.41**). It is important also to evaluate the laxity of the temporal region because this can have an impact on the lateral ptosis of the upper eyelids.

In some patients there is excessive skin in the lateral aspect of the upper eyelid which is evident as "hooding." In such circumstances and in the absence of the need for temporal lift or browpexy, the upper eyelid incision has to be modified. The lateral extremity instead of being the conventional ellipse has to be modified as depicted in the diagram in **Fig. 10.42**. This will result in correction of lateral hooding. The resultant scar will, of necessity, extend beyond the outer canthus and this can be carefully positioned so that it will fall into one of the natural crease lines or crow's feet in that area. Failure to use this modification will result in persistence of the hooding (**Fig. 10.43**).

In evaluating the upper eyelid for blepharoplasty, consideration is given to skin, muscle, fat, upper lip ptosis, lip crease, and the lacrimal gland.

Skin

With aging, the elasticity of the skin diminishes and the skin becomes loose and wrinkled. There can be real or apparent skin excess. Apparent skin excess can happen in the presence of brow ptosis. It is, therefore, important to place the brow in its correct position and then evaluate the excess skin. The lids should be evaluated with the eyes open and closed. The presence or absence of the lid fold should be evaluated.

Muscle

With aging, the orbicularis ocular muscle becomes lax and hypertrophic, particularly in the pretarsal area, resulting in the so-called "floppy lid." Floppy lid usually occurs in patients of advanced age and in obese patients.

Fat

Herniation of fat pads can occur in three compartments: medial, middle, and lateral compartments. The morphological appearance of fat in the three compartments is different from each other. The fat in the medial compartment is pale in color compared to the one in the middle and lateral compartments. Also, the three fat pads are compartmentalized.

In the past, it was customary to excise fat in every patient; however, currently, conservation of the fat is the trend. Fat

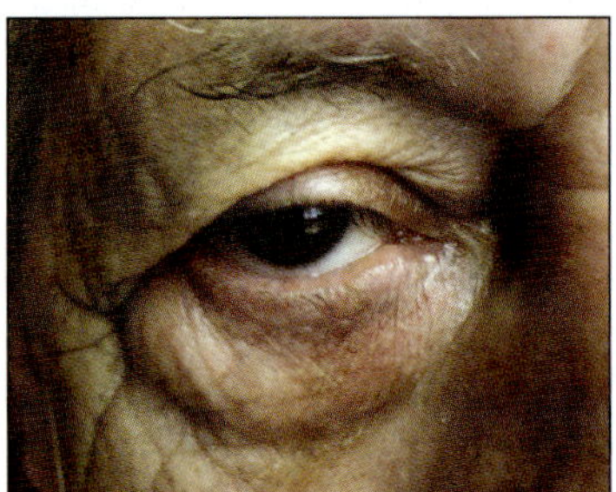

Fig. 10.40 Brow ptosis, herniated medial fat pad, and skin redundancy with lateral hooding.

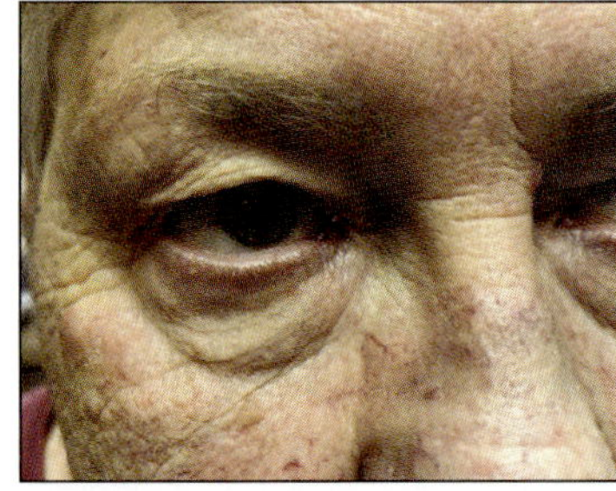

Fig. 10.41 Lateral fullness due to ptosis of lacrimal gland.

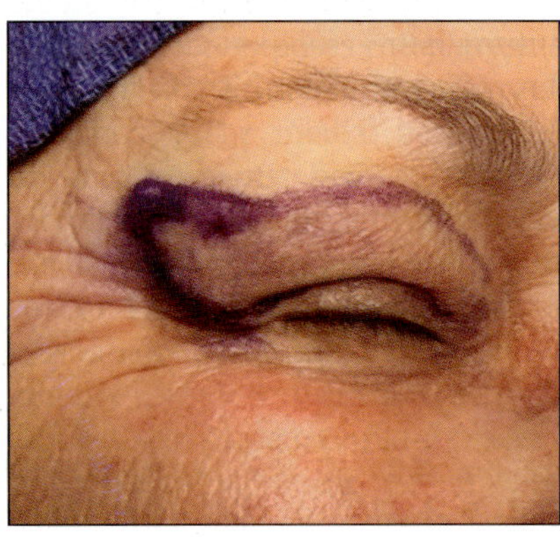

Fig. 10.42 Modified incision for upper blepharoplasty with lateral hooding.

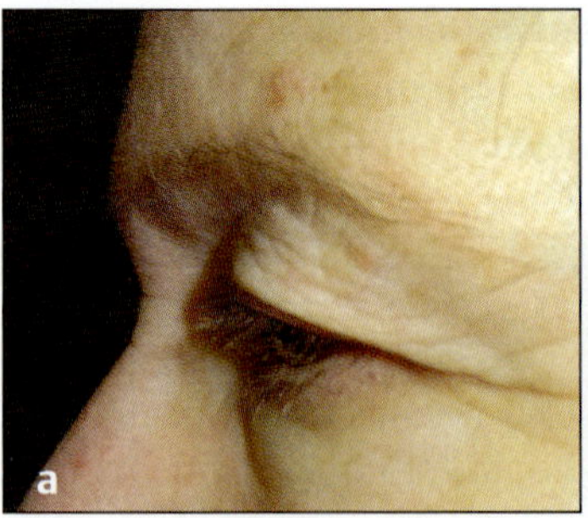

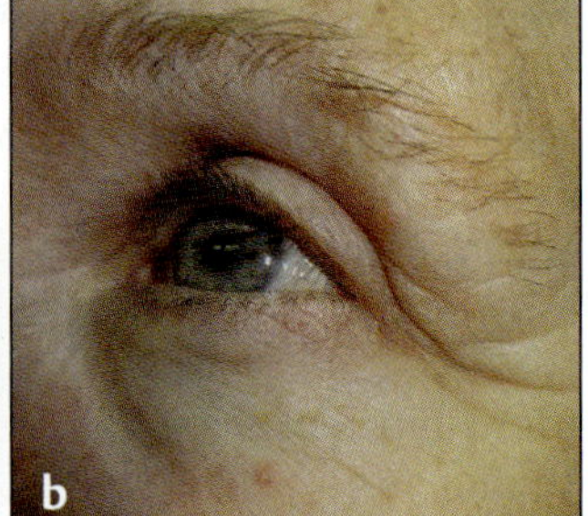

Fig. 10.43 (a, b) Persistence of lateral hooding without modified incision for upper blepharoplasty.

grafting to the upper eyelids is also in vogue in order to provide a more youthful appearance. Excessive resection of fat can result in a sunken eyelid appearance.

Lid Ptosis

It is important to evaluate for lid ptosis. Lid ptosis can be apparent or real. Apparent lid ptosis can occur due to brow ptosis and redundancy of upper eyelid skin. Real brow ptosis should be evaluated by comparing the position of the brow relative to the supraorbital rim. Brow ptosis and upper eyelid redundancy can coexist. It is important to recognize this as treating lid redundancy without attention to brow ptosis would result in a suboptimal result. Currently, brow ptosis can be easily corrected by doing transpalpebral browpexy at the time of the upper lid blepharoplasty.

Lid Crease

The lid crease should be carefully assessed. The lid crease is absent in the oriental eyelid due to absence of dermal extension of the levator aponeurosis into the skin. The lid crease may be asymmetric. High lid crease usually occurs due to levator dehiscence.

Lacrimal Gland

Ptosis of lacrimal gland will be evident as fullness laterally (**Fig. 10.44a**). If present, it can be corrected during blepharoplasty by repositioning it into the lacrimal fossa (**Fig. 10.44b, c**).

Applied Anatomy[19]

- Upper eyelid skin is very thin.
- Orbicularis oculi muscle has three components, (i.e., pretarsal, preseptal, and orbital).
- Lacrimal gland.
- Preaponeurotic fat.
- Orbital septum.
- Fat pads—nasal, central, lateral.
- Interpad septa.
- Medial palpebral artery.
- Levator palpebrae superioris muscle.
- Levator palpebrae superioris aponeurosis and dermal extensions.
- Muller muscle.
- Superior tarsal plate.
- Conjunctiva.
- Subbrow fat pad descent into the preseptal space.

Technique

Markings are made with the patient in the upright position. The lower incision should be placed just above and parallel to the upper border to the tarsal plate. This will determine the location of the prospective supratarsal crease. It is very important not to extend the incision medial to the lash line of the upper eyelid. Doing so can result in a bowstring or a bridle scar. With the patient's forehead relaxed, the upper eyelid can be grasped gently with a blunt forceps and the redundant skin outlined (**Fig. 10.45a, b**). Markings are made on both sides. Asymmetry should be taken into consideration.

Isolated upper blepharoplasty can be performed quite easily under local anesthesia as an outpatient. It is beneficial to ask the patient to take nonprescription pain killer such as acetaminophen or ibuprofen prior to surgery. This minimizes the pain during infiltration of the local anesthetic. After performing skin prep, preoperative markings are reinforced. A local anesthesia is then infiltrated into each upper eyelid. The most commonly used local anesthetic is 1% Lignocaine with 1/100, 000 epinephrine to allow for vasoconstriction. Equal amounts of local anesthesia should be infiltrated into each eyelid and this usually is no more than 1 mL. Excessive amounts of infiltration will result in distortion and swelling of the eyelids. After waiting for an appropriate period of time to obtain vasoconstriction and anesthesia, the lower skin incision is first made. Some surgeons prefer to use laser or electrocautery. The upper incision is then made along the markings described above. In most instances it is only necessary to remove the skin. However, when there is redundancy and attenuation of the ocular component of the orbicularis oculi muscle, such as in so-called floppy upper eyelid, then a strip of the muscle can also be excised (**Fig. 10.46**). The herniation of the fat pad is then addressed if necessary. Usually this is most prominent in the medial compartment. By gentle pressure on the eyeball, the herniation of the fat pads is accentuated and an incision is then

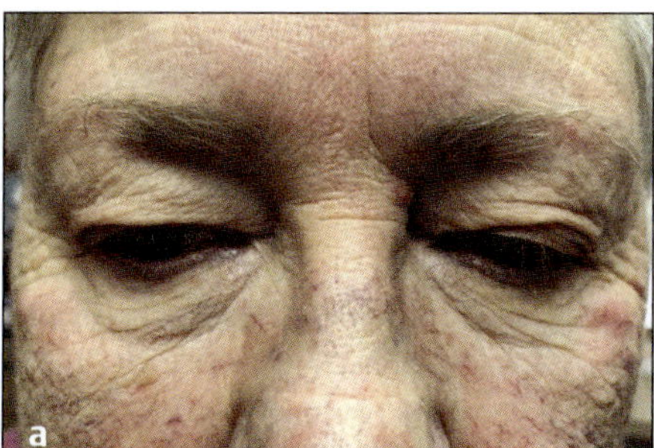

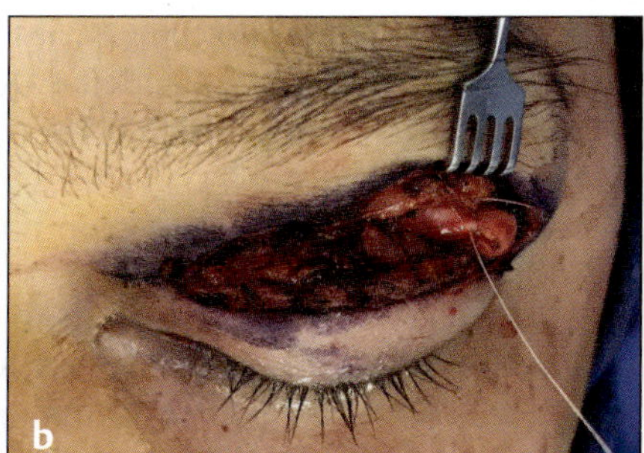

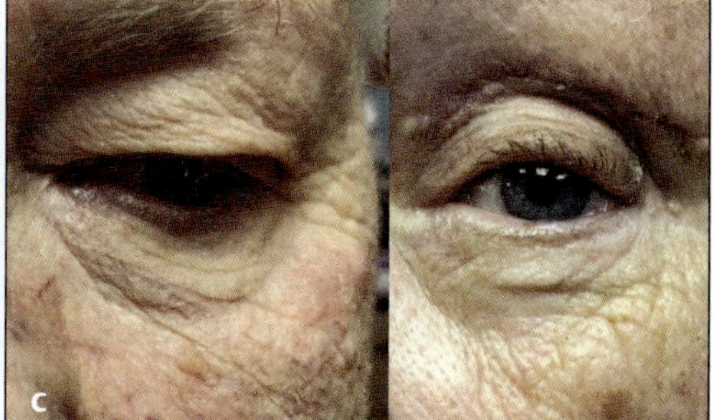

Fig. 10.44 (a) Ptosis of lacrimal gland. **(b)** Correcting lacrimal gland ptosis. **(c)** Correction of lacrimal gland ptosis.

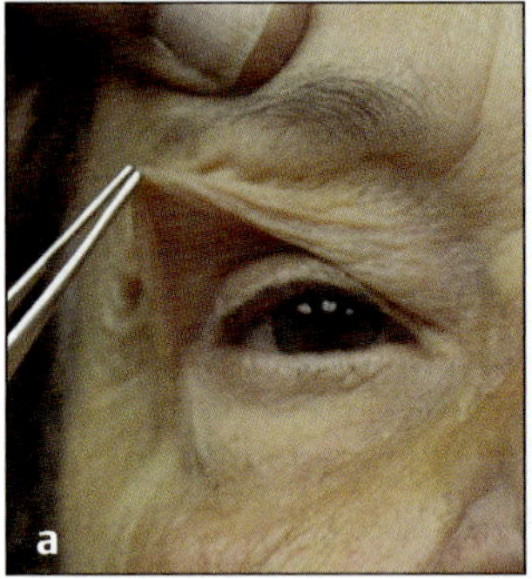
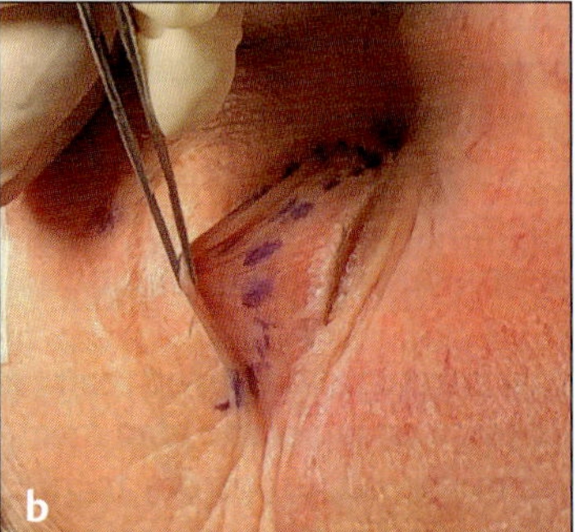

Fig. 10.45 **(a)** Grasping the upper eyelid with blunt forceps. **(b)** Upper and lower skin markings should approximate when lifted up with a blunt forceps.

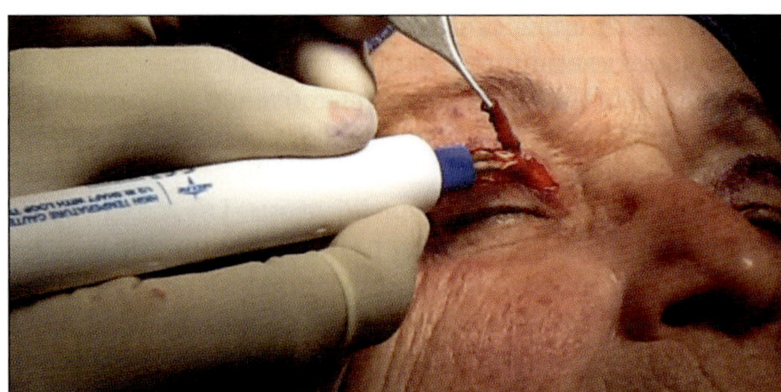

Fig. 10.46 Excision of redundant orbicularis oculi muscle in floppy lid.

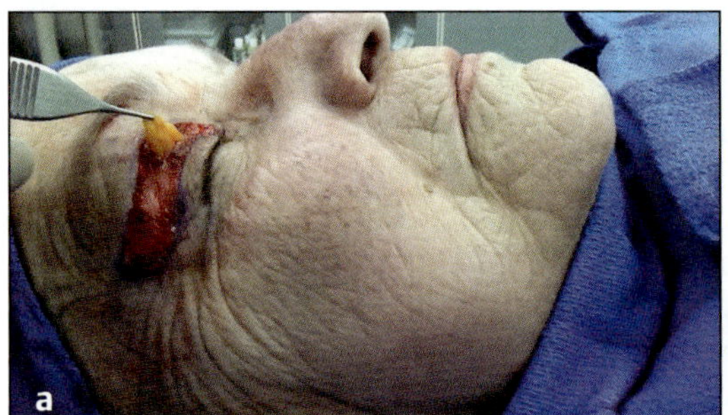
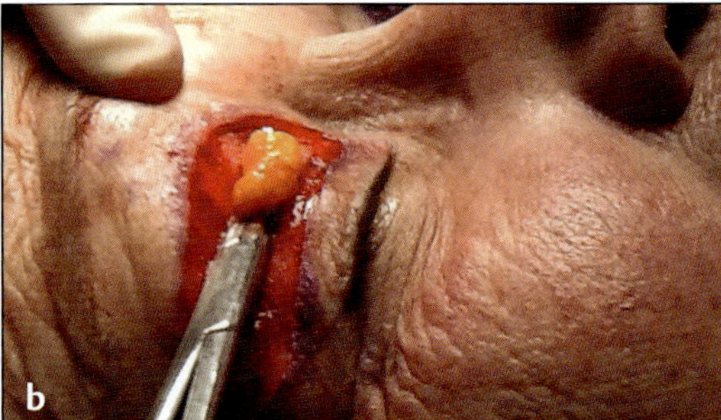
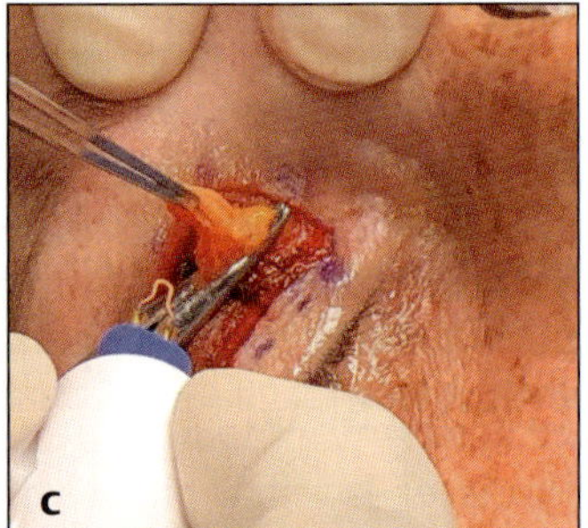

Fig. 10.47 **(a)** Fat pad dissected. **(b)** Fat pad clamped. **(c)** Fat pad excised with handheld battery-operated cautery.

made through the orbital septum (septum orbitale) and the fat pad usually bulges out. The fat pad is then carefully dissected, clamped, and transected with handheld cautery to establish hemostasis (**Fig. 10.47a–c**). The stump is then cauterized. There are usually three fat compartments in the upper eyelid. The fat in the medial compartment is usually pale in color compared to the other compartments. This fat pad is usually discrete and anatomically separate from the fat in the middle compartment which may be contiguous with the fat in the lateral compartment. If there is herniation of fat pads in the middle and lateral compartments, then the incision in the orbital septum can be extended and the fat pads can be resected as described above. Following excision of the fat pads the rent in the orbital septum is repaired with 6-0 Vicryl sutures.

If there is ptosis of the lacrimal gland or descent of the subbrow fat pad into the upper eyelids, this should be addressed (**Fig. 10.48a, b**). Ptotic lacrimal glands are corrected by doing a lacrimal pexy in which the gland is pushed up and maintained in place with nonabsorbable sutures anchored to the supraorbital rim periosteum.

Ptosis of subbrow fat pads can be addressed by dissecting the ptotic fat pad and clamping it and then excising it with electrocautery (**Fig. 10.49a**). The stump is also cauterized to ensure hemostasis. The skin is usually closed with a running and interrupted 6-0 nylon sutures. Sometimes there is a disparity between the upper and lower skin flaps, resulting in a dog ear at the medial extremity. There is usually redundancy of skin in the upper flap and it can be corrected by doing a small triangular skin excision, as shown in **Fig. 10.49b**. Some surgeons prefer to use a subcuticular running suture which is pulled out after 6 days or so. Fast absorbing chromic catgut sutures can also be used. Alternatively, for patients coming from far off places, 7/0 Vicryl can be used.[21] **Fig. 10.50** shows pre- and postop photographs of a patient with excision of subbrow fat ptosis.

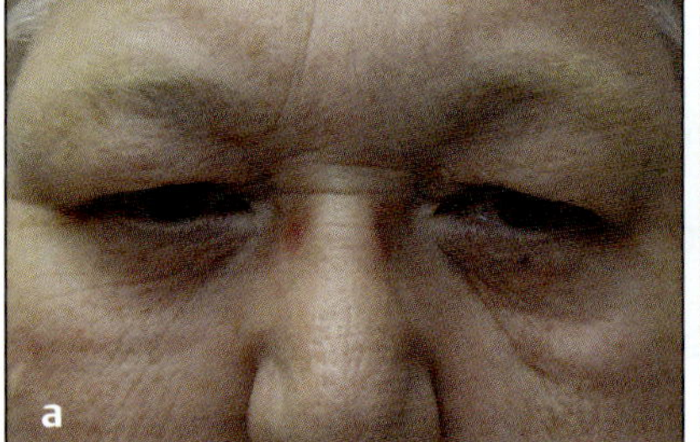
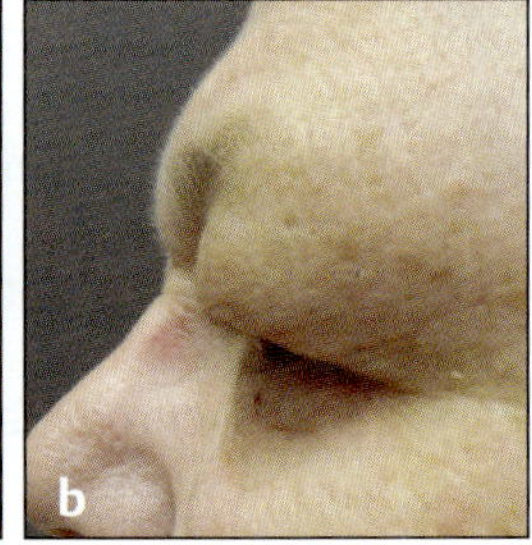

Fig. 10.48 **(a, b)** Subbrow ptosis and lateral fullness. **(a)** Front view. **(b)** Lateral view.

With the patient under anesthesia at the end of the procedure, the lids may be open and a gap of 2 mm is acceptable. When the procedure is performed under local anesthetic, it is important to make sure that the patient is able to close the eyelids without tension.

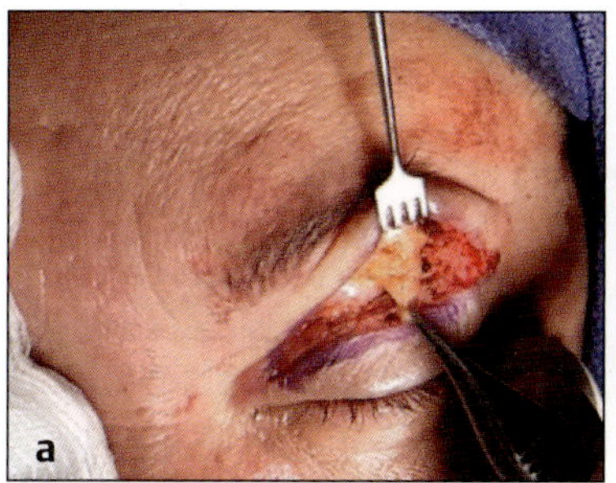
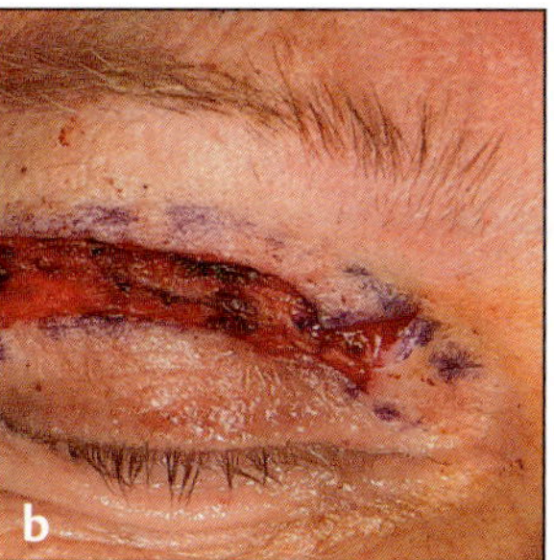

Fig. 10.49 (a) Excision of subbrow ptotic fat pad. **(b)** Triangular skin excision from the upper flap medially to prevent dog ear.

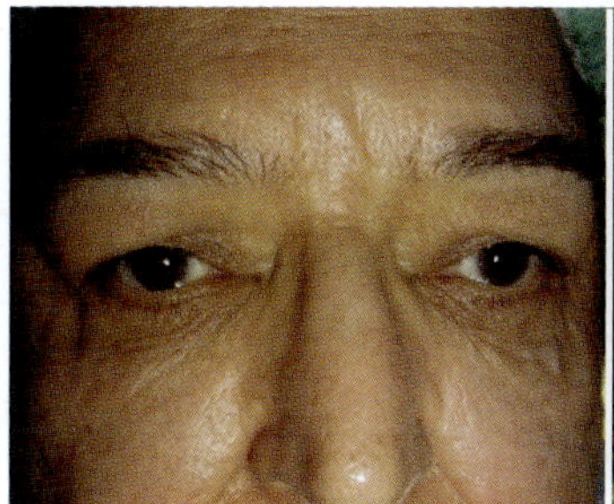
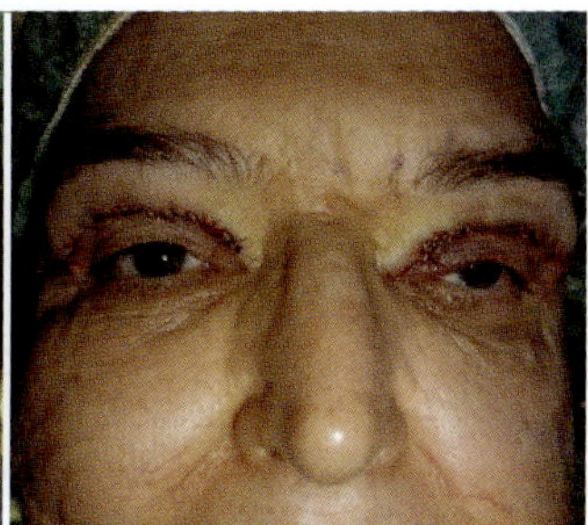

Fig. 10.50 Subbrow fat ptosis pre- and postop.

During excision of the upper eyelid skin, the author prefers to save this excised skin in sterile saline-soaked sponge until the end of the procedure. In the event that excessive skin has been removed as may happen when concurrent browpexy is also performed and if there is lagophthalmos, skin can be grafted to correct the ectropion. In the author's experience, these grafts have healed very nicely with hardly any residual scarring because of the native nature of the graft. Following the surgery, ophthalmic ointment is applied to the suture line. The patients are also advised to insert the antibiotic ointment into the eyes at night because the patients may not be able to close their eyes completely during their sleep due to swelling.

Postoperatively the patients are asked to apply ice packs over their eyes for 48 hours. They are advised to sleep with their head elevated. Suture lines are cleansed with sterile Q-tips twice a day so no scabs form on the incision line. For pain, oral nonprescription pain medications such as acetaminophen or ibuprofen are adequate. Sutures are removed in less than one week. If the sutures are left in for a longer period of time, it will result in multiple implantation cysts along the incision line.

Ptosis of Lacrimal Gland

Ptosis of the lacrimal gland usually occurs in elderly patients.[20] It is evident as fullness over the lateral aspect of the upper eyelid. **Fig. 10.44a** shows fullness of the lateral aspect of the upper eyelid due to ptosis of lacrimal gland. Intraoperative photograph (**Fig. 10.44b**) shows ptosis of the lacrimal gland. It can be corrected by elevating the gland by placing a suture through the periosteum of the supraorbital rim as shown in **Fig. 10.44b**.[21] Postoperative result shows correction of the ptotic lacrimal gland (**Fig. 10.44c**).

Absent Upper Eyelid Crease[22,23]

The supratarsal fold is frequently absent in the oriental eyelid. The absence of the supratarsal fold or the lid crease is due to absence of dermal extensions of the levator aponeurosis into the overlying skin. The lid fold can be created by incorporating the levator aponeurosis when approximating the skin edges of the upper lid following skin resection. This will result in the creation of the supratarsal crease (**Fig. 10.3**).

Complications of Upper Eyelid Blepharoplasty

Hematoma

Subcutaneous hematoma after upper eyelid blepharoplasty is rare because there is no undermining and no dead space. The more dreaded complication is retrobulbar hematoma which can occur following excision of the fat pads. This can be avoided by doing meticulous hemostasis at the time of fat pad excision. The author clamps the herniated fat pads after dissecting them and then excising the fat pads using electrocautery. This will result in hemostasis of the stump. If a retrobulbar hematoma occurs, it should be promptly recognized and addressed. The patient will usually complain of severe pain and also there will be proptosis of the eyeball. Unrecognized retrobulbar hematoma can lead to blindness due to compression of the central artery of the retina.

Ptosis

Ptosis can occur due to disruption of the levator aponeurosis. This sometimes occurs after excessive use of electrocautery to resect the fat pads. **Fig. 10.51** shows iatrogenic ptosis and the correction.

Corneal Injury

Corneal injury can occur intraoperatively due to excessive dryness of the eyeball. More frequently, it occurs due to injudicious use of cautery and transmission of heat through the attenuative lid structures to the cornea. This can be avoided by using a corneal shield.

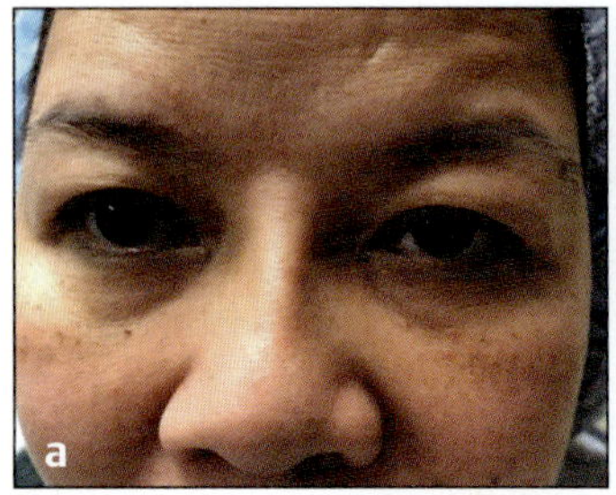
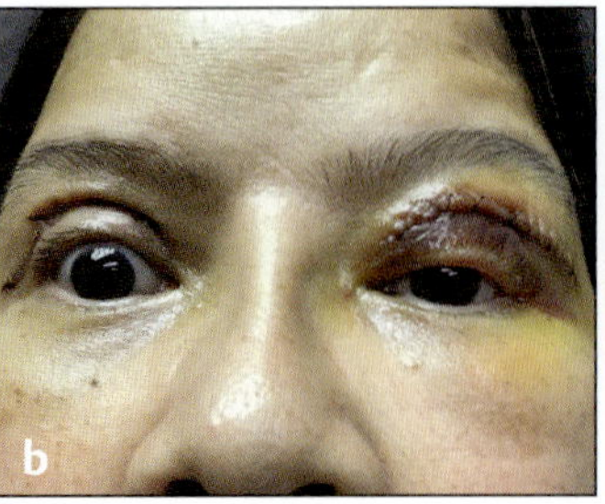
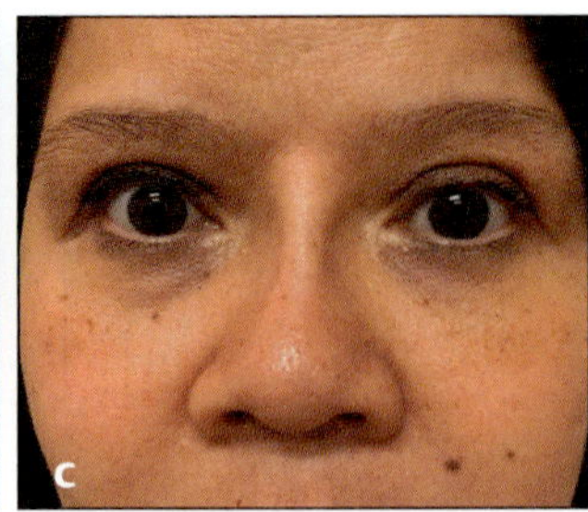

Fig. 10.51 **(a)** Preop absent lid fold and severe blepharochalasia. **(b)** Iatrogenic ptosis due to injury to levator aponeurosis. **(c)** Postop correction of iatrogenic ptosis.

Lagophthalmos and Ectropion

This results from excessive resection of skin. It can be prevented by evaluating excess skin preoperatively by pinching the skin with a blunt forceps and coapting the anticipated cut edges of the upper eyelid. It is a good practice to preserve the resected skin in saline until the end of the procedure. If deficiency of skin is noted at the end of the procedure as evidenced by lagophthalmos or ectropion then some of this resected skin can be reattached as a full-thickness skin graft. This usually heals very nicely without any perceptible scarring. To that end, it is a good practice to preserve the resected skin in saline until the very end of the operative procedure.

A-frame Deformity

This deformity is evident as an inverted V-shaped depression in the eyelid resulting from overresection of fat. It can be very distressing postoperatively, and every attempt should be made to avoid it.

Residual Fat Pads

Fig. 10.52a, b show residual medial fat pads that were not removed during the blepharoplasty.

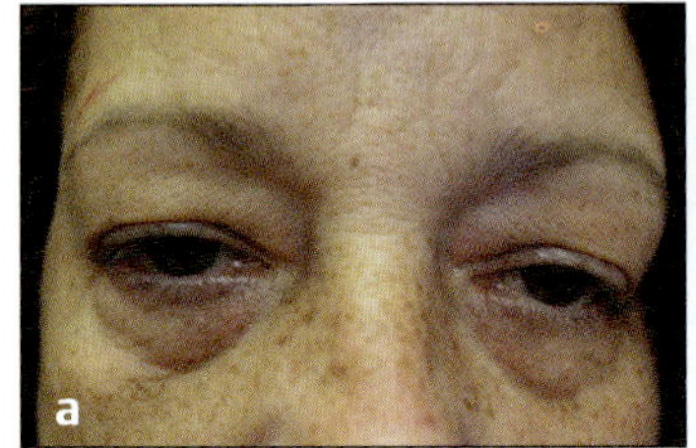
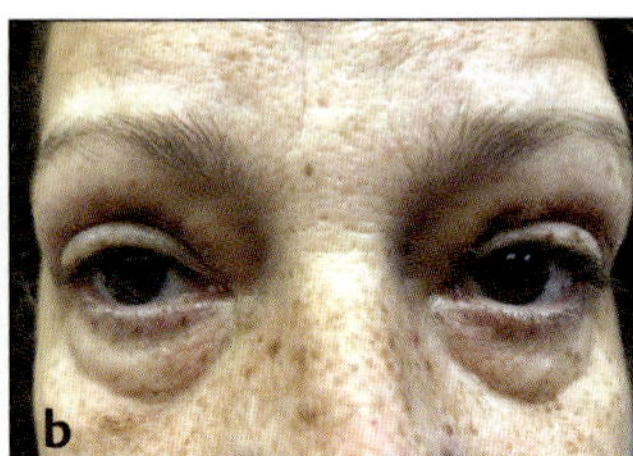

Fig. 10.52 **(a)** Preop upper blepharoplasty with fat excision. **(b)** Persistence of medial fat pads following upper blepharoplasty.

Blindness

Blindness, which is a dreaded complication, is extremely rare in upper blepharoplasty.[24] All reported cases have occurred in patients who have undergone resection of fat pads. The reason is obscure, but it is felt that it could be due to traction on the fat pads during resection and spasm of the central artery of the retina. Another reason could be the development of a retrobulbar hematoma following fat pad excision and compression of the central artery of the retina. It is, therefore, extremely important to ensure exacting hemostasis during fat pad resection and minimal traction.

References

1. Kaur M. Garg RK, Singla S . Analysis of facial soft tissue changes with ageing and their effects on facial morphology: A forensic perspective. Egyptian J Forensic Sci 2015;5:46-56
2. Dutton JJ. Surgical management of the floppy eyelid syndrome. Am J Ophthalmol 1985;99(5):557-560
3. Liu D. Oriental eyelids: Anatomic differences and surgical consideration. In Hornblass A (ed): Oculoplastic, Orbital and Reconstructive Surgery, vol 1. Baltimore, Williams and Wilkins, 1988; 513
4. Chen WPD. Asian blepharoplasty. Update on anatomy and techniques. Ophthalmic Plast Reconstr Surg 1987;3(3): 135-140
5. Modarressi A. Platlet rich plasma (PRP) improves fat grafting outcomes. World J Plast Surg 2013;2(1):6–13
6. Kaye BL. The forehead lift. Plast Reconstr Surg 1977;60(2):161-171
7. Javidnia H, Sykes J. Endoscopic brow lifts: have they replaced coronal lifts? Facial Plast Surg Clin North Am 2013;21(2): 191–199
8. Isse NG. Endoscopic forehead lift: Evolution and update. Clin Plast Surg 1995;22(4):661-673
9. Vasconez LO, Core GB, Gamboa-Bobadilla M, Guzman G, Askren C, Yamamoto Y. Endoscopic techniques in coronal brow lifting. Plast Reconstr Surg 1994;94(6):788-793
10. Daniel RK, Tirkanits B. Endoscopic forehead lift: An operative technique. Plast Reconstr Surg 1996;98(7):1148-1157, discussion 1158
11. Bostwick J III, Nahai F, Eaves F III. Endoscopic Brow Lift in Endoscopic Plastic Surgery. St Louis: Quality Medical Publishing, 1996
12. Ramirez O, Daniel R (eds): Endoscopic Plastic Surgery. NYork, Springer-Verlag, 1996, pp65-67
13. Rohrich RJ, Beran SJ. Evolving fixation methods in endoscopically assisted forehead rejuvenation: Controversies and rationale. Plast Reconstr Surg 1997;100(6):1575-1582
14. Graham HD III, Core GB. Endoscopic forehead lifting using fixation sutures. In Freidman M (ed): Operative Techniques in Otolaryngology-Head and Neck Surgery, Philadelphia, WB saunders Co, 1995;6(4):245-252

15. Holzapfel A, Mangat D. Endoscopic forehead-lift using a bioabsorbable fixation device. Arch Facial Plast Surg 2004;6(6):389-393
16. Gleason MC. Brow lifting through a temporal scalp approach. Plast Reconstr Surg 1973;52(2):141-144
17. Knize DM. Transpalpebral approach to the corrugator supercilii and procerus muscles. Plast Reconstr Surg 1995;95:52
18. Guyuron B, Michelow B, Thomas T. Corrugator supercilii muscle resection through blepharoplasty incision. Plast Reconstr Surg 1995;95(4):691-696
19. Zide BM, Jelks GW. Surgical Anatomy of the Orbit. New York: Raven Press; 1985
20. Smith B, Petrelli R. Surgical repair of prolapsed lacrimal glands. Arch Opthlamol 1978; 96(1):113-114
21. Horton CE, Carraway JH, Potenza AD. Treatment of a lacrimal bulge in blepharoplasty by repositioning the gland. Plast Reconstr Surg 1978;61(5):701-702
22. Sayoc BT. Surgery of the oriental eyelid. Clin Plast Surg 1974; 1(1):157-171
23. Sheen JH. Supratarsal fixation in upper blepharoplasty. Plast Reconstr Surg 1974;54(4):424-431
24. Anderson RL, Edwards JJ, Wood JR. Bilateral visual loss after blepharoplasty. Ann Plast Surg 1980;5(4);288-292

11

Surgical Rejuvenation of Midface and Lower Face including Neck Rejuvenation—Principles and Techniques

Ashish Davalbhakta

Introduction

The desire to look good is ingrained in our psyche since start of civilization. All historic art from Ajanta, Ellora, in India, and also other places of the world like Greece and Egypt show people with finest of jewelry, makeup, and aesthetics. The desire to look good continues as we age, and along with aging comes the desire to reverse the aging changes, to continue to look good. Plastic surgeons have evolved the science of antiaging and facelift is the cornerstone of all antiaging procedures.

The most obvious sign of aging is the increase in laxity of the skin and the first description of attempts at correcting this goes back to 1901 by Hollander. He wrote in a book published in 1912 that he had excised the skin in front of the ear and margin of hairline in a Polish Aristocrat.[1] Lexer reported that he had performed a facelift for an actress in 1906.[2] Along with these surgeons, Miller, Kolle, Passot, Bourget, and many others had started facelift procedures all around the world.[3–6] From 1900 to 1970 was the era of skin excisions for tightening the lax skin of the face. All the early facelift procedures were skin excision and wound closures only, without much subcutaneous undermining.

In 1927, Bames described subcutaneous face and neck undermining and, along with the continuous incision described by Bettman in 1920, formed the basis of the facelift procedure of the future.[7,8] Although this procedure gave effective tightening and early results, due to the viscoelastic properties of the skin and its inherent tendency to maintain the neutral tension in the skin, the results were not long lasting. There was also a higher incidence of skin necrosis due to extensive undermining of the skin. In 1976, Mitz and Peyronie described a fascial layer under the subcutaneous fat, called the superficial musculoaponeurotic system (SMAS), and using this information, Skoog described a technique to lift the skin and the superficial fascial layer of the face, pulling the myofascial layer in the upward and backward direction. He suggested that it could be used to give a tighter and more long-lasting lift to the facial tissues.[9] This started the era of SMAS facelift and many surgeons published modifications to improve on the problems or deficiencies of earlier techniques. There was a trend to be more extensive in SMAS mobilization with the hope to improve results, starting with deep plane facelift by Hamra.[10] Aston described FAME (finger-assisted malar elevation) lift, a way to lift the sagging malar fat pad with the finger.[11] Stuzin presented his extended SMAS dissection and Oscar Ramirez described endoscopic subperiosteal dissection in 1995.[12,13] Sam Hamra described composite facelift, where he proposed doing a deep plane facelift and moving the orbicularis oculi, malar fat pad, and skin as a composite unit to correct the midface sag.[14] More recently, Andrew Jocono has revisited the deep plane and extended it to lift the anterior midface more thoroughly and extending the dissection into the neck, for a better result.[15]

Each and every modification has been toward either improving results or reducing shortcomings and complications. Tim Marten recognized the need for adding volume along with the traditional tightening procedures and described fat grafting along with facelift.[16]

As the procedures started getting more elaborate and complex, some surgeons kept on looking at less elaborate and simple ways of meeting the goal of facial rejuvenation and reducing risk of complications. Baker in 1997 described the lateral SMASectomy, a technique to tighten the SMAS without any SMAS undermining, thus reducing the risk of facial nerve injury.[17] He further described short scar facelift, where the access incision was reduced to avoid retroauricular extension.[18] Minimal access cranial suspension (MACS lift) was described by Patrick Tonnard where the SMAS was plicated with sutures instead of elevation and repositioning.[19,20]

Conceptually, as the understanding of the descent of tissues has increased, there has been an evolution in the vectors of the lift as well. Skoog facelift, which lifted SMAS and skin together, pulled the skin laterally and backward.[9] With Baker's lateral SMASectomy and subsequent modifications, there has been a realization that the SMAS should move upward and backward, while the skin moves toward the upper pole of the ear.[21] With Tim Marten's high lamellar facelift, there is a rotation of SMAS on a pivot point in the anterior malar region. This lifts the SMAS backward and upward and increases the prominence at the pivot point in the malar region.[16] There has also been a change from excessive skin resection to minimal skin resection. Most of the tension is placed in the SMAS and less on the skin. This has reduced the complications resulting from excessive tightening of the skin. The facelift of today is more long lasting and harmonious. If the principles are followed, it is possible to give high level of satisfaction.

Relevant Anatomy

As the anatomy of the face has been discussed in detail in the previous chapter, we shall only discuss the relevant points pertinent to this chapter.

Tissues of the face are arranged in five layers as elsewhere in the body, (viz., the skin, subcutaneous tissue, superficial musculoaponeurotic layer, deep fascia, and loose areolar tissue).[22] The subcutaneous fat is mingled with the superficial fascia system. It is this layer and the skin that sags as aging progresses. It is held on to the face with condensations of the fascial structures called ligaments.[22] Facelifting is all about lifting these layers of the face.

Subcutaneous Tissue and Fascial Arrangement

This layer is composed of a uniform layer of fat, compacted in to a superficial subdermal zone and a deeper subscarpa zone. The superficial fat has globules in tiny size. The deeper fat has larger globules. The deeper fat contributes to the fat pockets of the face (**Fig. 11.1**) and also rests on the SMAS. Rohrich and Pessa studied the fat pockets of the face and found 56% of the fat superficial to the SMAS and 44% deep.

The forehead has one central and two medial and two lateral compartments/pads on either side. The lateral temporal fat pad extends down on the side of the face and is called the lateral temporal cheek fat pad. The lower lid has infraorbital fat pad. The cheek has a medial and middle cheek fat pad (**Fig. 11.1**), which corresponds to the commonly known malar fat pad.[23] The nasolabial fat pad is the medial most fat pad in the cheek. The jowl area has a superior and inferior fat pad. The chin has a premental fat pad.

The Deep Fat Pads

The deep fat is deep to the muscles of the face (**Fig. 11.2**). The infraorbital rim forms the superior border of the suborbicularis oculi fat (SOOF). It is deep to the orbicularis oculi. It is compartmentalized into medial and lateral SOOFs. The medial SOOF fat compartment is bordered medially by the pyriform aperture, superiorly by the orbitomalar-retaining ligament, laterally by the zygomatic major and buccal fat pad. The lateral SOOF fat pad lies lateral to the lateral canthus, and extends over the malar area under the orbicularis. The buccal fat pad is lateral to the deep medial fat pad and has extensions to the temporal fossa from under the arch of the zygoma.[24] For further details, refer to Chapter 6 on "Anatomy of Aging Face and Its Assessment" in Volume VI.

It is atrophy of the deep medial fat that causes the deflation of anterior and malar facial fat. The overlying skin and subcutaneous fat then sag over the deflated deeper fat, creating the classic inverted-V deformity over the anterior malar region. Loss of the SOOF fat pad results in tear troughs or reveals the preseptal fat bulge called under eye bags.

Fascial Ligaments

The superficial subcutaneous fat is separated into different compartments by fibrous septae. These are fibrous retinacular ligaments that pass from the deeper structures vertically, arborizing upward, fixing the skin to the deeper structures.[22] When these ligaments arise from the periosteum and anchor the skin, they are direct or true ligaments, (e.g., zygomatic, parotidomasseteric, and mandibular). Rest of the places they are indirect and originating from deep fascia or muscles, or might be adhesions of fascial layers, (e.g., the temporal ligaments, orbicularis-retaining ligaments, the midcheek ligament, etc).[23] At places where the thickness of subcutaneous fat is more, also called fat pockets of the face, the retention ligaments are few and less thick. This allows the fat to slide off the deep fascia and form gliding planes. These ligaments also stretch with gravity causing lengthening. The clinical relevance of this is to understand the plane of dissection and the plane in which skin shifts and sags. It also helps in understanding the zones of adherence and anchoring. One has to release these anchoring ligaments to effectively lift the face skin (**Fig. 11.2**).

Superficial Musculoaponeurotic Layer (SMAS)

First described by Mitz and Peyronie in 1970, this is a continuation of the platysma upward on the face.[25] It continues upward in the temporal region as the superficial temporal fascia, on to the forehead and scalp as the galea aponeurotica. In the face, the upward continuation of platysma muscle forms a condensation of fascia, forming a thin tough layer, interspersed with fat from the subcutaneous layer, called SMAS.

The thickness of the SMAS varies from person to person. The fuller, plumper the face is, the thicker the SMAS layer is. The leaner the face is, the thinner the SMAS layer is. The clinical implication of this is that in a fuller face, raising the SMAS is easy as it is a thicker substantial layer. In a leaner individual, one has to be more careful to avoid perforating the SMAS. The SMAS is closely linked to the skin due to the arborization pattern of the fascial ligaments. When you move the malar skin, the skin, the malar fat pad, and the SMAS move as a unit.[14] The part of the SMAS over the parotid is fixed to the deeper fascia, while the part over the muscles of the face is mobile. Usually sagging happens in the sub-SMAS plane in this mobile region.

Loose Areolar Tissue

Beneath the SMAS is the loose areolar tissue, which forms the gliding plane for tissues on top to slide down. It is also a natural plane of dissection. Very few structures pass through it and it is relatively avascular.

Deep Fascia

Beneath the loose areolar layer is the deep fascia. The deep fascia over the face is a continuation of the superficial layer of the investing layer of the cervical fascia. Over the parotid gland this is called the parotidomasseteric fascia. It continues over the facial muscles anteriorly, passing deep to the lip elevators and thus dividing the muscles of fascial animation into superficial and deep layers. The facial nerve lies deep to the deep fascia.[26] The superficial and deep fascia is firmly attached to each other in areas of the ligaments or zones of adhesion (**Fig. 11.3**).

Muscles of Facial Animation

From the anatomy what is relevant is to know that they are arranged in four layers as per Freilinger et al.[27] The first, second, and third layers form the superficial muscles. The superficial muscles are the frontalis, orbicularis, the platysma, corrugators, procerus, zygomaticus major, minor, levator labii superioris, depressor labii inferioris, and risorius. The deepest layer consists of the mentalis, levator anguli oris,

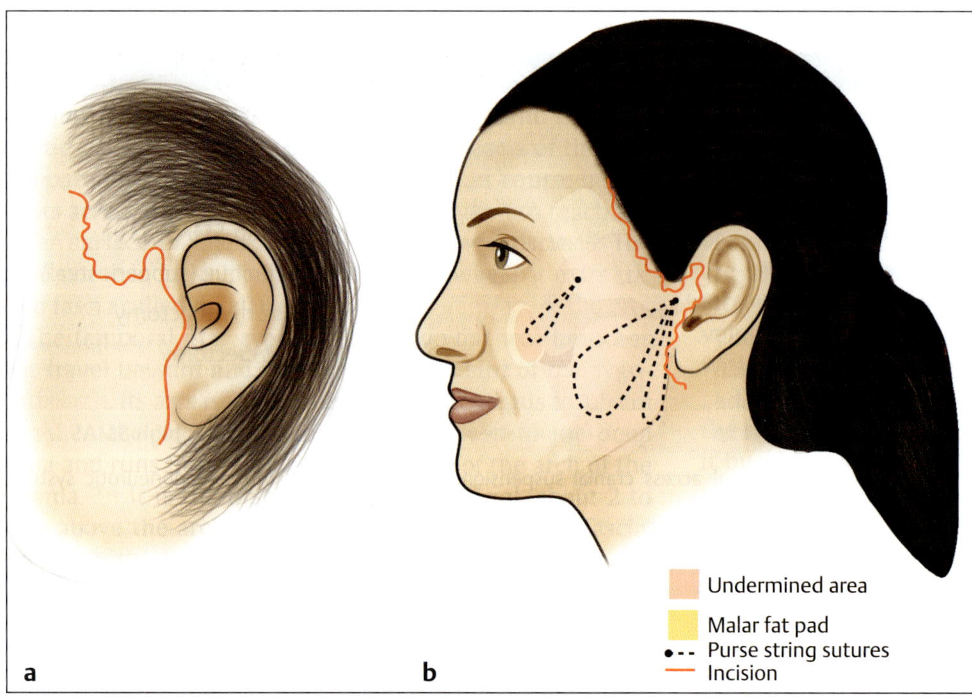

Fig. 11.5 (a, b) Access and suspension sutures of minimal access cranial suspension (MACS) lift. (Adapted from Tonnard et al 2005.[19])

Table 11.2 Pros and cons of the subcutaneous rhytidectomy technique

Pros	Cons
Simple technique	Skin tension and necrosis
Easy to learn	Does not correct sagging SMAS—jowls and NL folds
Immediate improvement visible	Horizontal vector
Quick	Lateral sweep/wind swept face
No risk of damage to nerves	Short-term results

Abbreviations: NL, nasolabial; SMAS, superficial musculoaponeurotic system.

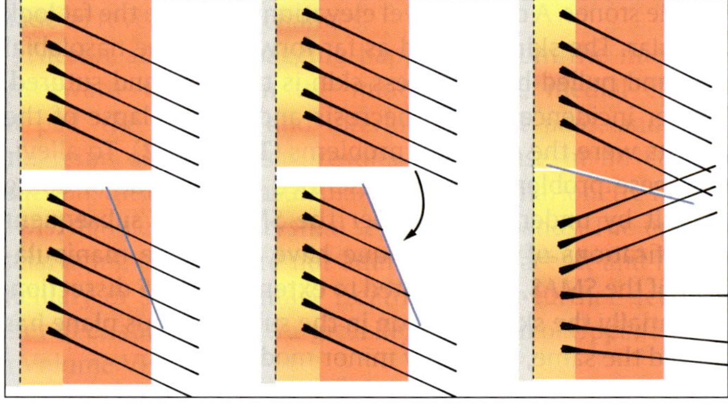

Fig. 11.6 Diagrammatic representation of trichophytic closure.

extended MACS lift, it goes up to the eyebrow level. This part of the incision is wavy as in a W-plasty and angled forward at 90 degrees to the shaft of the hair follicles, cutting the shafts so as to perform trichophytic closure which allows hair growth through the scar (**Fig. 11.6**).

The extent of the undermining is up to the angle of the mandible below, then curving forward 5 to 6 cm from the ear. In extended MACS lift, it goes across anterior cheek and malar area.

A 0.5 cm window is created in the SMAS in front of the helix and above the zygomatic arch to anchor the first and second stitch to the deep temporal fascia. They use three 1-0 PDS loop sutures passed from the temporal fascia downward taking small bites of the SMAS and looping back on itself. The first loop passes vertically downward in the pretragal region going up to the angle of the mandible. The second passes further forward in an O-shaped loop in the midpart of the face in the direction of the jowls. The third is more anterior and is anchored above the anterior end of the zygomatic arch, and passes through the malar mound (**Fig. 11.5b**). Small 0.5 cm deep bites are taken, 1 to 1.5 cm long, with the loop suture as it catches the SMAS in the loop. The loops are tightened at maximal tension and suspended from the deep temporal fascia. The SMAS gathers up with tiny imbrications. The skin is then redraped more vertically and excess excised.

The limitations of this technique were the inability to address the neck (**Table 11.3**) and this was subsequently addressed in another article wherein he described addition of liposuction for the neck, anterior cervicoplasty and posterior cervicoplasty,[19] and the longevity.[43]

Table 11.3 Pros and cons of MACS lift

Pros	Cons
Simple to learn	Lift is moderate as limited by ligaments
Lifts SMAS by imbrication	Ancillary treatments such as fat grafting and postauricular incision are required for advanced cases
Low risk of injury to important structures	Longevity is shorter
Quick recovery, shorter downtime	

Abbreviations: MACS, minimal access cranial suspension; SMAS, superficial musculoaponeurotic system.

Proximal SMAS-Elevating Techniques

Skoog Facelift

The main criticism of the subcutaneous rhytidectomy technique was the short duration of the results.

Tord Skoog in 1970 described a technique wherein the skin and SMAS are raised from the preauricular incision as a composite flap and are advanced cephaloposteriorly. Instead of undermining in the subcutaneous plane in the standard rhytidectomy of those times, he moved one layer down. This improved the vascularity of the skin, reduced the incidence of skin necrosis, and also improved the longevity of results.[9] The drawback of this technique was the vector in which the SMAS was moved. It was pulled backward toward the ear and often led to lateral sweep deformity. It also did not move the anterior face sag much.[10]

Deep Plane Facelift

Sam Hamra had been doing the Skoog facelift for years, but felt the results were incongruous, as the Skoog facelift would lift and pull the lateral part of the face well, without addressing the nasolabial folds and medial face.[10] Hence, he described his modification of Skoog technique in 1990. He limited the skin elevation, as in the subcutaneous rhytidectomy, to only a few centimeters. He would then lift the SMAS like in a Skoog technique but continue the elevation over and beyond the zygomaticus major and minor. He would raise the skin, fat, and SMAS of the anterior face as a myocutaneous flap, going beyond the nasolabial fold. After this extensive SMAS dissection, the SMAS was stitched to the deep temporal fascia with 3–0 Vicryl. He claimed significantly better improvement in anterior face, nasolabial, and malar eminence sag (**Table 11.4**).[10]

Composite Facelift

Sam Hamra understood the need to rejuvenate all areas of the face for a harmonious rejuvenation. He noted that the orbicularis oculi, cheek fat pad, and platysma all aged conjointly. Until 1992, all facelift methods focused on lifting the skin separately and the SMAS separately, disregarding the other aged structures. He stated that there was need to lift the sag in the orbicularis oculi muscle and the malar fat pad as well and described his technique to treat all the areas or zones of the face by doing a forehead lift, blepharoplasty, facelift, and neck lift at the same time. The forehead lift was done through a bicoronal incision (**Fig. 11.7**). The blepharoplasty and facelift dissections were connected from under the lower border of orbicularis oculi to under the deep plane dissection of the SMAS. The orbicularis oculi was lifted upward and medially, while the SMAS, malar fat pad, and skin was lifted upward and laterally in a composite manner. This was extensive and considered quite radical too. However, he did show that the results he achieved were quite harmonious and comprehensive (**Table 11.5**).[14]

Table 11.4 Pros and cons of the deep plane facelift

Pros	Cons
More effective effacement of NL folds and jowls	Extensive dissection, more time consuming
Good longevity of improvement	Risk of damage to facial nerves
	Longer recovery, more downtime

Abbreviation: NL, nasolabial.

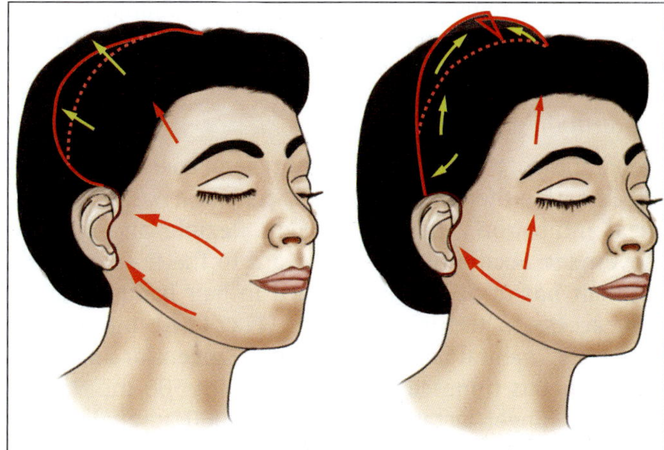

Fig. 11.7 Composite facelift. (Adapted from Hamra 1992.[14])

Cervicoplasty and Lamellar High SMAS Facelift

This is a technique which principally believes that the SMAS needs to rotate and lift vertically, while the skin moves in a posterosuperior direction, hence the word "lamellar." The SMAS and skin are moved as two separate lamellae.[16] The SMAS is divided high on the upper border of zygoma, higher than other techniques, hence called high SMAS. The sub-SMAS dissection is extended to cross the zygomaticus major, and this moves the SMAS up in the front of the face, more effectively correcting the undereye aging changes like in a mid-facelift. Tim Marten principally believes that sag and volume loss are two features that need to be addressed

Table 11.5 Pros and cons of composite facelift

Pros	Cons
Full face rejuvenation	Extensive surgery
Significant change in NL folds and jowls	Long operative time
Longevity of improvement good	Longer downtime and recovery

Abbreviation: NL, nasolabial.

during facial rejuvenation, and hence he popularized fat grafting for volume-deficient areas at the same time as the facelift.

Preparation and Anesthesia

Preparation of the patient: Usually general anesthesia is preferred with either an armored oral tube or a nasal endotracheal intubation. The tube is kept flexible and free for movement. Fixation is either upward to the nose or teeth. The hair has to be parted and tied in hair bands to allow easy access to the incision lines (**Fig. 11.8**). Infraorbital, zygomatic, mental nerve blocks can be given for analgesia. Subcutaneous tumescent infiltration with 500 mL Normal saline or Ringer lactate with 1 mL 1:1000 adrenaline and 20 mL 2% lignocaine/0.25% bupivacaine helps in giving an avascular plane while raising the skin flap. Fat grafting is done to the periorbital area, temple, midcheek, anterior cheek, nasolabial area, and marionette areas as per preoperative assessment.[45]

Treating the Neck

First determine if the fat is subcutaneous or subplatysmal. If subcutaneous, it can be removed by liposuction. If it is subplatysmal, it has to be removed while performing a cervicoplasty. Neckbands or hanging platysmal straps should be treated through a cervicoplasty approach.

Cervicoplasty

A 4 cm incision is taken 1 to 2 cm behind the mentocervical crease (**Fig. 11.9a**). Subcutaneous undermining in the submental region exposes the platysmal edge. The fat beneath the platysma in the submental region is surgically excised judiciously. The medial borders of platysma are sutured upward from just below the hyoid bone level with 4–0 Vicryl. It is then cut transversely, preferably completely, at the cricoid cartilage level, to relax the tension in the platysma and allow it to sit flush against the neck and mentocervical angle. The subsequent part of the neck lift is achieved when the SMAS is lifted and pulled back. The platysma works like a corset around the neck (**Fig. 11.9b**).

Skin Incision

Typically, the incision for facelifts is in front of the ear, skirting the anterior helical rim, passing behind the tragus in women, but in the front in men (**Fig. 11.8**).

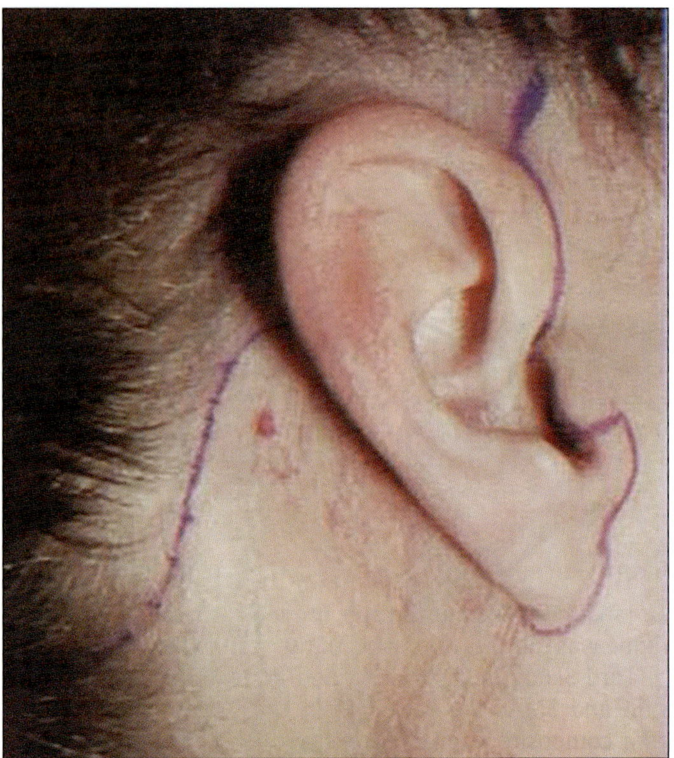

Fig. 11.8 Incision for lamellar high superficial musculoaponeurotic system (SMAS). (Adapted from Marten 2008.[16])

The incision skirts the earlobe, leaving a 1 mm rim at the inferiormost point. This is to prevent the appearance of the earlobe being stuck to the skin of the cheek after suturing, a complication commonly referred to as Pixie ear deformity. It then passes retroauricularly in the groove. If there is not much laxity in the neck skin, the incision can end in the retroauricular area as in a short scar modification described by Baker.[18] If lot of neck skin needs excision, then the incision is continued along the occipital hairline and then a transverse back cut into the hair (**Fig. 11.8**).

Whether to have a temporal extension of this incision or skirt the temporal hairline would depend on how much skin shift and temporal hairline shift is expected. If more than 2 cm shift is expected, it is better to stay anterior to the hairline. Shifting the temporal hairline more than 2 cm results in the typical facelifted look. The incision in this region has to be taken carefully respecting the directions of the hair follicles. Beveling the incision in the direction of the follicle allows trichophytic closure or tiny W-plasties help in concealing this scar.

A pretragal incision is preferred in men to avoid beard skin creeping on to the tragus. Alternatively, care should be taken to divide the bulb of the follicles of the skin creeping over the tragus, or treat this area with LASER hair removal.

Skin Elevation

While undermining in the subcutaneous plane, it is important to keep the skin flap thin. The fat should look like pavement

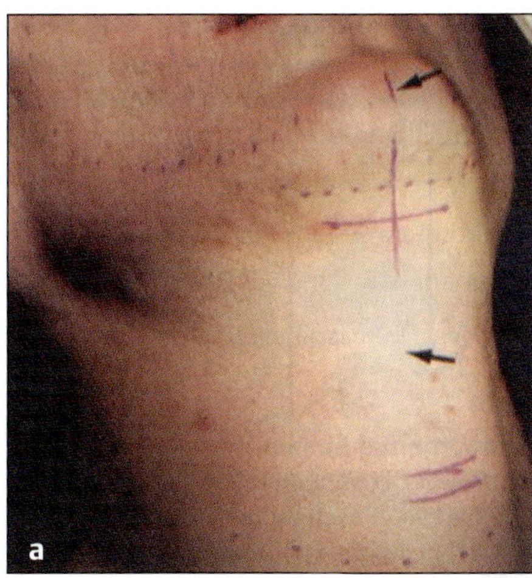

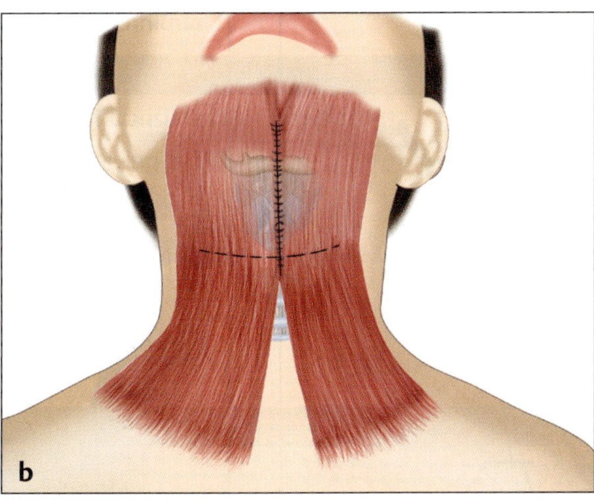

Fig. 11.9 **(a)** Neck incision. **(b)** Platysma corset.

of pebbles on transillumination. If fat looks globular, the skin flap is too thick. The undermining extends from the temple, lateral orbital rim, zygomatic prominence, lateral part of cheek (preserving the parotid cutaneous ligaments between the SMAS and skin), down to the chin and neck (**Fig. 11.10**). This allows the skin to move with the SMAS as one unit. It also preserves the blood supply to the skin.

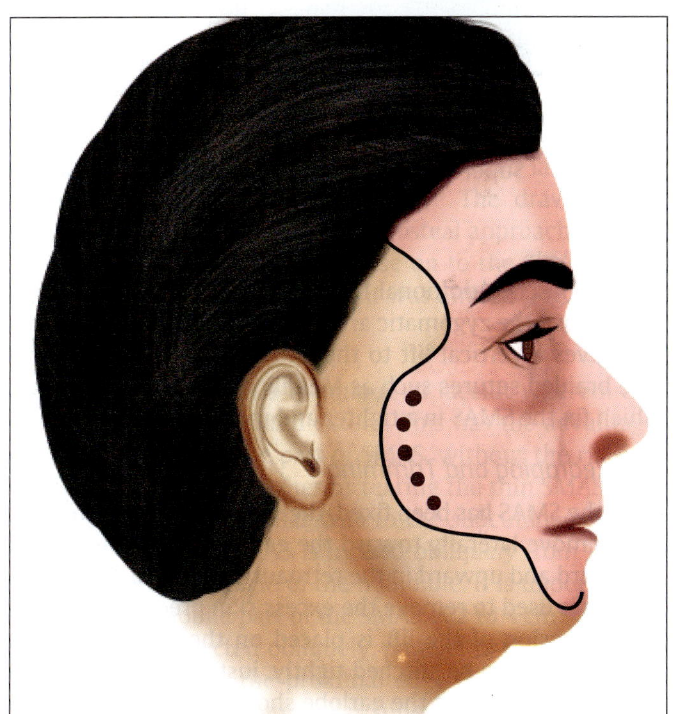

Fig. 11.10 Extent of skin undermining.

SMAS Elevation

Prior to lifting the SMAS, it often helps to infiltrate saline adrenaline under it. It balloons up the SMAS, makes the plane easy to lift, and also creates a relatively avascular plane. The SMAS is incised along the middle or upper border of the zygomatic arch right up to the malar prominence anteriorly (**Fig. 11.11**). This is higher than other variations. This incision has to be done gently with just the weight of the blade. The SMAS is lifted with forceps and scissors are opened in a vertically spreading fashion under the SMAS, snipping only at the fibrous bands. The frontal branch of the facial nerve is deep to the deep fascia along the central third of the zygomatic arch.

The facial nerve branches are deep to the parotidomasseteric fascia. As long as this fascia is not breached, and you stay flush to the under surface of the fibroareolar SMAS, the SMAS elevation is safe. The SMAS is elevated beyond the zygomaticus major muscle, dividing the zygomaticofacial and masseteric ligaments. The mandibular ligaments are released in the subcutaneous plane (**Fig. 11.12**). The SMAS moves freely once these ligaments are released. The mark of proper release is when the tug moves the alar base, upper lip, and lower lip together.

Vector of Lift

The most important component of this technique is the vector of movement. The SMAS should move posterosuperiorly and upward toward the temporal region (above the upper pole of the ear). More centrally, the movement would be vertical (a mid-facelift moves vertically). The axis of rotation of the high SMAS technique causes fullness at the malar prominence. This fills and rounds off the malar mound, exaggerating the ogee curve and improving the aesthetics of the face. It also lifts the sagging superficial, medial, and middle fat pad up, along with the superior and inferior jowl fat pads.

SMAS Fixation

When the lax SMAS is pulled back and up, the excess can be cut as an inferiorly based flap and transposed behind the ear (**Fig. 11.13**). The SMAS is pulled tightly and stitched to the deep temporal fascia above the zygomatic arch in the temporal fossa, with either 2–0 Ethibond or Mersilk. The second key stitch is to fix the posterior SMAS flap to the

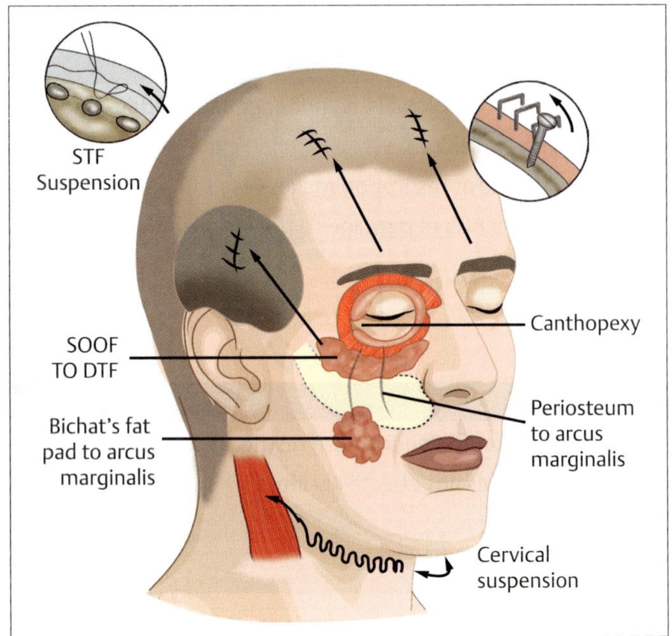

Fig. 11.15 Endoscopic facelift. DTF, deep temporal fascia; STF, superficial temporal fascia. (Adapted from Ramirez and Pozner 1996.[46])

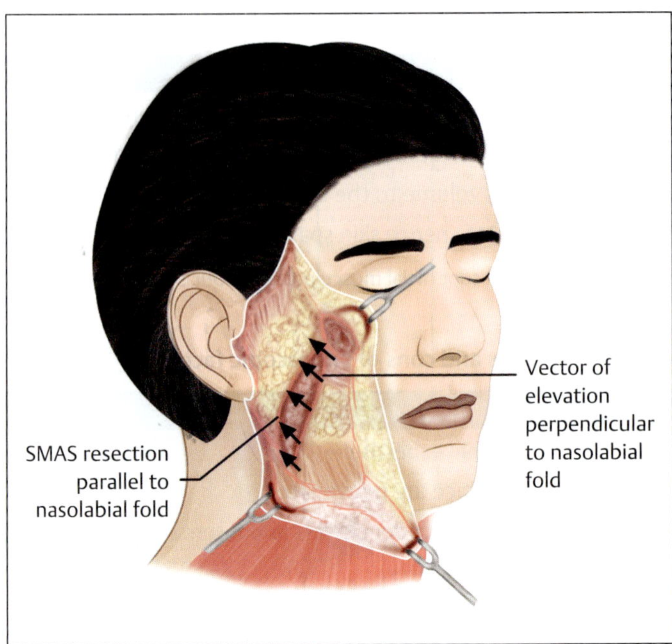

Fig. 11.16 Superficial musculoaponeurotic system (SMAS) resection in lateral SMASectomy. (Adapted from Baker 1997.[17])

Table 11.8 Pros and cons of the lateral SMASectomy procedure

Pros	Cons
Lifts the SMAS, giving improvement	May not completely correct the NL folds, jowls, and underchin sag
Less risk to damage of facial nerves	In case of severe laxity of skin, under correction possible
Short scar limited dissection, early recovery	Higher tuck-up rate at 2 years[43]

Abbreviations: NL, nasolabial; SMAS, superficial musculoaponeurotic system.

proximal edge. Andrew Jacono in 2011 described his modification wherein he approached the deep plane along a line drawn from the lateral canthus to the angle of the mandible, similar to the lateral SMASectomy approach, but dissected beyond the zygomaticus major and minor, on to the anterior midface, right up to the nasofacial groove and nasolabial fold.[44] This dissection was similar to Sam Hamra's deep plane facelift.

Marking and Incision

The skin incision in the extended deep plane technique starts from the temporal region, a few millimeters inside the hairline, cuts transversely across the sideburn to reach the upper edge of the superior helix of the ear. It then curves downward along the superior helical rim. It turns acutely backward to reach the posterior border of the tragus. It courses along the tragus to the intertragal notch, where it cuts sharply forward to reach the earlobe facial sulcus. It skirts this to leave a 2 to 3 mm cuff of skin on the earlobe at the apex. Behind the ear, the incision runs just inside the postauricular sulcus to prevent visibility of the scar, in case downward migration of the scar happens with age. The extent of postauricular incision would depend on the amount of neck laxity. For those who have a lot of laxity, the incision is carried down the occipital hairline.

Skin Elevation

Subcutaneous dissection in superficial fat is similar to any standard subcutaneous rhytidectomy. Its extent is a few millimeters anterior to the line drawn from the lateral canthus to the angle of the mandible. In the neck it extends at least to the cricoid cartilage level and anteriorly to the midline. Subcutaneous undermining on the anterior jawline is used to divide the mandibulocutaneous ligaments. For those who are going to need a cervicoplasty, they can have these ligaments divided from cervicoplasty approach as well. These ligaments are present at the lower edge of the mandibular border, at the anterior edge of the jowls, around 5 cm from the midline.

SMAS Elevation

The skin is lifted with lighted retractors under tension and an incision is made in the SMAS along the line from the mandibular angle to the lateral canthus. Vertical spreading scissor blades open the SMAS as we move along. First the orbicularis oculi is identified and then the zygomaticus major. While staying above the orbicularis oculi, the malar fat pad is lifted up bluntly. This approach has been described in the FAME technique of Sherrel Ashton.[11] Coming from below, a similar pocket is created by blunt dissection, which leaves only the zygomaticocutaneous ligaments attaching the SMAS to the zygoma. This is then divided sharply with scissors, exercising extreme caution to stay superficial and prevent injury to the zygomatic branches. Once the ligaments are divided, it is possible to bluntly dissect and lift the anterior cheek skin and fat pads off the underlying muscles easily. The dissection is continued downward along the zygomaticus muscles, staying on top, till the nasolabial fold. The SMAS dissection along the jaw line is limited anteriorly up to the anterior border of the masseter, or facial artery, thereby dividing the masseteric ligaments. The marginal mandibular nerve crosses from deep to superficial just distal to this point, so dissection should not be continued any further than this.

The SMAS dissection is continued inferiorly in to the neck. The posterior border of the platysma is incised at the anterior border of the sternocleidomastoid, dividing the cervical-retaining ligaments which hold the two together.[47] The cervical-retaining ligaments are divided sharply about 5 cm below the angle of the mandible and up to 1.5 cm in front. This frees the platysma and allows it to be pulled backward. The platysma is then transected at 5 cm below the border of the mandible and anteriorly up to the submandibular gland (**Fig. 11.17**).

SMAS Suspension and Vector

The lift is achieved by pulling the cuff of SMAS left on the distal skin in an upward and backward direction, 60 degrees to the Frankfurt horizontal plane.[48] The pull is vertically dominant near the angle of the mandible, and horizontally dominant near the orbit. Five to Seven 4–0 Nylon mattress sutures anchor the SMAS to the deep temporal fascia in the superior part, and to the parotidomasseteric fascia in the inferior part.

The posterior edge of the upper free border of the platysma in the neck is stitched to the gonial angle, which then forms a hammock to suspend and lift the submandibular gland. The posterior free edge of the lower free border of the platysma is anchored with a stitch to the mastoid process. This lifts the neck skin and recreates the mentocervical groove. The additional layer of SMAS at the gonial angle adds volume to the deflating mandibular angle. A few more anchoring stitches to the sternocleidomastoid fascia pull the horizontal component of the platysma posteriorly (**Fig. 11.17**).[49]

Skin Redraping and Distribution

The skin is redraped in the same direction as the SMAS pull, in an upward and backward direction. The excess skin is removed in a more vertical direction against the temporal skin edge and the preauricular skin edge. If there is neck laxity, it is adjusted behind the ear. 5–0 Ethilon mattress sutures are used over most of the suture line, except occipital hairline where 4–0 Ethilon is used.

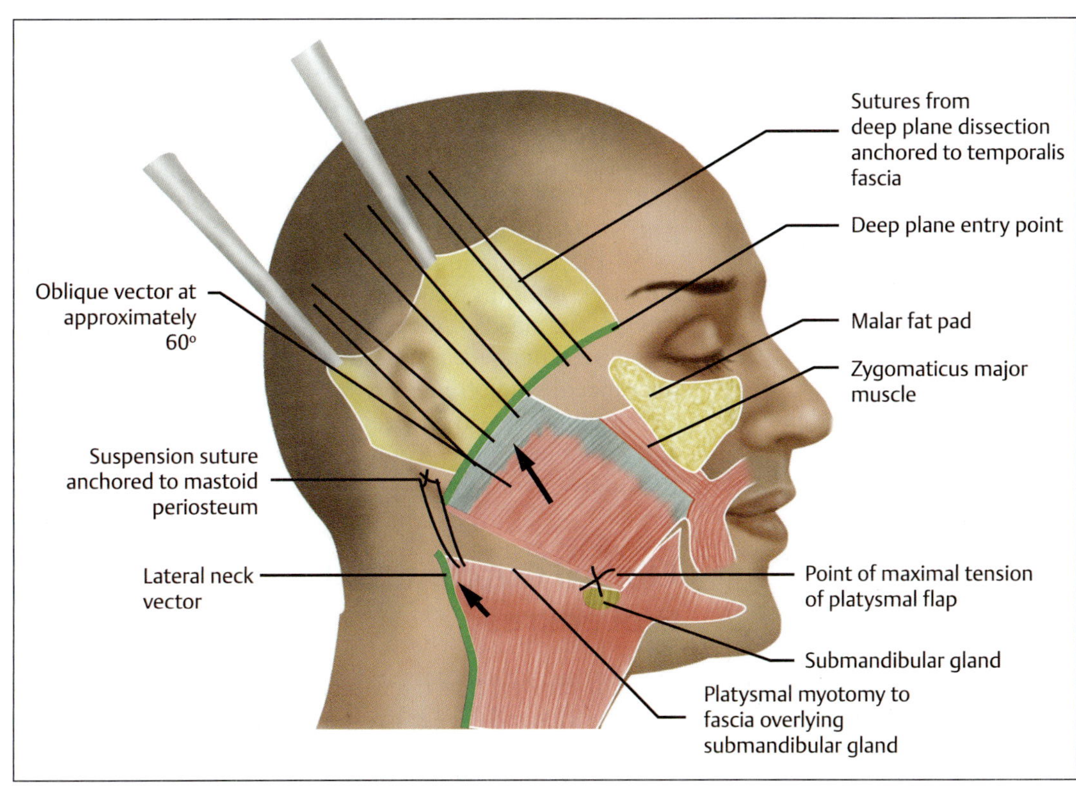

Fig. 11.17 Deep plane facelift. Incision in superficial musculoaponeurotic system (SMAS) and anchoring points. (Adapted from Jacone and Parikh 2011.[15])

Complications

Apart from the complications as a result of prolonged general anesthesia, complications specific to the procedure are hematoma 1.1%, infections, seroma, delayed healing, skin necrosis, and facial nerve paresis or paralysis (1.3%).[15,50]

Hematoma can manifest immediately overnight or be delayed over 5 days. The incidence of hematoma is higher in hypertensive patients.[51]

Auersvald and Auersvald described a hemostatic net stitched transcutaneously in the undermined areas, like a quilting suture using 5–0 Ethilon and has shown a statistically significant reduced hematoma rate (**Fig. 11.18**).[52] This stitch is removed on second postoperative day. Although it looks gruesome when swollen on second postop day, it does not leave a mark, although sufficient studies in Types IV to VI are lacking. There are various other means of reducing the incidence of hematoma, and preop proper control of blood pressure is one of them, avoiding postoperative high blood pressure spikes, coagulation screening, and rectifying clotting deficiencies are others.[53]

Necrosis of the edge of the skin, either during extensive dissection, too thin elevation of skin flap, or poor handling of the skin can be a disaster if large areas necrose. Minor edge necrosis can be managed conservatively.

Injury to the marginal mandibular nerve is one of the most dreaded complications and can cause paralysis or paresis of the depressor labii, depressor anguli oris, and mentalis,[54] thus causing weakness in retracting the lower lip while speaking. This is often a temporary phenomenon due to traction injury of the nerve and hence recovers in a majority of cases. Very rarely it could be permanently damaged. Injection of botulinum toxin in the contralateral depressor labii is an option to achieve some balance if that happens.

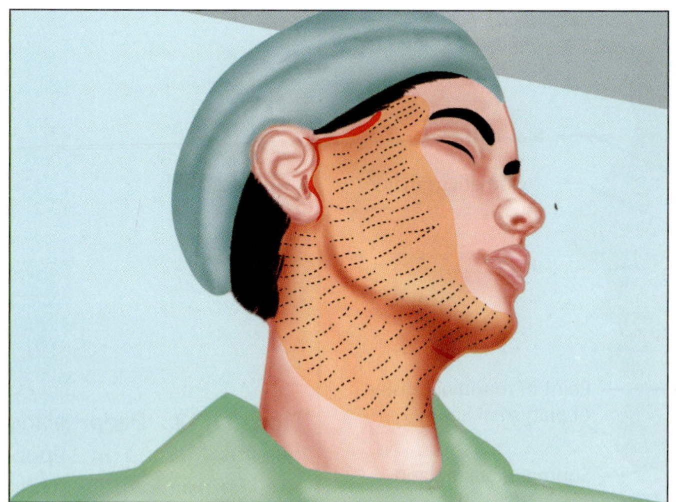

Fig. 11.18 Hemostatic net suturing. (Adapted from Auersvald and Auersvald 2014.[52])

Injury to the frontal branch or zygomatic branches of the facial nerve is even more rare, but reported in literature from 1 to 20% and can cause asymmetry on animation.[30]

Rarely the greater auricular nerve can get damaged, causing numbness to a part of the ear.[55]

Delayed healing is seen in the postauricular skin if it is thin and sutured under tension.

In an analysis of 11,300 patients, overall complications rate in facelift was 1.8%, out of which hematoma (1.1%) and infections (0.3%) were most common.[50] There was no statistically significant difference in complication rates in the study which compared the subcutaneous and minimally invasive to the SMAS techniques indicating that the SMAS techniques are equally safe with the added vascularity of the skin flaps.[56] Hematoma incidence varies from 0.9 to 6.5% with a statistically significant correlation to preoperative hypertension.[51,53] Facial nerve injury is one of the most dreaded complication in facelift surgery; however, it has been reported in between 1 and 2.6% of cases and recovery happens in 80% of these cases.[29,30] The incidence of facial nerve injury has not increased with the more extensive SMAS techniques, and Jacono reported a temporary facial nerve paralysis rate of 1.2% in the extended deep plane technique.[15]

Ancillary Techniques

The most commonly performed procedure along with facelift is fat grafting.[45,57–59] The areas where volume has depleted, if refilled with microfat, gives the best and most natural rejuvenation. Fat is harvested from any of the fat deposits such as abdomen, flanks lower back, or inner thighs. For facial fat grafting, it should be harvested with a smaller sized cannula, 2.4 to 2.1 mm. It can be sedimented or centrifuged, transferred to 1-mL syringes and then injected with 0.7- to 1.2-mm cannula. The commonly injected fat pockets are the retro-orbicularis oculi fat (ROOF), suborbicularis oculi fat (SOOF), medial cheek, middle cheek, temporoparotid cheek pad, NL fold, marionette lines, and lips.

All these techniques correct the structure of the face, but often the skin has aged and become thin, wrinkly, and callous, and needs rejuvenation. The quality of the skin can be rejuvenated with superficial peels, ablative lasers, or microneedle radiofrequency.[60–64]

Botulinum toxin is used for upper face rejuvenation and completes the comprehensive facial rejuvenation treatment.[65–67]

Clinical Outcome of Facelift Procedures

Ivy et al showed that the clinical outcomes are comparable at 6 months and 1 year irrespective of technique, whether MACS, lateral SMASectomy, or extended or deep plane.[64]

Prado et al compared the results between MACS lift and lateral SMASectomy and found outcomes were similar at 2 years, but both had a 50% tuck/revision rate.[43] So, minimal SMAS manipulation techniques show an improvement in the early period, but the results do not last in up to 50%. Kamer and Frankel in their study showed that the proximal SMAS techniques had an 11.4% tuck/revision rate, while the deep plane had a 3.3% tuck or revision rate.[68] This was statistically significant and implying that the deep and extended deep plane had an advantage over the proximal SMAS technique. SMAS manipulating techniques such as SMASectomy or plication have an average life of 9 years[69] while the SMAS lift techniques had a life of 11.9 years.[70]

Comments on Heavy Indian Faces

As per author's own experience, Indian faces, in the lower half, are often full with a thick dermis and subcutaneous superficial fat pad. In the upper half, near the periorbital area, the skin is thin and so is the superficial fat pads. The deep fat pad shrinks and hence the superficial structures sag. This type of aging change is best treated with some form of lift, along with filling of periorbital fat pad.

What we have learnt is that there is volume loss, there is a sag, and the skin becomes inelastic and thin. The earlier you start rectifying these, you can get away with lesser or relatively minor interventions. For example, radiofrequency skin tightening procedures, HIFU or threads, fillers, botulinum toxin, etc.[61,65,66,71–75] The more established the changes are, the more likely that only surgery will help.

Summary

Facelift works best for those who have sagging of malar cheek fat pad, jowls, deep nasolabial folds, marionette lines, and sagging neck skin. Any of the facelift techniques described aim to lift the sagging SMAS. Final result depends on the vector and extent of correction. One can use any technique that you are comfortable with, as long as the above-mentioned principles are followed to get a good result, and be proficient in it (**Figs. 11.19–11.22**). It is imperative to have a good understanding of the pathophysiology of aging, anatomy of the facial ligaments, the layers of the face, especially the SMAS and the important facial nerves.

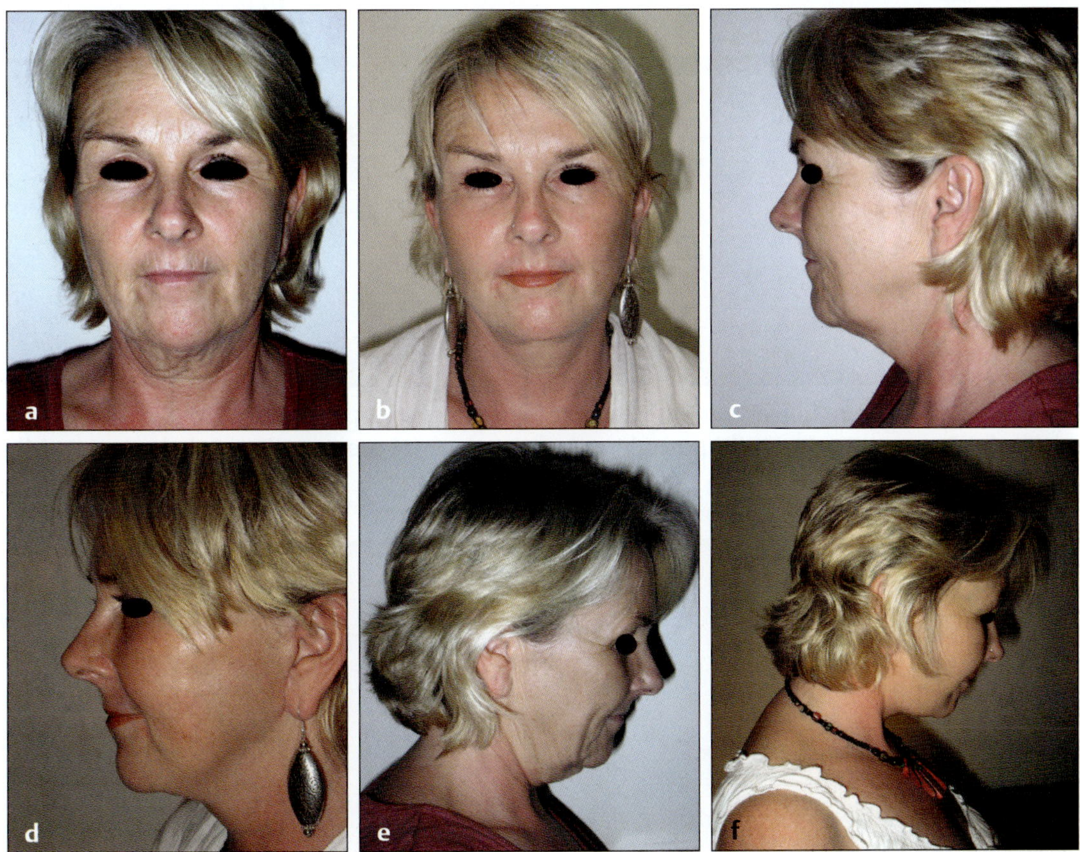

Fig. 11.19 Botulinum for forehead, frown, and crow's feet upper and lower blepharoplasty, facelift, neck lift. **(a)** Preoperative front, **(b)** postoperative front, **(c)** preoperative left side, **(d)** postoperative left side view, **(e)** preoperative neck down side, **(f)** postoperative neck down side.

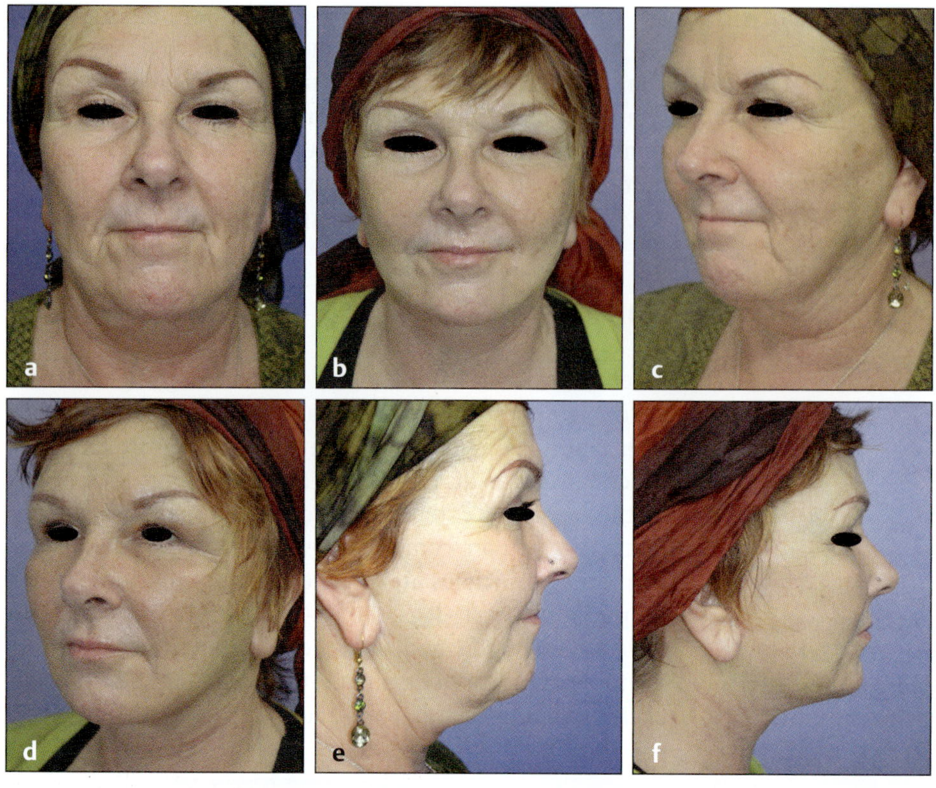

Fig. 11.20 Microfat grafting to periorbital, midface, nasolabial fold, and marionette areas plus extended high lamellar facelift. **(a)** Preoperative front, **(b)** postoperative front, **(c)** preoperative oblique, **(d)** postoperative oblique, **(e)** preoperative right side, **(f)** postoperative right side view.

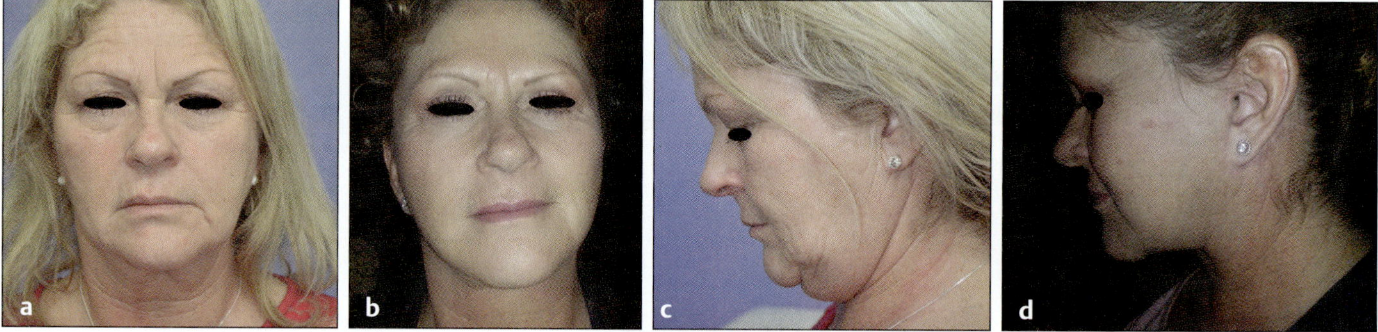

Fig. 11.21 Upper and lower blepharoplasty with extended high lamellar superficial musculoaponeurotic system (SMAS) facelift and neck lift. **(a)** Preoperative front, **(b)** postoperative front view, **(c)** preoperative neck down side, **(d)** postoperative neck down side view.

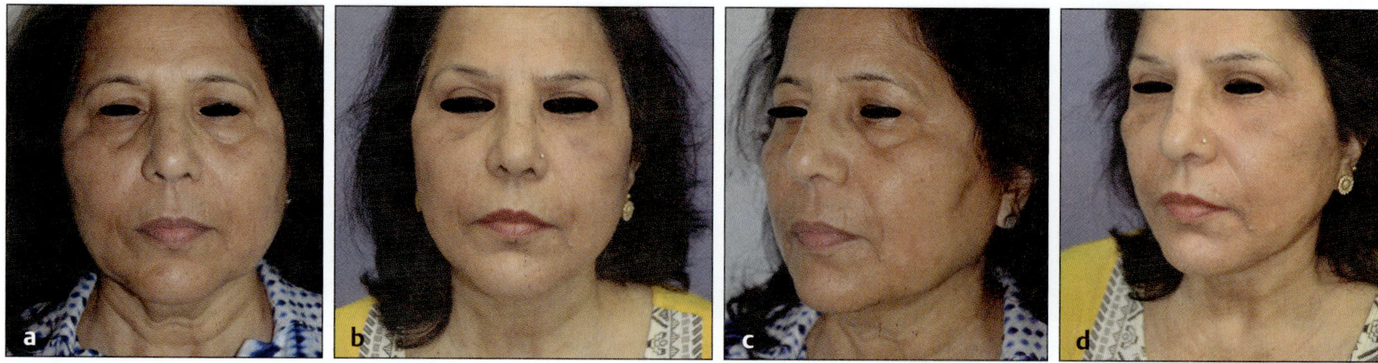

Fig. 11.22 Microfat grafting to temples, periorbital, malar, nasolabial fold, Marionette areas, plus lateral temporal brow lift, high lamellar extended sub-SMAS facelift and neck lift. **(a)** Preoperative front, **(b)** postoperative front view, **(c)** preoperative oblique, **(d)** postoperative oblique view.

References

1. Holländer E. Plastische (kosmetische) operation: Kritische Darstellung ihres gegenwärtigen Standes. Neue Dtsch Klin 1932;9:1–17
2. Locher WG, Feinendegen DL. The early days of aesthetic surgery: facelift pioneers Eugen Holländer (1867–1932) and Erich Lexer (1967–1937). Handchir Mikrochir Plast Chir Organ Deutschsprachigen Arbeitsgemeinschaft Handchir Organ Deutschsprachigen Arbeitsgemeinschaft Mikrochir Peripher Nerven Gefasse Organ V. Published online May 14, 2020. doi:10.1055/a-1150-7343
3. Miller CC. Cosmetic surgery: the correction of featural imperfections. Publisher not identified; 1908
4. Kolle: Plastic and cosmetic surgery. Google Scholar. Accessed July 17, 2020. https://scholar.google.com/scholar_lookup?title=Plastic%20and%20cosmetic%20surgery&author=FS.%20Kolle&publication_year=1911
5. Passot R. La cheirurgie esthetique des rides du visage. Presse Med 1919;27:258
6. Bourguet: La disparition chirurgicale des rides et plis du visage. Google Scholar. Accessed July 17, 2020. https://scholar.google.com/scholar_lookup?title=La%20disparition%20chirugicale%20des%20rides%20et%20plis%20du%20visage&author=J.%20Bourget&journal=Bull%20Acad%20Med&volume=82&pages=183&publication_year=1919
7. Bames HO. Truth and fallacies of face peeling and face lifting. Med J Rec 1927;126:86–87
8. Bettman AG. Plastic and cosmetic surgery of the face. Northwest Med 1920;19:205
9. Skoog TG. Plastic surgery: new methods and refinements. Saunders; 1974
10. Hamra ST. The deep-plane rhytidectomy. Plast Reconstr Surg 1990;86(1):53–61, discussion 62–63
11. Aston SJ. The FAME facelift: finger assisted malar elevation. In: Proceedings of The Cutting Edge: Aesthetic Surgery Symposium, New York, NY; 1998
12. Stuzin JM, Baker TJ, Gordon HL, Baker TM. Extended SMAS dissection as an approach to midface rejuvenation. Clin Plast Surg 1995;22(2):295–311
13. Ramirez OM. Endoscopic subperiosteal browlift and facelift. Clin Plast Surg 1995;22(4):639–660
14. Hamra ST. Composite rhytidectomy. Plast Reconstr Surg 1992;90(1):1–13
15. Jacono AA, Parikh SS. The minimal access deep plane extended vertical facelift. Aesthet Surg J 2011;31(8):874–890
16. Marten TJ. High SMAS facelift: combined single flap lifting of the jawline, cheek, and midface. Clin Plast Surg 2008;35(4):569–603, vi–vii
17. Baker DC. Lateral SMASectomy. Plast Reconstr Surg 1997;100(2):509–513
18. Baker DC. Minimal incision rhytidectomy (short scar face lift) with lateral SMASectomy: evolution and application. Aesthet Surg J 2001;21(1):14–26
19. Tonnard PL, Verpaele A, Gaia S. Optimising results from minimal access cranial suspension lifting (MACS-lift). Aesthetic Plast Surg 2005;29(4):213–220, discussion 221
20. Tonnard P, Verpaele A. The MACS-lift short scar rhytidectomy. Aesthet Surg J 2007;27(2):188–198
21. Baker D. Rhytidectomy with lateral SMASectomy. Facial Plast Surg 2000;16(3):209–213
22. Mendelson BC, Jacobson SR. Surgical anatomy of the midcheek: facial layers, spaces, and the midcheek segments. Clin Plast Surg 2008;35(3):395–404, discussion 393
23. Furnas DW. The retaining ligaments of the cheek. Plast Reconstr Surg 1989;83(1):11–16
24. Rohrich RJ, Pessa JE. The fat compartments of the face: anatomy and clinical implications for cosmetic surgery. Plast Reconstr Surg 2007;119(7):2219–2227, discussion 2228–2231
25. Mitz V, Peyronie M. The superficial musculo-aponeurotic system (SMAS) in the parotid and cheek area. Plast Reconstr Surg 1976;58(1):80–88
26. Stuzin JM, Baker TJ, Gordon HL. The relationship of the superficial and deep facial fascias: relevance to rhytidectomy and aging. Plast Reconstr Surg 1992;89(3):441–449, discussion 450–451
27. Freilinger G, Gruber H, Happak W, Pechmann U. Surgical anatomy of the mimic muscle system and the facial nerve: importance for reconstructive and aesthetic surgery. Plast Reconstr Surg 1987;80(5):686–690
28. Cardoso de Castro C. The value of anatomical study of the platysma muscle in cervical lifting. Aesthetic Plast Surg 1984;8(1):7–11
29. Owsley JQ, Agarwal CA. Safely navigating around the facial nerve in three dimensions. Clin Plast Surg 2008;35(4):469–477
30. Baker DC, Conley J. Avoiding facial nerve injuries in rhytidectomy: anatomical variations and pitfalls. Plast Reconstr Surg 1979;64(6):781–795
31. Castañares S. Facial nerve paralyses coincident with, or subsequent to, rhytidectomy. Plast Reconstr Surg 1974;54(6):637–643
32. Roostaeian J, Rohrich RJ, Stuzin JM. Anatomical considerations to prevent facial nerve injury. Plast Reconstr Surg 2015;135(5):1318–1327
33. Gosain AK. Surgical anatomy of the facial nerve. Clin Plast Surg 1995;22(2):241–251
34. Seckel BR. Facial danger zones: avoiding nerve injury in facial plastic surgery. Can J Plast Surg 1994;2(2):59–66
35. Mendelson B, Wong C-H. Anatomy of the aging face. In: Plastic Surgery. Vol. 2. 3rd ed. New York: Elsevier Saunders;2013:78–92
36. Pitanguy I, Ramos AS. The frontal branch of the facial nerve: the importance of its variations in face lifting. Plast Reconstr Surg 1966;38(4):352–356
37. Furnas DW. Landmarks for the trunk and the temporofacial division of the facial nerve. Br J Surg 1965;52:694–696
38. Agarwal CA, Mendenhall SD III, Foreman KB, Owsley JQ. The course of the frontal branch of the facial nerve in relation to fascial planes: an anatomic study. Plast Reconstr Surg 2010;125(2):532–537
39. Dingman RO, Grabb WC. Surgical anatomy of the mandibular ramus of the facial nerve based on the dissection of 100 facial halves. Plast Reconstr Surg Transplant Bull 1962;29:266–272
40. Daane SP, Owsley JQ. Incidence of cervical branch injury with "marginal mandibular nerve pseudo-paralysis" in patients undergoing face lift. Plast Reconstr Surg 2003;111(7):2414–2418
41. McKinney P, Gottlieb J. The relationship of the great auricular nerve to the superficial musculoaponeurotic system. Ann Plast Surg 1985;14(4):310–314
42. Mendelson B, Wong C-H. Changes in the facial skeleton with aging: implications and clinical applications in facial rejuvenation. Aesthetic Plast Surg 2012;36(4):753–760
43. Prado A, Andrades P, Danilla S, Castillo P, Leniz P. A clinical retrospective study comparing two short-scar face lifts: minimal access cranial suspension versus lateral SMASectomy. Plast Reconstr Surg 2006;117(5):1413–1425, discussion 1426–1427

44. Jacono A, Bryant LM. Extended deep plane facelift: incorporating facial retaining ligament release and composite flap shifts to maximize midface, jawline and neck rejuvenation. Clin Plast Surg 2018;45(4):527–554
45. Marten TJ, Elyassnia D. Fat grafting in facial rejuvenation. Clin Plast Surg 2015;42(2):219–252
46. Ramirez OM, Pozner JN. Subperiosteal minimally invasive laser endoscopic rhytidectomy: the SMILE facelift. Aesthetic Plast Surg 1996;20(6):463–470
47. Jacono AA, Malone MH. Characterization of the cervical retaining ligaments during subplatysmal facelift dissection and its implications. Aesthet Surg J 2017;37(5):495–501
48. Jacono AA, Ransom ER. Patient-specific rhytidectomy: finding the angle of maximal rejuvenation. Aesthet Surg J 2012; 32(7):804–813
49. Jacono AA, Bryant LM, Ahmedli NN. A novel extended deep plane facelift technique for jawline rejuvenation and volumization. Aesthet Surg J 2019;39(12):1265–1281
50. Gupta V, Winocour J, Shi H, Shack RB, Grotting JC, Higdon KK. Preoperative risk factors and complication rates in facelift: analysis of 11,300 patients. Aesthet Surg J 2016;36(1):1–13
51. Maricevich MA, Adair MJ, Maricevich RL, Kashyap R, Jacobson SR. Facelift complications related to median and peak blood pressure evaluation. Aesthetic Plast Surg 2014;38(4):641–647
52. Auersvald A, Auersvald LA. Hemostatic net in rhytidoplasty: an efficient and safe method for preventing hematoma in 405 consecutive patients. Aesthetic Plast Surg 2014;38(1):1–9
53. Ramanadham SR, Mapula S, Costa C, Narasimhan K, Coleman JE, Rohrich RJ. Evolution of hypertension management in face lifting in 1089 patients: optimizing safety and outcomes. Plast Reconstr Surg 2015;135(4):1037–1043
54. Stuzin JM, Rohrich RJ. Facial nerve danger zones. Plast Reconstr Surg 2020;145(1):99–102
55. Sharma VS, Stephens RE, Wright BW, Surek CC. What is the lobular branch of the great auricular nerve? Anatomical description and significance in rhytidectomy. Plast Reconstr Surg 2017;139(2):371e–378e
56. Rammos CK, Mohan AT, Maricevich MA, Maricevich RL, Adair MJ, Jacobson SR. Is the SMAS flap facelift safe? A comparison of complications between the sub-SMAS approach versus the subcutaneous approach with or without SMAS plication in aesthetic rhytidectomy at an academic institution. Aesthetic Plast Surg 2015;39(6):870–876
57. Buckingham ED, Smith SW. Incorporating fat grafting with facelift surgery: when, how, and where. Facial Plast Surg Clin North Am 2020;28(3):397–407
58. Molina-Burbano F, Smith JM, Ingargiola MJ, et al. Fat grafting to improve results of facelift: systematic review of safety and effectiveness of current treatment paradigms. Aesthet Surg J 2020
59. Rohrich RJ, Durand PD, Dayan E. The lift-and-fill facelift: superficial musculoaponeurotic system manipulation with fat compartment augmentation. Clin Plast Surg 2019;46(4): 515–522
60. Alhaddad M, Wu DC, Bolton J, et al. A randomized, split-face, evaluator-blind clinical trial comparing monopolar radiofrequency versus microfocused ultrasound with visualization for lifting and tightening of the face and upper neck. Dermatol Surg 2019;45(1):131–139
61. Ali YH. Two years' outcome of thread lifting with absorbable barbed PDO threads: Innovative score for objective and subjective assessment. J Cosmet Laser Ther 2018;20(1):41–49
62. Kaplan H, Kaplan L. Combination of microneedle radiofrequency (RF), fractional RF skin resurfacing and multi-source non-ablative skin tightening for minimal-downtime, full-face skin rejuvenation. J Cosmet Laser Ther 2016;18(8):438–441
63. Kwon HH, Lee W-Y, Choi SC, Jung JY, Bae Y, Park G-H. Combined treatment for skin laxity of the aging face with monopolar radiofrequency and intense focused ultrasound in Korean subjects. J Cosmet Laser Ther 2018;20(7-8):449–453
64. Ivy EJ, Lorenc ZP, Aston SJ. Is there a difference? A prospective study comparing lateral and standard SMAS face lifts with extended SMAS and composite rhytidectomies. Plast Reconstr Surg 1996;98(7):1135–1143, discussion 1144–1147
65. Sundaram H, Signorini M, Liew S, et al; Global Aesthetics Consensus Group. Global aesthetics consensus: Botulinum toxin type A—Evidence-based review, emerging concepts, and consensus recommendations for aesthetic use, including updates on complications. Plast Reconstr Surg 2016;137(3): 518e–529e
66. de Maio M, Swift A, Signorini M, Fagien S; Aesthetic Leaders in Facial Aesthetics Consensus Committee. Facial assessment and injection guide for botulinum toxin and injectable hyaluronic acid fillers: focus on the upper face. Plast Reconstr Surg 2017;140(2):265e–276e
67. Le Louarn C. Botulinum toxin: An important complement for facial rejuvenation surgery. Ann Chir Plast Esthet 2017; 62(5):495–519
68. Kamer FM, Frankel AS. SMAS rhytidectomy versus deep plane rhytidectomy: an objective comparison. Plast Reconstr Surg 1998;102(3):878–881
69. Beale EW, Rasko Y, Rohrich RJ. A 20-year experience with secondary rhytidectomy: a review of technique, longevity, and outcomes. Plast Reconstr Surg 2013;131(3):625–634
70. Sundine MJ, Kretsis V, Connell BF. Longevity of SMAS facial rejuvenation and support. Plast Reconstr Surg 2010;126(1): 229–237
71. Carruthers J, Carruthers A. A multimodal approach to rejuvenation of the lower face. Dermatol Surg 2016;42(Suppl 2): S89–S93
72. Casabona G, Kaye K. Facial skin tightening with microfocused ultrasound and dermal fillers: considerations for patient selection and outcomes. J Drugs Dermatol 2019;18(11):1075–1082
73. Sundaram H, Liew S, Signorini M, et al; Global Aesthetics Consensus Group. Global aesthetics consensus: hyaluronic acid fillers and botulinum toxin type A—Recommendations for combined treatment and optimizing outcomes in diverse patient populations. Plast Reconstr Surg 2016;137(5):1410–1423
74. de Maio M, DeBoulle K, Braz A, Rohrich RJ; Alliance for the Future of Aesthetics Consensus Committee. Facial assessment and injection guide for botulinum toxin and injectable hyaluronic acid fillers: focus on the midface. Plast Reconstr Surg 2017;140(4):540e–550e
75. de Maio M, Wu WTL, Goodman GJ, Monheit G; Alliance for the Future of Aesthetics Consensus Committee. Facial assessment and injection guide for botulinum toxin and injectable hyaluronic acid fillers: focus on the lower face. Plast Reconstr Surg 2017;140(3):393e–404e

12

Aesthetic Skeletal Surgery

Pramod Subash, Maria Kuriakose, and Arjun Krishnadas

Introduction

An attractive face is dependent upon the harmonious relationship between the skeleton and soft tissues. A hypoplastic or vertically elongated maxilla leading to nasal deformities and hypoplastic mandible with retrogenia causing incompetence of lips resulting in forceful closure and mentalis strain are examples of soft tissue dependence on good skeletal foundation. One should also bear in mind that symmetry between two halves of face and anteroposterior relationship between facial structures causing a "relative projection and relative retrusion" are factors that contribute to an attractive face. An aesthetic surgeon should have a thorough understanding about the effect skeleton and soft tissues have on each other in order to develop a diagnosis and treatment plan.

History of Orthognathic Surgery

Hullihen in 1849 performed a mandibular osteotomy to correct a protruding dentoalveolar segment. Toward the end of the 18th century, Blair performed a body osteotomy for the correction of mandibular prognathism. In the early 20th century, procedures like Blair's and Kostecka's were performed, in which the ramus was cut transcutaneously with patient under sedation and local blocks. But most of them were considered failures as the surgical results were not stable, due to poor bony contact. These were followed by few futile efforts to modify the osteotomy design. In 1925 Limberg proposed the oblique subcondylar osteotomy[1] followed by Caldwell and Letterman[2] by extraoral vertical ramus osteotomy.

Orthognathic surgery as we know today is considered to be born in the late 1960s. It was the work of Hugo Obwegeser,[3,4] who proposed a sagittal split osteotomy (SSO) of the mandible transorally, which revolutionized the basic concepts about deformity correction of the face and made orthognathic surgery a subspecialty in itself (**Fig. 12.1**).

The first modification of SSRO was proposed by Dal Pont who, after assisting Obwegeser, proposed the idea of changing location of osteotomy on the lateral cortex of the mandible from the horizontal cut on ramus to a vertical osteotomy on the body. Later Hunsuck and Epker advised that the osteotomy on medial/lingual cortex can stop just beyond the mandibular foramen, instead of carrying it back to posterior border of ramus. In 1968 Winstanely[5] proposed intraoral vertical ramus osteotomy (IVRO) which was later popularized by Hall.[6]

Le Fort osteotomy was practiced initially for gaining access to skull base and nasopharynx. During early 1930s maxillary osteotomies gained popularity in correction of occlusal problems. In mid 1930s Axhausen reported complete mobilization of maxilla after performing pterygoid disjunction and used this technique to correct cleft and posttraumatic deformities. Till 1960s there was no evidence about satisfactory advancement of maxilla, which left behind a suboptimal aesthetic outcome like a dish face to the patient. In 1970s the first simultaneous osteotomy of maxilla and mandibular sagittal split was done by Obwegeser.[7] Another revolutionary change was brought about by Hans Luhr in 1968 when he proposed internal fixation, which obviated the need for prolonged intermaxillary fixation and bone grafting.[8]

Converse in 1969 reported the importance of orthodontic collaboration during the planning stages for correction of dentofacial deformity with orthognathic surgery.[9] This paved way for surgical and orthodontic specialities to come together for the correction of dentofacial deformities and are now inseparable in sculpting occlusal harmony along with facial aesthetics.

Assembling Records and Clinical Examination

The evaluation and assessment of a patient with skeletal deformity starts as they walk in to the clinic. Attention

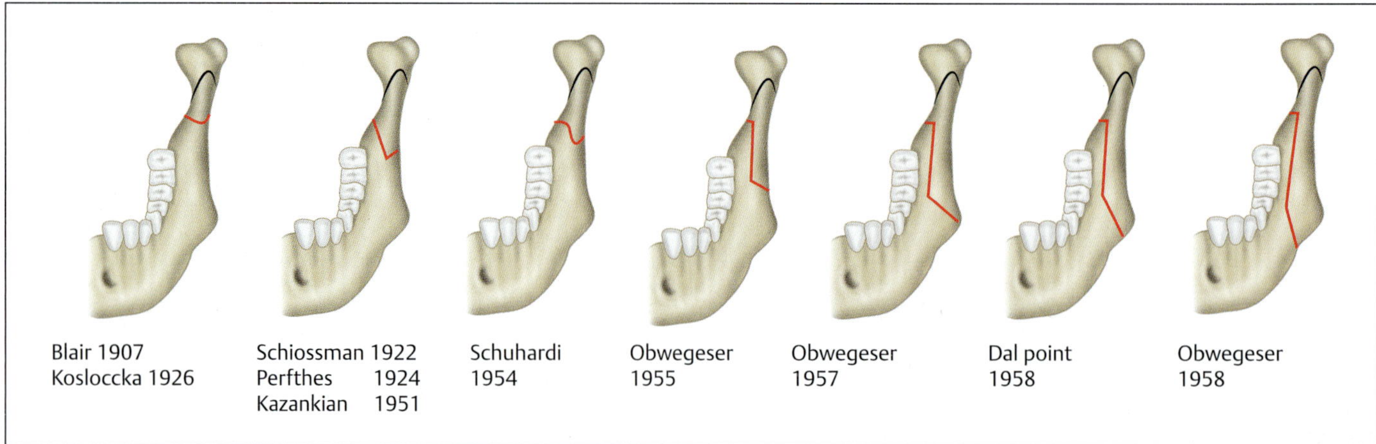

Fig. 12.1 Evolution of sagittal split osteotomy of the mandible. (Adapted from Obwegeser 2007.[4])

should be given to general structure of the body, gait, and neutral head position. "What would make the face appear symmetrical and aesthetically pleasing" is a very vital thought process that will help to identify deficiencies and formulate treatment plan. For example, in a patient with gummy smile and small chin, the thought process will be a vertically shorter maxilla and more prominent chin would bring balance between facial structures.

Facial deformity correction procedures usually require multiple stages and a multidisciplinary approach, and planning happens over multiple time points during the course of presurgical orthodontic treatment. Initial treatment plan is created as an outcome of the primary consultation in conjunction with the orthodontist and surgeon. Capturing patient records at these time points is integral to reassess clinical exam findings in greater detail, make measurements, observe progress of treatment, and make modifications in treatment plan as required and is a great tool in patient education. A complete set of records should include photographs (**Fig. 12.2**), dental study models, X-rays (orthopantomogram, lateral cephalogram, and PA cephalogram), and computed tomography (CT) scan.

Facial Examination

The goal of potential treatment can be functional, aesthetic or both. In conjunction with the patients' primary concerns, observations based on detailed clinical examination of facial and intraoral structures will help to create a problem list. Frontal evaluation should assess the vertical dimensions and proportions as well as the symmetry of skeletal soft and hard tissues. Examination should be done with the facial muscles at repose and in animation. Parameters should include height of forehead, slant of eyebrows and eyes, interpupillary and interorbital distance, presence of epicanthal folds, scleral show, deficiencies in malar and pyriform regions, width of nose, length and fullness of upper lip (18 +/– 2 mm), interlabial gap (competence of lips), incisor exposure at rest (3–4 mm), activity of mentalis, and length of neck. Incisor exposure and gum show should be measured again with a full animated smile. Asymmetry should be measured by assessing facial 1/5ths (**Fig. 12.3a**). Vertical cant and deviation of soft tissue, skeletal and dental midlines from facial midline at soft tissue, and skeletal and dentition level should be measured and quantified. Vertical proportion of facial 1/3rds (**Fig. 12.3b**) and angles (**Fig. 12.4**) between facial structures should be evaluated in profile examination. Lip competence, labiomental fold, hyperactivity of mentalis, and chin-neck-throat form should be carefully assessed at rest and in animation. Structure of nose should be assessed and recorded, keeping in mind the positive or negative influence of skeletal surgery on external nasal form.

Intraoral Examination

Basic knowledge about occlusion is paramount in understanding facial deformities, developing a treatment plan and executing surgical procedures accurately. The father of modern orthodontics, Edward Hartley Angle, in 1899 characterized occlusions as Class I, Class II, and Class III (**Fig. 12.5**) depending on the relationship of permanent first maxillary and mandibular molars. Though it is the most commonly

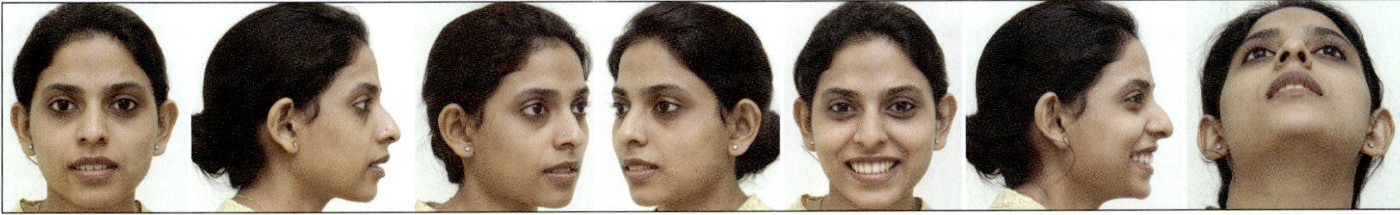

Fig. 12.2 Photographic record of face—frontal, profile, 1.3rd obliques right and left, frontal smiling, lateral smiling, worm's eye views.

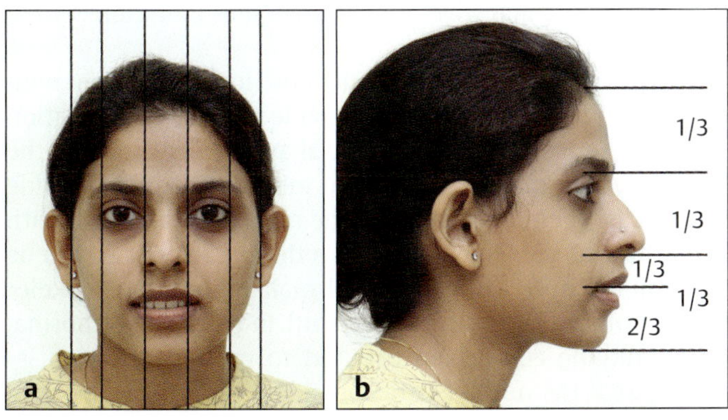

Fig. 12.3 Facial proportions. **(a)** Facial 1/5ths. **(b)** Facial 1/3rds.

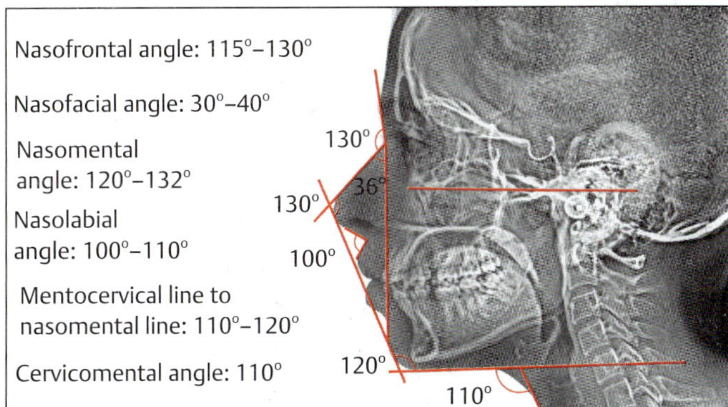

Fig. 12.4 Facial angles.

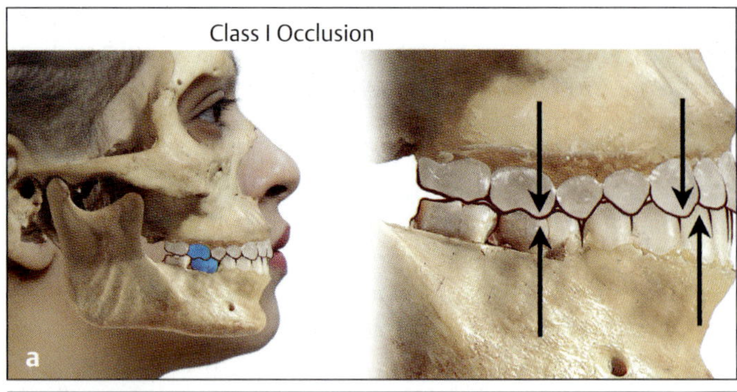

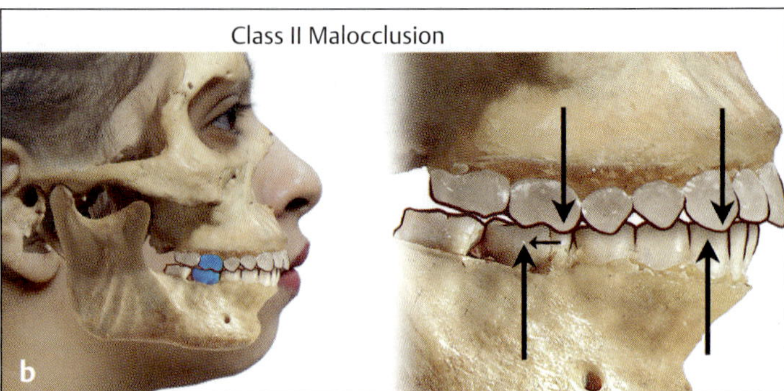

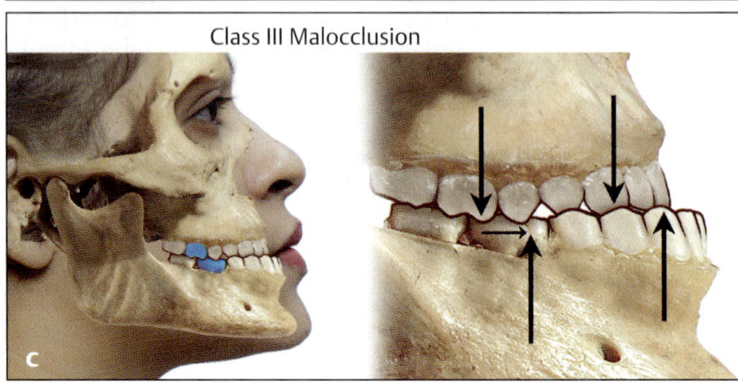

Fig. 12.5 Angle's classification of dental occlusion. **(a)** Class I malocclusion. **(b)** Class II malocclusion. **(c)** Class III malocclusion.

used classification for occlusion, one needs to be cognizant of the fact that it does not allow for transverse and vertical malocclusion considerations.

Class I Occlusion

The mandibular dental arch is in normal mesiodistal relation to the maxillary arch, with the mesiobuccal cusp of the maxillary first molar occluding in the buccal groove of the mandibular first permanent molar and the mesiolingual cusp of the maxillary first permanent molar occluding with the occlusal fossa of the mandibular first permanent molar, when the jaws are at rest and the teeth approximated in centric occlusion (**Fig. 12.5a**).

Class II Malocclusion

Mandibular dental arch and body are in distal relation to the maxillary arch. The mesiobuccal cusp of the maxillary first permanent molar occludes in the space between the mesiobuccal cusp of the mandibular first permanent molar and the distal aspect of the mandibular second premolar. Also, the mesiolingual cusp of the maxillary first permanent molar occludes mesial to the mesiolingual cusp of the mandibular first permanent molar (**Fig. 12.5b**).

Class III Malocclusion

The mandibular dental arch and body is in mesial relationship to the maxillary arch; with the mesiobuccal cusp of the maxillary first molar occluding in the interdental space between the distal aspect of the distal cusps of the mandibular first molar and the mesial aspect of the mesial cusps of the mandibular second molar (**Fig. 12.5c**).

Preliminary intraoral examination looks at the health of hard and soft tissues and general oral hygiene. Gingiva should be evaluated for inflammation, recession, or hypertrophy. Increase in size and anterior posture of tongue would suggest a tongue thrust habit that could be present in a patient with anterior open-bite deformity.

Hard tissue examination should include number, size, shape of teeth, missing teeth, and teeth in altered position. Evaluation of alignment of teeth should focus on inclination, rotation, malposition, presence of spacing, or crowding of teeth. Shape and position of the teeth have a bearing on the space required for aligning the teeth. Class I canine and molar dental relationships as well as positive overjet and over bite (2–3 mm) will suggest a normal dental alignment and skeletal base. An increased overjet could arise from exaggerated dental proclination, dentoalveolar protrusion or could be an indicator of hypoplastic mandible. An increased overbite or a deep-bite is suggestive of hypodivergent mandible with a short lower third of face.

Evaluation of dental midline and its correlation with facial midline (**Fig. 12.6**) will provide valuable information about presence and causes of facial asymmetry. Ideally, the maxillary and mandibular dental midlines should coincide with each other, the midline of the respective arch and with the center of the face. If there is a discrepancy, it has to be determined if it is due to dental malalignment or a skeletal deformity. A dental midline shift in presence of normal facial midline could be attributed to misaligned or missing teeth. If the midlines are coincident with the respective dental arch but not with the face, then the cause could be skeletal (**Fig. 12.7**).

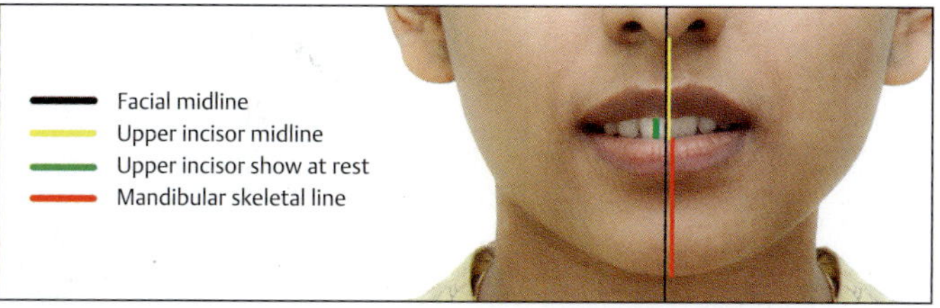

Fig. 12.6 Clinical assessment of dental and facial midlines at repose.

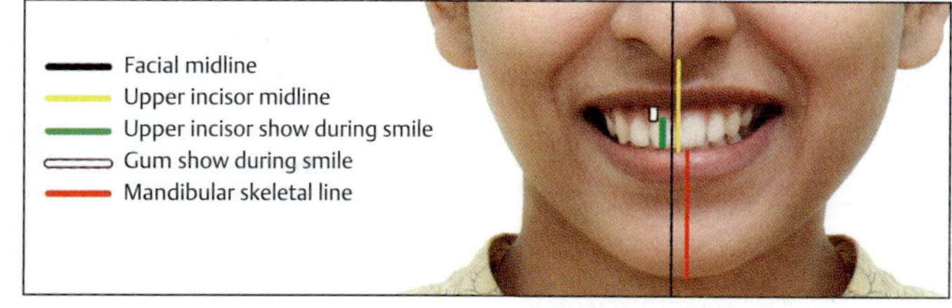

Fig. 12.7 Clinical assessment of dental and facial midlines during animation.

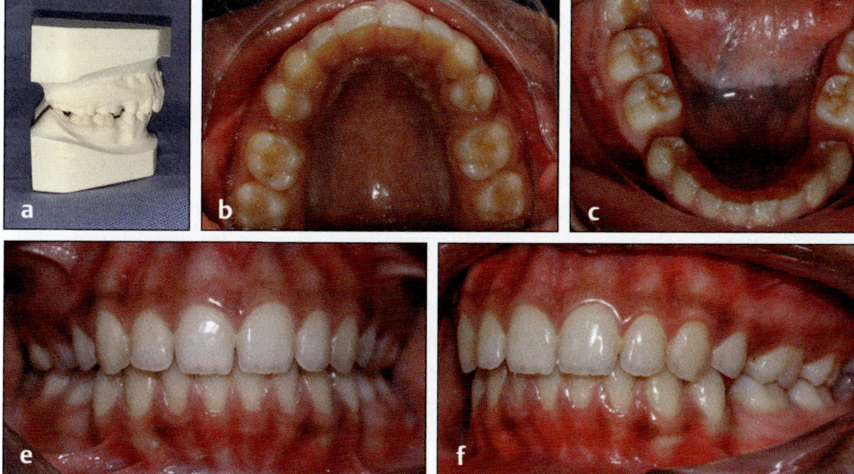

Fig. 12.8 Assessment of dental occlusion on model and clinical occlusal photographs. **(a)** Dental study models. **(b)** Maxillary occlusal view. **(c)** Mandibular occlusal view. **(d)** Right buccal occlusion. **(e)** Frontal occlusion. **(f)** Left buccal occlusion.

Variations in length, size, shape, and symmetry between maxillary and mandibular dentoalveolar arches will suggest transverse (width) discrepancy between the arches. Presence of posterior cross-bite, unilateral or bilateral, is an indicator of transverse arch discrepancies.

Evaluation of Diagnostic Dental Study Models

Study models are an invaluable tool in understanding the dentofacial deformity and treatment planning. Apart from corroboration of clinical examination findings, model analysis helps to quantify tooth size–arch length discrepancy and tooth size discrepancy (**Fig. 12.8**).

Bolton analysis measures the mesiodistal width of each tooth and determines the discrepancy in tooth material between maxillary and mandibular teeth. In patients with tooth size discrepancies, the space occupied by teeth in one arch will be greater than the space occupied by teeth in the opposing arch, producing suboptimal interarch relationship.

The difference between tooth material and available alveolar arch can be measured using Carey's analysis. If the tooth material available is less than space available on the arch, spacing results and an excess of tooth material causes crowding. A space requirement of more than 5 to 6 mm is considered severe crowding and will require extraction of teeth.

Curve of Spee is an anteroposterior curvature of mandibular occlusion measured from the tip of canine posteriorly along the buccal cusp tips till the terminal molar, in a sagittal plane. An exaggerated occlusal curve is similar to crowding and creates a need for space to align teeth on the available arch. Additional space can be created by expansion of arch, proclination of teeth, interproximal reduction of tooth material, or extraction.

Along with the clinical examination and radiographic findings, these assessments aid the surgeon and orthodontist to determine the pattern of teeth extractions required during presurgical orthodontics, in order to prepare the jaws for surgical movement (**Figs. 12.8 and 12.9**).

Determining Growth Pattern and Status of Growth in Facial Deformities

Skeletal development of the maxilla and mandible occur in three dimensions—anterior posterior, vertical, and transverse. Abnormalities in all the three planes can occur independently or in conjunction with other dimensions. Generally, deformities are referred to as Class II or Class III dentoskeletal malocclusions, which is indicative of growth discrepancy in anteroposterior dimension. Often anteroposterior malocclusions are compounded by discrepancies in the vertical and/or transverse planes. Deformities in the vertical plane are seen in hyperdivergent growth pattern (long face with skeletal open bite) and hypodivergent growth

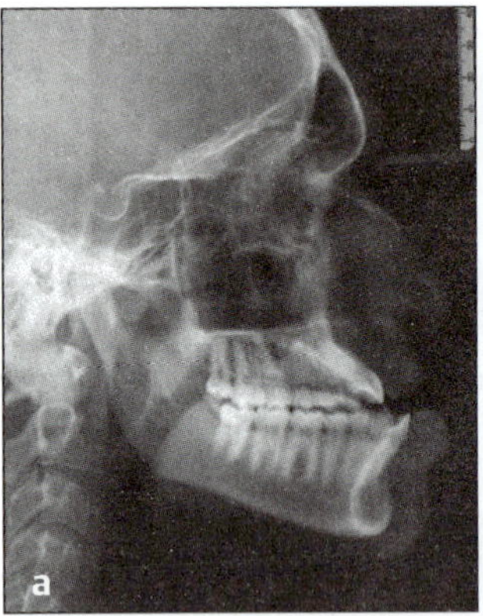

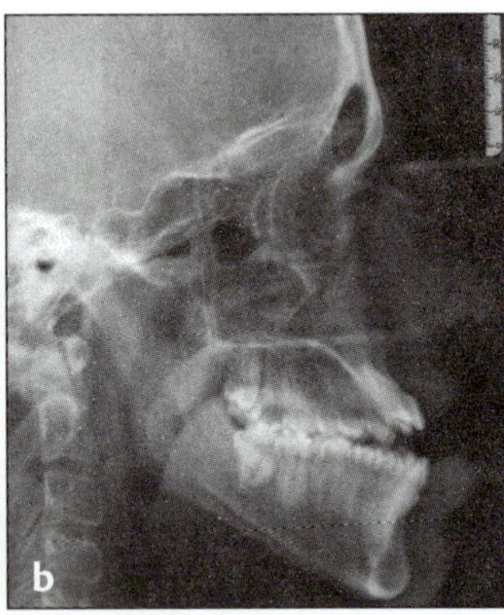

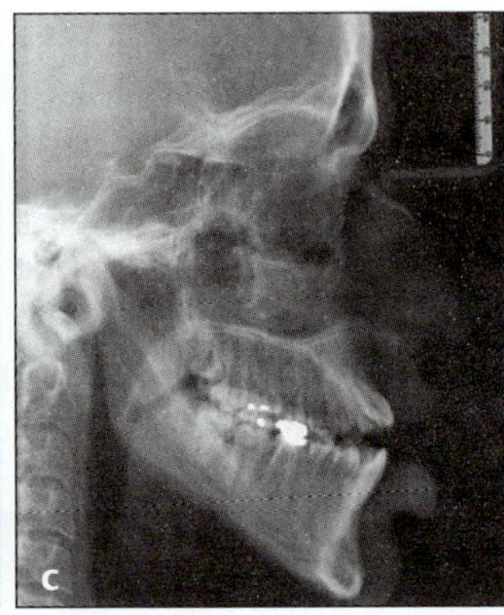

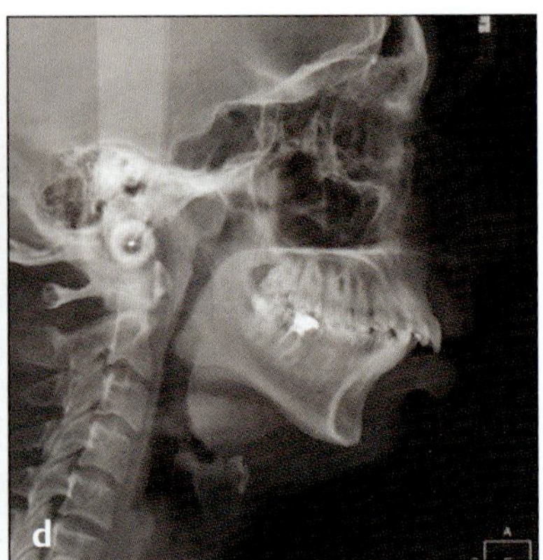

Fig. 12.9 Radiological assessment on lateral cephalometry. **(a)** Long mandibular body. **(b)** Open bite with horizontal palatal plane. **(c)** Exaggerated gonial angle—hyperdivergent growth. **(d)** Short mandibular arch-hypodivergent growth.

pattern (short face with skeletal deep bite). This growth pattern is also described as downward rotation of maxilla-mandibular complex for long faces and upward rotation of the maxilla-mandibular complex for short faces.

Although the most common cause for skeletal Class II malocclusion is lack of mandibular growth and retrusion of the mandible, it is also seen along with prognathic maxilla or as a combination of both. Class II skeletal malocclusions are very often associated with vertical plane discrepancies like skeletal open bite or deep bite which is a reflection of the facial growth pattern.

Class III malocclusion is characterized by a prognathic mandible and/or a retrusive maxilla. Growth pattern changes of the cranial base like backward alignment of posterior cranial fossa, decreased posterior cranial base length, and reduced cranial base angle can contribute to forward positioning of the mandible. Another major contributing factor is true horizontal growth of the mandible itself, causing increase in length of mandibular body.

In a growing patient, hand wrist X-ray is used to determine status of skeletal maturation by assessing ossification of sesamoid and hook of hamate.[10] Single-photon emission computed tomography (SPECT) scan with Technetium 99 methylene diphosphate (MDP) is a valuable investigation to determine active differential growth in patients with facial asymmetry.[11]

Cephalometrics in Orthognathic Surgery

Cephalometrics measures the position of maxilla and mandible (which are movable landmarks) against the stable points on skull base (immovable landmarks). The information derived can complement the clinical evaluation to develop a suitable treatment plan.

Individual variations in skull base anatomy can make the normative values in established analyses nondependable. A typical example would be a left or syndromic patient with short cranial base who could have cephalometric values as that of a bimaxillary protrusive patient even though there may be horizontal deficiency. The angulation of the Sella-Nasion (SN) plane is another aspect to be considered while taking cephalometric values into consideration. A cephalometric value derived from a horizontal SN plane will significantly alter the values of maxilla and mandible in comparison with the clinical examination findings. Hence, the clinician must identify the shortcomings and limitations of the cephalometric analysis and not base clinical decisions on cephalometric values alone; it should only be an adjunct to clinical assessment.

An added advantage of cephalometry is that it quantifies values and aids in communication with other clinicians, apart from assessing the progression of the treatment as well as monitoring the postsurgical stability and relapse. **Figs. 12.10 and 12.11** illustrate the commonly used cephalometric landmarks for lateral and posteroanterior cephalogram, respectively.

Recent advances in software technology allow merging of the conventional cephalometric radiography on CT scans which makes it possible to analyze soft and hard tissues in all three dimensions. Since 3D cephalometry is based on CT scan protocols, all the measurements are life-sized scale and allows comparisons of linear measurements in all planes. The image created from CT scan can be oriented in any plane, which negates the need for fixation of the skull during image acquisition, unlike the 2D cephalometry. Fusion of clinical photographs or 3D facial photographs enables more accurate prediction of surgical outcome in aesthetic facial surgery.

Presurgical Orthodontics (Compensation and Decompensation)

In ideal facial form, the alveolar process and dentition are aligned in an optimal position on the basal bone of mandible and maxilla. When this basal bone is overgrown or deficient, the position of alveolar process and the teeth are

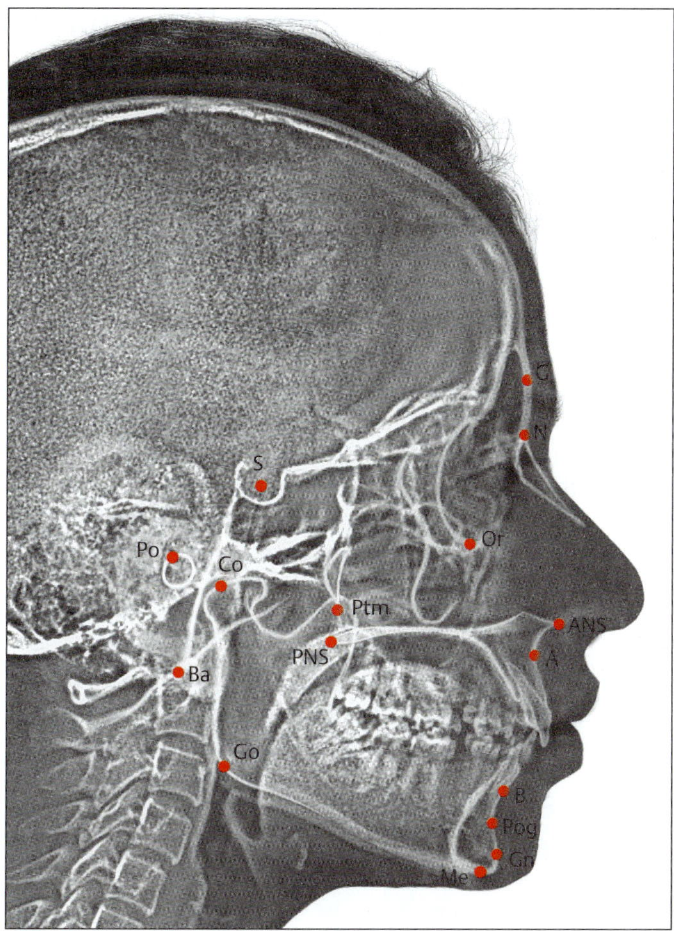

Fig. 12.10 Lateral cephalogram-Landmarks.

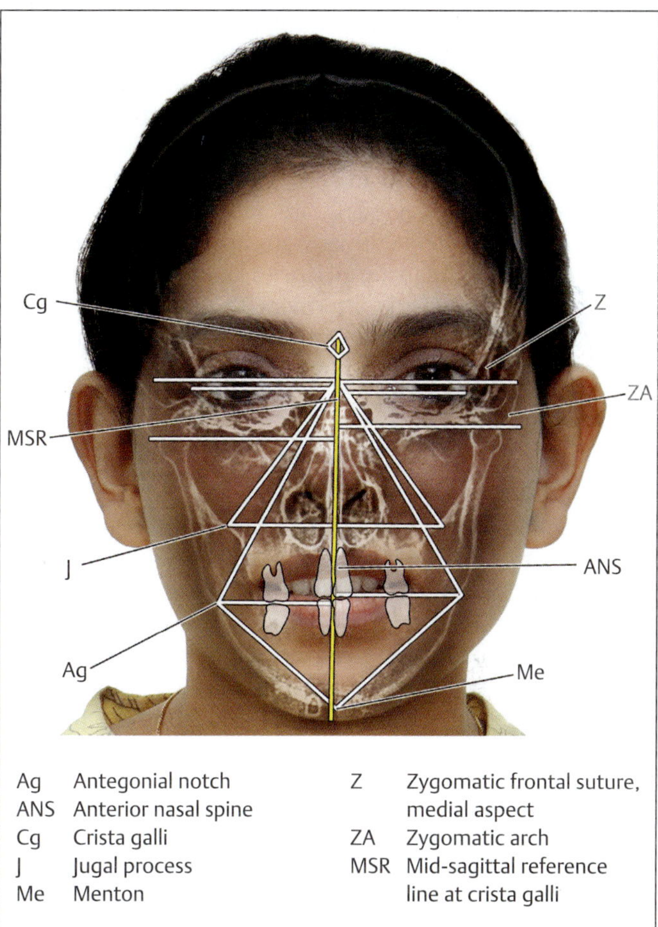

Fig. 12.11 Posteroanterior cephalogram-Landmarks.

unduly influenced and moulded by the forces exerted by tongue lingually and muscles of facial expression buccally. This causes compensatory changes and causes the dentition to be proclined/retroclined, crowded/spaced, and the maxillary/mandibular arches to be expanded or constricted. To camouflage the skeletal discrepancy, alveolus and teeth compensate to a position which is in equilibrium with each other. During presurgical orthodontics these compensations are removed and the teeth are repositioned within the basal bone so that the skeletal discrepancy is fully unmasked. Extractions of teeth are done during presurgical orthodontics to correct crowding, increased proclination of teeth, and exaggerated Curve of Spee. This process of decompensation creates a negative overjet in class III deformities, positive overjet in class II deformities, and allows movement of the jaws during surgery.

Facebow Transfer and Model Surgery

After a treatment plan is made from the clinical assessment and cephalometric analysis, the next step will be to replicate the exact 3-dimensional movements of the jaws in lab or on a virtual platform to fabricate intraoperative surgical splints. The most common method to fabricate splints is to perform model surgery which would also allow the surgeon to foresee any issues that can present during the operative procedure (**Box 12.1**).

Box 12.1 Steps in model surgery

- Creating anatomical plaster dental models
- Occlusal bite registration
- Face-bow transfer
- Mounting models on semiadjustable articulator
- Model surgery using model platform mimicking the jaw movements
- Surgical splint fabrication (intermediate and final)

Facebow transfer is an essential step in conventional orthognathic surgery and mandatory in bimaxillary procedures. Face bow is a device that is used to record the relationship of the jaws to the temporomandibular joints (TMJs) and to register the 3-dimensional relationship of the maxillary dental cast to a reference plane (Frankfort's horizontal [FH] plane) which represents the cranial base. The recorded relationship is then transferred to a semiadjustable articulator.

A model surgery platform is a useful tool for performing model surgery. It has a base, a model block, and an electronic caliper which is at 90 degrees to the platform and can make metric measurements accurate up to 0.01 mm. The dental cast is placed on to the model block in the same way as it is held on to the articulator. According to the treatment plan, the articulated models are moved in anteroposterior, vertical, transverse dimensions and even as segments. Measurements are made in all three planes and once desired movement is achieved, intermediate and final occlusal splints (occlusal wafer) are fabricated which determine the position of jaws during the surgery (**Fig. 12.12**).

Virtual Surgical Planning (VSP)

In the modern era, with the advancement in technology, it is possible to virtually recreate the entire laboratory-based planning and workflow (**Table 12.1**). VSP provides flexibility to try different treatment strategies and the ability to visualize the predicted treatment during planning. Surgical splints and guides can be designed virtually using 3D printing technology. These models are useful for educating the patients too (**Fig. 12.13**).

Maxillary and Mandibular Procedures

Though many variations like Le Fort II, III, Quadrangular or zygomatic wing osteotomies, and anterior/posterior/multisegmental osteotomies have been described, Le Fort I osteotomy is the most commonly performed procedure for correction of midface deformities. Due to its versatility in performing advancements and setbacks, bilateral sagittal split osteotomy (BSSO) is the workhorse among mandibular procedures. Intraoral vertical ramus subsigmoid osteotomy (IVRO) is a preferred procedure for mandibular setback owing to the reduced occurrence of neurosensory deficit and reduced operative time.[12,13] IVRO is more difficult to perform when the setback is more than 10 mm and in cases of mandibular advancement and rotation of maxillomandibular complex. Internal fixation following IVRO is technically demanding and can be avoided with long-term intermaxillary fixation (4–6 wk).

Patient Positioning and Anesthesia

The patient is placed supine and general anesthesia is administered with a north facing nasotracheal cuffed tube

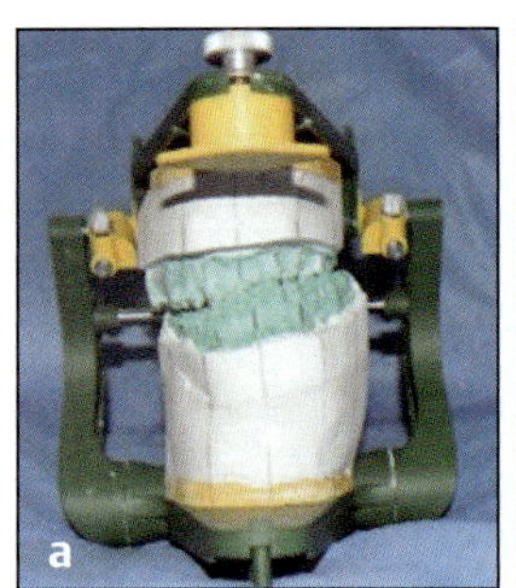

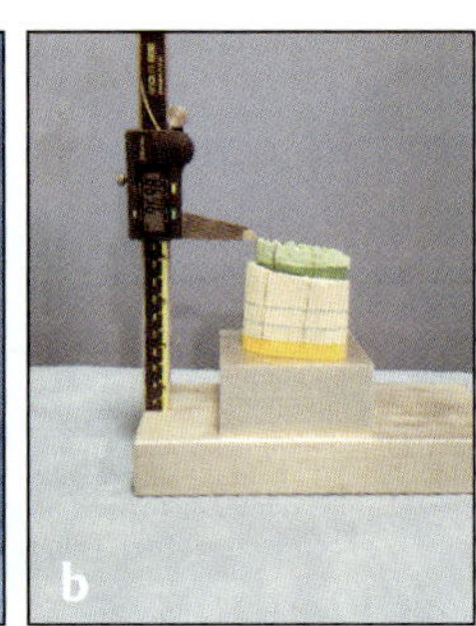

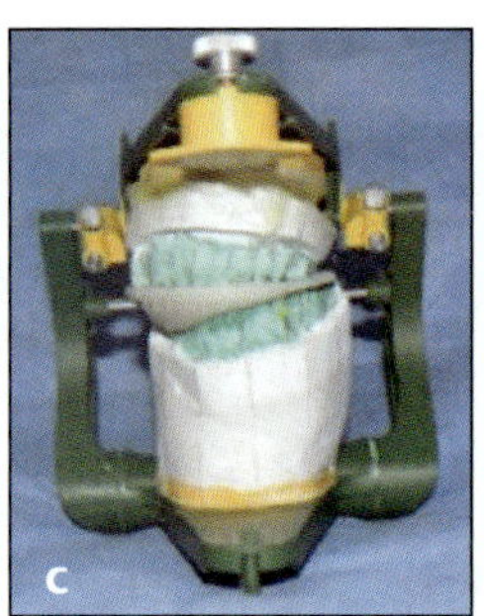

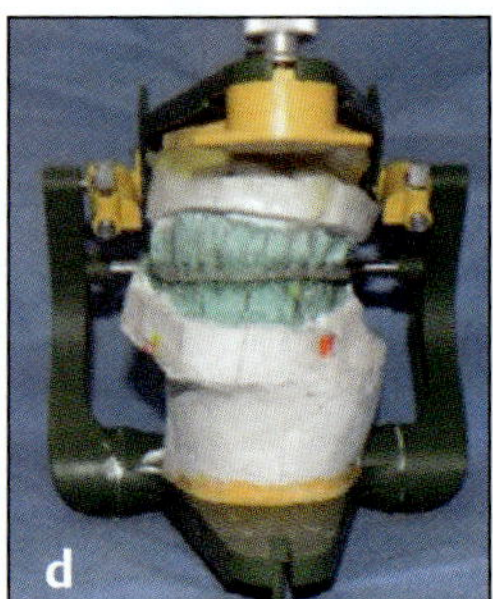

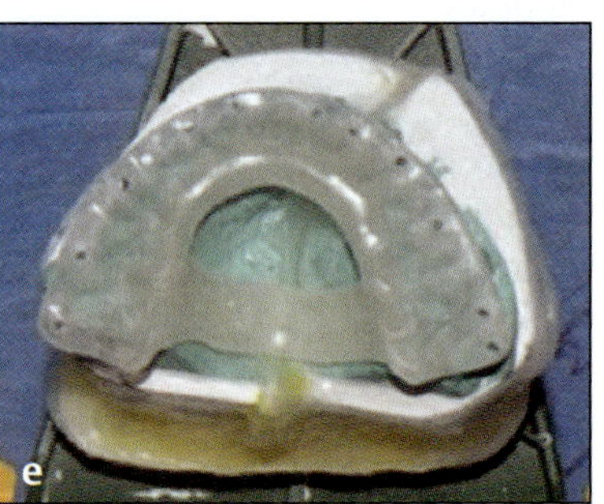

Fig. 12.12 Steps in model surgery. **(a)** Models mounted following face bow transfer. **(b)** Predetermined movements executed using model surgery platform. **(c)** Intermediate occlusal splint. **(d, e)** Final occlusal splint with transpalatal bar used specifically following segmental maxillary osteotomies.

Table 12.1 Virtual surgical planning: prerequisites and steps

Prerequisites of virtual planning	• VSP software • Patient's photographs/3D facial image • Dicom data (CBCT/conventional CT) • Dental model scanner/intraoral camera • 3D printer
Steps in virtual surgical planning	• Orienting the CT scan • Creation of orthopantomogram (OPG) • Superimposition of photographs and scanned dentition on CT • Defining segments (e.g., Le Fort I maxilla, BSSO mandible, genioplasty) • Marking the osteotomy lines • Hard and soft tissue cephalometric markings • Virtual movement of jaw segments to desired position (treatment) • Splint designing and printing

Abbreviations: BSSO, bilateral sagittal split osteotomy; CBCT, cone beam computed tomography; CT, computed tomography; VSP, virtual surgical planning.

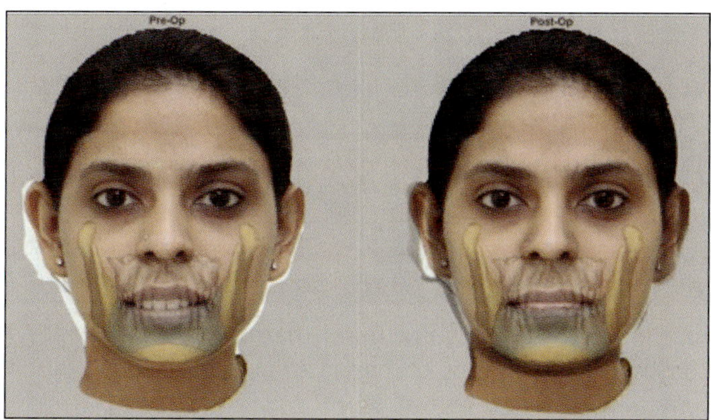

Fig. 12.13 Virtual surgical planning and predication using Dolphin Imaging software.

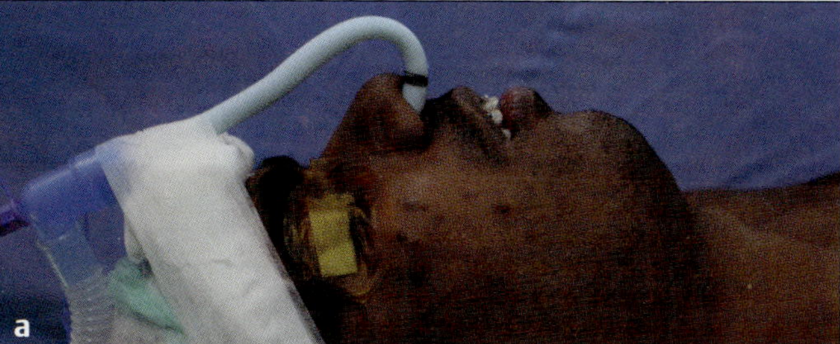

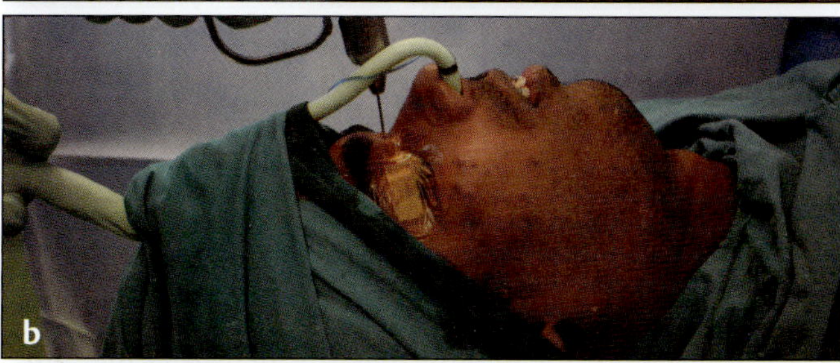

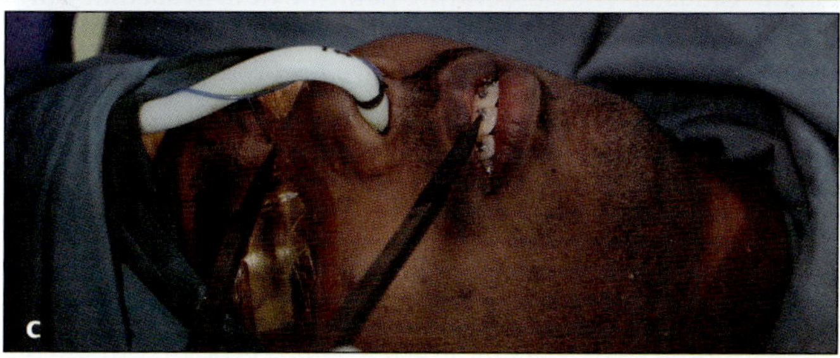

Fig. 12.14 Position and preparation on operation table. **(a)** "North facing" endotracheal tube fixed to forehead and sutured to nasal septum. **(b)** 1.5-mm K-wire placed as external reference point. **(c)** Preoperative measurement of midface height.

which is sutured to the cartilaginous septum (**Fig. 12.14a**). The nasotracheal tube is further fixed to the head in a neutral position, ensuring the nasal form is left undisturbed. Ophthalmic lubricant gel is applied to both eyes and taped with clear adhesive tapes. Anesthesiologist is requested to maintain hypotensive during the course of surgery with intraoperative mean arterial pressure (MAP) 20 to 30% below the patient's usual MAP.[14] Patient table is adjusted at 15 degrees reverse Trendelenburg position. Lidocaine solution (Xylocaine 1% with 1:100,000 epinephrine) is infiltrated into the surgical site.

The head and neck are prepped and draped to provide adequate exposure of the forehead, the eyes, external ears, the face, and the neck.

Le Fort I Osteotomy

A 20-gauge K-wire is inserted at the radix of nose using a K-wire driver, as an external reference point for vertical dimension measurements (**Fig. 12.14b**). With the use of a caliper, the distance between the K-wire and the cephalic surface of orthodontic bracket on the central incisors and canines is measured and recorded as a relative measure of the anterior vertical maxillary height (**Fig. 12.14c**).

Using micropoint electrocautery, a vestibular mucosal incision is placed from mesial of second premolars on either side (**Fig. 12.15a**). A minimum of 5 mm of mucosal cuff is left on the gingival margin to facilitate good closure. A subperiosteal dissection is carried out to expose the anterior nasal spine, pyriform rims, anterior and posterior walls of maxillary sinus, up to the pterygomaxillary junction. Careful dissection is carried out along the nasal floor and lateral wall of nose and nasal cartilaginous septum.

Toe-out retractors are placed subperiosteally along the posterior wall of maxilla in the pterygomaxillary space and osteotomy line is marked bilaterally. An elevator is placed along the lateral nasal wall to protect the nasal mucosa and a reciprocating saw is used to place the Le Fort I osteotomy cut through the posterior, anterior, and medial maxillary walls on each side. With a guarded chisel, the nasal septum, lateral wall of nose, and posterolateral walls of the maxillary sinus are cut through. A 4-mm osteotome is used on lateral wall of nose and the posterior wall of maxilla to complete the cut up to pterygomaxillary junction. The nasal septum can be dislocated from the palatal groove using an elevator, cut with a heavy scissor or with a nasal septal chisel. Pterygomaxillary disjunction is done using a curved pterygoid chisel. Alternatively, the maxillary disjunction can be performed through the maxillary third molar extraction socket as described by Trimble et al.[15]

If the osteotomies and pterygoid disjunction are complete, the maxillary down fracture can be performed with finger pressure. A bone hook placed on the anterior nasal floor and a Smith's spreader at the zygomatic buttress can be additionally used to facilitate downfracture of maxilla. The greater palatine neurovascular bundle is identified, protected during removal of skull base interferences as well as mobilization of maxilla, and is preserved except in very large advancements of maxilla (**Fig. 12.15b**).

A Tessier mobilizer is placed on the posterior wall of maxilla and controlled force in anterior direction is applied

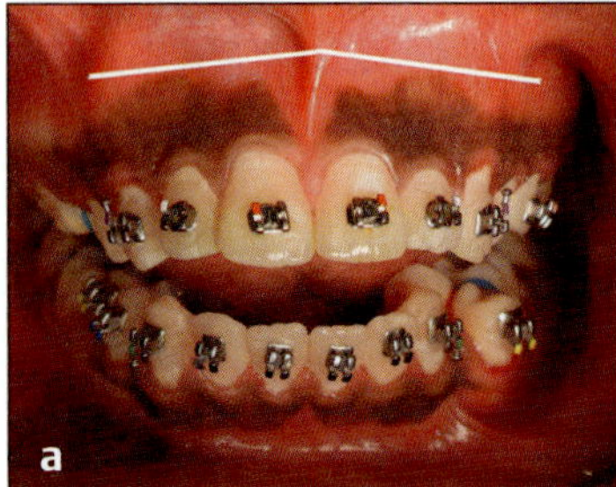
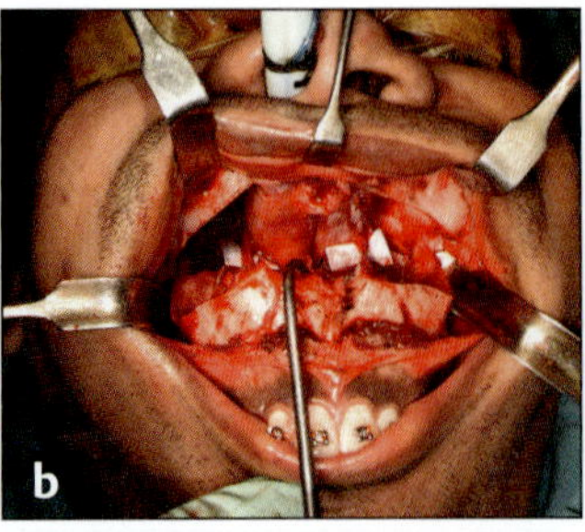
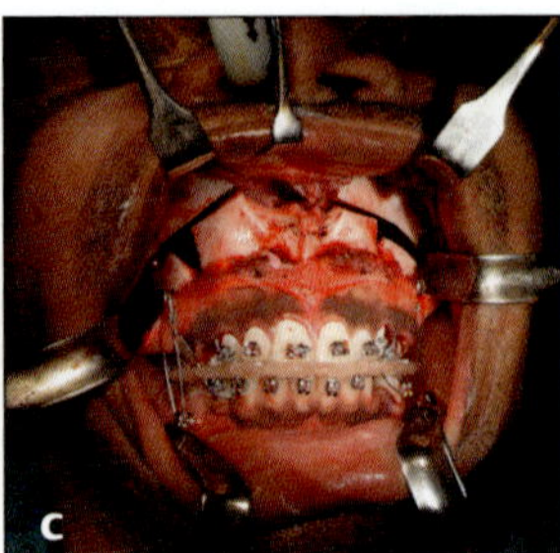
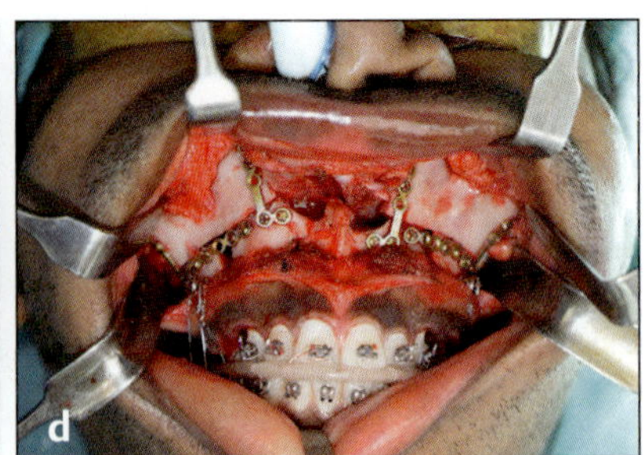

Fig. 12.15 Steps of Le Fort I maxillary osteotomy. **(a)** Vestibular incision. **(b)** Downfractured maxilla—arrow illustrating preserved greater palatine neurovascular bundle. **(c)** Three-piece segmental osteotomy of maxilla and intermaxillary fixation using surgical occlusal splint. **(d)** Fixation of segments using titanium miniplates and screws.

to mobilize the maxilla. Unlike the standard (Rowe) nasomaxillary disimpaction forceps, Tessier mobilizer assists mobilization of the maxilla without causing contusion of the palatal mucosa. The descending palatine neurovascular bundles are identified and preserved whenever possible. Bone from posterior sinus wall and pterygoid region is removed using a bone rongeur or an egg bur. In cases of excessive hindrance from skull base during superior impaction of maxilla, pterygoid plates can be fractured with an osteotome or cut with a reciprocating saw and pushed back in to the infratemporal fossa. In case of maxillary impaction, the nasal septum is trimmed using scissors to accommodate the superior repositioning of maxilla or alternatively a groove is made on the palatal floor to accommodate the septum.

Interferences at skull base and maxillary sinus walls are removed using bone rongeur or round bur and the maxilla is completely mobilized. Any preplanned segmental osteotomies are performed and the maxilla is passively moved into the predetermined position with the guidance of surgical occlusal splint and intermaxillary fixation is achieved with the mandible (**Fig. 12.15c**). Fixation of the repositioned maxillary segment is achieved using "L"-shaped plates and 4- to 5-mm-long screws (plates with profile thickness of 0.6 mm suited for screws with 1.5 or 1.7 mm diameter) at the pyriform rim and zygomatic buttress which form the vertical buttresses of maxilla. These sites are the vertical buttresses of maxilla and offer bone with adequate thickness for osseointegration of the screws (**Fig. 12.15d**).

Following maxillary superior impaction, pyriform-plasty to recontour anterior nasal floor using a rotary bur helps to recreate the normal anatomical contour of the pyriform aperture, anterior nasal floor, and anterior nasal spine. This measure, along with muscular cinch sutures using nonresorbable suture, prevents alar base flare of the nose. Closure of the mucosal incision is done using resorbable sutures.

Sagittal Split Osteotomy (SSO)

SSO of the ramus and body is primarily performed for anteroposterior movement of mandible, though it also permits a certain degree of rotation of the maxilla-mandibular complex in a clockwise or counterclockwise direction. The osteotomy consists of a horizontal cut on the medial surface of the ramus of mandible, a vertical cut on the lateral surface of the body of mandible, and an intermediate cut that runs medial to the external oblique ridge and the horizontal and the vertical osteotomy.

A medium-sized bite block is placed between the maxillary and mandibular molars on the contralateral side to maintain the mandible in an open and steady position during the procedure.

A curvilinear incision is placed in the vestibule starting from the first molar and extending posteriorly about 1 cm behind the third molar, with a sufficient cuff of attached and free alveolar mucosa facilitating closure (**Fig. 12.16a**). The incision extends both anteriorly and posteriorly for a total length of approximately 4 cm. While placing the incision, due consideration should be given to the presence of mandibular third molar. If simultaneous extraction is planned, the incision should be carried to the distobuccal line angle of third molar and then extended laterally and posteriorly. Incision is carried down to the bone. The mucoperiosteum is reflected to expose lateral surface of the body of mandible and the anterior ramus, the external oblique ridge, and the lower border of mandible in the molar region. Exposure of the medial surface of ramus is also done up to the posterior border in a plane superior to the lingula of mandibular foramen. The cut is initiated with a reciprocating saw from the medial ramus above the lingula at a 45-degree bevel. Extension of the medial osteotomy is limited just posterior to the mandibular foramen (**Fig. 12.16b**). The cut is carried forward anteriorly, parallel to the lateral border of the mandible, following the external oblique ridge and stopped where the external oblique ridge flows into the body of the mandible. An anatomic reference point for this would be the distal aspect of mandibular first molar where the external oblique ridge ends. Bite block is removed and a lower border retractor is placed to obtain adequate access and visualization. Reciprocating saw is used to cut the complete width of the lower border of the mandibular. The vertical cut is placed within to connect the intermediate and lower border cuts. A thin spatula osteotome is used to ensure a completeness of osteotomy through the cortex into the marrow along the horizontal cut (**Fig. 12.16d**). Further tapping is done

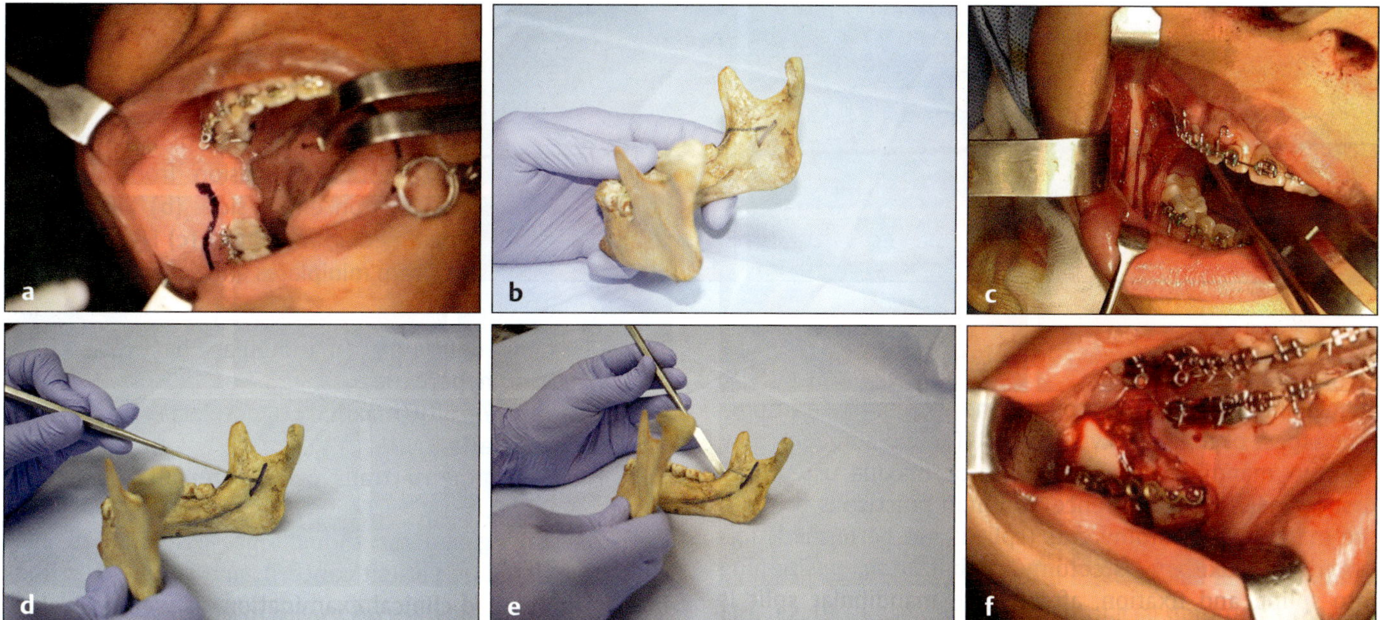

Fig. 12.16 Steps of sagittal split osteotomy of mandible. **(a)** Curvilinear incision. **(b)** Extent of horizontal osteotomy. **(c)** Intermediate osteotomy connecting horizontal and vertical cuts. **(d, e)** Direction of spatula osteotome to ensure completeness of osteotomy. **(f)** Fixation of mandibular segments using 2.0-mm miniplates and screws.

with the osteotome placed at the retromolar region with an angulation toward the angle of mandible (**Fig. 12.16e**) directed toward the lower border cut. The saw should go through the cortex (a thickness of 4–5 mm) into the marrow through the entire length of the osteotomy, which is the key step in preventing a bad split from occurring. Gentle prying of the bone is started at the lower border with an Obwegeser lower border spreader. Simultaneously, Smith's spreader is used at the superior border and progressive spreading of the segments is achieved with this maneuver. If the segments do not spread symmetrically, it may be necessary to check completeness of bone cuts throughout the osteotomy line. Gradual use of the spreaders in a posterior direction completes the split. Any attachment of the medial pterygoid muscle to the distal segment is done with a lower border "J" stripper to facilitate free anteroposterior movement.

Genioplasty

Local anesthetic with a vasoconstrictor is infiltrated into the lower vestibule. The incision is made through the lip mucosa extending from canine to canine, using a micropoint electrocautery (**Fig. 12.17a**). The incision traverses the mentalis ensuring an adequate cuff of the muscle is left attached to periosteum on the gingival margin for muscle resuspension during closure.

Subperiosteal dissection is carried out to expose the symphysis down to the inferior border. Elevate the periosteum and muscle overlying the incisor and canine roots on the anterior mandible to identify the root prominence. The dissection is further carried out posteriorly along the body of the mandible below the mental nerve. The dissection is finally carried out superiorly to identify and expose the mental nerve where it exits the foramen. The mental nerve is skeletonized to gain more access to place the posterior extent of the osteotomy behind the mental foramen and prevent avulsion of the nerve during retraction. These steps help to maintain adequate soft tissue attachment and thus blood supply to the advanced genial segment.

Symphyseal midline and two paramedian lines are marked above and below the intended osteotomy. This helps to keep the repositioned genial segment oriented to the midline (**Fig. 12.17b**). Osteotomy should be placed at least 5 mm below the apices of the canine teeth to avoid devitalization of the lower anterior teeth.

The osteotomy is initiated through the inferior border posterior to the mental foramen. The saw is uprighted as it is advanced anteriorly, to ensure that the osteotomy is bicortical. Awareness about variations in thickness of the symphyseal and parasymphyseal regions of mandible will help to control the depth of the saw and prevent injury to the sublingual soft tissues. Once osteotomy crosses midline, the saw is removed and the procedure is repeated from the opposite side.

Genial segment is repositioned three dimensionally according to the surgical plan, using the markings for guidance and fixed with 1.7-mm miniplates and screws (**Fig. 12.17c**). Mentalis muscle is carefully resuspended using interrupted 4-0 resorbable suture to avoid chin ptosis. Poor repositioning of mentalis can lead to inadequate muscle action eliciting patient complaint regarding inability to clear food accumulation in lower vestibule. The mucosa is closed with 4-0 resorbable suture.

Anterior Open-Bite Deformity

Anterior open-bite could be associated with class II and class III dentofacial deformities. Significant midface hypoplasia or severe class II facial growth pattern with a combination of maxillary and mandibular hypoplasia can reduce the tongue space in oral cavity leading to tongue thrust habit resulting in anterior open bite. True macroglossia should be ruled out which is not an uncommon finding in craniofacial syndromes.

A bonded tongue crib placed by the orthodontist to address tongue thrust habit helps to neutralize the hyperactivity of tongue and hasten presurgical orthodontic treatment. Premolar extractions are commonly performed to relieve crowding and align teeth. Alternatively, sectional orthodontics aid in leveling the maxillary arch in multiple segments when segmental osteotomies are planned in cases of severe dentoalveolar protrusion.

Cephalometrics will reveal presence of increased posterior vertical height with a reduced occlusal plane angle. Moving the dental study models into "a best possible occlusion" can be used to differentiate between true and relative transverse width discrepancy of maxilla. True transverse width reduction is seen more often in syndromic and cleft palate patients.

Counterclockwise rotation mandible against the submental and glossal muscular pull is an unstable movement to close an anterior open-bite (**Fig. 12.19**). A differential superior movement at Le Fort I level to impact the posterior maxilla more than the anterior to correct the occlusal plane, followed by a BSSO clockwise rotation of mandible, is a stable movement in comparison. An advancement genioplasty should be performed to restore the chin-throat length, obtain lip competence, and prevent a double chin. Two-piece or three-piece maxillary segmental osteotomies can be used to correct transverse width discrepancies in constricted maxilla and to level occlusal plane in severe dentoalveolar protrusion. Retaining the final surgical wafer for a period of 3 weeks helps to prevent relapse in segmental osteotomies by splinting the segments at the occlusal level as well as at the osteotomy sites and by allowing the soft tissue to stretch and adapt to the new position of bone.

Facial Asymmetry

Asymmetry is a common finding in patients with dentofacial deformities and is multifactorial. It could be congenital or developmental, pathological or acquired, and can manifest due to underdevelopment of one side or overgrowth of the other. Dental, skeletal, soft tissue deformity, or a combination of all factors can contribute to asymmetry. Obwegeser and Makek classified the overgrowth deformities as hemimandibular elongation due to condylar hyperplasia and hemimandibular hyperplasia causing a 3-dimensional enlargement of mandible or a combination of both.[17] Wolford et al reported a more descriptive classification system and management protocol for condylar hyperplasia based on occurrence rate and type of pathology.[18] Unilateral condylar hyperplasia (CH type 1A as per Wolford classification) can manifest during early adolescence, and it needs monitoring with serial X-rays and clinical examination of left side (**Fig. 12.20**). SPECT Bone scintigraphy is useful as an indicator but is not absolutely reliable in determining the activity of condyles.[11] High condylectomy in an active case of unilateral condylar hyperplasia is an established treatment modality to arrest worsening of deformity and can be combined simultaneously with orthognathic surgery to correct the facial deformity.[19] Relapse following mandibular setback surgery for mandibular prognathism is likely due to undiagnosed condylar hyperplasia.

Hemifacial microsomia (HFM) in its varying severity is a common congenital condition that causes asymmetry due

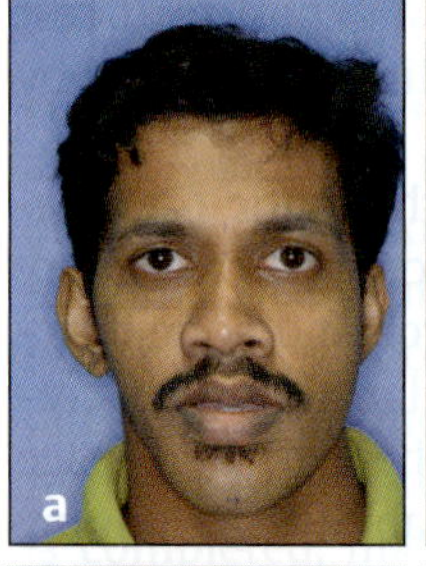
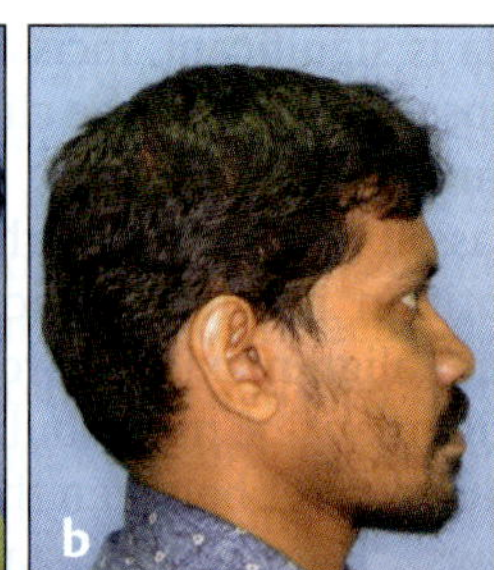
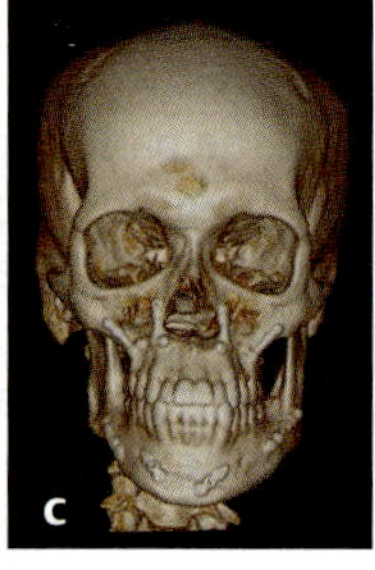
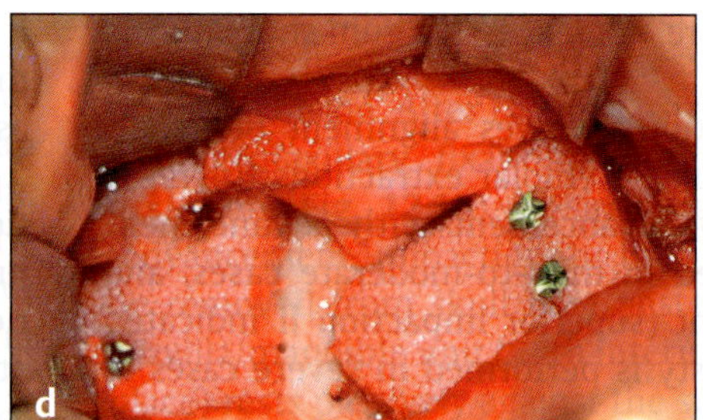
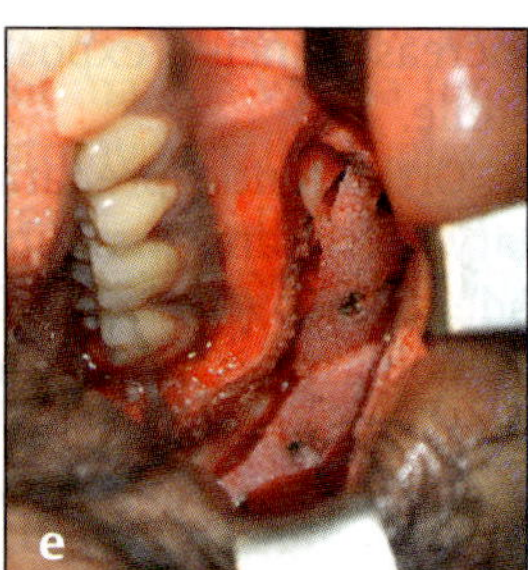
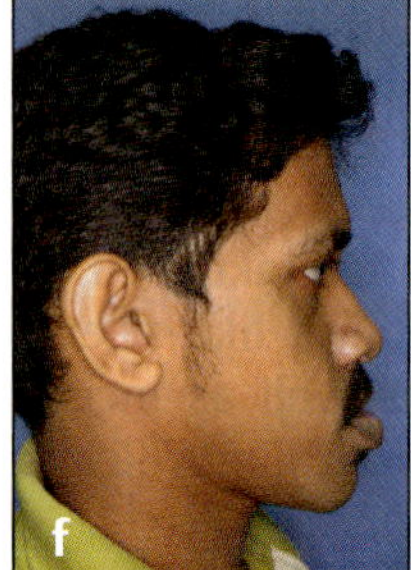
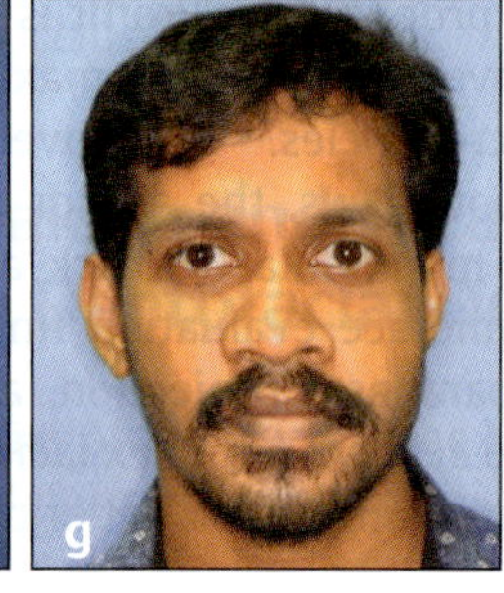

Fig. 12.20 Condylar hyperplasia type IA of left side with mandibular prognathism treated with Le Fort I osteotomy, bilateral sagittal split osteotomy (BSSO), and genioplasty. Alloplastic augmentation of malar and mandibular angle was performed secondarily to achieve optimal outcome. **(a)** Initial frontal image. **(b)** Post-treatment frontal image. **(c)** 3D computed tomography (CT) after orthognathic surgery illustrating morphological asymmetry of mandibular ramus and zygomatic prominence. **(d)** Alloplastic implant for malar augmentation. **(e)** Alloplastic implant for transverse augmentation of angle of mandible. **(f)** Initial profile image. **(g)** Post-treatment profile image.

to underdevelopment of craniofacial skeleton on affected side. Torticollis of neck and spine deformities can cause tilted neutral head position which complicates evaluation and formulation of treatment strategies. It is important to differentiate between hypoplasia and hyperplasia as the cause of asymmetry to institute a suitable treatment plan (**Table 12.2**).

A detailed understanding about asymmetry of all facial structures including the jaws is crucial in patient counseling, need for staged surgeries, and in generating realistic expectations about outcome. **Table 12.1** enumerates clinical and radiological features that help to differentiate between condylar hyperplasia and hypoplasia. The workhorse osteotomies, Le Fort I and bilateral sagittal split osteotomies, and a combination of condylectomy, lower border shave, or extended lateral sliding genioplasty and staged angle augmentation are the common treatment modalities for asymmetry. Alternate procedures like IVRO, distraction osteogenesis, and total alloplastic replacement of TMJ are often utilized in conditions that cause condylar hypoplasia.

Cleft Maxillary Hypoplasia

The stigmata of operated cleft lip and palate include midface hypoplasia, anteroposterior, transverse, and vertical maxillary deficiency causing severe crowding of teeth along with anterior and posterior crossbites, residual lip and nasal deformities, and speech issues. Challenges faced by the surgeon during skeletal surgery for a cleft maxilla are the severity of scarring from cleft palate repair, making mobilization of segments difficult, less predictable vascular supply, large extent of advancement, fixation of the advanced segments,

Table 12.2 Clinical and radiological differences between hypoplasia and hyperplasia of mandibular condyle

Condylar hypoplasia	Condylar hyperplasia
Clinical findings	
• Facial asymmetry	• Facial asymmetry
• Decreased lower facial height	• Increased lower facial height
• Vertical orbital dystopia	• Uncommon
• Vertically and horizontally offset ears	• Vertically and horizontally offset ears
• Malar flattening on affected side	• Midface deficiency with scleral show
• Soft tissue lip cant	• Rarely a soft tissue lip cant
• Deviated nose	• Deviated nose
• Chin deviated to the hypoplastic side	• Chin deviated to the unaffected side
• Flattening of angle region	• Flattening of angle region on to the unaffected side
• Soft and hard tissue transverse deficiency of the angle region on hypoplastic side	• Soft and hard tissue transverse excess of the angle region on hyperplastic side
• Reduced chin prominence	• Mandibular prognathism
• Normal incisal overbite relationship	• Reverse anterior incisal overjet
• Increased proclination of mandibular anterior teeth	• Retroclined mandibular anterior teeth
• Upward maxillomandibular occlusal cant on hypoplastic side	• Downward maxillomandibular occlusal cant on hyperplastic side (hemimandibular hypertrophy causes an upward cant on affected side)
• Reduced tooth show on the hypoplastic side during smile	• Increased gum/tooth show on the hyperplastic side during smile
Imaging findings	
• Hypoplastic mandibular condyle	• Hyperplastic mandibular condyle
• Reduced length of condylar neck	• Increased length of condylar neck
• Reduced height of ramus of mandible	• Increased height of ramus of mandible
• Transverse deficiency of ramus on the hypoplastic side	• Transverse excess (convexity) of ramus on the hyperplastic side
• Exaggerated antegonial notch	• Normal or flattened antegonial notch
• Dental crowding/impacted/missing teeth in hypoplastic side	• Increased vertical height of body of mandible on hyperplastic side
• Vertical axis of mandibular incisors tilted toward hypoplastic side	• Vertical axis of mandibular incisors tilted away from hyperplastic side

and increased possibility of postsurgical relapse. For further details refer to Chapter 8 on “Secondary Skeletal Deformities Associated with Cleft Lip and Palate” in Volume III.

Skeletal Surgery for Hemifacial Microsomia

Skeletal issues associated with HFM are malformed glenoid fossa, mandibular hypoplasia, maxillary hypoplasia, zygomatic hypoplasia, and occlusal canting. Compounding of tissue factors includes microtia, masticatory muscle hypoplasia, and macrostomia which produce a significant disparity in the tragus to commissure between the affected and normal sides of face.

Goals of treatment in HFM as described by Kaban et al are:[20]

- Increase the size of the malformed and underdeveloped mandible and soft tissues.
- Create an articulation between the mandible and the temporal bone.
- Correct the secondary deformities of the maxilla.
- Establish functional occlusion and optimal facial symmetry.

Clinical and radiological examination would reveal facial asymmetry, orbital dystopia, malar flattening, lip cant, deviated nose, transverse deficiency of the malar and ramus of mandible, deviated chin, exaggerated antegonial notch, and occlusal cant, causing reduced tooth show on the affected side during smile and a cant in the mandibular occlusal plane.

The inherent risk of relapse in conventional osteotomy for HFM is caused by the inability of muscles to be acutely stretched, often compromising the results. In addition, poor soft-tissue adaptation could lead to compromised function and esthetics.

Skeletal asymmetry caused by mild case of HFM is amenable to conventional orthognathic surgery. In moderate-to-severe situations, distraction osteogenesis of mandible is useful as a primary procedure to build up corpus of mandibular ramus and angle, level the mandibular occlusal table, and reduce the asymmetry (**Table 12.3**). Second stage Le Fort I osteotomy corrects the maxillary cant and achieve occlusion with optimal vertical positioning. Orthomorphic procedure as described by Salins et al while correcting the chin can be used to achieve transverse widening of the angle region on the affected side asymmetry creating symmetry (**Fig. 12.21**).[21]

Surgery First, Orthodontics After (SFOA) Approach

Presurgical orthodontic treatment is the key time-consuming element in conventional orthognathic surgery. Conventional orthognathic treatment plan would include presurgical orthodontic decompensation of average 10 months, surgery and postsurgical convalescence of 2 months followed by settling orthodontics for 6 to 8 months, with a total treatment period of close to 2 years. SFOA is a resurgence of the

Table 12.3 Management of dentoskeletal deformity associated with hemifacial microsomia

Development phase	Procedures performed
During growth phase	• Functional appliances—for mild class I cases • Growth center transplant—costochondral graft in Pruzansky class III mandible • Distraction osteogenesis of ramus of mandible
After growth completion	• Conventional orthognathic surgery • DO + conventional OGS + Orthomorphic procedure • Adjunct hard/soft tissue augmentation procedures • Alloplastic TMJ reconstruction

Abbreviations: DO, distraction osteogenesis; OGS, orthognathic surgery; TMJ, temporomandibular joint.

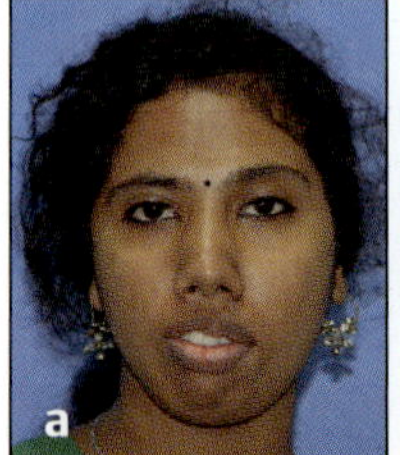
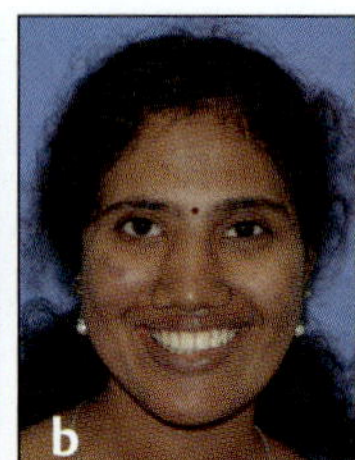
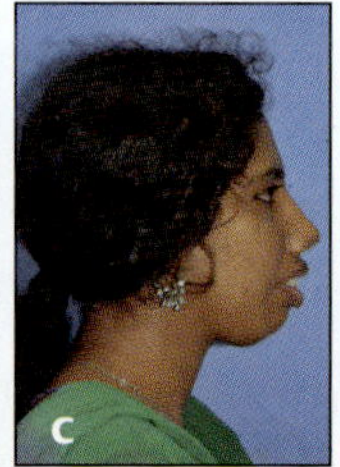
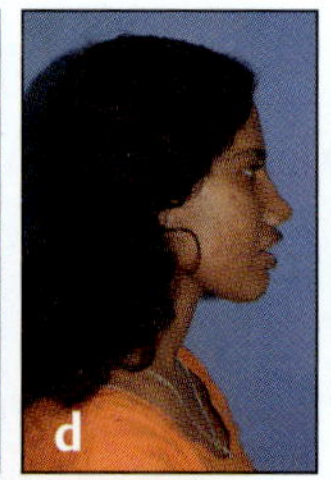
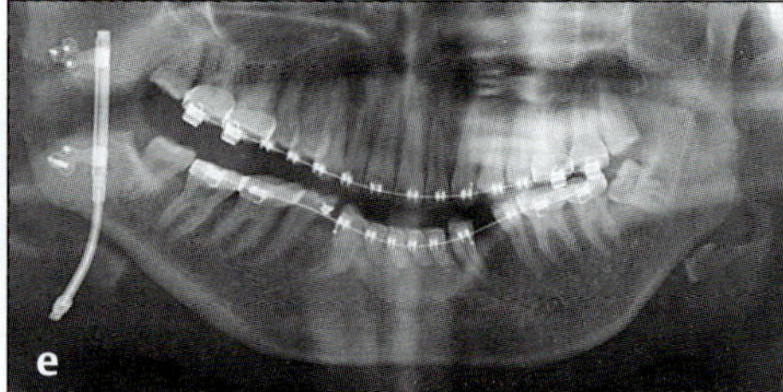
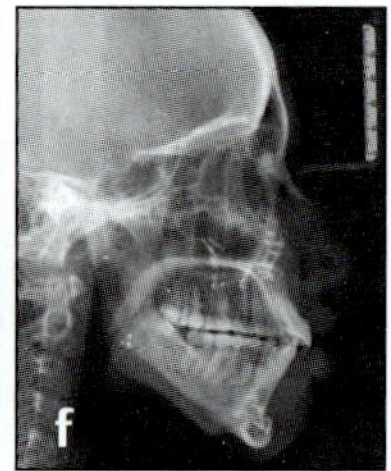
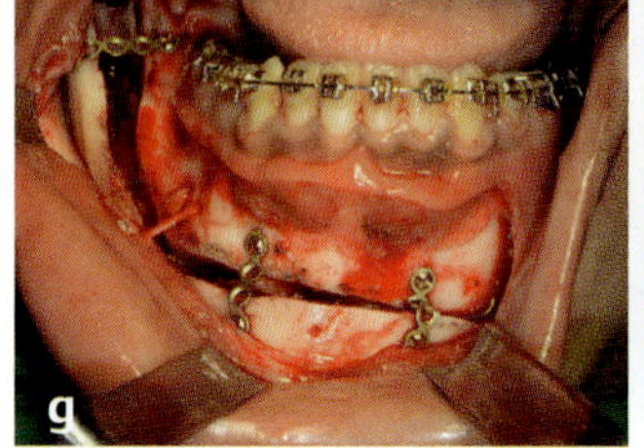
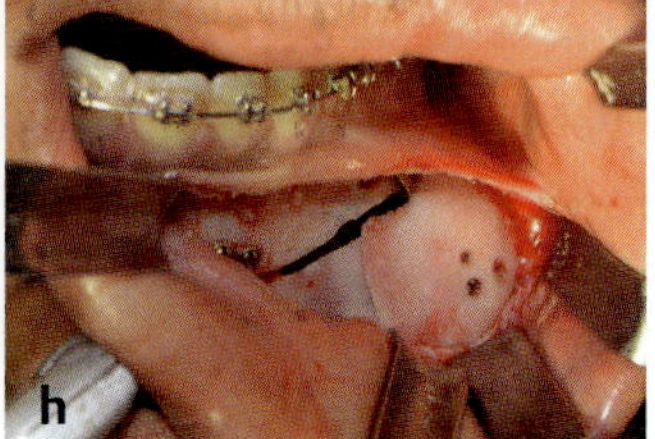

Fig. 12.21 Hemifacial microsomia with Pruzansky type 2A mandible. Distraction osteogenesis of ramus of mandible followed by Le Fort I osteotomy and orthomorphic procedure performed to obtain optimal outcome. **(a, c)** Preoperative images. **(b, d)** Post-treatment images. **(e)** Distractor device in situ. **(f)** Postoperative lateral cephalogram. **(g)** Orthomorphic procedure. **(h)** Alloplastic malar augmentation.

way in which orthognathic surgery was performed initially either without orthodontics or after orthodontic treatment was completed, without any oral appliances during surgery. Better understanding of deformities, refinement of orthodontic and surgical techniques, improved instrumentation and deeper understanding of bone healing paved the way for surgery-first technique.

SFOA can be performed in various ways. "Surgery only," as in a VME with a functional occlusion, is a situation where maxillary superior impaction and autorotation of the mandible can be performed without changing the occlusion, thus obviating the need for orthodontics treatment (**Fig. 12.18**). In patients with well-aligned arches, mild crowding, flat-to-mild curve of Spee, normal-to-mild proclination or retroclination of the incisors, and minimal transverse discrepancy, the situation is ideal for "Surgery-first." Orthodontic brackets are placed prior to the surgery. Active orthodontic treatment is initiated very soon after the surgical procedure to utilize the benefits of regional acceleratory phenomenon (RAP). Surgical procedure brings the skeletal base to a relatively normal position in relation to the skull base, which makes the postoperative orthodontic treatment similar to a nonsurgical scenario. At times, an upfront short-term orthodontic treatment (3 months) is done to convert the compensatory dental changes from moderate to mild, following which surgery is performed. This is the "early surgery" variant of SFOA.

Relative contraindications to patient's requiring orthodontic decompensation include severe crowding, severe vertical or transverse discrepancy, and severe proclination of upper and lower anterior teeth.

Dental study model analysis to check the best possible occlusion helps to ascertain the feasibility of SFOA procedure during initial patient evaluation (**Fig. 12.22**). Many technical variations are employed in SFOA procedure that contrasts conventional orthognathic surgery. Clockwise or anticlockwise rotation of maxillomandibular complex to address the maxillary incisor inclination and segmental osteotomies of maxilla and mandible are commonly employed to address transverse discrepancies and align the skeletal bases in a more natural position (**Fig. 12.23**). A more than normal anterior overjet between the upper and lower incisors is left behind after surgery to correct incisor inclination and aid in postsurgical orthodontic leveling and decrowding.

The period of presurgical orthodontics is minimal or absent as there are no extractions to decompensate dental arches preoperatively, which avoids the progressive deterioration of facial esthetics and dental function as seen in conventional orthognathic surgery. RAP, a byproduct of SFOA, is a tissue reaction to a noxious stimulus that increases the healing capacities of the affected tissues.[22] Once evoked, clinical evidence of the RAP typically lasts about 4 months in bone. Initial phase of RAP results in cortical bone porosity because of increased osteoclastic activity. The reduced bone density causes rapid tooth movement during the postsurgical period, accelerating the course of orthodontic settling and thus reducing the overall treatment time. SFOA has significant effect on functional outcome in patients with obstructive sleep apnea symptoms as the early surgical advancement causes immediate increase in the size of upper airway.

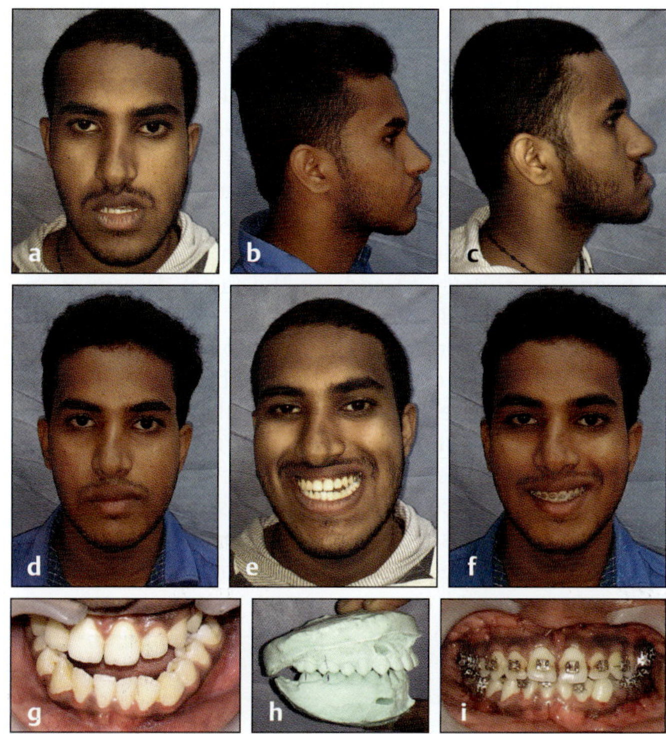

Fig. 12.22 Surgery first orthognathic approach (SFOA) for class III dentoskeletal deformity with facial asymmetry. Dental study model analysis helps to ascertain the feasibility of procedure. Orthodontic brackets are placed prior to the surgery and aids in intermaxillary fixation during surgery. **(a, c, e)** Preoperative images. **(b, d, f)**. Postoperative images. **(g)** Initial occlusion. **(h)**. Dental study models analysis showing feasibility of SFOA procedure. **(i)** On-table occlusion after planned jaw movements.

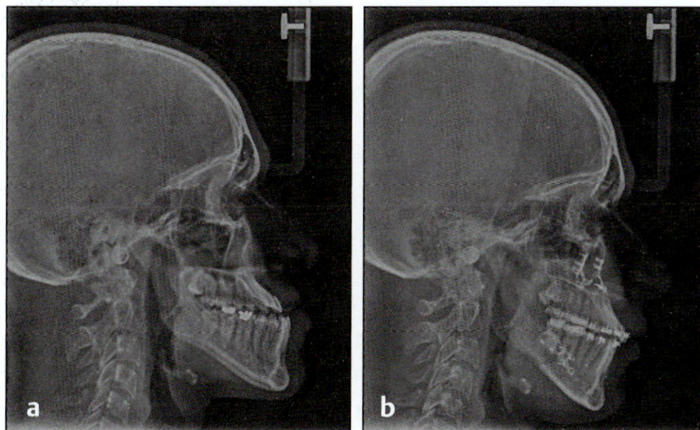

Fig. 12.23 **(a, b)** Pre- and postoperative lateral cephalograms illustrating clockwise rotation of maxillomandibular complex.

Concomitant Alloplastic TMJ Replacement (TJR) with Orthognathic Surgery

Temporomandibular joint (TMJ) disorders/pathology are known to coexist. Congenital absence of condyle or fossa and developmental conditions such as juvenile polyarthritis, childhood deformities trauma leading to ankylosis of TMJ, and idiopathic condylar resorption (ICR) are conditions that cause disturbance in growth and lead to dentofacial deformities. Apart from the congenital and developmental issues, acquired conditions like posttraumatic secondary deformities of face with associated TMJ ankylosis and tumors of mandibular condyle (osteochondroma, chondroblastoma, synovial chondromatosis, etc.) are situations that can warrant total alloplastic replacement of TMJ along with orthognathic surgery to address the facial deformity and TMJ pathology simultaneously.[23]

Complex variations in the bony morphology of mandible with compensatory changes in the neighboring craniofacial skeleton, complicated dentoalveolar malocclusion, obstructive sleep apnea due to obstruction of retrolingual airway are characteristic features of dentofacial deformity arising from disturbance of growth centers during childhood. Though osteotomies to create a pseudocondyle, transplantation of growth center, and distraction osteogenesis are conventional methods, alloplastic replacement of TMJ is the most predictable and definitive treatment modality to manage TMJ pathologies.

Though stock joints can be used for TJR, customized joints are more versatile while performing simultaneous TJR with orthognathic surgery. The alloplastic joint consists of a fossa component made from ultra-high molecular weight polyethylene (UHMWPE) and condylar component made from titanium in custom joints or chrome-cobalt-molybdenum alloy in stock joints (**Fig. 12.24**). Virtual planned and designed custom joints, surgical cutting guides, and occlusal splints provide accuracy and decrease operative time. Customized joints allow large advancement of mandible, complex 3-dimensional jaw movements bringing out overall improvement in facial aesthetics and function.[24]

Isolation of extraoral sites to prevent salivary contamination from the intraoral site is key in preventing postoperative infection of alloplastic joint. Hence due diligence should be given to sequencing the steps involved in TJR and jaw osteotomies. TMJ and ramus of mandible are accessed from a preauricular and submandibular incision. Glenoid fossa/skull base is then prepared to receive the fossa component by performing a condylectomy, tumor or ankylosis resection. Mandible is mobilized. At this point extraoral site is isolated and maxilla and mandibular are placed into intermaxillary

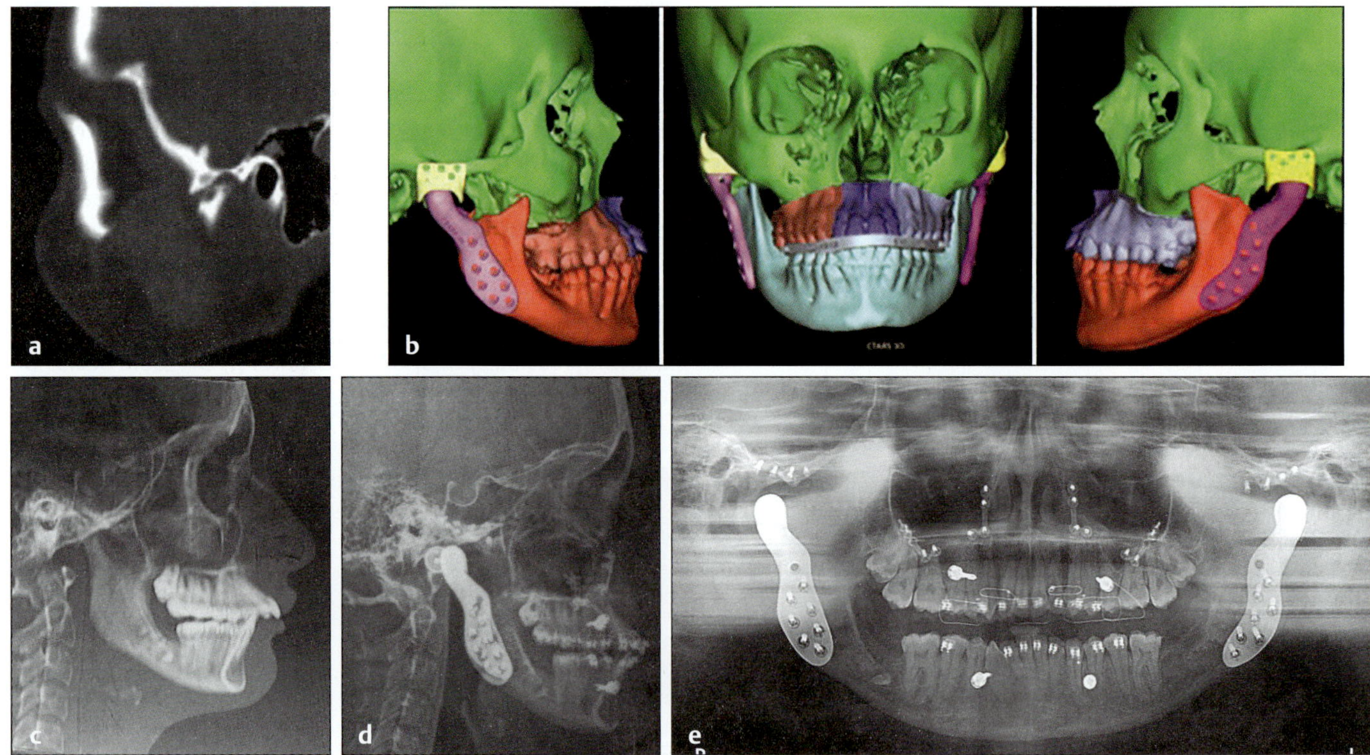

Fig. 12.24 Customized bilateral alloplastic temporomandibular joint reconstruction and three-piece segmental maxillary osteotomy in a case of severe, active, and symptomatic idiopathic condylar resorption to achieve occlusion and correct mandibular retrognathism. **(a)** Sagittal computed tomography (CT) image showing severe condylar resorption. **(b)** Virtually designed custom temporomandibular joint (TMJ), alloplastic joint, and occlusal splint for three-piece maxillary osteotomy. **(c)** Preoperative cephalogram. **(d, e)** Postoperative cephalogram and orthopantomogram (OPG).

fixation intraorally with the help of an intermediate occlusal splint. The oral cavity is isolated again and alloplastic joint components are fixed to skull base and the ramus of mandible. Facial incisions are isolated, IMF released and occlusion is checked at this point to ensure passive movement into the intermediate splint following which intermaxillary fixation is released. Maxillary osteotomy is performed and mobilized, jaws are placed into intermaxillary fixation with the help of final occlusal splint, and fixation is performed with miniplates. IMF is released and occlusion verified. Intraoral wounds are closed first and oral cavity isolated. Facial incisions are closed in layers with special attention given to recreation of the pterygomasseteric sling.

Complications in Aesthetic Facial Surgery

Aesthetic skeletal procedures comprise of precise planning and complex surgical techniques, thereby enhancing the chances of errors at multiple levels. For even the most experienced surgeon, unforeseen complications may arise, which consequently increases the surgical time, the risk of permanent deficiencies, and need for secondary procedures. **Flowchart 12.1** depicts the complications as per their occurrence in the preoperative, intraoperative (common and rare), and postoperative settings.[25–28]

Procedures Adjunct to Orthognathic Surgery

Soft tissue excess or deficiencies as well as contour irregularities owing to dysmorphology of skeleton and those created by the surgical procedures are often seen to persist after skeletal procedures. Augmentation or reduction and additional osteotomies as adjunct procedures are utilized to obtain more optimal outcome in such instances. Silicone implants for forehead augmentation[29] brings balance between upper third of face and the rest of facial skeleton in patients with short skull base. Severe midface hypoplasia with malar and infraorbital deficiency necessitates the use of infraorbital rim, malar, and pyriform rim augmentation using porous polyethylene or polyether ether ketone (PEEK) implants. Zygoma and zygomatic arch reduction reduces the midfacial width and mandibular angle ostectomy, and outer cortex ostectomy of the mandibular angle or inferior border resection are used to reduce the asymmetry left behind after

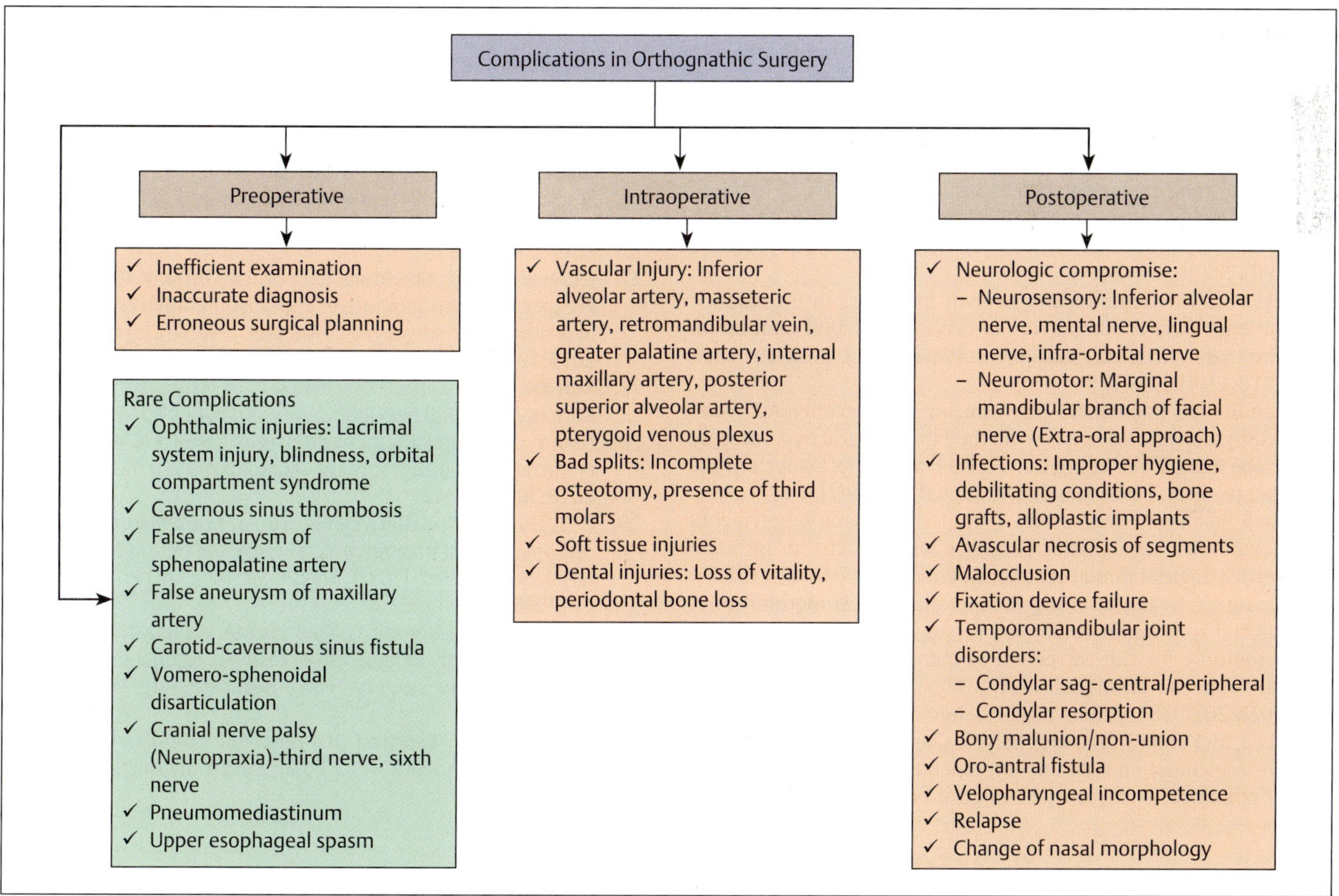

Flowchart 12.1 Complications in orthognathic surgery.

Le Fort I or sagittal split osteotomies.[30] Alloplastic augmentation to increase the width and height of ramus and chin is used alone or in conjunction with ostectomies to address transverse and sagittal discrepancies.[31] In addition, liporeduction of submental region and soft tissue volume augmentation using fillers are procedures used to complement the skeletal and adjunct procedures.[32]

References

1. Limberg A. Treatment of the open bite by means of plastic oblique osteotomy of the ascending rami of the mandible. Dent Cosmos 1925;67:1191–1197
2. Caldwell JB, Letterman GS. Vertical osteotomy in the mandibular raml for correction of prognathism. J Oral Surg (Chic) 1954;12(3):185–202
3. Trauner R, Obwegeser H. The surgical correction of mandibular prognathism and retrognathia with consideration of genioplasty. I. Surgical procedures to correct mandibular prognathism and reshaping of the chin. Oral Surg Oral Med Oral Pathol 1957;10(7):677–689
4. Obwegeser HL. Orthognathic surgery and a tale of how three procedures came to be: a letter to the next generations of surgeons. Clin Plast Surg 2007;34(3):331–355
5. Winstanley RP. Subcondylar osteotomy of the mandible and the intraoral approach. Br J Oral Surg 1968;6(2):134–136
6. Hall HD, Chase DC, Payor LG. Evaluation and refinement of the intraoral vertical subcondylar osteotomy. J Oral Surg 1975;33(5):333–341
7. Obwegeser H. The one time forward movement of the maxilla and backward movement of the mandible for the correction of extreme prognathism. SSO Schweiz Monatsschr Zahnheilkd 1970;80(5):547–556
8. Luhr HG. On the stable osteosynthesis in mandibular fractures. Dtsch Zahnarztl Z 1968;23(7):754
9. Converse JM, Horowitz SL. The surgical-orthodontic approach to the treatment of dentofacial deformities. Am J Orthod 1969;55(3):217–243
10. Litsas G, Ari-Demirkaya A. Growth indicators in orthodontic patients. Part 1: comparison of cervical vertebral maturation and hand-wrist skeletal maturation. Eur J Paediatr Dent 2010;11(4):171–175
11. Saridin CP, Raijmakers PG, Tuinzing DB, Becking AG. Bone scintigraphy as a diagnostic method in unilateral hyperactivity of the mandibular condyles: a review and meta-analysis of the literature. Int J Oral Maxillofac Surg 2011;40(1):11–17
12. He P, Iwanaga J, Matsushita Y, et al. A comparative review of mandibular orthognathic surgeries with a focus on intraoral vertico-sagittal ramus osteotomy. Cureus 2017;9(12):e1924
13. Leung YY, Wang R, Wong NSM, et al. Surgical morbidities of sagittal split ramus osteotomy versus intraoral vertical ramus osteotomy for the correction of mandibular prognathism: a randomized clinical trial. Int J Oral Maxillofac Surg 2020;S0901-5027(20)30384-2. doi: 10.1016/j.ijom.2020.06.023
14. Lin S, McKenna SJ, Yao CF, Chen YR, Chen C. Effects of hypotensive anesthesia on reducing intraoperative blood loss, duration of operation, and quality of surgical field during orthognathic surgery: a systematic review and meta-analysis of randomized controlled trials. J Oral Maxillofac Surg 2017;75(1):73–86
15. Trimble LD, Tideman H, Stoelinga PJ. A modification of the pterygoid plate separation in low-level maxillary osteotomies. J Oral Maxillofac Surg 1983;41(8):544–546
16. Proffit WR, Turvey TA, Phillips C. The hierarchy of stability and predictability in orthognathic surgery with rigid fixation: an update and extension. Head Face Med 2007;3:21–32
17. Obwegeser HL, Makek MS. Hemimandibular hyperplasia: hemimandibular elongation. J Maxillofac Surg 1986;14(4):183–208
18. Wolford LM, Movahed R, Perez DE. A classification system for conditions causing condylar hyperplasia. J Oral Maxillofac Surg 2014;72(3):567–595
19. Niño-Sandoval TC, Maia FPA, Vasconcelos BCE. Efficacy of proportional versus high condylectomy in active condylar hyperplasia: a systematic review. J Craniomaxillofac Surg 2019;47(8):1222–1232
20. Kaban LB, Padwa BL, Mulliken JB. Surgical correction of mandibular hypoplasia in hemifacial microsomia: the case for treatment in early childhood. J Oral Maxillofac Surg 1998;56(5):628–638
21. Salins PC, Venkatraman B, Kavarody M. Morphometric basis for orthomorphic correction of mandibular asymmetry. J Oral Maxillofac Surg 2008;66(7):1523–1531
22. Frost HM. The regional acceleratory phenomenon: a review. Henry Ford Hosp Med J 1983;31(1):3–9
23. Wolford LM. Concomitant temporomandibular joint and orthognathic surgery. J Oral Maxillofac Surg 2003;61(10):1198–1204
24. Movahed R, Wolford LM. Protocol for concomitant temporomandibular joint custom-fitted total joint reconstruction and orthognathic surgery using computer-assisted surgical simulation. Oral Maxillofac Surg Clin North Am 2015;27(1):37–45
25. Bays RA, Bouloux GF. Complications of orthognathic surgery. Oral Maxillofac Surg Clin North Am 2003;15(2):229–242
26. Sousa CS, Turrini RNT. Complications in orthognathic surgery: a comprehensive review. J Oral Maxillofac Surg Med Pathol 2012;24(2):67–74
27. Jędrzejewski M, Smektała T, Sporniak-Tutak K, Olszewski R. Preoperative, intraoperative, and postoperative complications in orthognathic surgery: a systematic review. Clin Oral Investig 2015;19(5):969–977
28. Kim YK. Complications associated with orthognathic surgery. J Korean Assoc Oral Maxillofac Surg 2017;43(1):3–15
29. Park Y-W. Frontal augmentation as an adjunct to orthognathic or facial contouring surgery. Maxillofac Plast Reconstr Surg 2016;38(1):37–42
30. Li Y, Hu Z, Ye B, Liu Y, Ren X, Zhu S. Combined use of facial osteoplasty and orthognathic surgery for treatment of dentofacial deformities. J Oral Maxillofac Surg 2016;74(12):2505.e1–2505.e12
31. Yaremchuk MJ, Doumit G, Thomas MA. Alloplastic augmentation of the facial skeleton: an occasional adjunct or alternative to orthognathic surgery. Plast Reconstr Surg 2011;127(5):2021–2030
32. Mohamed WV, Perenack JD. Aesthetic adjuncts with orthognathic surgery. Oral Maxillofac Surg Clin North Am 2014;26(4):573–585

13

Structural Considerations in Rhinoplasty

Uday Bhat and Amit R. Peswani

Introduction

Rhinoplasty is a unique operation as it involves both art and science. It is an epitome of expression of the word "plastic" (surgery) in its true sense. It entails putting art before science.

Although done routinely with good results the world over, some procedural concepts are still vague and not very clearly understood. In practice, we frequently come across terminologies which may sound right, but are conceptually wrong. Terms like "L strut" and "floating columellar strut" are grossly incorrect, but still find place in day-to-day practice and sometimes even in literature. Terms like "batten graft" or "buttress graft" are often used in a wrong context. There have also been instances where surgeons justify use of techniques which are not in sync with the structure and physiology of the nose, for example cantilever graft, which ideally should have been obsolete by now. Unfortunately, anachronistic concepts still prevail in modern day rhinoplasty.

It is an irony that while everyone chases an aesthetic outcome, the "structure" or the base on which this beauty is built does not get enough importance. To add to this, the related architectural terminologies are used with conflicting connotations, creating further confusion. There is a need to look into this topic afresh. We have attempted to clarify some concepts related to nasal structure, because attempts to enhance the aesthetics are futile when the structure is not taken into account.

In the last 30 years there has been a paradigm shift in our understanding of rhinoplasty. From the classical reduction model of the 1990s, we have today progressed to a variety of maneuvers, cartilage work, and addressing the functional components, the competence of valves in particular. The structural considerations command equal respect.

The importance of structural support is well established in reconstructive rhinoplasty. The standard plan for a defect of the nose involving loss of volume is replacement of not only the envelope but also the framework underneath. Unless the framework is restored, a proper contour, function, and aesthetics would not be established. For example, consider a defect involving the lobule, columella, and membranous septum (**Fig. 13.1a**).

If the defect is perceived as involving only the skin, the result will certainly be suboptimal. The three-dimensional nature of the defect must be taken into account and the plan must include restoration of the framework as well. In this instance, the costal cartilage was used to provide support adding grafts for alar cartilages, the dorsum, spreader graft for the right side of the septum, and a columellar strut (**Fig. 13.1a–c**). This assembly was covered by a forehead flap at the same sitting (**Fig. 13.1d**).

The pleasing result obtained (**Fig. 13.2**) was possible only because due consideration was given to the three-dimensional nature of the defect. Had it been perceived as only a two-dimensional defect and corrected without adding the framework, the outcome would have been far inferior, resulting in a flat lobule, lack of definition and contour, and ill functioning nasal valves. The vital component of the reconstruction is the framework that not only provides the shape, but also prevents collapse of the transferred skin.

These structural considerations perhaps do not receive the same importance in aesthetic rhinoplasty. Our categorizing mind mistakenly tends to classify rhinoplasties as either purely reconstructive or purely aesthetic. The structure and aesthetics go hand-in-hand and are inseparable. It is logical that only when the structural support is ensured, aesthetics will follow!

Structural Support

Structural support is the component/constituent of a construction, responsible for bearing the load and maintaining the shape. When a construction is planned, the architect designs the building keeping the aesthetics and the utility in mind, while the structural engineer ensures it is strong

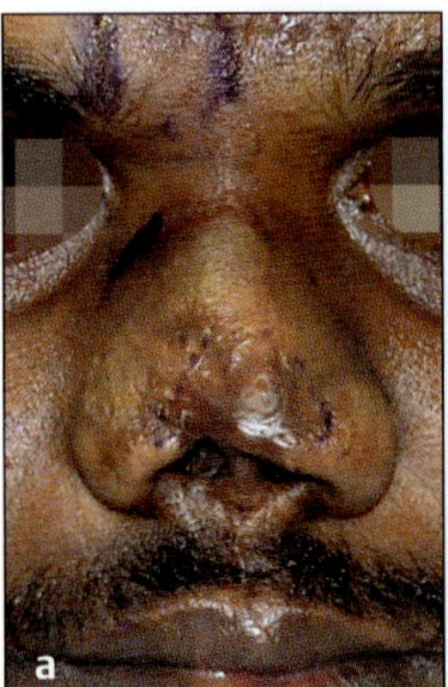

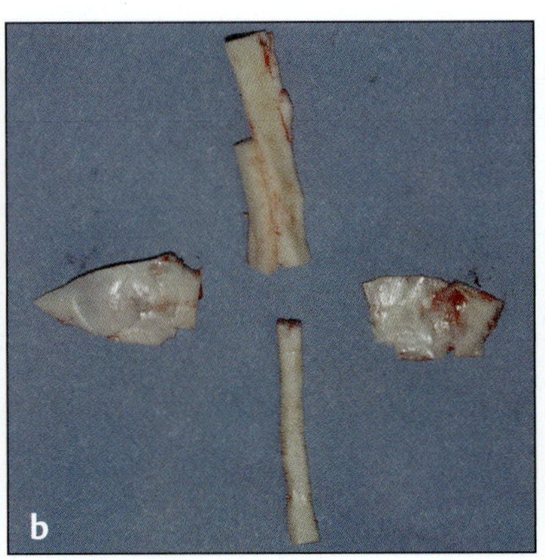

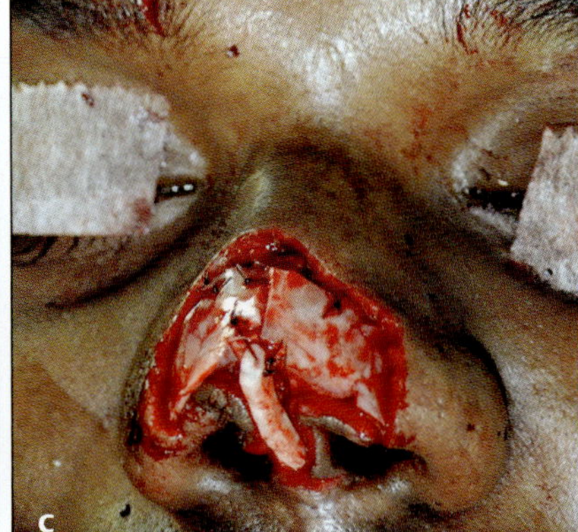

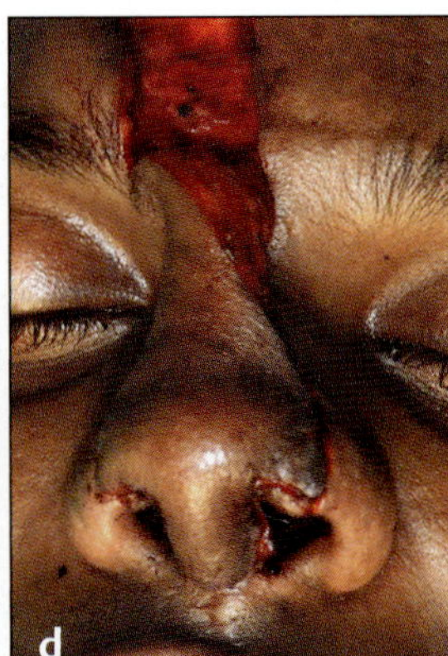

Fig. 13.1 **(a)** A 25-year-old with defect of lobule, columella, and membranous septum. **(b)** Costal cartilage carved for onlay graft, alar cartilages, and columellar strut. **(c)** The recreated defect with restored cartilage framework in place. **(d)** A paramedian forehead flap has been transferred to cover the framework.

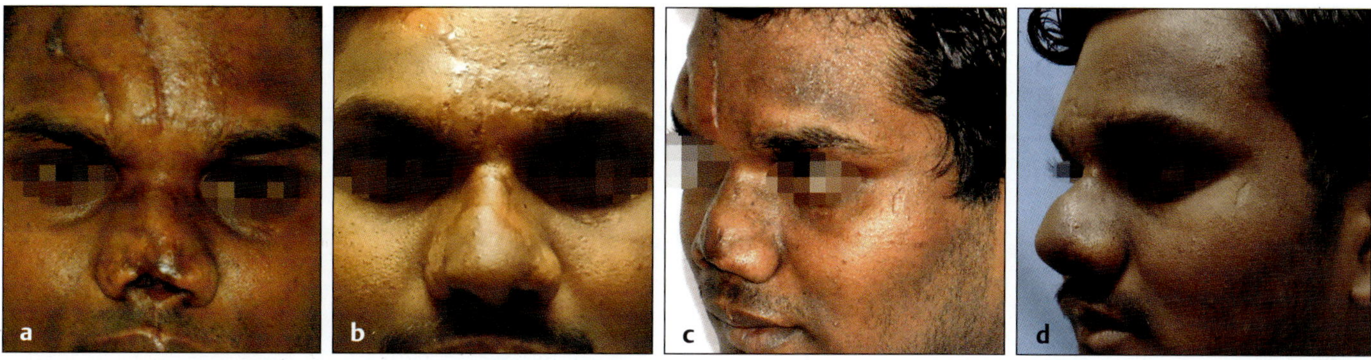

Fig. 13.2 Good contour and adequate projection at 2-year follow-up. **(a, b)** Frontal pictures—preoperative and postoperative. **(c, d)** Lateral views—preoperative and postoperative.

enough to stand up.[1] We, as plastic surgeons, should take up the responsibility of both.

The term "structural support" is loosely applied in rhinoplasty, creating confusion. Two different concepts of support provision are clubbed together in a single term "structural support." The two concepts individually do fit in the broad term "structural support," but they are fundamentally diverse and merit a classified, stand-alone recognition.

The two types of support are:

- Load-bearing support: Counters gravity, carries the load, and transfers the weight to the ground.
- Shape-holding support: This type of support maintains shape of an object by providing the necessary potential energy. It is not related to gravity, as it is not involved in load bearing.

An example of a load-bearing support is the raise provided by body of a man to a bag being carried astride the shoulders (**Fig. 13.3**). The weight of the bag is borne and transmitted to the ground by the legs that act as supporting elements resting on terra firma.

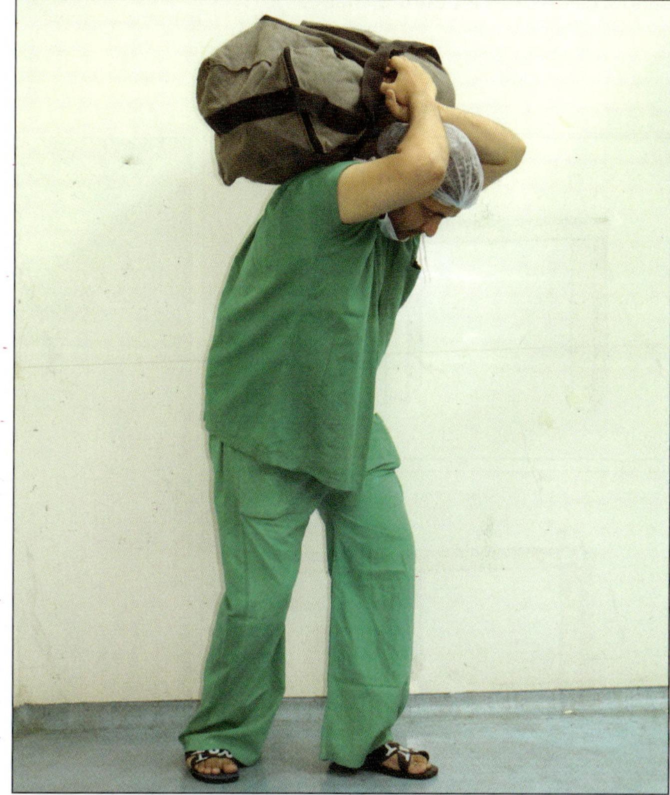

Fig. 13.3 A man carrying a bag (load) on his shoulders, demonstrating a load-bearing support.

In contrast to this, imagine a rubber balloon, which does not have any definite shape in deflated condition (**Fig. 13.4a**). When this balloon is inflated, it assumes a definite shape. The blowing force is converted into a potential energy of the luminal air, resulting in an outward thrust that prevents collapse (**Fig. 13.4b**). The luminal air is not involved in any transfer of load, but simply provides shape-holding support.

The distinguishing factor is that the load-bearing type of support actually transmits load and prevents fall, while the shape-holding support utilizes potential energy to prevent collapse and thus maintain shape. Also the load-bearing structural elements must directly or indirectly rest on terra firma, while the shape-holding elements need not.

Related Architectural Terminologies

Load-Bearing Structural Elements[1]

Column

A column is a vertical load-bearing structural element that resists longitudinal compression or *a pushing force* applied along or *parallel to the axis*. The terms "column," "strut," and a "pillar" are synonymous. Column is the fundamental load-bearing element, supports beams and/or other columns above, and is responsible for final transfer of the load to the ground (**Fig. 13.5a**). A jack post or a prop is a like a thin column used for temporary support in construction (**Fig. 13.5b**).

Beam

A beam is a structural element that resists a bending load that applies a *lateral force* or a force *perpendicular to the axis*. Beams transmit their loads horizontally across a space to

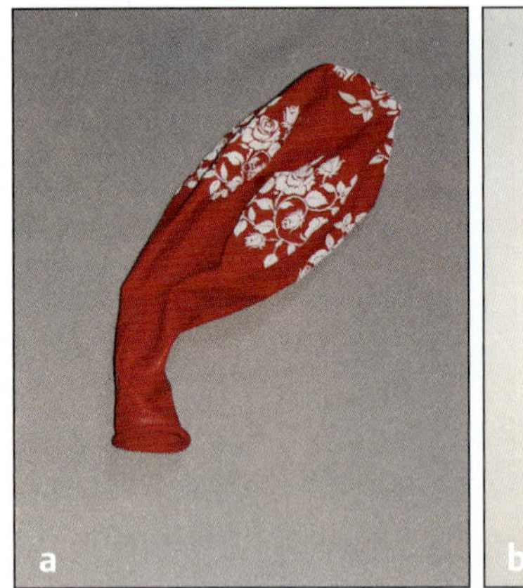

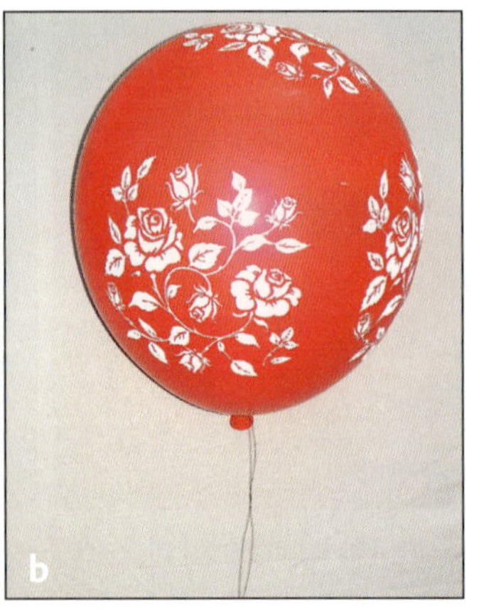

Fig. 13.4 **(a)** A deflated balloon. **(b)** On blowing air into the balloon, it attains a definite shape.

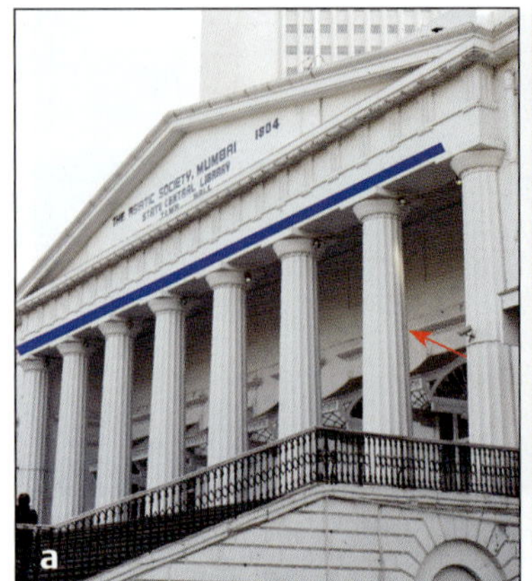

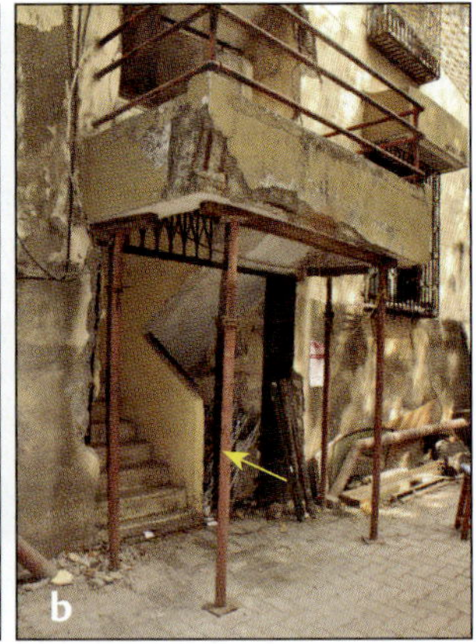

Fig. 13.5 **(a)** A series of columns at the façade, one of which is highlighted by *red arrow* and a beam (*blue line*) at the State Central Library, Mumbai. **(b)** Jack posts used for temporary support (*yellow arrow*).

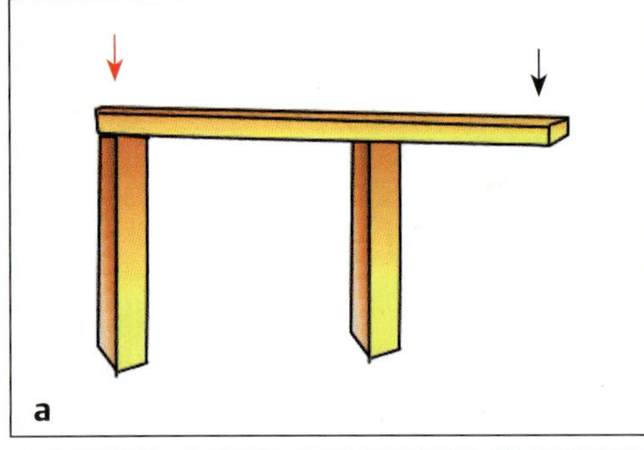

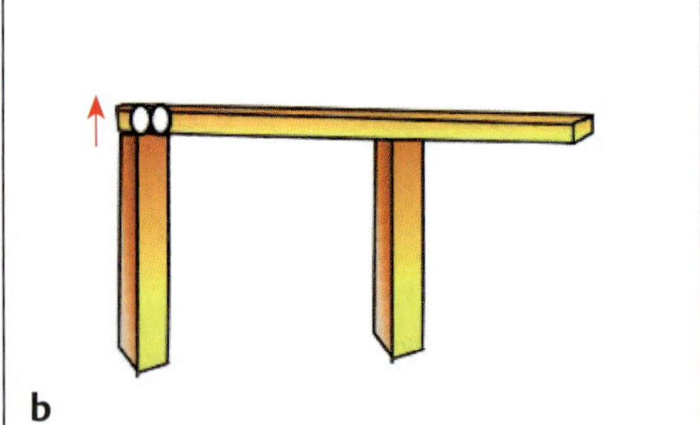

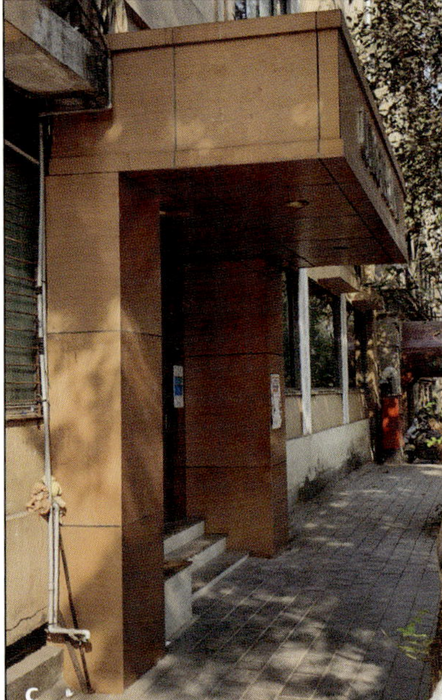

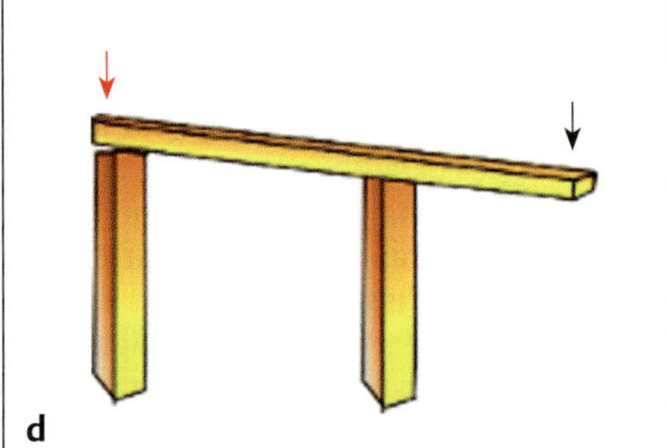

Fig. 13.6 **(a)** A cantilevered beam with a supported end (*red arrow*) and an unsupported part (*black arrow*). **(b)** The unsupported load creates a shearing force (*red arrow*) at the point of fixation. **(c)** A cantilevered construction. **(d)** When subjected to a heavy load (*red arrow*), the fixation may disrupt leading to a collapse (*black arrow*).

another vertical supporting element, either column or load-bearing walls, and eventually to the base[2] (**Fig. 13.5a**).

Beams may be simply supported, or cantilevered. A simply supported beam rests on supports, usually located at each end of the beam. A **cantilever** (**Fig. 13.6a**) is a beam with a rigid structural element anchored at one end and it has an unsupported part extending beyond the column. To avoid collapse, the supported part of the beam should preferably be longer and must be rigidly fixed at one end (**Fig. 13.6b**). The purpose of having a cantilevered structure is to have unobstructed movement below it (**Fig. 13.6c**). The disadvantage is that it is subjected to shear force, a cutting or slicing action which causes a beam to break. A heavy load located near the unsupported end of the beam might cause a shear failure to occur (**Fig. 13.6d**).

Tie/Tendon

A tie or a tendon is a structural element that is employed when the load has to be suspended from above. This element resists *longitudinal tension* or distraction or subjected to a "*pull*" force. The ropes of a suspension bridge are an example of a tie (**Fig. 13.7**).

As discussed earlier, for effective load transmission these elements must rest on terra firma, either physically or indirectly. Both the tie and the beam eventually transfer the weight to a vertical element which in turn transfers the weight to the ground.

It is interesting to see how these elements behave following a transverse break (fracture). A transverse break in a beam leads to its collapse (**Fig. 13.8a**).

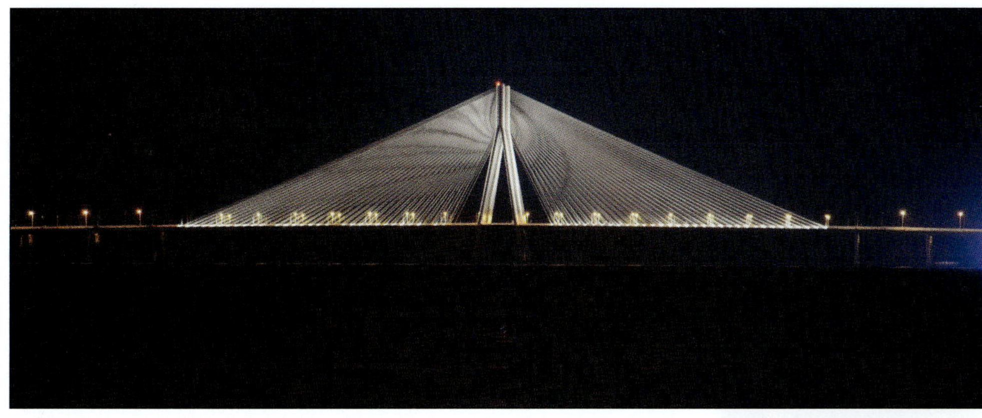

Fig. 13.7 Example of a tie or suspension ropes supporting the Bandra–Worli sea link, Mumbai, Maharashtra, India.

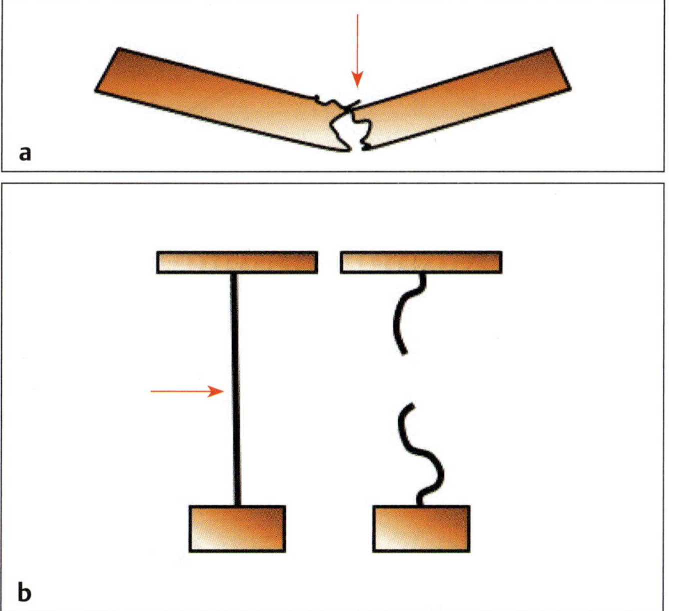

Fig. 13.8 A load of magnitude beyond the critical limit (*red arrow*) results in **(a)** a break (fracture) in a beam and **(b)** disruption in a tie.

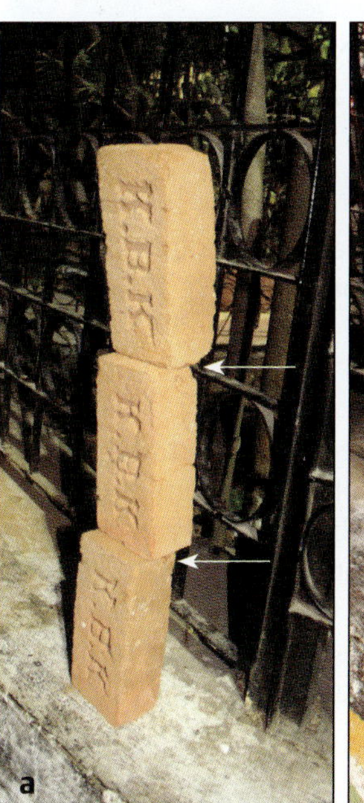

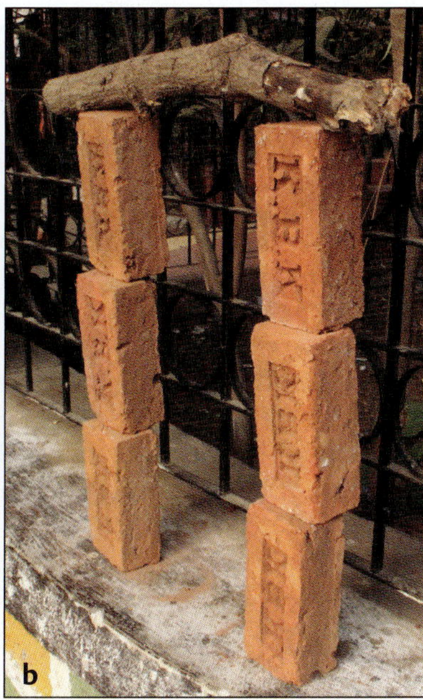

Fig. 13.9 **(a)** An assembly of bricks arranged vertically, even without an adhesive and with an imperfect alignment (*arrows*). This composition mimics a column. **(b)** Despite the multiple discontinuities, the assembly is stable enough to transmit the load.

Similarly, a fracture in the tie will result in a disruption (**Fig. 13.8b**). In contrast to this, a transverse break in the continuity of the column may not always lead to a collapse. An assembly of bricks arranged vertically as a column (**Fig. 13.9a**) that has multiple discontinuities in its alignment is still stable enough to transmit weight to the ground (**Fig. 13.9b**). This is because in this case the direction of the force along the axis, and gravity acts as a binding force maintaining the integrity of the column. If one has to draw an analogy, a transverse break in the column can be likened to a favorable fracture of mandible, where despite the discontinuity, the deformity is minimized by favorable vector of the muscle pull. This concept of controlled discontinuity or a favorable fracture is made use of while performing osteotomies in rhinoplasty.

The two common combinations of beam and column are an "arch" and a "truss" (**Fig. 13.10**). A truss, which is relevant in nasal structure, is meant to carry only small loads like that of a roof or a single story.

Truss

A truss is a two- or three-dimensional framework composed of linear members. The horizontal components or the "tie-beams," the vertical components or the "posts," and the oblique or inclined components or the "rafters" are assembled by the peak joint (at the apex) and the heels (**Fig. 13.11a**). It is interesting to note that if an additional support in the form of a "brace" is provided at the peak joint and at the heels, both the beam and columns can be safely removed with the rafters alone left to balance the

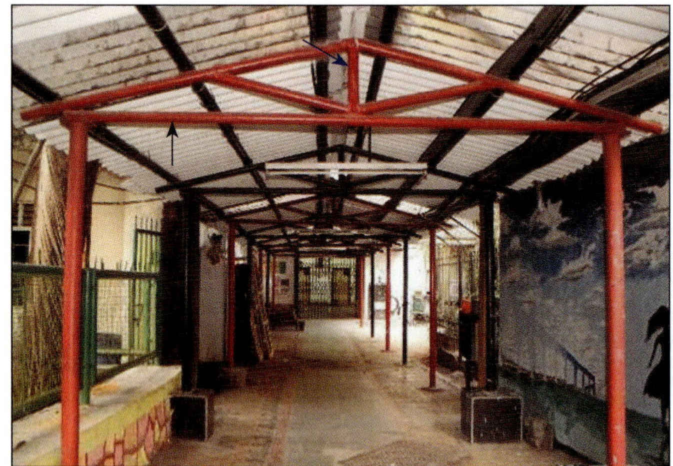

Fig. 13.10 A truss at *Arogya Path*, Nair hospital is composed of vertical structures (*blue arrow*) and horizontal elements (*black arrow*).

weight (**Fig. 13.11b**). In short, the beam and column components of a truss are expendable, provided the peak and heels are supported well.

Brace

A brace is a supporting element used to connect things or to make an assembly stable and stronger by immobilization. Stability can be added to an unstable assembly of columns by adding a brace of a horizontal bar (**Fig. 13.12a, b**). A brace can also be applied to the junction of a column and a beam to lend stability (**Fig. 13.12c, d**). In short, unstable or broken pieces can be held together by a brace.

Buttress

A buttress is an architectural structure built against a wall, to provide support to act against its outward thrust or the lateral (sideways) forces (**Fig. 13.13a**).

Sometimes instead of a solid buttress, a flying buttress is used (**Fig. 13.13b**). It consists of a column and a segmental arch (**Fig. 13.14a**). The configuration of lateral bony wall of nose along with its maxillary base resembles a flying buttress and is appropriately named as "nasomaxillary buttress" (**Fig. 13.14b**).

Shape-Holding Structural Elements

Wedge

A wedge prevents collapse by occupying space (**Fig. 13.15**). In rhinoplasty, the junction of the septum and upper lateral cartilages (ULCs) may have to be dissected and spread out for better functioning of the internal valves. To prevent the collapse of the valves, use of interposition grafts between ULCs and septum is recommended. These "spreader grafts" function just like a wedge to increase the cross-sectional area of the internal nasal valve by displacing the ULCs laterally.

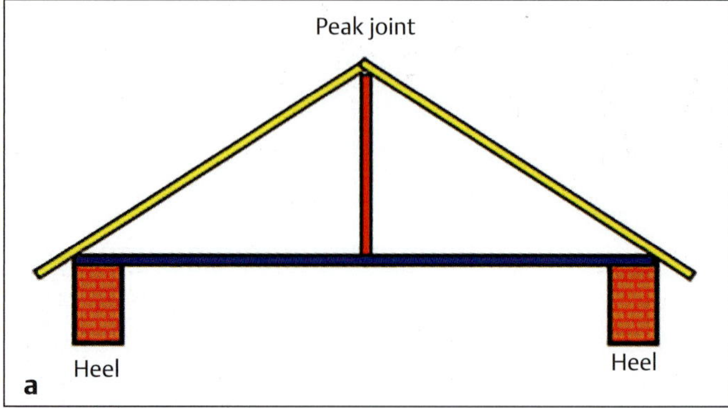

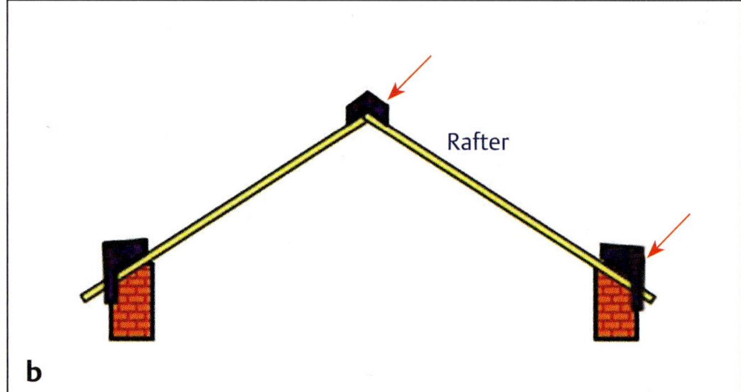

Fig. 13.11 **(a)** A simplified composition of a truss showing its basic elements, a vertical post (*red*) and a horizontal tie beam (*blue*). **(b)** If the peak joint and heels are adequately braced (*purple blocks marked with red arrows*), the load can be carried by only the oblique rafters.

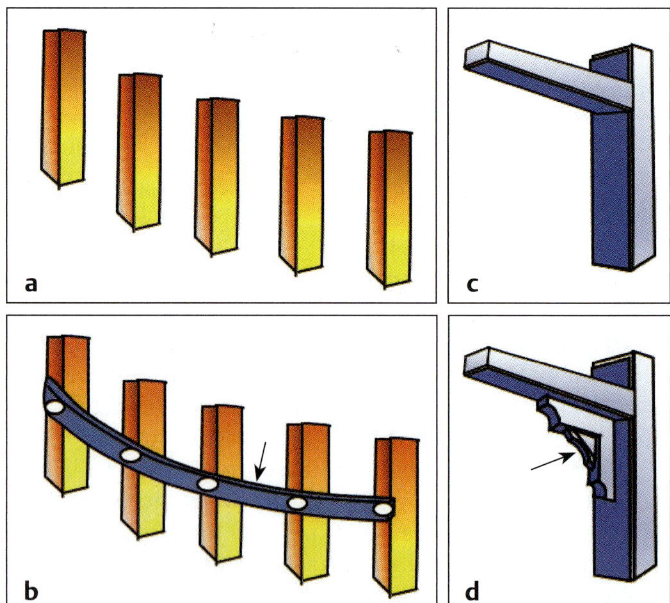

Fig. 13.12 **(a)** An unstable assembly of columns stabilized using **(b)** a brace in the form of a horizontal bar (*arrow*). **(c)** An unstable assembly of a beam and a column stabilized using a **(d)** brace (*arrow*).

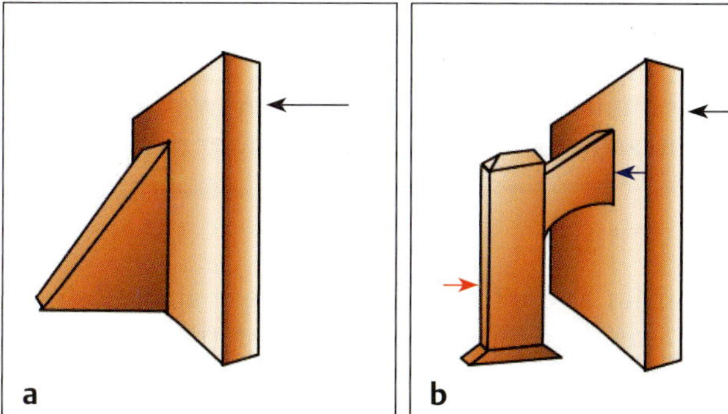

Fig. 13.13 **(a)** A buttress which is used to resist the lateral forces (*black arrow*) and **(b)** a flying buttress which is composed of a column (*red arrow*) and segmental arch (*blue arrow*) resisting the lateral forces (*black arrow*).

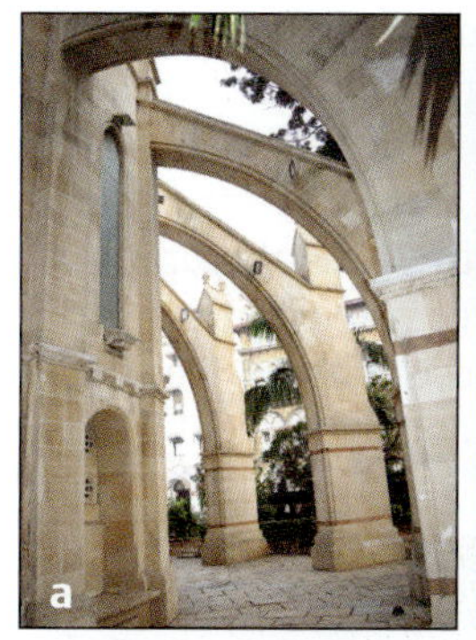

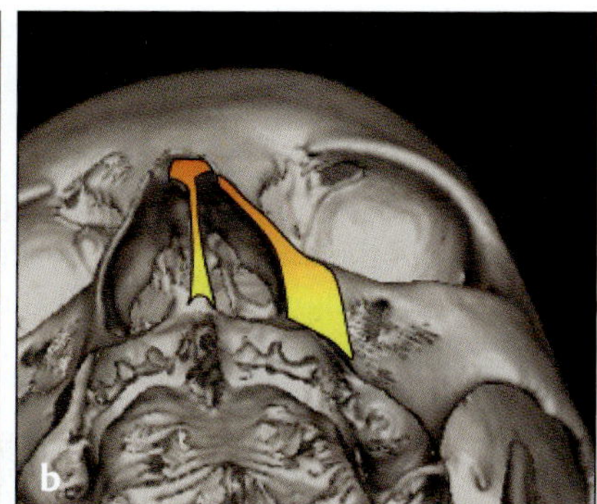

Fig. 13.14 **(a)** A flying buttress at St. Thomas cathedral, Mumbai. **(b)** 3D reconstruction CT scan of face with the nasomaxillary buttress highlighted along with the septal wall to show its resemblance to the architectural flying buttress.

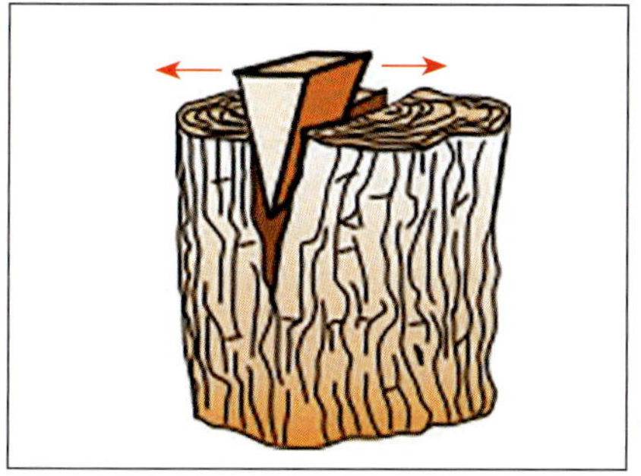

Fig. 13.15 Shape-holding property of a wedge: It prevents collapse of the spread-out parts (*red arrows*).

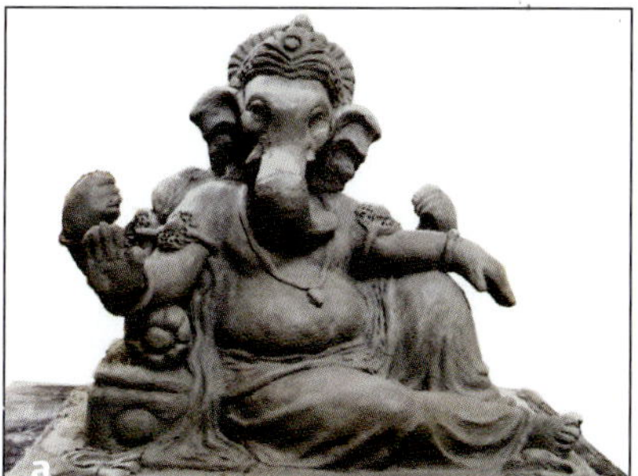

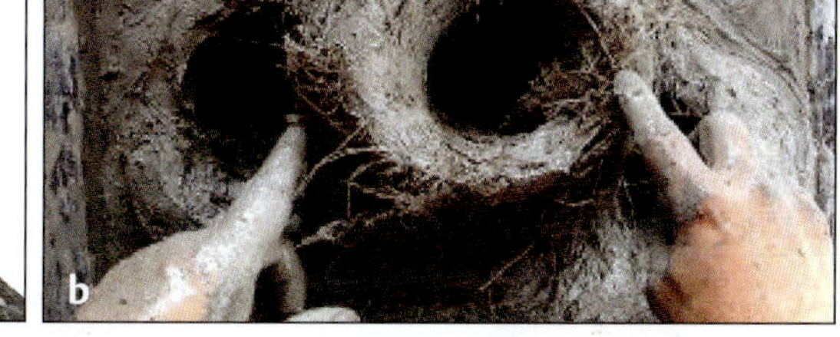

Fig. 13.16 **(a)** A clay sculpture which is hollow from within. **(b)** Same sculpture at an initial stage of construction showing grass scaffolding.

Scaffolding

Scaffolding is usually a hidden frame inside a wall or sometimes against it.[3] Most of the clay sculptures are hollow from within, to reduce the weight and quantity (**Fig. 13.16a**) of raw material used. The shape of the hollow construction is maintained by a grass scaffolding (**Fig. 13.16b**). In the human nose, the alar cartilage, which maintains the shape of the lobule without transmitting the weight, works in similar lines.

Volume Augmentation

If we consider a packet of detergent half filled, it has a loose shape. When it is stuffed with more detergent, the additional volume provides the potential energy which stretches the bag and maintains an inflated shape. An onlay graft stretches the skin envelope and supports the internal valve in similar manner (**Fig. 13.17**). Earlier example of an air-filled balloon is alike in principle.

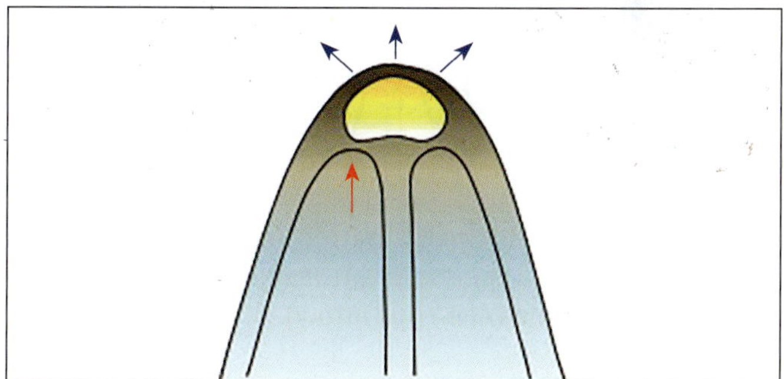

Fig. 13.17 A dorsal onlay graft (*yellow*) by sheer volume applies an outward force and stretches (*blue arrows*) the overlying skin envelope. In addition, it also supports the internal valve.

Batten

A batten is used to make a fence strong and secure. It does not rest on the ground and hence cannot take the load. In fact, it puts its own load on the bars and the poles, yet provides bolstering to the fence (**Fig. 13.18**). The example of such a support is an alar batten graft.

The terms "batten" and "strut" are different in principle (**Fig. 13.19**). A strut, as we have seen before, is synonymous with "column" which is a load-bearing structure and hence it rests on terra firma. In contrast, a batten being a shape-holding support may be hanging or floating. Thus, the term "floating columellar strut" often used in literature is a contradiction. As a strut rests on the ground, the columellar strut must rest on the anterior nasal spine (ANS) (it may or may not be fixed). If it is floating, it should be termed as a columellar "batten." Similarly, a floating lateral crural graft is batten and the one resting on pyriform aperture is a strut.

It is interesting to note that all these concepts have profound applications in nasal anatomy and dynamics.

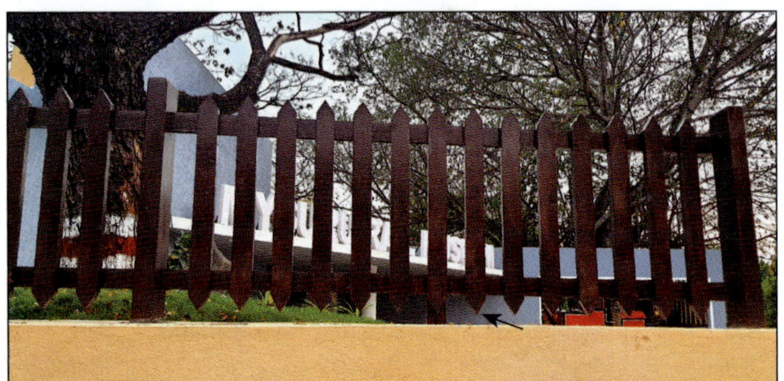

Fig. 13.18 The arrow points to a batten, a support element used to make the fence strong. In contrast to the strut, it does not rest on the ground and hence is not load bearing in nature.

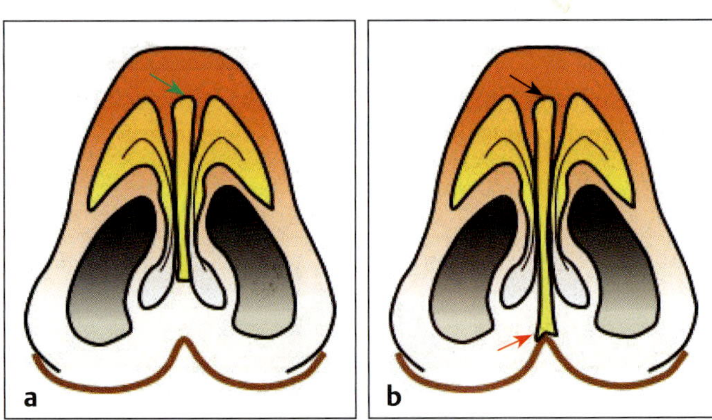

Fig. 13.19 **(a)** A columellar batten (*green arrow*) graft is floating while **(b)** a columellar strut (*black arrow*) rests on **anterior nasal spine** (ANS) (*red arrow*).

Anatomy of Nose

The skin is thinner and mobile in the upper two-thirds of the nose and it is thick and adherent in the lower third.

Blood Supply

The two main arteries supplying the nose are the supratrochlear artery and the facial artery. The former is a branch of internal carotid artery while the latter is a branch of external carotid artery. These arteries have branches which cross the midline, and thus between these two systems there is an extensive collateral network that provides robust vascularity to the nose.[4]

The supratrochlear branch gives rise to lateral nasal, descending external nasal, and angular vessels (**Fig. 13.20**). These vessels course directly below the dermis, superficial to the intrinsic nasal muscles.

The facial artery travels superiorly. It gives off the superior labial artery and continues upward to connect with the angular vessel (**Fig. 13.20b**). The superior labial gives rise to the philtral arteries, which provide the main contribution to the ascending columellar arteries. It also gives a small artery to the sill. The lateral nasal artery courses 2 to 3 mm above the alar groove. Hence it is advisable to restrict the extent of alar wedge excision within a distance of 2 mm from the groove.

The commonly used approaches for rhinoplasty include:

- The closed approach: Using the intercartilaginous incision (**Fig. 13.21a**).
- Bipedicled flap incision (**Fig. 13.21b**).
- The open approach: Using the infracartilaginous incision connected by a columellar incision in a stepladder or an inverted-V pattern (**Fig. 13.21c**).

When the open approach is used, the columellar artery is likely to be transected. However, this has little effect because of the intact lateral nasal artery and multiple branches that perfuse the region of the nasal dome.

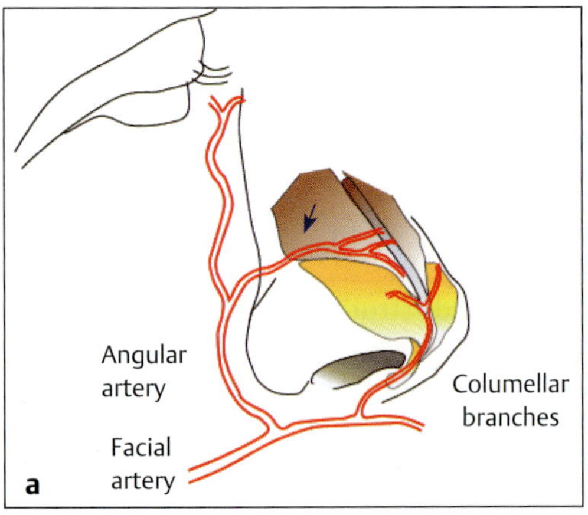

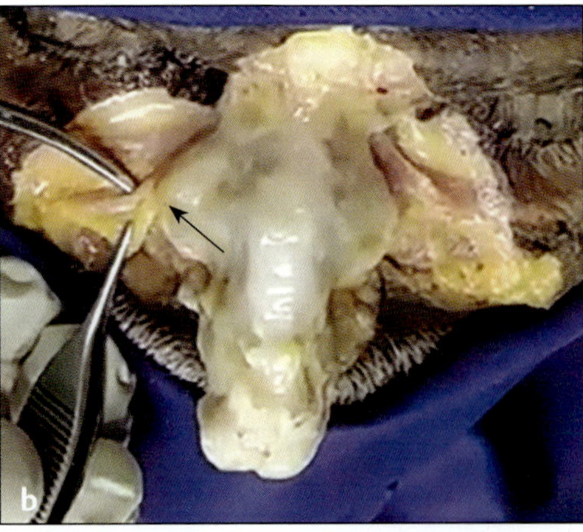

Fig. 13.20 **(a)** Blood supply of the nose. The columellar branches get transected in an open approach. The lateral nasal artery (*blue arrow*) courses 2 to 3 mm above the alar groove. **(b)** The course of angular artery shown in a cadaver.

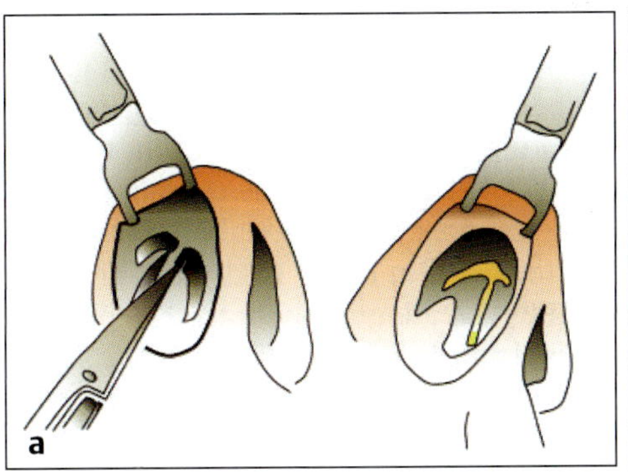

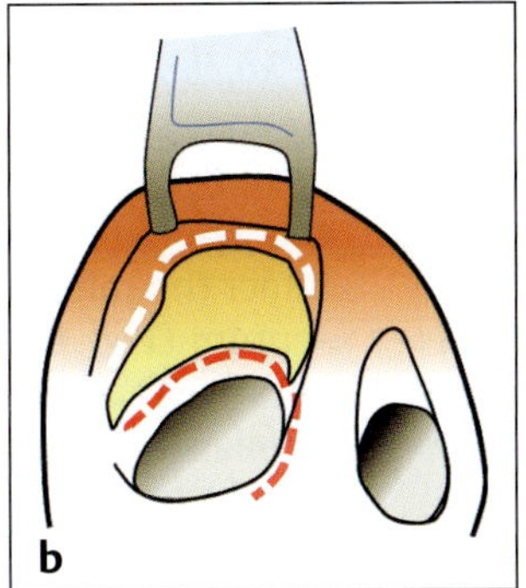

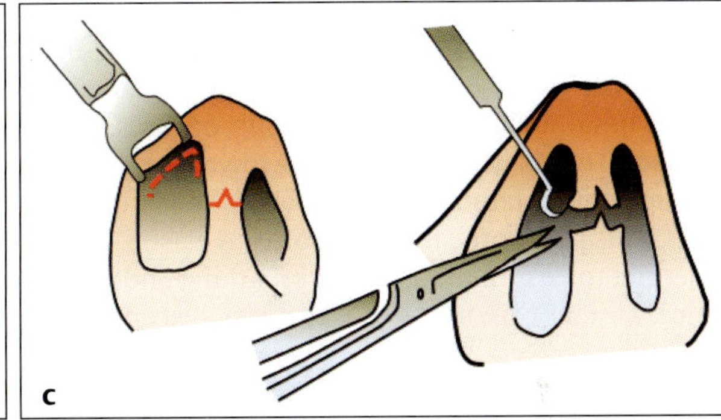

Fig. 13.21 **(a)** Intercartilaginous incision used in closed approach. **(b)** The bipedicled flap incision combining intercartilaginous and infracartilaginous approaches. **(c)** Incision for an open approach rhinoplasty with an inverted-V columellar incision.

Muscles of the Nose

There are several nasal muscles, but not all are clinically significant.[5] The muscles are a part of the superficial musculoaponeurotic system (SMAS) layer. The relevant ones are:

- Levator labii alaeque nasi (**Fig. 13.22**): Helps to keep the external nasal valve open.
- Depressor septi nasi: Pulls the upper lip up and can decrease tip projection on animation.
- Procerus (**Fig. 13.22**): Expression of anger.

Periosteum and Perichondrium

This layer once thought to be not relevant from surgical point of view can be used judiciously to our advantage. A technique has been described by Nazim Cerkes to elevate the perichondrium of the ULC and the periosteum of the nasal bones concurrently, as a single flap on both sides.[6] A midline incision is used for this (**Fig. 13.23**). This maneuver exposes bare cartilage and bone throughout the nasal dorsum.

The advantages of this perichondro-periosteal flap are:

- Excellent visualization of the nasal bones, ULC, and most important, the keystone area.
- Deformities of dorsum can be determined more accurately and correction of the deformities is easier.
- The extra layer of connective tissue helps to smoothen minor irregularities of the nasal dorsum, particularly in the keystone area. This is important in patients with thin nasal dorsal skin, in whom miniscule dorsum irregularities can become visible in the long-term.

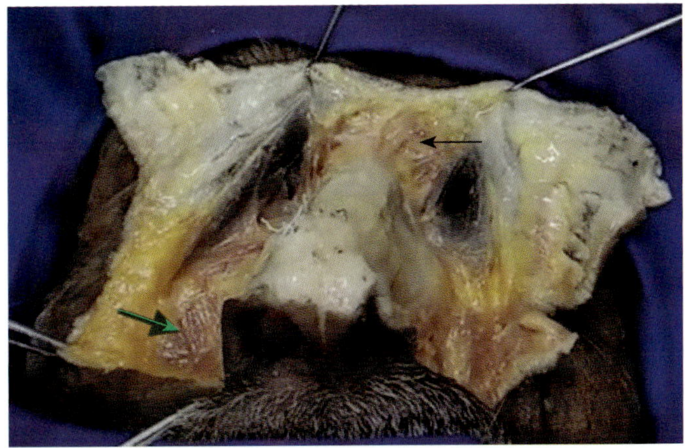

Fig. 13.22 Cadaveric dissection showing Procerus (*black arrow*) and Levator labii alaeque nasi (*green arrow*).

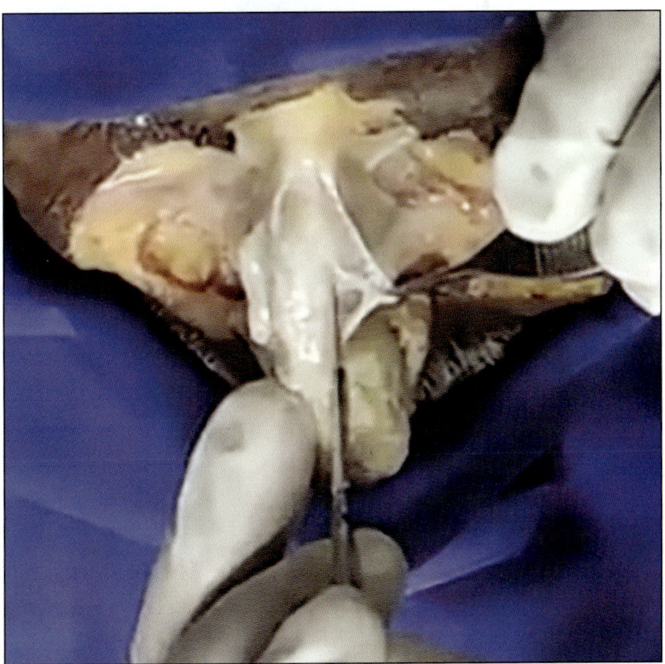

Fig. 13.23 Elevation of perichondroperiosteal flap in a cadaver.

Architecture of the Nose

The nose has a unique, yet simple architecture. It is a single-story structure, and hence it is not required to carry too much load. It is composed of two units. The rigid or semirigid unit of the osseocartilaginous vault in the upper two-third; and the mobile unit of lobule with alar cartilages in the lower one-third. The upper part of osseocartilaginous vault is bony, made up of nasal bones and frontal process of maxilla on lateral sides and the perpendicular plate of ethmoid in midline. The lower part of the vault or the middle third of the nasal architecture is made up of ULCs laterally and the septal cartilage in midline. The lower third is made up of a pair of lower lateral cartilages (LLCs) and accessory cartilages. This part or the lobule is soft and elastic. This nature is essential to ensure mobility for breathing and valve competence. Besides this, it also makes it less susceptible to effects of trauma.

The architecture of the nose is built around a bottomless cavity (pyriform aperture) meant for the air passage. The circumferential plinth is made up by the alveolar and frontal processes of the maxilla and partly by the frontal bone (**Fig. 13.24**); and in the midline, there is a partition wall (**Fig. 13.25**).

This midline wall is load bearing by nature and forms the main supporting element of the nasal architecture. It does not have a ground for to rest on; it rests on the sidewalls; it is attached to frontal bone and skull base cranially and to the seam of maxillae and palatine bones caudally. It is made up of the ethmoid plate, the vomer, and the septal cartilage (**Fig. 13.25**).

This midline wall has flying buttresses formed by the lateral walls on either side, which are part bony and part cartilaginous (**Fig. 13.26a, b**). The contributing bones are frontal process of maxilla and the nasal bones, and the cartilaginous part is made up of ULCs. These buttresses constitute the lateral walls of the osseocartilaginous vault (**Fig. 13.26**).

As the central wall carries the load of only the roof or the skin soft tissue envelope (SSTE) along with the lobular framework, it can safely be converted into a truss or a *"kaichi."* If we brace the truss at the peak and heel joints, we may simply leave behind only the rafters, removing everything else. In the septum, this has an implication that we can safely remove most of the cartilage as a graft, leaving intact the rafters along the dorsal and caudal borders of the septum (**Fig. 13.27**). However, in order to do this, the corners (peak and heel) must be adequately braced to prevent a collapse. Hence the incision should be curved at the septal angle to ensure there is additional support at this point. It must also be ensured that the dorsal and caudal rafters are strong enough; the recommended width is 8 to 10 mm.

The term "L strut" is frequently used in literature which is a contradiction, as a "strut", by definition, is same as a "column" which is a linear structure. Another application of this concept is while reconstructing a new septum in post-traumatic septal collapse, as discussed later.

Changes after Osteotomies

Osteotomies are routinely used in rhinoplasty and the indications range from broad nose to asymmetry. The maneuver of osteotomy is a planned surgical weakening of the bone induced to manipulate it from an existing undesirable position to an acceptable position.

As we have seen earlier, the lateral wall of the nose acts as a buttress. When lateral and medial osteotomies are performed, this buttress support is weakened. However, the midline wall remains unaffected (**Fig. 13.28**) and is stable enough to adequately support the vault.

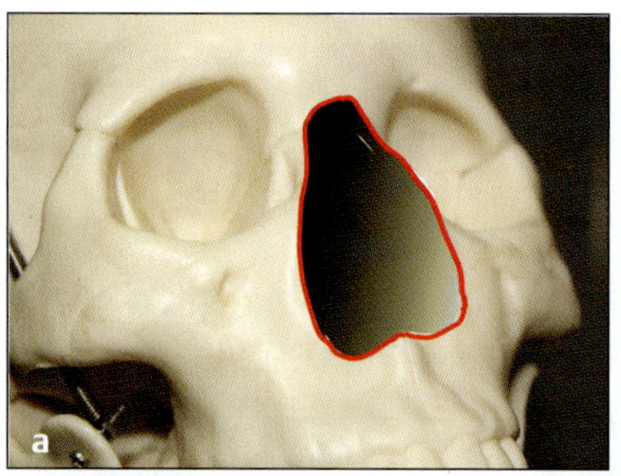

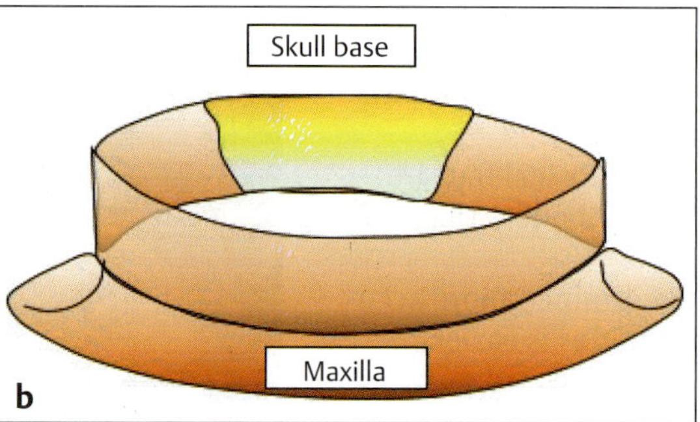

Fig. 13.24 (a) A skull model showing the air passage and the base on which nasal framework rests. **(b)** The circumferential plinth formed by the maxilla and the skull base.

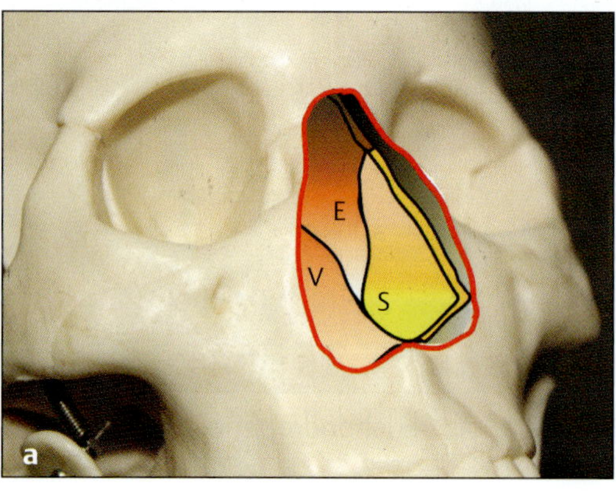

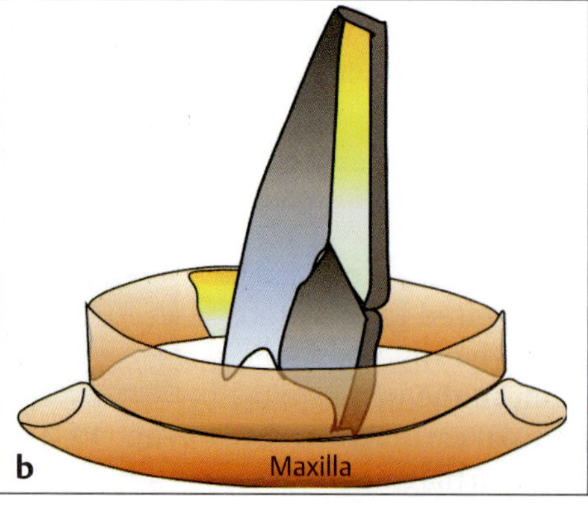

Fig. 13.25 (a, b) Diagrammatic representation of circumferential plinth along with central septum. E, ethmoid plate; S, septal cartilage; V, vomer.

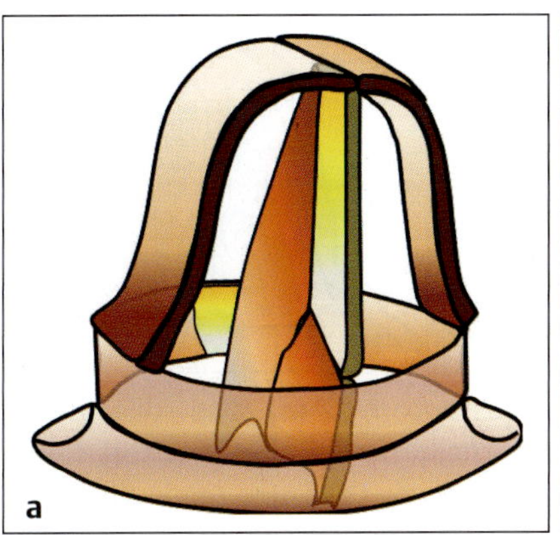

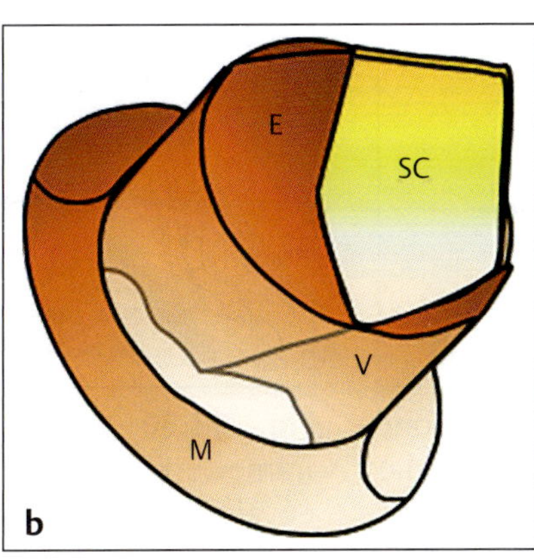

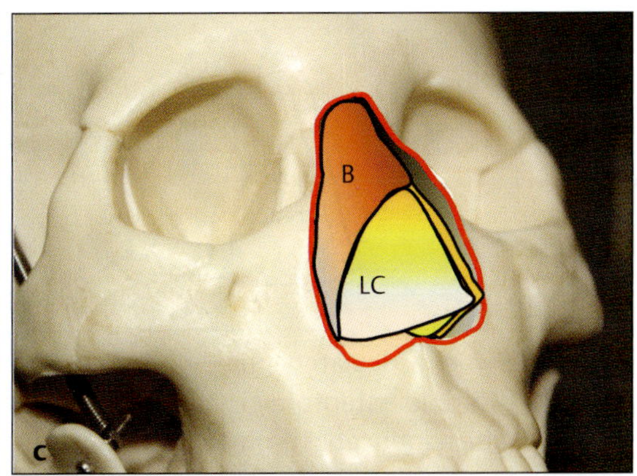

Fig. 13.26 **(a)** The plinth, central septum, and the lateral walls of the nose. **(b)** The upper part of the lateral buttress is bony while the lower part is made of upper lateral cartilage. **(c)** The architecture of the nose highlighted on a skull model. Lateral wall on the opposite side has been omitted for clarity in **(b)** and **(c)**. Abbreviations: E, ethmoid; SC, septal cartilage; V, vomer; M, maxilla; B, bone; LC, lateral cartilage.

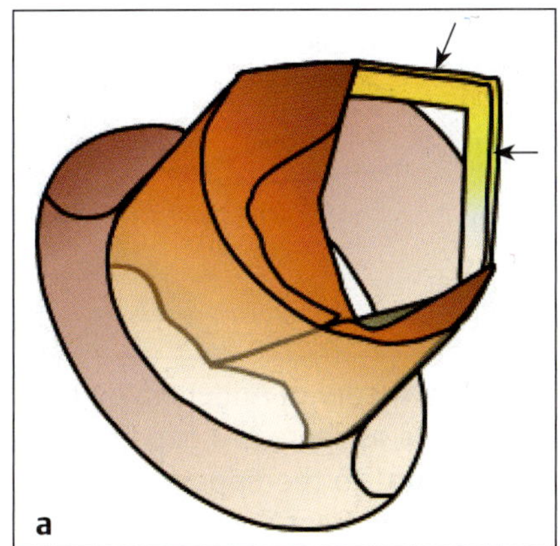

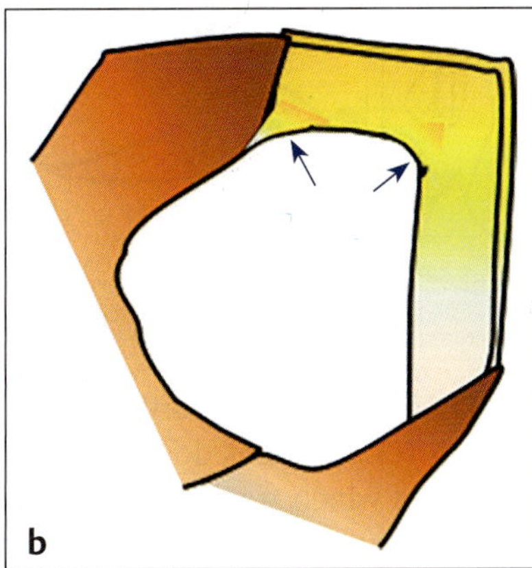

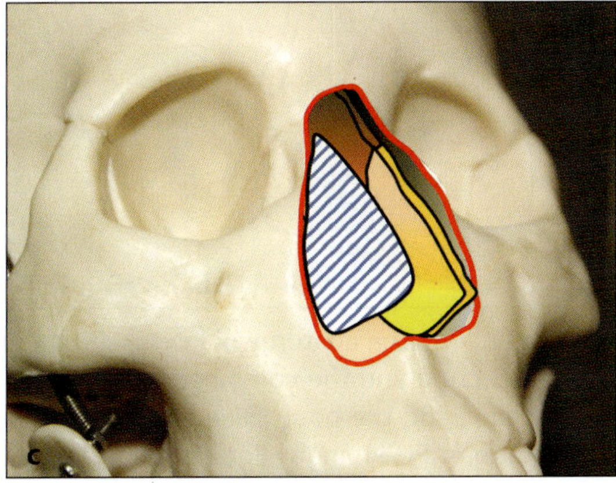

Fig. 13.27 **(a)** A truss of nasal septum with only oblique rafters (*black arrows*). **(b)** The peak joint and the heels of the truss have been effectively braced by modifying the incisions at these junctions, shown by *blue arrows*. **(c)** The septal braced truss in situ after harvest of septal cartilage (from *shaded area*).

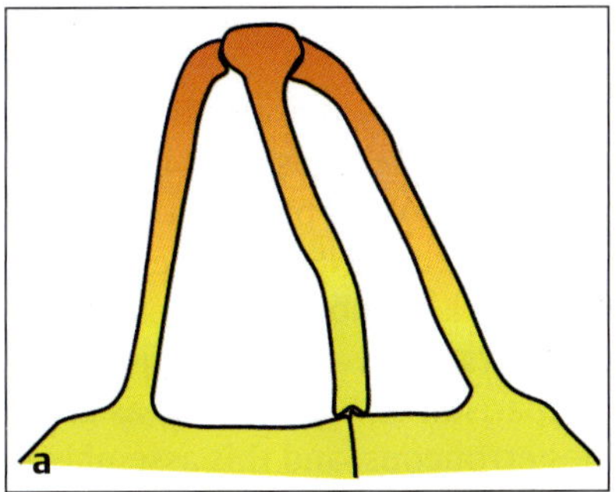

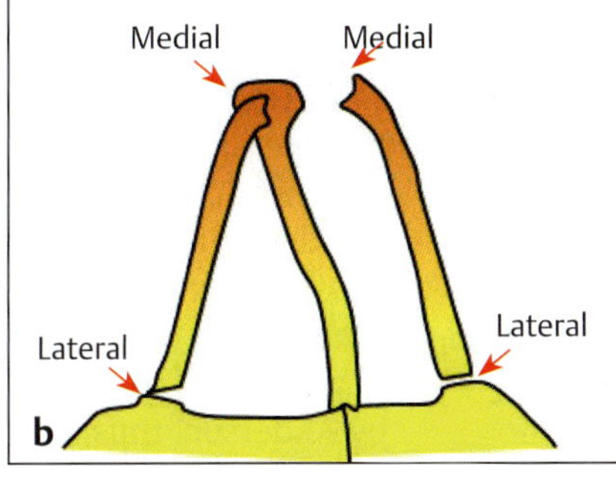

Fig. 13.28 **(a)** A cross-sectional view of a deviated nose. **(b)** The lateral and medial osteotomies result in weakening of the lateral buttress. However the central load-bearing wall remains unaffected.

In a deviated nose with an asymmetric bony vault, in addition to the lateral and medial osteotomies, it is necessary to perform the ethmoid osteotomy as well to counter the asymmetry. When we break the ethmoid, the central wall is also fractured and the whole structure becomes dilapidated (**Fig. 13.29**).

As we have discussed earlier, a transverse break in the column need not always lead to collapse, as this type of a fracture is a favorable fracture. Secondly, preservation of septal volume reduces the dead space and adds to the stability. Hence it is important to restrict the amount of harvested septal graft to minimum, and "brace" the septum, if required.

In addition to this, another factor which holds the framework together is the inner lining which drapes it from within. The percutaneous "postage stamp osteomy" does not cut the

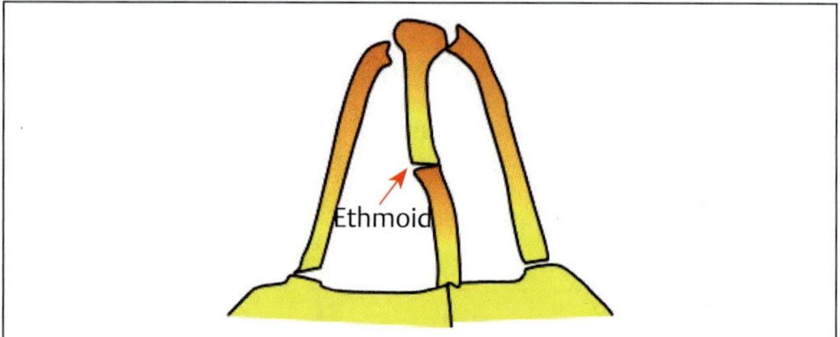

Fig. 13.29 In a deviated nose with an asymmetric bony vault, an ethmoid osteotomy is also performed. Despite the discontinuities induced surgically, the whole assembly of framework is stable enough to transmit the load. This can be likened to the assembly of bricks in **Fig 13.9b**.

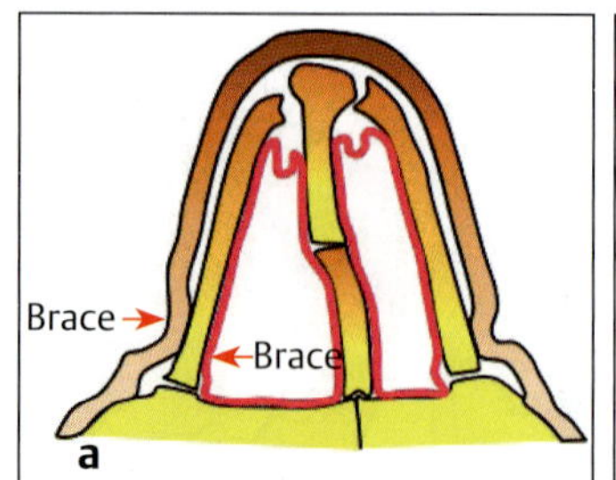

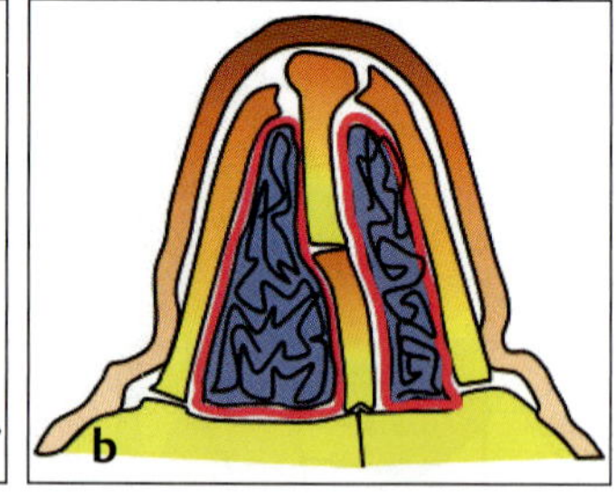

Fig. 13.30 After an osteotomy, **(a)** the dilapidated framework is braced externally by the skin and soft tissue envelope (*brown*) and internally by the lining (*pink*). **(b)** Nasal packing (*blue*) supports the assembly and acts as a temporary jack post for the weakened structure, like in **Fig. 13.5b**.

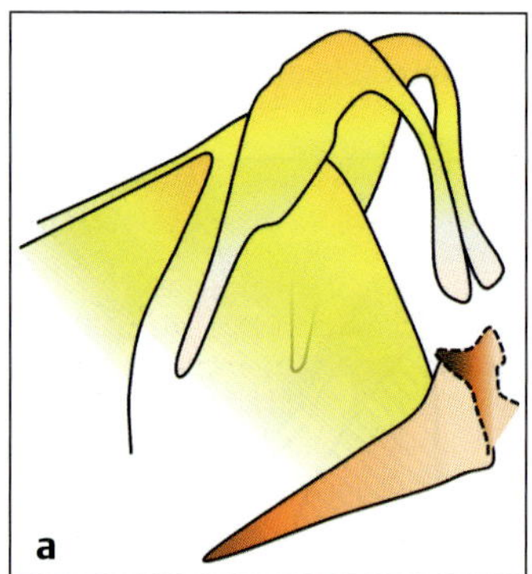

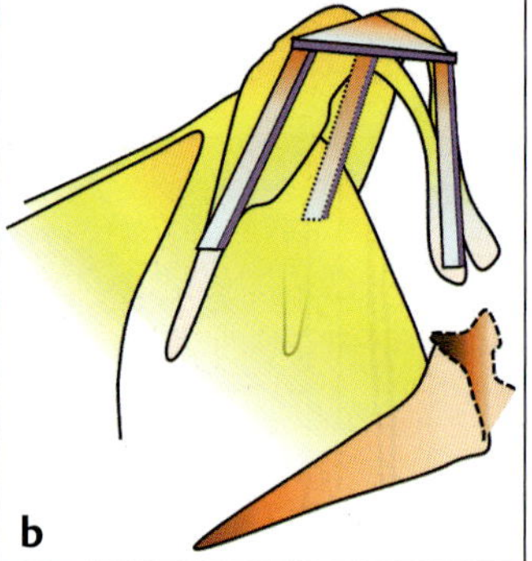

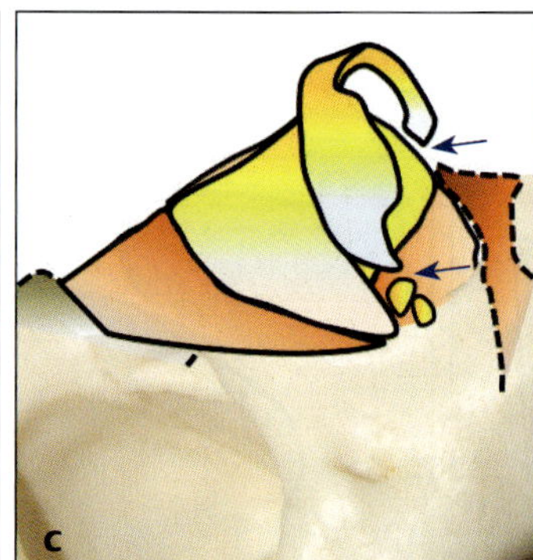

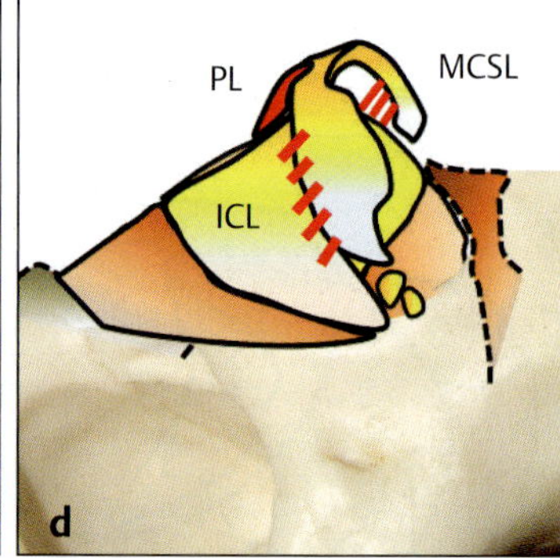

Fig. 13.31 **(a)** The anatomy of lateral and medial crura of lower lateral cartilage. **(b)** The tripod theory of Anderson equates the lateral crura and the combined medial crura to pods. **(c)** The pods do not rest on terra firma as there is a gap between the cartilage and the bone (*blue arrows*). **(d)** The ligaments which transmit the load of lower third to the upper two-thirds. Abbreviations: PL, Pitanguy ligament; ICL, intercartilaginous ligament; MCSL, medial crural septal ligament.

lining all along, it creates only perforations, maintaining the continuity of the lining. The outer skin and soft tissue envelope may also retain some attachments with the bone. The attachments of the lining and the envelope together act as a brace that holds the unstable bones (**Fig. 13.30a**). Besides this, the use of nasal packing functions as a temporary jack post to stabilize this weakened assembly (**Fig. 13.30b**).

Osteotomy is a delicate maneuver, and when performed carefully does not result in vault collapse. However, in an unfortunate situation when that happens, the technique described later for correction of total collapse following trauma may be employed.

Architecture of the Lobule

The lobule is the mobile part of the nose, hanging from the vault and has a scaffold of alar cartilages. The accepted theory vis-à-vis dynamics of the alar cartilages is the tripod theory proposed by Anderson.[7] This popular theory likens the cartilaginous framework to a tripod, or a three-legged *column assembly that bears the load* ("pod": from Ancient Greek podóς or podós resembling a foot or limb).[8] That essentially conveys the meaning that the lateral crura and the combined medial crura provide the tip the limbs to stand on; or these are the pillars which bear the load of the lobule (**Fig. 13.31**). In a nutshell, this theory categorizes alar cartilages as load-bearing elements.

In reality, the LLC does not directly rest on the maxilla. Despite the presence of accessory cartilages, the lateral crus does not actually rest on the border of the pyriform aperture, nor does the medial crus rest on the ANS. Because of these gaps, the lateral and medial crura cannot be likened to columns, as they do not rest on terra firma and are not involved in transfer of load. The comparison to legs or pods as given by Anderson, thus, becomes erroneous, and this assembly is not a real tripod because it offers no load-bearing support.

The role of LLCs is explained by the elastic spring model of Westreich and Lawson.[9] The cartilages act like a scaffold, and their elasticity provides the potential energy that holds the cartilages expanded and prevents their collapse (**Fig. 13.32**). It is important to remember that the LLCs provide the shape-holding support only.

If the LLCs are hanging, without limbs or columns, what does the lobule rest on? The hanging lobule along with its cartilage framework is *cantilevered* on the weight bearing

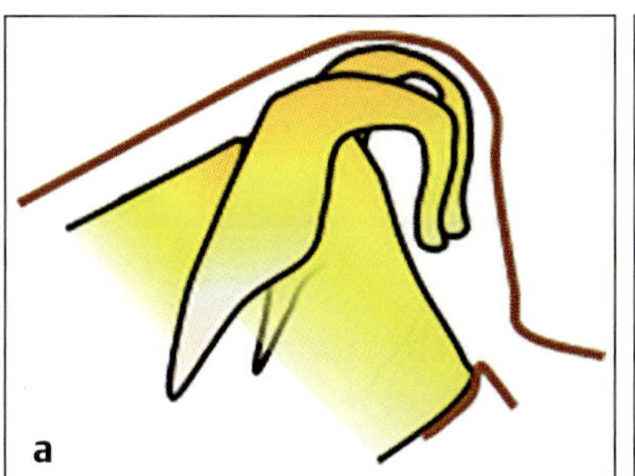

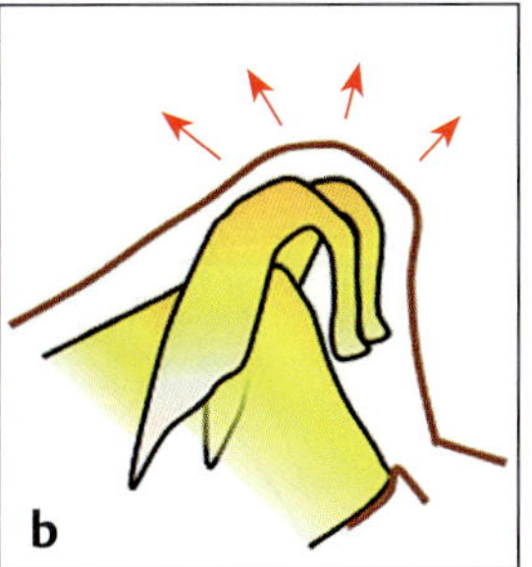

Fig. 13.32 **(a)** The potential energy within the lower lateral cartilage (LLC) maintains its shape and the shape of the lobule. **(b)** As these cartilages are non-weight-bearing, they are shape holding (*red arrows*) by nature.

upper two-thirds or the vault. Three important ligaments that attach the framework to the vault are used for the cantilever effect. The three ligaments are the Pitanguy ligament (PL) which was originally described by Pitanguy as a "dermocartilaginous ligament" occurring in the noses of blacks and in bulbous noses, but Sadan et al found it to correspond to the deep medial layer of nasal SMAS that runs between the anterior septal angle and the interdomal ligament. It runs in the membranous septum, between the caudal border of the septum and the medial crura of the LLC, toward the anterior nasal spine and thus binds the two alar domes to each other and also to the septal angle.[10] Besides this, the intercartilaginous ligament (ICL) binds the lateral crus to the ULC on either side, and the medial crural septal ligament (MCSL) binds the medial crura to the caudal border of the septum (**Fig. 13.31d**).

The SMAS layer of the nose acts as an additional tie rope/suspension. To summarize, the quasi-tripod of the lobule does not rest next to the vault as shown in **Fig. 13.33a**, but is suspended at a higher level because of the cantilever effect as shown in **Fig. 13.33b**.

What Happens after Surgical Exposure?

In closed approach for rhinoplasty, the intercartilaginous incision divides the ICL. When the incision is extended between the caudal border of the septum and the membranous septum (transfixion), the Pitanguy ligament and the MCSL are also divided (**Fig. 13.34a**). This results in sagging of alar cartilages with loss of tip projection by 2 to 3 mm (**Fig. 13.34b**).[11] Some surgeons recommend not to extend the septal incision all the way down to the ANS, conserving the MCSL .[12] Similarly, intercartilaginous incision can be restricted laterally to partially conserve the ICL.

During open approach ICL and Pitanguy ligament are lost during cephalic trim of the alar cartilages, extensive mobilization for their relocation, or upward or downward rotation of the tip. The MCSL is lost during caudal resection of the septum. Whenever possible, the Pitanguy ligament and the ICL should be meticulously sutured.[12] Hitching the LLC to ULC with multiple sutures is also recommended. The sagging can be partly compensated by meticulous closure. In addition, a pack in the nostrils can hold the tip up and use of adhesive tape will act as a tie-rope (**Fig. 13.35**).

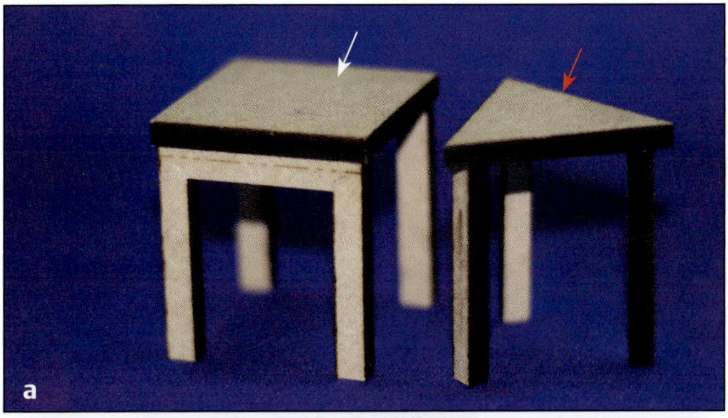

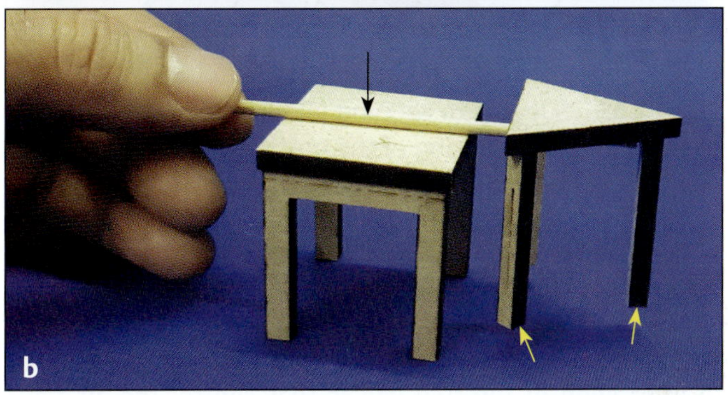

Fig. 13.33 **(a)** General (erroneous) perception about the nose is that the two units (*white* and *red arrows*) are independent of each other. **(b)** Representative illustration of two distinct units of nose where the lower third is shown cantilevered (*yellow arrows*) to the upper two-third with the help of ligaments (*black arrow*).

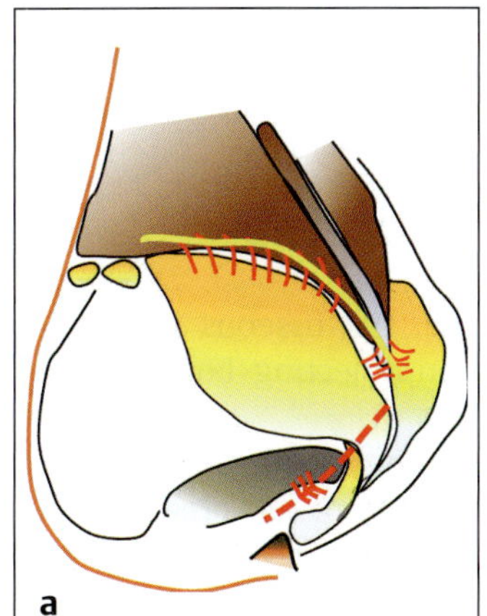

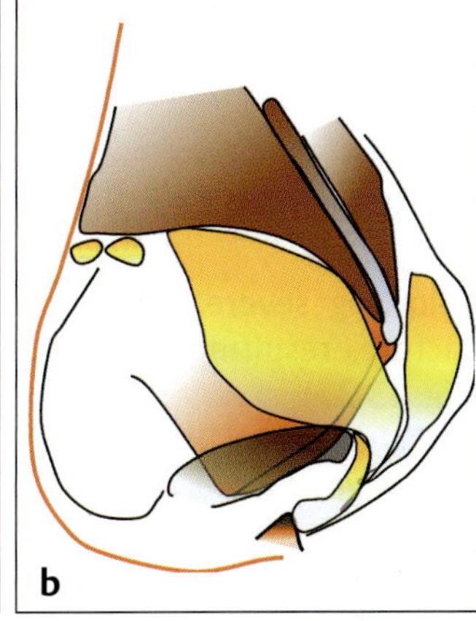

Fig. 13.34 **(a)** The intercartilaginous incision of the closed rhinoplasty cuts through the ligaments which support the lobule resulting in **(b)** sagging of the lobule.

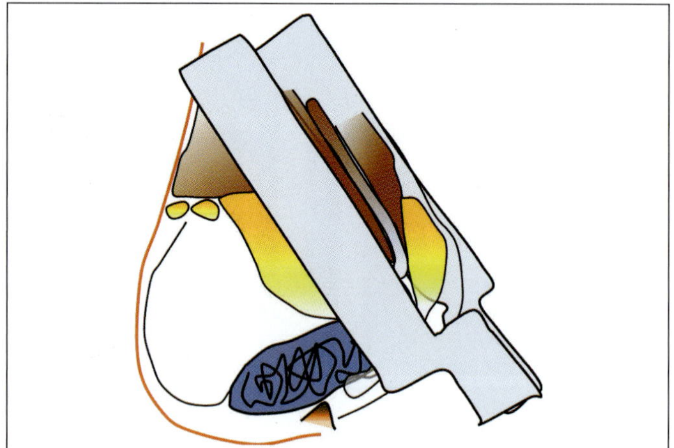

Fig. 13.35 Support to sagging lobule following disruption of ligaments with packing of the nostril cavity (*blue*) and use of adhesive tape.

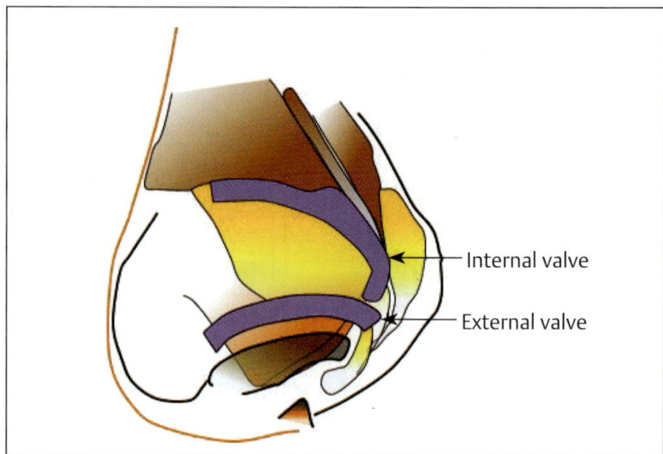

Fig. 13.36 Locations of the internal and external valves.

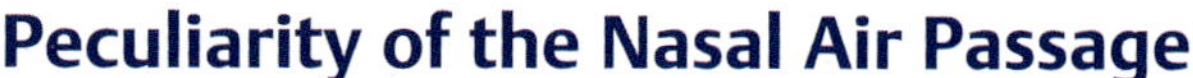

Peculiarity of the Nasal Air Passage

The air passage is not uniform throughout. It is narrower in the region of the two valves that control the air flow. Competence of the valve that allows regulation of air volume is important for proper airway. The external valve is located at the nostril rim while the internal valve is located at the confluence of intercartilaginous region, junction of ULCs, and the septum (**Fig. 13.36**). Some maneuvers used in rhinoplasty may affect the integrity of the framework at these crucial sites. The competence of the valves depends upon the integrity of the cartilages and the elastic potential energy they provide. Hence, these junctions should be adequately supported.

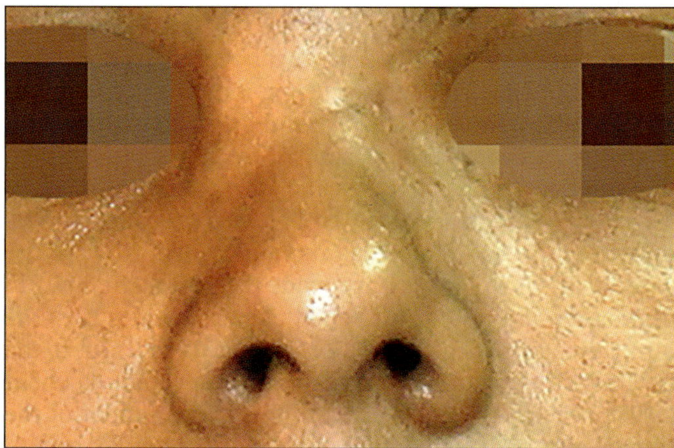

Fig. 13.37 The deformity following a severe frontal impact with a flat, nonprojecting bony dorsum.

Changes after Severe Trauma

Following severe frontal trauma, the osseous vault may fracture, resulting in a flat, nonprojecting bony dorsum (**Fig. 13.37**).

If the impact is restricted to bony vault, it becomes a favorable situation because deformity of this area does not interfere with air flow. With the cartilaginous vault still intact, the deformity is aesthetic in nature, and the valves and the lobule are well supported. This deformity is amenable to grafts to the dorsum and the side walls.

With injury to the cartilaginous vault, the deformity is more complex. The septum buckles and if the accompanying septal hematoma is not drained, the cartilage may resorb.[13] Loss of cartilage results in lowering and flattening of cartilaginous septum. Eventually the ULCs also weaken, resulting in total structural loss to the middle third support. The loss of cartilage volume is attributed to the septal hematoma with or without infection.[14] They may have airway obstruction as the internal valve is not well supported.

When there is trauma to the middle third of the nose with a force of substantial magnitude (**Fig. 13.38a**), there is a very high chance of septal collapse. Deformity occurs due to compression injury to the cartilaginous part of the septum, and if not adequately treated, it may lead to collapse of the midvault (**Fig. 13.38b**).[14]

Constantian has given a detailed description of the deformity following septal collapse.[15] The hallmark of this deformity includes flattened appearance of the nasal dorsum, which can be seen on the frontal view (**Fig. 13.39a**) with accentuation or development of a dorsal hump and narrowing of the middle third of the nose with a blunt tip and a hollow supratip region (**Fig. 13.39b**).[16] This happens because of the collapse of a critical part (dorsocaudal truss) of the septum. There may be a change in the nasal length, the apparent increase in the nasal base size, and apparent bony vault widening. Loss of caudal septal support may result in sharpening of the subnasale, upper lip retrusion with flattening, and posterior displacement of the upper lip. The airway obstruction in these patients is usually due to lack of

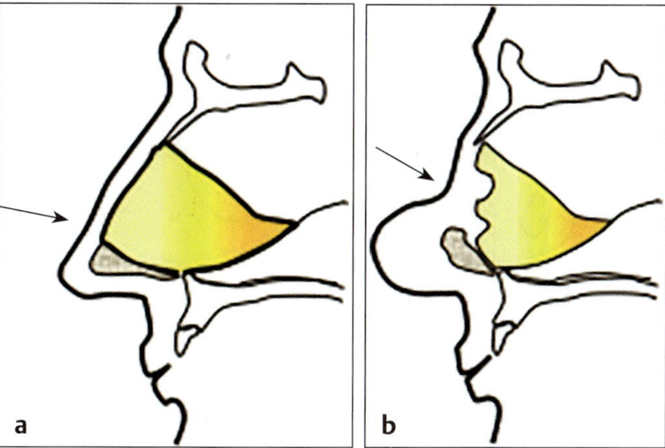

Fig. 13.38 (a) A powerful blow (*black arrow*) to the middle third of the nose results in **(b)** compression injury of the cartilaginous septum leading to collapse of the midvault (*black arrow*).

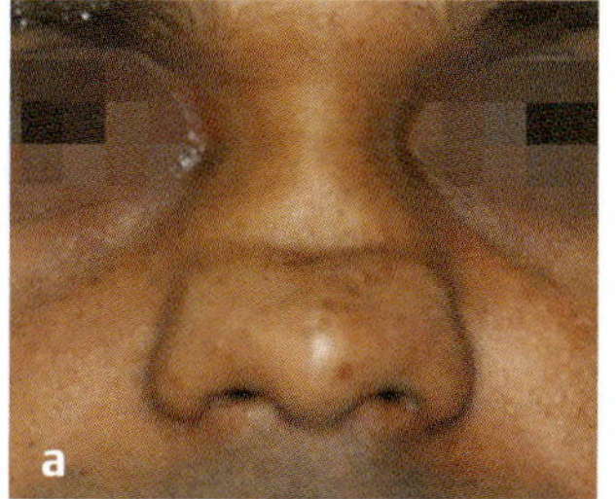

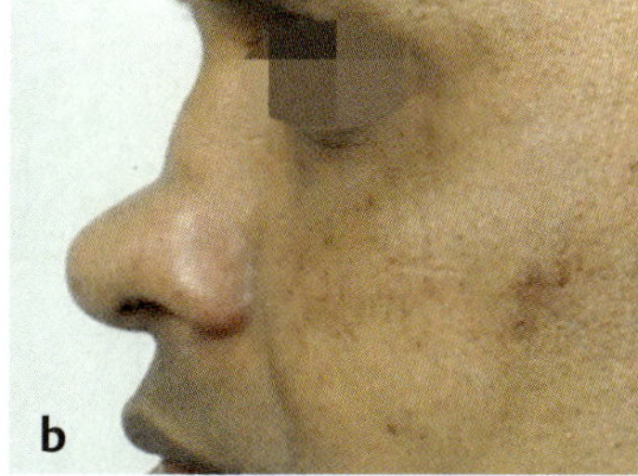

Fig. 13.39 (a) The deformity on frontal view appears as flattened appearance of the dorsum. **(b)** Profile shows accentuation of a dorsal hump and narrowing of the middle third of the nose with a blunt tip and a hollow supratip region. (Reproduced with permission from Bhat et al 2017[17].)

support to the internal valve and not because of deviation of residual septum.

Following septal collapse there is total structural loss to the upper third of the nose. But this loss of support has a secondary effect. As the lobule or the lower third depends on the upper two-thirds for its load bearing, there is loss of support to the lobule as well (**Fig. 13.40**).

There are some clinical tests which support the diagnosis of a septal collapse. The septal support test of Daniel states that when the lobule is compressed, it offers no resistance (**Fig. 13.41**).[16]

The senior author has also mentioned the following diagnostic signs of total septal collapse:[17]

- Shadow sign: On frontal view, a horizontal linear shadow is visible in the middle of the nose (**Fig. 13.42a**). This is a pathognomonic sign of septal collapse.
- Tip-touch sign: When a gentle pressure is applied on the nasal tip, the edge of the pyriform aperture may become visible (**Fig. 13.42b**).

Material for Structural Support

A typical Indian nose is broad and lacks projection. Often, there is a need for augmentation by a significant volume.[18] A severe saddle nose or a cleft lip nose deformity may require still a larger volume. The autologous cartilage has distinct advantages over alloplastic materials.[19] It withstands functional stress better, can survive in a scarred bed, and chances of resorption are less.

The costal cartilage is the best material among the options simply because it provides volume in abundance. The popular diced grafts may not be suitable for structural support as they are loose, yield to pressure, and can neither bear load nor provide the potential energy for support. The structural grafts, either for load bearing or shape holding must be compact or noncollapsible (**Fig. 13.43**).

The costal cartilage is criticized for its quality of warping. However, techniques are available to overcome this problem. "Precision carving technique" allows warping to happen and uses the phenomenon to advantage.[20] As stated by Gibson and Davis, surface incisions on a cartilage make the surface expand, inducing a curvature.[21] Similarly, incisions on the concave surface would make the surface expand, neutralizing the curvature and straightening the piece. Thus, by making surface incisions of different depths and spacing (scoring) on the given surface, or if required on both the surfaces, the desired contouring can be affected in a cartilage graft. "Oblique section" and the "Namaste" techniques are other techniques to prevent warping.[22,23]

Support Provision to Upper Two-Thirds or Osseocartilaginous Vault

Depending on the mode of trauma, we may encounter cases with varied presentations. The involvement patterns may be grossly classified as upper (bony) and middle (cartilaginous) with or without secondary lower third structural loss. In addition, we also should assess whether the deformity involves isolated loss of buttress, isolated septal collapse, or a combination of both. In such cases, the requirement of cartilage is more and therefore costal cartilage is used.

Loss of upper third bony vault causes decreased projection of tip indicating structural loss. A clay template can be used for estimation of volume loss and thus the desired dimension of grafts (**Fig. 13.44b**).

When there is a structural loss of middle third cartilaginous vault with secondary structural loss of lower third lobule, the deformities are traditionally corrected by either a cantilever graft or an L-graft. A cantilever bone graft is fixed rigidly to the nasal bones using a screw. This gives an unnatural result as it uses only a single rigid piece of framework, which tends to be displaced outward. Alternatively,

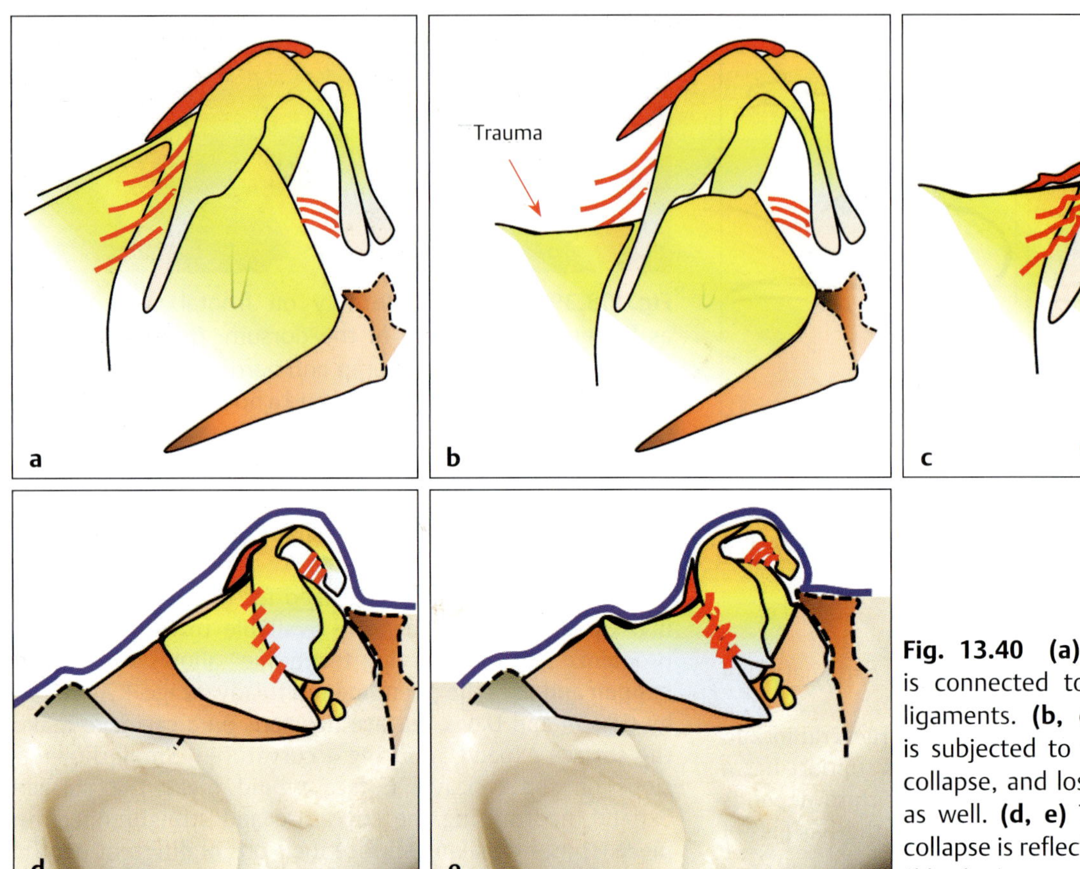

Fig. 13.40 **(a)** The lower third of nose is connected to the upper third by the ligaments. **(b, c)** When the upper third is subjected to trauma which results in a collapse, and loss of support to the lobule as well. **(d, e)** This secondary framework collapse is reflected on the envelope as well (*blue line*).

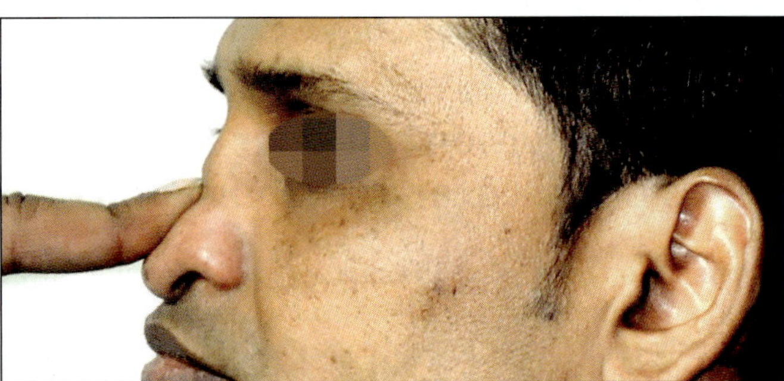

Fig. 13.41 On septal support test, compression of the lobule by digital pressure to the supratip region offers no resistance. (Reproduced with permission from Bhat et al 2017[17].)

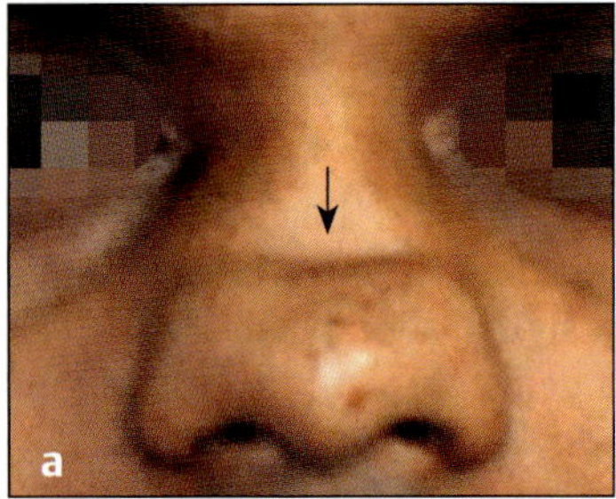

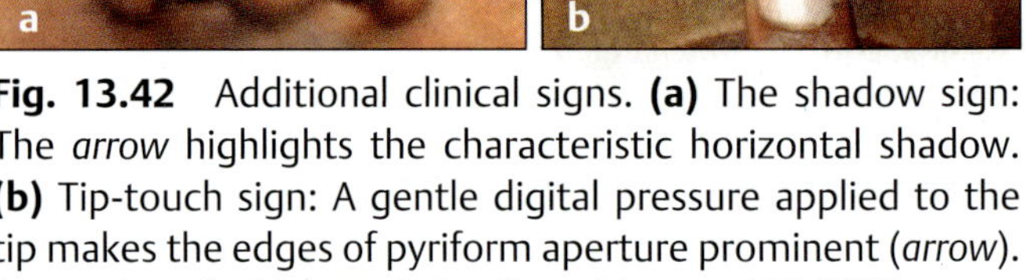

Fig. 13.42 Additional clinical signs. **(a)** The shadow sign: The *arrow* highlights the characteristic horizontal shadow. **(b)** Tip-touch sign: A gentle digital pressure applied to the tip makes the edges of pyriform aperture prominent (*arrow*). (Reproduced with permission from Bhat et al 2017[17].)

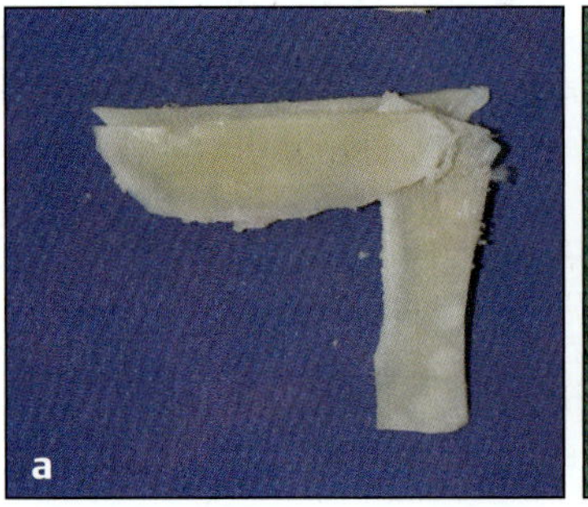

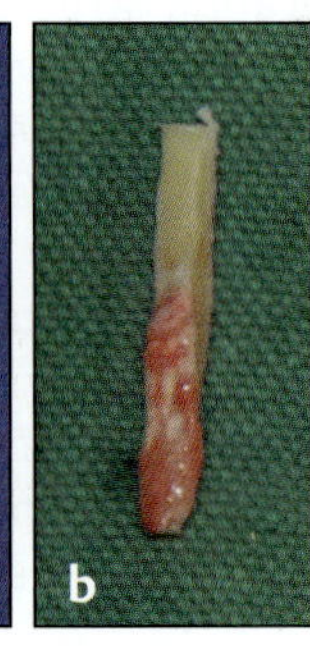

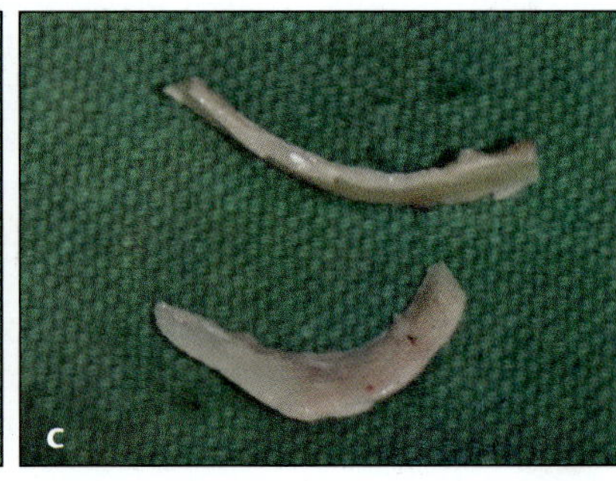

Fig. 13.43 Cartilage grafts for load-bearing support. **(a)** A septal construct and **(b)** columellar strut. **(c)** Alar cartilage grafts for alar support.

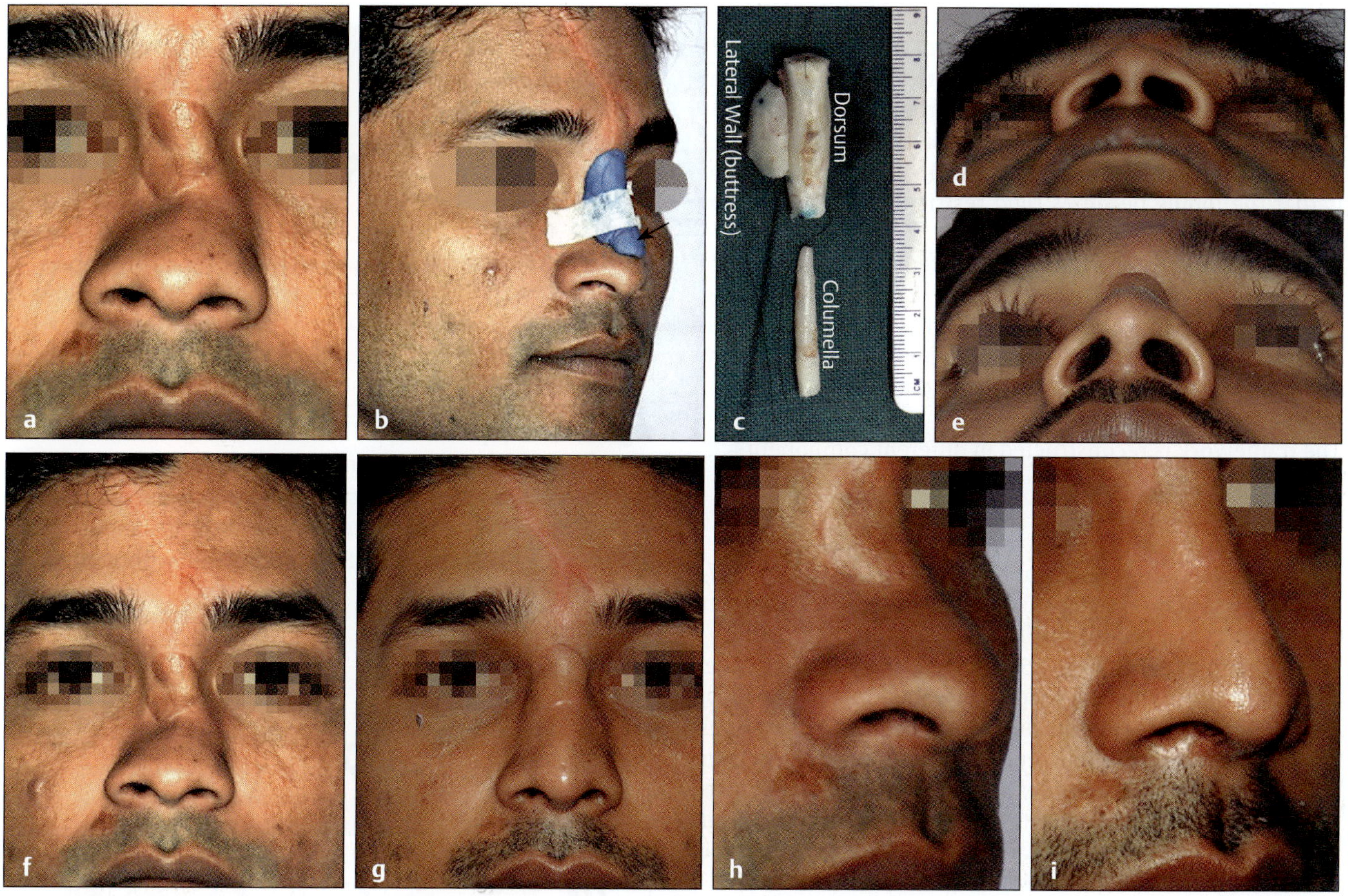

Fig. 13.44 **(a)** The telltale deformity seen in collapse of buttress after trauma to the bony framework. **(b)** Use of clay template (*arrow*) to assess the size and volume of the defect to accurately estimate the cartilage requirement. **(c)** Use of eighth costal cartilage to carve the dorsal onlay graft, columellar strut, and the lateral buttress graft. **(d, e)** The frontal view shows the volume deficit has been adequately corrected. **(f, g)** The oblique views shows an aesthetic appearance and **(h, i)** the projection appears good on the worm's eye view. (Reproduced with permission from Bhat et al 2014[20].)

graft is used which consists of two components, the dorsal graft which extends to the tip and the caudal graft which lies below the membranous septum in the columellar region (**Fig. 13.45**).

Both these methods may provide some support, but do not take into consideration the resemblance of the septal support to a truss. Both the methods result in a single rigid framework and disregard the basic two component nature of nasal structure: a rigid or semi-rigid upper two thirds and a soft and elastic lower third. Hence, the result obtained may be compromised.

In the cantilever graft technique, the bony or cartilage graft is used as a cantilevered beam, usually fixed at the cranial end to the nasal bone with a stainless-steel wire or a screw (**Fig. 13.45a**). The free, unsupported caudal end of the graft extends right up to the tip with no caudal supporting strut. The downside of a cantilever fixation is the shear force and hence the area around the hardware is under stress, which may lead to loosening up of the framework and subsequent collapse. Besides this, if bone is used as a graft,

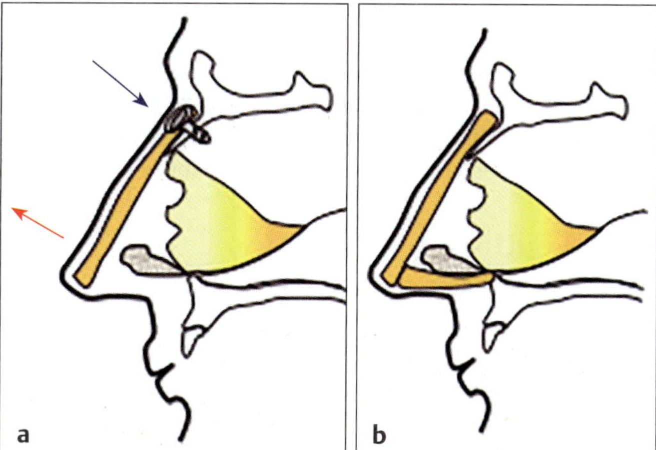

Fig. 13.45 Traditionally used structural support techniques. **(a)** Cantilever graft technique, *blue arrow* indicates screw fixation and *red arrow* indicates risk of outward displacement. **(b)** L-graft consisting of two components: dorsal and caudal grafts. (Reproduced with permission from Bhat et al 2017[17].)

it may get resorbed, leading to an unacceptable appearance. The unsupported end is prone to trauma and fracture too.[24]

The conventional "L-graft" has both dorsal and caudal limbs, but the caudal limb is placed in the columella and not in the caudal septal area. The dorsal limb extends from the radix to the tip of the nose (**Fig. 13.45b**). The disadvantage is that the lobule becomes rigid restricting the mobility of the tip.

To overcome these problems, a better way of reconstruction is to support the vault and the lobule by providing separate frameworks as recommended by Daniel et al.[16] We must provide a truss for the septum, a buttress for the lateral walls, and a strut for the columella and a dorsal onlay graft when needed.

The framework is reconstructed in different components.

Septal Construct or a "truss"

Approximately 1 cm width of the dorsocaudal truss is sufficient to maintain the structural integrity.[25,26] This construct consists of two pieces of cartilage:

- A strip of graft, 20 to 25 mm long, 10 to 12 mm wide, and 3 mm thick, is braced on either side by a pair of slightly longer pieces on either side. The three pieces together mimic the septum braced by the spreader grafts and thus provides support to the internal valve. In a situation of shortage of cartilage, two thicker pieces are enough instead of three. This constitutes the dorsal rafter (**Fig. 13.46a**) of the truss.
- A graft 20 to 25 mm long, 10 to 12 mm wide, and 2 to 3 mm thick, serving as the caudal septal strip or the caudal rafter, fits into the assembly of dorsal rafter at a suitable angle. The caudal rafter graft is split at the posterior end for anchoring to the ANS (**Fig. 13.46c**).

The septal component or the truss is L-shaped, like any other truss, but it is different from the conventional "L-graft" (**Fig. 13.45b**). The dorsal component or the "dorsal rafter" extends only till the septal angle area and not up to the tip. Unlike the conventional "L-graft", the caudal part of this construct mimics the natural caudal area of the septum. It keeps the membranous septum free as it lies cranial to the membranous septum and not in the columella.

Lateral Buttress Graft

Along with the septum, if there is loss of buttress as well, reconstructing the septum alone will result in a compromised result, not just aesthetically but functionally as well, as the lateral grafts provide additional reinforcement to the internal valve (**Fig. 13.47**).

Columellar Strut

This is used to provide tip support. The graft is approximately 2 to 3 mm in thickness so that it does not encroach on the membranous septum (**Fig. 13.47**).

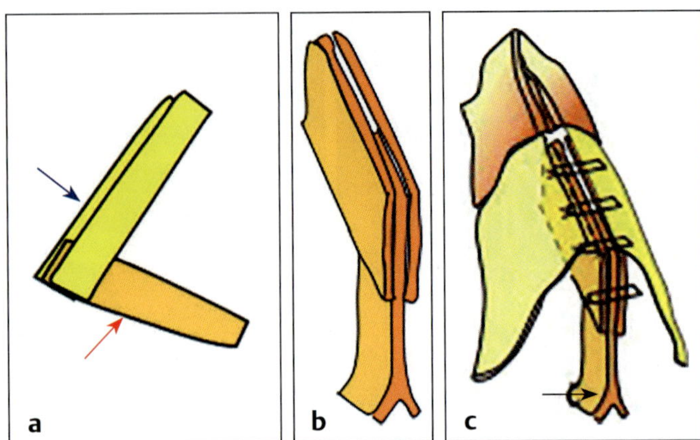

Fig. 13.46 **(a)** The septal construct consists of a pair of dorsal grafts (*blue arrow*) and one caudal graft (*red arrow*). **(b)** The construct acts as a truss. **(c)** The caudal graft is split at its posterior end (*black arrow*) so that it fits snugly on to the anterior nasal spine (ANS). (Reproduced with permission from Bhat et al 2017[17].)

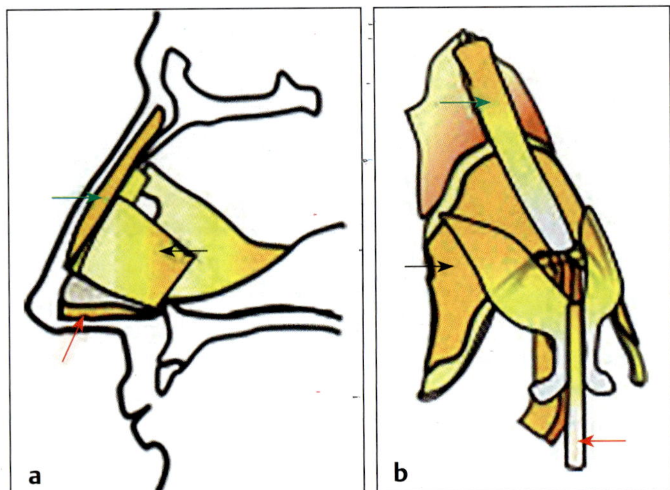

Fig. 13.47 **(a)** The lateral buttress grafts (*black arrow*) provides reinforcement to the internal valve. The columellar strut (*red arrow*) should be placed in a compartment separate from the septal construct and the dorsal onlay graft (*green arrow*) imparts projection and definition to the dorsum. **(b)** An oblique view illustrating the lateral buttress grafts (*black arrow*), the columellar strut (*red arrow*), and the dorsal onlay graft (*green arrow*).

Dorsal Onlay Graft

The dorsal onlay graft provides additional framework to support the internal valve by volume augmentation.[27] Secondly, the dorsal rafter of the septal construct alone may not always be sufficient to provide an aesthetic profile line. For adequate projection, definition, and width of the nasal dorsum, an onlay graft may be tailored as per the requirement (**Fig. 13.47**).

These different compositions of framework should be judiciously used (**Fig. 13.48**). All the components may not be required in some cases of structural loss of lesser severity.

This technique has distinct advantages over the traditional techniques:

- It maintains pliability of the lobule as the framework is constructed as separate components.
- It ensures better support to the internal valve as it incorporates three different ways of valve support: the septal construct that mimics spreader grafts, the dorsal onlay graft, and the ULC support grafts, thus minimizing the chances of failure.
- The dorsal onlay component also offers better control of aesthetic needs.

Provision of Support for a Weakened Septum (Scoring after Septoplasty) and the Internal Valve

A deviated septum is a commonly encountered condition in practice. However, if principles of structural restoration are not adhered to, the consequences can be catastrophic. This is because in such cases, the septum has to be exposed by releasing most of its attachments. This obviously results in an iatrogenic weakness of the framework as its integrity has been disturbed.

Usually, the septal cartilage is separated from the ULCs and the vomerine groove. The curvatures may be neutralized

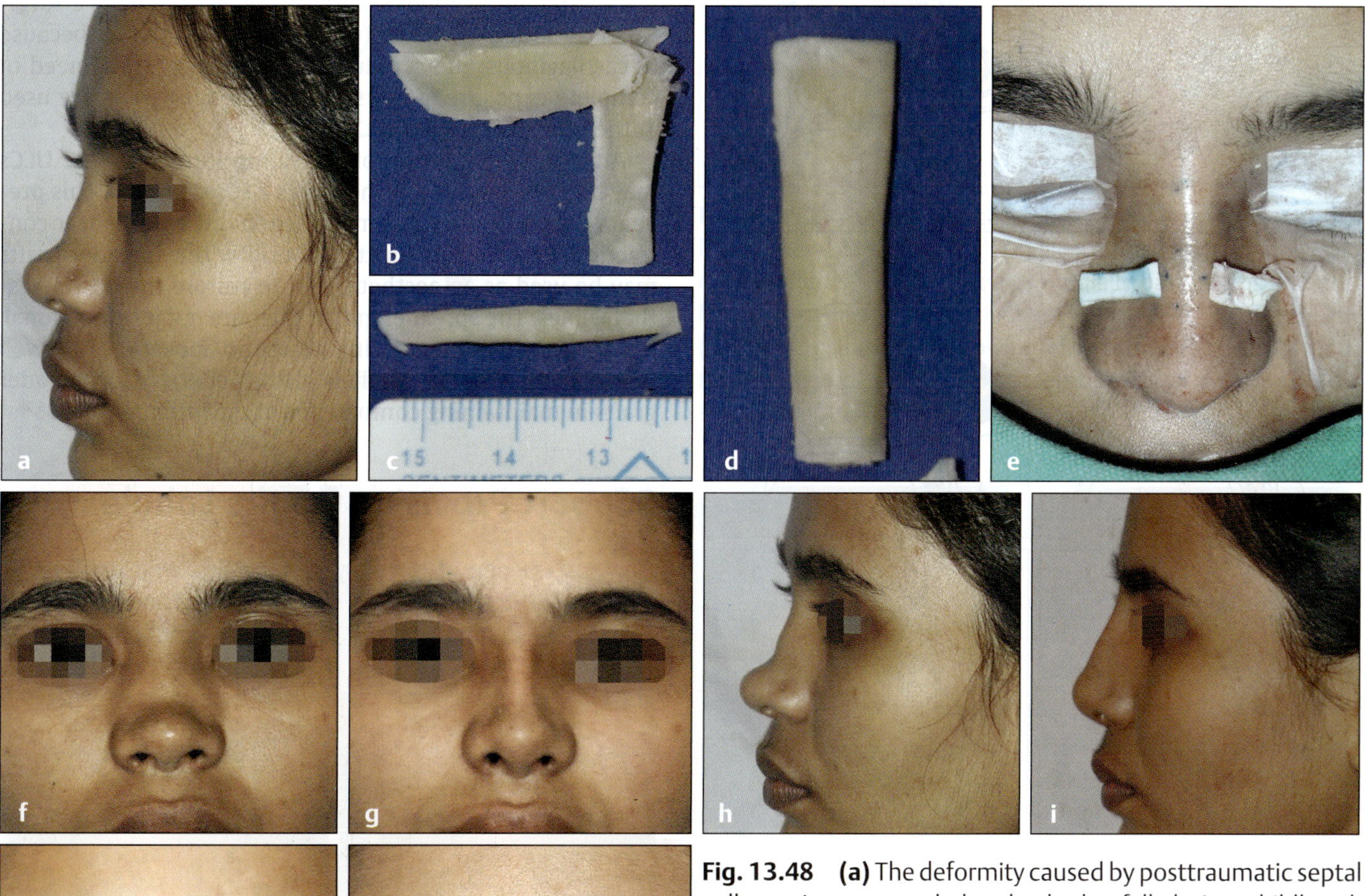

Fig. 13.48 **(a)** The deformity caused by posttraumatic septal collapse in a young lady who had a fall during childhood. **(b)** The septal construct shaped as a truss. Although it is L-shaped like a conventional "L-graft", the dorsal rafter extends only till the septal angle and not up to the tip. **(c)** The lateral buttress grafts. **(d)** The columellar strut, and **(e)** a dorsal onlay graft to improve the profile. **(f, g)** The change in frontal view which postoperatively shows narrow slender appearance with dorsal aesthetic lines. **(h, i)** Profile shows adequate projection and a well-defined profile line. **(j, k)** The pliability of the lobule can be appreciated. (Reproduced with permission from Bhat et al 2017[17].)

Tebbetts has described a septal-medial crural suture for support of the medial crura.[32] This suture is placed between the caudal edge of the septum and the medial crura, going across the membranous septum, and tied with adjustable tension (**Fig. 13.54**). As discussed earlier, the septum rests on the bony platform. The MCS suture acts as a tie or suspension rope hitching the medial crura to the caudal septum. Thus it provides a load-bearing support to hanging or a floating assembly of the medial crura. The suture can be effectively used for correction of hanging columella (**Fig. 13.55**).

Just like a columellar strut provides the medial pod of the tripod, the lateral limbs can be made to rest on the terra firma using a lateral crural strut graft (**Fig. 13.56**). This graft stabilizes the cartilage from the lateral side, making it rest on the pyriform region.

The method is useful in cases where the alar cartilages are weak or damaged; and in cleft lip nose correction (**Fig. 13.57**).

Suture Techniques for Lobule Support

The above-mentioned maneuvers describe different methods of the load-bearing support to the lobule. The shape-holding support is best provided by suture modification of the tip. The transdomal, interdomal, lateral crural mattress sutures and intercrural sutures provide potential energy that moulds the cartilages in a better shape (**Figs. 13.58 and 13.59**).

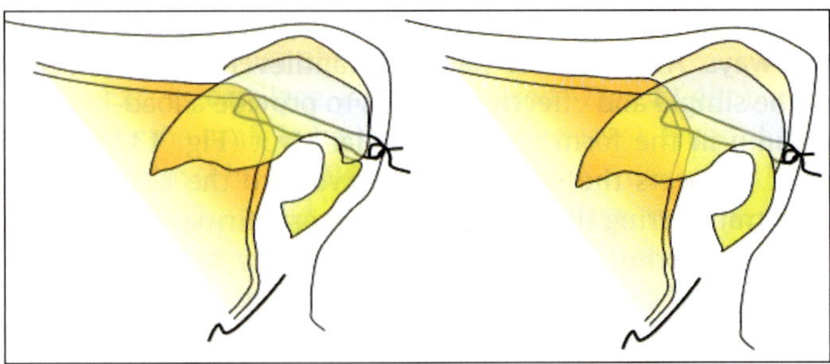

Fig. 13.54 The medial crural septal suture (*blue*) acts as a suspension which hitches the medial crura to the septum.

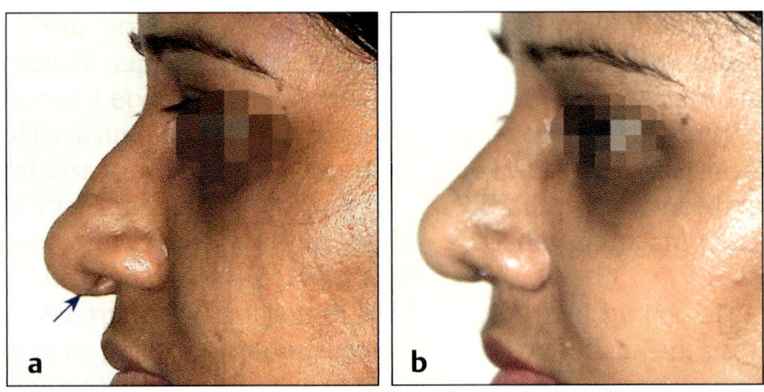

Fig. 13.55 **(a)** Profile showing a hanging columella (*blue arrow*). **(b)** The deformity was effectively corrected using medial crural septal suture. (Reproduced with permission from Bhat et al 2019[30].)

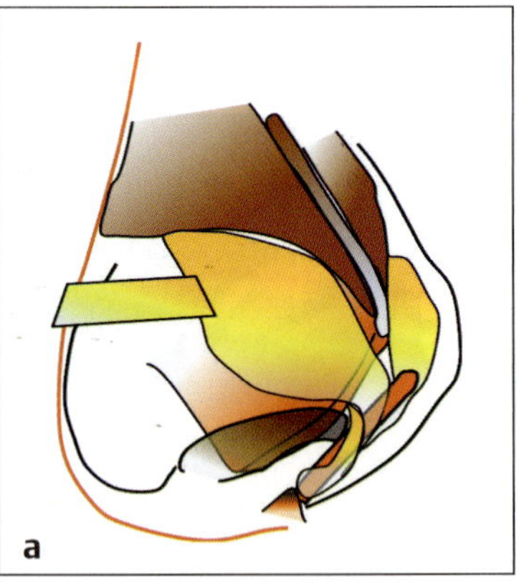

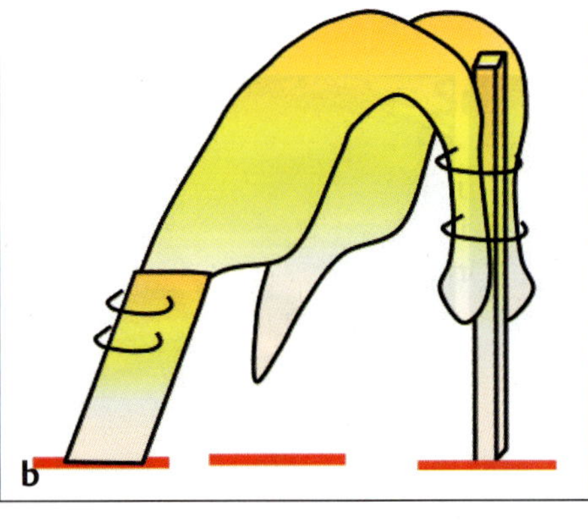

Fig. 13.56 **(a)** The lateral crural strut graft is a load-bearing support which connects the lateral crura of alar cartilage to the pyriform aperture. **(b)** Columellar strut and a lateral crural strut graft convert a floating pseudotripod to a true tripod.

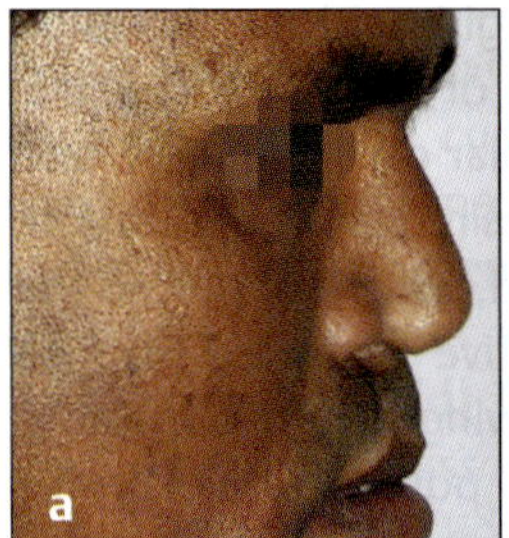

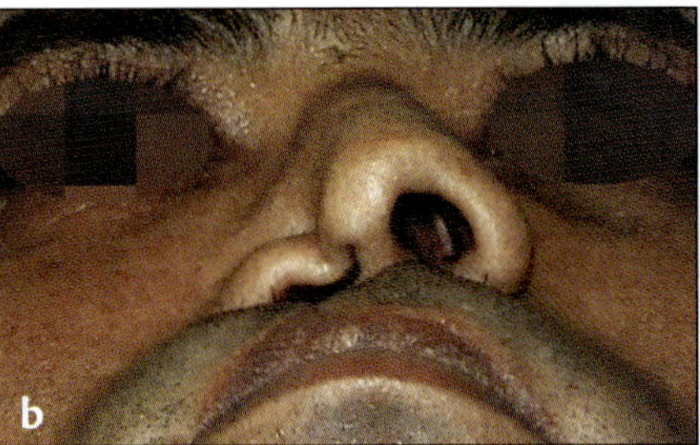

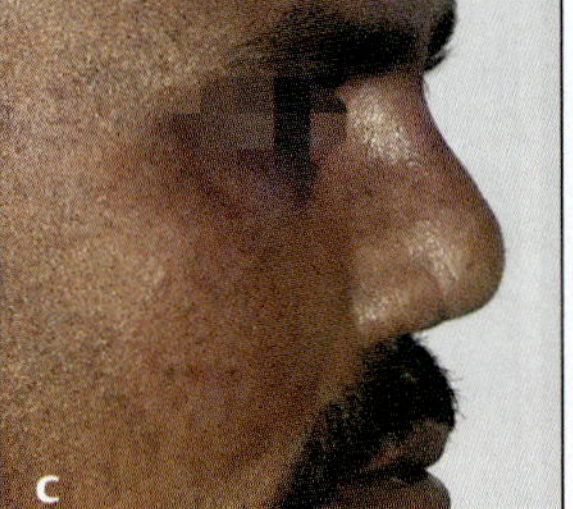

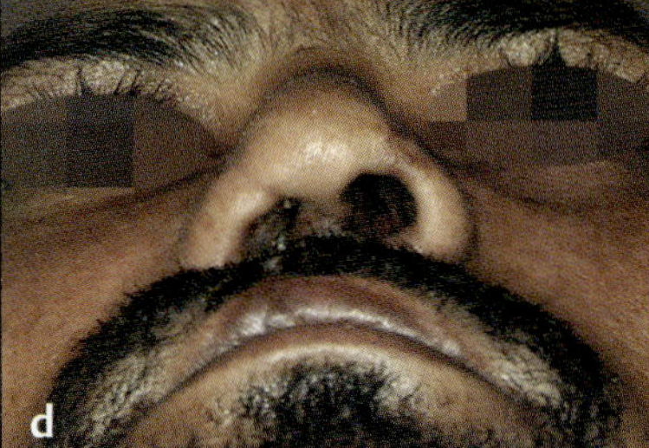

Fig. 13.57 Use of lateral crural strut, columellar strut, and dorsal onlay grafts in the correction of unilateral cleft lip nose deformity. **(a, b)** Preoperative profile and basal views showing collapse of the framework on the cleft side. **(c, d)** Postoperative profile and basal views with the use of cartilage struts and dorsal graft.

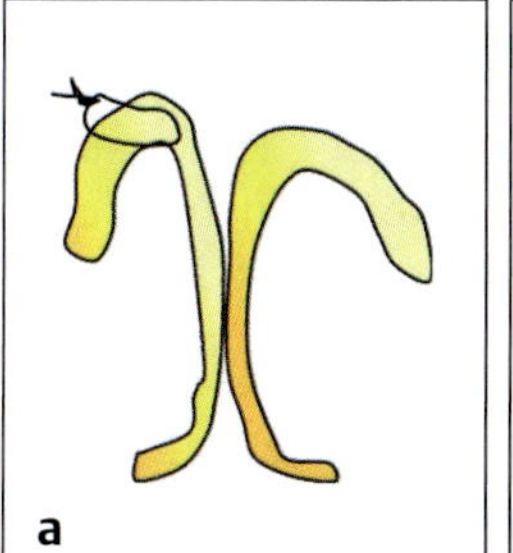
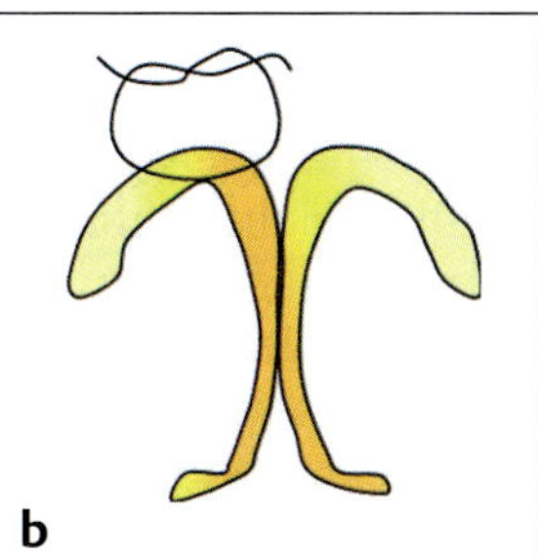
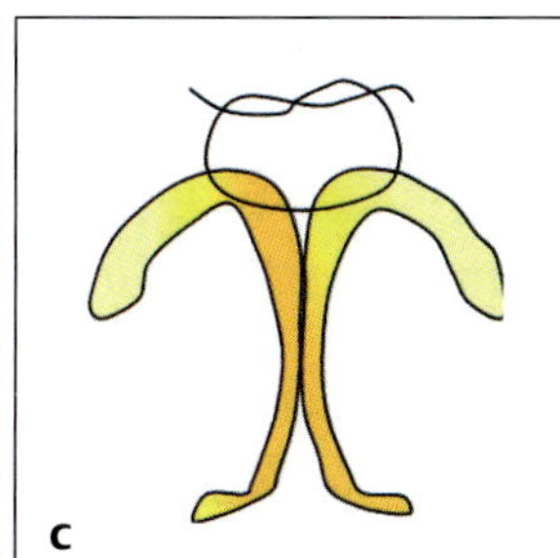
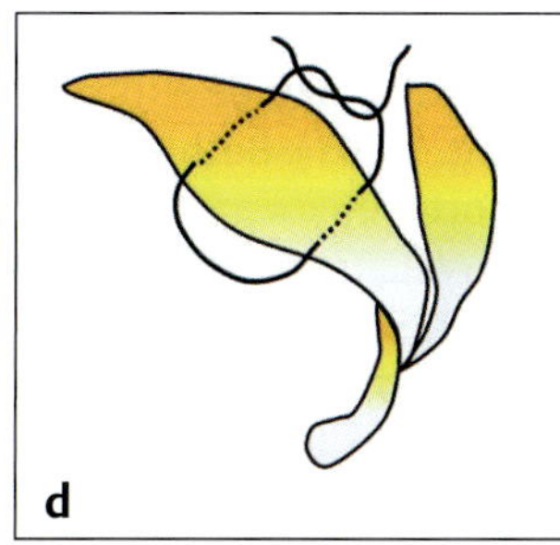
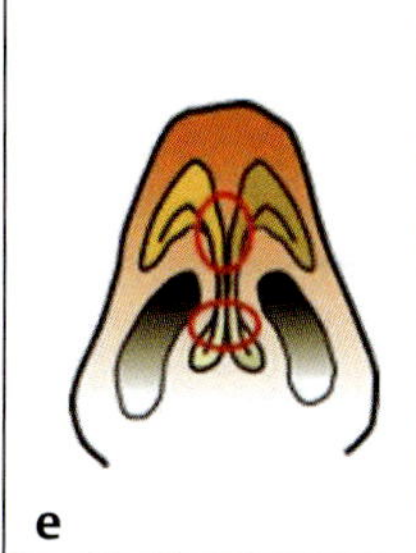

Fig. 13.58 Suture modifications on alar cartilages in the form of **(a, b)** effect obtained with transdomal sutures. **(c)** Interdomal suture. **(d)** Lateral crural mattress sutures, and **(e)** intercrural sutures offer shape-holding support by providing potential energy.

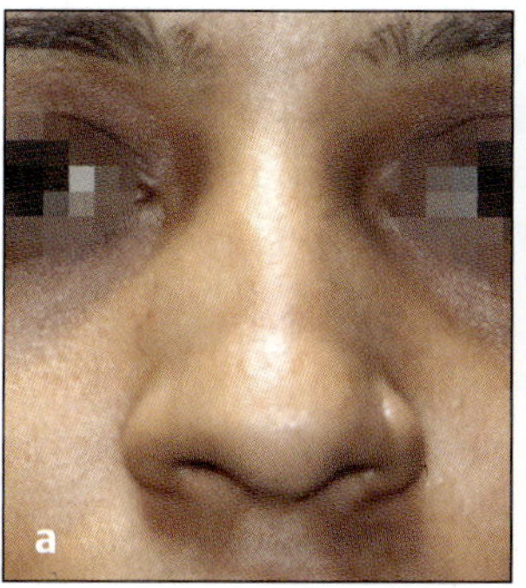
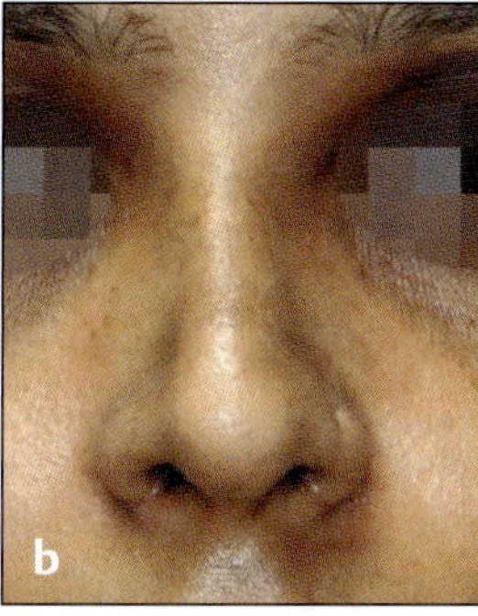
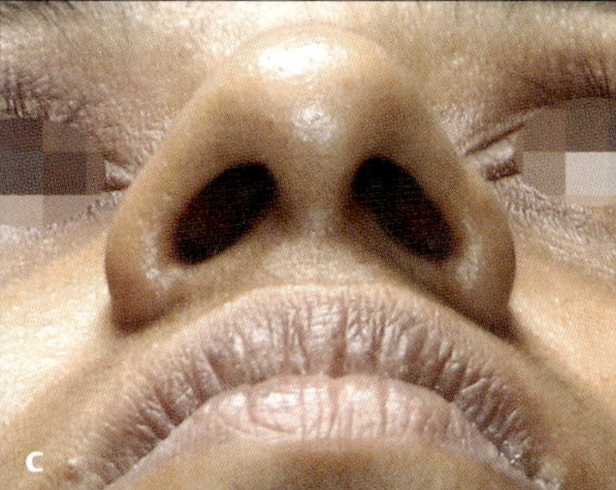
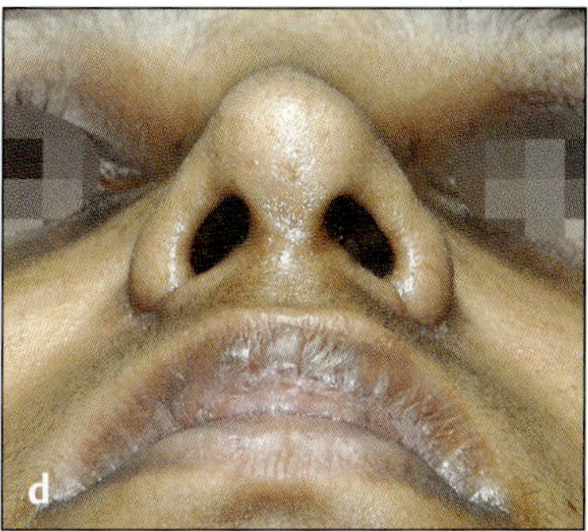

Fig. 13.59 A young lady with deviated nasal septum and poorly defined tip. **(a)** Front and **(c)** worm's view preoperatively. **(b)** The tip was modified using transdomal and interdomal sutures and the tip defining points can be appreciated on the frontal view. **(d)** The gain in projection can be seen on the basal view. Alar wedge resection and alar cinch suture were also used.

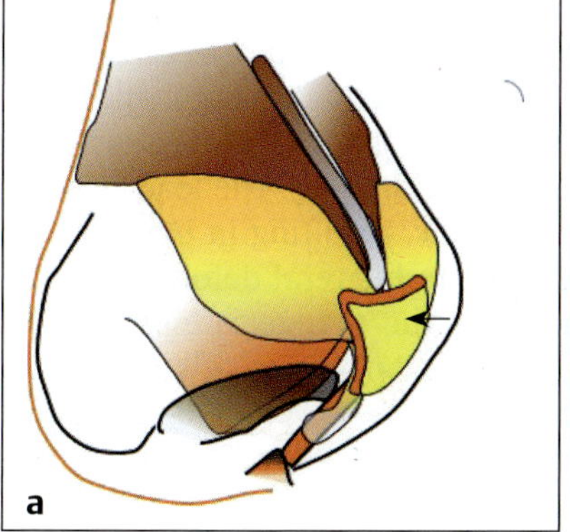
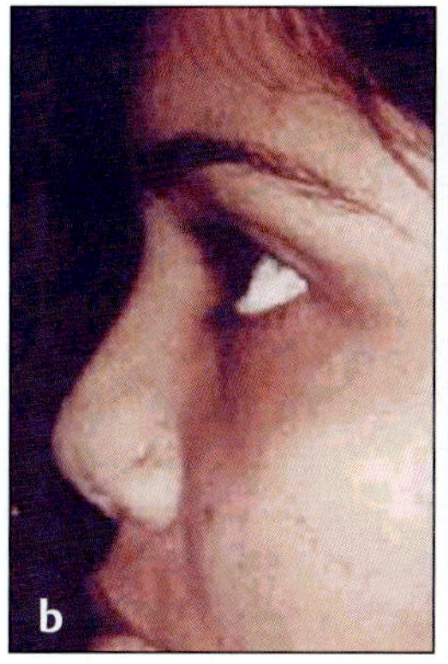
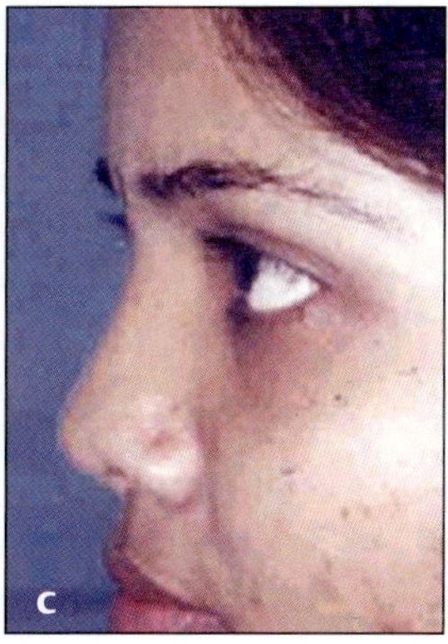

Fig. 13.60 **(a)** Illustration showing position of a tip graft (*black arrow*). **(b, c)** The result obtained by using a tip graft: pre- and postoperative profile pictures showing a well-defined tip.

Cartilage Grafts for Tip Support

In addition to these, tip grafts may also be used (**Fig. 13.60**). These grafts utilize the potential energy to stretch the skin envelope, thus providing shape-holding support.

Extrinsic Methods of Lobule Support

Temporary support can be provided by extrinsic means as well. A simple way to provide support postoperatively is to use an adhesive tape till healing occurs (**Fig. 13.35**). Silastic splint kept in the nostrils for a short period is also useful to maintain alar configuration, particularly after correction of cleft lip nose.

Rohrich et al have recommended a graduated approach for tip/lobule support.[33] Load-bearing support is the first option, using a columellar strut. This should be followed by shape-holding support of suture modification. Tip graft may be added, if further projection is required.

Support Provision for the External Valve

External valve problems may occur in posttraumatic deformities or because of excessive cephalic trim of the alar cartilages. The conventional columellar strut lifts the tip up and thus in a way supports the external valve to some extent. In addition, the external valve may be supported using rim grafts or batten grafts (**Fig. 13.61**). Both of these grafts provide shape-holding support.

In cases where there is collapse of the nostril (**Fig. 13.62a**), an alar batten graft (**Fig. 13.62b**) can restore integrity of the framework and prevent closure of nostril during inspiration (**Fig. 13.62c**).

The alar cartilages may be inherently weak or deformed, resulting in pinched appearance of the nose (**Fig. 13.63a**). The alar cartilages are concave in shape, instead of the usual convexity (**Fig. 13.63b**). The lower 6 to 7 mm of alar cartilages are sufficient to maintain the integrity of the framework.[34] In such cases, the incision used for cephalic trim is carried through only half the depth of the cartilage and the cephalic portion of the LLCs is used as a "turned-in" flap. This turned-in flap acts like a batten, supporting the rest of the alar cartilage from the inner side (**Fig. 13.63c**). This maneuver, coupled with the domal sutures, creates the natural convexity of the alar cartilages (**Fig. 13.63d, e**). It also improves breathing apart from pleasing aesthetic result.

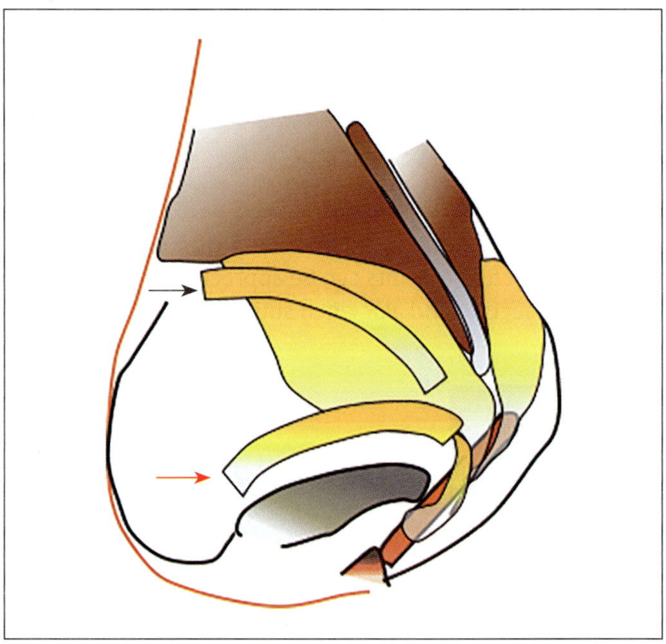

Fig. 13.61 The external valve region may be reinforced by use of either an alar batten graft (*black arrow*) or a rim graft (*red arrow*).

Structural Support in Cleft Lip Nasal Deformity

The nasal deformity associated with cleft lip is one of the most challenging ones faced by plastic surgeons. The pinched appearance of alar cartilage continues to be a stigma even after the lip has been corrected (**Fig. 13.64**).

The deformity is resistant to correction and has been rightly attributed to deficiency of envelope as well as the framework. The deficiency or underdevelopment of the framework is severe when the cleft extends into the alveolus and the palate and in patients who missed nasoalveolar molding (NAM) or preoperative orthodontics. The alveolar and maxillary platform on the cleft side are deficient (**Fig. 13.65**), situated more posteriorly. In a unilateral deformity, this results in tilting of the base and the cleft-sided buttress, or the lateral wall is shorter, due to sagging of its foundation. This results in tilting of the pyramid, including the septum. The deviation coupled with inherent deficiency of the septum results in loss of projection and tilting of the tip. The asymmetry gets reflected in the lobule and the upper two-thirds. The cleft-sided alar cartilage is smaller, does not have enough potential energy, and loosens the shape-holding support, having a flatter cartilage with pinched appearance (**Fig. 13.65a–d**). The load-bearing cantilevering ligaments are weak, resulting in inferoposteriorly dislocated alar cartilage. In bilateral deformity, there is a semblance of symmetry, as the changes are present on both the sides; however, the deficiency is equally severe. On adding to this the deficiency of the envelope, particularly the columella, the correction of the deformity becomes a challenge (**Fig. 13.65e, f**)

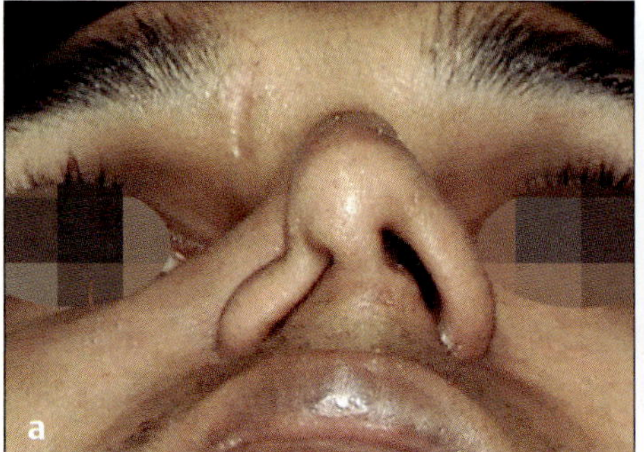

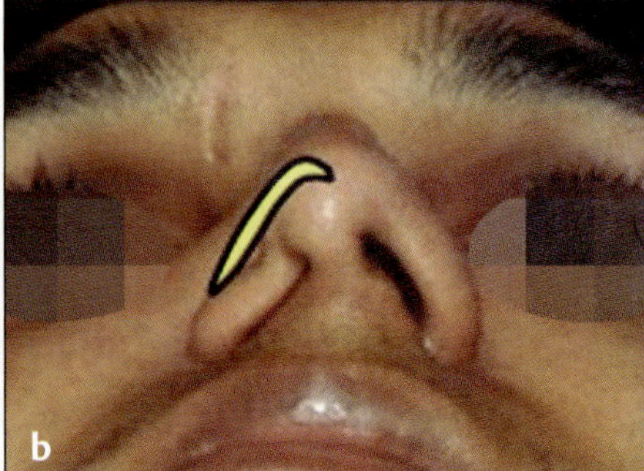

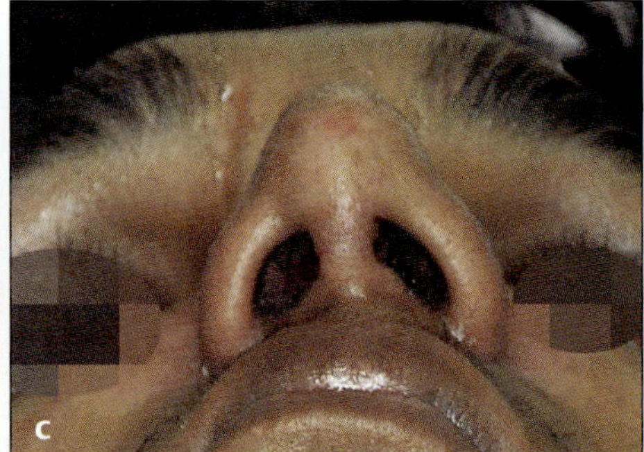

Fig. 13.62 **(a)** A young boy with posttraumatic collapse of the external valve. **(b)** Planning of the proposed alar batten graft. **(c)** Postoperative result shows corrected deformity and an acceptable shape of nostril. The patient did not experience closure of the nostril during inspiration.

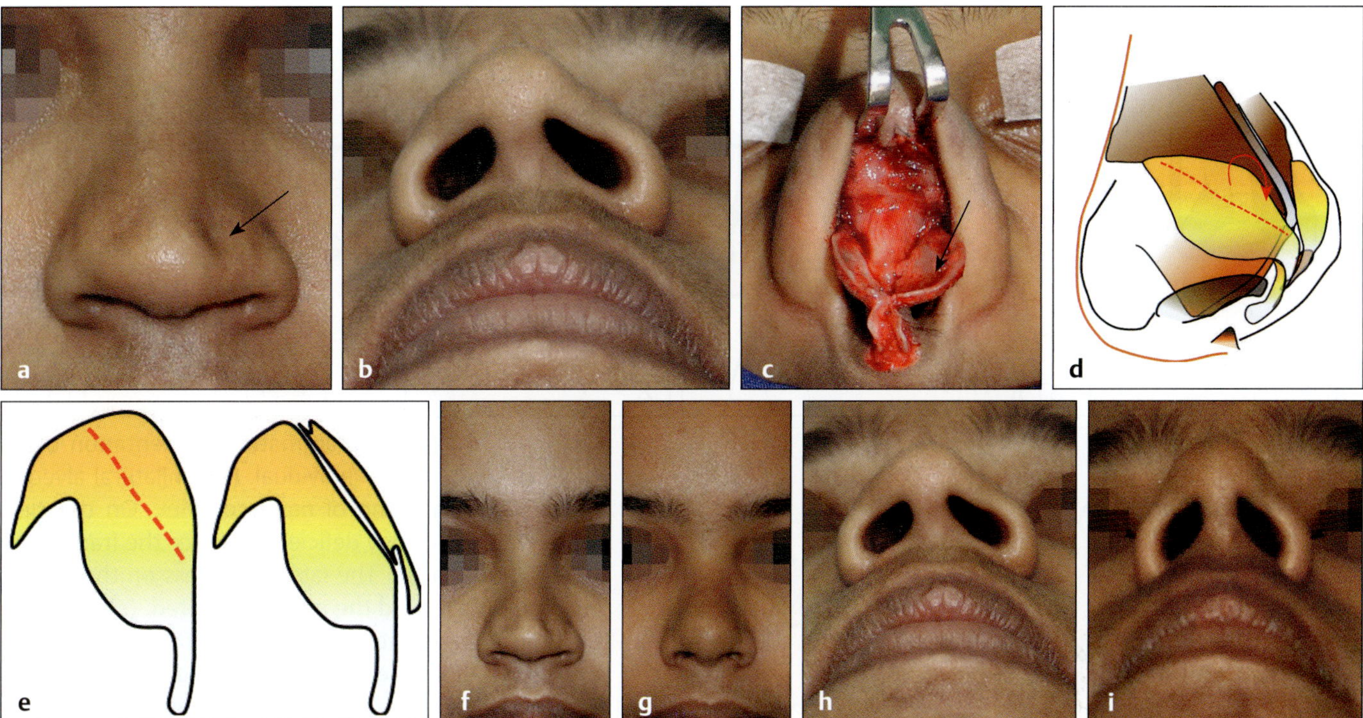

Fig. 13.63 **(a)** An inherent weakness of alar cartilages presenting as pinched appearance of the nostrils (*black arrow*). **(b)** The deformity on the worm's view. **(c)** The alar cartilages were found to be concave instead of the usual convex orientation. **(d, e)** The cephalic portions of the alar cartilages were used as turn-in flaps to reinforce the weakened cartilages (movement denoted by *red arrow*). **(f, g)** This restored the natural convexity of the cartilages resulting in an aesthetic appearance of the lobule. **(h, i)** The result can be appreciated on the worm's eye view as well.

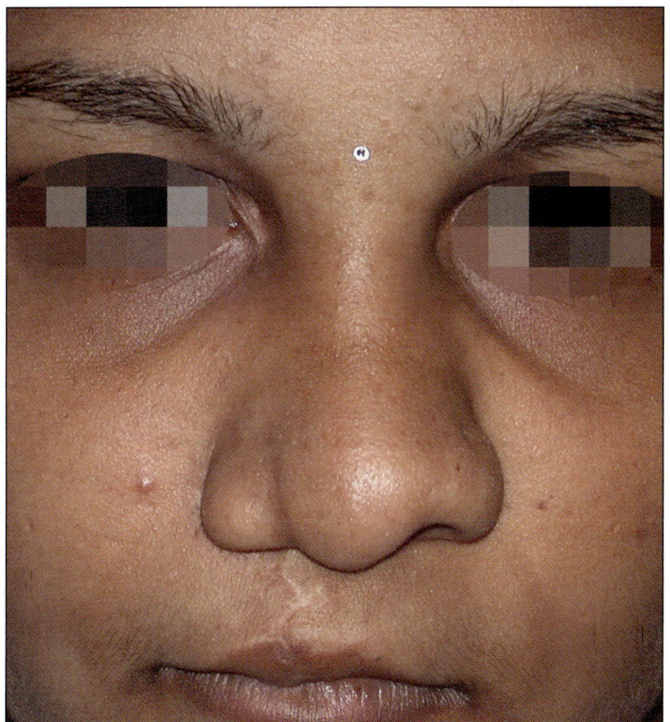

Fig. 13.64 The stigmata of a cleft lip nasal deformity remain even after correction of the lip deformity.

The principles of correction include raising the maxillary platform by arch preparation, alveolar bone grafting, maxillary osteotomy, or pyriform border augmentation by graft under the alar base, depending on the indication. The pyramid must be straightened by septal correction and osteotomies. The framework may be strengthened by addition of a septal truss, brace grafts, onlay grafts, and buttress grafts when indicated. The potential energy of alar cartilage is augmented by suture modification, alar batten graft, or lateral crural strut graft. The columella may be lengthened by V-Y advancement (**Fig. 13.66**).

Structural Support in Binder Syndrome

Like in the correction of cleft lip nasal deformity, another challenging scenario is the correction of nose in a patient with Binder syndrome (**Fig. 13.67a**). In these cases not only the framework, but the soft tissue envelope also is inadequate, particularly the columellar.[35] The plinth of the architecture is deficient, in the form of retruded maxillary platform. In addition, the septal projection is less, with a flattened septal angle. The alar cartilages may have an obtuse curvature. The prospective plan of correction includes augmentation of

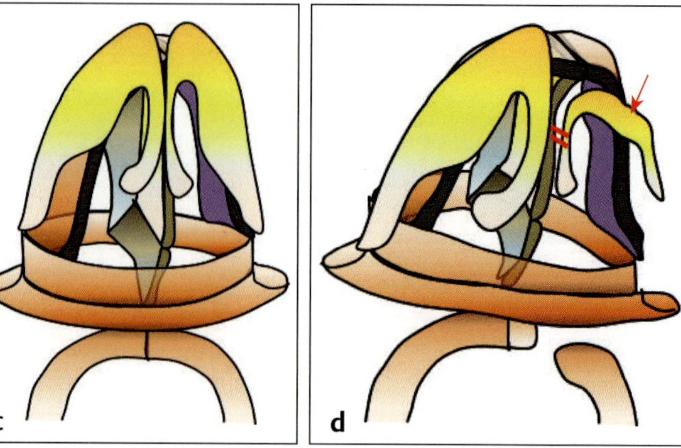

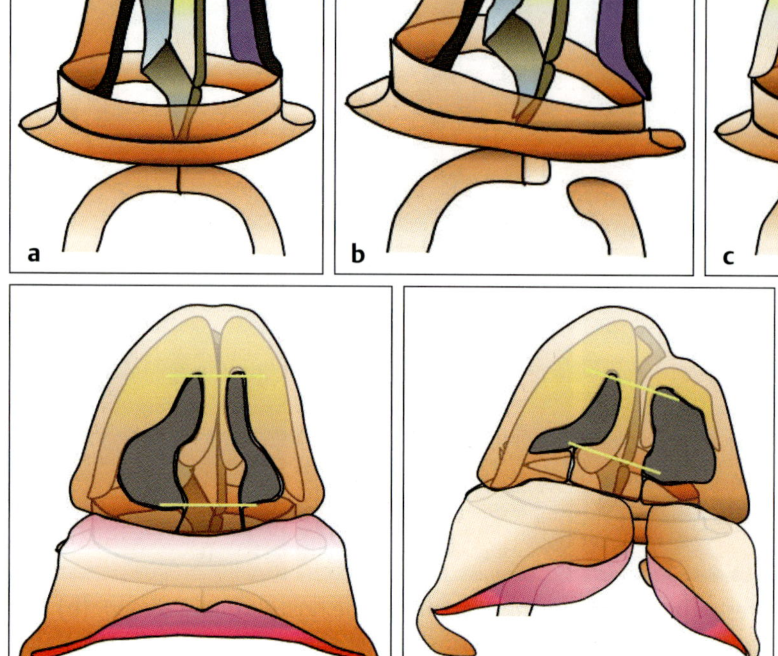

Fig. 13.65 **(a)** Diagrammatic representation of lip and nose in normal individual. **(b)** Unilateral alveolar cleft showing tilting of nasal complex. On the cleft side, there is a bony deficiency. Hence the framework is retro displaced. The lateral buttress on the side of cleft is smaller and the pyramid is tilted. **(c)** Anatomy of normal lower lateral cartilages. **(d)** The lower lateral cartilage is smaller on the cleft side with reduced potential energy, is flatter in shape, and has a pinched appearance (*red arrow*). **(e)** Normal anatomy of skin envelope of nose and lip. **(f)** In unilateral cleft patients, the envelope is asymmetric, the tip is deviated, and the columella on the cleft side is short.

the maxillary platform using a graft and a crescentic graft on either alar base. Besides this, the deficient septum should be augmented, using the septal construct of a cartilaginous truss with dorsal and caudal rafters. The truss not only improves the stability, but also corrects the flattened septal angle improving the projection. The columellar strut is used for tip support and desirable projection. An additional dorsal onlay graft improves the profile line, with an aesthetically pleasing result. The anticipated augmented framework must have an envelope that can accommodate it without tension (**Fig. 13.67b**).

Conclusion

The anatomy of the nose can be better understood if one applies basic principles of structural engineering and architecture to it. A lot of concepts in plastic surgery can be explained on the basis of these sciences. This correlation between architectural terms and their importance in rhinoplasty is summarized in **Table 13.1**.

With this analogy and the architectural background for the terms, we hope this correlation helps to curb usage of unscientific terms like floating columellar strut and L-strut, found in literature.

To simplify the nasal architecture, the upper two-thirds or the osseocartilaginous vault is rigid/semirigid with a well-supported framework and the lower third or the lobule, although provided with good shape-holding support, has inadequate load-bearing support. In our experience, the best way to provide structural support is by use of compact cartilage grafts. Reconstruction or restoration should always be planned in terms of individual components: septum, lateral buttress, columella, etc. The structural and functional diversity of the two units should be maintained, converting the nose into a single stiff unit should be avoided.

The structural support options for various conditions are summarized in **Table 13.2**.

Anticipating the insufficiency of the envelope equally is important. The bottom-line in achieving a satisfactory result is: *Restore the structure, aesthetics follows!*

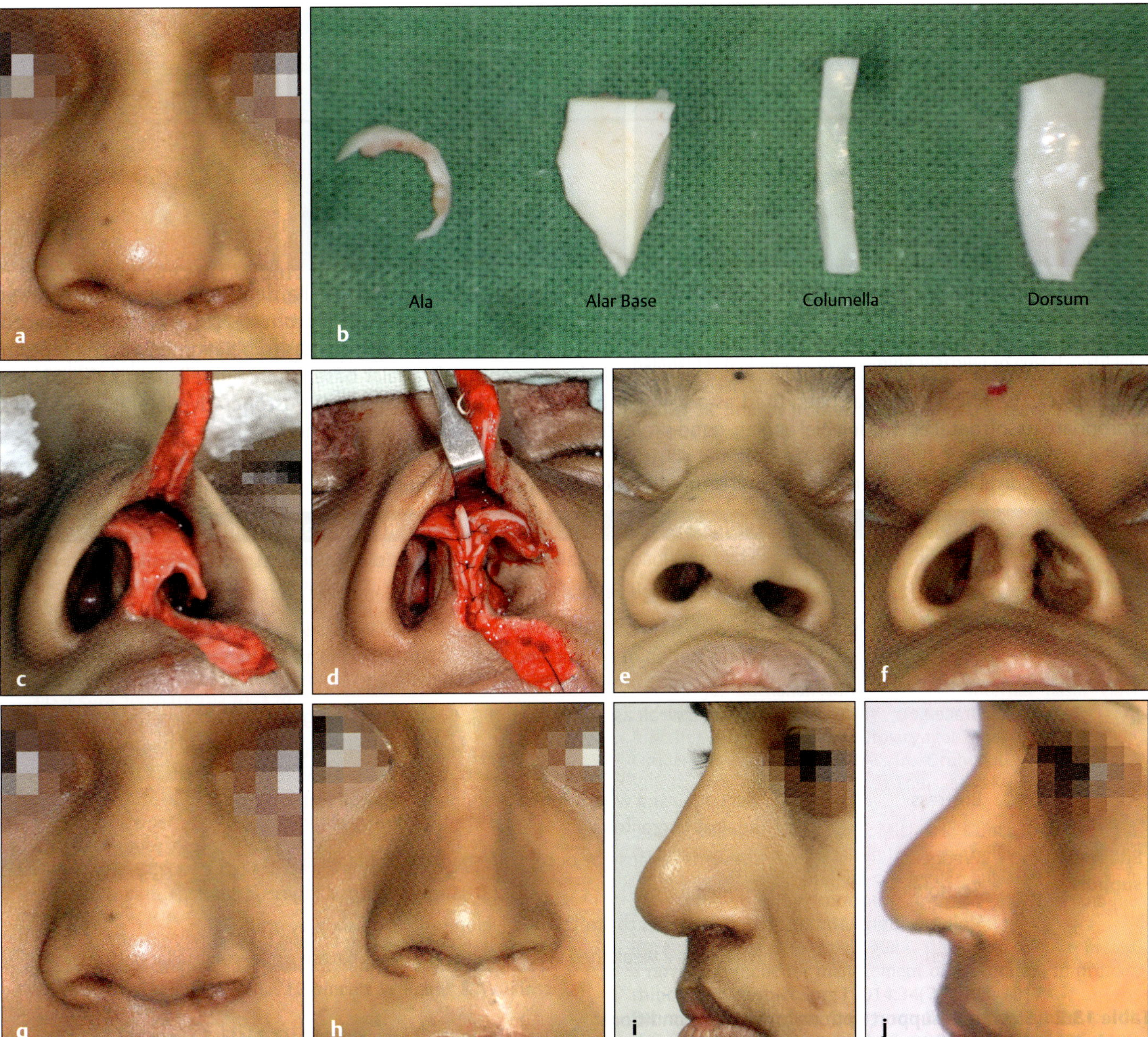

Fig. 13.66 **(a)** The characteristic features of a cleft lip nasal deformity can be appreciated in this young lady. Her nose is asymmetric and also has a slightly masculine appearance because of a broad osseocartilaginous vault. **(b)** Costal cartilage was used to carve alar cartilage, alar base, columellar graft, and the dorsal onlay graft. **(c)** Use of scar from previous surgery as a flap to lengthen the short columella **(d)** The grafts have been positioned, restoring the integrity of the framework **(e)** Besides the underdeveloped framework, the preoperative basal view shows a short columella on the cleft side, indicating the skin envelope is also deficient **(f)** The deficiency of columella has been corrected post-operatively; the teardrop shape of nostrils is obtained and the projection of the lobule is good on the basal view **(g)** The pre-operative frontal view **(h)** Post-operatively, the nose appears narrow with feminine features and the symmetry is acceptable. **(i)** The nasion was relatively high preoperatively **(j)** Post-operative profile shows an aesthetic dorsal line with adequate tip rotation. (Reproduced with permission from Bhat et al 201420.)

Introduction

The combination of form and function is a pillar for modern rhinoplasty techniques. In the quest to achieve the most aesthetic result, long-term considerations of the airway are often either not recognized or, perhaps worse, neglected by inexperienced rhinoplasty surgeons. Often, simple techniques can be employed to minimize issues with function although it is important to recognize potential pitfalls with cosmetic techniques. Equally, in many cases breathing difficulty is the more pressing problem for many patients so having a broad ability to deal with this problem is imperative for those undertaking such surgery. This chapter will seek to feature how to analyze nasal function based on patient symptoms, good clinical examination with endoscopy, and possible use of objective measures. It will also highlight common potential causes for nasal obstruction and how to deal with these. Preventative measures to avoid postoperative functional problems will also be detailed. On occasion, a discussion of the relative importance of function over form needs to be had with the patient because some techniques, as detailed below, can affect the external appearance. It can often be a fine balancing act to correct both fully to a patient's satisfaction.

Anatomy

The nasal airway contains both dynamic and rigid structures; it relies on the relationship between the soft tissues and the supporting osteocartilaginous structures. The bony vault of the nose is pyramidal in shape; it includes a pair of nasal bones and the ascending frontal process of the maxilla (**Fig. 14.1**).[1,2]

The cartilaginous nasal frame is comprised of a pair of upper and lower lateral cartilages. The upper lateral cartilages are rectangular in shape and join the septum medially while providing support to the lateral nasal wall. The lower lateral cartilages consist of four crura: the medial crus, the middle crus, the lateral crus, and the dome (**Fig. 14.2**).

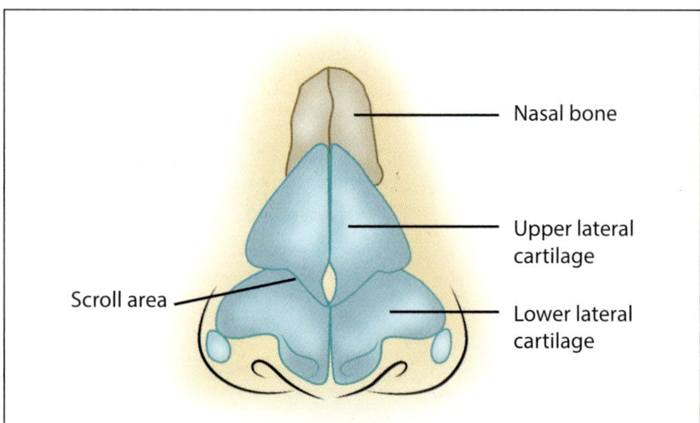

Fig. 14.1 Frontal view of the bony and cartilaginous nasal frame.

The curled junction where the inferior edge of the upper lateral cartilage and the superior edge of the lateral crus of the lower lateral cartilage join is termed the scroll area (**Fig. 14.1**).[1,3]

The nose is divided into two passages by the septum. The nasal septum is composed of the perpendicular plate of the ethmoid, the vomer, the crest of the maxillary bone, and the quadrilateral or septal cartilage (**Fig. 14.3**). The septum does not only give the nose important structural support but it also plays a major role in determining its shape. Deviations in the septum can affect the nasal airflow and have a significant impact on the nasal airway.[1,2,4]

The nasal turbinates are three shelf-like, bony projections along the lateral nasal wall: the superior, middle, and inferior turbinates (**Fig. 14.4**). These are covered with a ciliated respiratory epithelium that has a rich vascular supply which can lead to engorgement. Caudal to each turbinate is the sinus opening. Deviations in the septum can allow for compensatory turbinate hypertrophy and displacement which can have a significant impact on the nasal airway. In these cases improvement in the nasal airway would require both the septum and the turbinate to be addressed.[1–3]

The middle turbinate is an important landmark anatomically both when endoscopically examining the nose and when performing endoscopic sinus surgery. It forms part of the ethmoid bone and can sometimes be pneumatized. This pneumatization is referred to as a concha bullosa and can lead to obstruction of the middle meatus.[5,6]

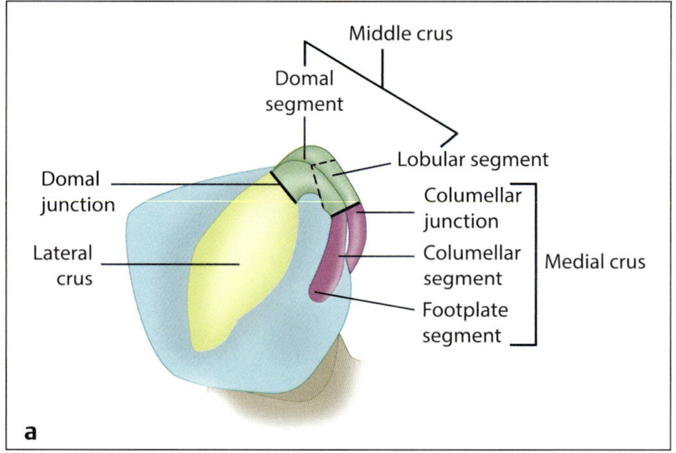

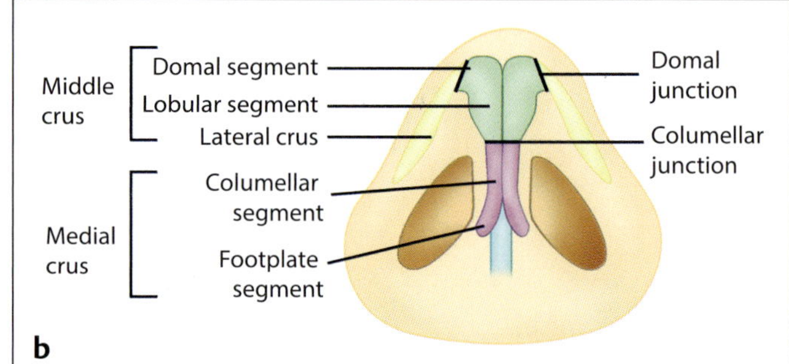

Fig. 14.2 **(a, b)** Overview of the alar cartilages.

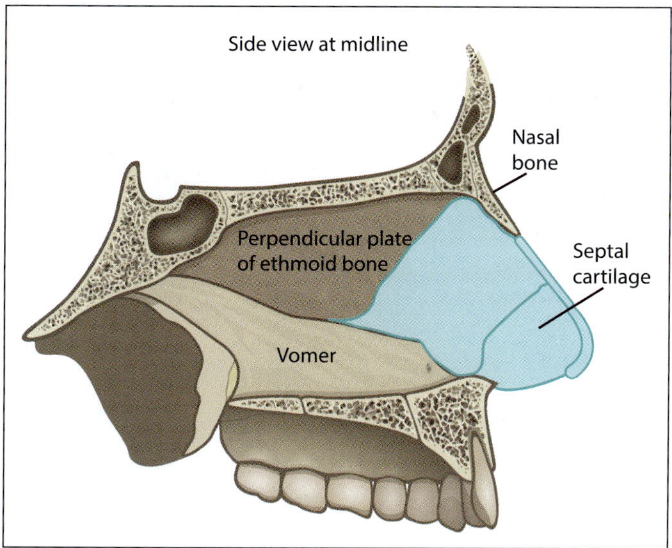

Fig. 14.3 Septal anatomy.

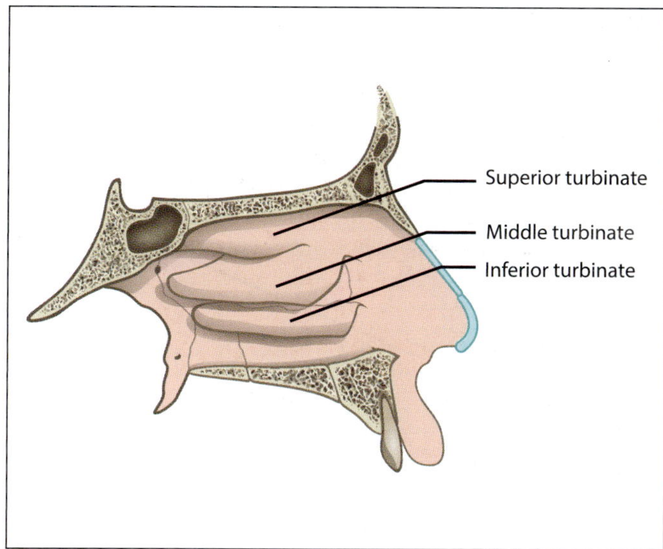

Fig. 14.4 Schematic diagram showing the anatomy of the turbinates.

The inferior turbinate is a separate bone attached to the nasal wall inferolaterally. Its anatomical dimensions are approximately 50 to 60 mm in length, 7 to 10 mm in height, and can vary in its width.[7] The inferior turbinate can lead to nasal obstruction by hypertrophy of its soft tissue, alteration of its bony anatomy, or a mixture of both. Soft tissue hypertrophy can occur as a reciprocal expansion with septal deviation as well as allergic or nonallergic rhinitis. Bony hypertrophy can be congenital, traumatic, or secondary to ossification.[5,6]

The Nasal Valves

The external nasal valve is defined as the angle between the lateral and medial crus of the lower lateral cartilage. The internal nasal valve is the narrowest part of the upper airway and is the angle between the caudal upper lateral cartilage, the septum, and the anterior face of the middle turbinate. This angle is reported to be between 10 and 15 degrees (**Fig. 14.5a, b**).[1,2,8]

Analysis of the Airway as Part of Rhinoplasty Examination

Good preoperative analysis is the cornerstone of all rhinoplasty practices, and examination of the internal nose to assess airway and function is key to a successful long-term result.

History

As part of a detailed history about cosmetic concerns, patients should be questioned specifically about any breathing and sinus-related issues. This will include asking about the side of obstruction, how long it has been there, its severity, a history or prior surgery or trauma, whether it is worse at any time of the day, and any specific triggering factors such as known environmental or seasonal sensitivities. There may also be associated taste or smell disturbances. Symptom and quality-of-life questionnaires may be used.[1,4] Patients often will relate their blockage to positional changes such as lying on one side or the other during the night. It is important to realize that much of functional obstruction may be associated with mucosal issues rather than specific structural problems.

External Evaluation

The facial proportions, symmetry, and geometry are carefully assessed first by inspection. The nose should be viewed from all angles including a basal view. Close attention should be paid to the skin thickness and texture as well as the nasal cartilage and bones. The face and nose can be palpated to feel for scarring, skin elasticity, trauma, or previous surgery. Palpation along the nasal dorsum from the nasion to the nasal tip can allow the surgeon to check the structural integrity of the septum allowing for inferences about the anterior septal angle and tip support. The patient should be asked to take a gentle breath in and the alar cartilage assessed for any signs of collapse on inspiration.[1,2,4,9]

Internal Inspection

Anterior rhinoscopy using a thudicum speculum and a headlight is performed to establish a baseline view of the nose and examine the caudal septum's position and attachment at the maxillary crest. The surgeon should assess the condition of the mucosa, the septum, the inferior turbinates,

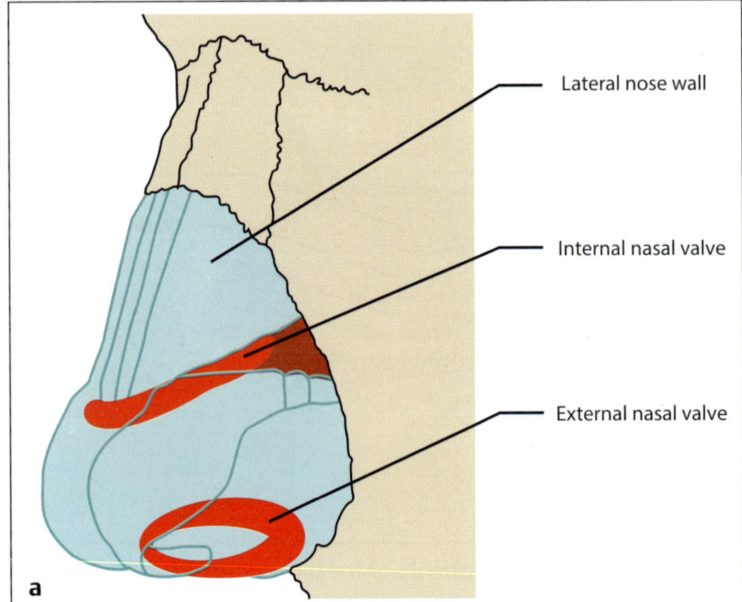

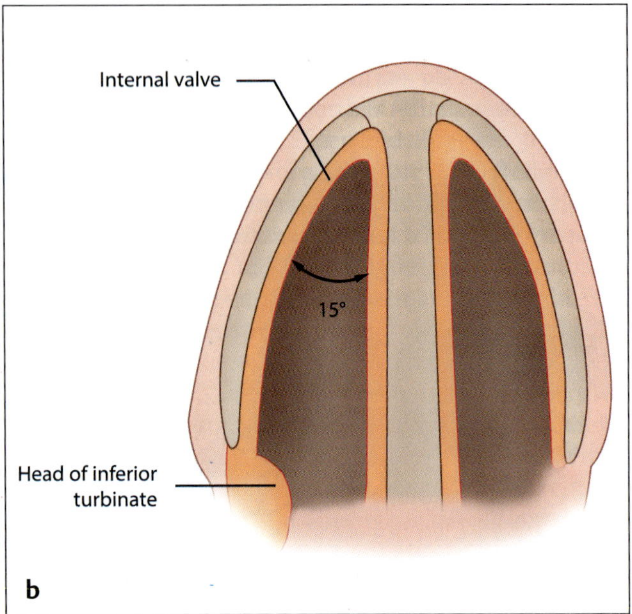

Fig. 14.5 (a, b) Diagrams to illustrate the internal and external nasal valves.

and any other visible structures while considering if these features could restrict the airway. The thumb and the index finger can be gently placed in each vestibule to assess the caudal septum's thickness, position, and mobility while also allowing the surgeon to manipulate the membranous septum.[2–4,10]

It is important to check if there is alar collapse on normal inspiration but in its absence, valve collapse cannot be excluded. Assessment with Cottle maneuver is often advocated to assess internal nasal valve obstruction but can be nonspecific. The cheek is pulled laterally and the patient is asked to report if this improves nasal airflow on the same side. If it does improve nasal airflow the test is positive and denotes obstruction at the external nasal valve, although this is often found even with normal patients (**Fig. 14.6**).[1] The modified Cottle test may thus be a better evaluator. This involves placing a cerumen hook on the internal aspect of the lower lateral cartilage and gently lateralizing it, the patient is then asked to report if this improves the airflow on that side. An improvement in airflow signifies a positive test and obstruction at both nasal valves.[4,9]

Nasal Endoscopy

Endoscopic evaluation of the internal structure of the nose looking at the nasal septum, the turbinates, and any mucosal change is invaluable and should be part of routine practice of a rhinoplasty surgeon and will act to complement examination of the external nose. It may elucidate other causes of obstruction including sinonasal problems such as nasal polyps or rarely even tumors, benign or otherwise. This examination provides detailed information about the intranasal anatomy and the structural relationships within the nasal cavity. It allows hidden areas of the nose that cannot be assessed during anterior rhinoscopy to be easily visualized and the internal nasal valve can be inspected without distortion. Ideally a 30-degree, 4-mm diameter, rigid telescope should be used but a flexible nasal endoscope can also be used. The endoscope is inserted parallel to the floor of the nose with the patient seated or in a supine position; care should be taken to avoid forceful advancement or trauma to the nasal mucosa. The nose is then examined using a three-pass technique.[5,11]

The first pass is parallel to the floor of the nose, the inferior meatus can be seen here; this is also the region where the nasolacrimal duct drains. Advancement of the endoscope posteriorly in this position will allow visualization of the nasopharynx. The orifice of the Eustachian tube can be seen laterally and the fossa of Rosenmüller superiorly. The size and mucosa of the inferior turbinate, any growths or pus, or nasopharyngeal discharge should be noted.[10,11]

The second pass commences at the anterior nasal valve at an angle of 45 degrees between the middle and superior turbinates. The maxillary antrum is inspected. Note should be made of any polyps, discharge, or accessory ostia. The endoscope can then be advanced medially and posterior to the middle turbinate to view the sphenoethmoidal recess.[10,11]

In the third pass, the endoscope is advanced lateral to the middle turbinate so the middle meatus can be viewed. This also enables visualization of the infundibulum, uncinate, and the ethmoid bulla.[10]

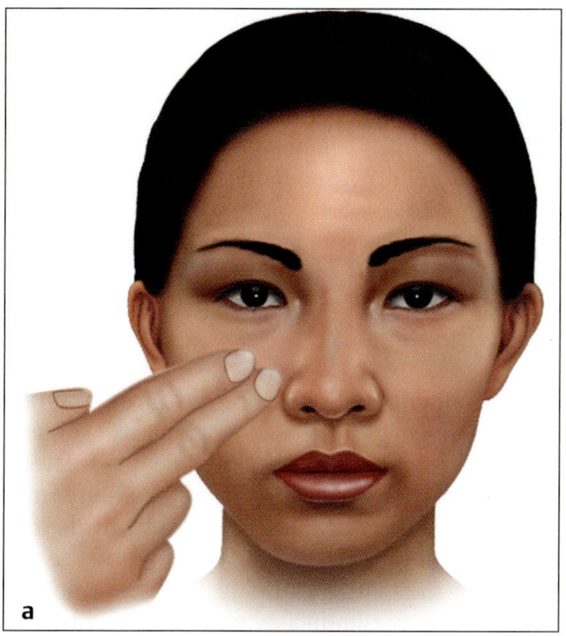

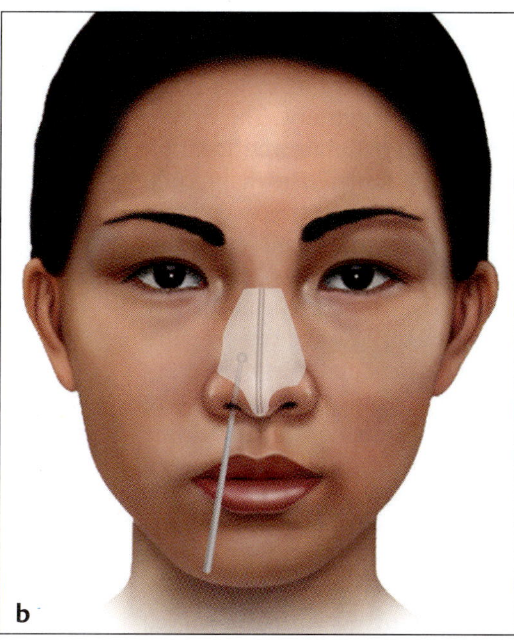

Fig. 14.6 (a, b) Cottle test and modified Cottle test.

Meticulous examination involves looking at the intranasal structures and assessing for both subtle and obvious abnormalities then considering their impact on nasal airway and function. Common findings include mucosal pathology such as rhinitis, nasal discharge, (e.g., mucopus, nasal polyps, septal deviation, hypertrophy of the nasal turbinates, and adenoidal hypertrophy). If signs of paranasal sinus disease are observed, a CT scan of the nose and paranasal sinuses should be performed for further evaluation.[3,5]

Rhinitis is an extremely common symptom that can be associated with allergic or environmental causes but equally can be idiopathic in origin (nonallergic).

Examination of the external aspects may further suggest causes for functional issues, such as weakening or collapse of the cartilaginous framework including the midvault area or indeed the lower laterals in the tip which may lead to internal or external nasal valve problems, respectively.

Diagnosis of the underlying anatomic deformity is essential prior to embarking upon a surgical plan. Both inspection and palpation of the integrity of lower lateral support are equally important. It may not be possible to assess whether there is an intact strip of the lower lateral cartilage and prior operative notes if performing a revision may be helpful in this regard.

Some authors have advocated routine CT scanning, and with the advent of cone beam technology with limited radiation, there may be more justification for this, particularly with specific problems such as a significantly deviated posttraumatic nose, or with a cleft lip patient. An argument may also be made for having a CT scan showing bone thickness if sculpture of the bony pyramid is anticipated with powered instrumentation such as piezoelectric or drills. It has been suggested that it may also provide an adjunct when assessing the internal nasal valve.[12,13]

It is generally not routinely required, however, and ideally should not be used in lieu of, but rather guided by proper endoscopy, particularly if sinonasal pathology is seen.

Functional Studies

Objective testing of nasal function remains somewhat controversial and underutilized, particularly in routine practice.

Optimal nasal airflow requires patent nasal passages and normal mucociliary function. Nasal airway obstruction is defined as poor or absent airflow, unilaterally or bilaterally, which can be constant or fluctuating. This may be structural, physiological, or both. Nasal obstruction following rhinoplasty is one of the most common indications for revision rhinoplasty with reports ranging from 15 to 85%.[14–16]

Nasal obstruction can be assessed subjectively using symptom scores or visual analog scales and on the basis of the clinical examination and experience of the surgeon. There are also objective assessment techniques. Evidence to support correlation between these techniques is weak.

Acoustic rhinometry (AR), rhinomanometry (RM), and peak nasal inspiratory flow (PNIF) look at different parameters of nasal airflow and obstruction. They can be utilized for the clinical evaluation of nasal obstruction, research in nasal physiology, allergy challenge testing, assessment of pre- and posttreatment with either surgical or medical therapy, and evaluation of patients with sleep apnea.[15,17]

Peak nasal airflow can be easily measured using an expiratory flow meter to assess the nasal airway. This is a fast, easy, and cost-effective method that has the potential to be useful; however, there are questions regarding its reproducibility.[3,18]

Acoustic rhinometry, first described by Hillberg in 1989, is a noninvasive objective test to assess nasal geometry using sound waves. The cross-sectional area of the nose is measured from the nostril. Sound waves that enter the nose are analyzed using a machine, and distortions to the wave occur as a result of variations in nasal anatomy. The timing of these deflections can be used to estimate the location within the nose as distance from the nostril. The magnitude of the deflection estimates the impact on the cross-sectional area. The sound wave is then digitally translated into a rhinograph for analysis.[2,19,20]

Rhinomanometry measures nasal pressure and airflow during breathing. By measuring the airflow and the pressure gradient, nasal resistance can be calculated. Airflow occurs during inspiration and expiration because of the pressure difference between the nose and the outside world. Multiple factors can influence nasal airflow including transnasal pressure, cross-sectional area, and the length of the nose.[19,20]

Airflow is measured using a pneumotachometer and a pressure transducer, the output is then read by a digital recording device (**Fig. 14.7**). Three different techniques of rhinomanometry may be used to measure transnasal pressure: anterior, posterior (per oral), and postnasal (per nasal). The difference lies in the location of the pressure transducer.[3,19,20]

It is important to be aware of the objective techniques available for the measurement of nasal airflow. However, they are not routinely used worldwide due to a lack of consensus about validity and reproducibility. There are also implications related to their cost and availability. Objective methods are not essential for the assessment of nasal obstructive symptoms, but they provide valuable objective information in keeping with the practice of evidence-based medicine and allow for pre- and postoperative comparison.[19–22]

A review of the literature also finds growing interest in the use of 3D modeling and computational fluid dynamic simulations in nasal obstruction for their potential use in virtual surgery planning. Three-dimensional nasal models can be reconstructed from cone beam computer tomography scans and subsequently used for airflow simulations.[23]

Specific Functional Problems

Septal Pathology

Nasal septal deviations are likely to be the most common functional problem encountered in rhinoplasty surgery. Most issues arise from caudal deviation of the quadrilateral cartilage rather than more posterior deviation when symptoms are far less problematic. Similarly, dorsal deviations may compromise the internal nasal valve area and cause significant obstruction. It is important that such deviations are dealt with as part of any rhinoplasty procedure and indeed often dictate the shape externally. While it is beyond the scope of this chapter to detail all aspects of septal surgery, some salient points are described below.

Incision

Access to the cartilage and bone aspects of the septum is via either a hemitransfixion or, less preferably, a Killian incision. The former is made on either side adjacent to the caudal border of the native cartilage and allows access to the whole cartilaginous septum facilitating correction of caudal deformities as well as further more posterior deviations (**Fig. 14.8**). The soft tissue in this area is generally more adherent to the underlying cartilage and hence dissection

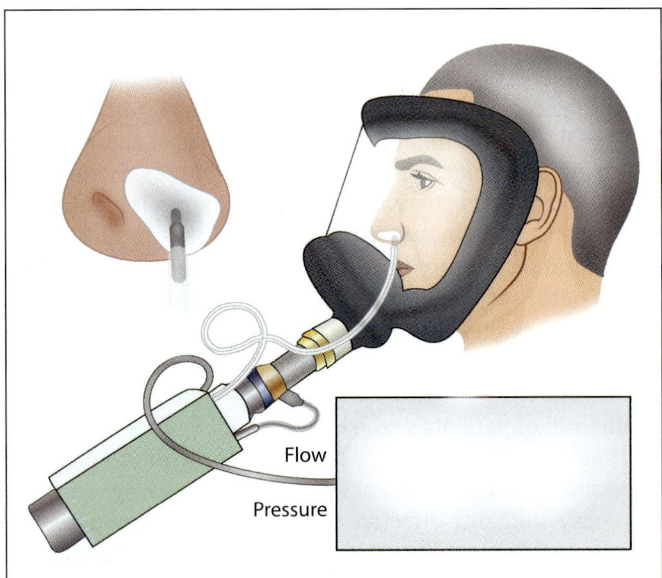

Fig. 14.7 Equipment required for rhinomanometry.

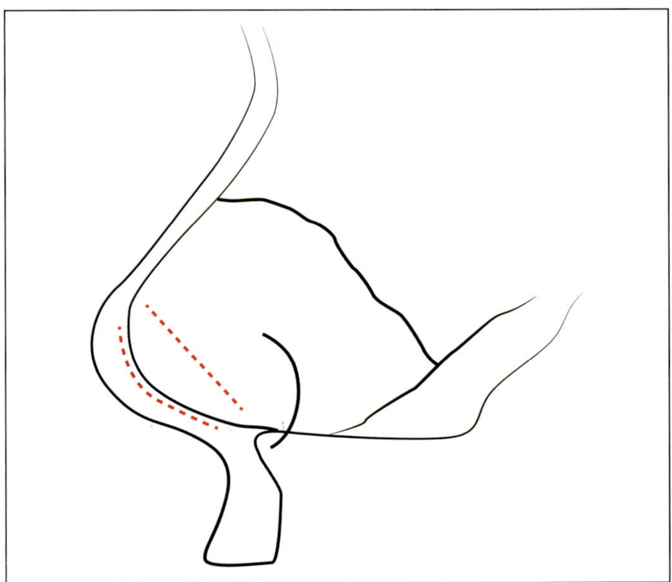

Fig. 14.8 Hemitransfixion and Killian septal mucosal incisions.

into the submucoperichondrial layer can prove more difficult than with a Killian incision which is made at a distance behind the caudal edge of cartilage. Here, it is easier to enter the correct plane which is generally bloodless. A further option is by dissection between the medial crura if performing an open approach effectively dividing through the membranous septum to access the most caudal part of quadrilateral cartilage (**Fig. 14.9**). This will, however, disrupt one of the minor tip support mechanisms so may be best avoided if no cartilaginous material is available to provide structural support to maintain postoperative tip projection. Sharp dissection with a tip of an Iris-type scissor will aid the dissection and once the correct plane is entered, the mucoperichondrium is lifted effortlessly with a Freer elevator.

It is important to avoid tears in the mucosa where possible and particularly bilateral opposing tears as this may lead to a perforation. If bilateral opposing tears are noted, attempted closure with mobilization and reapposition of the mucosal edges and placement of an interpositional graft is best performed at the primary procedure rather than risking it and having to deal with a long-term perforation with all its inherent complexities. Whether to lift one or both mucosal flaps is often debated and there are clearly advantages and disadvantages with each. Lifting a single flap reduces the risk of tearing both mucosal flaps but often will not allow full appreciation of the septal deformity as the mucosa remains firmly attached to one side and this could also cause differential healing between the two sides.

Cartilaginous Mobilization

Cartilaginous deviations may occur secondary to posterior bony deviations and can be dealt with by a simple chondrotomy with detachment of the cartilage from the perpendicular plate of the ethmoid and vomer posteriorly plus maxillary crest inferiorly: the so-called "swing door" septoplasty. It is important to extend the chondrotomy as far superiorly as possible to avoid leaving a dorsal deviation, but equally be aware of the region just below the keystone area where the cartilage must remain attached to bone to avoid downward movement creating a saddle deformity. A supratip depression may also occur as a result of when the caudal septum has been detached from the anterior nasal spine as part of the septal mobilization as in the case of a caudal septal dislocation or an overlong cartilage generally. If this area is not reconstituted, the quadrilateral cartilage may have a tendency to rock backward, thereby losing its dorsal support to the middle third of the nose. Reattachment of the cartilage to the nasal spine can be achieved either with a 3.0 PDS suture placed through a drilled hole in the spine or through the periosteum immediately surrounding this. Saddling of this nature is best dealt with by reattaching the posterior septal angle back into its correct place, thereby re-establishing two-point support of the septum between the anterior nasal spine and the keystone area (**Fig. 14.10**).

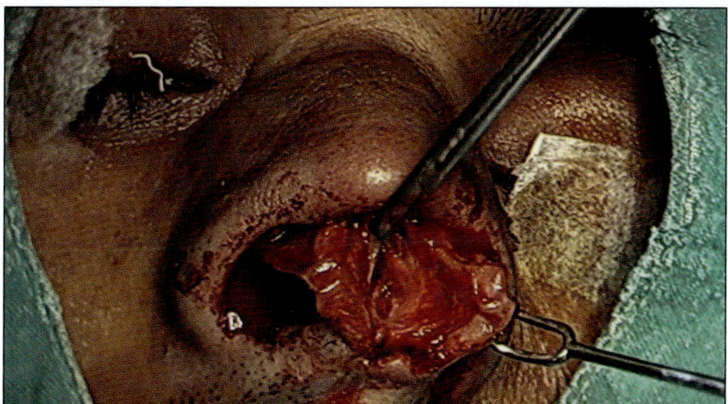

Fig. 14.9 Access to caudal nasal septum by division between medial crura.

Cartilaginous Correction

Inherent cartilaginous septal deformity is perhaps more challenging and may require scoring techniques (**Fig. 14.11**), although these alone are not sufficient as postoperative scar contracture will cause further recurrent septal buckling. Using batten grafts can help keep the cartilage straight. Thin bony perpendicular plate grafts with multiple drilled holes are ideal in this regard and allow for rigid fixation of cartilage into a straighter position using mattress sutures. Other options include using other septal cartilage but this can cause some overall thickness of the area. PDS plate grafts have been advocated,[24] but these should be used judiciously as they can cause inflammation and granulation tissue to form.[25]

Further more complex, multiple deviations may necessitate an extracorporeal septoplasty, either with removal of the whole septal cartilage[26] or subtotal removal in a modified approach.[27] The cartilage can then be divided between fracture lines or deviations, straightened and a L-shaped type framework fashioned from the various cartilage pieces (either sewn directly together or by building a construct) often with attached spreader grafts. An alternative is to attach the cartilages to a supporting scaffold with small pieces of PDS plate.[28]

The cartilage is then reimplanted back into the nose and held to the upper lateral cartilages dorsally, attached to the anterior nasal spine caudally, and the keystone area reconstituted by drilling into the nasal bones and a suture placed in a crisscross fashion to support the cartilage in the correct anatomical position.[29] Even with such accurate and robust placement, extracorporeal techniques may risk a step deformity creating a shallow saddle in the dorsal region. Often finely diced cartilage, placed freely, wrapped in fascia, or held with glue can help efface such issues.[30,31] The modified extracorporeal approach leaves behind a strip of cartilage attached at the keystone area. This can be used to reattach the straightened cartilage pieces, thereby negating the need for reconstitution of the keystone area and avoiding the risk of saddle deformity.[27] These methods should be

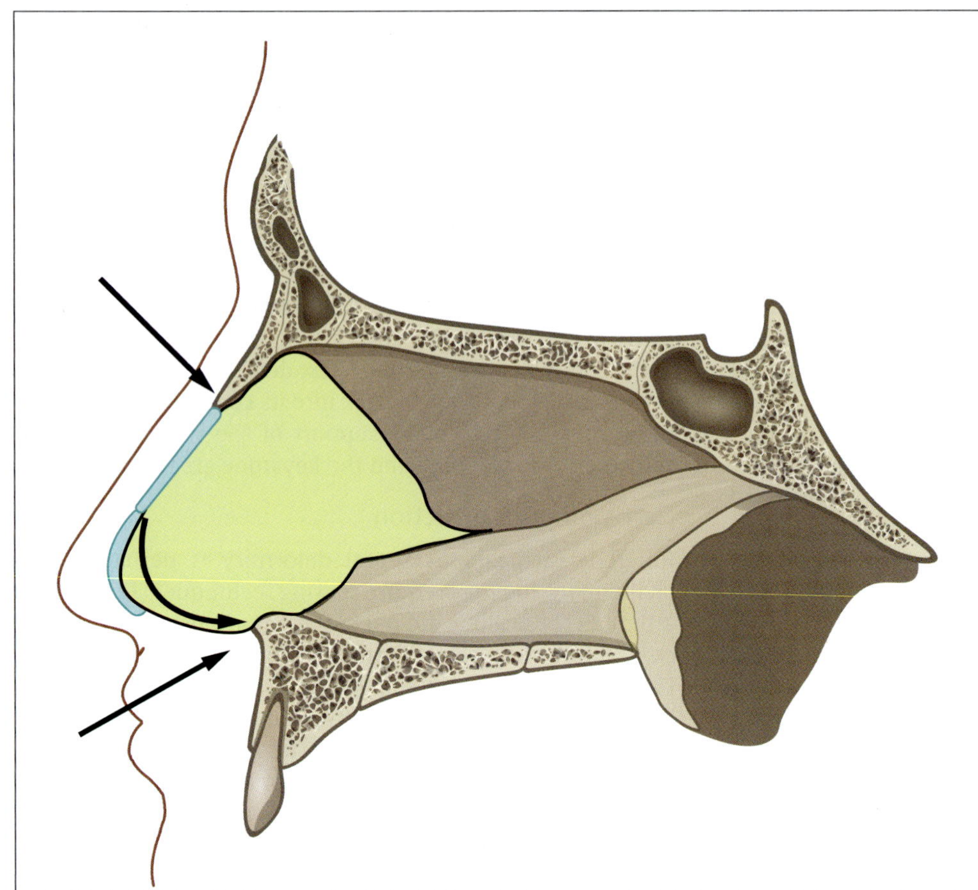

Fig. 14.10 Importance of two-point fixation of the quadrilateral cartilage at the keystone area and anterior nasal spine to ensure no rotation backward of the cartilage.

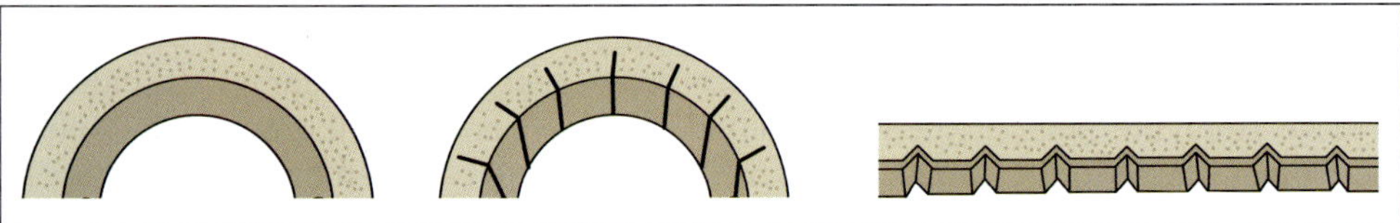

Fig. 14.11 Principles of scoring cartilage. But scoring alone may not be enough, so adding a batten graft to strengthen the cartilage is ideal.

used sparingly in general rhinoplasty practice as the vast majority of septal correction can be achieved without the need for extracorporeal removal.

Septal deviations can cause many of the functional airway issues within the nose. Good techniques for correction can not only improve the airway but may equally be a major part of the solution when straightening a deviated nose.

Turbinate Hypertrophy

Two-thirds of the nasal airway resistance can be attributed to the inferior turbinates. If medical management fails to address symptoms or does not have a role, there are a number of surgical techniques available for inferior turbinate reduction. The goal is to decrease their size by targeting the submucosal soft tissue or *(less frequently)* the bony tissue, while maintaining the overlying mucosa. Techniques vary from mechanical outfracture and lateralization, intramural bipolar diathermy, laser, microdebridement, and more recently coblation.[4,14,15,32]

Reduction of the inferior turbinates can be achieved with bipolar or monopolar or bipolar cautery under general anesthesia, which causes a deep thermal lesion. Healing occurs following this and fibrosis results in shrinking of the surrounding tissue.[3,32]

The microdebrider may also be used to treat the inferior turbinates. The inferior turbinate is incised anteroinferiorly and the microdebrider is used in the submucosal plane. Care must be taken to remain in the plane to prevent mucosal trauma.[33]

Other methods include excision of the turbinate in the form of total or partial turbinectomy, submucosal turbinectomy, or turbinoplasty. These are more invasive techniques and were used conventionally. They offer improved symptomatic relief compared to medical therapy alone but are associated with increased complications such as bleeding, postoperative pain, synechia, crusting, and atrophy of the inferior turbinates.[4,33]

Coblation, short for "controlled ablation," is a relatively new technique that can be used to treat the turbinates. Radiofrequency energy is passed through a conductive medium, usually saline, producing a plasma field that results in vaporization of the tissue without the use of thermal energy.[34]

Nasal Valve Pathology

Internal Nasal Valve

The "internal nasal valve area" represents the smallest cross-sectional area in the nasal airway. It is bounded by the caudal end of the upper lateral cartilage, the head of the inferior turbinate, the floor of the nose, the nasal septum, and the intervening mucosal tissue surrounding the pyriform aperture. Traditional rhinoplasty techniques with removal of a dorsal hump can compromise the nasal valve, particularly in patients with short nasal bones, a high bony/cartilaginous hump, and weak upper lateral cartilages.[35] Frequently, there is an additional corresponding aesthetic defect of a "sunken" or "pinched-in" middle third. Such an inverted V-type deformity is a consequence of either excessive resection or collapse of the upper lateral cartilages inferomedially due to inadequate support after removal of a dorsal hump. The nose displays a "washed-out" appearance with prominence of the caudal edge of the nasal bones. There may be associated internal nasal valve collapse giving rise to nasal obstruction.[36]

Spreader Grafts

Placement of "spreader grafts" to open up the nasal valve area and angle has been described via an endonasal approach, thereby improving both function and cosmesis (**Fig. 14.12**).[37,38] The external approach allows easier and more precise placement and suture fixation of such spreader grafts, minimizing risk of displacement.[36] These cartilaginous strips are placed longitudinally between the upper lateral cartilage and septum. The mucosa between these cartilages is often divided but, based on Sheen's original work[38] this should be avoided and rather the spreader graft placed extramucosally. The functional improvement has been difficult to quantify objectively but subjective improvement is to be anticipated. Placement via an external approach (**Fig. 14.13**) allows for accurate visualization but, when required, can be equally well placed endonasally[39] into tight submucoperichondrial pockets and held with tissue glue or with percutaneous trans-septal sutures if needed. Unilateral placement of spreader grafts may also correct asymmetries of the dorsum.

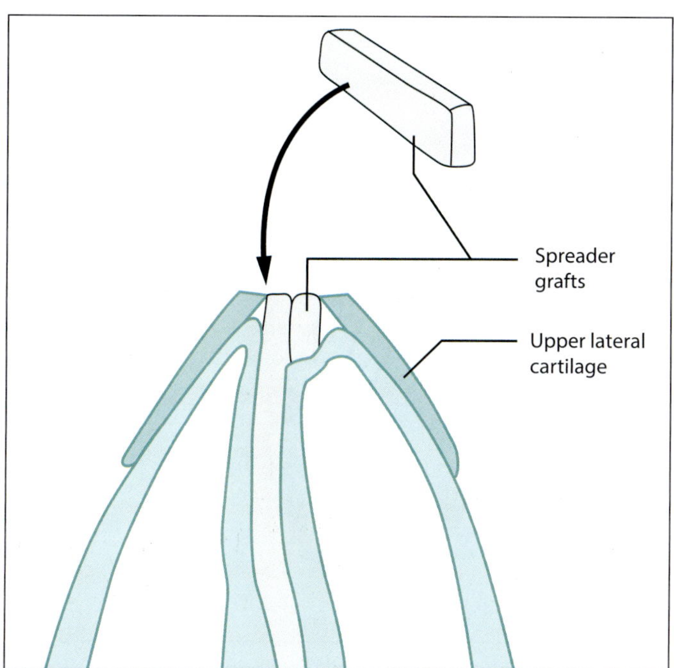

Fig. 14.12 Placement of spreader grafts.

Autospreader/Spreader Flaps

The use of spreader flaps (**Fig. 14.14**) has been popularized and proven to be an effective and simple alternative that negates the need for a separate cartilaginous source. It is particularly useful in a cartilage-depleted patient.[40,41]

While the described "en-bloc" resection of the bony and cartilaginous dorsum has been the preferred option of many authors in prior years, the risk of collapse of the mid-third of the nose caused by over-resection of the upper lateral cartilages has led to thought about how to strengthen the midvault area. An alternative to the traditional method is deconstruction of the cartilaginous dorsum with sequential segmental lowering. The upper lateral cartilages can be divided from the quadrilateral septal cartilage extramucosally initially and the most superior aspect of its cephalic edge dissected off the underside of the bony vault cap, if this is not already lowered. The midline septal cartilage is then lowered alone to the desired level. The upper laterals are thus left intact and at this point the bony cap can be lowered

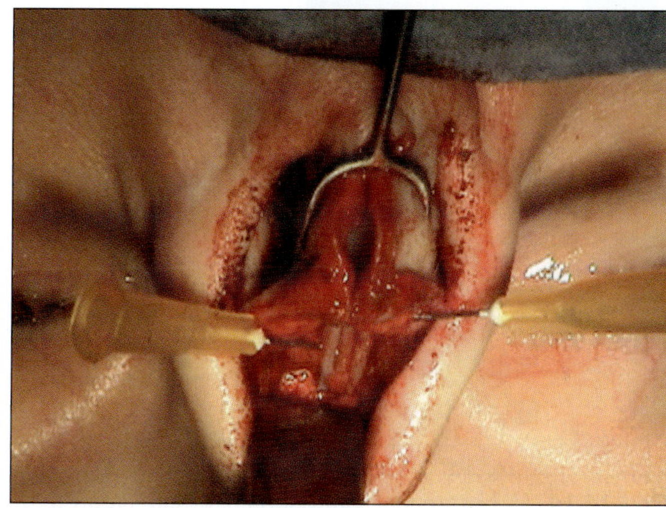

Fig. 14.13 Securing spreader grafts to the dorsal septum.

by the usual methods: with a rasp or powered instrument. The upper lateral cartilages will now remain proud and can be infolded and sutured to the septal cartilage in a horizontal mattress fashion to create spreader flaps mimicking the effect of spreader grafts, thus protecting against long-term collapse in this area. It is inadvisable to score the cartilage before infolding as this reduces any mechanical spring advantage. These can be an effective way of avoiding midvault narrowing but alone are unlikely to proffer any significant functional benefit. They can be used in combination with traditional spreader grafts if the midvault needs to be strengthened or widened further.[42]

Upper Lateral Flaring Suture

This permanent suture, placed in a horizontal mattress fashion through the upper later cartilages in the region of the internal nasal valve, causes lateral eversion of the cartilages, thereby increasing the nasal valve angle.[43] This represents a useful adjunct to the use of spreader grafts and has the potential to markedly improve the airway, although there is risk of some widening and flaring of the mid-third of the nose externally. Discussion with the patient about the potential risk of this is clearly advised. In effect, this suture emulates the effect of the widely available external nasal strips that are placed on the skin over the mid-third area to help improve the airway **(Fig. 14.15)**.

Titanium and Cartilaginous Mid-Third Implants

So-called cartilaginous butterfly grafts have been described to improve the airway and are generally placed on top of the upper lateral cartilages, tucked just under the lower laterals (**Fig. 14.16**).[44] These also are used to elevate the upper laterals into a more favorable position for functional purposes. An alternative is to use a titanium implant placed over the upper lateral cartilage area, and this has been advocated as an excellent way of improving the airway.[45] There is potential for patients to see and feel the rigidity of the metal so this technique, while effective, may be best reserved for patients with thicker skin type (**Fig. 14.17**).

External Nasal Valve

It is important to consider the anatomy of the external nasal valve region. The ideal aesthetics of the basal view of the nasal tip is that of an equilateral triangle. The lateral crura should have a flattened but slightly outward convexity of the posterior alar rims and gentle rounding in the dome region. Specifically, there should be no pinching of the lateral alar walls. Various factors including thickness of the overlying skin, musculature (dilators), strength, and position of the lower lateral cartilages can directly influence the tip shape and dynamics.[46]

The caudal margin of the lateral crus should ideally lie in a horizontal plane such that it lies just inferior to the cephalic margin. If the cartilage is angulated such that there is a significant superior-to-inferior relationship between the cephalic and caudal margins, this may predispose to loss of support in the lateral alar region and consequent pinched tip deformity[47] with its corresponding functional issues.

Inherent or postoperative weakness in the lateral crus can cause the anterior and midportion of the tip to collapse, as there is direct cartilaginous support in this portion. Posterolaterally, there is thick alar soft tissue and skin so less problems are likely in this area (**Fig. 14.18**).

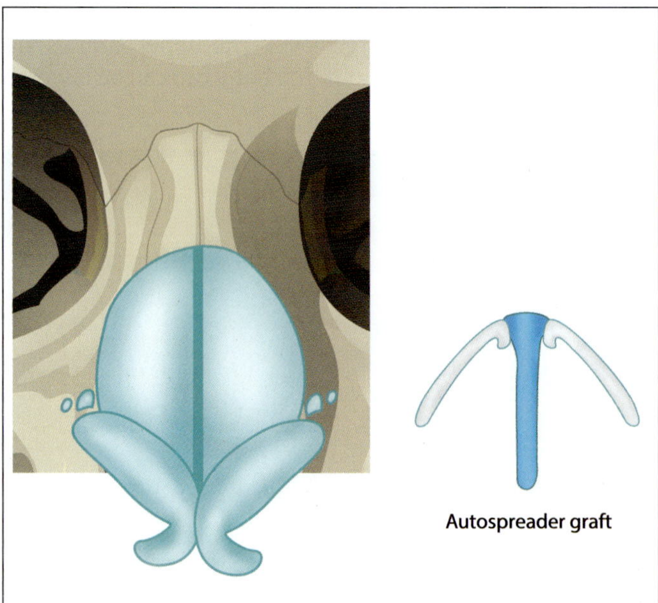

Fig. 14.14 Autospreader graft/spreader flap created by turn-in of upper lateral cartilages.

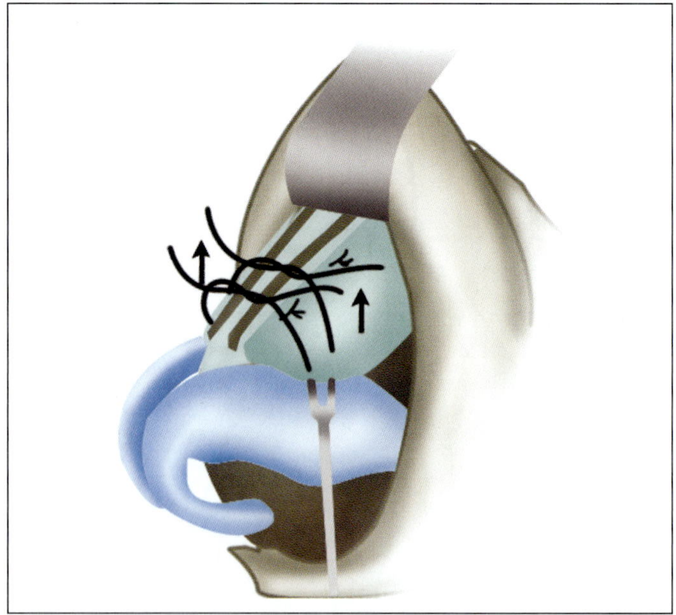

Fig. 14.15 Upper lateral cartilage flaring suture.

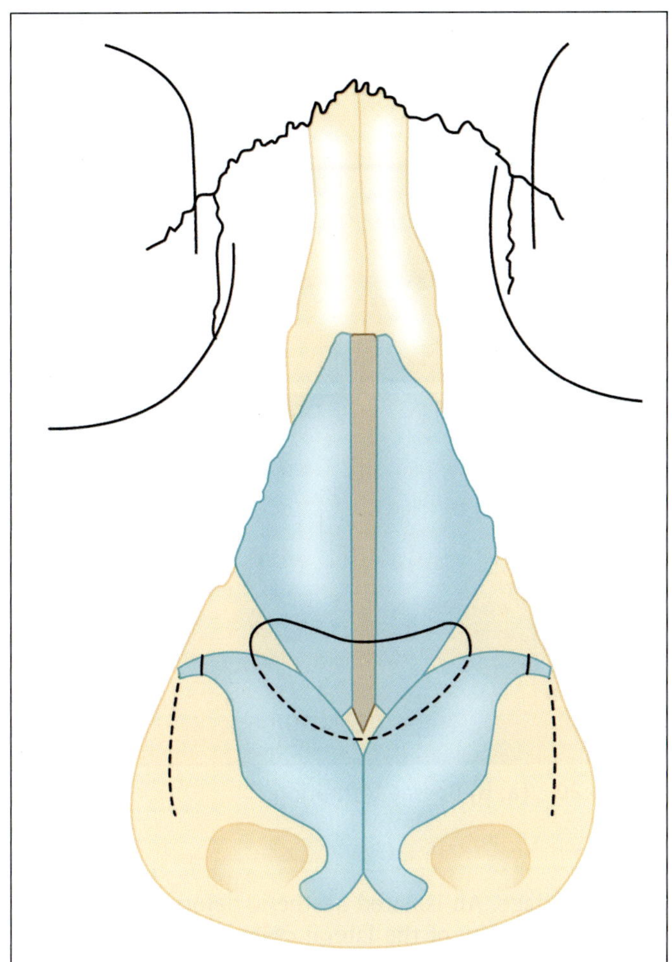

Fig. 14.16 Cartilaginous butterfly graft placement.

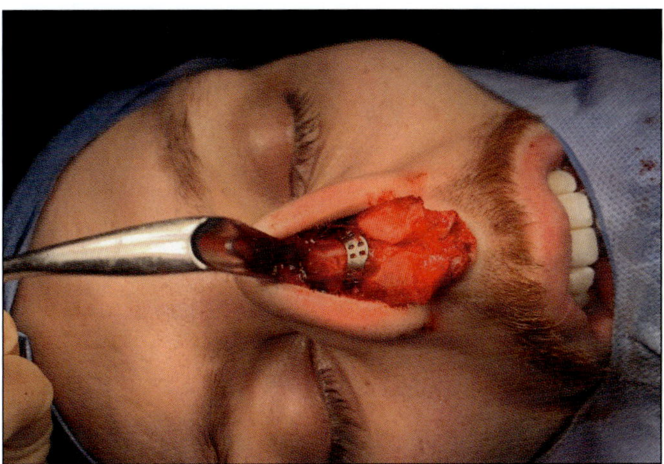

Fig. 14.17 Placement of a titanium implant to improve internal valve function.

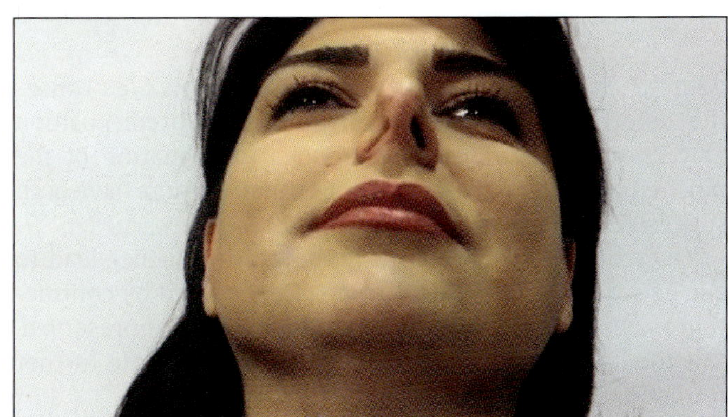

Fig. 14.18 External valve collapse on mild inspiration.

The so-called "pinched nasal tip" is a deformity caused primarily by collapse of the lateral crura of the lower lateral cartilages. Such collapse may be congenital secondary due to inherent hypoplasia, weakening, or malposition of the cartilaginous support. It is, however, often secondary to acquired, with commonly iatrogenic causes. The resultant pinching effect gives an unaesthetic appearance characterized by an alar groove, which extends to the alar rim, causing shadowing between the tip and alar lobules. Such shadows give rise to a ball-shaped tip and the basal view exhibits a typical pinched appearance. An inward curvature of the lateral crural cartilage can further impinge into the airway. At its worst, narrowing can lead to severe knuckling and bossae formation in the nasal dome region with resultant nasal obstruction by impedance of the airflow on inspiration.[48] Correction of the functional and aesthetic components to this problem is achieved with restoration of the alar cartilaginous strength and structure and requires appropriate, ideally autogenous, grafting material.

Weakness of the lateral cartilaginous support leads to the nostril rim contracting inwards under the weight of the thick alar skin and soft tissue envelope. Inspiration may exacerbate this collapse. The basal view (**Fig. 14.19**) exhibits a typical appearance resembling a teat on a baby's bottle.[36]

Congenitally weak lower lateral cartilages predispose to this deformity. The lateral nasal rim is typically convex and its most severe form can buckle in so dramatically that it can restrict the nasal airway even in the resting state.

The most common cause for this deformity is due to iatrogenic weakening of the lower lateral cartilages due to over-resection of the cephalic edge of the lower lateral cartilages with subsequent weakening of intact rim strip. The useful edict of leaving behind more cartilage than that resected should always be remembered, although the authors recommend an absolute minimum of 6-mm cartilaginous support but leaving more may be favorable.

Knuckling of the lower lateral cartilages, in the domal area, form bossae (**Fig. 14.20**). The inexperienced rhinoplasty surgeon may not be aware of the triad of thin skin, strong alar cartilages, and bifidity of the tip, which together predispose to their formation when there is an excess cephalic strip reduction and inadequate narrowing of the

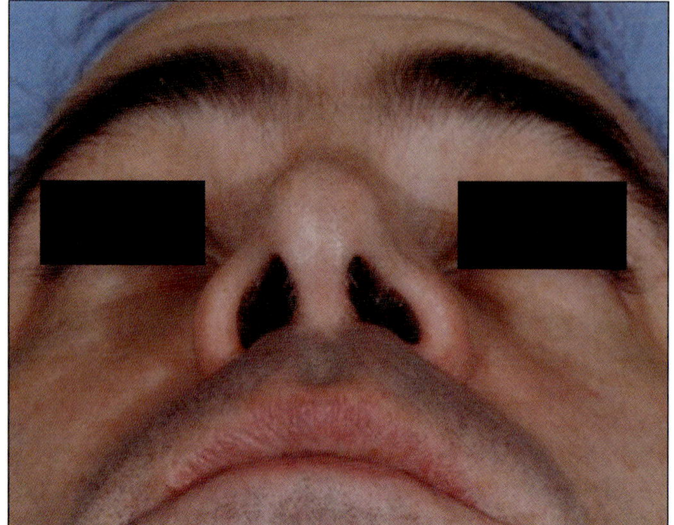

Fig. 14.19 "Baby bottle teat" appearance to nasal tip.

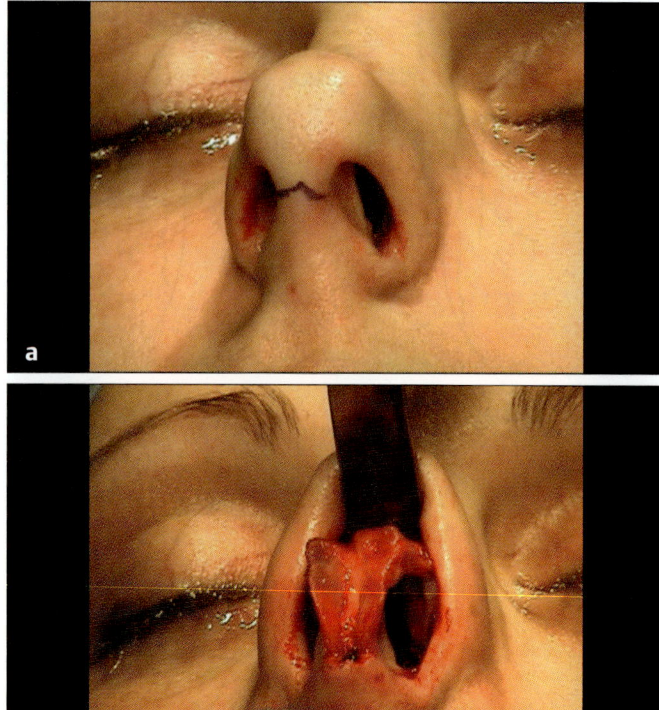

Fig. 14.20 **(a, b)** Bossae formation.

domes.[46] Postoperative scar contracture in this area causes the deformity. Controversy surrounds the predisposition of vertical dome division techniques to formation of the pinched tip and bossae, and distinguished authors have both suggested and refuted this possibility.

Overzealous cephalic strip resection can further lead to alar retraction due to the visoring effect caused by contraction as healing occurs. If vestibular mucosa is not preserved, this too can contribute to contracture and promote further retraction.

Aggressive domal suturing with its resultant alteration in tip orientation and dynamics can cause notching in the dome region predisposing to a pinched tip effect. The curvature of the lateral crus into the airway can contribute significantly to nasal obstruction postoperatively and is important to assess perioperatively.

Other more unusual causes of this deformity include collapse of the alar cartilaginous region following inflammatory conditions such as Wegener granulomatosis but may also occur following cocaine abuse.

Operative Techniques for the External Nasal Valve

Endonasal Approach

Correction of the pinched tip deformity can be achieved in a variety of ways. For minor deformity, an endonasal approach may prove adequate for placement of supporting grafts in primary surgery or to correct prior overzealous tip suturing. Marginal incisions may allow delivery of the lower lateral cartilages that can be repositioned and modified as required. Small specific pockets can also allow batten grafts to be inserted to correct concavities caused by weakness of the cartilage. An isolated aesthetic deformity caused by inherent concavity of the lateral crus may be corrected by complete mobilization of the lower lateral cartilage from the vestibular skin. An incision is then made just lateral to the domal area and the lateral crus flipped over such that the concavity now becomes a convexity. The rotated crus is then sutured reconstructed to the medial segment.

External Approach

It is our preference to employ the external approach for most revision cases. This allows accurate evaluation of the orientation, integrity, and strength of the alar cartilages.

Cartilaginous Augmentation

Restoration of cartilaginous support is paramount with this deformity. The firmness and straightness of septal cartilage may be an advantage for alar batten and lateral crural strut grafting but auricular cartilage can be carved to shape very well even if it is a little weaker. Rib cartilage may be the preferred option in severe postinflammatory contraction and in the presence of multiple other grafting needs. Other nonautogenous material is generally not advocated by the authors.

Batten Grafts

Cartilaginous batten grafts can help strengthen the lateral wall of the mid-third of the nose in cases of upper lateral cartilage weakness. These can be taken from any suitable cartilaginous source, although conchal cartilage sometimes does not afford enough rigidity. Such grafts need to extend to the bony pyriform aperture to ensure there is a lateral anchor so that inward displacement does not occur. They are often fashioned to be triangular in shape with the pointed part extending laterally to lie in a pocket overlying the bone. They act to stabilize and prevent inward movement of the weakened cartilaginous area into the airway, thereby preventing obstruction on normal nasal inspiration. Care to feather graft edges is particularly important in the thinner skinned patient as such grafts may have a degree of visibility with time and can certainly increase the width of the midthird somewhat. Both issues need to be discussed with the patient preoperatively, especially in the aesthetically sensitive patient.

These grafts can be easily placed endonasally in a "hand-in-glove" fashion into a dissected pocket and held with a percutaneous suture if needed. Otherwise, an open approach will facilitate accurate visualization and direct suturing onto the underlying structures.

The graft may need to extend to the caudal lateral crus. A more anatomically placed graft extending along the weakened lateral crus to the pyriform aperture is termed a lateral crural graft. The convex side of the graft is placed laterally to help correct the pinch deformity. It is important to maintain as much skin and soft tissue cover to reduce the risk of the graft showing postoperatively. If inserted in a specific "hand-in-glove" manner, fixation may not be necessary particularly if performed via an endonasal approach. When an open approach is preferred, the grafts can be suture fixated to the lateral crus (**Fig. 14.21**).

Lateral Crural Strut Grafts

Lateral crural strut grafts are placed in a pocket between the lateral crus and vestibular skin such that they extend laterally to the pyriform aperture. They are not to be confused with lateral crural grafts, which are positioned between the external skin and lateral crus (see alar batten section). While they essentially have the same function as alar battens, they have the advantage of causing less visible distortion externally in thin skin patients. Such grafts are also used to provide support when cephalically malpositioned lateral crura are repositioned caudally in patients with a "parenthesis"-type tip deformity.

Careful dissection is required between the vestibular skin and lateral crus, making this technically more difficult than alar battens. Care has to be taken to avoid the graft protruding into the airway.

Dome suturing is used to narrow the domal angle but may also cause significant concavity or occasionally convexity of the lateral crus in the process. If such deformity cannot be resolved by repositioning of the sutures, lateral crural strut grafts can effectively flatten this area giving rise to an aesthetic contour (**Fig. 14.22**).

Alar Rim Grafts

Alar rim grafts are fashioned from thin, soft cartilage. They are approximately 2 to 3 mm wide. A pocket is created between the external skin and vestibular skin along the caudal margin of the marginal incision along the alar rim border. Care is taken to remain as close to the vestibular skin as possible to avoid any risk of puncture through the

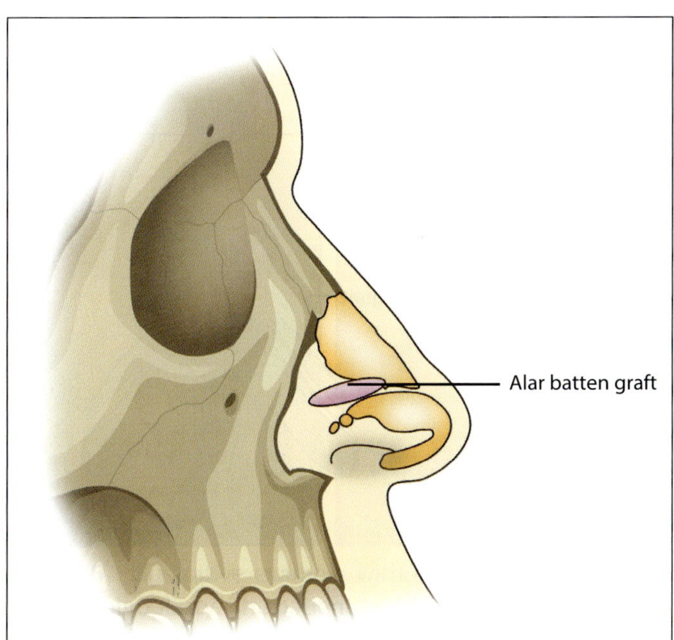

Fig. 14.21 Alar batten graft anchored laterally over the pyriform aperture.

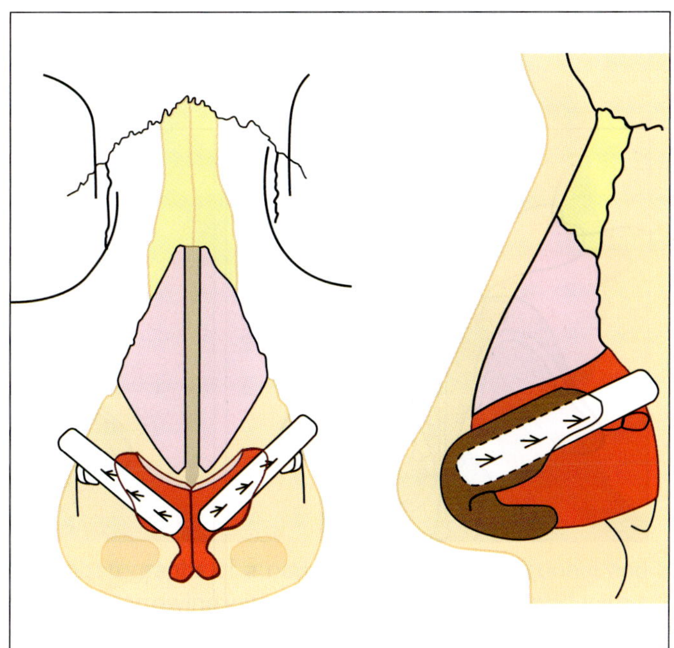

Fig. 14.22 Lateral crural strut grafts.

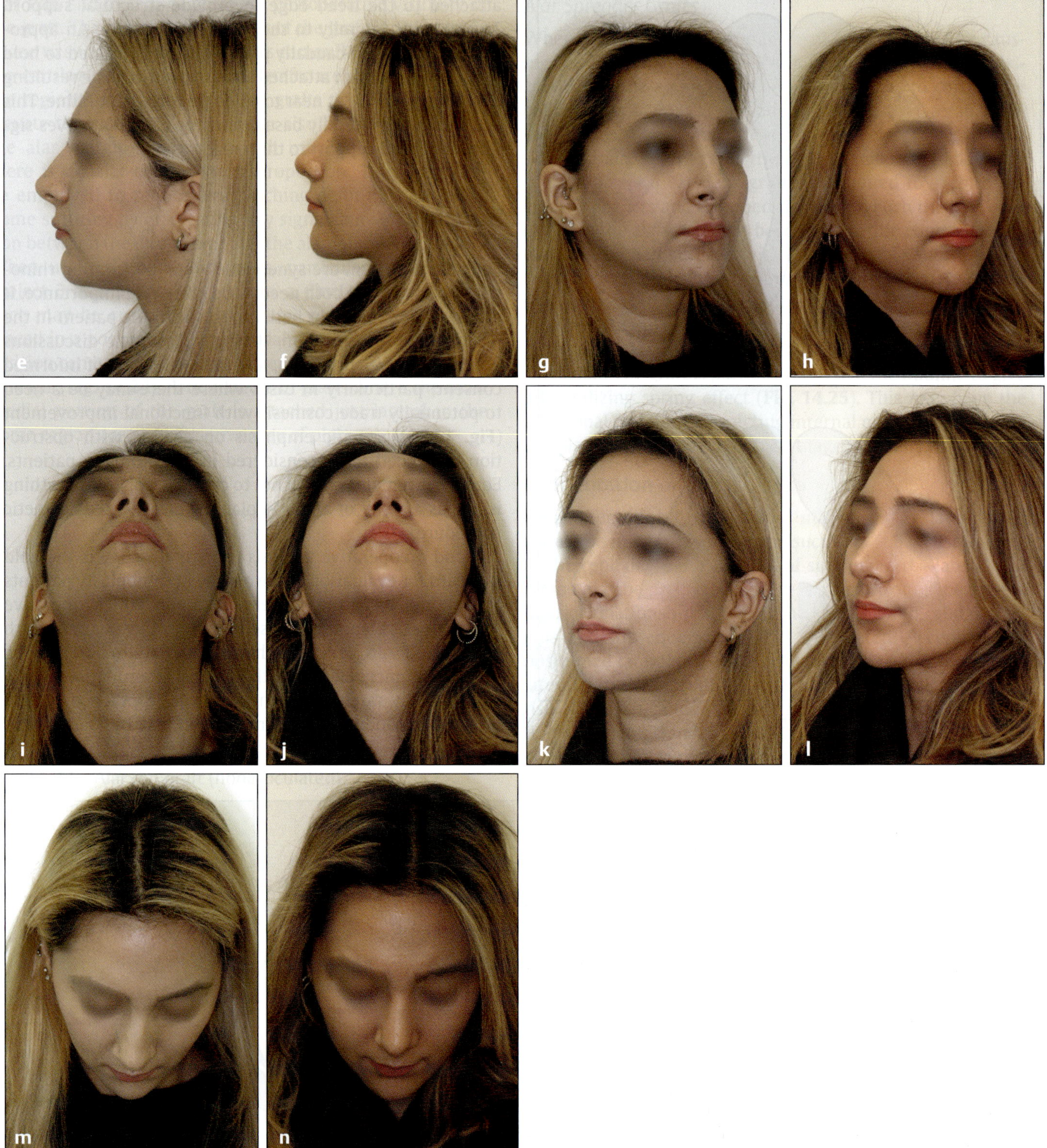

Fig. 14.26 (*Continued*) **(e, g, i, k, m)** Preoperative and **(f, h, j, l, n)** postoperative images in various views.

regulators or insurance providers to demonstrate objective need for surgical intervention.

Surgical correction with the described methods can help correct septal deformities, internal and external nasal valve issues, and deal with turbinate hypertrophy if required. Equally, protection against long-term functional compromise can be had with robust technique, and most importantly, aforethought after recognition of potential pitfalls in standard rhinoplasty techniques.

References

1. Guyron B. Rhinoplasty. New York: Elsevier; 2012
2. Daniel R, Palhazi P. Rhinoplasty: an anatomical and clinical atlas. Springer International; 2018:114
3. Kennedy D, Hwang P. Rhinology diseases of the nose, sinuses and skull base. New York: Thieme; 2012
4. Behrbohm H, Tardy M. Essentials of septorhinoplasty. New York: Thieme; 2012
5. Casiano R, Herzallah I, Eloy J. Endoscopic sinonasal dissection guide. New York: Thieme; 2017
6. Chavan SS, Khond AD, Saple P, Kurle VR. Comparative study between diathermy and microdebrider for inferior turbinate reduction surgeries. Rhinology Online 2020;3:1–7
7. Lund VJ, Stammberger H, Fokkens WJ, et al. European position paper on the anatomical terminology of the internal nose and paranasal sinuses. Rhinol Suppl 2014;24:1–34
8. Nigro CE, Nigro JF, Mion O, Mello JF Jr. Nasal valve: anatomy and physiology. Rev Bras Otorhinolaringol (Engl Ed) 2009;75(2): 305–310
9. Sclafani A. Rhinoplasty: the experts' reference. New York: Thieme; 2015
10. Sethi N, Pearson A, Bajaj Y. Key clinical topics in otolaryngology. London: JP Medical Ltd; 2017
11. Wormald PJ. Endoscopic sinus surgery: anatomy, three dimensional reconstruction, and surgical technique. New York: Thieme; 2012
12. Robotti E. Shaping the nasal dorsum. HNO 2018;66(2):92–102
13. Bloom JD, Sridharan S, Hagiwara M, Babb JS, White WM, Constantinides M. Reformatted computed tomography to assess the internal nasal valve and association with physical examination. Arch Facial Plast Surg 2012;14(5):331–335
14. Afifi AM, Kempton SJ, Gordon CR, et al. Evaluating current functional airway surgery during rhinoplasty: a survey of the American Society of Plastic Surgeons. Aesthetic Plast Surg 2015;39(2):181–190
15. Wright L, Grunzweig KA, Totonchi A. Nasal obstruction and rhinoplasty: a focused literature review. Aesthetic Plast Surg 2020 Apr 23. Online ahead of print
16. Tanna N, Nguyen KT, Ghavami A, et al. Evidence-based medicine: current practices in rhinoplasty. Plast Reconstr Surg 2018;141(1):137e–151e
17. Ottaviano G, Fokkens WJ. Measurements of nasal airflow and patency: a critical review with emphasis on the use of peak nasal inspiratory flow in daily practice. Allergy 2016;71(2):162–174
18. Duygu D, Cingi C, Cakli H, Kaya E. Use of rhinomanometry in common rhinologic disorders. Expert Rev Med Devices (London) 2011;8(6):769–777
19. Roithmann R, Cole P, Chapnik J, Shpirer I, Hoffstein V, Zamel N. Acoustic rhinometry in the evaluation of nasal obstruction. Laryngoscope 1995;105(3 Pt 1):275–281
20. Cole P, Fenton RS. Contemporary rhinomanometry. J Otolaryngol 2006;35(2):83–87
21. Eccles R. A guide to practical aspects of measurement of human nasal airflow by rhinomanometry. Rhinology 2011;49(1):2–10
22. Hirschberg A. Rhinomanometry: an update. ORL J Otorhinolaryngol Relat Spec 2002;64(4):263–267
23. Borojeni AAT, Garcia GJM, Moghaddam MG, et al. Normative ranges of nasal airflow variables in healthy adults. Int J CARS 2020;15(1):87–98
24. Boenisch M, Nolst Trenité GJ. Reconstructive septal surgery. Facial Plast Surg 2006;22(4):249–254
25. Wang LL, Frankel AS, Friedman O. Complications of polydioxanone foil use in nasal surgery: a case series. Facial Plast Surg 2018;34(3):312–317
26. Gubisch W. Zwanzig Jahre Erfahrung mit der extrakorporalen Septumkorrektur. (20 years' experience with extracorporal septoplasty). Laryngorhinootologie 2002;81(1):22–30
27. Most SP. Anterior septal reconstruction: outcomes after a modified extracorporeal septoplasty technique. Arch Facial Plast Surg 2006;8(3):202–207
28. Bönisch M, Mink A. Septumrekonstruktion mit PDS-Folie. (Septum reconstruction with PDS implant). HNO 1999;47(6): 546–550
29. Rezaeian F, Gubisch W, Janku D, Haack S. New suturing techniques to reconstruct the keystone area in extracorporeal septoplasty. Plast Reconstr Surg 2016;138(2):374–382
30. Daniel RK, Calvert JW. Diced cartilage grafts in rhinoplasty surgery. Plast Reconstr Surg 2004;113(7):2156–2171
31. Tasman AJ. Advances in nasal dorsal augmentation with diced cartilage. Curr Opin Otolaryngol Head Neck Surg 2013;21(4):365–371
32. Sinno S, Mehta K, Lee Z-H, Kidwai S, Saadeh PB, Lee MR. Inferior turbinate hypertrophy in rhinoplasty: systematic review of surgical techniques. Plast Reconstr Surg 2016; 138(3):419e–429e
33. Cingi C, Ure B, Cakli H, Ozudogru E. Microdebrider-assisted versus radiofrequency-assisted inferior turbinoplasty: a prospective study with objective and subjective outcome measures. Acta Otorhinolaryngol Ital 2010;30(3):138–143
34. Bhattacharyya N, Kepnes LJ. Clinical effectiveness of coblation inferior turbinate reduction. Otolaryngol Head Neck Surg 2003;129(4):365–371
35. Gillman GS, Simons RL, Lee DJ. Nasal tip bossae in rhinoplasty. Etiology, predisposing factors, and management techniques. Arch Facial Plast Surg 1999;1(2):83–89
36. Paun S. External rhinoplasty. Ch. 82. In: Watkinson JC, Clarke RW, eds. Scott Brown's otolaryngology and head and neck surgery. 8th ed. Boca Raton: CRC Press; 2018:1143–1160
37. Sheen JH. Spreader graft: a method of reconstructing the roof of the middle nasal vault following rhinoplasty. Plast Reconstr Surg 1984;73(2):230–239
38. André RF, Paun SH, Vuyk HD. Endonasal spreader graft placement as treatment for internal nasal valve insufficiency: no need to divide the upper lateral cartilages from the septum. Arch Facial Plast Surg 2004;6(1):36–40
39. Tardy ME. Cartilage autografts reconstruction of the nose. In: Rhinoplasty, the art and the science. Volume II. Philadelphia: W.B. Saunders; 1987:648–724
40. Oneal RM, Berkowitz RL. Upper lateral cartilage spreader flaps in rhinoplasty. Aesthet Surg J 1998;18(5):370–371
41. Gruber RP, Park E, Newman J, Berkowitz L, Oneal R. The spreader flap in primary rhinoplasty. Plast Reconstr Surg 2007;119(6):1903–1910

42. Paun S. Rhinoplasty in patients from South Asia. In: Cobo R, ed. Ethnic considerations in facial plastic surgery. New York: Thieme; 2016:231–240
43. Park SS. The flaring suture to augment the repair of the dysfunctional nasal valve. Plast Reconstr Surg 1998;101(4): 1120–1122
44. Clark JM, Cook TA. The "butterfly" graft in functional secondary rhinoplasty. Laryngoscope 2002;112(11):1917–1925
45. van den Broek SJAC, van Heerbeek N. The effect of the titanium butterfly implant on nasal patency and quality of life. Rhinology 2018;56(4):364–369
46. Paun SH, Nolst Trenité GJ. Revision rhinoplasty: an overview of deformities and techniques. Facial Plast Surg 2008;24(3): 271–287
47. Toriumi DM, Checcone MA. New concepts in nasal tip contouring. Facial Plast Surg Clin North Am 2009;17(1):55–90, vi
48. Cottle M. Changing concepts in rhinoplastic surgery. Ann Otol Rhinol Laryngol 1955;64(2):632–633
49. Ballin AC, Kim H, Chance E, Davis RE. The articulated alar rim graft: reengineering the conventional alar rim graft for improved contour and support. Facial Plast Surg 2016;32(4):384–397

15

Primary Rhinoplasty

Lokesh Kumar

Introduction

The word "rhinoplasty" originates from Greek word *Rhis* which means the nose and *Plassein* which means to shape. In common language it is known as the nose job. Out of all cosmetic operations it is one of the most complex, trickiest, and poorly understood procedure. It is difficult to master even after many years of experience. It is sometimes frustrating to see your own results crumbling before your eyes over a period of time—if you have courage to follow them up for long. Poor understanding of anatomy, surgical cause and effect relationship, and failure to visualize three-dimensional nature of the deformity contribute to poor outcomes of rhinoplasty surgery.

Results that might look good on the operation table may distort over a period of time because of forces of healing. Despite various teaching tools available today, this is the operation where one would much rely on self-learning. Careful maintenance of surgical records and comparable clinical photographs at various stages of follow-up is an important self-learning tool. Rhinoplasty techniques also have undergone a sea change in the past decade or so. Cartilage conservation and optimum utilization through suture modification have given way to resection and rejection. The trend is more toward conserving native anatomy.[1] The conservative approach to gain subtle results has given way for more radical approach for better refinement and long-lasting results. Preoperative assessment of nasal anatomy and nasofacial analysis helps in determining the operative plan which should be adhered to, with minor deviations in the operating room.

This operation is aimed at restoring form and function both and involves a variety of operative steps to achieve this. Therefore, the rhinoplasty surgeon needs firm knowledge of functional and aesthetic aspect of this surgery.

Historical Perspectives

Even though the history of rhinoplasty dates back to several centuries before Christ, most earlier descriptions in Indian and Egyptian writings relate to the reconstructive rhinoplasty for lost or broken nose.[2] This trend continued in the Roman era till as late as 16th century with description by Gaspare Tagliacozzi (1546–1599) of flap reconstruction of nose.[3]

The first available account of rhinoplasty purely for cosmetic reasons is by American otolaryngologist John Orlando Roe (1848–1915)[4] for correction of saddle nose deformity which he termed as pug nose in his original article published in 1887. This seems to be the first case of endonasal rhinoplasty as per resources available today.

Jacques Joseph, an orthopaedic surgeon from Germany in the year 1898 developed many revolutionary concepts in rhinoplasty which still stand ground, and for this reason he is rightly credited to be the father of modern rhinoplasty. His techniques were carried on by many American surgeons, such as Gustav Aufricht, Joseph Safian, Samuel Fomon, and many others, who further refined them. In early 20th century, surgeons like Freer and Killian contributed to the refinement of septum work with the description of many concepts like mucoperichondrial flaps, resection of cartilage, bone, vomer, ethmoid, etc., which were new at that time.

Even though described quite early in 1921 by Rethi,[5] the "open rhinoplasty approach" was lost to the archives till it was rediscovered by surgeons like Goodman (1973)[6] who with his publication "External approach to rhinoplasty" in the year 1973 popularized the open approach. His views were further strengthened by Jack Anderson (1982)[7] in an article "Open rhinoplasty: an assessment." He was a big critic of open rhinoplasty but later changed his stance and became an ardent supporter of the open technique. Gunter further popularized the technique with his two publications: "External approach to secondary rhinoplasty" and "The merits of open approach in rhinoplasty" in the PRS journal in 1987 and 1997.[8,9]

Many rhinoplasty surgeons have emerged in recent times, who are contributing to the understanding of this intricate operation to the benefit of both patients and surgeons.

Surgical Anatomy

A thorough knowledge of nasal anatomy is of paramount importance for the rhinoplasty surgeon. The nose is a unique organ in the human body because of intricate cause-and-effect relationship of nasal skeleton with the external appearance. Even a slight change made in skeletal tissues has a profound effect on appearance, which can be exploited by learned surgeons to their advantage to achieve better shape of the nose. On the other hand, incorrect manipulation can lead to disastrous results.

Similarly, functional anatomy is also important since any change made on nasal skeleton has far-reaching consequences vis-à-vis the breathing functionality of nose. Breathing mechanism of the nose of a person can vastly be improved through a correctly done rhinoplasty operation, and the reverse of this statement is also true. A detailed description of nasal anatomy is beyond the scope of this chapter. However, it is pertinent to mention a few important practical points.

Nasal soft tissues deserve special mention because it has a direct bearing on the outcome, especially in ethnic noses. The nasal soft tissues comprise of nasal skin, subcutaneous fibrofatty tissue and underlying muscles, and submusculoaponeurotic system (SMAS).

Skin evaluation plays an important role in predicting the outcome of surgery as thick skin will not drape well over the modified cartilaginous framework as compared to thin skin.[10] The quality and thickness of nasal skin varies as per the ethnicity of an individual. The skin has varying thickness and characteristics in various parts of the same nose. It is thickest and overtly inelastic in nature in the lower portion of the nose, and is closely adherent to the underlying cartilaginous frame work. Together they form a mobile structure of the nose, which can move and glide over the fixed upper portion formed by the bony and cartilaginous skeleton. The skin gradually becomes thin and elastic over middle portion of the nose, and again acquires moderate thickness in the glabellar region. In most Caucasians the skin is soft, thin, and elastic, and generally covers a strong bony and cartilaginous framework. Reverse is true in South-East Asian noses, where the skin is thick and sebaceous and compensates the support mechanism to the nose in the absence of a strong cartilage framework. The thickness in the lower third is attributed to the presence of sebaceous glands and a thick musculoaponeurotic system, which lies over lower half of the nose.

Clinical examination is accurate and good enough as compared to a high-resolution computed tomography (CT) scan; therefore, it is quite unnecessary to conduct any radiographical examination just for this purpose.[11] However, Zein Obagi has highlighted the importance of ultrasound in skin assessment and has given an algorithm of pretreating various skin types before rhinoplasty.[12] This is important since there is very little we can do to alter skin surgically, as compared to the underlying soft tissues which have manipulability during surgery.

Aesthetic segments of the nose are analyzed in relation to the rest of the face. Segmental examination does not leave any scope of missing important points in nasal anatomy. A systematic analysis of not only the nose but the whole face can reveal information hitherto unknown to the patient and useful for surgeons (**Fig. 15.1**).

Blood supply to the nasal tip is an arcade of blood vessels from angular artery which is a branch of facial artery and columellar arteries which are branches of superior labial artery. This has bearing in open rhinoplasty cases in which the columellar branches are divided as a consequence of the transcolumellar incision leaving the blood supply solely coming from branches of angular artery. The alar resection in such cases is carefully planned; otherwise, it may compromise the blood supply to the tip (**Fig. 15.2**).

Most *nerves* supplying the nose are located in deep subcutaneous fatty layer.[13] The correct plane of undermining is loose areolar tissue superficial to perichondrium which protects these nerves. This is a relatively bloodless plane as the blood vessels are also located in the same layer as nerves (**Fig. 15.3**).

Bony and cartilaginous skeleton should be assessed preoperatively. This helps in making crucial decisions during surgery. Length of the nasal bones in particular has bearing upon the type of osteotomy chosen. Long bones are accompanied by a hump, which is mostly bony and requires power tools for reduction. In such cases, usually the upper lateral cartilages are very short and greater portion of them lie buried under the nasal bones.

Functional anatomy gives important information about the nasal airway. External and internal nasal valves should be studied, and appropriate measures should be taken during surgery to prevent any collapse of airway. Corrective steps should be part of operative plan, if collapse is already present. For further details, refer to Chapter 14 on "Functional Septorhinoplasty" in Volume VI.

Patient Selection

Evaluation of Psychological Status

A patient seeking rhinoplasty should be carefully scrutinized for behavioral anomalies, and for this reason a rhinoplasty surgeon should adopt the role of a psychologist. He should be able to recognize and segregate those who have frank body dysmorphic disorder (BDD), need consultation with a psychiatrist. By doing so, he may save lots of future troubles which come with treating such patients. The prevalence of BDD may be as high as 13% for all patients seeking facial plastic surgery[14] and up to 43% in patients who present for a cosmetic rhinoplasty consultation.[15]

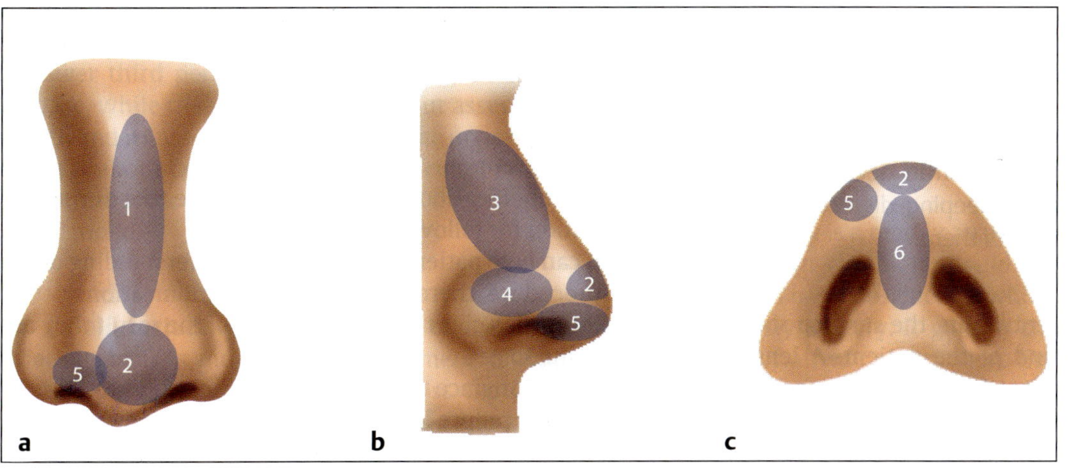

Fig. 15.1 (a–c) Aesthetic segments of the nose: 1, dorsal nasal segment; 2, hemilobule segment; 3, lateral nasal wall segment; 4, alar segment; 5, soft tissue triangle segment; 6, collumelar segment.

Open versus Closed Rhinoplasty

Open versus closed rhinoplasty is a never ending debate. There are die-hard proponents of both these approaches. In author's opinion both the procedures are same in terms of technical alterations, albeit executed differently.

External or open approach is executed via a transcolumellar incision combined with marginal incision. The potential to cause prolonged tip edema, destabilization of cartilage framework, increased operating time, and columellar scar are some of the factors due to which critics of this technique argue against this approach. Except the prolonged tip edema which is a firm reality, other objections are very relative. The cartilage framework is carved and stabilized more effectively in open technique. Operating time depends on the experience of the surgeon and the extent of work requirement in a particular case. The incision if placed and sutured carefully gives a virtually nonexistent scar. All these factors should not be a deterrent in view of tremendous advantage open rhinoplasty gives in terms of 3D visualization and bilateral comparison of native nasal anatomy and its possible modification.[25] Majority of the patients (98%) are not "disturbed" by their external rhinoplasty scar, with 90% considering them to be invisible or barely perceptible.[26]

Closed rhinoplasty, which should be more correctly called endonasal rhinoplasty, in comparison, gives us limited access and exposure of nasal framework. However, it is more demanding and puts the surgeon's capability of visualization imagination to test. Proper modification of nasal framework may require many incisions, with the potential to scar and disturb the function of the nose. At the most, the technique can be used for a limited step rhinoplasty, and should be avoided for extensive corrections of middle vault and tip. Similarly, cases requiring extensive septal work also should be avoided by endonasal approach.

Most surgeons recognize the preference of one technique over the other in a particular case. But still there is a large gray area where either technique could be applied, and the surgeon's comfort in his choice for one over another should be respected.

Operative Techniques

For many years rhinoplasty was considered a reduction operation and for this reason the operative techniques, in most literature of that time, subscribed mostly to Caucasian noses. There has been very little space allocation to the ethnic considerations in rhinoplasty. Even the books especially written on the subject like *Ethnic considerations in facial plastic surgery* by Roxana Cobo[27,28] has failed to address this issue properly.

Ethnic variations of African, Mediterranean, Latin, South-East Asian, Oriental, and Indian noses should be thoroughly studied by the surgeons depending on the demography of the practicing area. Even though the basic techniques of reduction, augmentation, and structural support remain same, it is the minor differences in application of these techniques in different ethnic subgroups which set them apart from a typical Caucasian rhinoplasty. Surgeons must remember that most ethnic patients want a better looking ethnic nose, rather than converting their nose into a Caucasian nose. Rhinoplasty surgery in Indian patients can be a challenging task because of a wide variety of nasal shapes and sizes found in different regions. While the noses from extreme north may mimic Caucasians and from extreme east to Orientals, the noses from southern most states have Dravidian traits in them. All other parts of India have a mix of all these characteristics. Any rhinoplasty surgeon dealing with diverse demographic population should be versatile enough to deal with all the problems associated with them and yet maintain their ethnicity.

Anesthesia

Adequate anesthesia is crucial for the success of this operation. Rhinoplasty has changed in the past decade and so has its anesthesia. Earlier, surgeons preferred local anesthesia and sedation for this operation, which is now not considered a safe option any more. Due to the extended length of operation in view of structural buildup and use of multiple grafts, this operation is best executed safely under general anesthesia by an anesthetist aware of specific needs of this operation. Adequate hypotension during the entire length of operation should be the goal. Labetalol, a β-blocker with alpha-blocking activity, works well in trained hands to reduce blood pressure safely in nonasthmatic patients or those without severe cardiac conduction defects like AV block. If need be, it can be combined with dexmedetomidine/propofol infusion. As these drugs work indirectly by deepening the level of anesthesia, they should be used sparingly. Various studies comparing labetalol with remifentanil, nitroglycerine, and dexmedetomidine have established superiority of labetalol for induced hypotension as judged by the absence of reflex tachycardia, faster induction of hypotension, faster recovery from anesthesia, and less postoperative sedation. It is recommended to use labetalol infusion after bolus doses, for induced hypotension.[29,30] Premedication with oral labetalol is also found to be an effective method to blunt induction and intubation-induced pressor reflex.[31,32]

Among inhalational anesthetic agents, sevoflurane is found to be most suitable due to lack of sympathetic cardiac stimulation. Desflurane, another agent, induces hypotension by peripheral vasodilation. This in turn causes reflex tachycardia which can be effectively countered by concomitant use of labetalol.[33]

Skilled anesthetist always prefers to use these antihypertensive agents at induction before surgeon injects adrenaline solution in operative area. Sympathetic cardiac stimulation, once established requires higher doses of these agents.

Incisions

Irrespective of the approach, there are six different incisions used in rhinoplasty in different permutations and combinations. Endonasal approach, in particular, needs a surgeon's dexterity to select the type and number of such incisions and will largely depend on the problem and surgical maneuver needed to correct it (**Fig. 15.4**).

Intercartilaginous Incision

This is a universal incision used in the endonasal technique. The incision is placed in the groove between upper lateral and lateral crus of lower lateral cartilages (LLC). This incision when joined with incision in the membranous septum gives sufficient exposure to dorsum and septum for normal reduction rhinoplasty and harvesting septal graft but is limited in application when extensive septal or tip work is needed. The incision preserves the intercartilaginous ligament at the cost of giving limited tip exposure. It also violates the scroll area which is a very vital area of internal nasal valve and any scarring can compromise function (**Fig. 15.5a, b**).

Transcartilaginous Incision

This incision is given in the lateral crus of LLC at the proposed line of cephalic resection. This has less risk of scarring in the internal nasal valve area, but is applicable to only those reduction rhinoplasties where LLC is very prominent and contributing to the bulk of the tip. In most ethnic rhinoplasties where we need to conserve as much cartilages as possible and there is need to augment the existing weak cartilages, this incision has very little utility.

Infracartilaginous or Marginal Incision

This incision is given at the distal margin of LLC. It has very little or no use when used alone but is of great value when it is combined with intercartilaginous incision in endonasal approach. This helps in delivery of LLC as a bipedicle flap which gives a greater visibility to both LLCs simultaneously for their modification. This is also an important part of open rhinoplasty incision when combined with transcolumellar incision.

Hemitransfixation

This incision is given at the distal margin of the septum in the membranous septum. This is mostly combined with intercartilaginous incision to provide wide exposure in endonasal approach.

Killian Incision

This incision is given in septal mucoperichondrium approximately 5 mm above the free margin of septum. It has advantage of approaching the area of septum where the

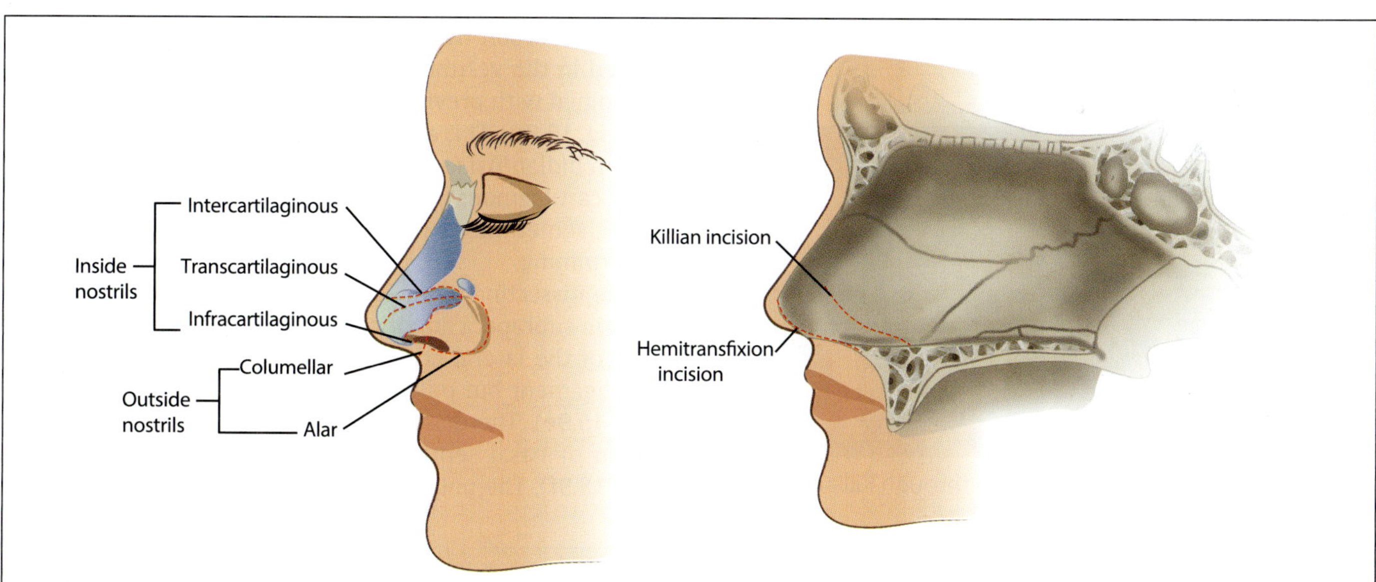

Fig. 15.4 Various incisions used in rhinoplasty.

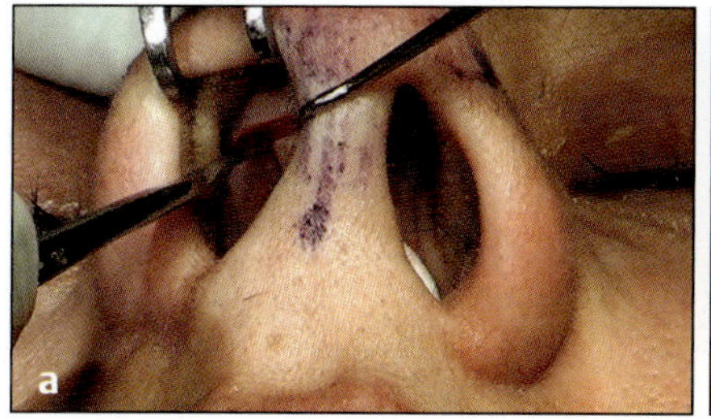

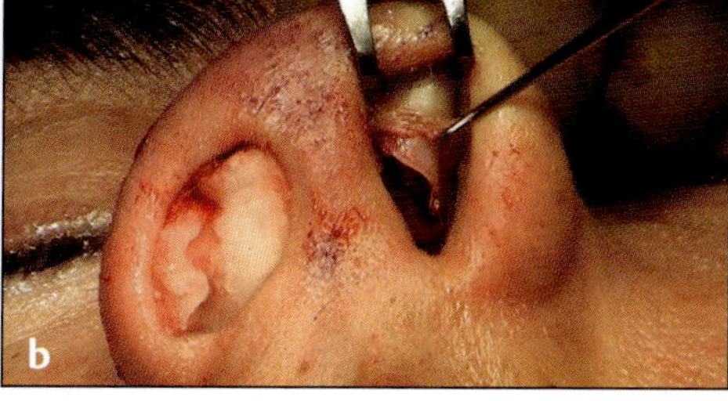

Fig. 15.5 **(a, b)** Intercartilaginous incision and exposure of lower lateral cartilage (LLC) through eversion technique in closed rhinoplasty.

mucoperichondrium is not densely adhered and gives a quick clean plane of access to septum. This was quite commonly used in earlier days when septoplasty was considered a separate operation from rhinoplasty. It has advantage of preserving the important support mechanism of tip. This has limited value today and can be utilized for harvesting septal graft in those few cases of tip plasty which do not need septal or dorsal modification (**Fig. 15.6a, b**).

Transcolumellar Incision

Transcolumellar incision combined with the marginal incision is the most common approach in open rhinoplasty. The incision has three distinct segments: marginal incision, transcolumellar segment across columella, and a vertical portion of incision on the side of columella joining these two. While the marginal and vertical portions remain same in all cases, the transcolumellar portion may differ in design as per the surgeon's preference (**Fig. 15.7a–c**).

The biggest criticism of this incision is the visible scar in columella. Various designs in the visible portion of columella can be stair step, chevron shape, straight cut at lip columella junction, V shape or inverted-V shape, W shape, etc. There are various studies in literature comparing stair step to inverted-V, transverse to inverted-V, and W to inverted-V. The chevron or transverse scars produce worst scars and should not be used. "W" incision and inverted-V incision provide good guide for suture placement and have similar scar quality. Stair step incision has been found to be inferior as compared to inverted-V.[34–36]

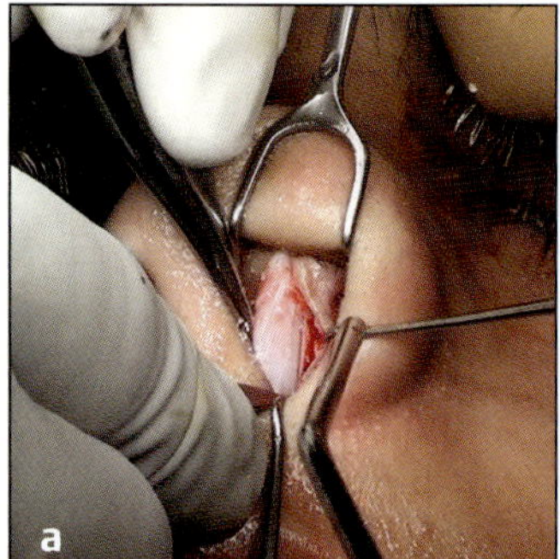

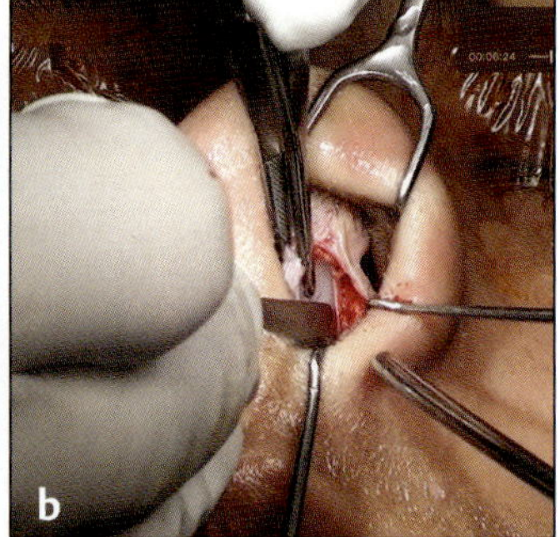

Fig. 15.6 **(a,b)** Exposure of septum through Killian incision.

Exposure

Surface markings are useful for predicting abnormalities in underlying skeletal structures. This also helps in post correction assessment of anomalies on operating table (**Fig. 15.8**).

Out of various transcolumellar incisions described for open approach, there is more or less consensus among well-known rhinoplasty surgeons on use of inverted-"V" incision. This is bilaterally symmetrical giving an equal view of both the nostrils and gives symmetry to both sides after closure. Underlying edge of medial crura provides support to the scar and prevents scar contraction (**Fig. 15.9a**). Injection of local anesthetic with 1:100,000 epinephrine, deep to SMAS layer, helps bloodless dissection in correct plane (**Fig. 15.9b**).

The *incision* is placed at the narrowest part of the columella. It is deepened in the center of "V" and kept superficial as one goes across the columella to reach the lateral side of the columellar pillar. The vertical portion of the incision is carefully deepened to expose the surface of medial crus of LLC (**Fig. 15.9c**). This incision is placed approximately 2 to 3 mm behind the distal free edge of medial crura. This bares about half width of the medial crura for placement of sutures which will be covered with the mucosa on final closure and do not stand chance of exposure. The final scar is also in the hidden portion of columellar mucosa. The mucosa in this region is thin and one has to be careful not to injure underlying cartilage. The whole columella is thus lifted till the region of soft triangle. The second part of incision is now started in the vestibule at the distal margin of lateral crus and joined with previous incision in the region of soft triangle (**Fig. 15.9d**). This approach of columella first gives advantage in Indian/Asian patients who have narrow nostrils and weak cartilaginous framework. Because of abundance of soft tissue, sometimes it is difficult to find the correct plane of undermining.

The dissection plane is kept very close to the alar cartilages in supraperichondrial plane till one reaches the upper limit of the lateral crus. Pitanguy ligament which is not a true ligament but only thickening of SMAS is now divided (**Fig. 15.9e**). The dissection plane now sharply dips in the region of nasal septal angle to stay close to the dorsum (**Fig. 15.9f**). The undermining is limited to the central area

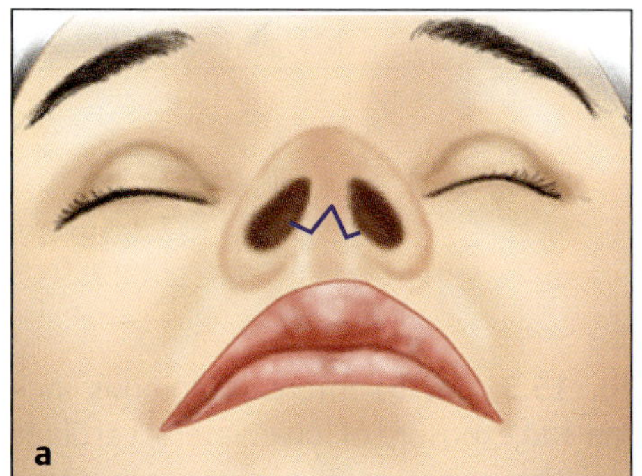

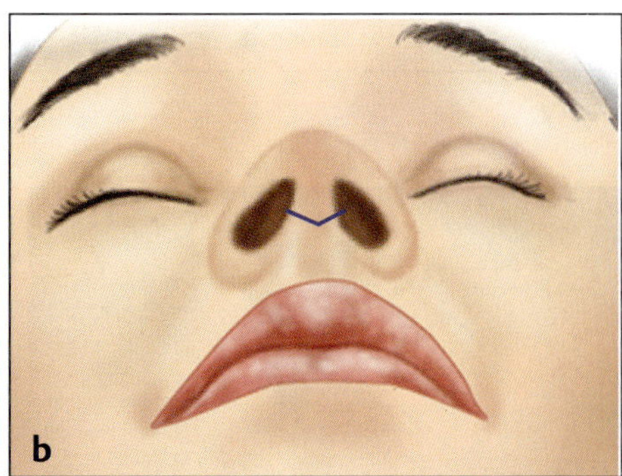

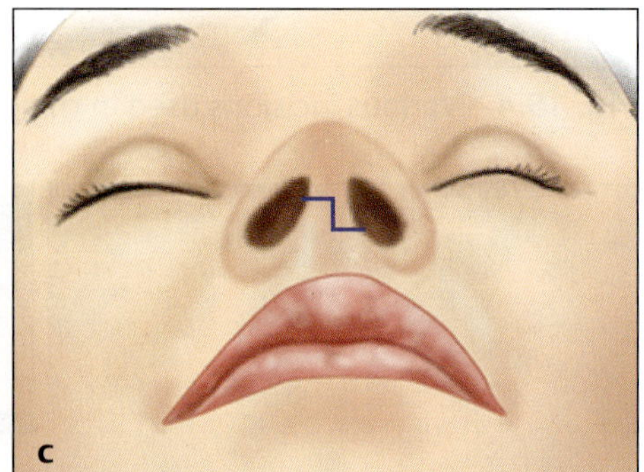

Fig. 15.7 Various columellar incisions. **(a)** Inverted-V. **(b)** Chevron. **(c)** Stair step.

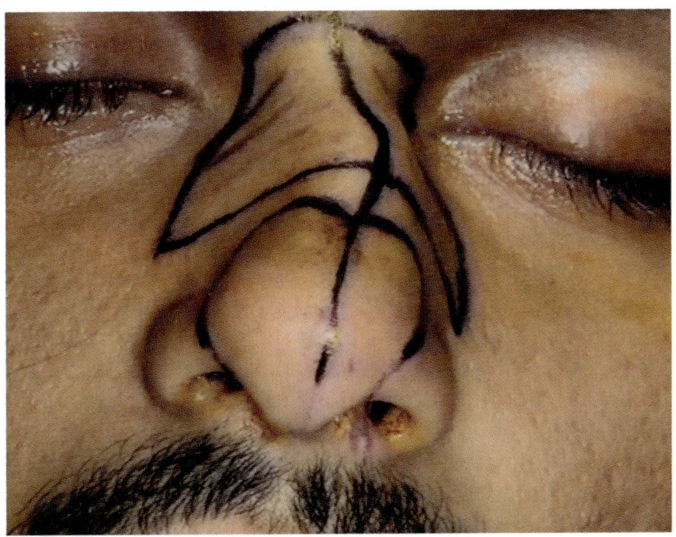

Fig. 15.8 Surface markings.

in this region and one should avoid going too far laterally if not needed (**Fig. 15.9g**). This dissection avoids blood vessels and nerves which are located in a fatty plane above SMAS of nose. The dissection stops at the lower margin of nasal bones. Midline vertical incision is given in the perichondrium on the dorsum (**Fig. 15.9h**). The upper end of the incision is merged with subperiosteal dissection over the nasal bones, which is undermined in the limited area on the dorsum. Extensive undermining of nasal bone periosteum should be avoided. Bilateral perichondral flaps are now raised over upper lateral cartilages for about 7 to 8 mm to give a clear view of upper lateral cartilage junction with the septum (**Fig. 15.9i**).

Septal exposure is done at this stage by midline approach. Sharp dissection in between medical crura is carried till the distal edge of septum, which may not always be in the midline and may be displaced into either of the nostrils (**Fig. 15.9j**). The distal most perichondrium on the septum is

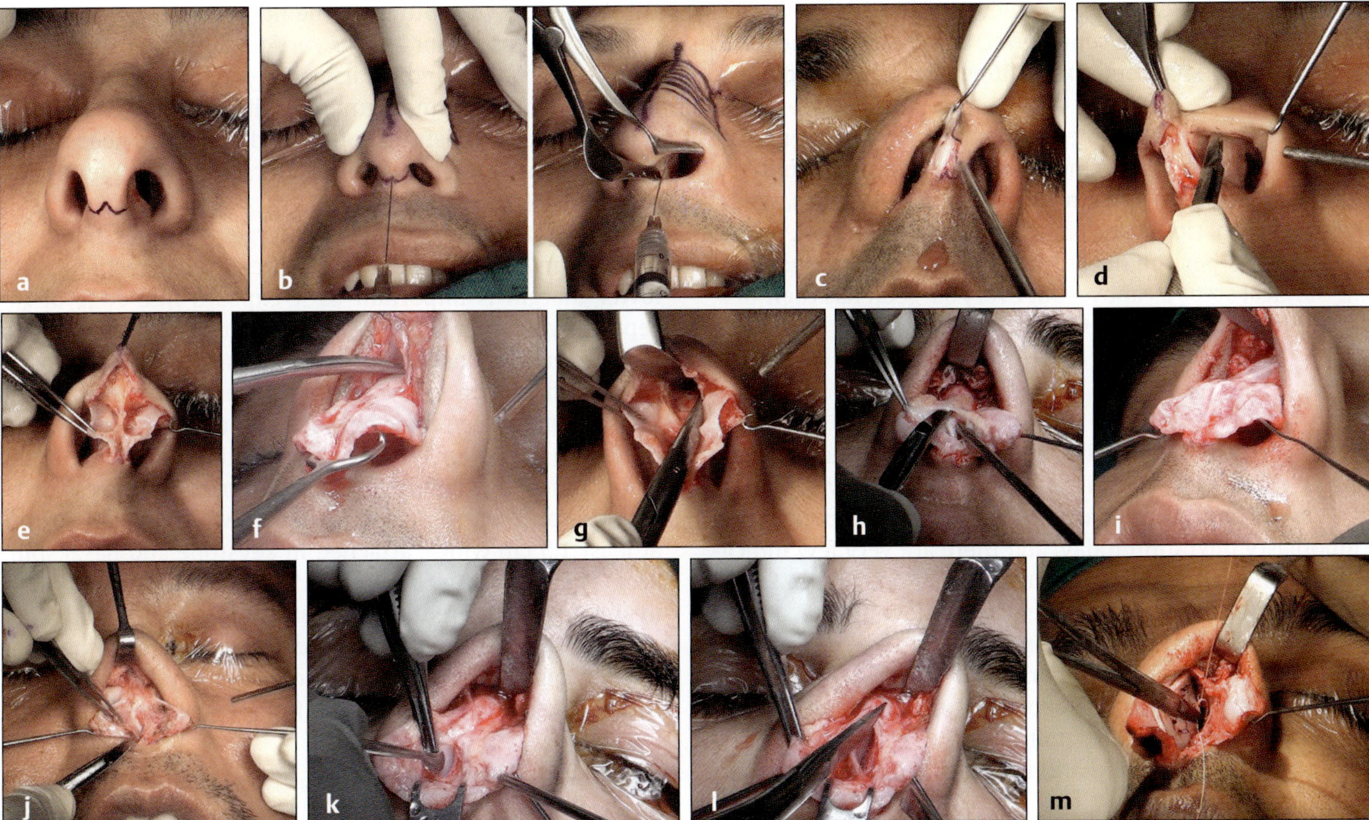

Fig. 15.9 **(a)** Inverted-V incision in open rhinoplasty. **(b)** Injection plane should be deep just over perichondrium. **(c)** Vertical limb of the incision is placed 2 to 3 mm behind the distal-free edge of medial crura to expose its surface. **(d)** Lifting the columella exposes the distal margin of lateral crus for vestibular part of incision. **(e)** Pitanguy ligament. **(f)** Dissection plane kept close to the perichondrium. **(g)** Lateral dissection is limited as per the need. **(h)** Dorsal perichondrium can be raised as flaps which can be closed over the dorsum after closure of the dorsum. **(i)** Degloving dorsal and distal exposure completed. **(j)** Septum is approached through intercrural space with sharp dissection till distal end of septum is encountered. **(k)** Perichondrium over the distal margin of septum is elevated with sharp dissection till glistening white cartilage surface is exposed. **(l)** Dissection is carried till junction of upper lateral cartilage (ULC) with septum and ULC is separated from septum. **(m)** Repair of mucosal tears before reconstructing septum.

densely adherent and should be separated by sharp dissection till one reaches glistening white cartilage (**Fig. 15.9k**). The mucoperichondrium on either side of the septum is now lifted with relative ease. The mucoperichondrium is separated in the uppermost part till the junction of upper lateral cartilage with septum. The upper lateral cartilages are now separated from the septum, keeping mucoperichondrial flaps on upper lateral cartilage side, using cartilage scissors or no.11 scalpel blade (**Fig. 15.9l**). Special care is taken while exposing septum in the lower most portion as mucoperichondrium is densely adherent in this area, and there may be bony spurs. The septum may not be in the vomerine groove, but may be deflected into either of the nostrils. This is the area most vulnerable to buttonholing which should be avoided at all costs. Any inadvertent disruption in the mucoperichondrium should be approximated with interrupted absorbable sutures (**Fig. 15.9m**). The degree of septal exposure needed varies from case to case. Sometimes only partial exposure is required, just to fix the spreader grafts in the dorsum or a septal extension or batten graft at the distal end. In any case of septal deviation or distortion, or if one needs to procure a septal graft, the wider area needs to be exposed. Medial osteotomies if needed are carried out at this stage.

Once exposure is complete it is important to sequence the operation at this stage. One needs to perform septoplasty, dorsal modification and closure of roof, osteotomies, dorsal augmentation, tip plasty, closure, and alar resection, in that order and as per the need. Most of the surgeons sequence the surgical steps as above, but every surgeon has their personal preferences.

Modification of Septum (Septoplasty)

Septal correction is the first and foremost step undertaken in any rhinoplasty as this forms the base on which nasal skeleton is built. Septoplasty is an essential component of a rhinoplasty operation today, and there are very few indications of this being done as a stand-alone procedure. Septal manipulation is needed for one of the following indications:

- Correction of crooked nose.
- Deprojection of nasal dorsum.
- Providing structural support in augmentation cases.
- Harvesting cartilage graft.
- Greater tip manipulation-projection, deprojection, or rotation.

Technique of Septal Correction

After exposure, the septum should be assessed for its size, shape, and anomalies. We may encounter hypoplastic or overgrown septum in some individuals.

Hypoplastic Septum

Hypoplastic septum is the characteristic of noses which require significant amount of structural support. It is rarely crooked but is weak and deficient in anteroposterior or vertical directions (**Fig. 15.10**). In both circumstances it needs strengthening with grafts like batten, spreader, or septal extension graft, or a combination, depending on the need. Hypoplastic septum which is straight and in midline should be exposed enough to fix the grafts for structural support. Opening the roof by separating upper laterals from septum is quite unnecessary in such cases. This keeps the nasal valve intact preserving its function, and saves surgical time. Presuming hypoplastic septum requiring structural support and augmentation, the surgeon should choose a suitable extranasal donor site for the graft. The costal cartilage provides abundant graft material. It should be harvested quite early during the operation or even before starting rhinoplasty. Very thin slices of this graft should be cut with the help of a dermatome blade and left in antibiotic solution. This allows time for any warping, which can be taken care of during final carving and preparation of graft before insertion (**Fig. 15.11a, b**).

Large Overgrown Septum

Large overgrown septum on the other hand is in excess in either anteroposterior and/or vertical directions. It is either crooked, deviated, and/or displaced into one of the nostrils and frequently not in alignment with anterior nasal spine (**Fig. 15.12**). Even if straight, this kind of septum needs exposure for hump removal or simple dorsal trimming for deprojection of a large nose (**Fig. 15.13**).

Unlike hypoplastic septum, large septum should be exposed in its entire length and breadth. Dissection at the lower margin is important as it exposes free edge of the septum which may have displaced into one of the nostrils. This extensive undermining removes all extrinsic forces causing distortion in the shape of the septum. If it is still bent it is presumed to be because of intrinsic forces. Author prefers to assess and remove any cartilage including hump from dorsal edge first. Next step is to trim any excess cartilaginous portion of septum from below, leaving a L-strut of at least 1.5 cm width, attached in keystone and nasal spine area (**Fig. 15.14**). Any bony reduction over dorsum to bring it in alignment with reduced septum should precede this step, as the septum is now very delicately attached to the bony septum only. Dorsal bony reduction in keystone area further weakens this support and if one is not careful enough,

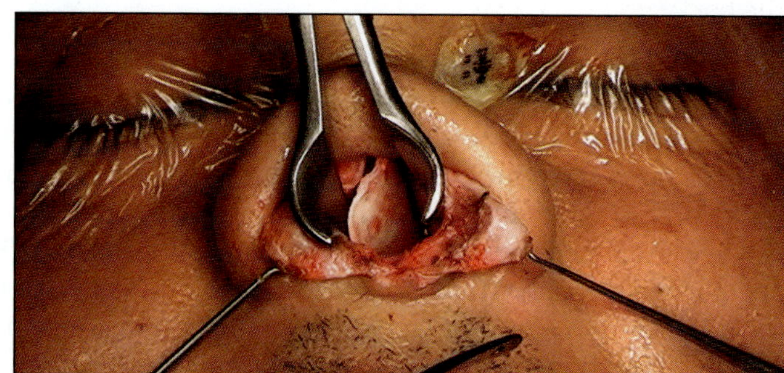

Fig. 15.10 Hypoplastic septum.

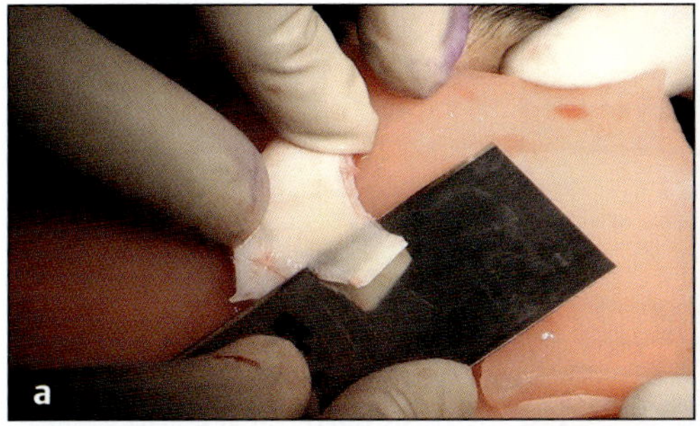

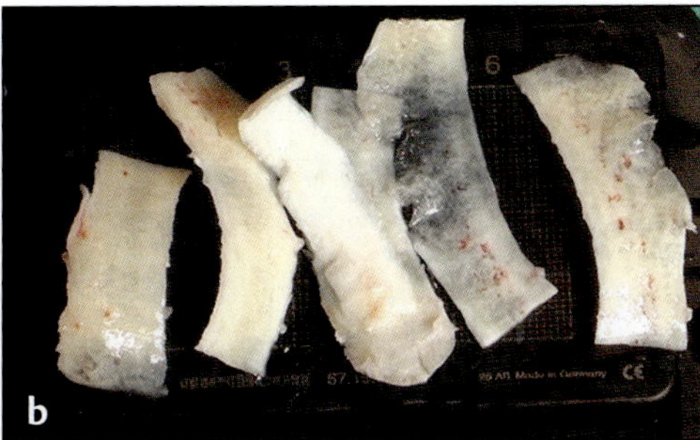

Fig. 15.11 (a, b) Cartilage graft is carved into thin slices and left in saline.

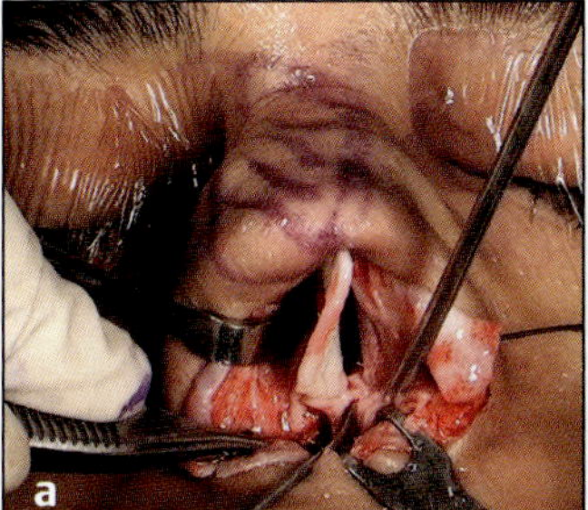

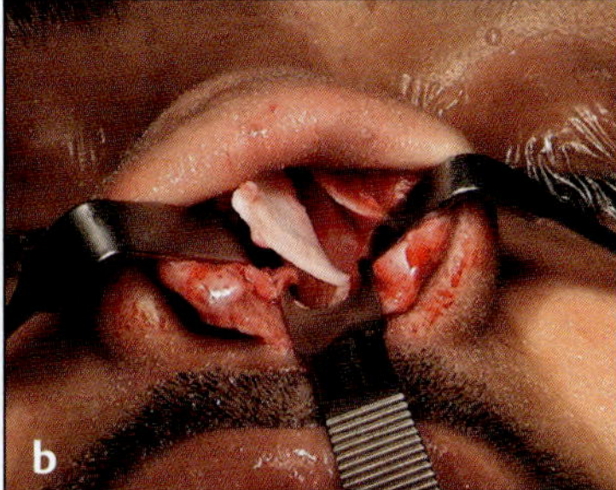

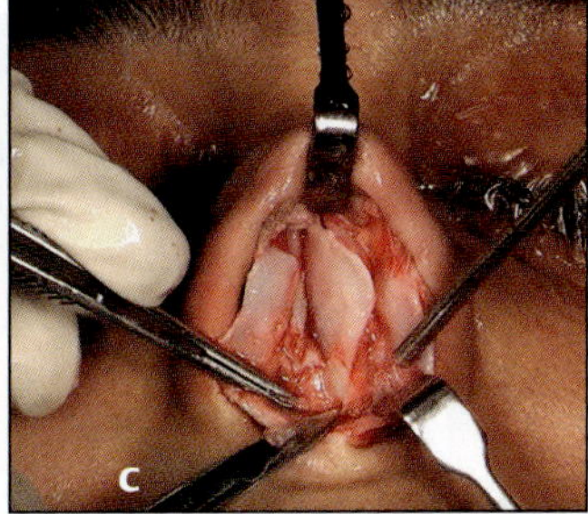

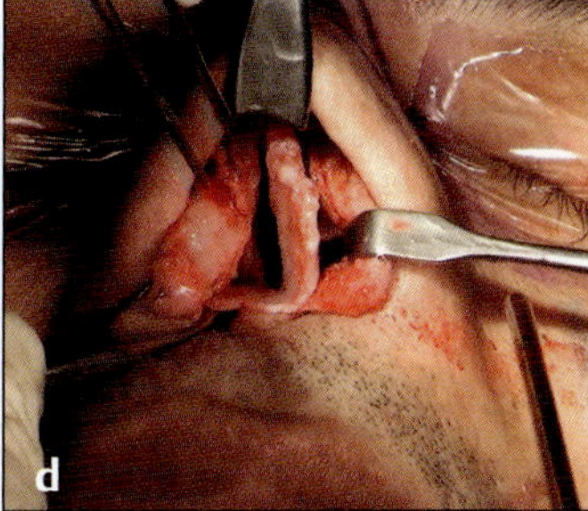

Fig. 15.12 (a–d) Large overgrown septum gets distorted/displaced in multiple directions.

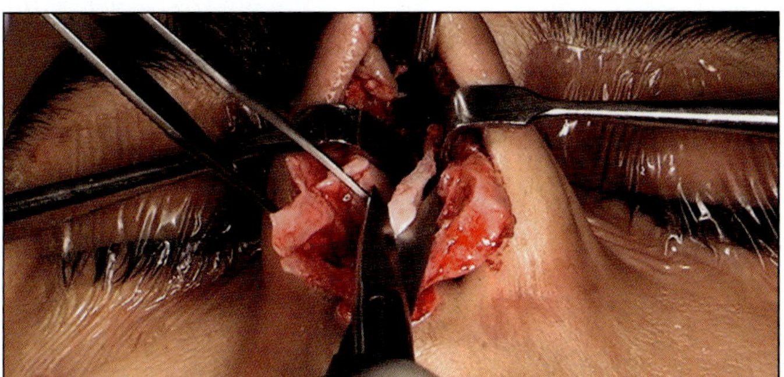

Fig. 15.13 Dorsal height reduction should precede the septal graft harvest.

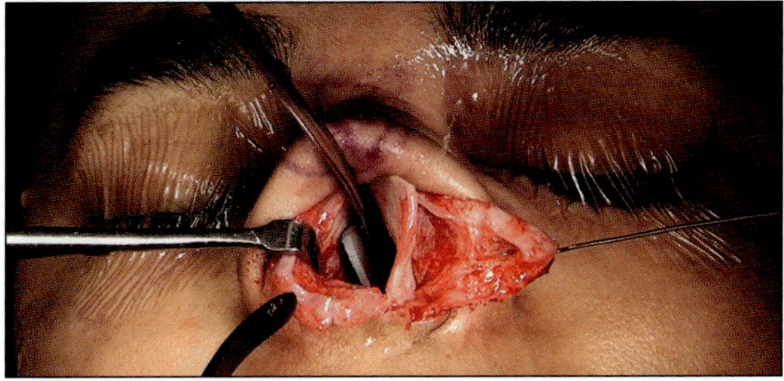

Fig. 15.14 Septal graft is harvested leaving L-strut of atleast 1.5 cm width of cartilage in the dorsum and caudal border.

the septum may get detached from all around and become free. If this happens accidentally, one has to convert it to the "extracorporeal" septoplasty procedure.

Removal of cartilage provides sufficient graft to strengthen leftover septum and gives a clear view to the surgeon of any spurs in bony portion causing obstruction. If the bony septum is tilted in cases of extreme deviation, then a fine 3-mm sharp osteotome is used to create an osteotomy between the vomer and perpendicular plate of ethmoid under vision. This will help in better alignment and straightening of the nasal tilt after lateral osteotomies.

Finally, the leftover septum is assessed for any tendency toward buckling. If buckling is in the vertical limb of L then there are two ways to correct it. If the septum is subluxated from nasal spine to one side, it is freed of distal attachment and reattached to the nasal spine after trimming excess portion (**Fig. 15.15**). If the lower end is central and attached to nasal spine then it is better to transect the vertical limb in middle, and cut ends are allowed to telescope over each other, fixed and strengthened with extra strip of septal graft. If the horizontal limb of L is buckled, it can be splinted with spreader grafts on both sides as it is or after transection in the middle depending on the excess. If the leftover septum is not in excess, it should still be splinted with grafts removed from septum only, which should be fixed in the appropriate new position as a batten graft, spreader graft, or a septal extension graft as per the need (**Fig. 15.16**).

Batten Grafts

First reported by Dingman in 1956,[37] they are small pieces of strong and thin grafts either from septum or slices of rib cartilage which can be used to strengthen the hypoplastic septum, leftover L-strut of septum, or as a splint to correct curvature of the septum. Perpendicular plate of ethmoid can also be harvested for this purpose and used by drilling multiple holes through it (**Figs. 15.17 and 15.18**).

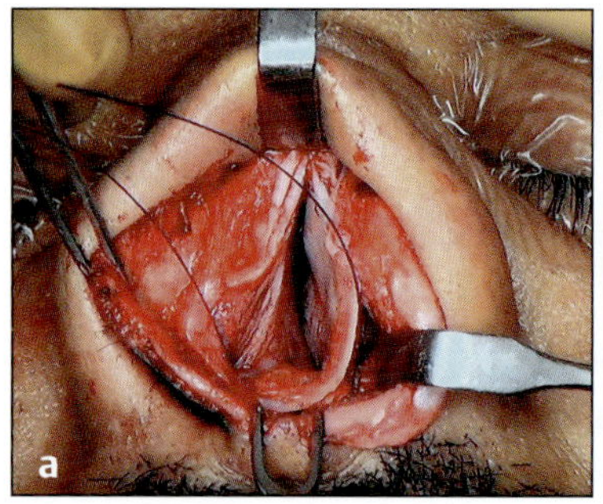
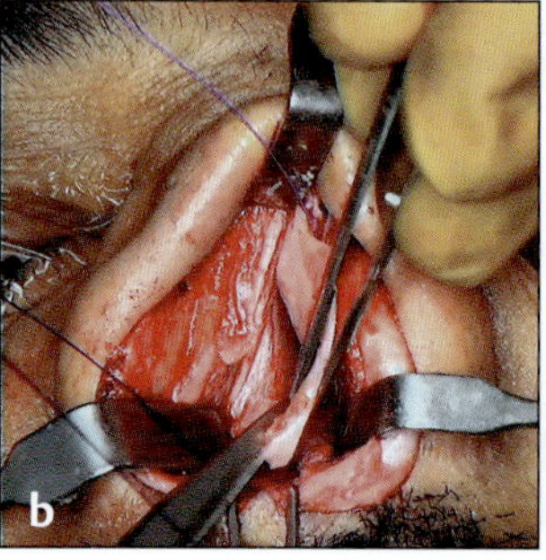
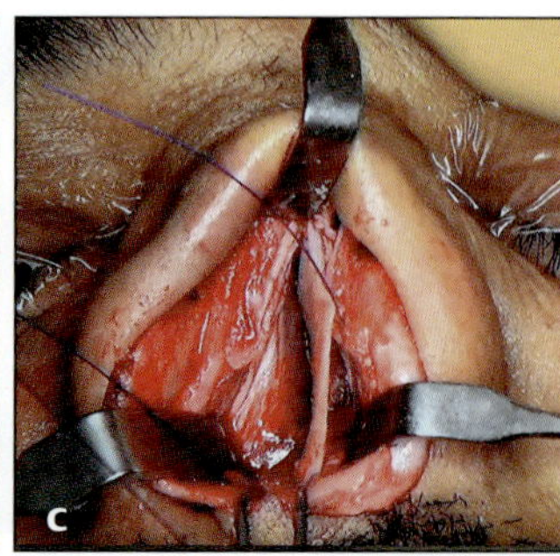

Fig. 15.15 (a–c) Transection of vertical limb of L-strut and fixation with nasal spine.

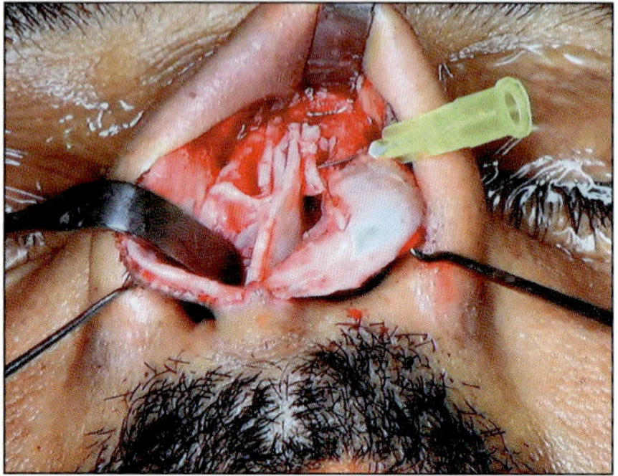

Fig. 15.16 Transection and fixation of horizontal limb of L-strut.

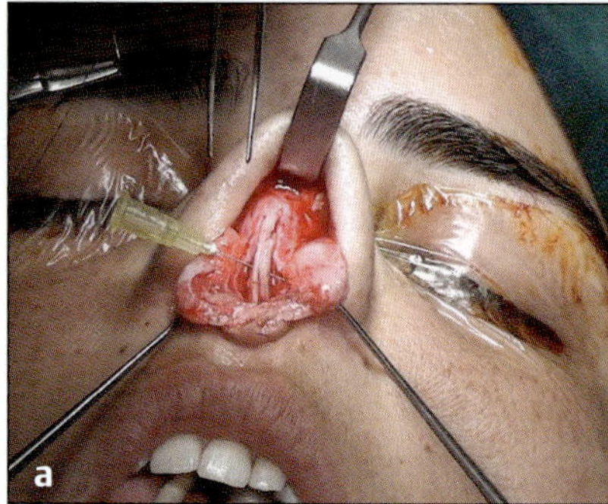
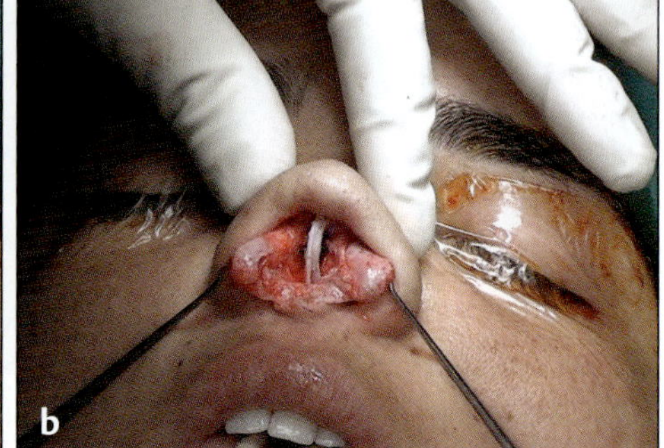

Fig. 15.17 (a, b) Classical Batten graft for structural septal support.

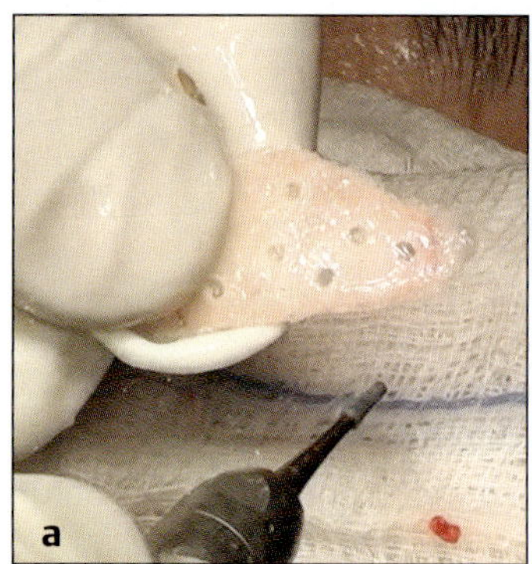
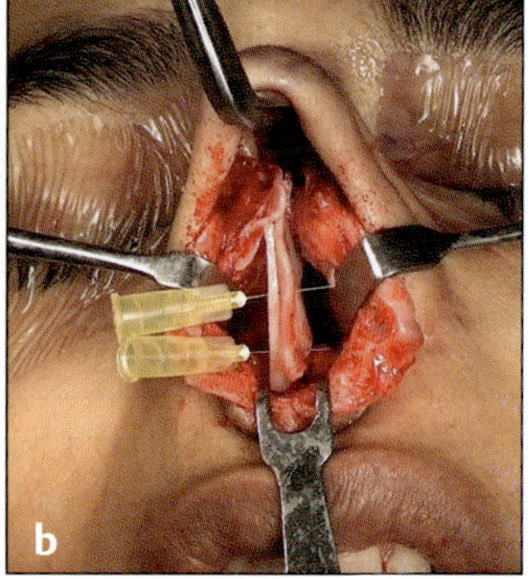

Fig. 15.18 (a, b) Ethmoid plate should be harvested when possible and can be used as a stable graft.

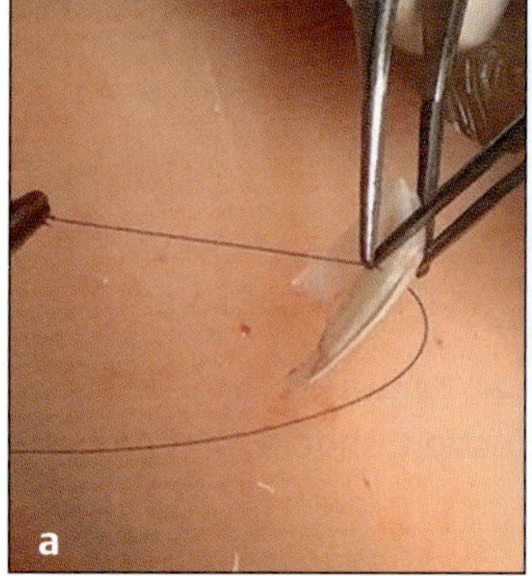
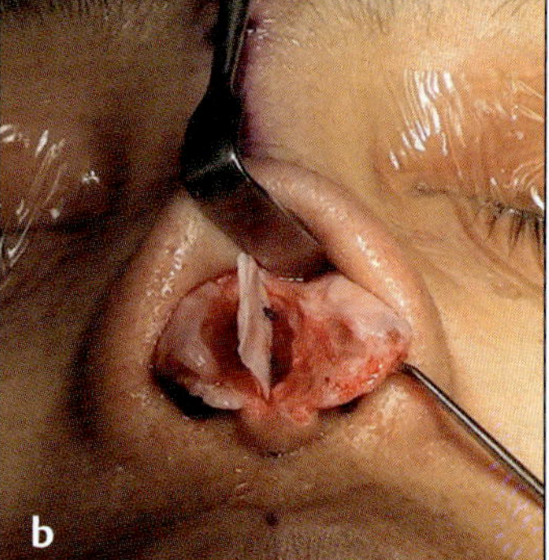

Fig. 15.19 (a, b) End on fixation of double-layer septal extension graft.

Caudal Septal Extension Grafts

These are the thin slices of grafts that are used at the caudal end of septum to provide support to plunging tip, for correction of retruded and overhanging columella, and correction of the tip.[38,39]

It should either be fixed with 4-0 polydioxanone at the lower end of caudal septum, on concave side if the caudal end is curved and displaced from midline with at least 1 cm overlap on the septum, or alternatively it can be fixed end-on, if the septum is straight. The caudal edge of the straight septum could be sandwiched between two thin quadrangular pieces of graft and fixed together with 4–0 PDS sutures (**Fig. 15.19a, b**). If the L-strut is not of sufficient length to reach nasal spine, extension graft is fixed with nasal spine. The fixation point should not be end-on, but about a cm behind the distal edge to leave sufficient length of graft projected beyond nasal spine, to reach and lie comfortably in between medial crura for fixation in tongue-in-groove manner (**Fig. 15.20**).

Spreader Grafts

First described by Sheen in 1984 to widen a narrowed internal valve, they have become invaluable tools in modern rhinoplasty.[40] They improve airway by lateralizing the lateral nasal wall, thereby creating more space. Traditionally used spreader grafts in endonasal rhinoplasty were of fixed dimensions of approximately 2 to 3 mm wide and 1.5 to 2 cm long and were placed in a tight submucosal pocket at the junction of upper lateral cartilage with septum, mainly in secondary rhinoplasty cases with middle vault collapse. Their use and indications increased with the advent of open rhinoplasty techniques in the last couple of decades. They are now used for splinting the dorsal septum and correcting its curvature.[41–43] Their size and shape also vary, depending on the need (**Fig. 15.21a–d**).

Extracorporeal Septoplasty

It was first reported by King and Ashley in 1952[44] and has been recently popularized by Wolfgang Gubisch.[45] It is reserved only for complex septal deformities with multi-directional curvatures particularly a bend in the keystone area at the junction of bony and cartilaginous septum. For achieving the correction, the septum is detached from bony septum and keystone area and is removed out of cavity in its entirety. This gives adequate exposure and unhindered view of the bony septum. The distorted portion of the bony septum can be removed now from below using sharp osteotomes. While doing so one must preserve most of the septum near nasal bones to prevent collapse. The cartilage which is removed earlier is shaped on the table using extra pieces of grafts. This is helped by making a template of the exact size and shape of the septum needed. This neoseptum is then reinserted into a slot made in between the nasal bones with fisher burr. If medial osteotomies are done this step is not necessary as there is already a gap in between the nasal bones to fit the septum. The septum is sutured in the keystone area by drilling holes on the distal edge of nasal bones, and taking 3-0 PDS suture through both nasal bones with septum in between.

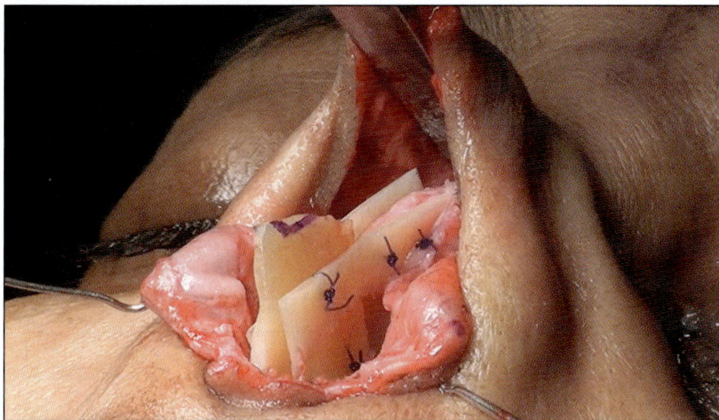

Fig. 15.20 Caudal septal extension graft is fixed to nasal spine 1 cm behind the distal end.

Another fixation point for septum is at nasal spine. First it is ascertained whether the nasal spine is located in the midline or not. If not, then the septum is fixed to the side of the spine, to counter distal curvature of septum. A drill hole through the nasal spine and figure-of-eight suture of 3-0 PDS is appropriate for this purpose. The fixation point should not be the distal most point of the septal edge, but is approximately 7 to 8 mm behind it as this much of septum projects beyond the nasal spine (**Fig. 15.22a–g**).

A simple algorithm has been designed for decision making on various procedures on septum during primary or secondary rhinoplasty (**Flowchart 15.1**).

Closure of Dorsum

The dorsum is now closed by approximating upper lateral cartilages to the septum. Upper edge of upper lateral cartilage can be folded as *spreader flaps*[46] to bring it to the level of reduced septum. These flaps are created by dissecting the mucosa away from the inner aspect of upper lateral cartilages for approximately 5 mm along the entire length. Upper edge of upper lateral cartilages is also released from underneath the nasal bones. Now the upper edge of upper lateral cartilage (ULC) is folded on to itself and approximated with the septum. One should avoid using mattress suture for fixation as it may lead to pinching of internal nasal valve. Instead one should use simple sutures by taking the bite through folded edge of upper lateral cartilage from inside out so that the final knot remains buried. The suture is tied by taking a bite through the septum. If a mattress suture is unavoidable, it should not be tied too tightly. Spreader flaps can only be used in reduction rhinoplasty (**Fig. 15.23a–d**). In augmentation rhinoplasty we use spreader grafts if needed.

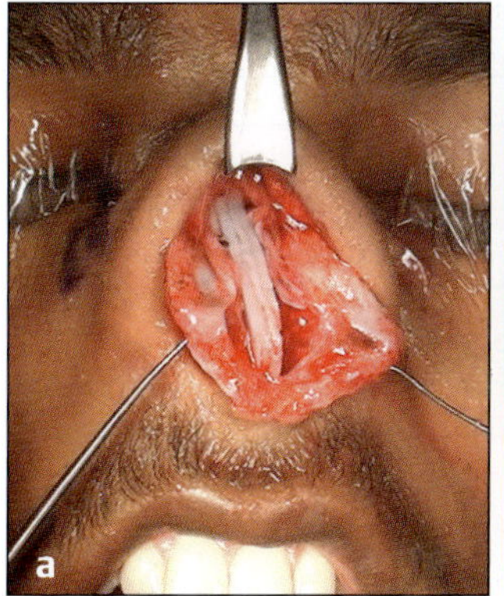

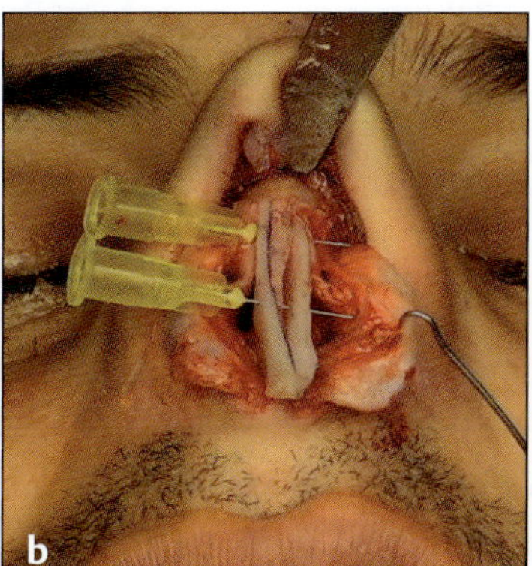

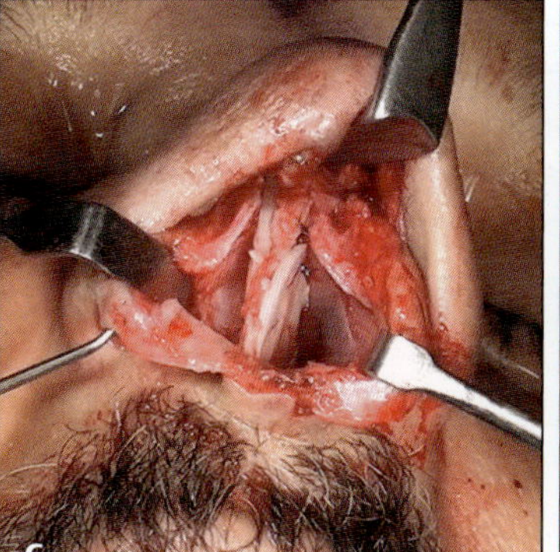

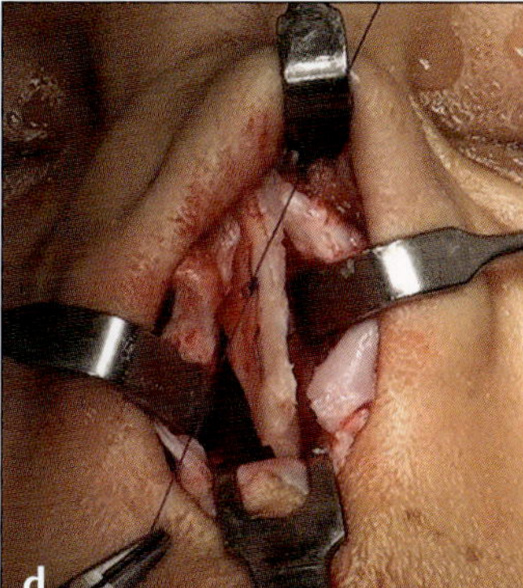

Fig. 15.21 **(a)** Classical spreader grafts. **(b)** Extended spreader grafts to support septal extension graft. **(c)** Differential spreader grafts. **(d)** Unilateral spreader graft.

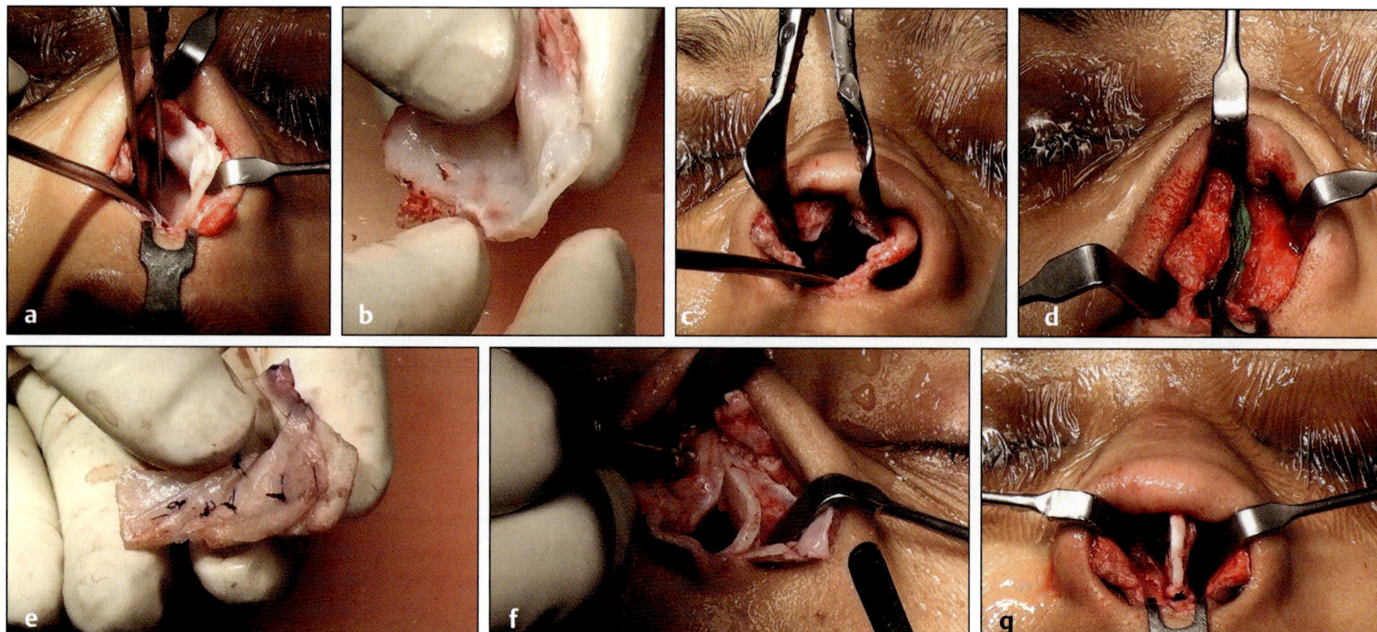

Fig. 15.22 **(a)** Severly deformed septum, which needs extracorporeal septoplasty. **(b)** Crooked septum after removal. **(c)** Empty nasal cavity after removal of the septum gives access to posterior bony segments which can be now modified under vision. **(d)** Slot is created in the nasal bones and template is used for measurement of defect. **(e)** Extracorporeal creation of neoseptum. **(f)** Neoseptum is fixed at keystone area by drilling holes in nasal bones. **(g)** Fixation of neoseptum at nasal spine.

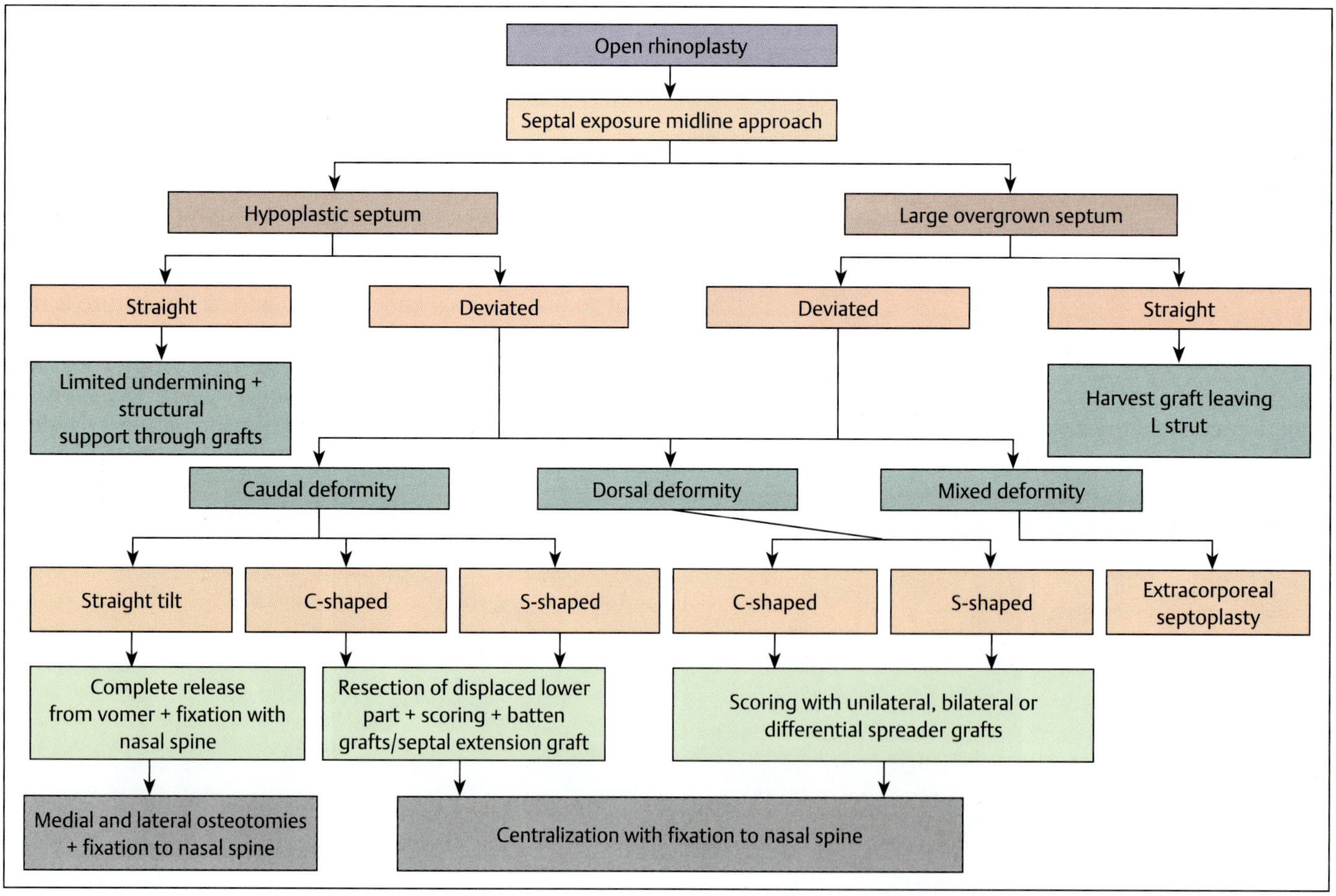

- Open rhinoplasty
  - Septal exposure midline approach
    - Hypoplastic septum
      - Straight
        - Limited undermining + structural support through grafts
      - Deviated → Caudal deformity / Dorsal deformity / Mixed deformity
    - Large overgrown septum
      - Deviated → Caudal deformity / Dorsal deformity / Mixed deformity
      - Straight
        - Harvest graft leaving L strut
- Caudal deformity
  - Straight tilt
    - Complete release from vomer + fixation with nasal spine
      - Medial and lateral osteotomies + fixation to nasal spine
  - C-shaped / S-shaped
    - Resection of displaced lower part + scoring + batten grafts/septal extension graft
      - Centralization with fixation to nasal spine
- Dorsal deformity / Mixed deformity
  - C-shaped / S-shaped
    - Scoring with unilateral, bilateral or differential spreader grafts
      - Centralization with fixation to nasal spine
- Mixed deformity
  - Extracorporeal septoplasty

Flowchart 15.1 Algorithm for septoplasty.

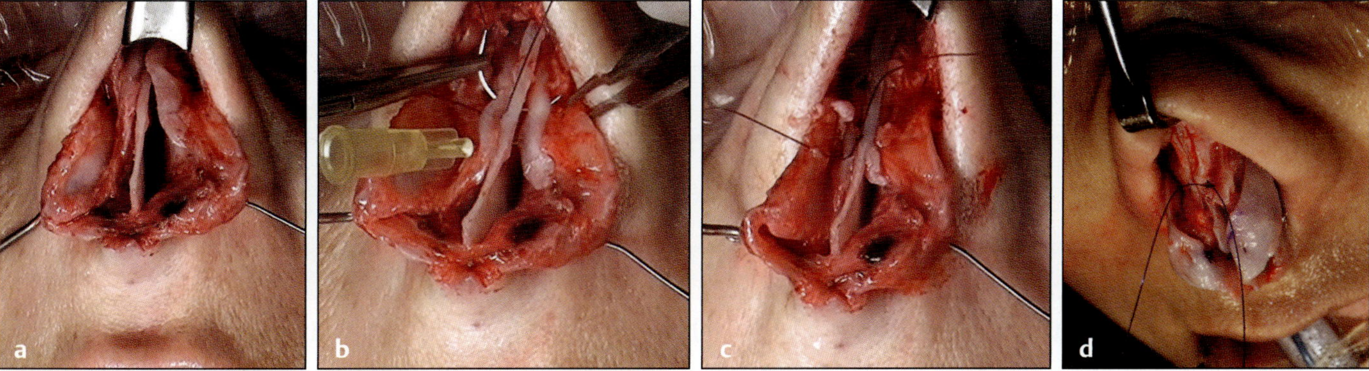

Fig. 15.23 (a–c) Closure of dorsum with spreader flaps. **(d)** Closure of perichondral flaps with simple sutures.

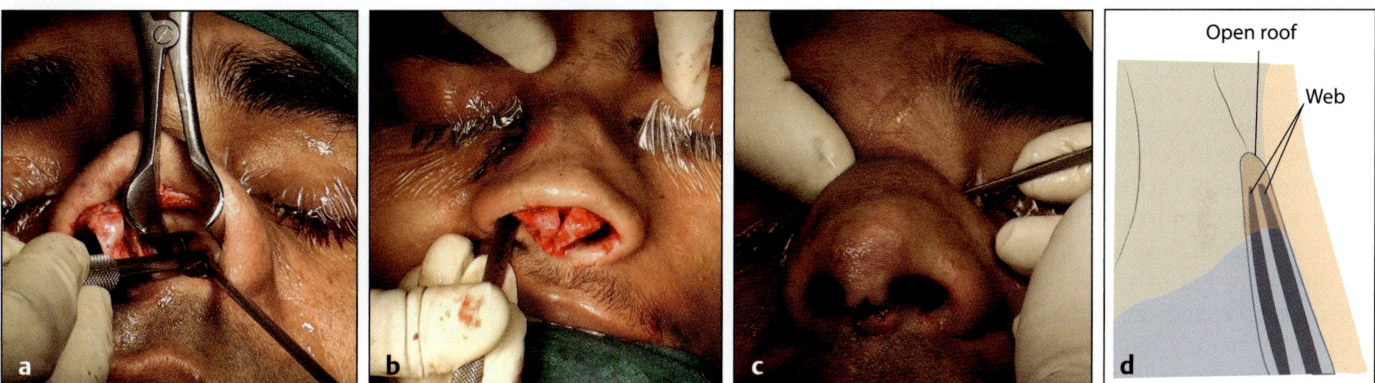

Fig. 15.24 (a) The incision for the lateral osteotomy is anterior to the level of inferior turbinate. **(b)** Lateral osteotomy is done in high low and high manner. **(c)** Transverse osteotomies are done sometimes with 2 mm osteotome through external approach. **(d)** Web between the nasal bone and bony septum.

Osteotomies if indicated are performed at this stage. Closure of the dorsum always precedes osteotomies; otherwise you will end up dismantling the entire nasal framework which will then be difficult to control.

Osteotomies

Medial osteotomies have already been executed while dealing with the septum, and so is the osteotomy detaching the bony septum from vomerine groove, while correcting the septum in severe bony deviation cases. Lateral osteotomies have the following definitive indications:

- To close the open roof in reduction cases.
- To correct the deviation.
- For narrowing a wide nasal base.

Lateral osteotomies are rarely required in pure augmentation cases where the septum is straight. Even an apparently broad nasal base in a saddle deformity will give illusionary effect of narrow base once the height of nasal pyramid is increased.

Osteotomy in most cases is performed in a high-low and high manner where the starting point and mucosal incision is just anterior to the inferior turbinate. A local anesthetic with epinephrine injection 10 minutes prior to osteotomy helps in minimizing bleeding. This injection should be deep over the osteotomy line and also inside the nostril cavity to balloon up the mucosa to prevent any inadvertent injury. The periosteum is not lifted as was practiced earlier. This helps in stabilization of bones after fracture as well as reduces postoperative swelling. Using a guarded 4-mm osteotome is a safer option for this purpose. Any larger osteotome is hazardous and produces more ecchymosis and edema. The osteotomy should stop at the canthal level as the nasal bones are thickest above this level and there is a danger of producing rocker deformity if it is extended any further. If there is a significant web between nasal bones and the bony septum, it should be burred at the time of septum correction or else it would prevent medialization of the osteotomized nasal bones (**Fig. 15.24a–d**).

Modification of the Dorsum and Middle Vault

Modification of the dorsum plays a crucial role in both reduction and augmentation rhinoplasties. After exposure we encounter four different types of dorsal problems (**Fig. 15.25**):

- High dorsum with or without a hump (**Fig. 15.25a, b**).
- Low dorsum with low tip height (**Fig. 15.25c**).

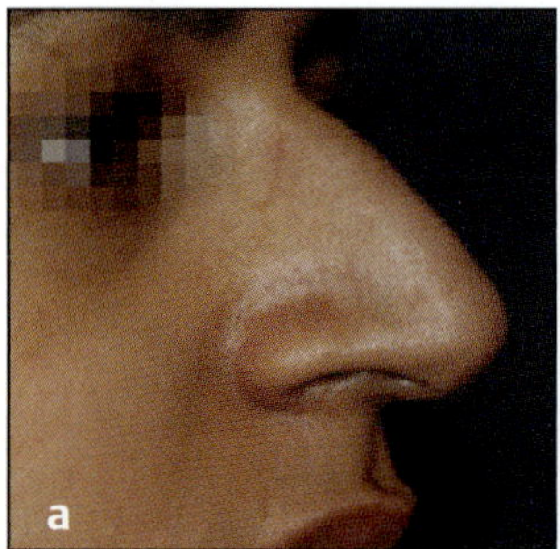

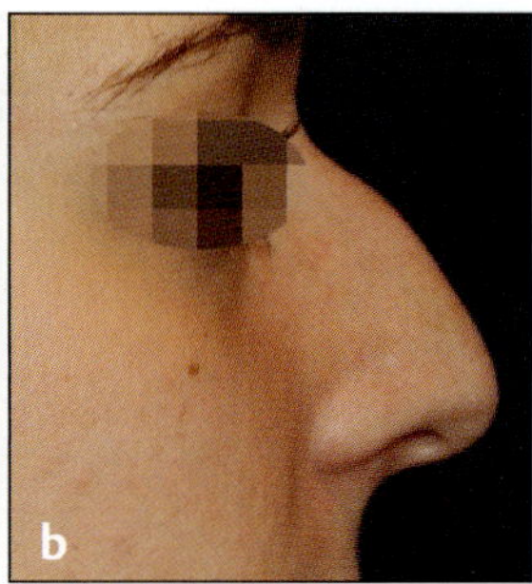

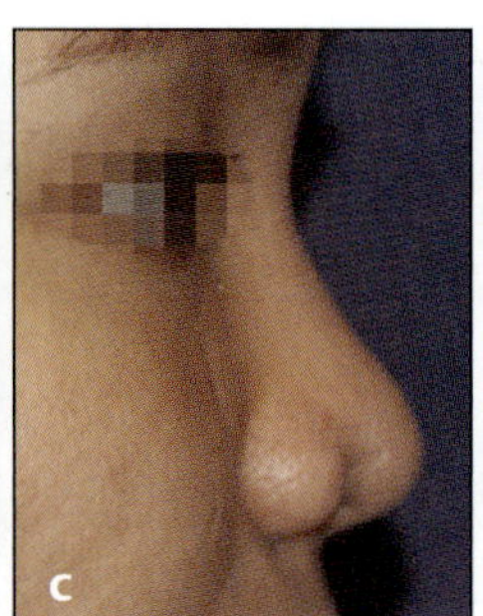

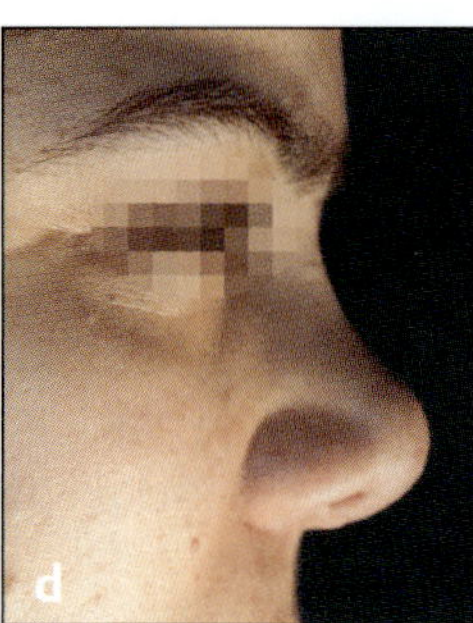

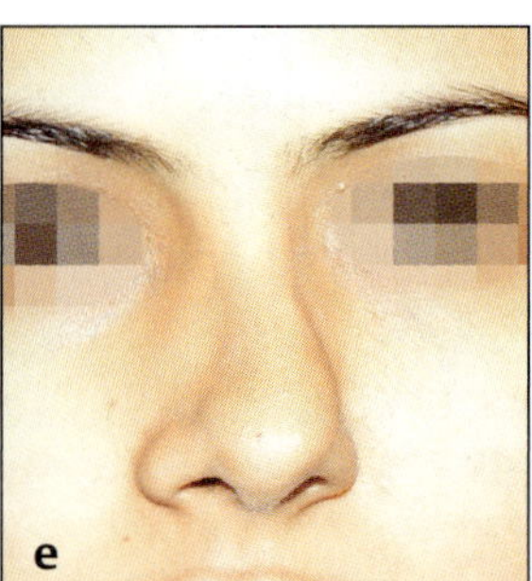

Fig. 15.25 **(a)** High dorsum. **(b)** High dorsum with hump. **(c)** Low dorsum. **(d)** Saddle dorsum. **(e)** Crooked dorsum.

- Saddle type of dorsum with normal or low tip height (**Fig. 15.25d**).
- Dorsum associated with a crooked nasal deformity (**Fig. 15.25e**).

High dorsum in a Caucasian type of large nose is modified while approximating the upper lateral cartilages with the septum. In this type of nose there is enough excess of the upper lateral cartilages to be used as spreader flaps, to create a smooth dorsum. The cartilages in these cases are strong enough to support the nose. Grafts on the dorsum are rarely needed in such cases. Irregularities if any are in keystone area and are mostly imperceptible through the thick skin, or may require soft tissue as camouflage graft. Soft tissue saved from thinning of the tip area or the perichondrium separated from costal cartilage can be used for this purpose. Alternatively, mastoid fascia can be harvested. Middle vault problems are taken care of simultaneously. A wide middle vault is because of inadequate mobilization of the nasal bones. Inverted-V deformity also occurs for the same reason and can be prevented by adequate mobilization of nasal bones and use of spreader grafts when indicated.

A *low dorsum* requires building up from the base. It is quite unnecessary to open the septum and separate it from upper lateral cartilages unless there is an indication. Exposing the dorsum is good enough with adequate mobilization of the tip structures as tip has to be simultaneously augmented to match the dorsum. Once exposed, a slight area of hump is noticed in the bony dorsum in the keystone region even if the dorsum looks straight from outside. This is because the differential thickness of skin and subcutaneous tissues in the Asian noses makes up for minor undulations in the bony dorsum. A single piece of graft or implant extending from the root of the nose to the tip is not the best way of augmenting the nose. Long graft or implant rocks at keystone area as a pivot point. Stronger force at the tip pulls distal end down and proximal end does not remain in contact with the bony base. This gives an unnatural wide appearance to the tip which on all accounts still remains depressed as compared to the dorsum.

The *dorsal graft* should be tailored to occupy the space from nasal root to the septal angle only. Accurate measurement of the length of graft should be made preoperatively (**Fig. 15.26**). The tip area should be augmented separately with various tip supports in such a way that it is 4 to 5 mm higher than the new dorsum. The author prefers to use a small cartilage graft underneath the distal edge of dorsal graft which is fixed to the septal angle area. The overlying distal edge of the graft is fixed over it with 4-0 PDS suture. This keeps the proximal portion of the dorsal graft in close contact with the nasal bone. The graft remains stable in its place without rocking. This strategy works irrespective of graft material used for augmentation. Even the implant used in such a way works well with less complication (**Fig. 15.27**).

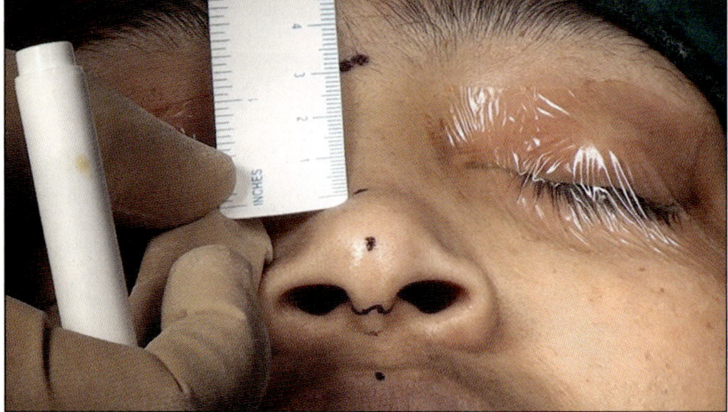

Fig. 15.26 Measuring exact length of graft needed for augmentation.

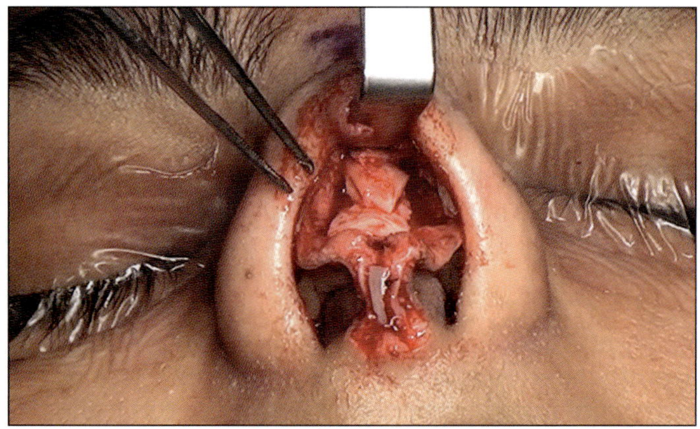

Fig. 15.27 Supporting cartilage under distal end of graft in the region of septal angle.

Saddle type deformity is corrected on similar lines. The graft material used should be sturdy enough to withstand the counter force by tight skin envelope. The skin envelope should be undermined in wider area to make enough room for augmentation material. The tip if under-projected is elevated first or at least temporarily held in elevated position with the help of skin hooks applied at the domes for judging the amount of augmentation required in relation with the tip height.

A *crooked dorsum* is built from the base. The septal correction is the key. It should be centralized and strengthened with grafts so that the bony dorsum is absolutely straight. The dorsal correction follows with or without dorsal graft. Attempts at camouflaging the twisted dorsum with dorsal grafts without working on septum at best fail and result in unsatisfactory outcome.

For a better understanding and for treatment purpose, it is important to classify the deviated and crooked nasal dorsum before venturing in to it.

Rod Rohrich proposed a simple classification to treat deviated noses in 2002.[47] Later, Jang Y.J., gave a more practical classification to help understand the deviated nasal deformity. He categorized deviated noses into five different types, dividing the nasal dorsum into bony and cartilaginous parts (**Fig. 15.28**).[48]

- Type I: Straight tilted bony pyramid and cartilaginous vault in the opposite direction.
- Type II: Straight tilted bony pyramid with bent cartilaginous vault (concave/convex).
- Type III: Straight bony pyramid parallel to the facial midline and tilted cartilaginous vault.
- Type IV: Straight bony pyramid parallel to the facial midline and bent cartilaginous vault.
- Type V: Straight tilted bony pyramid and cartilaginous vault in the same direction.

All these types can be successfully treated with techniques described earlier. However, one should be ready to face residual deformity. Sometimes these defects are real, and sometimes apparent in relation to the rest of the face. The patients should be counseled for the residual deformity as well as adjuvant procedures like genioplasty and fat grafting for better results.

Choice of the Graft

Potential graft donor site should be carefully chosen preoperatively, and should be consented for. If there is no clarity on this at this point of time then it is good practice to consent for all possible options. This is especially true in secondary rhinoplasty cases, which throw lots of surprises upon exploration. The choice of the donor site depends on the quantity of the graft material needed.

Septum

Septum as graft donor site is the first choice if the amount of graft needed is minimal. However, this only works well in primary cases where septum is large enough to act as donor and still left with sufficient amount after harvest not to cause

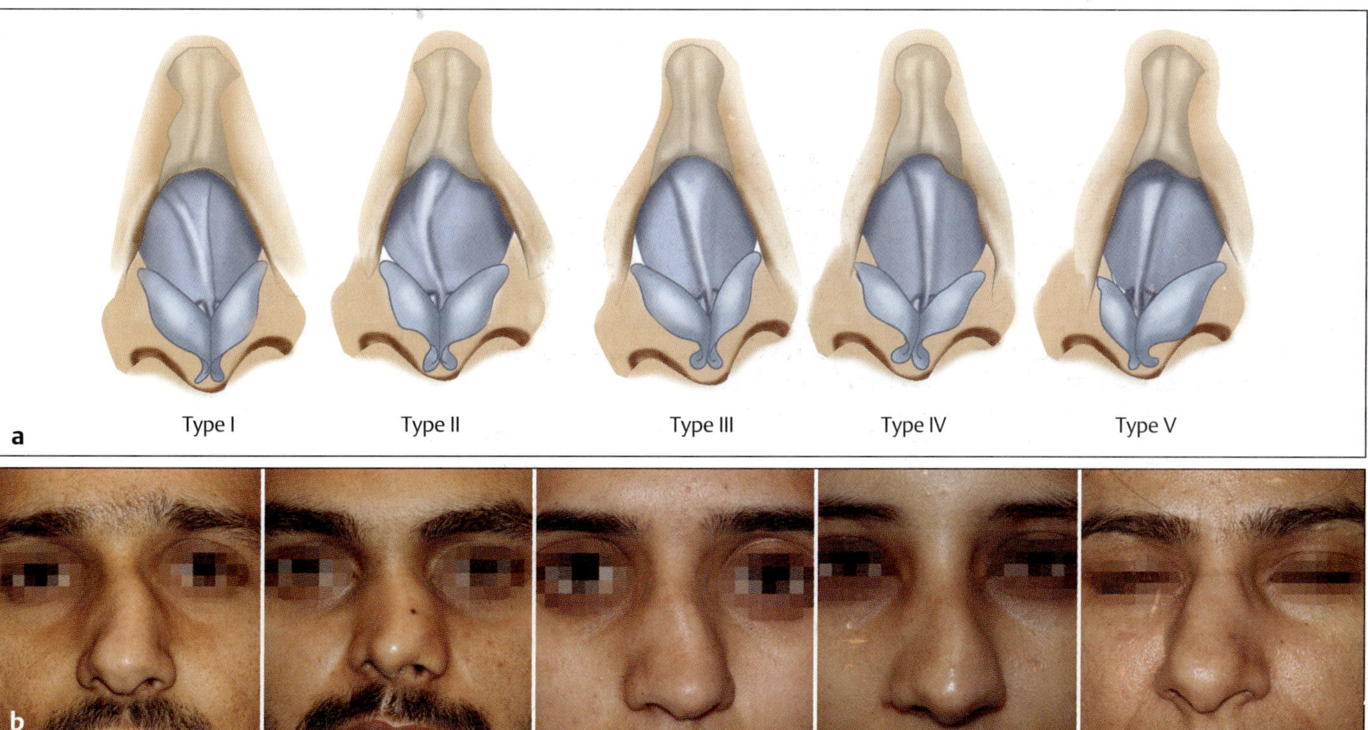

Fig. 15.28 Classification of deviated nasal deformity. **(a)** Illustrative representation of skeletal deformities of various types (Adapted from Jang et al, 2008)[48], **(b)** clinical examples of type I to type V nasal deviations.

collapse of nasal support. Straight and thin graft is the distinct advantage, which does not warp with time and is ideal for use as septal extension, batten or spreader graft, and as columellar strut. This case scenario fits well with reduction rhinoplasty cases which do not require any dorsal graft.

Conchal Cartilage

In augmentation rhinoplasty, the requirement of graft is considerably more than that septum may contribute. The conchal cartilage is the next preferred site which may be sufficient enough on its own or in combination with septal graft. The concha can supply enough graft to create a double layer dorsal graft. Hidden donor scar behind the ear and the potential to harvest mastoid fascia through the same incision are advantages with this donor site (**Fig. 15.29**).

Rib Cartilage

This donor site is used when a large amount of graft is needed. Abundance of graft material and hidden donor scar are clear advantages, and so is the potential to harvest perichondrium and rectus fascia through the same incision. Pain at the donor area and potential for warping are definite disadvantages. Any rib can be used as per the convenience of surgeon. The procured cartilage is modified in various ways to suite the individual need and to prevent it from warping (**Fig. 15.30**).

Graft Alternatives

Alloplastic Materials

Several alloplastic materials like Silicon, Dacron, Porex, Gore-tex, etc., have been used by various authors. Their use has some merits especially in Asian augmentation rhinoplasty. The main complication associated with their use is high extrusion rate. This is especially true with silicone implants, which is in most common use. The reason for this seems to be the use of oversized L-shaped implant. The blunt dissection for creation of a pocket is never in correct plane, leaving a thin cover of soft tissue over the implant. Constantly mobile L-implant in absence of structural support creates pressure points on the skin and leads to extrusion.

If one follows the principles of modern rhinoplasty and use implant as one will use graft, there are less chances of complications. The length of an implant should be from nasal root to the septal angle and it should be fixed to the dorsum. Certain materials like Gore-tex are more suitable for their pliability and softness while others like Porex should be avoided as they allow soft tissue ingrowth and cause lots of damage to surrounding tissue in case they have to be removed for any reason. Alloderm which is not exactly an alloplastic material is useful in secondary cases which have lost soft tissue thickness because of previous surgery.[49,50]

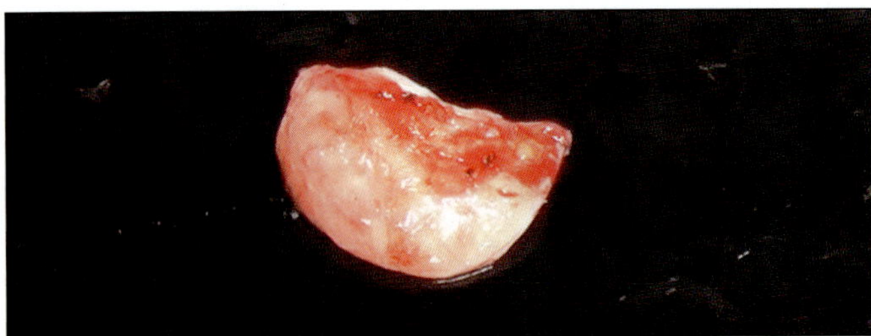

Fig. 15.29 Significant amount of conchal cartilage can be harvested.

Preparation of Grafts

The cartilage and fascia thus harvested are to be prepared as per the need (**Figs. 15.29–15.32**). There are a number of ways these grafts can be used for dorsal augmentation as beautifully illustrated by Rollin K. Daniel[51] viz.:

- Fascia.
- Diced cartilage.
- Diced cartilage in fascia (DCF).
- Diced cartilage and fascia.

Following are the additional methods to use the grafts for augmentation, especially in Asian rhinoplasty:

- Stacked cartilage graft.
- Stacked cartilage with fascia.
- Stacked cartilage with DCF.
- Diced cartilage in a pocket of fascia over cartilage base.

Use of diced cartilage especially the diced cartilage in fascia or DCF as it is commonly known, has caught the fancy of rhinoplasty surgeons the world over since its introduction in the last decade (**Fig. 15.31**). Erol was the first to report use of diced cartilage in the year 2000. But his technique of wrapping in Surgicel soon fell out of favor because of very high absorption rate and inconsistent results.[52] Later, many researchers through their excellent work proved that it perhaps induces an inflammatory reaction, which causes

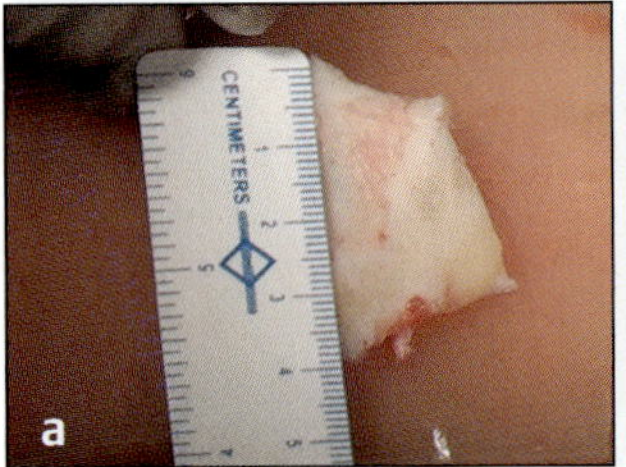

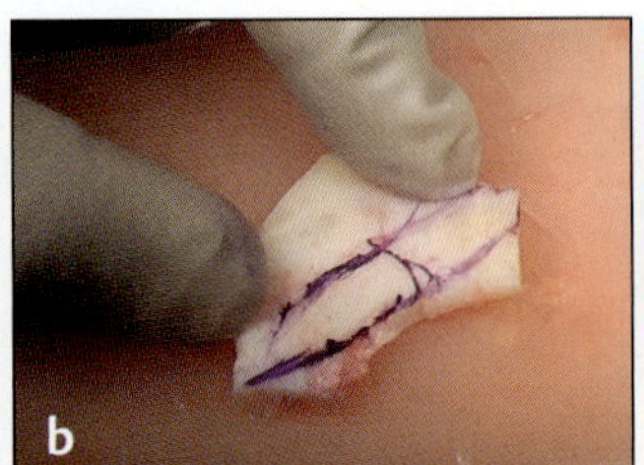

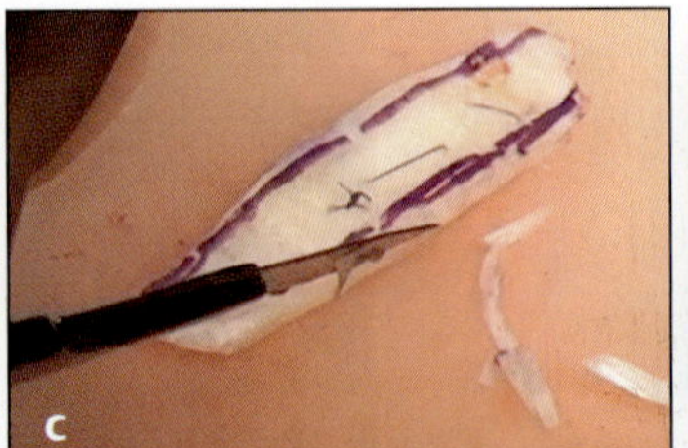

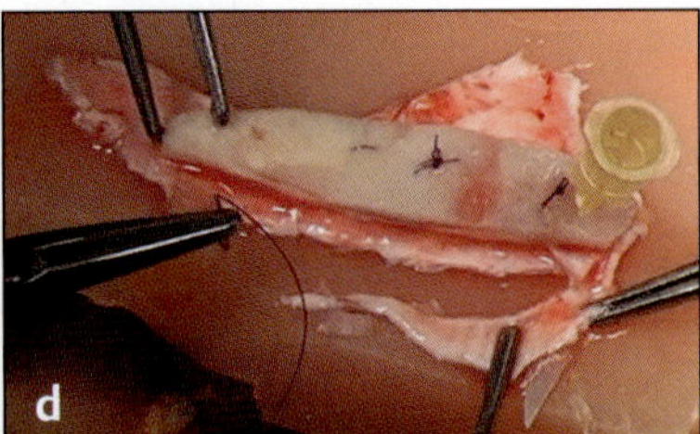

Fig. 15.30 **(a, b)** Rib cartilage graft. **(c, d)** Rib cartilage is split and opposing surfaces are stitched together to prevent warping. Graft thus prepared is lined with fascia.

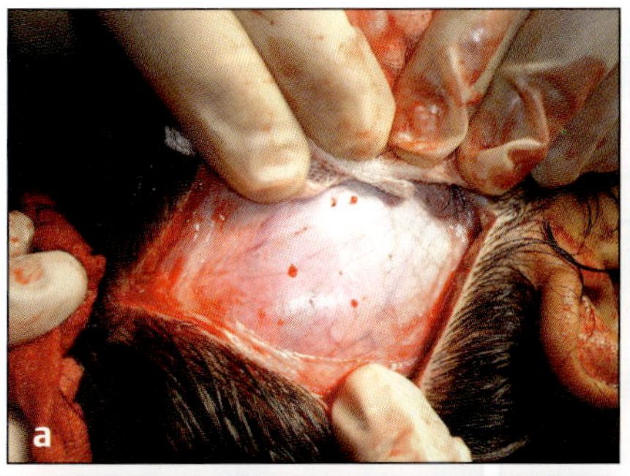
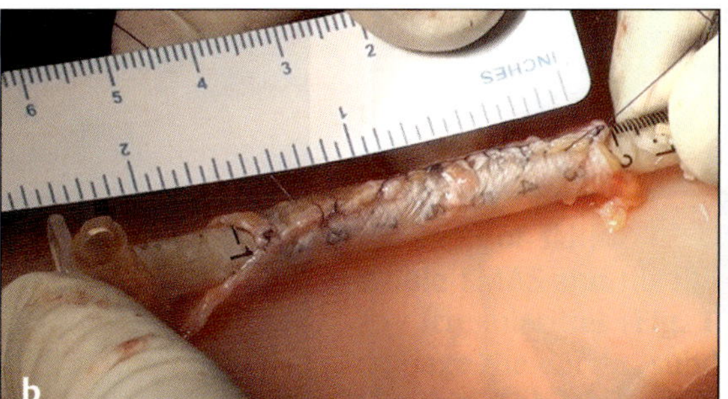
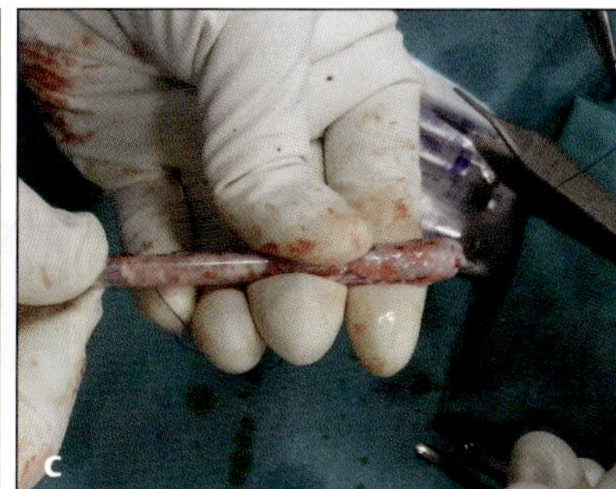
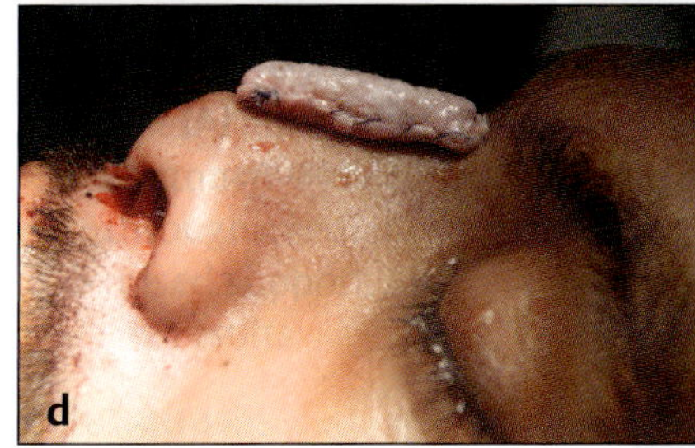

Fig. 15.31 **(a)** Harvesting deep temporal fascia. **(b)** Preparing sleeve over a disposable insulin syringe. **(c)** Filling diced cartilage. **(d)** Final diced cartilage in fascia (DCF) ready for insertion.

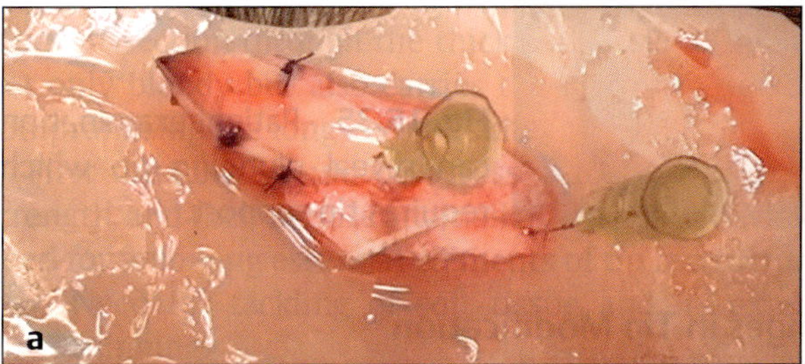
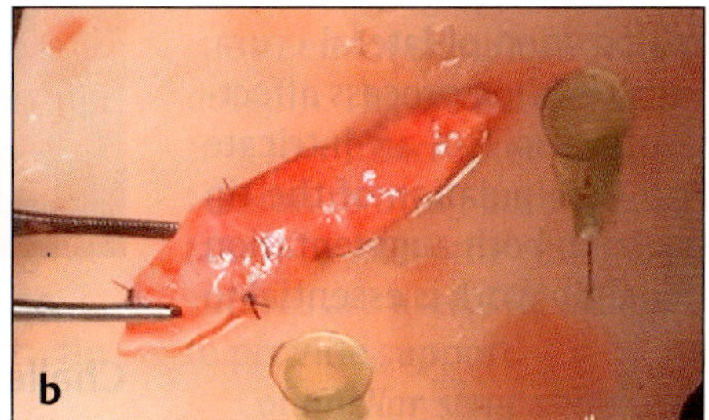

Fig. 15.32 **(a, b)** Conchal cartilage is lined with fascia.

absorption of cartilage and fibrosis. Rollin Daniel's excellent landmark paper[53] compared diced cartilage alone, diced cartilage wrapped in Surgicel which he later abandoned, and diced cartilage wrapped in fascia. Diced cartilages when used alone or when used in fascia survived in all cases and were very well vascularized to give long-term consistent results. Dicing of the cartilage has been found to be a much superior method for graft preparation than crushing as the latter destroys the chondrocytes and hence is not reliable.[54,55]

The initial enthusiasm with DCF is fading albeit for different reasons. In the west, surgeons are using it less and less because it gives an appearance of a rounded dorsum, with loss of vertical lines which is the hallmark of a good Caucasian nose. It works in Asian noses, if it is not used for structural support. In noses which have a very tight skin envelope, it invariably flattens out under pressure from skin above, especially if it is not tightly filled and closed at the distal end. Nevertheless, this is a good technique in suitable cases with either inherent or built-up structural support.

Stacked cartilage either from concha or rib should be more often used with fascia, either as top layer or diced cartilage in a pocket of fascia over stacked graft (**Fig. 15.32**). These are good choices in Asian augmentation rhinoplasty. It provides enough resistance under the tight skin to give long-lasting results. Stacking of thin slices of rib graft or concha should be wisely used in counterbalancing to prevent warping and distortion.

Irrespective of the type of graft used, the key point is fixation of the graft. The proximal end of the graft should be inserted under the periosteal pocket over nasal bones. Two absorbable sutures tied to the two sides of proximal end of the graft coming out through skin at the root of the nose should keep the proximal end in position. This suture is trimmed flush with the skin a week later. The distal end should lie over the septal angle and should be fixed using a mattress suture. An additional piece of graft may be placed under the distal end if needed as described earlier (**Fig. 15.33**).

Modification of Nasal Tip

The nasal tip has received great attention in the past decade or so, especially with the gain in popularity of open rhinoplasty, with many techniques being discovered and rediscovered. Most of these techniques are described for Caucasian noses, where the cartilages are strong and invariably need reduction and reshaping. Overlying skin is also thin and pliable and drapes well over the modified tip. These techniques are aimed at getting an ideal tip through cartilage manipulation. Suture manipulation of the tip is a perfect example of this.

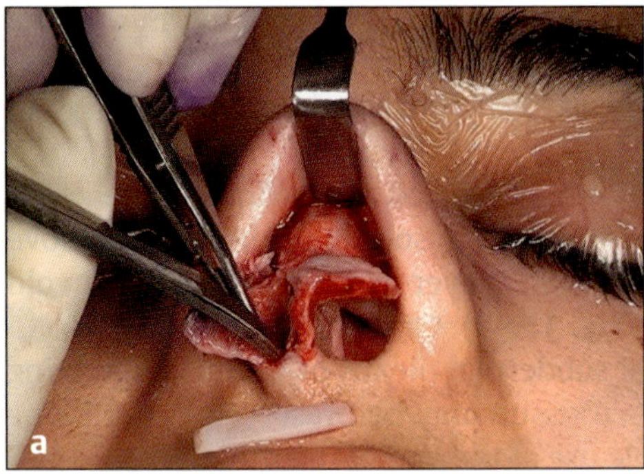
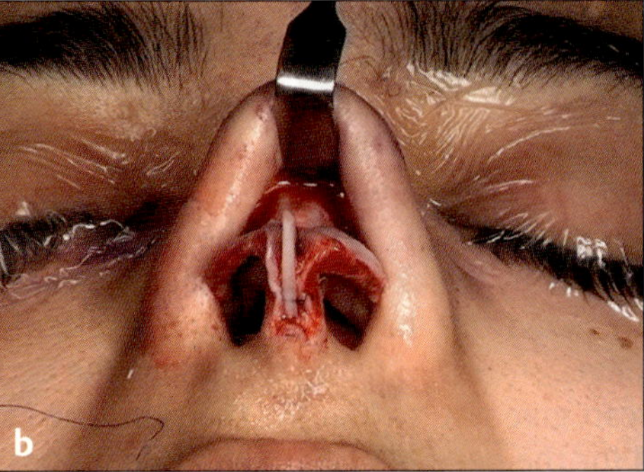
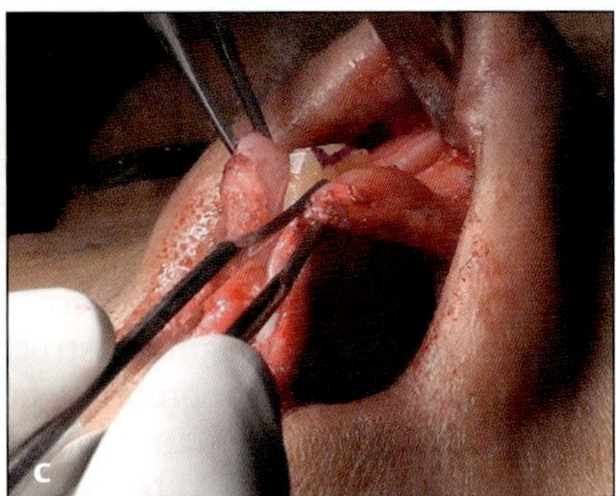

Fig. 15.37 **(a)** Dissection of pocket for columellar strut. **(b)** Columellar strut inserted in the pocket. **(c)** Height of the tip is adjusted as much soft tissue allows and is fixed to the columellar strut or septal extension graft.

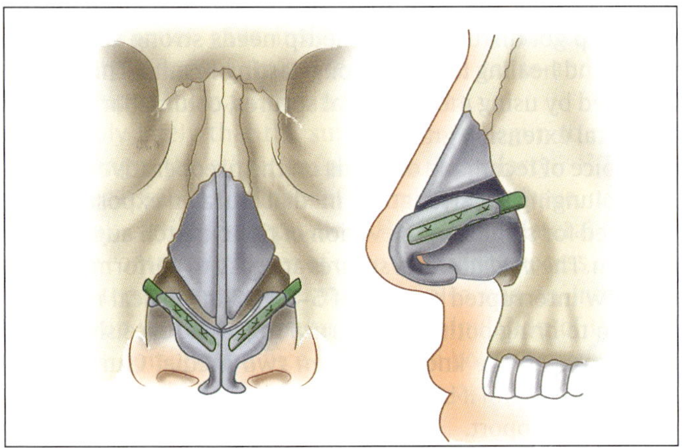

Fig. 15.38 Drawing of lateral crural support graft.

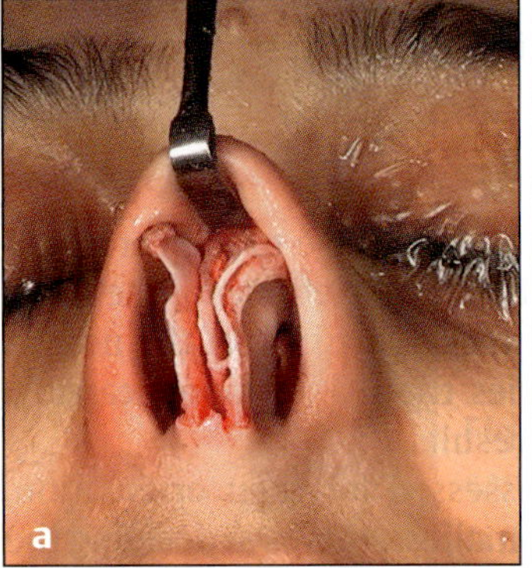
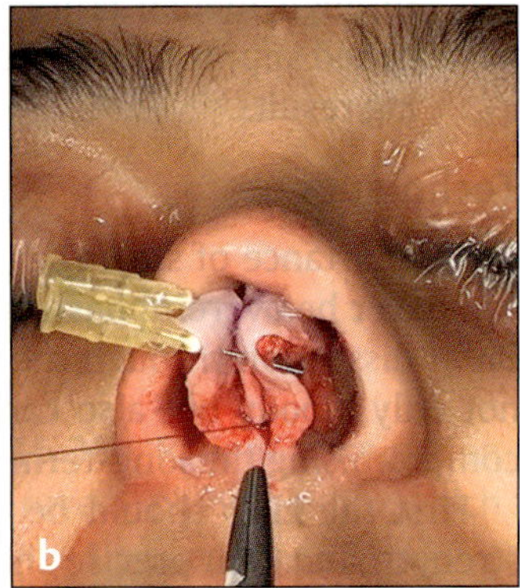

Fig. 15.39 **(a, b)** Classic tongue-in groove where both medial crura are shifted up and sutured with septum sandwiched in between them.

If the tip is to be significantly elevated, or it is to be rotated up or down, columellar strut is not the best choice. In such cases *septal extension graft* provides a solid pillar to support the tip. Its use was first proposed by Byrd in 1997.[59] The septal extension graft should be of sufficient length to comfortably lie in between the medial crura in a tongue-in-groove fashion and fixed with 5–0 PDS sutures. One can take the liberty of adjusting the tip height as much as soft tissue pliability allows. Final tip height should be 3 to 4 mm above elevated dorsum. If the tip needs more projection, lateral crural strut grafts may give additional support to the tip (**Fig. 15.38**).[60–63]

The retruded or overhanging columella if diagnosed preoperatively should also be corrected by proper placement and fixation of medial crura over distal septal margin at this stage (**Fig. 15.39**).

Modification with Tip Sutures

Much work has been done on tip sutures in the past decade or so and they have become an integral part of modern open rhinoplasty. If not for reshaping the tip, they are most needed to put together the tip structures which are taken apart for approaching the upper part of nose.

Traditional cephalic excision of lateral crura of LLC should be avoided at all cost in cases which have thin and pliable

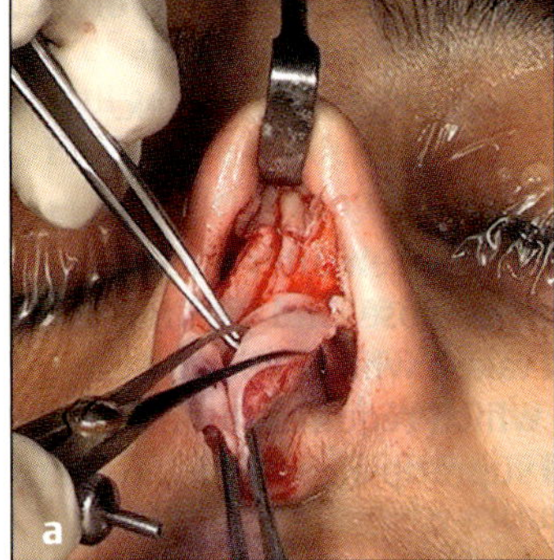
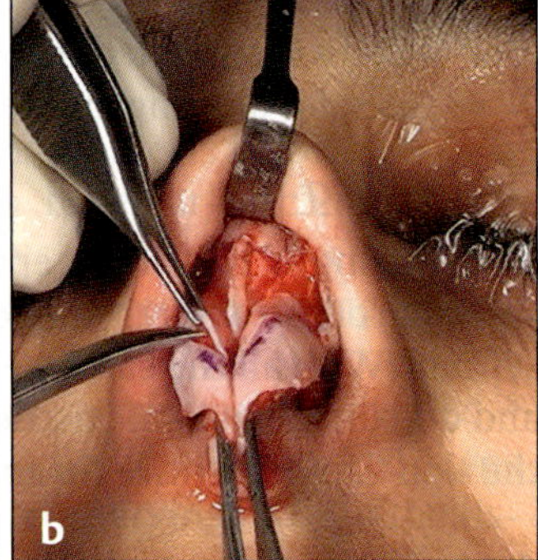

Fig. 15.40 **(a, b)** Measured cephalic resection with the help of caliper.

LLC, and should only be done in those cases that have strong Caucasian-like cartilage features (**Fig. 15.40**). Even in those cases, cartilage excision remains very conservative. In all other cases, it is better to conserve and use the cephalic portion intended for excision and use it to give strength to the lateral crus. This portion is folded on to itself by creating a pocket between LLC and mucosa for 3 to 4 mm. This folded portion is then fixed with multiple 5–0 PDS mattress sutures.[64] This doubling provides enough strength and support to the lateral crus (**Fig. 15.41**).

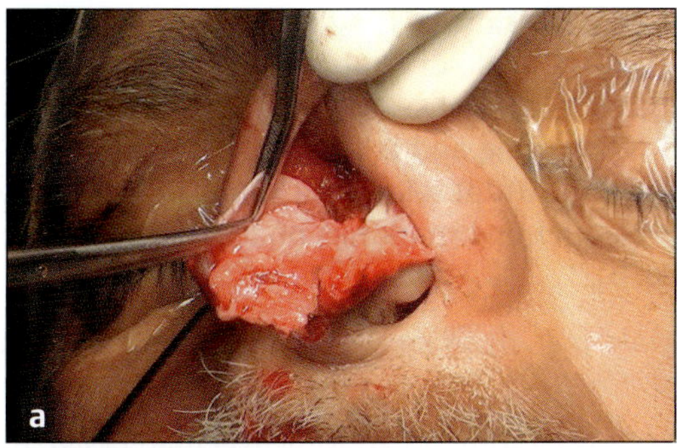

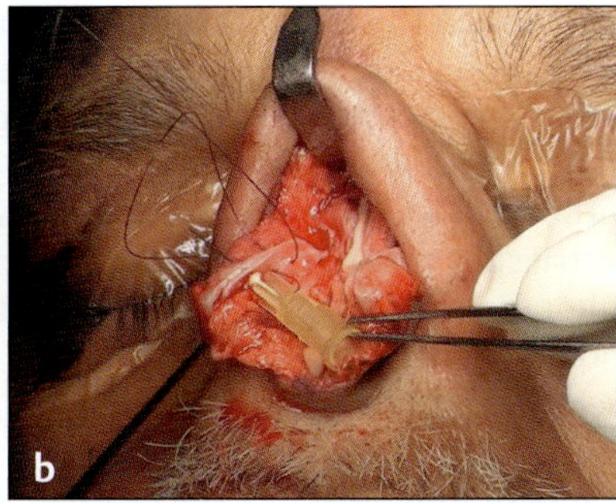

Fig. 15.41 **(a, b)** Lower lateral cartilage (LLC) flap.

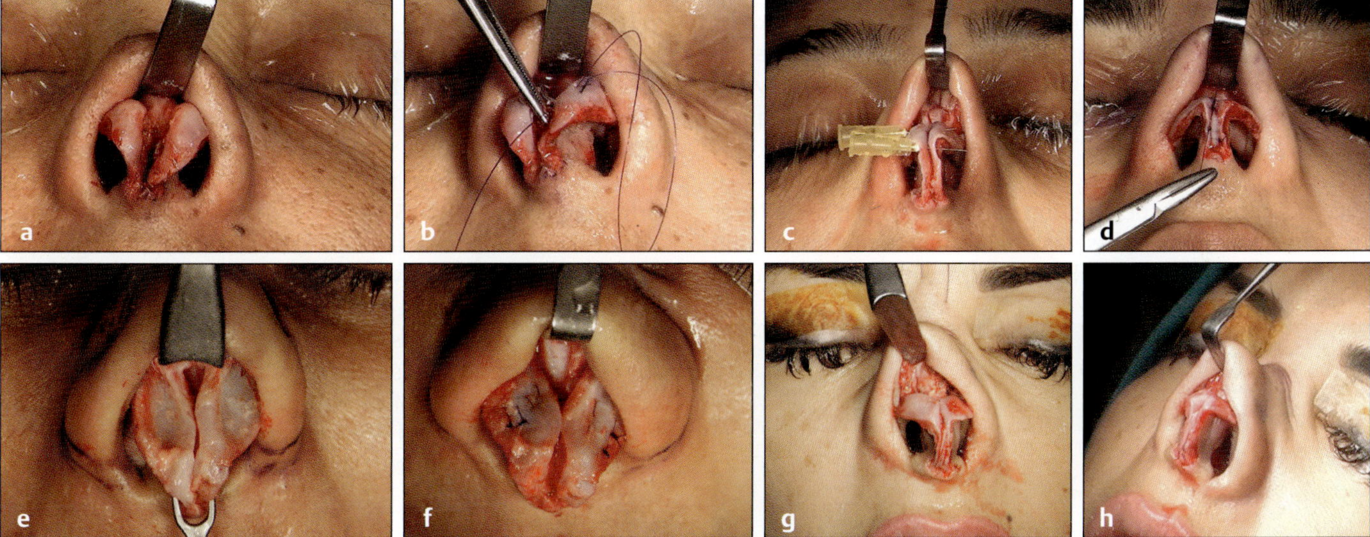

Fig. 15.42 **(a, b)** Domal creation sutures in an ill-defined dome. **(c)** New domal height is judged by application of needles before final suture creation of domes. **(d)** Domal approximation sutures. **(e, f)** Concave lateral crus can be flattened with the use of sutures. **(g)** Lateral crura should ideally be straight after application of sutures. **(h)** Ideal tip after suture modification.

Domal creation sutures of 5–0 PDS in a mattress configuration are now either applied at the cephalic end of an existing dome or a new dome is created at an appropriate place. Both the alar cartilages are now brought together with suture placement at the upper end of medial crura. If needed, a last cinching suture is inserted to bring domes in close approximation with each other. This suture is carefully tightened just enough to keep lateral crus straight.[65–67] Too tight suture may produce concavity of lateral crus which manifests itself on the surface as a crease in the ala. Lateral or medial crural steal and overlay are achieved for deprojection and projection of tip with the use of sutures in appropriate manner. Concave lateral crus of LLC can be straightened with appropriate use of sutures (**Fig. 42a–h**).[68]

A temporary columella closure with 6–0 Ethilon suture at the inverted-V gives an opportunity to assess the nose. One can assess the alar base in view of newly positioned tip and alteration in its relationship with the tip tripod. It gives an opportunity to assess the tip, dorsum, columella, alar rim, and overall appearance of the nose before final closure (**Fig. 15.43**).[69,70]

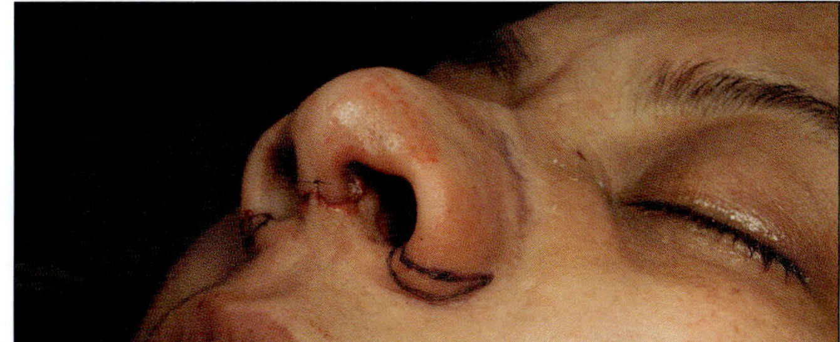

Fig. 15.43 Temporary suture at inverted-V and alar reduction marking.

Alar Wedge Resection

Alar base modification should be carefully planned and conservatively executed since there is no going back after incision is made and the procedure is entirely irreversible.

Decision on the type and amount of resection is based on the nostril shape and sill width, and the overall alar width in relation to intercanthal distance. Alar width is measured at the alar crease and alar flare at the widest point on the ala (**Fig. 15.44**). The first incision for alar base resection should not be exactly in the alar groove, but is offset about 2 mm on the alar side to preserve this important landmark which should not be obliterated as a result of suturing. Both incisions should converge and stop short of nostril sill if nostrils are of adequate size and do not need any alteration.

The incision for alar wedge resection should be skin deep only and stop short of the underlying muscle layer. The skin should be excised with sharp knife just deep to the dermis. Full-thickness excision of alar base is the cause of trouble as putting it back in original position can seldom be executed accurately and does not work even in experienced hands. Extending incision in the nostril sill takes care of excess mucosa if present. Leaving the muscle layer intact keeps the ala in proper anatomical position for suturing. Following this strategy, a major irreversible complication in rhinoplasty can be avoided.

For suturing, the one and only buried suture of 4–0 Vicryl is applied at the junction of dermis with muscle layer in a horizontal mattress fashion. When tied this should rotate and advance the ala and approximate it in proper alignment, with two incisions kissing each other. Final skin closure is achieved with use of simple 5–0 Ethilon sutures (**Fig. 15.45a–g**).

If nostril sill is too wide and is to be reduced, it should be marked as inverted trapezoid. Both limbs of trapezoid should join the parallel line markings of alar wedge resection (**Fig. 15.46a, b**).[71]

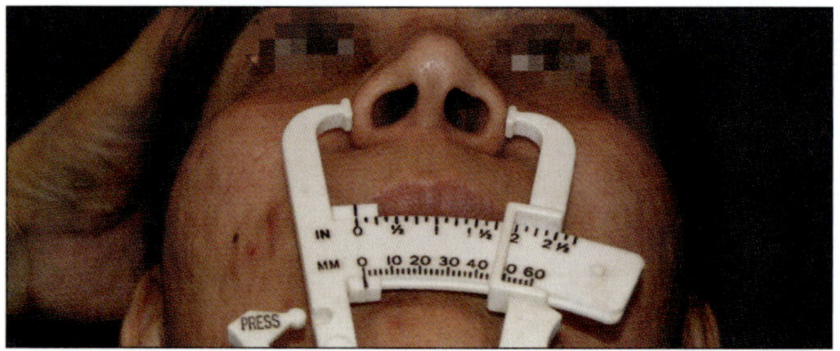

Fig. 15.44 Alar width measurements at the widest part of the alar curvature which should be equal to the intercanthal distance.

Closure

The last part of this operation is carefully executed to get an imperceptible scar. All the tattooed ends in visible portion of columella are first approximated with 6–0 Ethilon, and then vertical portion of the incision in columellar mucosa and part of incision in the nostril are approximated with absorbable Vicryl Rapide (**Fig. 15.47**). Apparently use of absorbable sutures over columellar skin does not alter the scar quality.[72] Finally few interrupted 3–0 Vicryl Rapide sutures are used in the septum to close the dead space and promote better primary healing (**Fig. 15.48**).

Dressing: ¼ inch skin strips are used for splinting on the skin in the manner shown in **Fig. 15.49**. Two long strips on the side of the nose are joined together distally near dorsal edge. Cut pieces of strips cover whole dorsum starting at the root of the nose and finishing in the supratip area. A thermoplastic splint in cases of osteotomy and intranasal packs in both nostrils completes this operation. Overpacking should be avoided as it may distort the nasal framework (**Fig. 15.49**).

Postoperative Care

Antibiotic prophylaxis is important in all rhinoplasty cases for two reasons: First, surgery is being performed on potentially contaminated area which harbors many pathogens,

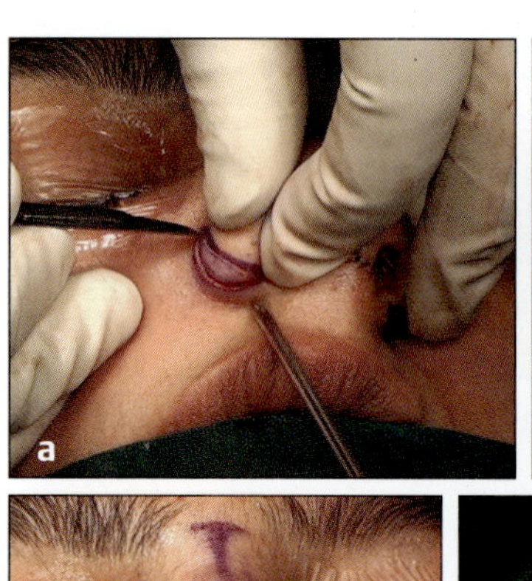

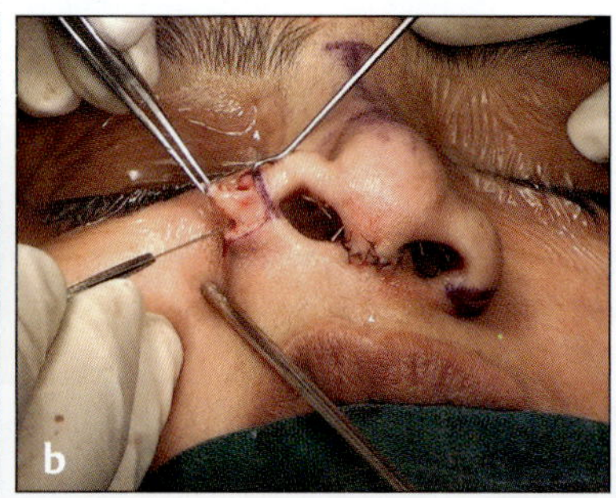

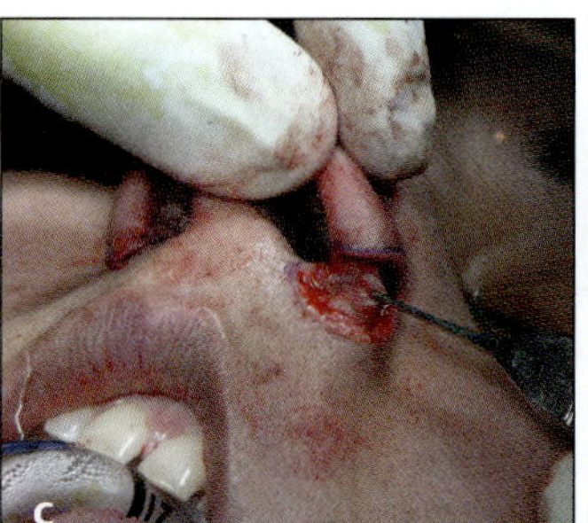

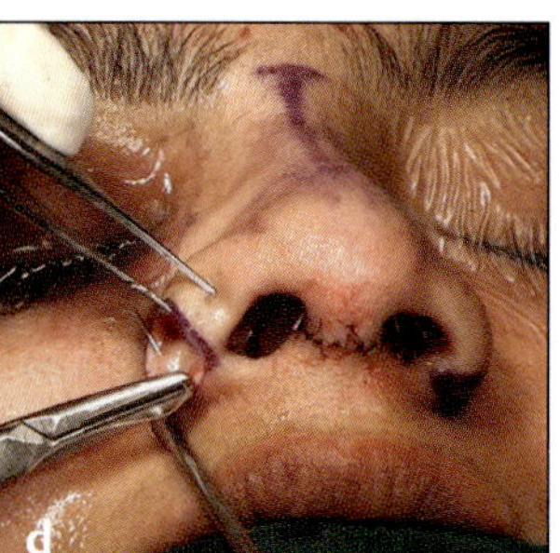

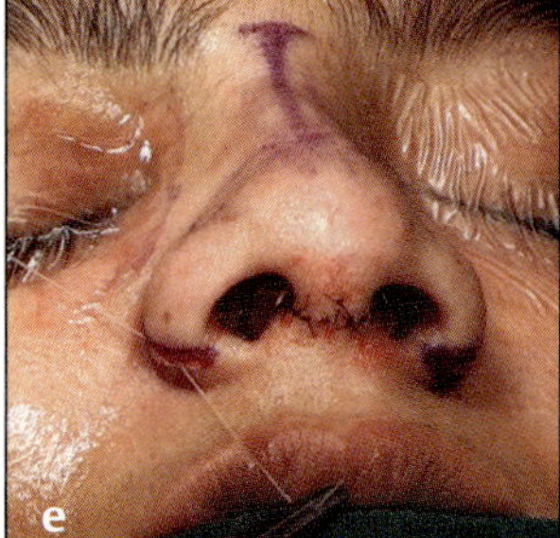

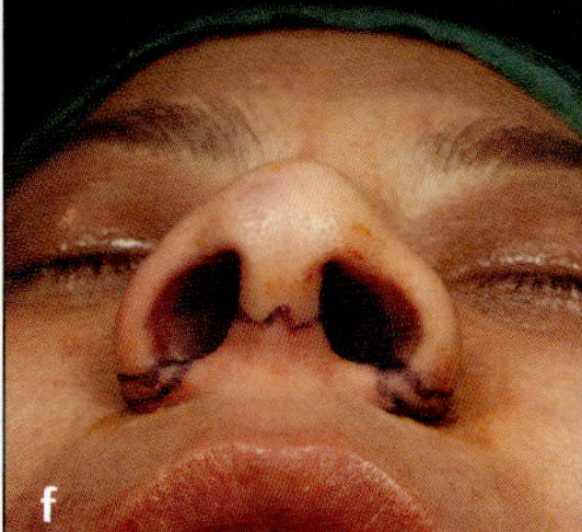

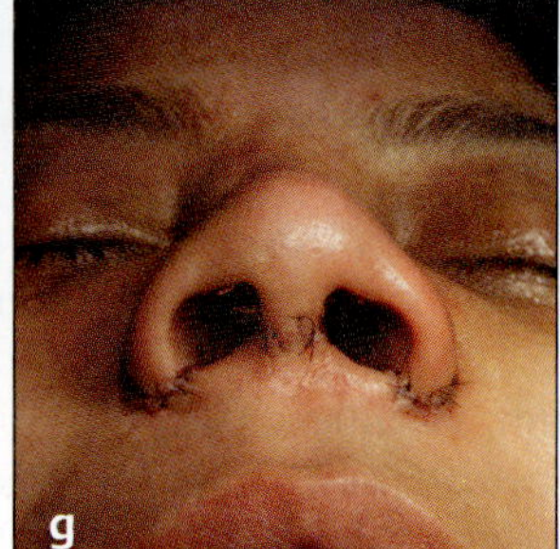

Fig. 15.45 **(a)** Incisions for alar wedge resection should be parallel to each other and about 2 mm away from alar groove. **(b, c)** Alar skin resection is done at dermis fat junction sparing the underlying muscle. **(d, e)** Subdermal alar suture. **(f)** Preoperative view. **(g)** Appearance after closure of the incisions. and skin closure.

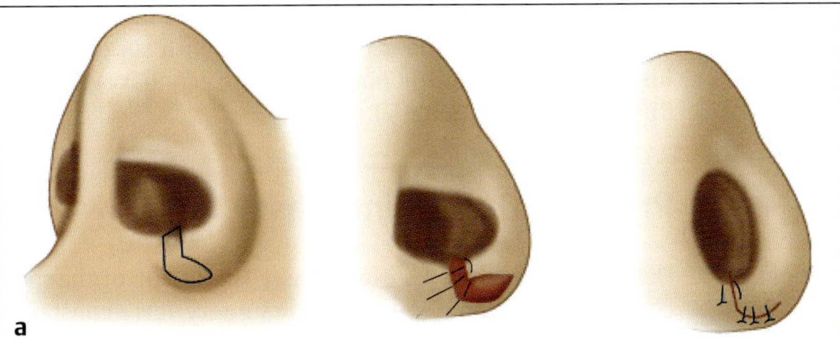
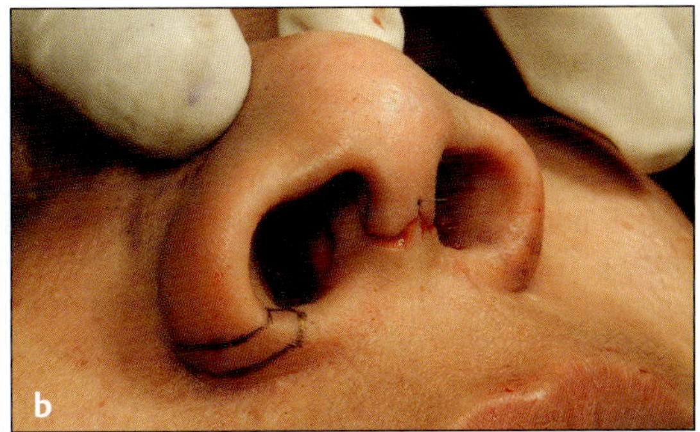

Fig. 15.46 **(a)** Inverted trapezoid excision for nostril floor reduction. **(a)** Drawings illustrating trapezoid excision: Marking, defect following excision and sutured defect, **(b)** clinical example of marking for inverted trapezoid excision of nostril floor and alar base.

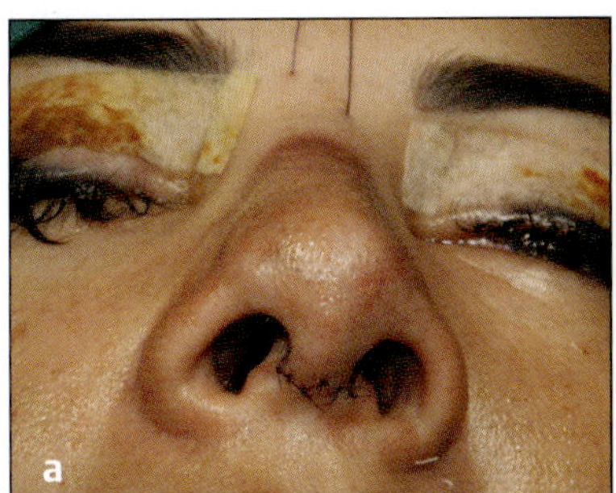
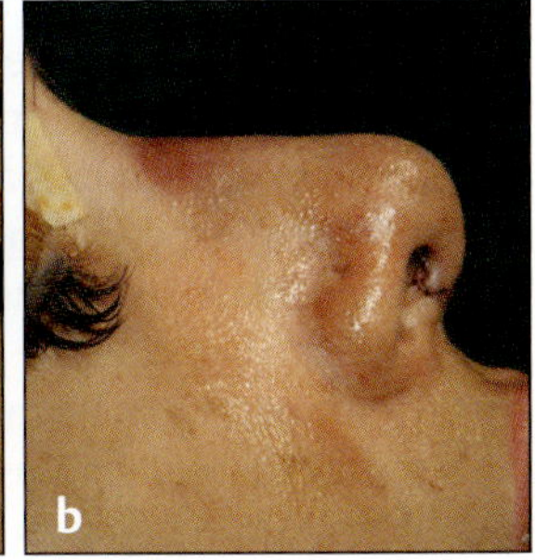

Fig. 15.47 **(a, b)** Final closure is achieved by carefully approximating the angles of incision.

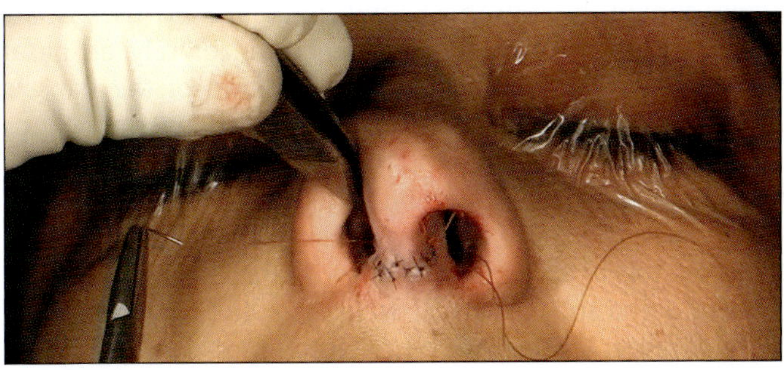

Fig. 15.48 Mattress septal sutures fix the mucoperichondrial flaps against the septum to minimize dead space.

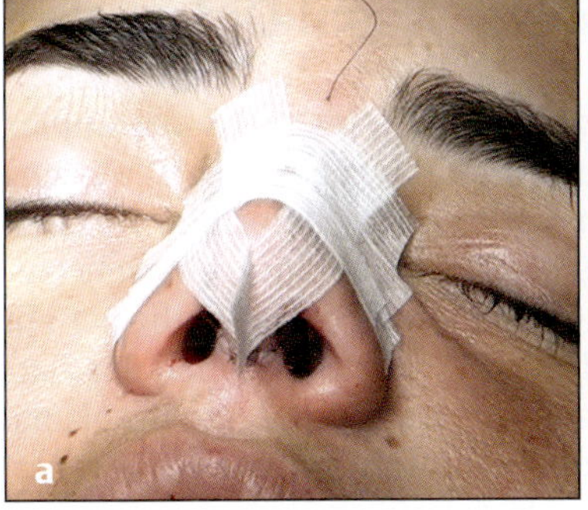
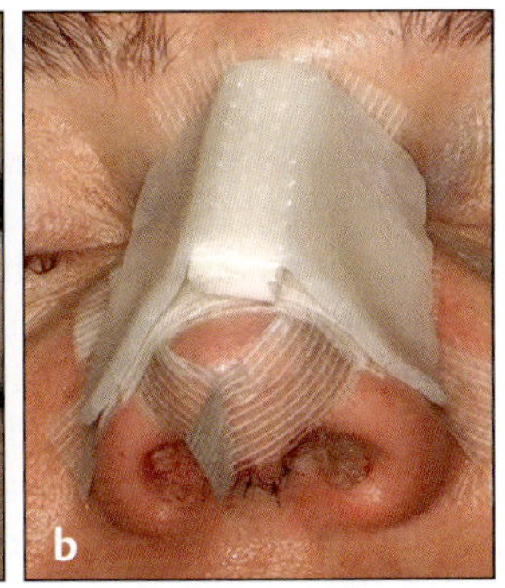

Fig. 15.49 **(a)** Two long skin tapes stabilize tip area. **(b)** Thermoplastic splint is used in all those cases where osteotomies are performed.

and second, use of grafts which act as foreign body until they are vascularized. Inj. dexamethasone 8 mg intravenously during the operation acts as an antiemetic, and also helps in postop recovery by easing out laryngeal edema which might occur because of prolonged intubation and throat pack.

It is advisable for patients to use pillows to elevate head by about 30 degrees to minimize the postoperative congestion. Strenuous activity, lifting heavy weight, and exercises are put off for 3 to 4 weeks.

Patients are usually discharged home the next day of surgery after removal of the nasal pack. Postoperative cold compresses over the eyes and face that minimize ecchymosis are to be continued for 48 hours. Plain saline spray should be used frequently to keep the nostrils clean and to prevent crusting. Nasal decongestants like oxymetazoline can be used at night for a week to reduce edema and better breathing.

The first return visit is planned after 6 days of surgery. All sutures are removed on this day. Skin tapes and splint are removed and reapplied for a week. Patient returns after another week for cleansing and postoperative pictures for records. Later visits are scheduled at 1 month, 3 months, 6 months, and then 1 year.

Complications

Serious complications of primary rhinoplasty are rare.[73] Their prevention lies in careful preoperative assessment, counseling and planning, a meticulous intraoperative technique, and a careful postoperative monitoring of the patient.

Immediate Complications

Postoperative Bleeding

Bleeding can occur immediately after surgery or any time following for up to 2 weeks. Periorbital ecchymosis is usually seen in immediate postoperative period and can be reduced by use of cold packs. Osteotomy performed during a rhinoplasty may cause excessive bleeding in immediate postoperative period due to damage to the branches of the facial or anterior ethmoidal artery. The incidence of excessive bleeding reported in the literature ranges from 2 to 4%.[74] Treatment is usually conservative with endonasal packing for 48 hours. In order to prevent this complication, minimizing trauma with the utilization of micro-osteotomes for lateral and oblique osteotomies is recommended.[75] Late bleeding is usually due to secondary infection and should be treated with appropriate antibiotics.

Septal Hematoma

Wide undermining of the mucoperichondrium on both sides of the septum is a routine part of any rhinoplasty operation. At the end of the procedure the mucosal flaps should be put back and fixed either with mattress quilting sutures across the septum or rely on nasal packing to do this job. When the fixation of the flaps is insufficient, bleeding between the two mucoperichondrial flaps can create a septal hematoma. It is usually evident 3 to 5 days after surgery. Significant septal hematoma may block the nasal cavities causing airway obstruction. Treatment is in all cases surgical, with incision and drainage of hematoma and endonasal packing for 48 hours, combined with parenteral broad-spectrum antibiotics.

Infection

Infection following rhinoplasty is rare. Intra- and perioperative broad-spectrum antibiotics prevent the serious infection. Early recognition and aggressive treatment can prevent serious sequelae like tissue necrosis, toxic shock syndrome, cavernous sinus thrombosis, etc. Nasal septal abscess is rare but may be the sequel of untreated septal hematomas.[76] It requires immediate surgical intervention with drainage of pus, nasal packing, and treatment with parenteral broad-spectrum antibiotics.

Prolonged Edema

Prolonged edema is because of scar tissue and its remodeling. Usually organized hematoma under the skin may cause long inflammatory response. It is more common in secondary rhinoplasty cases and those with thick skin. It is recommended to use injection triamcinolone in doses of 3 to 5 mg prepared by mixing triamcinolone 10 mg/mL with lignocaine 2% in 1:1 ratio and is injected subcutaneously. It can be repeated at 4 to 8 weeks interval.

Late Complications

Late complications in rhinoplasty are usually because of poor surgical technique. They can manifest as functional or cosmetic problems or as a combination of both. Complications like dorsal irregularities, dorsal mucous cysts, overresection, underresection, pollybeak deformity, overrotated tip, inverted-V deformities, open roof, alar insufficiency, and many others are better prevented with diligent surgical techniques. If they happen, they are subject matter of secondary rhinoplasty and should be dealt with surgically. For further details, refer to Chapter 16 on "Secondary Aesthetic Rhinoplasty" in Volume VI.

Preservation Rhinoplasty

Despite many advances, rhinoplasty is still one of the most challenging procedures in aesthetic surgery. It is a constantly evolving operation. Closed techniques gave way to open techniques, which gave a better understanding of anatomy, and led the way to structural nature of this operation. One of the drawbacks of extensive structural correction is disturbance of keystone area which loses its integrity. If not reconstructed satisfactorily, it leads to compromise in the final outcome. Techniques are evolving in reduction rhinoplasty to preserve this important structure, and reduce the nasal pyramid from its base. These techniques are not new but are being revived in a new way. The hump area can also be pushed back by reducing the underlying septum from base. All this has become possible with inclusion of piezo in the armamentarium of rhinoplasty surgeon. It is possible to create precise and fine osteotomy lines under vision without either loosing or disturbing the adjacent bone. Whether these techniques will become the holy grail of reduction rhinoplasty, only time will tell (**Fig. 15.50**).[77,78]

Rhinoplasty in Binder Nasal Deformity

Binder syndrome or maxillonasal dysplasia is a complex developmental anomaly of midface consisting of varying degree of nasomaxillary hypoplasia. The deformity was first described by Noyes[79] in 1939 but later comprehensively elucidated by Binders[80] in 1964. The presentation of the patient includes underdeveloped maxilla marked by perialar flatness, absent anterior nasal spine, flat nose, acute nasolabial angle, an apparently short columella, and absent frontal sinus. Nasofrontal angle is almost obliterated and upper lip is convex. The occlusion is normal in many cases but several others have class III malocclusion as a result of maxillary retrusion. Lower jaw appears protruded as a result of relative mandible prognathism (**Box 15.1**).[81]

Box 15.1 Facial anomalies associated with Binders

- Maxillary hypoplasia
- Absent nasal spine
- Convex upper lip with acute nasolabial angle
- Flat vertical nose with nasofrontal angle of almost 180 degrees
- Proinclination of upper incisors with very thin anterior vestibular plate
- Semilunar nostrils
- Relative mandibular prognathism

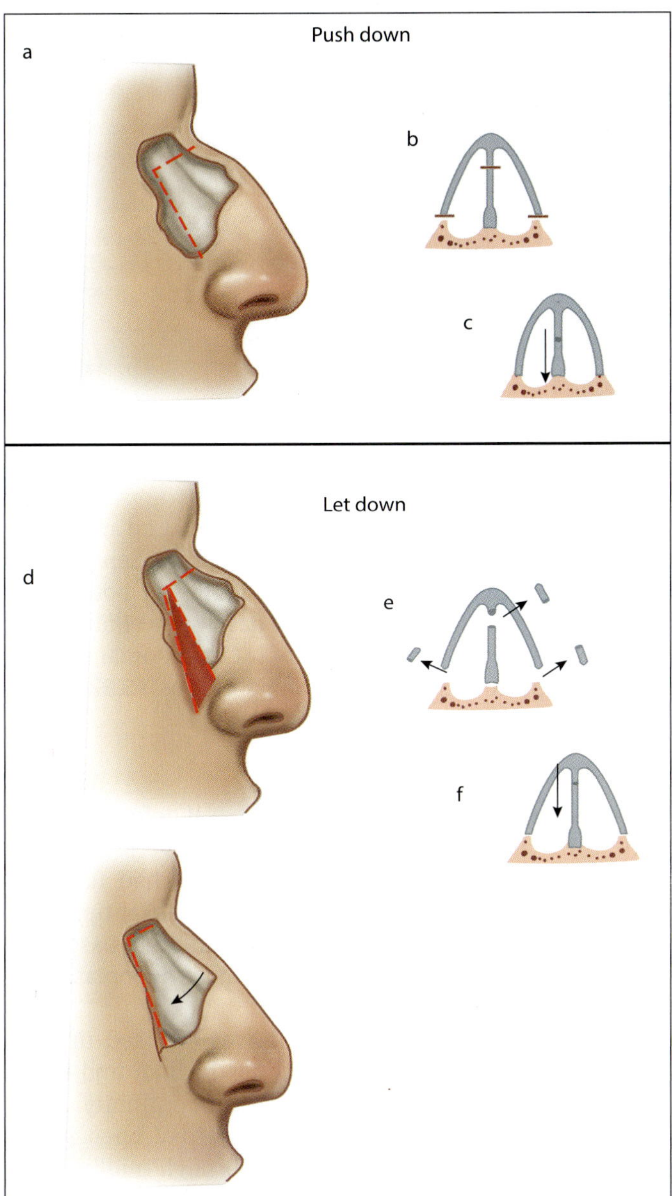

Fig. 15.50 (a–f) Preservation rhinoplasty. (Adapted from Saban et al[78].)

Surgical Planning

Operating on Binder nasal deformity is a frustrating experience. Nasal lining seems to have stuck down to the hypoplastic maxilla and the augmentation efforts do not give desired results as the nose refuses to come out of face despite our best efforts. There appears to be a shortage of columella as well as mucosa but in fact there is no shortage of both these structures as previously thought. There are many reports in literature of procedures aiming to directly lengthen these structures like V-Y plasty and even composite graft.[82] But with our better understanding of underlying pathology we now know that these procedures are likely to do more harm than good. Effective release of columella is obtained by detaching it from nasal spine. For it to stay, a strong structural support with septal extension graft is required.

There are several techniques described in literature for correction of this deformity. Perhaps none of them give satisfactory results. Holmström described intraoral approach for subperiosteal release and bone grafting. He advocated two procedures for nasal correction done simultaneously. The first procedure used L-shaped bone graft to lift the nose and in second procedure he describes releasing the septum from all sides and hinging it in keystone area by separating it from bony septum. He claimed to achieve 6- to 10-mm advancement of nasal tip with this procedure, although it is difficult to comprehend how advancing septum will advance the nasal tip. It will only enhance the dorsum till supratip area.[83] Ian Jackson recommended use of cantilever graft of calvarial bone fixed at nasal root with wires to augment the nose.[84] He also justified doing Leforte II osteotomy in severe variety of cases with class III malocclusion. This may not be necessary for those cases with normal occlusion or mild occlusal problems correctable with orthodontics.

Modern principles of structural rhinoplasty if used judiciously along with midface augmentation can give a good and lasting result in most of these cases.

Principles of procedures as followed by the author:

- Effective release of lining from nostril floor in continuity with septal mucoperichondrium and pyriform aperture through gingival incision.
- Release and undermining in subperiosteal plane around pyriform aperture.
- Complete septal release from vomerine groove in its entire length.
- Augmentation of nostril floor.
- Septal lengthening, strengthening, and support in new position with strong cartilage grafts.
- Caudal rotation and strong tip support with septal extension graft.

Operative Steps

The first step is to approach the nostril floor and pyriform aperture through periodontal/gingival approach. A no. 15 blade is used to run at the gingival edge to dig the gingival papillae in between teeth. The whole gingiva is lifted with subperiosteal dissection up to nasal spine area and going peripherally around the pyriform aperture. This incision as compared to the vestibular sulcus incision avoids going through the muscle which is left intact over the periosteum (**Fig. 15.51**). The dissection continues along the nostril floor lifting the mucosa from floor, going laterally inside the pyriform aperture, and continuing medially over the vomer. The mucoperichondrium is dissected off the lower part of the septum. Thus an extensive undermining is performed in subperiosteal plane.

The septum is dissected through routine open rhinoplasty inverted-V incision. And the mucoperichondrium is separated from both the sides. This dissection joins the

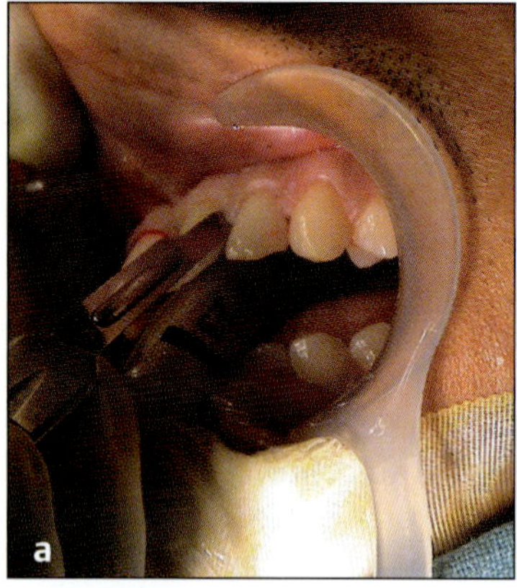
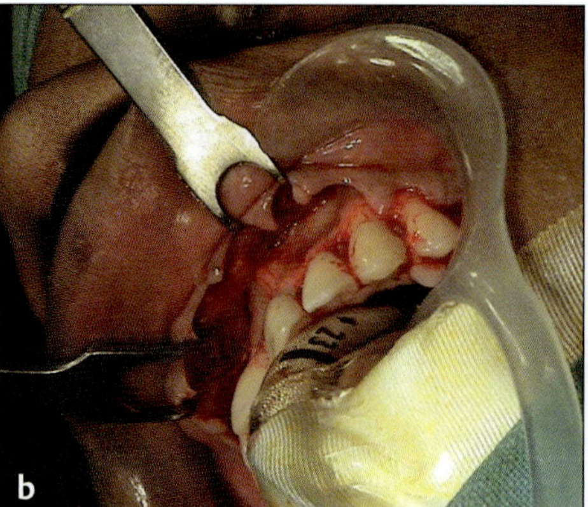
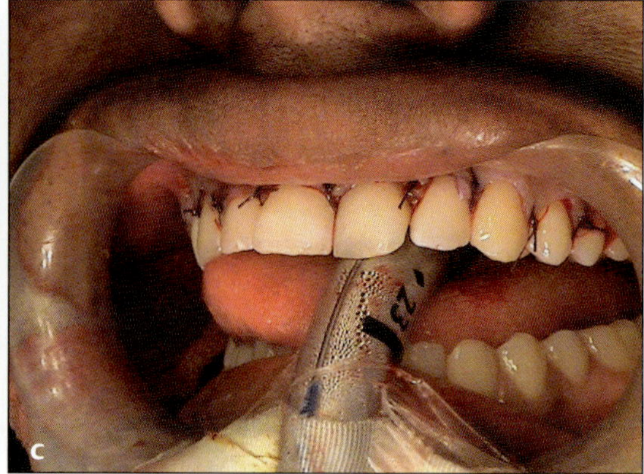

Fig. 15.51 **(a)** Gingival incision. **(b)** Dissection of the pocket. **(c)** Closure of gingival incision.

earlier dissection of nostril floor. Septum is released from the vomerine attachment with the help of a 3-mm osteotome anteroposteriorly in its entire length. This allows the nose to come out of the face. Nostril floor is augmented with diced cartilage graft and pyriform aperture is augmented with solid bone or costal cartilage grafts. Gingival incision is closed with interrupted 4–0 Vicryl sutures fixing the apices of gingiva in between teeth. The incision heals well and provides good soft tissue cover to the graft for good vascularization.

Routine rhinoplasty steps are then followed. The released septum is held in new position with septal extension graft which is wide enough to rest on the nostril floor. The septal extension graft should also be long enough to reach beyond nasal spine area to give support to the columella. Additional cartilage grafts can be used in nasal spine area to improve columellar labial angle. The septal extension graft is now used to relocate the tip in elevated position and provide adequate tip support.

Case Studies on Primary Rhinoplasty

Case 1

A 26-year-old man approached with nasal deformity and difficulty in breathing from left nostril. He had nasal deviation, small dorsal hump, and left-side nasal obstruction.

Open rhinoplasty was done through inverted-V incision. Bilateral septal exposure and separation from ULC were done. Bony hump reduction was done using power tools and rasp. Cartilaginous septum was minimally trimmed. Septum was thoroughly mobilized including bony portion. Lower portion of the septum was found to be deflected in left nostril. There was acute bend in the distal portion of the septum. Lower deflected portion of the septum was excised. Septal cartilage graft was harvested leaving 1.5-cm L-strut. Deviated ethmoid bone was also excised and used as a batten graft to straighten the bent portion of septum. Septum was further strengthened with cartilage grafts on both sides. Septum was centralized and fixed to nasal spine. Bulbous tip was corrected with cephalic trim of LLC and domal sutures. Columellar strut was used for tip support (**Fig. 15.52**).

Case 2

A 24-year-old women presented with nasal deformity since birth. On examination she was found to have Binder syndrome with nasomaxillary hypoplasia. She had flat nose with obtuse nasofrontal angle and bulbous nasal tip. There was apparent shortening of columella with acute nasolabial angle. Dental occlusion was normal. Midface hypoplasia was accompanied by perialar flattening.

Nasal floor and anterior maxilla was exposed through gingival incision. Mucosal lining in nostril floor and inside the pyriform aperture was mobilized in continuity. Nasal framework was exposed through inverted-V open rhinoplasty incision. Septum was exposed through midline with undermining mucoperichondrium on both sides. These mucoperichondrial flaps were joined with undermined nostril floor mucosa by dividing the dense bony adhesions at the junction. Septum was detached from vomerine groove through oral incision.

Nostril floor was filled with diced costal cartilage graft. Small cartilage grafts were used for augmenting maxilla in perialar region and gingival incision was closed. Septal extension graft was fixed to the distal septum and both septum and extension grafts were strengthened with extended spreader grafts. Extension graft was fixed with nasal spine, leaving enough graft projected to lie in between medial crura. Nasal tip was projected and both medial crura were fixed to septal extension graft giving a new height to the tip. Dorsum was augmented with cartilage graft and tip projection was further enhanced with tip graft (**Fig. 15.53**).

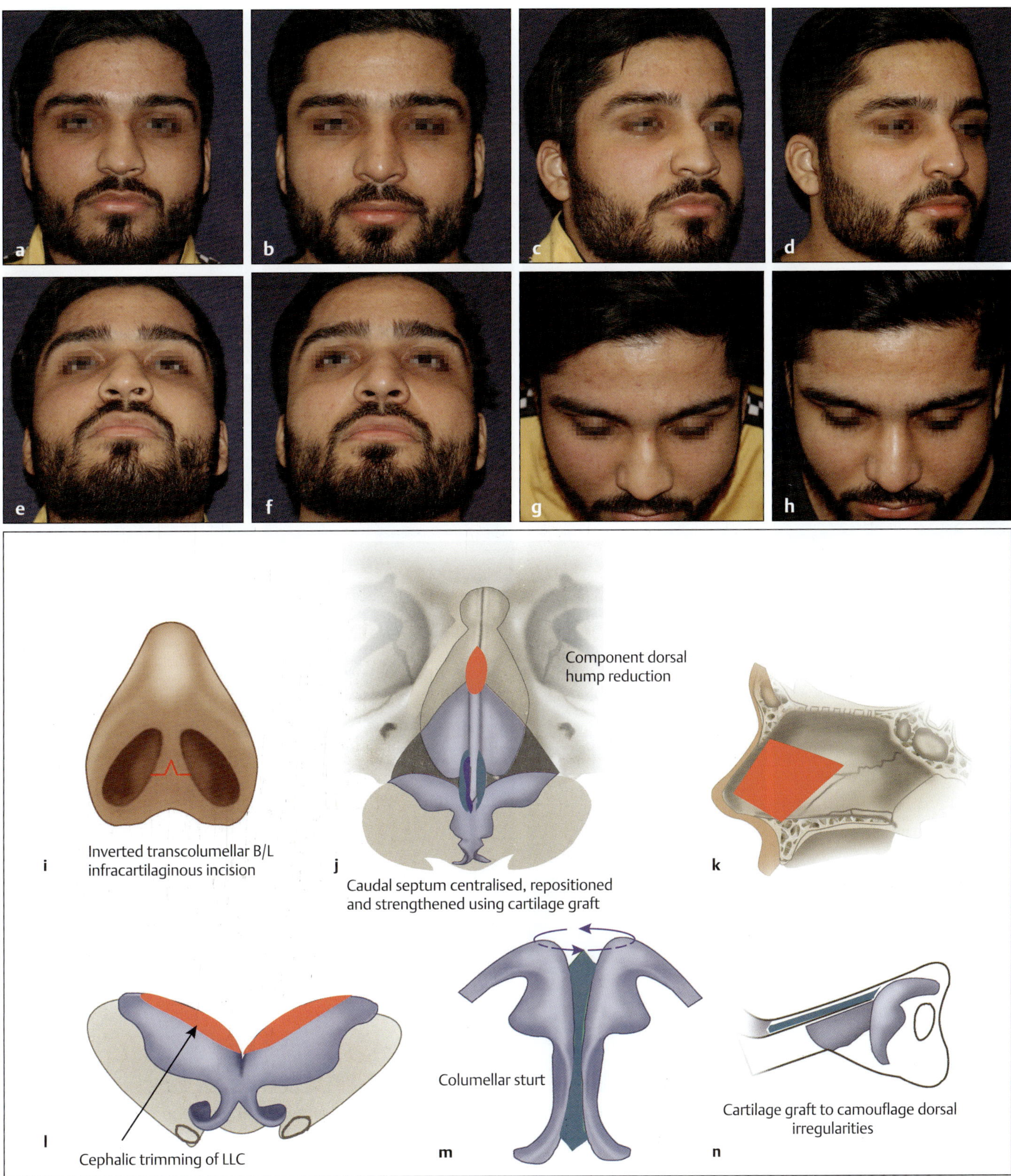

Fig. 15.52 Open rhinoplasty performed for nasal deviation, dorsal hump and left side nasal obstruction. **(a–d)** Preoperative and postoperative pictures front, left oblique, bird's eye and looking down views. **(i)** Inverted V transcollumellar infracartilaginous incision placed. **(j)** Component dorsal hump removed. Caudal septum straightened and strengthend using cartilage and bone grafts. **(k)** Septal cartilage graft and vertical plate of ethmoid graft harvested. **(l)** LLC cephalic trimming done. **(m)** columellar strut placed and suture tip plasty done. **(n)** Cartilage graft placed over dorsum to camoflage the irregularities.

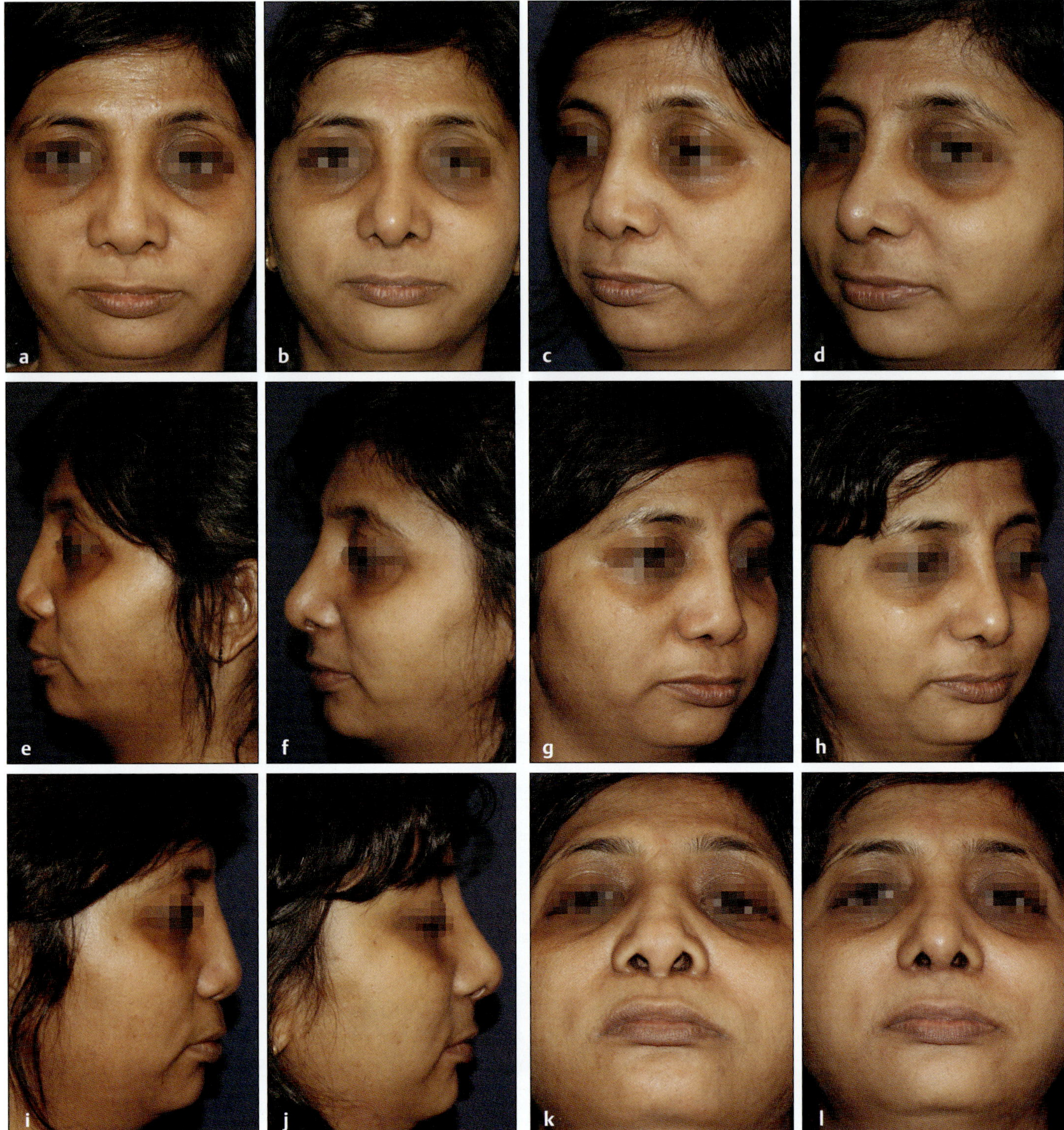

Fig. 15.53 (a–l) A case of Binder syndrome with nasomaxillary hypoplasia. Preoperative and postoperative pictures. The surgical details are diagrammatically presented. *(Continued)*

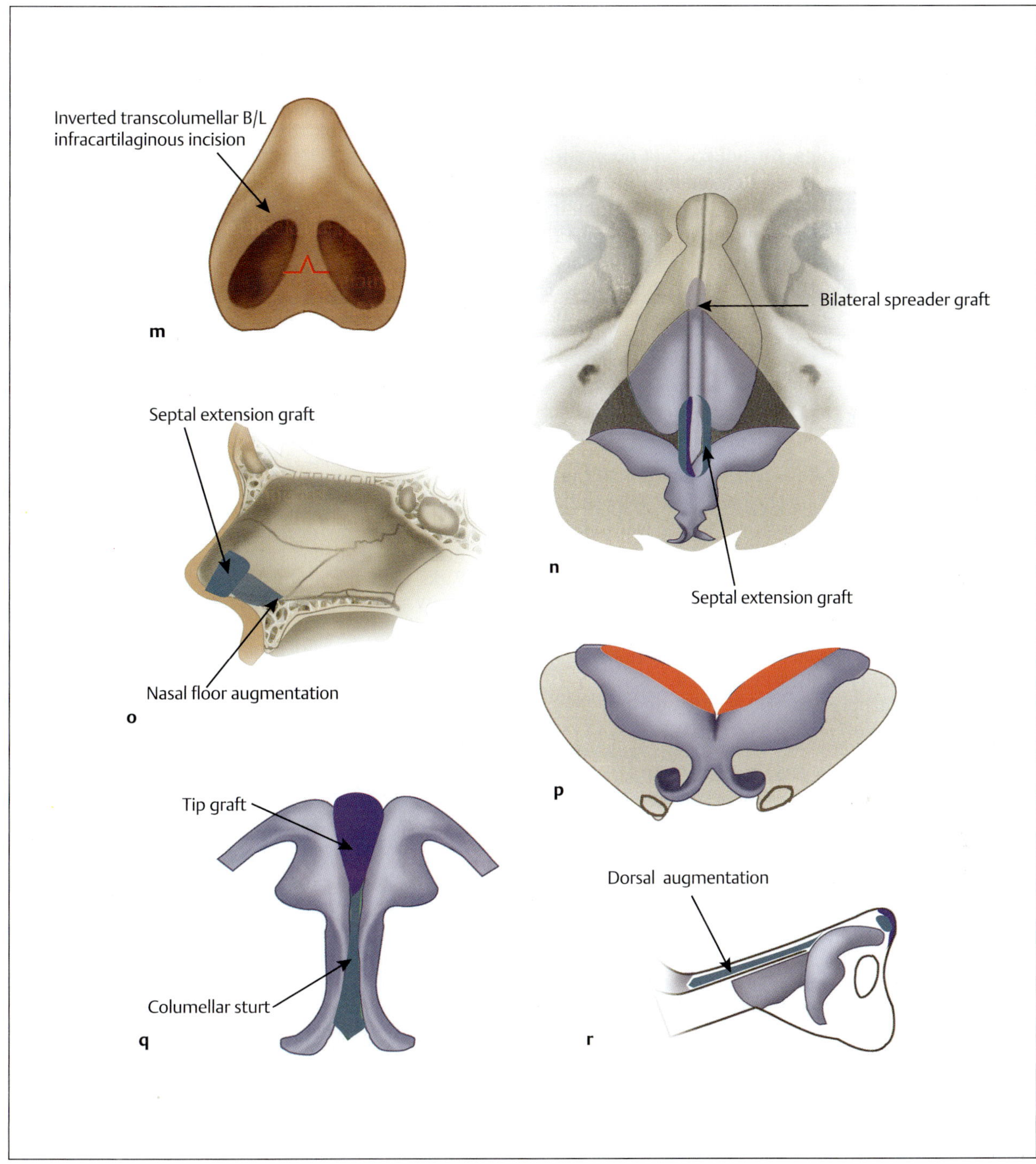

Fig. 15.53 *(Continued)* Diagrammatic representation of the procedure. **(m)** Open rhinoplasty performed with inverted V transcolumellar incision. **(n)** After septal dissection septal extension graft and bilateral spreader grafts were placed. **(o)** Nasal floor, alar base and dorsal augmentations are done using costal cartilage. **(p)** Cephalic trimming of lower lateral cartilages done. **(q)** Columellar strut and tip graft placed to create new tip. **(r)** Finally dorsal augmentation is done using long thin cartilage graft.

Conclusion

Rhinoplasty is one of the most difficult operations in aesthetic surgery. It is difficult to learn and even more difficult to master. There is long learning curve as this operation is both challenging and demanding. Introduction of open rhinoplasty techniques has made things easier for those who are performing this operation and those who are learning it. Accurate assessment of nasal anatomy and its modification is possible with open techniques, leading to its popularity. Those who aspire to be good rhinoplasty surgeons should learn all possible techniques available and apply them judiciously to achieve long-term good results.

Acknowledgment

I acknowledge and thank Dr Rajesh Tope, Senior Consultant, Department of Anesthesia, Apollo Hospital New Delhi India, for his contribution and help in writing anesthesia part of this chapter.

References

1. Daniel RK. Preservation rhinoplasty: a new rhinoplasty revolution. Aesthet Surg J 2018;38(2):228–229
2. Saraf S. Sushruta: Rhinoplasty in 600 BC. J Plastic Surg 2006; 3(2). https://ispub.com/IJPS/3/2/7839
3. Zimbler MS. Gaspare Tagliacozzi (1545–1599): renaissance surgeon. Arch Facial Plast Surg 2001;3(4):283–284
4. Lam SM. John Orlando Roe: father of aesthetic rhinoplasty. Arch Facial Plast Surg 2002;4(2):122–123
5. Rethi A. Operation to shorten excessively long nose. Rev Chir Plast 1934;2(85)
6. Goodman WS. External approach to rhinoplasty. Can J Otolaryngol 1973;2(3):207–210
7. Anderson JR, Johnson CM Jr, Adamson P. Open rhinoplasty: an assessment. Otolaryngol Head Neck Surg 1982;90(2):272–274
8. Gunter JP, Rohrich RJ. External approach for secondary rhinoplasty. Plast Reconstr Surg 1987;80(2):161–174
9. Gunter JP. The merits of the open approach in rhinoplasty. Plast Reconstr Surg 1997;99(3):863–867
10. Ha RY, Nojima K, Adams WP Jr, Brown SA. Analysis of facial skin thickness: defining the relative thickness index. Plast Reconstr Surg 2005;115(6):1769–1773
11. Dey JK, Recker CA, Olson MD, et al. Assessing nasal soft-tissue envelope thickness for rhinoplasty: normative data and a predictive algorithm. JAMA Facial Plast Surg 2019;21(6):511–517 https://www.liebertpub.com/doi/abs/10.1001/jamafacial.2019.0715
12. Kosins AM, Obagi ZE. Managing the difficult soft tissue envelope in facial and rhinoplasty surgery. Aesthet Surg J 2017; 37(2):143–157
13. Han SK, Shin YW, Kim WK. Anatomy of the external nasal nerve. Plast Reconstr Surg 2004;114(5):1055–1059
14. Joseph AW, Ishii L, Joseph SS, et al. Prevalence of body dysmorphic disorder and surgeon diagnostic accuracy in facial plastic and oculoplastic surgery clinics. JAMA Facial Plast Surg 2017;19(4):269–274
15. Picavet VA, Prokopakis EP, Gabriëls L, Jorissen M, Hellings PW. High prevalence of body dysmorphic disorder symptoms in patients seeking rhinoplasty. Plast Reconstr Surg 2011;128(2): 509–517
16. Koch RJ, Chavez A, Dagum P, Newman JP. Advantages and disadvantages of computer imaging in cosmetic surgery. Dermatol Surg 1998;24(2):195–198
17. Agarwal A, Gracely E, Silver WE. Realistic expectations: to morph or not to morph? Plast Reconstr Surg 2007;119(4):1343–1351, discussion 1352–1353
18. Punthakee X, Rival R, Solomon P. Digital imaging in rhinoplasty. Aesthetic Plast Surg 2009;33(4):635–638
19. Fung E, Hong P, Moore C, Taylor SM. The effectiveness of modified Cottle maneuver in predicting outcomes in functional rhinoplasty. Plast Surg Int 2014;2014:618313
20. Daniel RK. Mastering rhinoplasty. 2nd ed. Springer Publication; 2010:59
21. Wotman M, Kacker A. What are the indications for the use of computed tomography before septoplasty? Laryngoscope 2016;126(6):1268–1270
22. Aksoy MH. Preoperative evaluation of paranasal computed tomography reports of patients requesting rhinoplasty for the presence of septal deviation and inferior turbinate hypertrophy. Austin J Surg 2019;6(3):1–4
23. Parks ET. Cone beam computed tomography for the nasal cavity and paranasal sinuses. Dent Clin North Am 2014;58(3): 627–651
24. Khojastepour L, Mirhadi S, Mesbahi SA. Anatomical variations of ostiomeatal complex in CBCT of patients seeking rhinoplasty. J Dent (Shiraz) 2015;16(1):42–48
25. Rohrich RJ, Afrooz PN. Rhinoplasty refinements: the role of the open approach. Plast Reconstr Surg 2017;140(4):716–719
26. Foda HMT. External rhinoplasty for the Arabian nose: a columellar scar analysis. Aesthetic Plast Surg 2004;28(5):312–316
27. Cobo R. Ethnic considerations in facial plastic surgery. Thieme Publishers; 2015
28. Kumar L. Book review: ethnic considerations in facial plastic surgery. Aesthet Surg J 2016;36(10):NP324
29. Eghbal A, Modir H, Moshiri E, Khalili M, Barsari FZ, Mohammadbeigi A. Hypotensive effect of labetalol and dexmedetomidine blood loss and surgical conditions in functional endoscopic sinus surgery. Formosan J Surg 2018; 51(3):98–194
30. Sajedi P, Rahimian A, Khalili G. Comparative evaluation between two methods of induced hypotension with infusion of Remifentanil and Labetalol during sinus endoscopy. J Res Pharm Pract 2016;5(4):264–271
31. Salem AE, Hagras AM, Abo-Ragab HA. Labetalol hypotensive anesthetic protocol paves the way to safe open abdominal myomectomy. J Anesth Intensive Care Med 2017;3(2):1–5
32. Said AM, El-Serwi HB. Labetalol preoperative oral and intraoperative infusion overrides nitroglycerine infusion for hypotensive anesthesia during functional endoscopic sinus surgery. Res Opinion Anesth Intensive Care 2019;6(2):194–199
33. Gupta N, Talwar V, Prakash S, Deuri A, Gogia AR. Evaluation of the efficacy of desflurane with or without labetalol for hypotensive anesthesia in middle ear microsurgery. J Anaesthesiol Clin Pharmacol 2017;33(3):375–380
34. Hassanpour SE, Mahmoudvand H, Rouientan A, Asgarzadeh MR, Niazi M. Comparison between step incision and inverted-V incision in columellar scar in open rhinoplasty. J Res Med Dental Sci 2018;6(6):257–263

35. Aksu I, Alim H, Tellioğlu AT. Comparative columellar scar analysis between transverse and inverted-V incision in open rhinoplasty. Aesthetic Plast Surg 2008;32(4):638–640
36. Ihvan O, Seneldir L, Naiboglu B, Verim A, Cetiner S. Comparative columellar scar analysis between w incisions and inverted-V incision in open technique nasal surgery. Indian J Otolaryngol Head Neck Surg 2018;70(2):231–234
37. Dingman RO. Correction of nasal deformities due to defects of the septum. Plast Reconstr Surg (1946) 1956;18(4):291–304
38. Sazgar AA, Kheradmand A, Razfar A, Hajialipour S, Sazgar AK. Different techniques for caudal extension graft placement in rhinoplasty. Rev Bras Otorrinolaringol (Engl Ed) 2019; S1808-8694(19)30096-5. Online ahead of print
39. Toriumi D. Caudal septal extension graft for retracted columella. Oper Tech Otolaryngol: Head Neck Surg 1995;6(4):311–318
40. Sheen JH. Spreader graft: a method of reconstructing the roof of the middle nasal vault following rhinoplasty. Plast Reconstr Surg 1984;73(2):230–239
41. Boccieri A, Macro C, Pascali M. The use of spreader grafts in primary rhinoplasty. Ann Plast Surg 2005;55(2):127–131
42. Palacín JM, Bravo FG, Zeky R, Schwarze H. Controlling nasal length with extended spreader grafts: a reliable technique in primary rhinoplasty. Aesthetic Plast Surg 2007;31(6):645–650
43. Toriumi DM. Management of the middle nasal vault in rhinoplasty. Operative Tech Plast Recon Surg 1995;2:16–30
44. King ED, Ashley FL. The correction of the internally and externally deviated nose. Plast Reconstr Surg (1946) 1952;10(2): 116–120
45. Gubisch W. Extracorporeal septoplasty for the markedly deviated septum. Arch Facial Plast Surg 2005;7(4):218–226
46. Barone M, Cogliandro A, Salzillo R, et al. Role of spreader flaps in rhinoplasty: analysis of patients undergoing correction for severe septal deviation with long-term follow-up. Aesthetic Plast Surg 2019;43(4):1006–1013
47. Rohrich RJ, Gunter JP, Deuber MA, Adams WP Jr. The deviated nose: optimizing results using a simplified classification and algorithmic approach. Plast Reconstr Surg 2002;110(6):1509–1523, discussion 1524–1525
48. Jang YJ, Wang JH, Lee BJ. Classification of the deviated nose and its treatment. Arch Otolaryngol Head Neck Surg 2008;134(3):311–315
49. Kim CH, Park SC. Homologous tissue for dorsal augmentation. Facial Plast Surg Clin North Am 2018;26(3):311–321
50. Jackson IT, Yavuzer R. AlloDerm for dorsal nasal irregularities. Plast Reconstr Surg 2001;107(2):553–558, discussion 559–560
51. Daniel RK. Rhinoplasty: dorsal grafts and the designer dorsum. Clin Plast Surg 2010;37(2):293–300
52. Erol OO. The Turkish delight: a pliable graft for rhinoplasty. Plast Reconstr Surg 2000;105(6):2229–2241, discussion 2242–2243
53. Daniel RK. Diced cartilage grafts in rhinoplasty surgery: current techniques and applications. Plast Reconstr Surg 2008;122(6): 1883–1891
54. Cakmak O, Bircan S, Buyuklu F, Tuncer I, Dal T, Ozluoglu LN. Viability of crushed and diced cartilage grafts: a study in rabbits. Arch Facial Plast Surg 2005;7(1):21–26
55. Cakmak O, Buyuklu F, Yilmaz Z, Sahin FI, Tarhan E, Ozluoglu LN. Viability of cultured human nasal septum chondrocytes after crushing. Arch Facial Plast Surg 2005;7(6):406–409
56. Toriumi DM, Pero CD. Asian rhinoplasty. Clin Plast Surg 2010; 37(2):335–352
57. Rohrich RJ, Bolden K. Ethnic rhinoplasty. Clin Plast Surg 2010;37(2):353–370
58. Park SS. Fundamental principles in aesthetic rhinoplasty. Clin Exp Otorhinolaryngol 2011;4(2):55–66
59. Byrd HS, Andochick S, Copit S, Walton KG. Septal extension grafts: a method of controlling tip projection shape. Plast Reconstr Surg 1997;100(4):999–1010
60. Akkus AM, Eryilmaz E, Guneren E. Comparison of the effects of columellar strut and septal extension grafts for tip support in rhinoplasty. Aesthetic Plast Surg 2013;37(4):666–673
61. Sawh-Martinez R, Perkins K, Madari S, Steinbacher DM. Control of nasal tip position: quantitative assessment of columellar strut versus caudal septal extension graft. Plast Reconstr Surg 2019;144(5):772e–780e
62. Toriumi DM. Discussion: control of nasal tip position: quantitative assessment of columellar strut vs caudal septal extension graft. Plast Reconstr Surg 2019;144(5):781e–783e
63. Gunter JP, Friedman RM. Lateral crural strut graft: technique and clinical applications in rhinoplasty. Plast Reconstr Surg 1997;99(4):943–952, discussion 953–955
64. Murakami CS, Barrera JE, Most SP. Preserving structural integrity of the alar cartilage in aesthetic rhinoplasty using a cephalic turn-in flap. Arch Facial Plast Surg 2009;11(2):126–128
65. Gruber RP, Friedman GD. Suture algorithm for the broad or bulbous nasal tip. Plast Reconstr Surg 2002;110(7):1752–1764, discussion 1765–1768
66. Behmand RA, Ghavami A, Guyuron B. Nasal tip sutures part I: the evolution. Plast Reconstr Surg 2003;112(4):1125–1129, discussion 1146–1149
67. Gruber RP, Weintraub J, Pomerantz J. Suture techniques for the nasal tip. Aesthet Surg J 2008;28(1):92–100
68. Foda HMT, Kridel RW. Lateral crural steal and lateral crural overlay: an objective evaluation. Arch Otolaryngol Head Neck Surg 1999;125(12):1365–1370
69. Guyuron B, Bigdeli Y, Sajjadian A. Dynamics of the alar rim graft. Plast Reconstr Surg 2015;135(4):981–986
70. Boahene KD, Hilger PA. Alar rim grafting in rhinoplasty: indications, technique, and outcomes. Arch Facial Plast Surg 2009;11(5):285–289
71. Ishii CH. Current update in Asian rhinoplasty. Plast Reconstr Surg Glob Open 2014;2(4):e133
72. Alinasab B, Haraldsson PO. Rapid resorbable sutures are a favourable alternative to non-resorbable sutures in closing transcolumellar incision in rhinoplasty. Aesthetic Plast Surg 2016;40(4):449–452
73. Layliev J, Gupta V, Kaoutzanis C, et al. Incidence and preoperative risk factors for major complications in aesthetic rhinoplasty: analysis of 4978 patients. Aesthet Surg J 2017;37(7):757–767
74. Tamerin JA. Management of hemorrhage post rhinoplasty. NY State J Med 1967;67(4):550–551
75. Tardy ME Jr, Denneny JC. Micro-osteotomies in rhinoplasty. Facial Plast Surg 1984;1:137–145
76. Rettinger G, Kirsche H. Complications in septoplasty. Facial Plast Surg 2006;22(4):289–297
77. Santos M, Rego AR, Coutinho M, Sousa CAE, Ferreira MG. Spare roof technique in reduction rhinoplasty: prospective study of the first one hundred patients. Laryngoscope 2019;129(12): 2702–2706
78. Saban Y, Daniel RK, Polselli R, Trapasso M, Palhazi P. Dorsal preservation: the push down technique reassessed. Aesthet Surg J 2018;38(2):117–131
79. Noyes FB. Case report. Angle Orthod 1939;9:160–165
80. Binder KH. Maxillo-nasal dysostosis: an arhinencephalic malformation complex (author's translation) [in German]. Dtsch Zahnarztl Z 1962;17:438–444

81. Defraia E, Camporesi M, Conti G, Zoni V, Marinelli A. Oral and craniofacial findings of Binder syndrome: two case reports. Cleft Palate Craniofac J 2012;49(4):498–503
82. Draf W, Bockmühl U, Hoffmann B. Nasal correction in maxillonasal dysplasia (Binder's syndrome): a long term follow-up study. Br J Plast Surg 2003;56(3):199–204
83. Holmström H. Surgical correction of the nose and midface in maxillonasal dysplasia (Binder's syndrome). Plast Reconstr Surg 1986;78(5):568–580
84. Jackson IT, Moos KF, Sharpe DT. Total surgical management of Binder's syndrome. Ann Plast Surg 1981;7(1):25–34

16

Secondary Aesthetic Rhinoplasty

Kapil S. Agrawal

Introduction

The primary aim of secondary rhinoplasty is to obtain a properly functioning, aesthetically pleasing, and natural looking nose. Rhinoplasty, in general, is considered as one of the most challenging aesthetic procedures. Postoperative nasal deformities requiring secondary corrections pose greater challenge to a surgeon and demand analytical and technical artistry as distorted or altered anatomy, scarred/deficient tissues, and compromised vascularity cannot be managed by mere scientific knowledge of rhinoplasty steps. Deformities may vary in severity from mild irregularity of dorsum or asymmetry of nostrils to total collapse of nasal skeleton.

Exhaustion of primary source of cartilage graft (septal and conchal) is a common occurrence in secondary cases. Conchal cartilage, if intact, is neither enough in quantity nor structurally strong to support a collapsed skeleton. Secondary surgeon has to look for secondary source of cartilage to correct difficult aesthetic and functional deformities. The usual secondary source of cartilage is costal cartilage which fulfills requirements of both quantity and strength needed to rebuild, augment, and support the deformed nasal skeleton. Success in secondary rhinoplasty, therefore, relies on accurate clinical diagnosis and analysis of the nasal deformities, a thorough operative plan to address each abnormality, and a meticulous surgical technique. Restoration of skeletal framework is essential to get an aesthetically pleasing and a normally breathing nose.

Rhinoplasty is a balance of art and science. Scientific knowledge is needed to understand and learn the techniques, but it is a surgeon's inherent artistic and aesthetic vision by which he/she turns these techniques into great skills to produce a natural looking nose.

The incidence of secondary rhinoplasty in the practice of an established rhinoplasty surgeon is around 25 to 30%.[1] The percentage of revisions of a surgeon's own cases is around 5 to 15%.[2]

An agglomeration of techniques in use and few new techniques which have predictably and reliably been producing desired results in secondary noses is being presented.

The common causes of secondary nasal deformities are as follows:

- Improper or imperfect analysis leading to residual deformities is the most common cause of reoperation.
- Graft displacement or warping causing obvious dorsal deformity.
- Underresection/undercorrection causing dorsal, supratip, or tip deformity.
- Overresection leading to collapse or saddle nose.
- Too short or too long nose and columellar deformities.
- Faulty suturing of incisions causing asymmetry of nostrils and a visible columellar scar.

Definitions

Secondary rhinoplasty is a term given to corrective reshaping of a nose which was operated earlier once or multiple times by different surgeons.[3,4]

Revision rhinoplasty is done by the same surgeon in order to improve the results of a previous attempt.[3,4]

Secondary noses may present with deformities of:

- Bony pyramid.
- Cartilaginous pyramid.
- Nasolabial angle.
- Tip.
- Alae.
- Columella.
- Septum.
- Nostrils.
- Nasal skin.

Patient Presentation

Consultation

Convincing a patient with secondary nasal deformities is comparatively easier than primary because the patient is more realistic and usually concerned about the deformities rather than seeking for a perfect nose. For primary rhinoplasty the patients are excited and demand very specific changes. They occasionally bring photos of their favorite celebrity and ask the surgeon for exact replica.

The scene is completely different during consultation for secondary rhinoplasty. Patients with secondary nasal deformities usually behave in two different ways: one set is very suspicious about the abilities of the surgeon, is hard to convince, is unpersuasive, and is reluctant to take additional scars or to consent for any autograft harvest; the second set is well prepared for any kind of graft harvest and surrenders to the surgeon. This set asks the surgeon to do whatever he/she feels right and requests the surgeon to give him/her a normal nose as pleasing as possible. Recording the patient's complaints and examination findings is the most important step in the process of reaching a decision on how to deal with the case. As a rule all anatomical and functional problems are noted in detail and discussed with the patient. What can be improved or corrected and what cannot be is the most important point to be discussed with the patient.

Scars over nose are a difficult proposition and patients usually come with an impression that they can be erased by plastic surgery. They should be informed clearly that "scars cannot be erased, but can only be made better." A detailed discussion regarding an open approach, an open or extra corporeal septoplasty, ancillary procedures like alar reduction, mid face augmentation, or chin augmentation, and harvest of conchal, costal cartilage, and/or temporal fascia graft must be done during consultation only.[4,5]

Recording of Detailed History

Recording of past medical and surgical history is very important to avoid any untoward incident during or after surgery. History of allergic disorders, (e.g., asthma, vasomotor rhinitis, and sinusitis, must be obtained and recorded). History of trauma to nose, rhinoplasty, septoplasty, septorhinoplasty, and sinus or turbinate surgeries must be noted. Any addiction and drug abuse, and present medications including aspirin or any other blood thinners which may cause excessive bleeding must be recorded.[4,5]

Clinical Analysis

Clinical evaluation begins by defining the deformity, which is accomplished by a detailed history, physical examination, and complete aesthetic facial and nasal analysis. A thorough analysis of nose and anatomic diagnosis of each deformity is a key step for achieving optimal results in secondary rhinoplasty. All analytical points are noted and all deformities are marked systematically over the diagrams in the worksheet in **Fig. 16.1**.[4]

External Nasal Examination

The nose should be examined and analyzed either below upward or above downward (top to bottom) (**Box 16.1**). Starting from above, the shape of radix, and the height, width, and symmetry of the dorsum are noted. Normally, the nasofrontal angle starts from supratarsal crease but it may be obliterated by wrongly placed, oversized, or displaced dorsal strut. Collapse of middle vault presents as "inverted-V" deformity. Supratip area is inspected for depression or abnormal thickening ("poly-beak") and presence or absence of supratip break. The tip is examined and its projection, rotation, shape (bulbous, boxy, ill-defined), and symmetry is noted. The position and width of lower lateral cartilages (LLCs) change the configuration of tip.

Apart from alar flaring, the alae may be hanging or retracted. Similarly, columella may be retracted or hanging (decreased or increased show) and may be scarred. The columellar-tip and columellar-lip angles (nasolabial angle) are noted. Nostril asymmetry is a common finding **(Box 16.2)**. Three angles a rhinoplasty surgeon must note are nasofrontal (115–130 degrees), nasolabial (90–120 degrees), and nasofacial (35–55 degrees) angles, as these are the most important angles to be restored to achieve desired results.

After this topographical inspection, palpation is done to evaluate the thickness and pliability of nasal skin, bony and cartilaginous irregularities, and integrity of bony vault and septum. Gentle ballottement of nasal tip is done to evaluate the tip support.[4,5]

Box 16.1 Area of assessment

- Radix
- Nasofrontal angle
- Dorsum
- Supratip
- Tip
- Alar cartilage shape
- Bilateral ala and alar base
- Nasofacial angle
- Columella height and condition of medial crura
- ANS projection
- Columellar lip angle
- Septum
- Turbinates
- Upper lip projection
- Chin
- Bilateral angles of mandible
- Cheek bones
- Forehead slant
- Cottle's test in cases of breathing problems

Internal Nasal Examination

Position of vestibular scars, condition of nasal valves and mucosa, any hypertrophy of turbinates, and position and integrity of septum are noted. Bidigital palpation of septum is not only important to ensure its integrity but to have a rough idea as to how much graft could be harvested.[4,5]

Photographic Recording and Analysis

Photographs are a critical component of the medical record for preoperative analysis and planning, for postoperative audit, and for medicolegal purpose. Photographs of the patient must be taken during first consultation. The areas of concern must be discussed with the patient and what can be addressed or corrected and what may persist after surgery must be made clear to avoid any postoperative disappointments.

Photographs must include full-face frontal view, lateral, oblique, basal (worm's eye view), and a "text-neck" view.[6] All these views have their own importance. The technical details and clinical importance of all views are described in Chapter 24 on "Photography in Plastic Surgery", in Volume I. Here author would like to stress upon the ideal clinical views and the sequence in which the photographs should be taken.[6,7]

The sequence must be frontal (straight gaze), text-neck view (looking down), and basal view (looking up). In all these three views, patient stands straight facing the camera and only position of head changes. Now paired oblique (three-quarter view) and lateral views and smiling view (smiling in lateral view) are taken **(Fig. 16.2a–h)**.

Analysis/Planning /Operative Worksheet

Name Age / Sex OPD no. / IPD no. Date

Procedure: Rhinoplasty / Septorhinoplasty Approach: Open / Closed

Tip: Cephalic trimming

Columellar struts

Tip Suturing: Domal creation / Interdomal / Other

Tip grafts: Shield / Cap / Umbrella / Other grafts

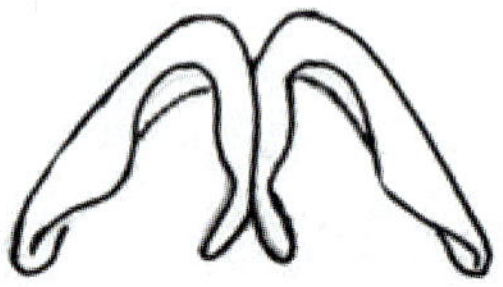

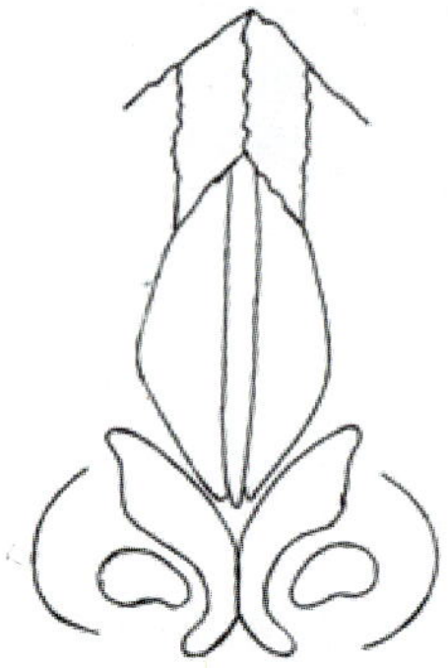

Septum: Septoplasty: Open / Extracorporeal / Endonasal

Septal graft harvest

Middle vault: Spreader grafts: U/L, B/L

Spreader flaps

Radix: Augmented / Rasped

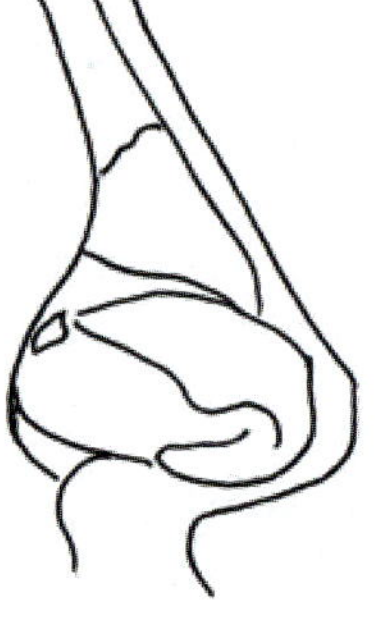

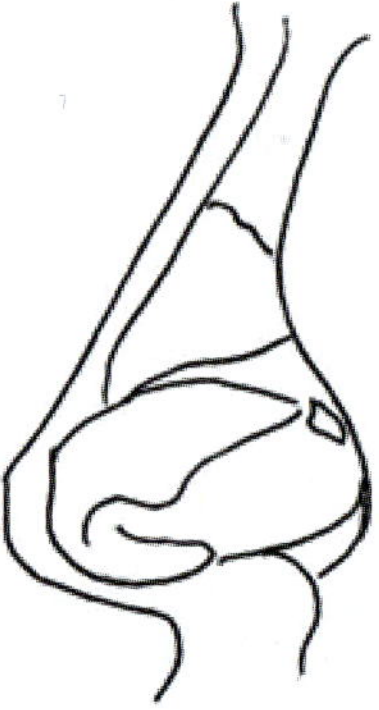

Dorsum: Reduction / Rasped

Augmentation: Cartilage; Solid / Stacks/

DCUP / DCF / Implant

Osteotomies: Not done

Done: Lateral / Intermediate /

Medial / Paramedian

Ala: Combined ala & sill reduction / Alar cinch

Ala reduction / Base excision / Sill excision

Ala rim graft / Batten graft

ANS: Reduction / Augmentation

Mid face: Augmentation / Nil

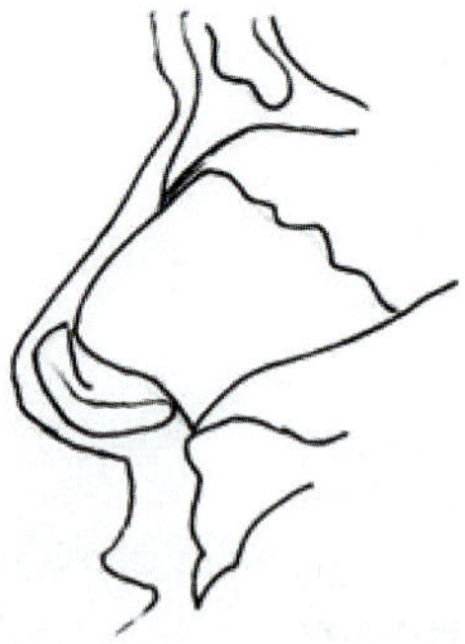

Chin: Augmentation / Reduction

Auto graft harvest: Costal cartilage (L/R/rib no.) /

Chonchal cartilage (L/R) / Septal cartilage / Temporalis fascia

Fig. 16.1 Worksheet. (Adapted from Rollin Daniel's operative sheet and modified.)

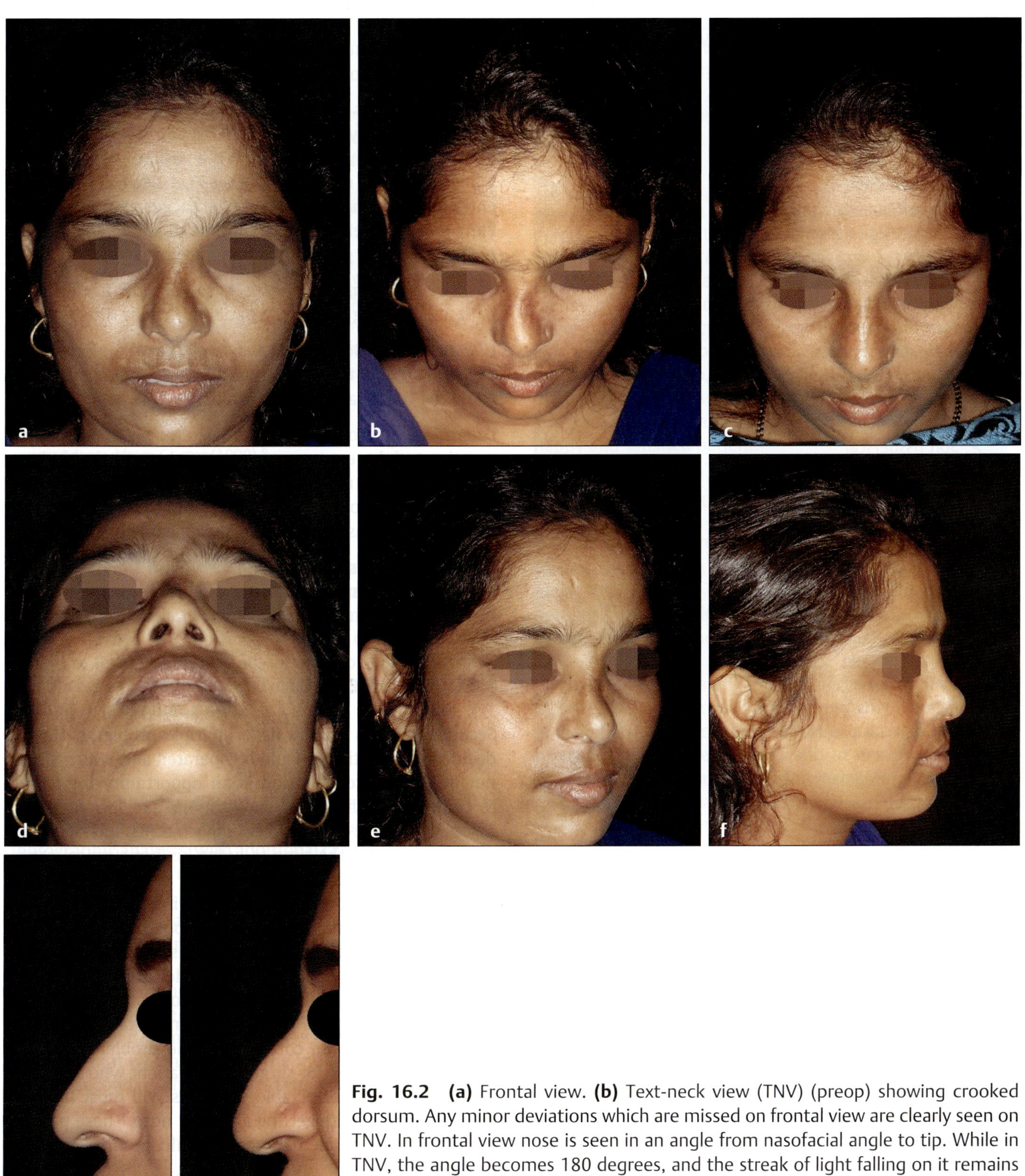

Fig. 16.2 **(a)** Frontal view. **(b)** Text-neck view (TNV) (preop) showing crooked dorsum. Any minor deviations which are missed on frontal view are clearly seen on TNV. In frontal view nose is seen in an angle from nasofacial angle to tip. While in TNV, the angle becomes 180 degrees, and the streak of light falling on it remains in midline and follows the shape of the dorsum. **(c)** TNV (postop) showing straight dorsum. **(d)** Basal or Worm's eye view. **(e)** Oblique view: this shows dorsal deviation but not optimal for proper analysis. **(f)** Lateral view: it is elusive as it is not showing any deviation. **(g)** Smiling view (before smile normal tip). **(h)** Drooping of tip on smile.

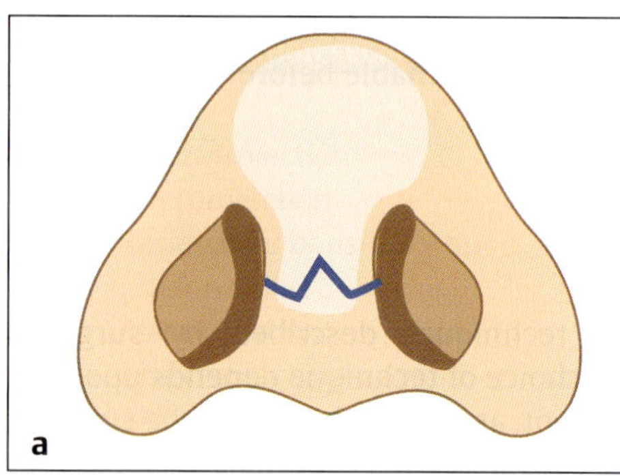

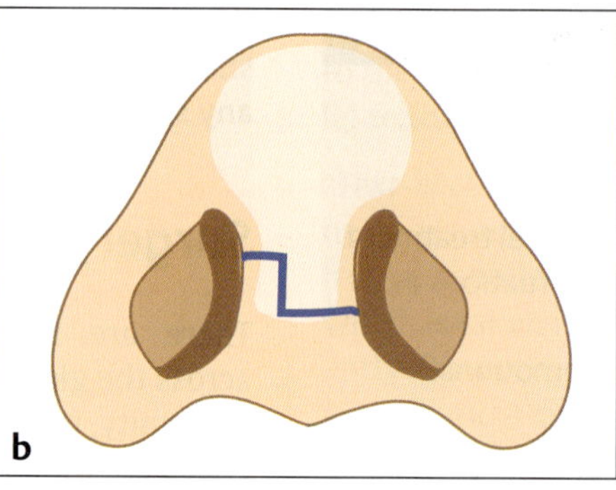

Fig. 16.3 **(a)** Inverted–V incision with wings. **(b)** Stair step incision.

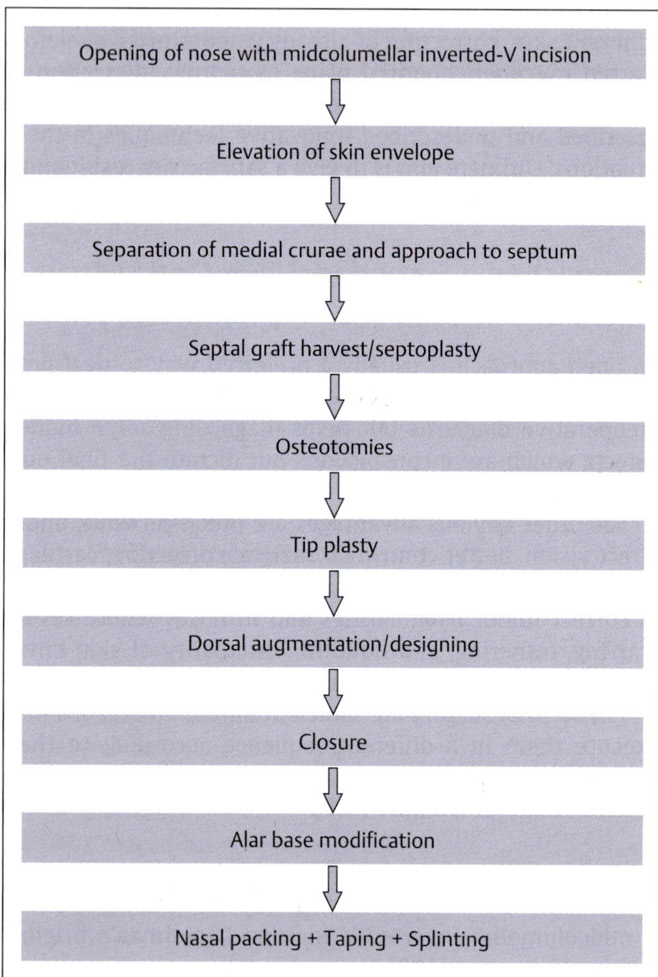

Flowchart 16.1 Operative steps followed by the author.

Dissection and Elevation of Skin Envelope

Opening a secondary nose is always difficult because of fibrosis and ensuing loss of natural planes. Careful dissection is important to protect skin as well as tip cartilage. A careful sharp dissection is done with scissors in close contact with crura. If dissection seems difficult, hydrodissection with normal saline helps at all stages of nasal opening. Once lobule is dissected, dorsal skin is infiltrated with normal saline to facilitate elevation of skin carefully without any damage. The subperichondrial and subperiosteal plane of dissection serves many purposes: (1) dissection is comparatively easier as this plane is virgin, (2) no damage to blood supply of skin envelope, (3) no chances of irregularity of skin envelope, (4) no chance of inadvertent thinning or button holing of the skin which is very common with sharp dissection mainly in the area of bony dorsum. Careful explantation of adherent implant or graft is done in a similar way.

Exposure of Septum, Graft Harvest/ Septoplasty

Opening a septum in secondary noses where septum was not touched earlier is a challenging task and doing secondary septoplasty in the noses where either septal graft was harvested or septoplasty was done is a nightmare even for an experienced surgeon. Opening a septum through dorsal approach is always difficult in secondary cases due to distorted anatomy. Dissection from caudal end (septal angle) is preferred. Medial crura are separated to gain excess of caudal septum. If there is loss of plane between medial crura, a midline incision helps in reaching caudal end of septum. A careful subperichondrial dissection is done to expose septum. Frequent hydrodissection must be used to facilitate elevation of adherent and frail mucoperichondrial flaps. Complete mucoperichondrial flaps are elevated in cases where septal cartilage is intact and needs correction or for graft harvest. A 10 mm of caudal and dorsal septal cartilage L-strut must be maintained for adequate support **(Fig. 16.4a)**. Partial elevation is done in cases where septoplasty is already done and septum either needs to be splinted to correct deviation or to correct internal valve collapse (inverted-V deformity of dorsum with breathing difficulty). Septoplasty in secondary cases should only be attempted in case of specific indication. Septal surgery should be avoided if there is history of septoplasty or septal graft harvest and patient has no septum-related complaints.[13]

Septal deformity in a secondary nose may be a deformity which was not addressed primarily, a residual deformity or iatrogenic. Only aesthetic deformity can be camouflaged, but when function is impaired because of septum then one needs to address the septal deformity irrespective of the difficulty.

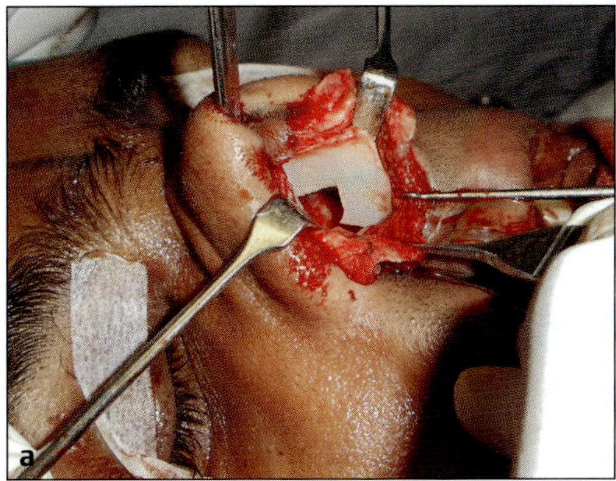

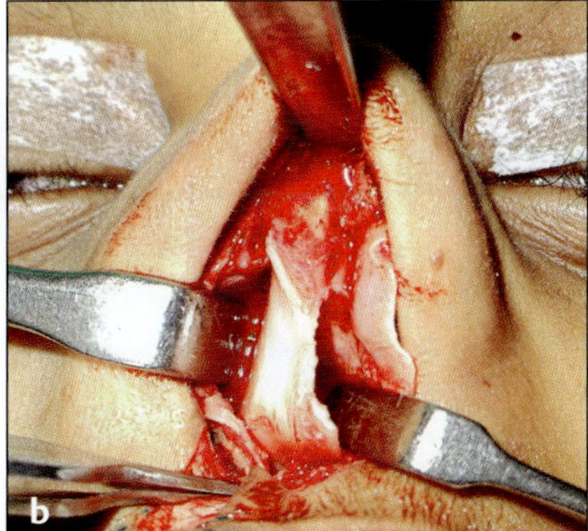

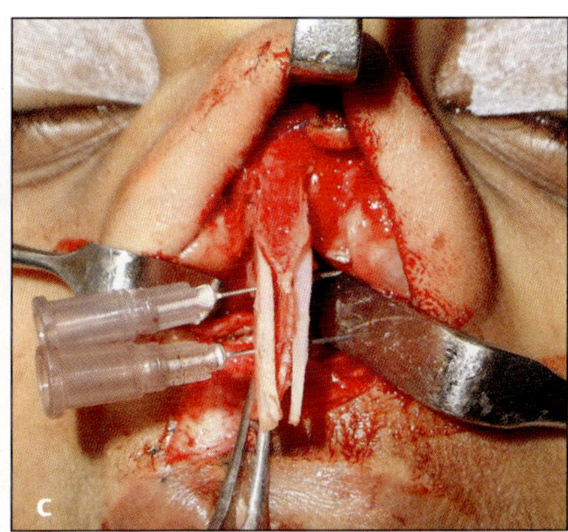

Fig. 16.4 **(a)** A sacrosanct L-strut of 1-cm width portion of the dorsal and caudal septal segment for fundamental support of the nose after septal graft harvest. **(b)** Crooked septum. **(c)** Splinting of crooked septum inside the nose with spreader grafts.

There are various methods to deal with difficult secondary septum.

Open septoplasty: Mild-to-moderate deformities can be tackled without disturbing the cephalic attachment of septum. Splinting of septum from both sides with septal cartilage spreader grafts **(Fig. 16.4b,c)**. When septal cartilage is not enough then spreader grafts can be made by bony septum or costal cartilage grafts.[13]

Extracorporeal and modified extracorporeal septoplasty: In rare cases, where severe septal deformities do not allow corrections inside the nose, extracorporeal septoplasty may be considered. L-strut is prepared by septal cartilage only or with a combination of cartilage and bony septum **(Fig. 16.5a–d)**. It is difficult to achieve stable fixation of a totally removed septum in all cases; hence, wherever possible modified extracorporeal septoplasty must be done. Here 5 mm to 1cm cephalic part of septal cartilage at keystone area is left attached, to which reconstructed L-strut can be fixed securely.[14–16]

PDS plate septoplasty: In more severe cases of secondary septoplasty where residual cartilaginous septum is severely distorted or fractured which is beyond repair and bony septal plate is either absent or is fractured in pieces, a PDS plate can be used to build a stable septal reconstruct. PDS plate is sized and designed according to the given nose and small pieces of cartilages are sutured to one side of it. Later PDS plate gets resorbed and the cartilage pieces provide adequate support.[17]

Total septal reconstruction using costal cartilage: Complete septum can be reconstructed with seventh costal cartilage using "counterbalancing technique."[18,19] This procedure is of immense value in difficult secondary septoplasty when there is paucity of native tissues **(Fig. 16.6a–c)**.

Osteotomies

The concept of osteotomies in rhinoplasty was first advocated by Jacques Joseph in 1898. He used a saw to make a low, continuous osteotomy (low to low), in which lacrimal sac was reported to be injured in a high proportion.[20,21] Sheen came out with the concept of low-to-high osteotomy, high in the region of the root of the nose to save the lacrimal sac injury.[22]

Osteotomy in rhinoplasty is a frequently performed step. A surgeon must know the implications of changes/modifications in bony vault on nasal function as well as on aesthetics. Osteotomy is performed only when it is indicated. One should keep in mind that as cephalic margins of upper lateral cartilages (ULCs) are closely adherent to the caudal part of nasal bones and together form the lateral wall of nose, any narrowing of the bones causes inward movement of ULCs resulting in narrowing of the middle vault which may lead to airway obstruction and/or undesired change in shape. There are four types of nasal osteotomies: lateral, intermediate, medial, and paramedian.

Lateral Osteotomies (Infracture)

- *Two approaches:*
  - Endonasal.
  - Extranasal (percutaneous).
- *Two techniques:*
  - Linear (continuous).
  - Perforating (postage stamp technique).
- *Three common variants:*
  - Low-low (Joseph, 1898).
  - Low-high (Sheen, 1976).
  - High-low-high (Webster, 1977).

Author prefers percutaneous "high-low-high" lateral osteotomy with postage stamp technique using 2-mm osteotome. "High-low-high" lateral osteotomy is widely accepted.[23,24] In this the lateral osteotomy starts few mm above the base of pyriform aperture, leaving a small triangle of bone at or slightly above the level of the insertion of the inferior turbinate. This small triangle of bone (Webster triangle) at the pyriform aperture is left intact to preserve the lateral attachments of the suspensory ligaments which prevents vestibular stenosis and prevents the medialization of inferior turbinates.[24–26] Next, the osteotomy is continued along the

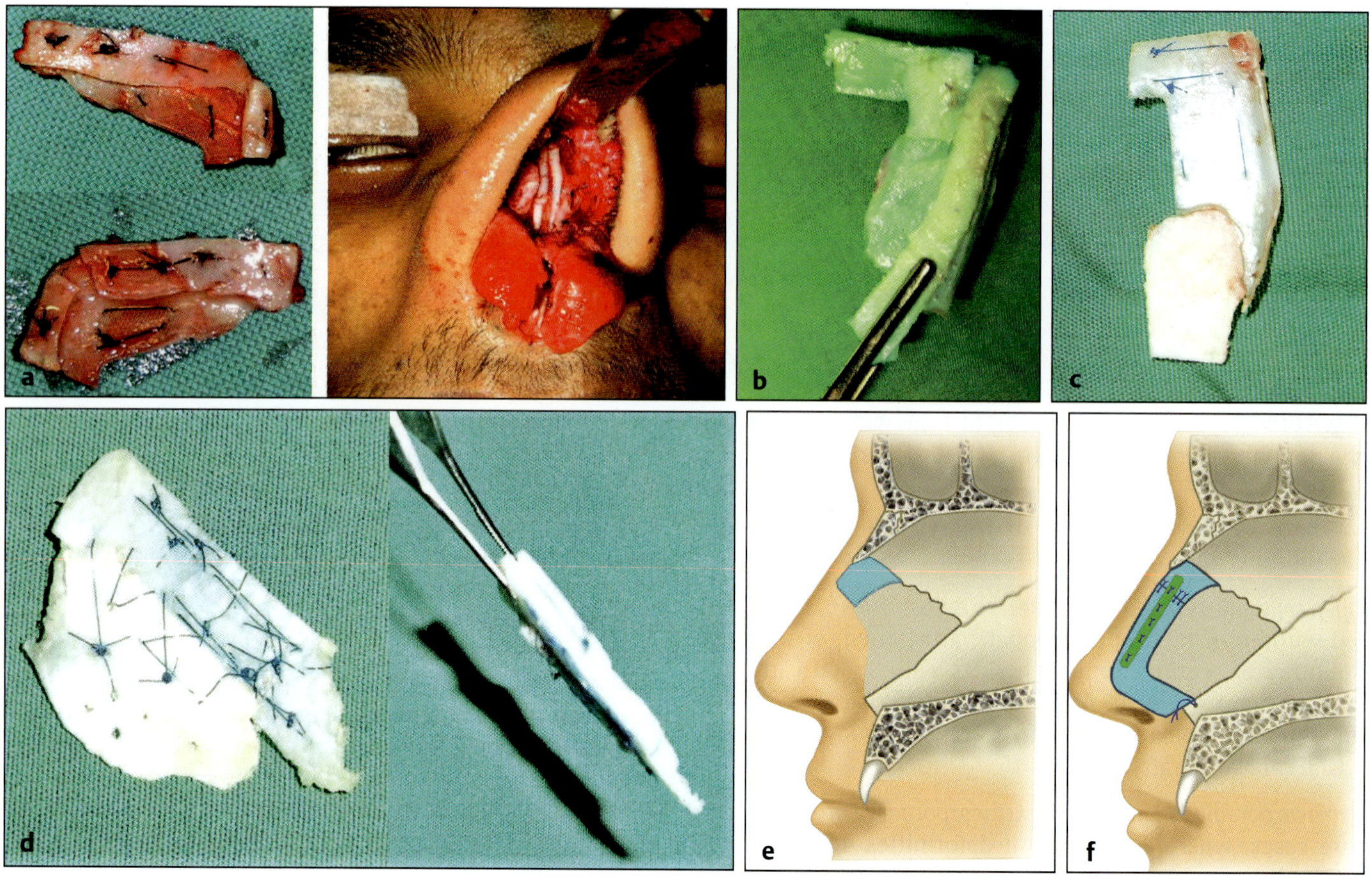

Fig. 16.5 Extracorporeal septoplasty. **(a)** L-strut of septal cartilage splinted with spreader grafts of septal cartilage and replantation of septum. **(b)** L-strut of septal cartilage splinted with spreader grafts of costal cartilage (composite). **(c)** L-strut with combination of cartilage and bony septum (hybrid). **(d)** Septal reconstruct fabricated with bony septum. **(e)** Diagram showing stump of cephalic part (0.5–1 cm) of septal cartilage attached to keystone area. **(f)** Diagram showing the reconstructed L-strut sutured to the cartilage stump and splinted with bilateral spreader grafts.

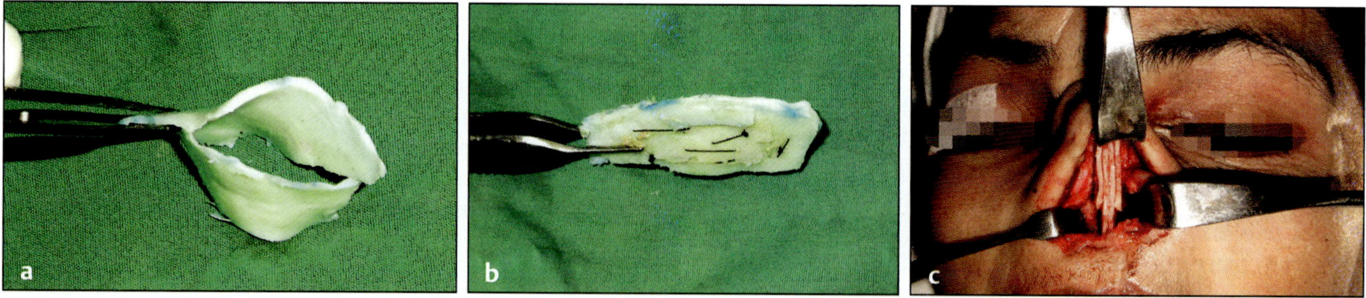

Fig. 16.6 Total septal reconstruction with costal cartilage graft. **(a)** Thin curved slices of seventh costal cartilage. **(b)** Reconstructed septum using counterbalancing technique. **(c)** Replanted septum with bilateral spreader grafts.

nasal facial groove until it curves superiorly and anteriorly into the thinner aspect of the nasal bone at the level of the inferior orbit. The cut is then terminated at the level of the medial canthus **(Fig. 16.7a)**.

Clinical Applications

- To close an open roof after hump reduction.
- To narrow a broad bridge.
- To straighten a crooked nose or posttraumatic deformity.
- To correct a collapsed nasal bone deformity using lateral osteotomy.

Intermediate/Double Lateral Osteotomy

An osteotomy between the medial and lateral osteotomies is called intermediate osteotomy. The intermediate osteotomy

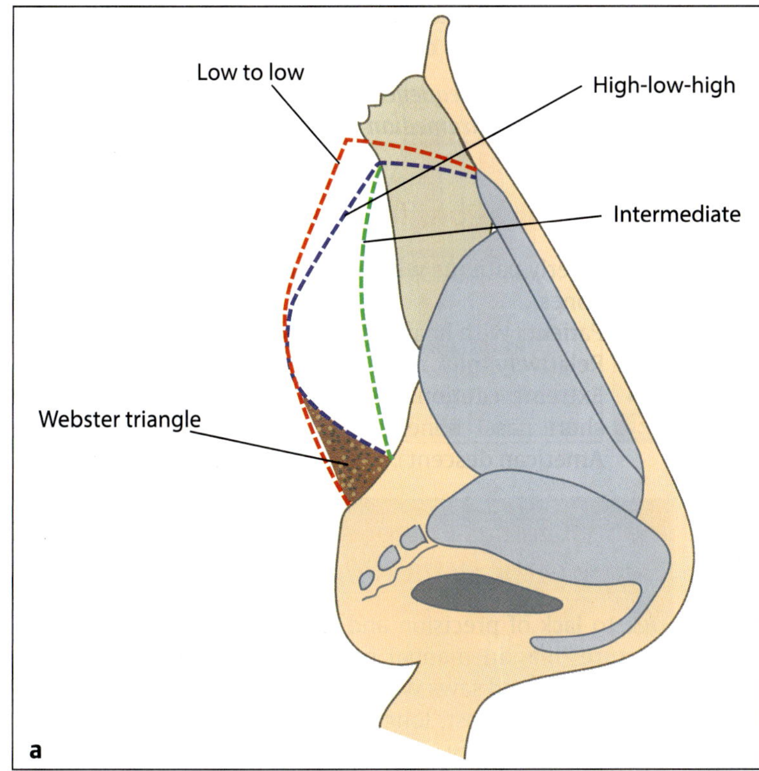

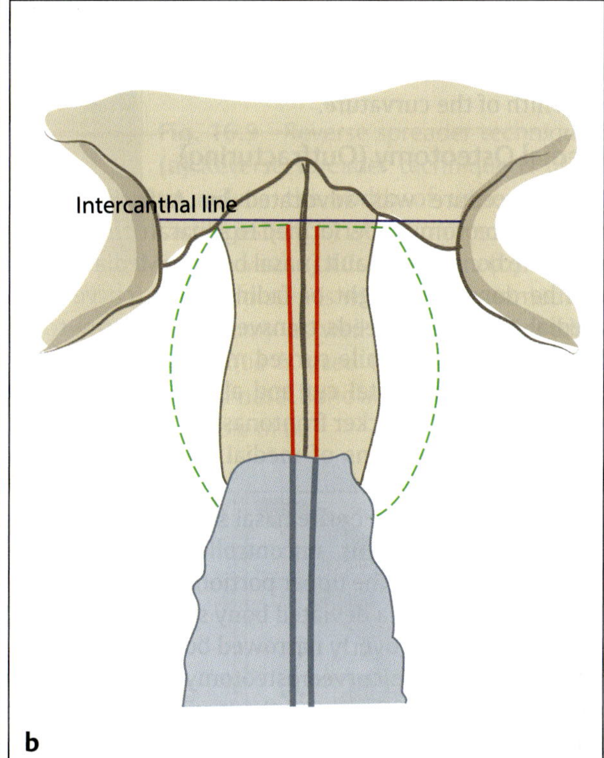

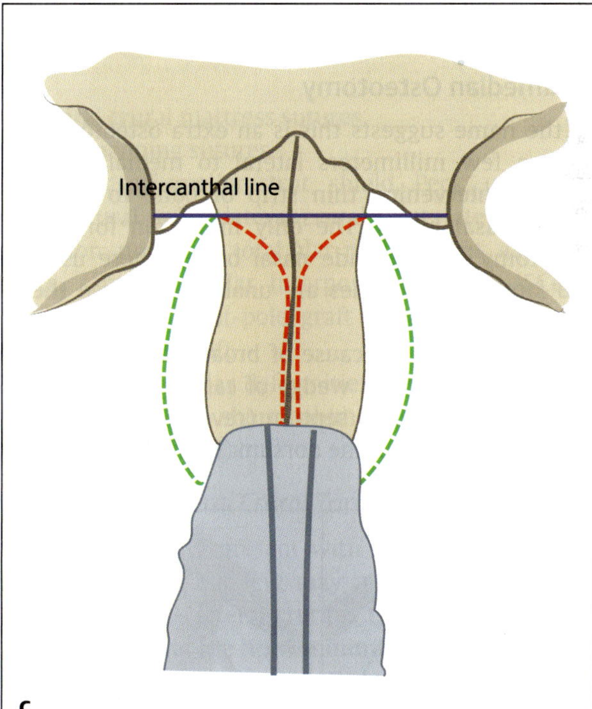

Fig. 16.7 Osteotomies. **(a)** Lateral, intermediate, transverse osteotomies and Webster triangle. **(b)** Medial straight osteotomy with transverse osteotomy to meet lateral cuts. **(c)** Medial oblique osteotomy does not need separate transverse osteotomy.

is made parallel to the lateral osteotomy somewhere along the midportion of the nasal sidewall. The exact placement of the osteotomy along the lateral nasal wall may vary depending on the anatomy of nasal bone and the surgical goals. In simple words, it is *double lateral osteotomy*.[27,28] It is occasionally indicated **(Fig. 16.7a)**.

Clinical Applications

- To narrow the extremely wide nose that has good height (bilateral osteotomy).
- To correct the deviated nose with one sidewall much longer than the other.
- To straighten a markedly convex/concave nasal bone.

Tip Suturing Technique

Irrespective of the number of surgeries, the suturing technique helps molding virgin or reconstructed LLCs. Nonabsorbable suture is preferred (5–0 polypropylene or nylon).

Intradomal or domal creation sutures: A horizontal mattress suture is taken through each dome. The knots are kept in between the two domes. Intradomal suture narrows and elevates the dome and accentuates the tip-defining points[37–39] **(Fig. 16.11a, b)**.

Interdomal or domal equalization suture is a single mattress/simple suture which traverses both the domes in their cephalic part. This suture approximates the cephalic corners of the narrowed domes to create a 30-degree angle of convergence to define the three-point projection of the tip. It keeps the cephalic ends converged and lower than the tip-defining points[37–39] **(Fig. 16.11a, b)**.

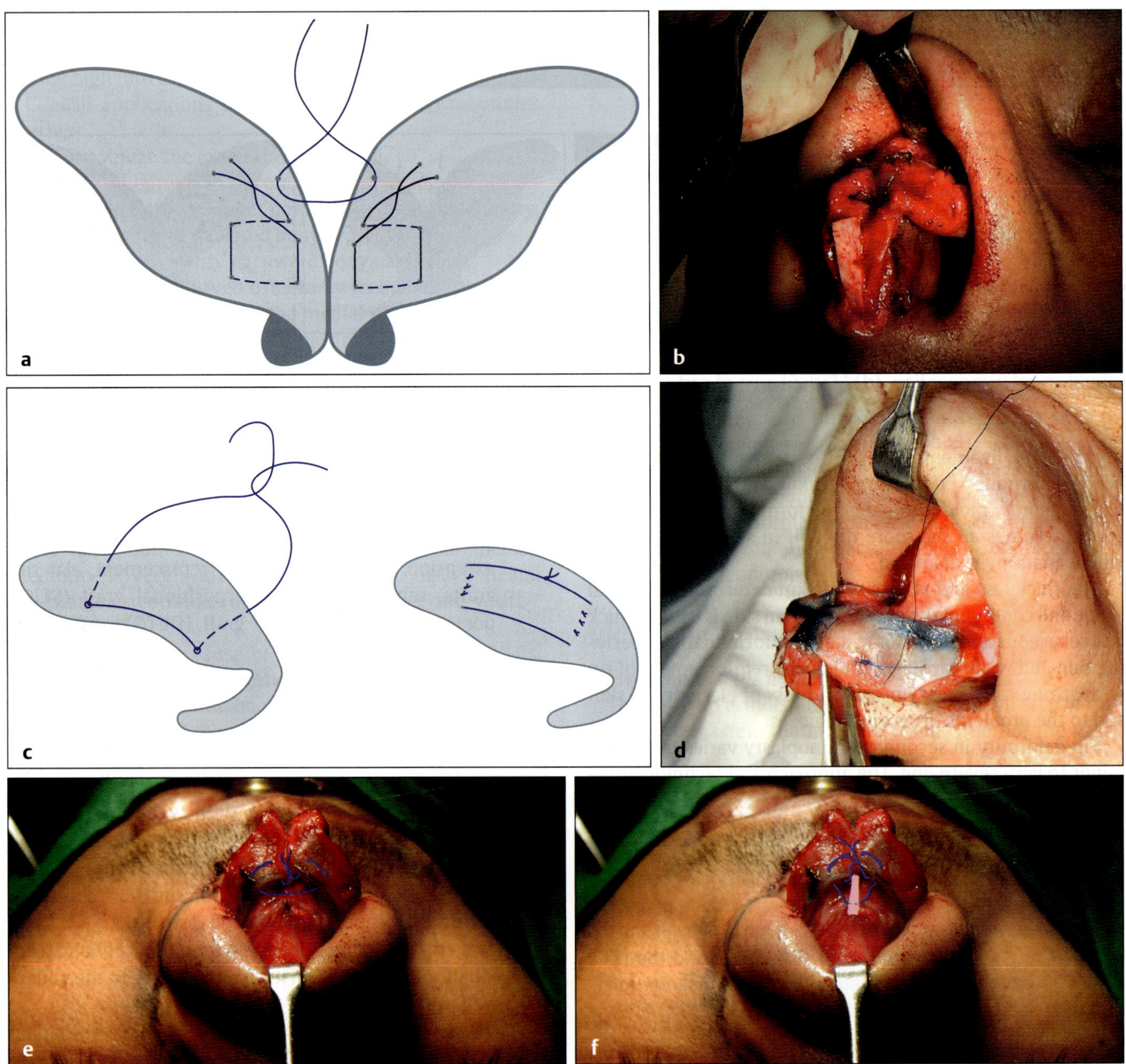

Fig. 16.11 Suturing technique. **(a)** Diagram showing dome creation and dome equalization sutures. **(b)** Intraoperative photograph showing dome creation and dome equalization sutures. **(c)** Diagram showing lateral crural mattress suture. **(d)** Intraoperative photograph showing lateral crural mattress suture. **(e)** Photograph showing alar-spanning suture. **(f)** Modified alar-spanning suture.

Lateral crural mattress suture is a horizontal mattress suture which converts convexity to concavity/flattening and vice versa. Suture is taken at the point of maximum convexity and is tightened gradually to achieve desired flattening of crura[40,41] **(Fig. 16.11c, d)**.

Alar-spanning suture is a horizontal mattress suture placed at the medial border of the lateral crus. It brings both crura medially and reduces the flaring[42] **(Fig. 16.11e)**.

The *modified alar-spanning suture* also takes a bite through the septum that is why along with reducing flare it also acts as tip suspension suture and prevents drooping of the tip[43] **(Fig. 16.11f)**.

Clinical applications: Boxy, bulbous, and ill-defined tips are corrected using cephalic trimming and various suturing techniques **(Fig. 16.12a, b)**.

Tip Grafts

Tip grafts are used very frequently in secondary rhinoplasties to improve tip projection. Indian noses have peculiar combination of thick skin and weak alar cartilages. Tip refinement by suturing technique is possible only in select cases. Most of the Indian noses and especially secondary noses need add-on grafts to build and refine the tip.

Commonly used tip grafts in secondary rhinoplasty are:

Columellar strut: It is an essential tip graft to support weak tip and must always be considered in open rhinoplasty[44,45] **(Fig. 16.13a–d)**.

- Floating: In closed approach when a piece of cartilage is put into the space between medial crurae. It is neither fixed to the medial crurae nor to the Anterior nasal spine (ANS).
- Fixed floating: In open rhinoplasty when strut is sutured to the medial crurae but it is not fixed to the ANS.
- Fixed: Fixed to the ANS.

Clinical application: Support and tip projection.

Shield graft (infralobular): First described by Sheen in 1975. He would prepare it by vomer or septal cartilage. It is sutured to the caudal margins of the medial and intermediate crura and usually rises over the existing domes by 1 or 2 mm or more as per need[44,46,47] **(Fig. 16.14a, b)**.

Clinical applications: Tip projection, tip refinement, and correction of tip asymmetry.

Peck graft (transdomal cap graft): The cap graft was first described by Peck to form and refine the tip. The cap graft is a small piece of cartilage that is precisely carved and placed across the domes of alar cartilages and secured with suture[48,49] **(Fig. 16.14c)**.

Clinical applications: To increase intrinsic projection of tip lobule and to camouflage irregularities and asymmetries of the domes.

Umbrella graft: It is an onlay tip graft which is a combination of columellar strut and Peck graft on top. It is constructed as a unit and fixed between the medial crurae.

Clinical application: Support and tip projection[50–52] **(Fig. 16.14d)**.

Lateral crural onlay grafts: These onlay grafts are used to correct contour deformities of an intact lateral crus. It strengthens and shapes the ala and may improve external valve function[53] **(Fig. 16.15a–c)**.

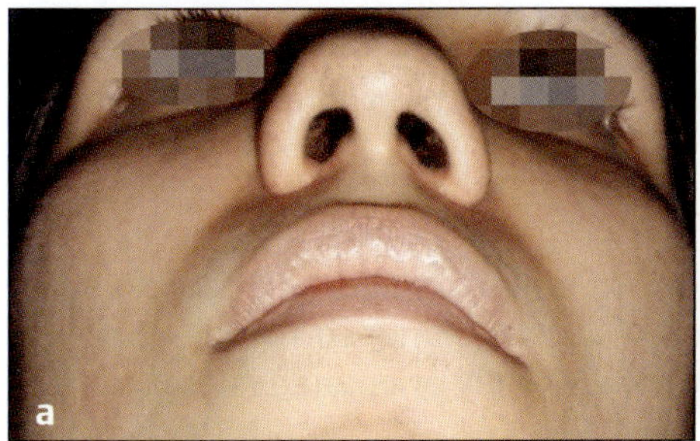

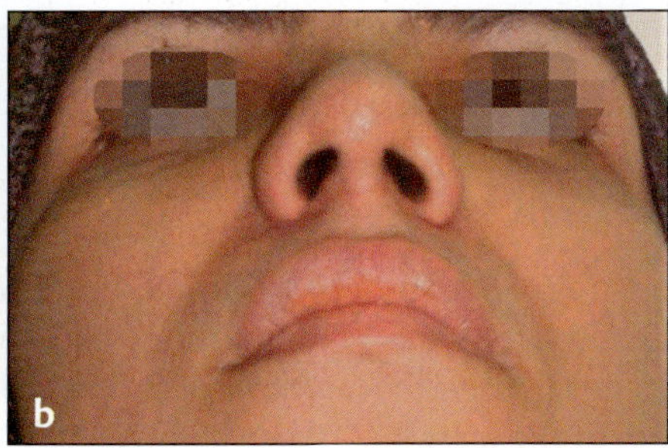

Fig. 16.12 Boxy tip. **(a)** Preoperative boxy tip deformity. **(b)** Correction of boxy tip deformity using cephalic trim, dome creation, dome equalization, and alar-spanning sutures.

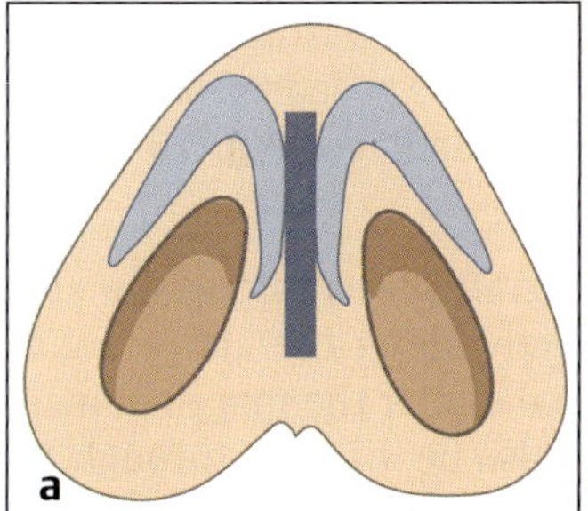

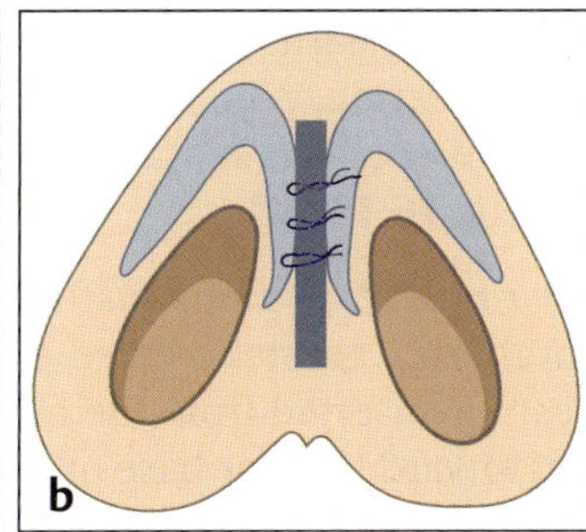

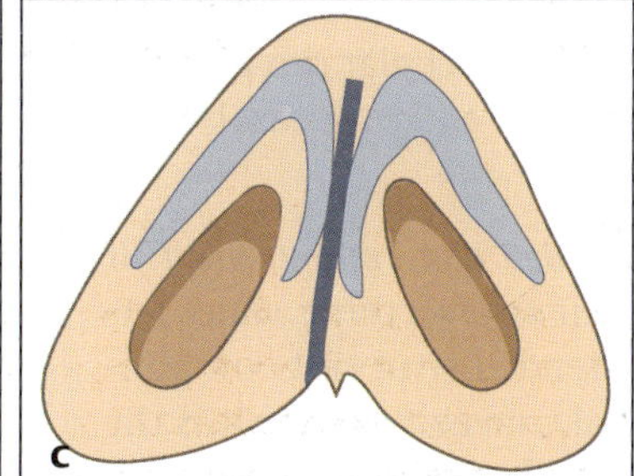

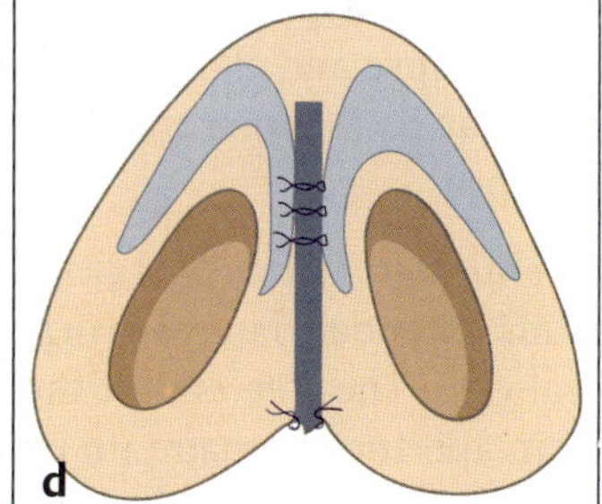

Fig. 16.13 Columellar strut: **(a)** Floating. **(b)** Fixed floating. **(c)** A long floating strut produces clicking sound and may cause deviation of tip when sits on one side of Anterior nasal spine (ANS). **(d)** Fixed columellar strut.

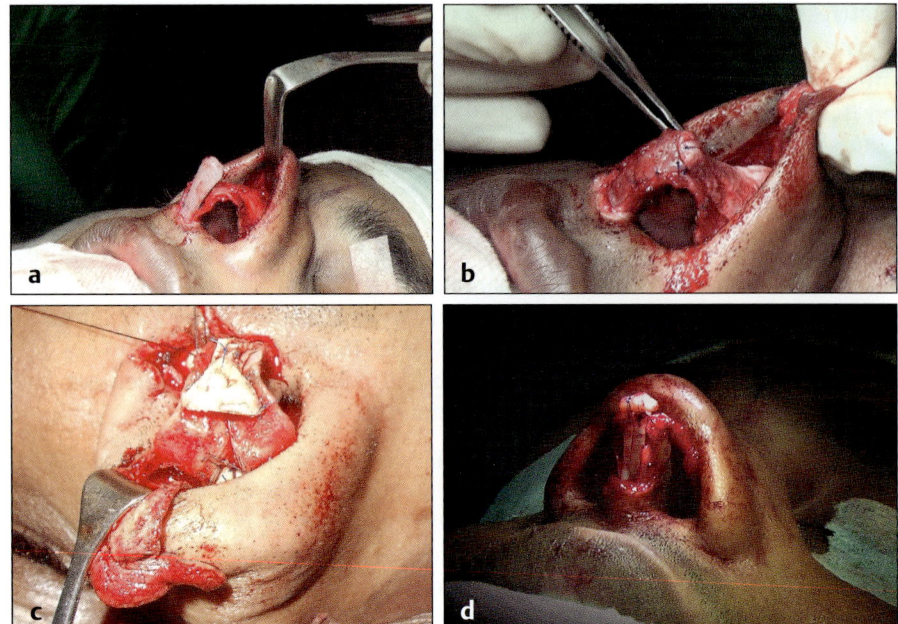

Fig. 16.14 Grafts for tip projection. **(a)** Shield graft. **(b)** Shield graft covered with fascia to avoid visibility of graft. **(c)** Peck (cap) graft. **(d)** Umbrella graft.

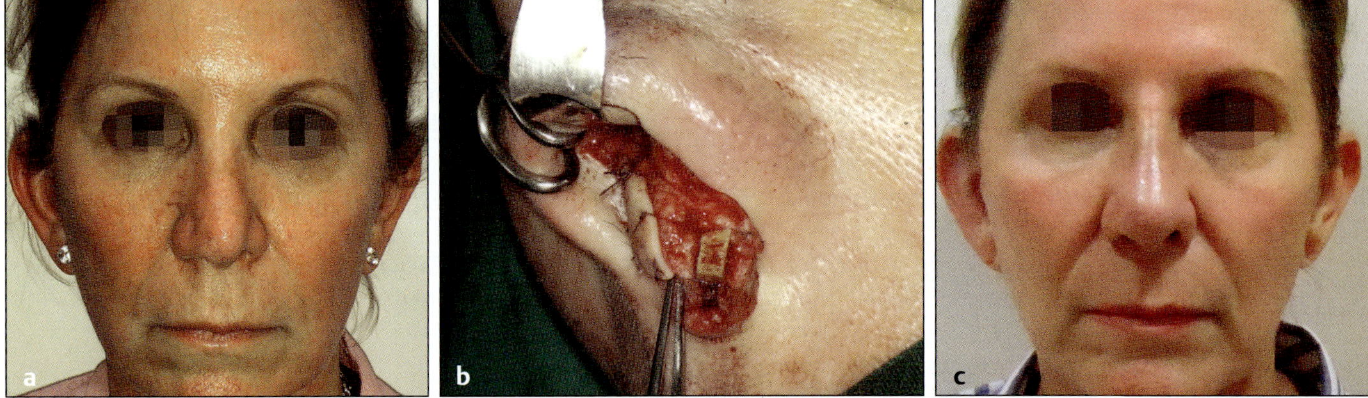

Fig. 16.15 Lateral crural onlay graft. **(a)** Photograph showing concave deformity of right ala. **(b)** Intraop photograph showing lateral crural onlay graft. **(c)** Postop result.

Lateral crural strut grafts:[44,46] These grafts are strips of autogenous cartilage that are sutured to the deep surface (ventral) of the lateral crura. Lateral crural strut graft is used to strengthen a weak ala and to reduce concavity of the lateral crura.[54,55]

Clinical applications: Prophylactically to prevent alar rim collapse and alar retraction; to correct alar rim collapse and alar retraction; and correction of external nasal valve collapse.

Lateral crural extension graft/extended alar contour graft: It is an extended lateral crural strut to overcome short lateral crus. The free end of the extended strut rests on pyriform aperture to maintain natural convexity of ala. It is the most commonly used graft in unilateral secondary cleft lip nose deformity to correct buckling of ala on cleft side[56] **(Fig. 16.16a–c)**.

Clinical applications: Secondary short and concave lateral crura; correction of alar notching; correction of parenthesis deformity: overly vertically orientated lateral crura of LLC.

Partial or total LLC reconstruction: Severe damage to the LLCs during earlier surgery may demand partial or total tip reconstruction. Whole set of LLCs can be prepared using thin strips of conchal, septal, or costal cartilage (**Fig. 16.17a–d and Fig. 16.18a–f**).

Alar rim graft is a nonanatomic graft placed along the alar margin in a tunnel created directly along the alar margin. It can be inserted from the medial end of the marginal incision toward the alar base or can also be inserted through an external incision taken on vestibular alar margin.[57,58]

Clinical applications: Corrects alar rim deformities (mild alar retraction); improves nasal base contour; additional

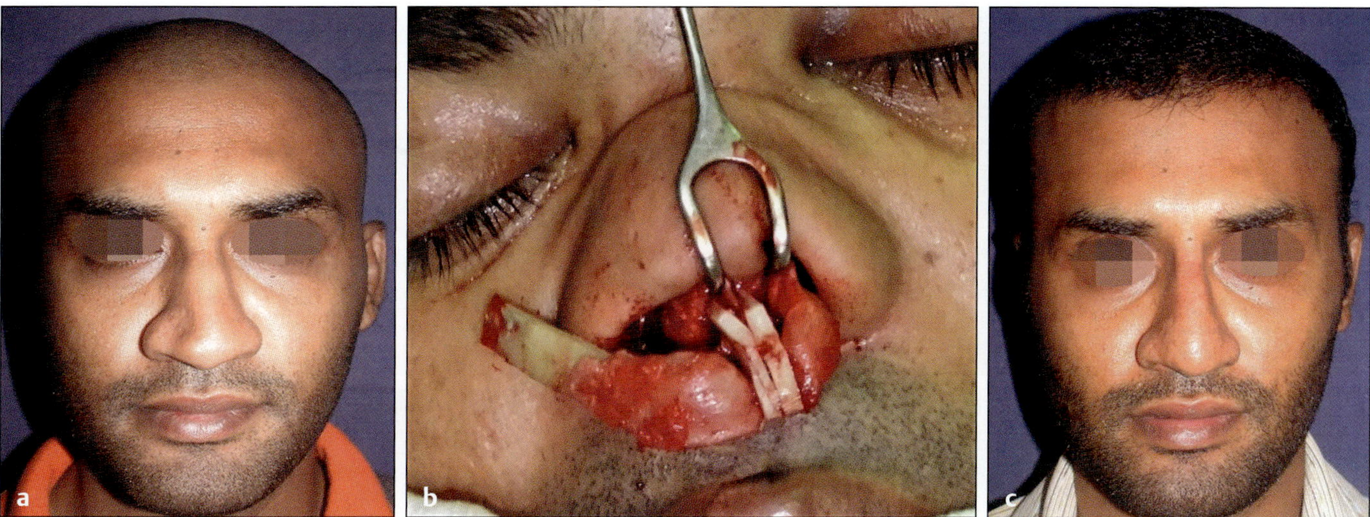

Fig. 16.16 Lateral crural extension graft. **(a)** Photograph showing buckling of right ala. **(b)** Intraoperative photograph showing strengthening and lengthening of shortened right ala with lateral crural extension graft. **(c)** Correction of concavity and buckling of right ala.

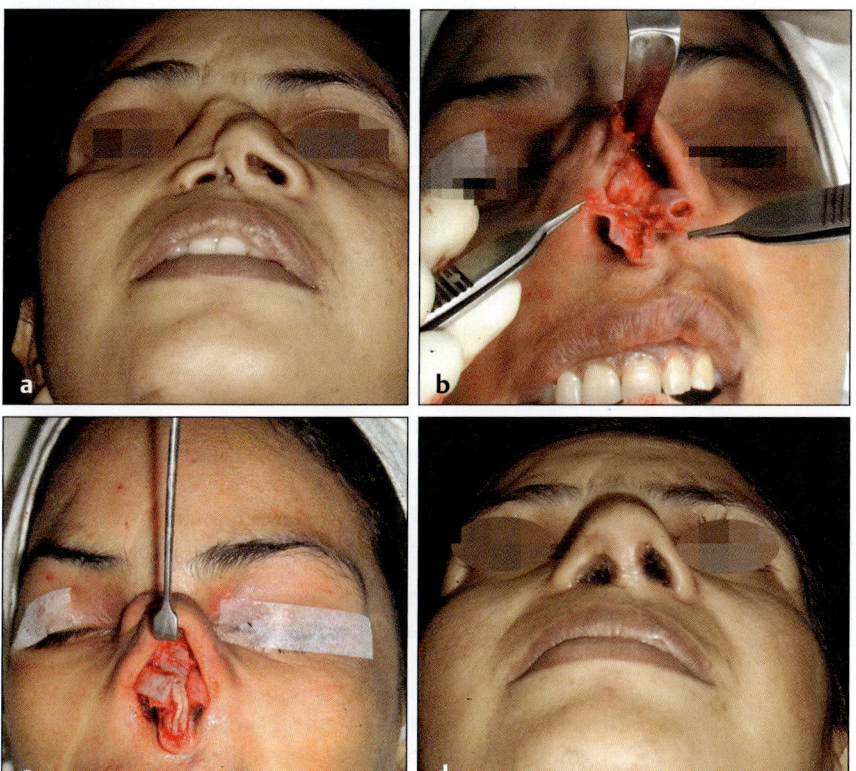

Fig. 16.17 Partial lower lateral cartilage (LLC) (lateral crus) reconstruction. **(a)** Preoperative deformity of ala. **(b)** Intraoperative photograph showing loss of right lateral crus. **(c)** Reconstruction of lateral crus with thin costal cartilage graft. **(d)** Postoperative photograph showing correction of deformity.

support to the external nasal valve; and lateral transitional camouflage for shield grafts.

Septocolumellar interpositional grafts (SCIG) are placed between the septum and ULCs and are similar to long spreader grafts. A columellar strut is sutured to the SCIGs. The length of the septocolumellar interposition graft may be varied to control tip rotation[59] (**Fig. 16.19**).

Clinical applications: To lengthen the short nose and to control inferior tip rotation and resultant tip projection.

Dorsocolumellar "tent-pole" graft (DCTG) works similar to SCIG, but here, there is no need to dissect or separate ULCs from septum to fix the grafts. This graft is akin to fixing a bamboo of a tent in position. A piece of cartilage is fixed to columellar strut in a desired position and then the best

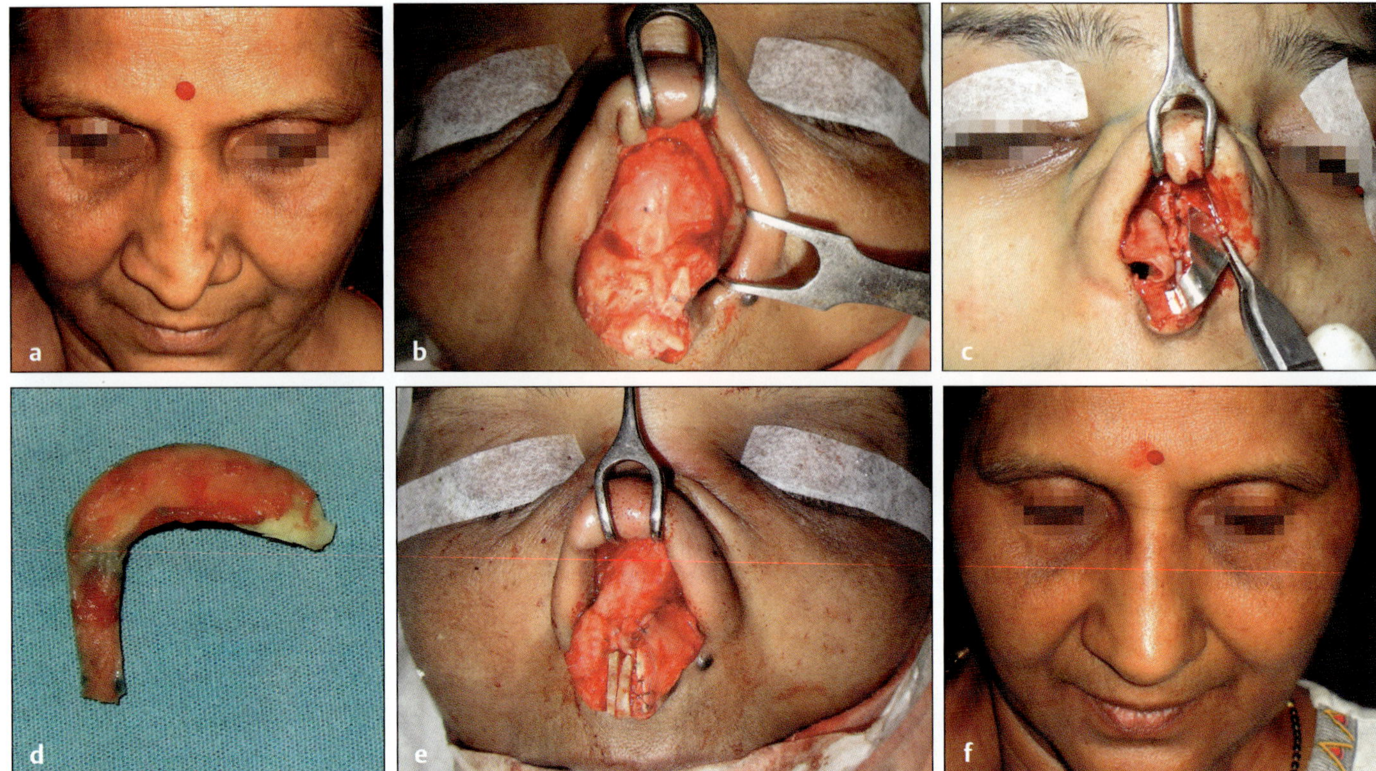

Fig. 16.18 Complete lower lateral cartilage (LLC) reconstruction. **(a)** Preoperative photograph showing notching of left ala. **(b)** Intraoperative photograph showing loss of one side of dome. **(c)** Pattern designed on aluminum foil by contralateral cartilage. **(d)** Designed conchal cartilage. **(e)** Dome reconstructed. **(f)** Postoperative photograph showing correction of deformity.

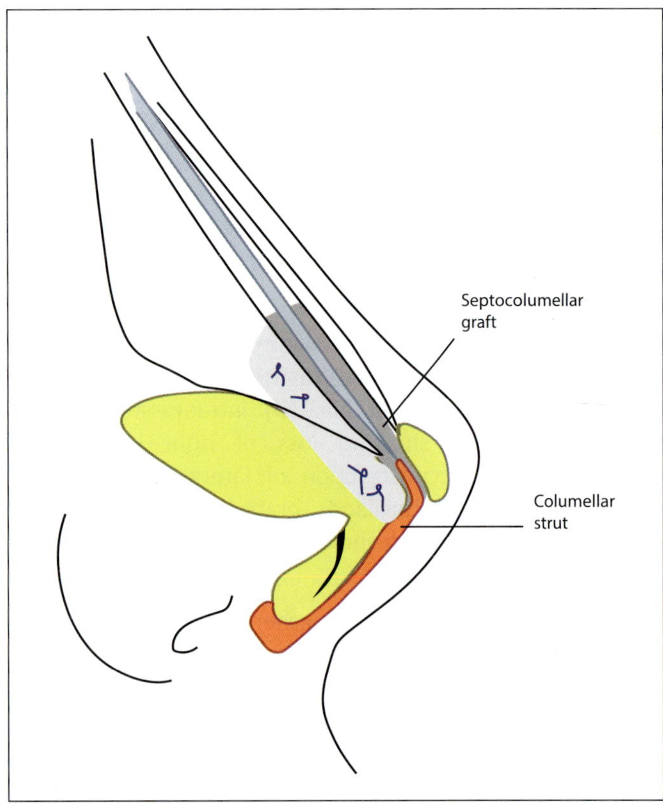

Fig. 16.19 Septocolumellar interpositional graft (SCIG).

possible angle is chosen by fixing the posterior end of graft temporarily with a needle to supratip cartilaginous dorsum. Once sure of the angle, the graft is sutured to the dorsum[60] (**Fig. 16.20a–d**).

Clinical applications: Author uses this graft in difficult secondary noses where maintaining the position of tip is difficult and dissection of caudal septum is not feasible. Its application includes: To set a nasolabial/columellar-lip angle of choice; to stabilize long columellar strut (does not allow the tip to fall back); and to lengthen the short nose.

Caudal septal extension graft: The graft is usually harvested from septal cartilage and is sutured to the caudal margin of the nasal septum. It is then secured between the medial crura by tongue-in-groove technique[61,62] (**Fig. 16.21a–c**).

Clinical applications: To correct a retracted columella; to Lengthen a short nose; and correction of an overrotated tip (closing the nasolabial angle/converting an obtuse angle into acute one). "Tongue-in-groove" method can also be used where septum is long enough and nose needs subtle corrections for[63,64] (**Fig. 16.22a–d**):

- Opening up the nasolabial angle (converting an acute angle into an obtuse one).
- Change in tip rotation or projection (correction of plunging tip).
- Mild shortening of nose.
- Reduction of columellar show.

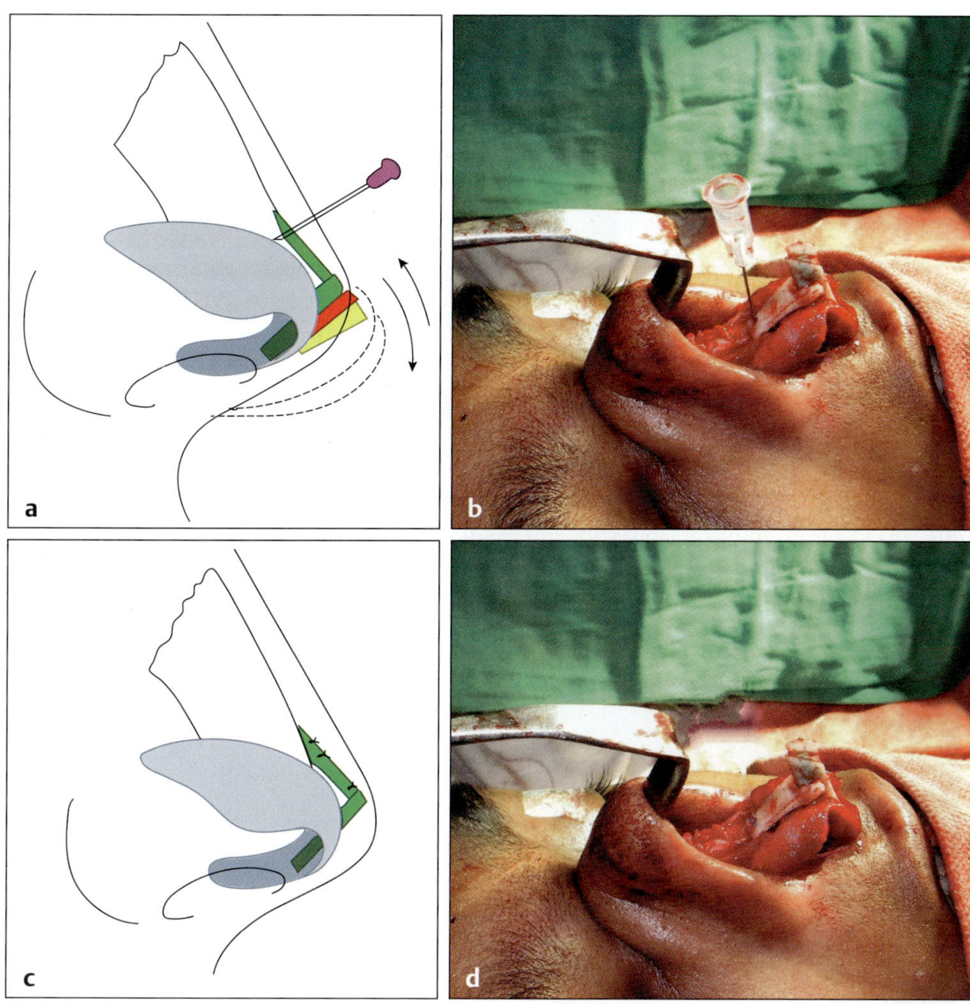

Fig. 16.20 Dorsocolumellar Tentpole graft (DCTG). **(a)** Temporary fixation of dorsal graft with needle while adjusting the nasolabial angle of choice. **(b)** Intraoperative photograph showing temporary fixation. **(c)** Diagrammatic representation of fixation of dorsal graft with permanent sutures. **(d)** Intraop photograph with permanent sutures.

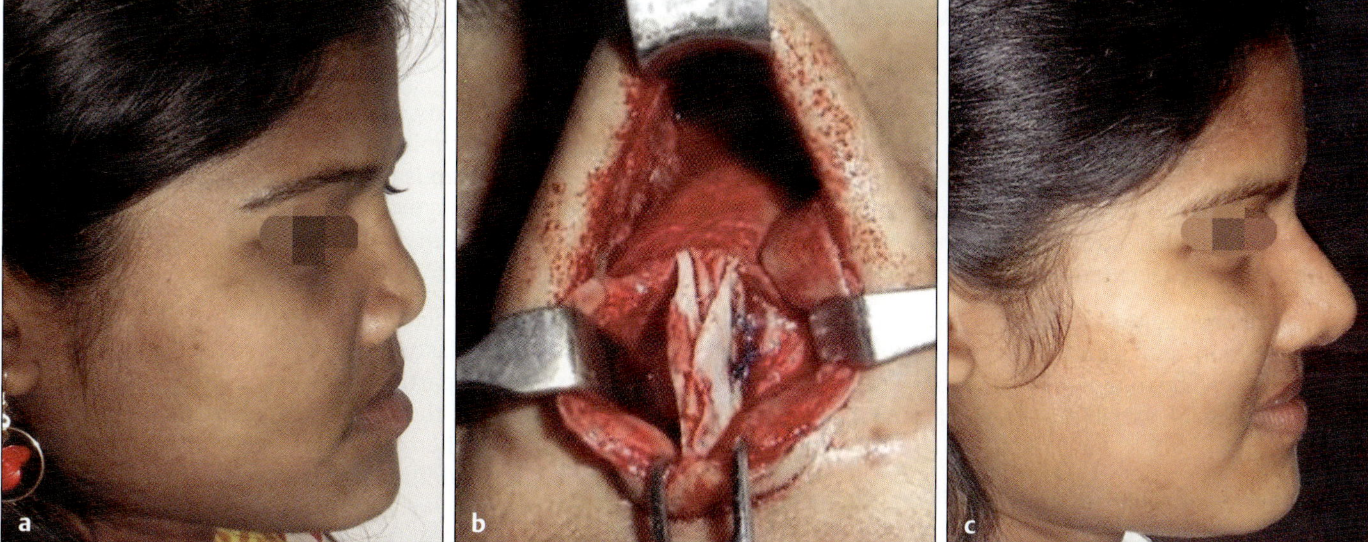

Fig. 16.21 Septal extension graft. **(a)** Short nose with obtuse nasolabial angle. **(b)** Intraoperative picture showing bilateral thin costal cartilage grafts as caudal septal extension. **(c)** Postoperative result showing increased nasal length and corrected nasolabial angle.

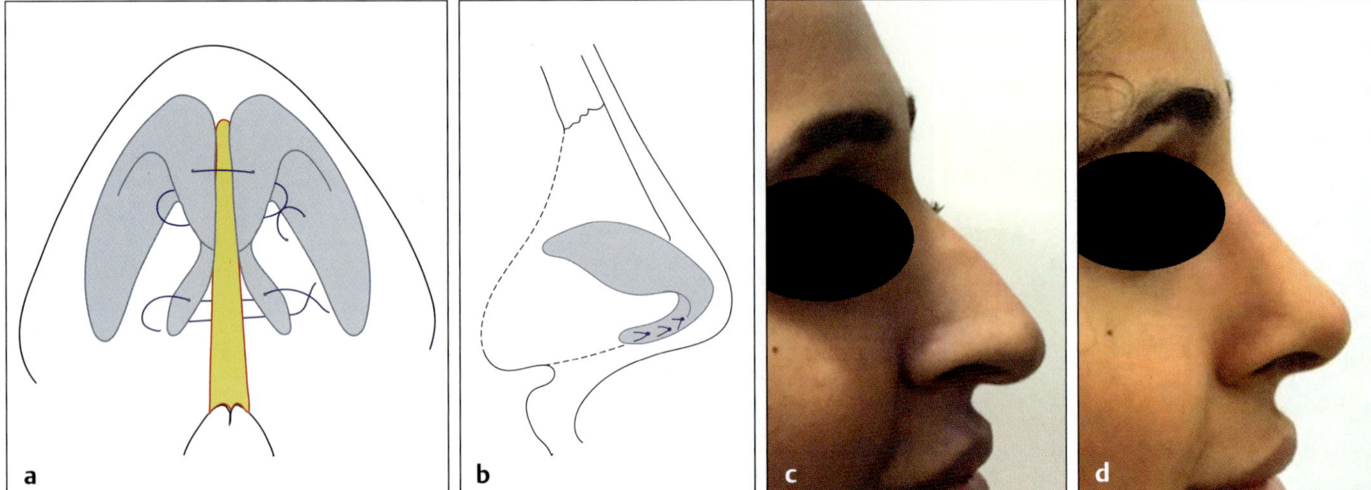

Fig. 16.22 Tongue-in-groove technique. **(a)** Diagram in basal view showing medial crura being sutured to caudal septum. **(b)** Diagram in lateral view showing medial crura sutured to caudal septum. **(c)** Drooping tip with acute nasolabial angle (closed angle). **(d)** Good tip projection and opening up of nasolabial angle using tongue-in-groove technique.

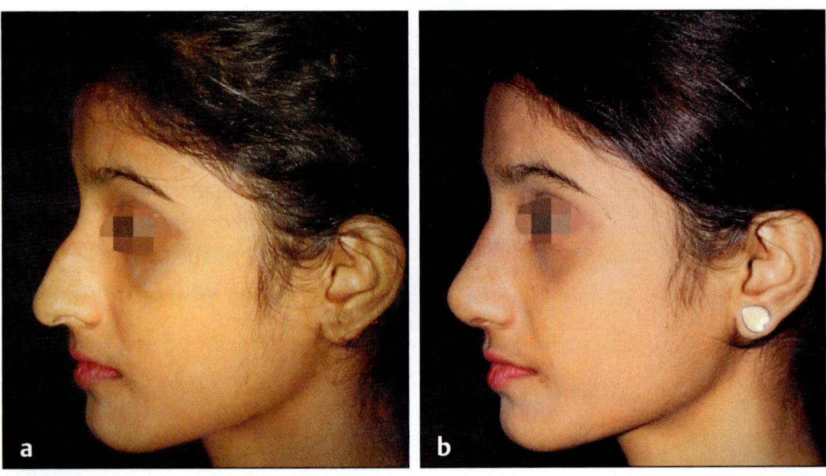

Fig. 16.23 Retracted columella. **(a)** Preoperative photograph showing retracted columella. **(b)** Corrected deformity with caudal septal modification.

Addressing Secondary Deformities of Columella

Retracted columella: Mildly retracted columella can be corrected by columellar strut graft. More severe cases may require caudal septal extension graft[65,66] **(Fig. 16.23a, b)**.

Hanging columella: Most often an ellipse of membranous septal resection and suturing is enough, moderate cases can be corrected by tongue-in-groove, but severe cases may need trimming of variable amount of caudal septum[66–68] **(Fig. 16.24a, b)**.

Short columella without previous incision: Lengthening of columella is done by adding skin from lip[69] **(Fig. 16.25a, b)**.

Short columella with previous midcolumellar incision: This is a difficult situation as blood supply of skin inferior to the incision is uncertain and lengthening of columella will surely lead to necrosis, which will be a catastrophe. Author uses flap-delay technique here. The delay is done under local anesthesia. Flap is elevated from marked area up to 2 mm beyond previous incision and incision is closed. After a week, once sure of survival of the extra skin, definitive rhinoplasty is done **(Fig. 16.26a–c)**.

Partial or complete loss of columella: This is a perplexing problem for rhinoplasty surgeon. A severe aesthetic deformity results from its partial or complete loss. Though the size of skin flap needed to reconstruct columella is really small (1–1.5 cm), it is a herculean feat to reconstitute the same without inflicting additional scars on face. Patient who seeks aesthetic correction of secondary deformity of columella never accepts a plan of reconstructing it either with nasolabial or forehead flap. The myriad surgical options available for columella reconstruction include tube pedicle flaps, upper lip flaps, forehead flap, alar margin flaps, internal

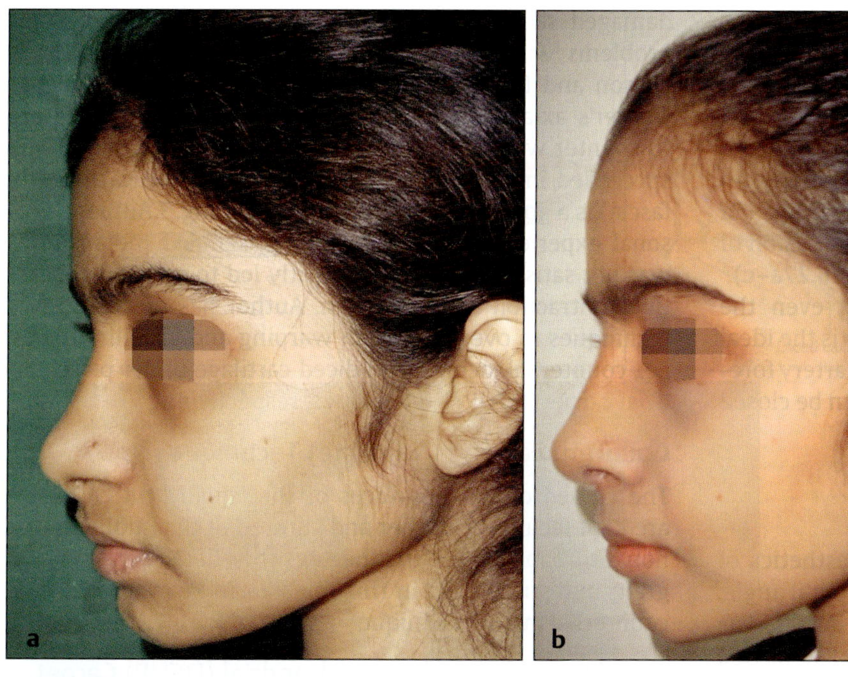

Fig. 16.24 Hanging columella. **(a)** Photograph showing hanging columella. **(b)** Correction of deformity using tongue-in-groove technique by suturing medial crura to caudal septum.

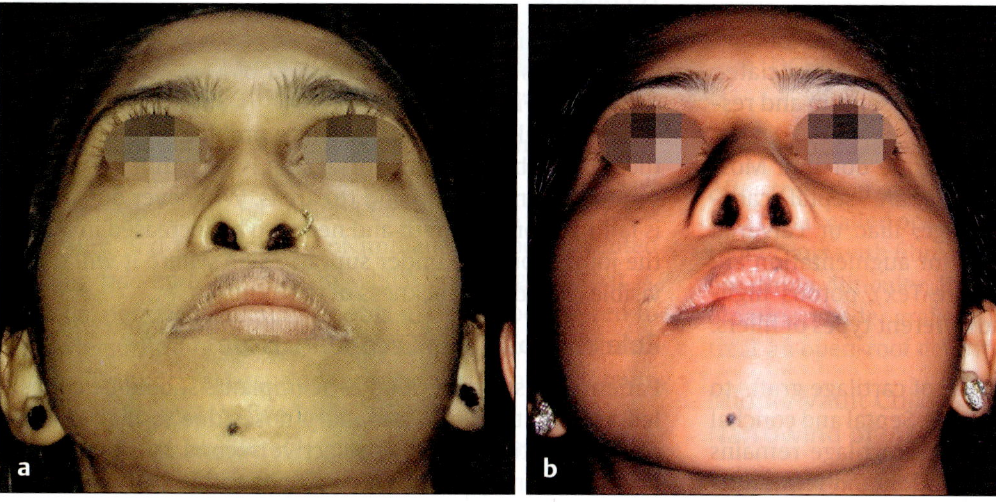

Fig. 16.25 Primary short columella. **(a)** Short columella. **(b)** Lengthening of primary short columella using lip skin.

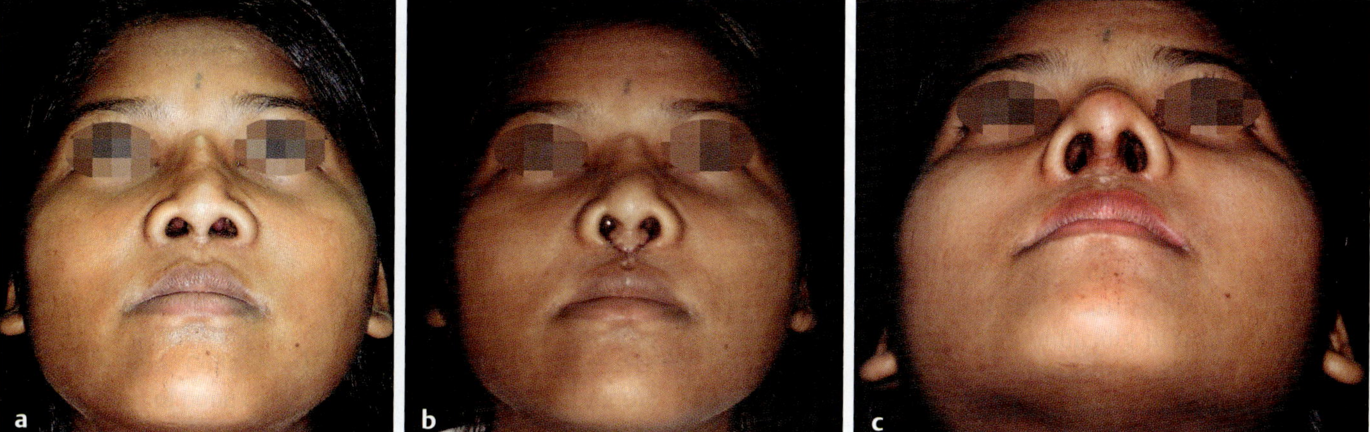

Fig. 16.26 Secondary short columella having midcolumellar scar. **(a)** Photograph showing midcolumellar incision. **(b)** Delay of flap. **(c)** Postoperative photograph showing lengthened columella using the delayed upper lip flap.

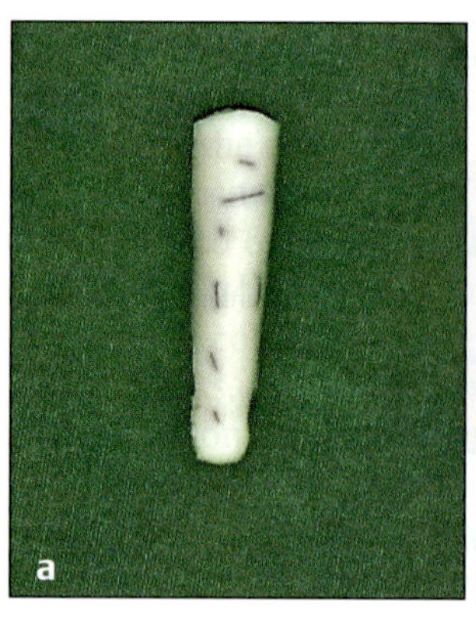
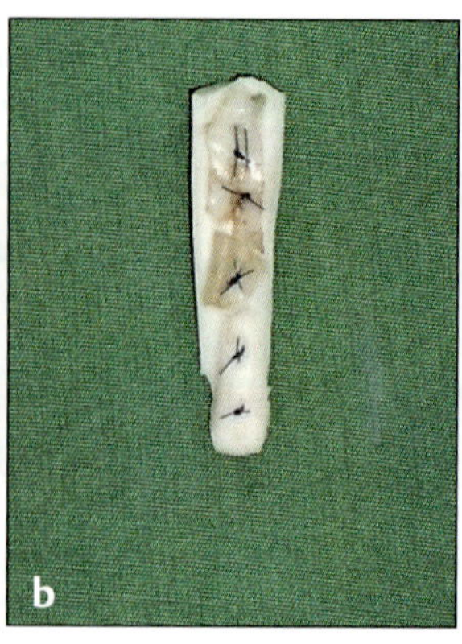
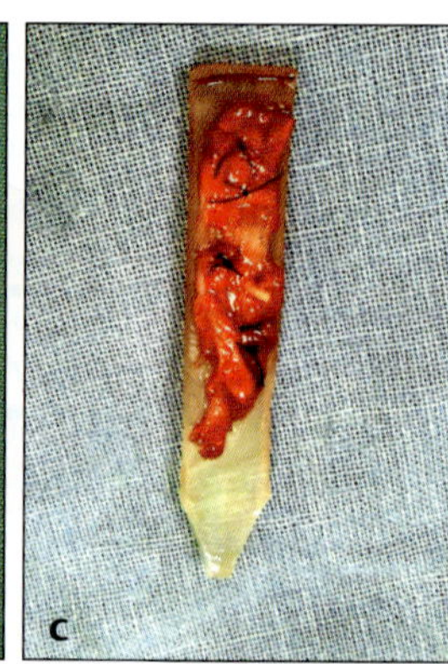

Fig. 15.29 Ride-on technique. **(a)** Dorsal surface of implant with sutures. **(b)** Ventral surface showing cartilage graft and knots of permanent sutures. **(c)** Ventral surface showing perichondrial graft and knots of permanent sutures.

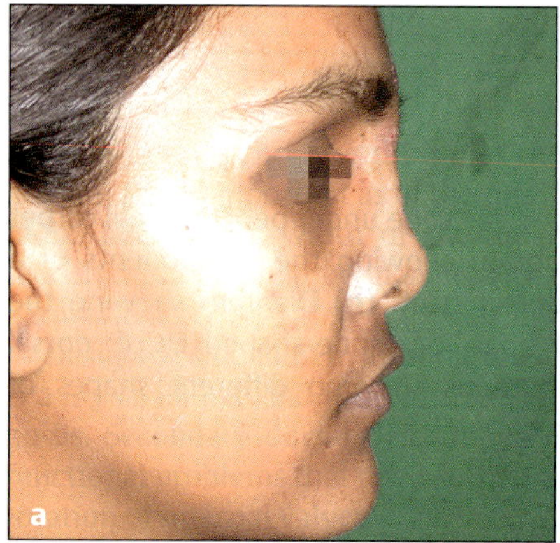
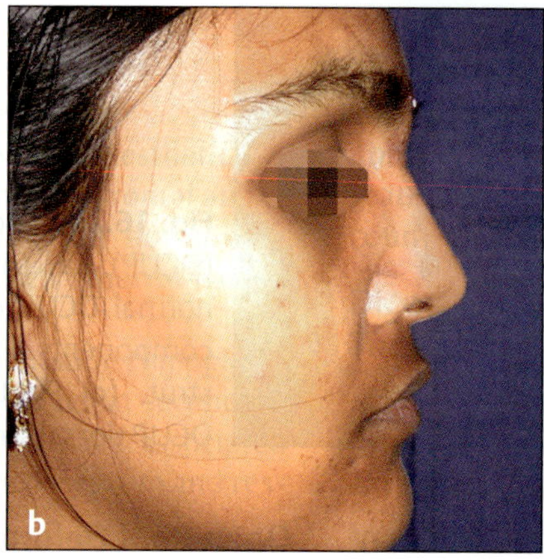

Fig. 16.30 Obliteration of nasofrontal angle. **(a)** Photograph showing the obliteration of nasofrontal angle. **(b)** Secondary correction of deformity by removal of graft and augmentation with precisely carved diced cartilage under perichondrial carpet (DCUP) strut.

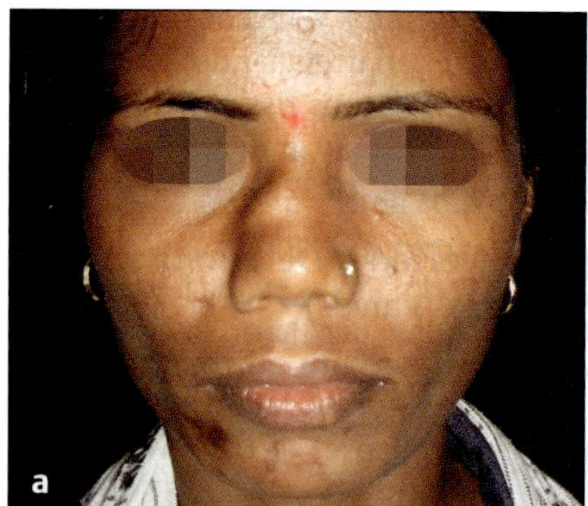
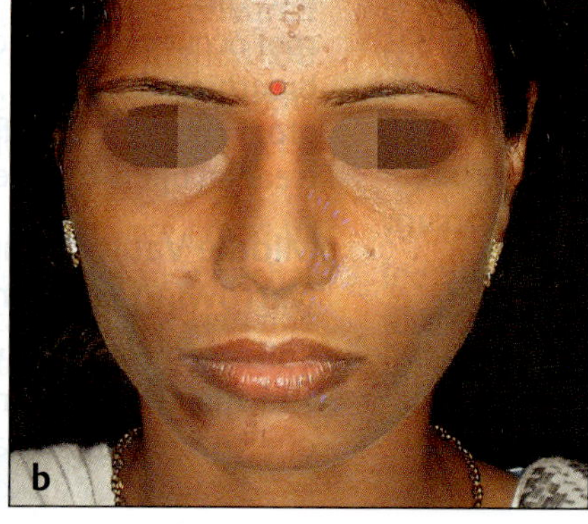

Fig. 16.31 Lateral wall deformity. **(a)** Photograph showing irregular dorsum and right lateral wall deformity. **(b)** Correction done with bilateral osteotomy, lateral wall camouflage grafts, and diced cartilage under perichondrial carpet (DCUP) strut.

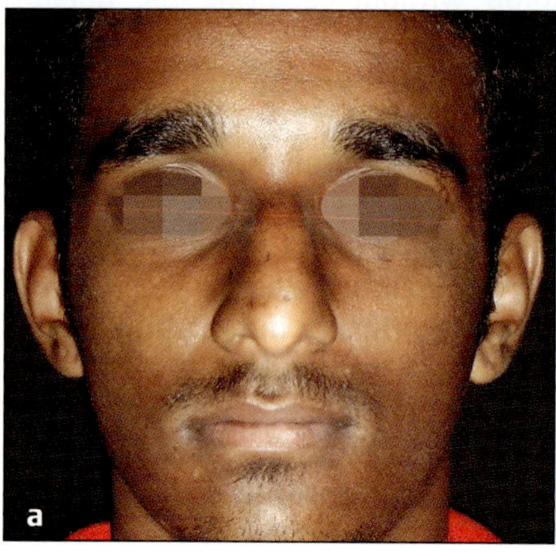
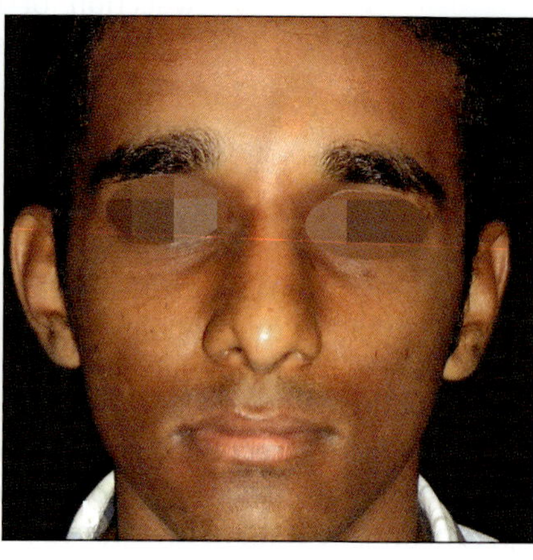

Fig. 16.32 Open-roof deformity. **(a)** Photograph showing flat and irregular dorsum. **(b)** Correction done with bilateral spreader grafts.

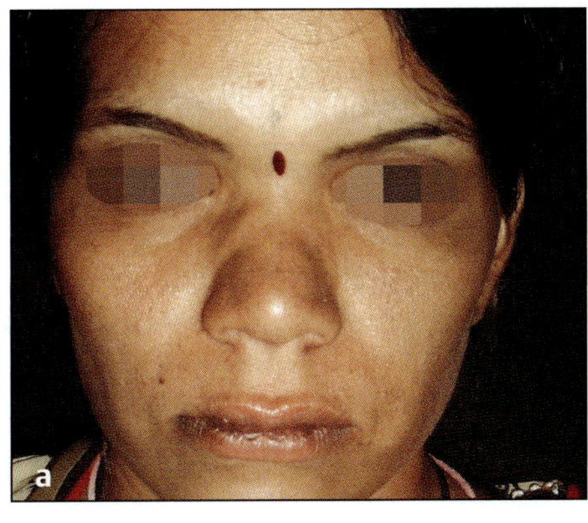

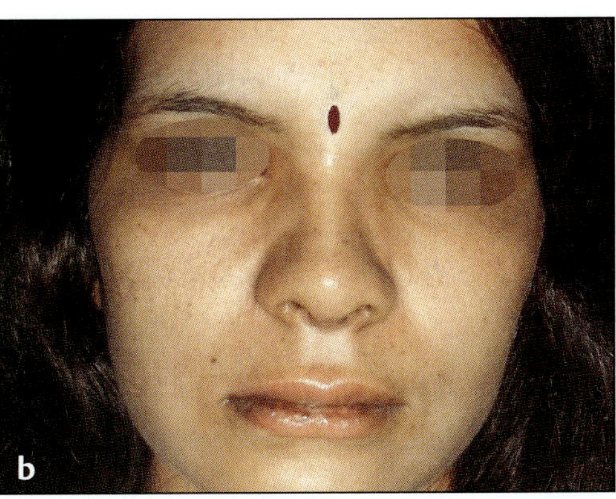

Fig. 16.33 Inverted-V deformity. **(a)** Photograph showing inverted-V deformity. **(b)** Correction done with bilateral osteotomy, spreader grafts, and dorsal camouflage graft.

Spreader Grafts

Sheen, Constantian, and Clardy established the importance of preserving the internal valve area and reconstructing the middle one-third of the nose by spreader grafts[81–83] **(Fig. 16.4c)**.

Preparation

Spreader grafts can be prepared using septal or costal cartilages or bony septum. The size and thickness of grafts may vary according to the need of a given patient. Usual dimensions range from:

- Length: 20 to 35 mm.
- Width/height: 3 to 6 mm.
- Thickness: 2 to 3 mm.

Functions

Spreader grafts correct the dorsal asymmetry and maintain the width. They prevent an inverted-V deformity and maintain straight and strong middle vault by splinting a weak or deviated nasal septum. Aesthetically they maintain the aesthetic dorsal lines. And functionally they spread the ULCs outward, restoring the open angle of the internal valve.

Clinical Applications

- To reconstruct open roof following resection of dorsal hump.
- To correct collapsed middle vault due to inverted-V deformity.
- To restore internal nasal valves in patients with no external deformity but difficulty in breathing due to narrowing of the valves.
- Whenever there is a need to separate the ULCs from septum.
- To splint/buttress a high, dorsally deviated, crooked septum in crooked noses.
- To increase the width of the dorsum without augmentation of dorsum.
- To recreate the dorsal aesthetic lines.

Problems

If the graft is not fixed properly, the graft may displace causing dorsal irregularity. If not designed well, it may cause widening of the dorsum.

Extended Spreader Grafts

Spreader grafts are usually kept up to or short of septal angle, but if the lengthening of the nose is desired or columellar strut needs rigid support, the caudal ends of the grafts are extended past the septal angle.[84]

Spreader Flaps

This has very little role in secondary procedures because of scarring, difficulty in dissection, and nonavailability of adequate native tissue. This is also termed as "autospreader" or "turnover flap." The indication of spreader flap is during reduction of the hump. In this technique after desired reduction of nasal septum, the medial edge of the ULCs is folded inside on itself bilaterally and sutured to the septum.[85–88]

Alar Base Modification

Deformities of alar base are a common finding in secondary rhinoplasty. It may be a primary deformity which was not addressed or might have developed as a secondary deformity, (e.g., excessive alar flaring developed after reduction of tip projection). Preoperative asymmetry in the alar base region or nostrils must be identified, discussed with the patient, and counseled regarding postoperative scar. The deformities encountered are alar flaring, increased interalar distance, wide nostril, or asymmetry of ala.

Alar flaring is defined as the lateral aspect of the ala extending significantly beyond the alar-facial groove (convex curve of the ala as seen on frontal and basal views).[89–93]

Interalar width is the distance between the alar creases or distance from columellar midline to alar crease.[89–93] Sheen modified alar base excision and divided on the basis of their objectives.[94]

- *Type I*: Alar wedge excision decreases alar flare seen on frontal view, but true interalar width remains unaffected as seen on a basal view.
- *Type II*: Combined alar base and nostril sill excision decreases alar flare and nostril size.
- *Type III:* Only sill excision reduces nostril size.
- *Type IV*: Combined alar base nostril sill and nostril floor excision decreases alar flare, nostril size, and interalar width.

Surgical correction is indicated when there is excessive interalar width, and there is enlarged nostril and has a horizontal axis. This is performed either by direct sill and/or floor excision. Alternatively, more so in secondary cases, a modified alar cinch is done using a de-epithelialized lateral flap using nostril sill-and-floor segment which is advanced medially to the caudal septum and sutured. Both the techniques decrease the interalar width effectively.[94]

Triangular Flap and Skin-Only Excision Technique

This technique is a modification in surgical technique of combined alar wedge and sill excision. No through-and-through cut is made; only skin is excised from the marked area. The forces responsible to maintain the convexity and inward rotation of ala lie in fibrofatty tissue of ala and the lining of nose. Cutting the ala through-and-through damages these forces and when it is sutured back it becomes unnaturally straight. Skin-only excision and a triangular flap on alar rim helps in maintaining normal curvature of ala and normal alar facial groove, preserves blood supply, prevents scarring and chances of nostril stenosis, and saves time and energy in suturing inside the nose[95] **(Fig. 16.34a–j)**.

Overzealous postoperative massage is likely to widen the scar at the alar base and a well-hidden scar is likely to become prominent. Hence author prohibits massage of alar crease scar[95] **(Fig. 16.34k)**.

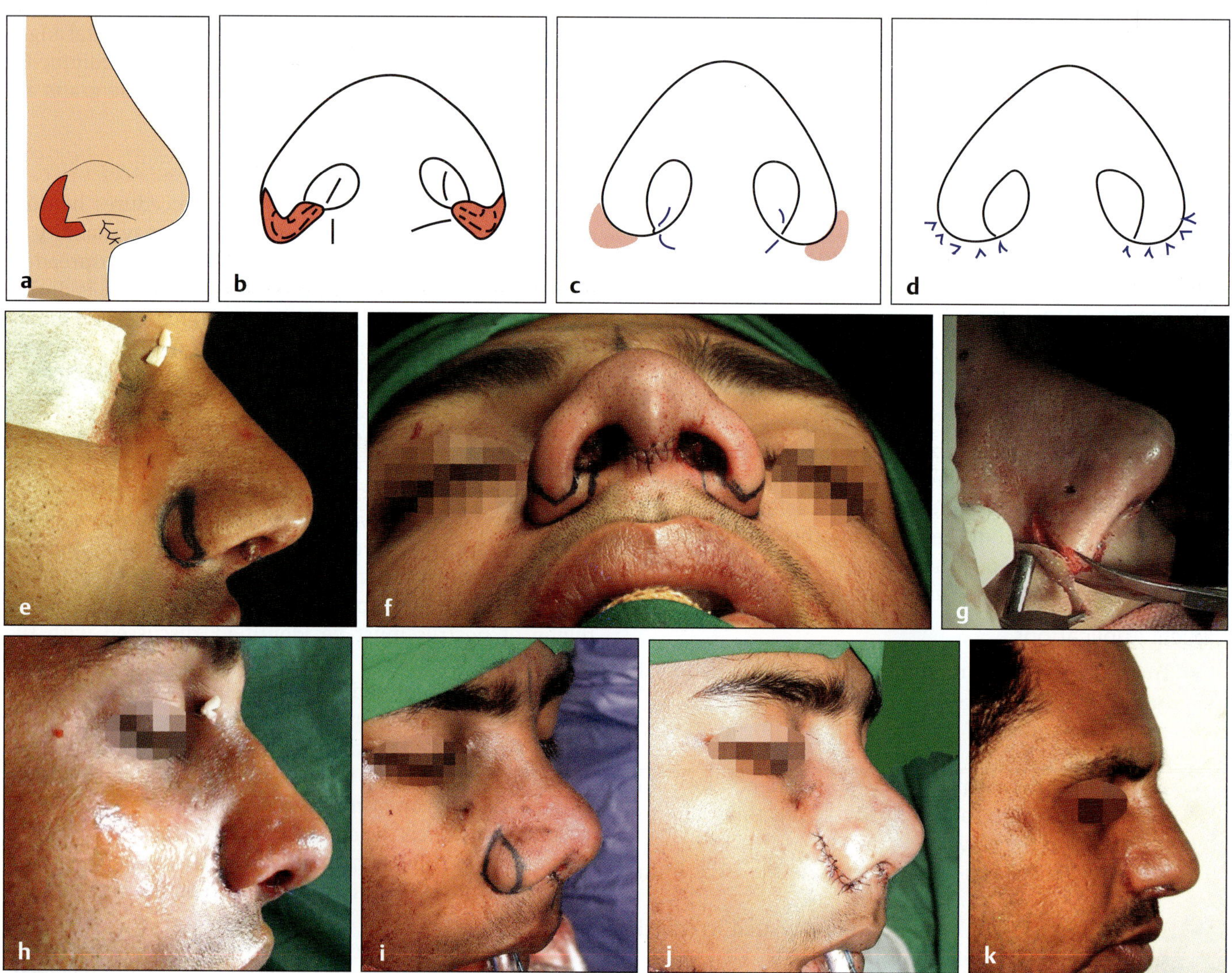

Fig. 16.34 Alar base modification. **(a)** Lateral view showing concavoconvex excision markings. **(b)** Basal view showing triangular alar rim flap and excision marking limited to nasal sill. **(c)** Basal view showing raw areas over alar base after medialization of triangular flaps into inverted-V incision in nasal sill. **(d)** Complete closure. **(e)** Markings on patient, lateral view. **(f)** Markings on basal view. **(g)** Photograph showing only skin excision. **(h)** Creation of a natural alar facial groove after concavoconvex (semilunar) skin excision. **(i)** Photograph showing a biconvex, elliptical skin markings. **(j)** An unnatural straight alar facial groove after biconvex, elliptical skin excision. **(k)** A widened scar after overzealous massage.

Final Steps of the Procedure

After completing the surgery the skin flap is put back to its normal place and all the details are checked several times. Photos are taken in profile, basal, and frontal views to see any minor fault. When the surgeon is sure that the desired result is achieved, closure is done.

Closure of incisions: The tissues in secondary surgery have already been traumatized and scarred. Any further mishandling will certainly cause problems. The columella must always be handled with the utmost gentleness. Columellar incision is closed with 6–0 prolene or nylon suture. Infracartilaginous incisions are closed with 4–0 or 5–0 vicryl.

Nasal packing: To avoid compromising the blood supply of already frail septal mucoperichondrial flaps, author avoids taking mattress sutures for preventing septal hematoma in secondary noses where extensive dissection was done. Light nasal packing is done using ribbon gauze soaked in sterile liquid paraffin or nicely smeared with Neosporin ointment. Packs are removed after 48 hours.

Taping: Nose is then taped with half-inch micropore tapes. Two to three horizontal strips are applied on dorsal skin from radix to supratip and then two vertical tapes on sides and pinched together over tip. These tapes help draping the skin well and play a very important role in healing of tissues (**Fig. 16.35a, b**).

Splint: A cone-shaped, 8- to 10-layered Plaster of Paris splint is prepared. Eyes are covered by applying micropore tape from medial to lateral canthus. Extra strips of tapes are applied over the forehead to avoid direct contact of splint to the skin. Splint should not cover the tip and this end of the splint should be folded up to create a small space between splint and supratip skin to avoid friction injury and inadvertent scarring to numb supratip region (**Fig. 16.35b–d**).

Splint is usually kept for 1week to 10 days when only dorsal augmentation is done, and for 2 weeks in cases where osteotomies are performed. More than 2 weeks of splintage is needed in a difficult crooked or secondary nose where extensive osseocartilagenous manipulations are done, or when DCF is used for dorsal augmentation.

Implant-Related Secondary Deformities

- Mobile implant.
- Deviation.
- Displacement.
- Infection.
- Thinning of skin, scarring.
- Capsular contracture and shortening of nose.
- Tip/dorsal skin/mucosal necrosis and exposure of implant.

Single most important problem with silicone implant is its mobility, which leads to almost all complications related to it. Using an L-implant over the tip and columella adds in to the problems. The capsular contracture leads to shortening of nose and extrusion of implant.[96] Secondary noses with complications of implants need implant removal and further management needs to be decided.

Explantation of Silicone Implants and Reaugmentation with Autografts

Explantation of silicone implants is a simple task but when to reaugment remains a dilemma specially when implant is exposed and infected. Augmenting the dorsum by directly putting autograft strut into the capsular tunnel leads to a mobile strut and complications related to capsular contracture. One should not try to excise the capsule as it may

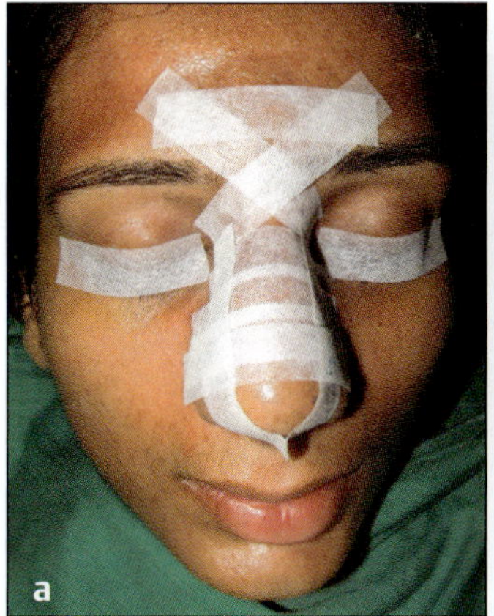
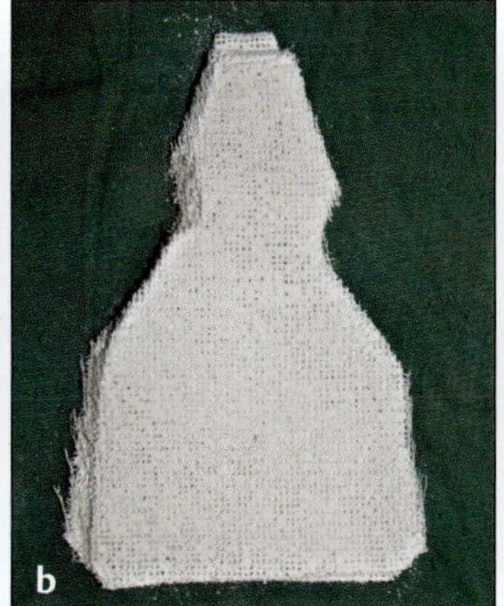
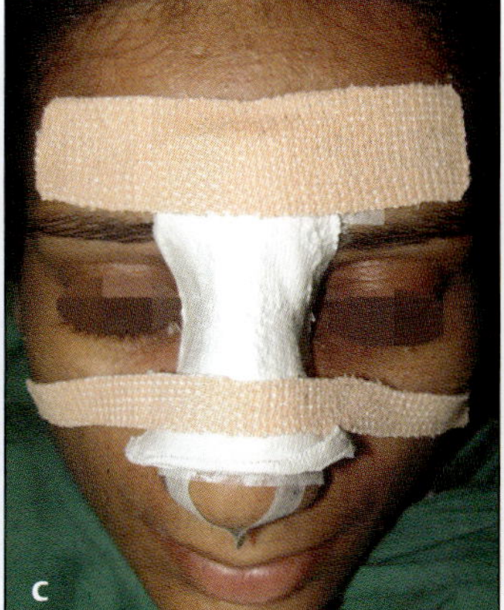
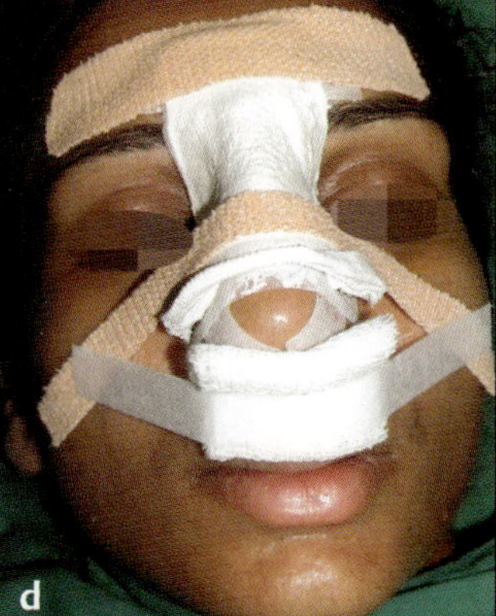

Fig. 16.35 Taping and splinting. **(a)** Photograph showing taping pattern, eyes are covered to avoid seepage of plaster fluid or dry powder during splint application. **(b)** Design of a plaster of paris (POP) splint. **(c)** POP splint with rolled-up distal edge to avoid friction injury to supratip region. **(d)** Photograph showing gap between POP splint and supratip.

damage the skin. The right way is to incise the capsule bilaterally over the dorsum, leaving half capsule attached to the dorsum and other half to the overlying skin. The pocket must be enlarged laterally, and part of the capsule attached to the dorsum may either be rubbed with file or excised completely. Rubbing the capsule with file removes its shiny smooth upper layer and autograft adheres nicely. In cases with severely contracted, thick, and deformed capsule, the capsule must be totally removed and the soft tissues must be reinforced with a fascial graft.[97] Human acellular dermis graft can be used similarly in place of fascial graft, if available. The resorption is more common with allografts.[96]

When to reconstruct these noses depends on the presence or absence of infection and any external wound.

Deviation and/or displacement without infection: Nose can be reaugmented with autograft in the same sitting after explantation of a noninfected implant **(Fig. 16.36a–c)**.

Infected cases with silicone implants with normal dorsal skin: Nose can be augmented secondarily, 6 months after explantation. In patient who can't afford to live with depressed nose and is willing to take risk, an early augmentation in 1 to 2 weeks can be planned after an IV antibiotic treatment for a week.[98,99]

Infection and exposure of implants through dorsal skin: These noses if left for secondary correction usually pose problems in dissecting the adherent, thin, and damaged dorsal skin. Author prefers using a dermafat graft as a filler and spacer until definitive augmentation surgery is done after 4 to 6 months. The dermafat graft provides temporary support and avoids dorsal depression in the intervening period. It also prevents adhesion of the thinned-out dorsal skin to the dorsum; the dermis of the dermafat graft provides good thickness to the dorsal skin and helps in healing of hole/holes in skin. It allows the resolution of the infection and, during the later surgery, provides an easy dissecting plane between the dorsum and fat[98,99] **(Fig. 16.37a–d)**.

Explantation of a Polyethylene Implant

It is a big challenge. L-implant with vertical limb adherent to columellar skin tests the patience of a surgeon. Traditionally, the implants are removed by sharp dissection using a scalpel

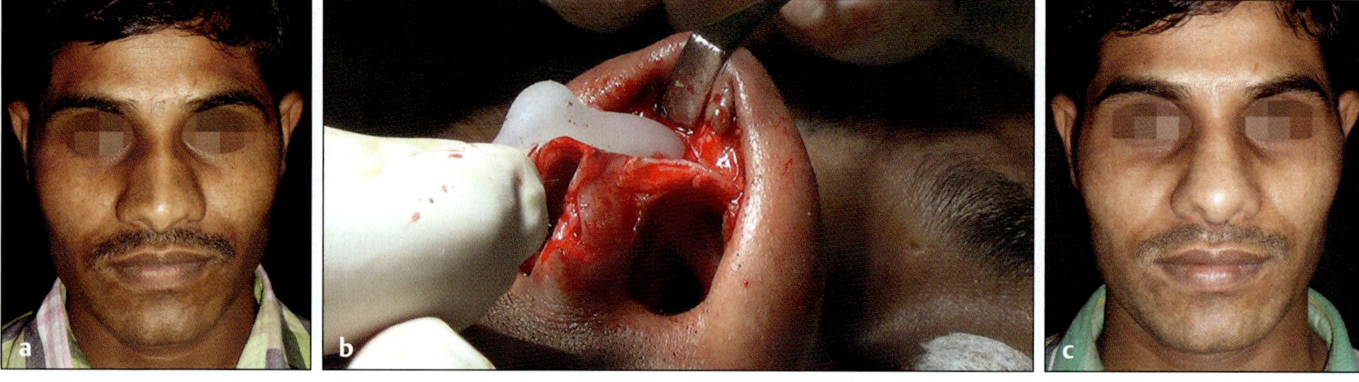

Fig. 16.36 **(a)** Noninfected silicone implant: patient having mobile implant and tip deformity. **(b)** Intraoperative photograph showing explantation of L-shaped implant. **(c)** Postoperative photograph after secondary surgery with cartilage grafts.

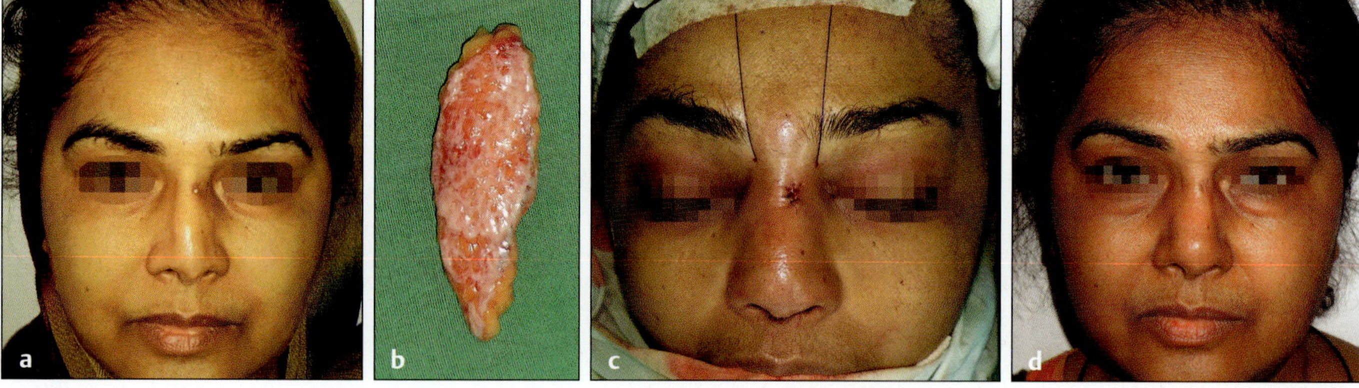

Fig. 16.37 **(a)** Photograph showing exposure of infected silicone implant through dorsal skin and capsular contracture causing deformity of nose. **(b)** Photograph showing dermafat graft. **(c)** Dermafat graft inserted and secured with pull-through sutures and closure of skin defect with sutures. **(d)** One-year postsurgery photograph showing survival of dermafat graft and good healing of skin defect.

or scissors. Author uses scalpel only to incise the fibrous covering of the indwelling implant at the tip and then implant is separated from the incorporated fibrous cover using a Freer's elevator akin to raising perichondrium off the costal cartilage. Frequent hydrodissection helps. Avoiding sharp dissection and leaving behind sufficient connective tissue on the undersurface of dorsal skin serves many purposes[99] (**Fig. 16.38a–d**):

- No button holing and irregularity of dorsal skin.
- Additional cushioning.
- Preserves vascularity.
- Minimal bleeding.

An Uncommon Secondary Case

A patient presented with pus discharging sinus over supratip region for 3 years. She was operated for bulbous tip in which conchal cartilage was used. During secondary surgery, a tuft of hair was retrieved from sinus. Conchal cartilage excised in toto with sinus. A piece of skin was found attached to conchal cartilage which led to the formation of this sinus (**Fig. 16.39a–c**).

Postoperative Management

Head is held in high position and cold compression over the eyes is given for 2 days. In view of extensive surgery as well as plenty of grafts and sutures used, IV antibiotic for 3 to 5 days and oral for another week should be given to prevent any chance of infection. Suture lines are cleaned regularly and antibiotic ointment is applied. Majority of the patients are discharged on day 3 after removal of nasal pack.

At discharge, patient is given oral antibiotics and anti-inflammatory drugs for a week, vitamin C for 4 weeks, and antihistamines on SOS basis, and is advised not to move out in dusty and dirty areas for 2 weeks, no blowing and picking of the nose, no use of spectacles for 6 weeks, and are asked to keep mouth opened while sneezing. Patients are asked to avoid moderate sport activities for 6 weeks and vigorous activities such as contact sports or professional exercises for 10 to 12 weeks. No columellar scar massage should be performed for first 6 weeks, and strictly no massage of scar of alar reduction forever.

Complications

Complications are more common with secondary rhinoplasty than with primary. All complications known for rhinoplasty can also happen after secondary surgery. Here emphasis will be given only on few specific complications which are common with secondary noses. The reasons are:

- Compromised or doubtful vascularity in presence of scar tissue.
- Compromised skeletal framework.
- Lack of cartilage and tissues to work.

Compromised or Doubtful Vascularity in Presence of Scar Tissue

Loss of normal planes and excessive scarring are the commonest reasons for complications in secondary rhinoplasty which may lead to disturbing complications.

Skin changes, buttonholing, bleeding, prolonged swelling, and ecchymosis: Patience, frequent use of hydrodissection, meticulous subperichondrial and subperiosteal plane of dissection are needed to prevent these complications.[100]

Tip, supratip ischemia: The reason is excessive defatting and debulking in tip and supratip region. Only defatting should be attempted. Defatting without injury to subdermal plexus can be done using balloon technique (**Fig. 16.40a, b**). An open approach, excessive debulking, and through-and-through

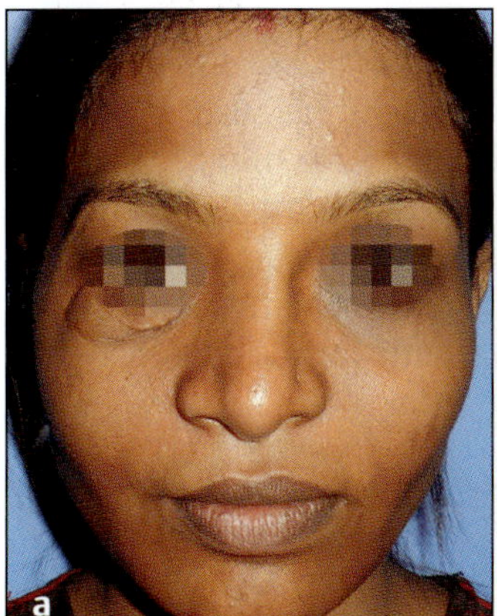
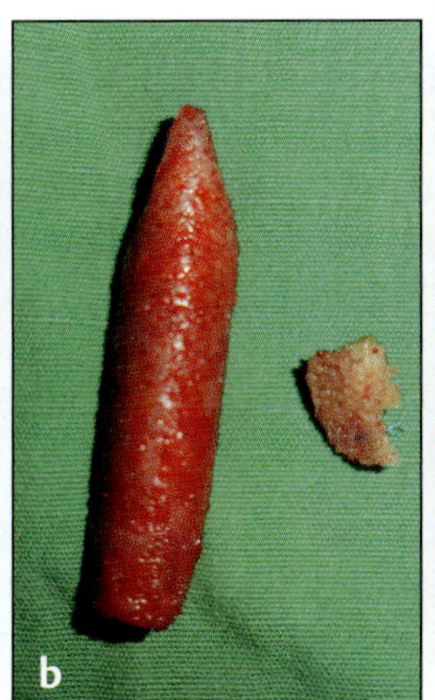
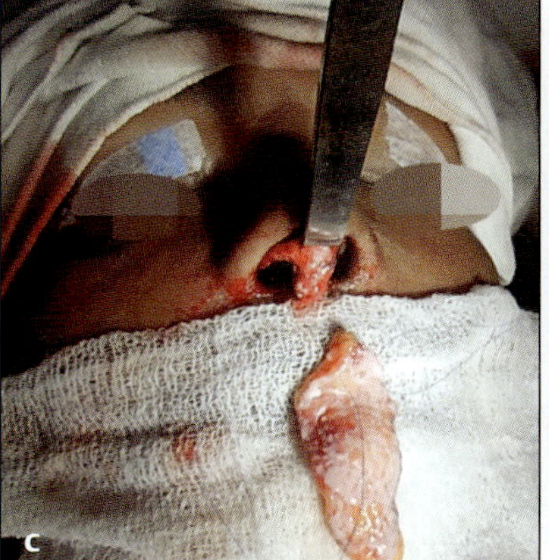
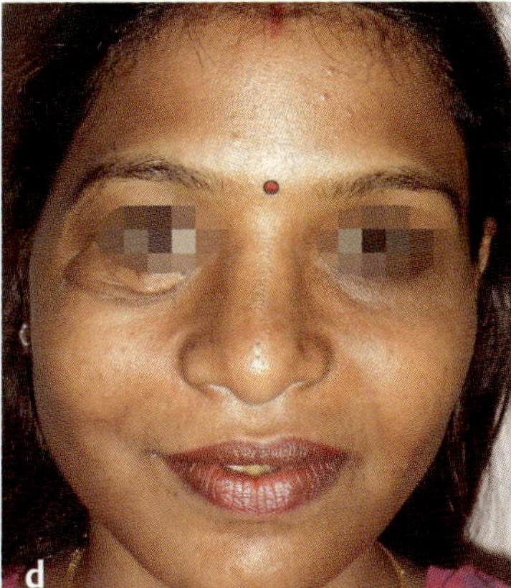

Fig. 16.38 **(a)** Photograph showing deviated and infected polyethylene (Medpor) implant. **(b)** Removed implant. **(c)** Intraoperative photograph showing insertion of dermafat graft. **(d)** Ten-months postsurgery photograph showing survival of dermafat graft.

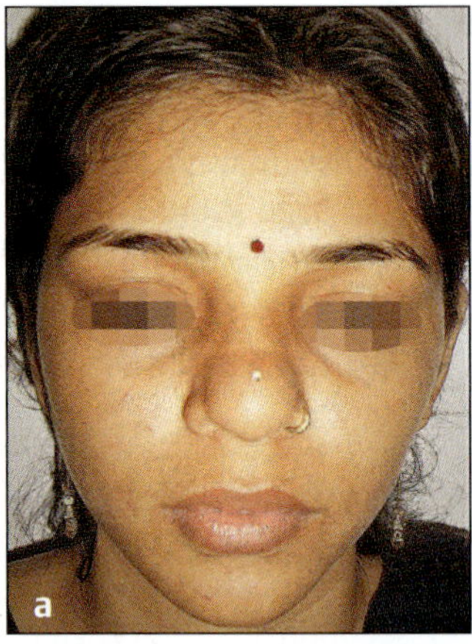
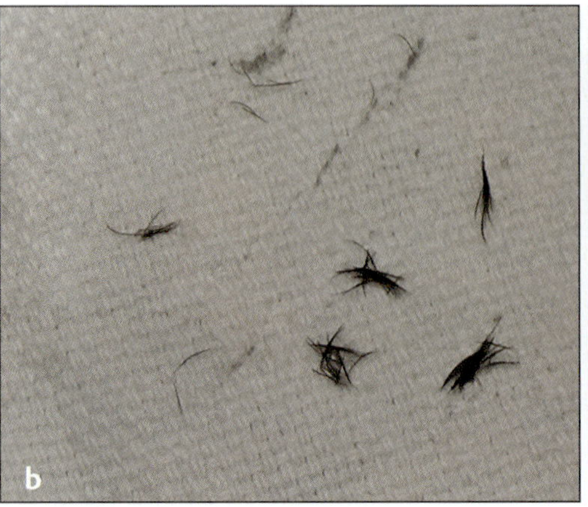
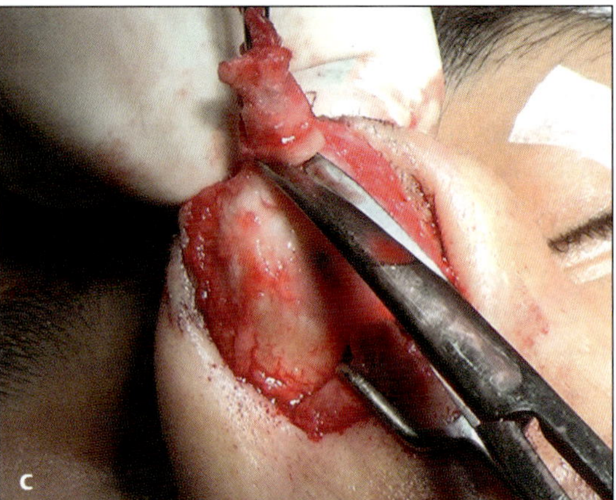

Fig. 16.39 Unusual secondary case. **(a)** Photograph showing sinus with pus discharge over supratip region. **(b)** Hair retrieved from sinus. **(c)** Excision of sinus and reconstruction of tip using conchal cartilage graft.

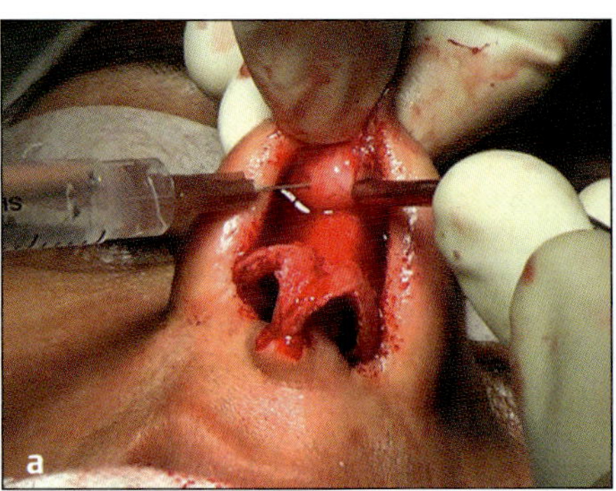
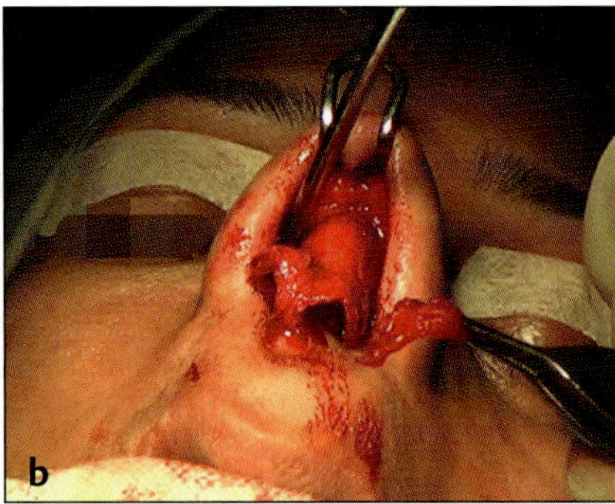

Fig. 16.40 **(a)** Photograph showing saline injection making a balloon of fatty tissue. **(b)** Excised fatty tissue.

alar reduction in secondary rhinoplasty may interfere with the blood supply of nasal tip and this will disrupt the blood supply from lateral nasal artery too, leading to tip necrosis and bad scarring[101,102] (**Fig. 16.41**).

Septal perforation: Unilateral tears of mucoperichondrial septal flap usually heal without incident, but bilateral aligned tears may result in a septal perforation. Bilateral tears of mucoperichondrial flaps must be sutured at the time of surgery with an intervening cartilage graft.[103–105]

Synechiae formation: Bilateral opposing tears of the septum and lateral wall may lead to synechiae formation and subsequent nasal obstruction. Silicone nasal dilators in early postoperative period prevent synechiae formation. Symptomatic synechiae will need surgical release and long-term use of silicone dilator.[105]

Compromised Skeletal Framework

This may lead to collapse of bony pyramid during osteotomies. A cautious approach is needed while tackling secondary nose in which excessive osseocartilaginous manipulation was done during primary surgery. In case of collapse, a careful approximation of the segments and adequate internal and external splint support is required for 3 to 4 weeks.[106]

Lack of Septal and Conchal Cartilage Grafts

This may lead to a substandard result or this forces the surgeon to use costal cartilage graft which may have additional donor-site complications like hemo- or pneumothorax pain and donor-site infection.

Other Common Complications

Infection: Infection is more common after extensive secondary surgery. Three to five days of IV antibiotics are must for a secondary or a revision case where a large number of grafts and sutures have been used. Autografts usually withstand few days of infection without losing support or shape but delay in treating the infection leads to softening and resorption of cartilage grafts, losing both form and function[105] (**Fig. 16.42**).

Plastic smile: Weak smile is a common complain post extensive septorhinoplasty. Author has termed it as "Plastic smile." Return of normal smile usually takes 4 to 8 weeks.

Polybeak deformity: Postoperative supratip bulge may occur due to organized hematoma. This is prevented with subdermal supratip suture. Regular taping is also helpful. In persistent cases, local triamcinolone injection in a deep plane is

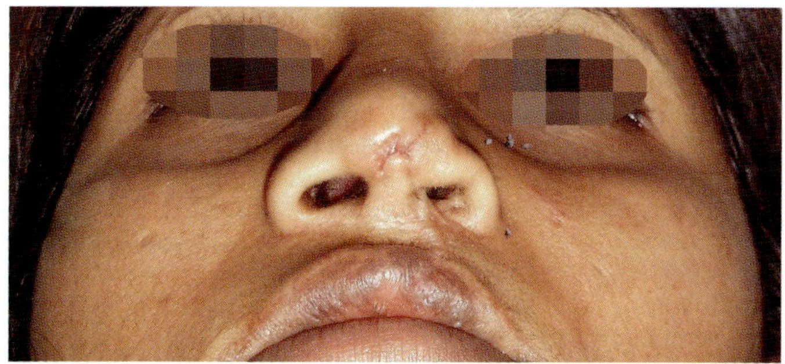

Fig. 16.41 Scarring of tip due to inadvertent thinning of tip skin.

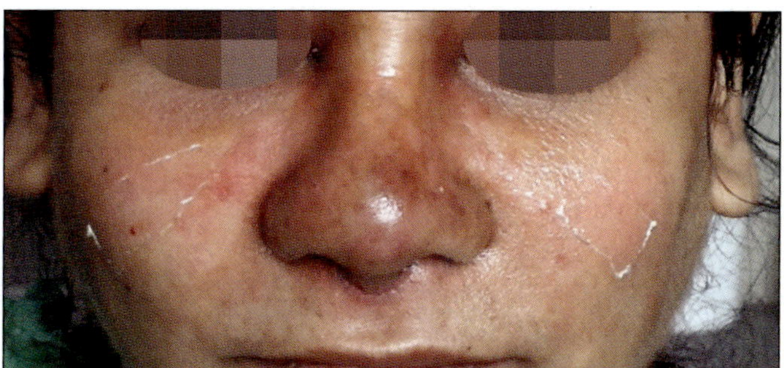

Fig. 16.42 Photograph showing early infection.

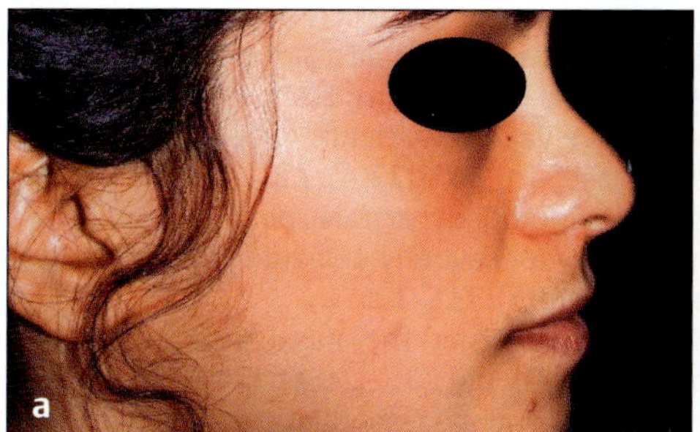

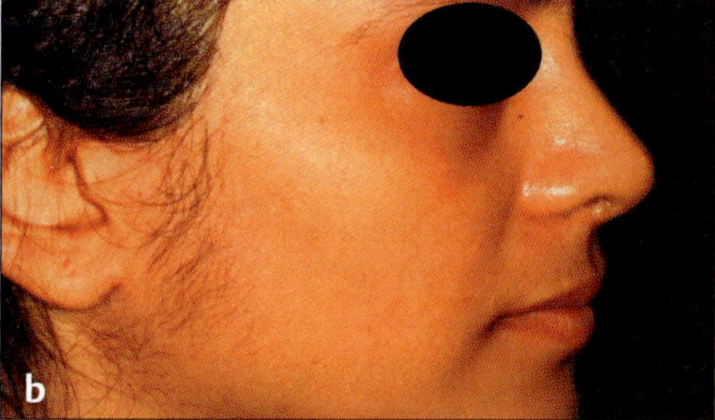

Fig. 16.43 **(a)** Secondary polybeak deformity. **(b)** Postoperative correction of polybeak deformity by excision of supratip fibrous tissues, tip plasty, and elevation of dorsum using diced cartilage under perichondrial carpet (DCUP) strut.

useful. An intradermal injection may cause skin atrophy[107,108] (**Fig. 16.43a, b**).

Lack of sensation over tip and supratip region: This is a common complain after open rhinoplasty due to transaction of external nasal nerves which are terminal branches of anterior ethmoidal nerves.[2] Complete return of sensation may take 6 to 18 months.[106,109]
Considering this fact, the caudal edge of plaster splint should be rolled up to avoid friction injury to the numb supratip region (**Fig. 16.44**).

Fig. 16.44 Scar over supratip due to friction injury caused by caudal edge of plaster of paris (POP) splint.

Summary

Secondary rhinoplasty throws challenges at every step from first consultation till last follow-up meeting with the patient. Keen analysis, thorough planning, and ability of a surgeon to quickly adapt and innovate on facing unforeseen difficulties during execution are the ways forward. The key points to keep in mind during primary and secondary rhinoplasty are almost same; however, some of the surgical tips to keep in mind are:

- Avoid use of forceps to hold columella or alae during rhinoplasty, it may cause terminal necrosis and bad scarring.
- Repeated use of hydrodissection and use of periosteal elevator should be done to protect severely adherent skin from inadvertent button holing or necrosis. Same is applicable for adherent porous polyethylene implant.
- Thick tip and supratip skin must not be thinned out arbitrarily; it may jeopardize the blood supply leading to necrosis and permanent scarring.
- Cephalic trimming of lateral crura is not an essential step. A cookie-cutter approach may lead to suboptimal result.
- When both septal cartilage harvest and reduction of hump are required, hump reduction should be done first so that the surgeon gets an idea about how much to leave behind for support while harvesting the cartilage graft.
- Osteotomies of nasal bones are not an essential step; these should only be executed for strong indications.
- Dorsum must be roughened with file or rasp for better adhesions of the dorsal strut.

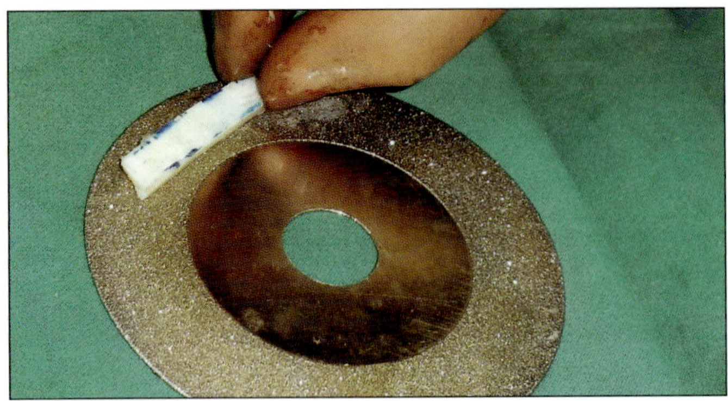

Fig. 16.45 Glass polishing disc being used to smoothen cartilage graft.

- Cephalic end of the dorsal strut should always be covered under procerus muscle to avoid visibility.
- If dorsal strut needs a joint to increase the length then the joint should be under the thick supratip skin to avoid visibility.
- Do not fall into the trap/resist the temptation of using a costal cartilage which is straight on table. Consider every single piece as a potentially warped cartilage and use any technique or trick which you feel is capable of keeping it straight.
- It is difficult to negotiate suture needle through partially ossified costal cartilage. It becomes softer by either rubbing with power-assisted burr or polishing disc[110] **(Fig. 16.45)**.
- Completely ossified costal cartilage shows no warping; hence, there is no need to use technique to prevent warping.[111]
- Through-and-through alar reduction should be avoided as it may lead to straightening of alae, nostril stenosis, and unnatural appearance.
- Strictly no massage should be advised to alar facial groove after alar correction. Overzealous massage may turn an inconspicuous scar into a visible one.

References

1. Shubailat G. Secondary rhinoplasty. Indian J Plast Surg 2008; 41(Suppl): S80–S87
2. Neaman KC, Boettcher AK, Do VH, et al. Cosmetic rhinoplasty: revision rates revisited. Aesthet Surg J 2013;33(1):31–37
3. Gruber RP, Wall SH Jr, Kaufman DL, Kahn DM. Secondary rhinoplasty. Aesthetic: textbook of plastic surgery by Neligan PC, Vol. 2, 3rd ed. New York: Elsevier Saunders; 2012:466–484
4. Daniel RK. Secondary rhinoplasty. In Mastering rhinoplasty, 2nd ed. London: Springer Heidelberg Dordrecht; 2010:349–406
5. Rohrich RJ, Sheen JH. Secondary rhinoplasty. In: Rohrich RJ, Sheen JH, Budget GC, BudgetDE Jr.Secondary rhinoplasty and nasal reconstruction .ST. Louis, Missouri, Quality Medical Publishing. 1996, Ch. 1, P-1-15
6. Agrawal KS, Singla S, Shrotriya R. Text neck view: a new photographic tool for assessment of nasal dorsum in crooked noses. Plast Reconstr Surg 2016;138(1):165e–167e
7. Jennes ML. Photography in rhinoplasty: an office technique. AMA Arch Otolaryngol 1954;60(6):695–701
8. Gunter JP. Rhinoplasty. In: EH Courtiss, ed. Male aesthetic surgery, 2nd ed. St. Louis, MO: Mosby; 1990: 1071–85
9. Gorney M. Criteria for patient selection: an ounce of prevention. Presented at the Residents and Fellows Forum, Aesthetic Plastic Surgery Annual Meeting, Boston, MA, May 16, 2003
10. Goodman WS. External approach to rhinoplasty. Can J Otolaryngol 1973;2(3):207–210
11. Goodman WS. Recent advances in external rhinoplasty. J Otolaryngol 1981;10(6):433–439
12. Adamson PA, Smith O, Tropper GJ. Incision and scar analysis in open (external) rhinoplasty. Arch Otolaryngol Head Neck Surg 1990;116(6):671–675
13. Becker DG. Septoplasty and turbinate surgery. Aesthet Surg J 2003;23(5):393–403
14. Gubisch W. Extracorporeal septoplasty for the markedly deviated septum. Arch Facial Plast Surg 2005;7(4):218–226
15. Gubisch W. Twenty-five years experience with extracorporeal septoplasty. Facial Plast Surg 2006;22(4):230–239
16. Jang YJ, Kwon M. Modified extracorporeal septoplasty technique in rhinoplasty for severely deviated noses. Ann Otol Rhinol Laryngol 2010;119(5):331–335
17. Simon P, Sidle D. Augmenting the nasal airway: beyond septoplasty. Am J Rhinol Allergy 2012;26(4):326–331
18. Agrawal KS, Shrotriya R. Total nasal septal reconstruction using costal cartilage in difficult cases of secondary septoplasty. Plast Aesthet Res 2016;3:306–310
19. Agrawal KS, Bachhav M, Shrotriya R. Namaste (counter-balancing) technique: Overcoming warping in costal cartilage. Indian J Plast Surg 2015;48(2):123–128
20. Joseph J. Die Hypertrophie der starren Nase: Nasenplastik und sonstige gesichtsplastik über smammaplastik und einige weitere Operationen aus dem gebiete der ausseren Korperplastik. Leipzig, Germany: Kabitzsch; 1931
21. Flowers RS, Anderson R. Injury to the lacrimal apparatus during rhinoplasty. Plast Reconstr Surg 1968;42(6):577–581
22. Sheen JH. Aesthetic rhinoplasty. St. Louis: C.V. Mosby Company; 1978
23. Murakami CS, Younger RAL. Managing the postrhinoplasty or post-traumatic crooked nose. Facial Plast Surg Clin North Am 1995;3:421–448
24. Webster RC, Davidson TM, Smith RC. Curved lateral osteotomy for airway protection in rhinoplasty. Arch Otolaryngol 1977;103(8):454–458
25. Becker DG, McLaughlin RB Jr, Loevner LA, Mang A. The lateral osteotomy in rhinoplasty: clinical and radiographic rationale for osteotome selection. Plast Reconstr Surg 2000;105(5):1806–1816, discussion 1817–1819
26. Anderson JR. A new approach to rhinoplasty. Trans Am Acad Ophthalmol Otolaryngol 1966;70(2):183–192
27. Larrabee WF Jr. Open rhinoplasty and the upper third of the nose. Facial Plast Surg Clin North Am 1993;1:23–38
28. Parkes ML, Kamer F, Morgan WR. Double lateral osteotomy in rhinoplasty. Arch Otolaryngol 1977;103(6):344–348
29. Fanous N, Amar YG. Narrowing of the wide nasal dorsum in the 'minimal-hump' nose: A simplified universal approach. Can J Plast Surg 2005;13(3):139–143
30. Prendiville S, Zimbler MS, Kokoska MS, Thomas JR. Middle-vault narrowing in the wide nasal dorsum: the "Reverse Spreader" technique. Arch Facial Plast Surg 2002;4(1):52–55
31. Davis RE, Raval J. Powered instrumentation for nasal bone reduction: advantages and indications. Arch Facial Plast Surg 2003;5(5):384–391

32. Gerbault O, Daniel RK, Kosins AM. The role of peizoelectric instrumentation in rhinoplasty surgery. Aesthet Surg J 2016; 36(1):21–34
33. Cochran CS, Roostaeian J. Use of the ultrasonic bone aspirator for lateral osteotomies in rhinoplasty. Plast Reconstr Surg 2013;132(6):1430–1433
34. Fomon S. Cosmetic surgery—principles and Practice. Philadelphia: Lippincott co.; 1960:329–332
35. Johnson CM, Toriumi DM. Open structure rhinoplasty. Philadelphia: W.B. Saunders; 1990:91–94
36. McCollough EG, Fedok FG. The lateral crural turnover graft: correction of the concave lateral crus. Laryngoscope 1993;103 (4 Pt 1):463–469
37. Tardy ME Jr, Patt BS, Walter MA. Transdomal suture refinement of the nasal tip: long-term outcomes. Facial Plast Surg 1993;9(4):275–284
38. Daniel RK. Rhinoplasty: creating an aesthetic tip. A preliminary report. Plast Reconstr Surg 1987;80(6):775–783
39. Daniel RK. Rhinoplasty: a simplified, three-stitch, open tip suture technique. Part I: primary rhinoplasty. Plast Reconstr Surg 1999;103(5):1491–1502
40. Gruber RP, Nahai F, Bogdan MA, Friedman GD. Changing the convexity and concavity of nasal cartilages and cartilage grafts with horizontal mattress sutures: part I. Experimental results. Plast Reconstr Surg 2005;115(2):589–594
41. Gruber RP, Nahai F, Bogdan MA, Friedman GD. Changing the convexity and concavity of nasal cartilages and cartilage grafts with horizontal mattress sutures: part II. Clinical results. Plast Reconstr Surg 2005;115(2):595–606, discussion 607–608
42. Perkins SW, Sufyan AS. The alar-spanning suture: a useful tool in rhinoplasty to refine the nasal tip. Arch Facial Plast Surg 2011;13(6):421–424
43. Hussein WKA, Ismail AS, Ibrahim AA, Omran AA. Modified lateral crural spanning suture of the nasal tip: suspension element. Egypt J Ear Nose Throat Allied Sciences 2017. http://dx.doi.org/10.1016/j.ejenta.2016.12.019
44. Toriumi DM. New concepts in nasal tip contouring. Arch Facial Plast Surg 2006;8(3):156–185
45. Gunter JP. Personal approach. In: Gunter JP, Rohrich RJ, Adams WP Jr, eds. Dallas rhinoplasty: nasal surgery by the master. St Louis: Quality Medical Publishing; 2002:1049
46. Sheen JH. Achieving more nasal tip projection by the use of a small autogenous vomer or septal cartilage graft. A preliminary report. Plast Reconstr Surg 1975;56(1):35–40
47. Whitaker EG, Johnson CM Jr. The evolution of open structure rhinoplasty. Arch Facial Plast Surg 2003;5(4):291–300
48. Peck GC. The onlay graft for nasal tip projection. Plast Reconstr Surg 1983;71(1):27–39
49. Rohrich RJ, Deuber MA. Nasal tip refinement in primary rhinoplasty: the cephalic trim cap graft. Aesthet Surg J 2002; 22(1):39–45
50. Mavili ME, Safak T. Use of umbrella graft for nasal tip projection. Aesthetic Plast Surg 1993;17(2):163–166
51. Peck GC Jr, Michelson L, Segal J, Peck GC Sr. An 18-year experience with the umbrella graft in rhinoplasty. Plast Reconstr Surg 1998;102(6):2158–2165, discussion 2166–2168
52. Erdogan B, Ayhan M, Görgü M, Deren O. Umbrella graft of columella tip: 20 years' experience. Aesthetic Plast Surg 2002;26(3):167–171
53. Watson D, Toriumi DM. Structural grafting in secondary rhinoplasty. In: Gunter JP, Rohrich RJ, Adams WP Jr, eds. Dallas rhinoplasty: nasal surgery by the masters. St. Louis: Quality Medical Publishing; 2002:705
54. Gunter JP, Friedman RM. Lateral crural strut graft: technique and clinical applications in rhinoplasty. Plast Reconstr Surg 1997;99(4):953–955
55. Gruber RP. Lateral crural strut graft: technique and clinical applications in rhinoplasty. Plast Reconstr Surg 1997;99(4): 943–52 [Discussion: 53–5].
56. Cochran CS, Sieber DA. Extended alar contour grafts: an evolution of the lateral crural strut graft technique in rhinoplasty. Plast Reconstr Surg 2017;140(4):559e–567e
57. Rohrich RJ, Raniere J Jr, Ha RY. The alar contour graft: correction and prevention of alar rim deformities in rhinoplasty. Plast Reconstr Surg 2002;109(7):2495–2505, discussion 2506–2508
58. Toriumi DM. Structure approach in rhinoplasty. Facial Plast Surg Clin North Am 2005;13(1):93–113
59. Dyer WK II. Nasal tip support and its surgical modification. Facial Plast Surg Clin North Am 2004;12(1):1–13
60. Agrawal K, Shrotriya R. Use of "tent-pole" graft for setting columella-lip angle in rhinoplasty. Plast Aesthet Res 2018; 5:13–17
61. Byrd HS, Andochick S, Copit S, Walton KG. Septal extension grafts: a method of controlling tip projection shape. Plast Reconstr Surg 1997;100(4):999–1010
62. Toriumi DM. Caudal septal extension graft for correction of the retracted columella. Oper Tech Otolaryngol--Head Neck Surg 1995;6:311–318
63. Ponsky DC, Harvey DJ, Khan SW, Guyuron B. Nose elongation: a review and description of the septal extension tongue-and-groove technique. Aesthet Surg J 2010;30(3):335–346
64. Kridel RW, Scott BA, Foda HM. The tongue-in-groove technique in septorhinoplasty. A 10-year experience. Arch Facial Plast Surg 1999;1(4):246–256, discussion 257–258
65. Flowers RS, Smith EM Jr. Technique for correction of the retracted columella, acute columellar-labial angle, and long upper lip. Aesthetic Plast Surg 1999;23(4):243–246
66. Gunter JP, Rohrich RJ, Friedman RM. Classification and correction of alar-columellar discrepancies in rhinoplasty. Plast Reconstr Surg 1996;97(3):643–648
67. Armstrong DP. Aggressive management of the hanging columella. Plast Reconstr Surg 1980;65(4):513–516
68. Adamson PA, Tropper GJ, McGraw BL. The hanging columella. J Otolaryngol 1990;19(5):319–323
69. Draf W, Bockmühl U, Hoffmann B. Nasal correction in maxillonasal dysplasia (Binder's syndrome): a long term follow-up study. Br J Plast Surg 2003;56(3):199–204
70. Pan K, Pan B. Columellar reconstruction in children. Oper Tech Otolaryngol—Head Neck Surg 2018;29(2):61–65
71. Mavili ME, Akyürek M. Congenital isolated absence of the nasal columella: reconstruction with an internal nasal vestibular skin flap and bilateral labial mucosa flaps. Plast Reconstr Surg 2000;106(2):393–399
72. Agrawal KS, Shrotriya R, Pabari M. An innovative technique for columellar reconstruction using "flip-over" buccal mucosa flap. J Clin Diagn Res 2016;10(7): PD05–PD06
73. Gibson T, Davis WB. The distortion of autogenous cartilage grafts: Its cause and prevention. Br J Plast Surg 1957–1958; 10:257–274
74. Gunter JP, Clark CP, Friedman RM. Internal stabilization of autogenous rib cartilage grafts in rhinoplasty: a barrier to cartilage warping. Plast Reconstr Surg 1997;100(1):161–169
75. Daniel RK, Calvert JW. Diced cartilage grafts in rhinoplasty surgery. Plast Reconstr Surg 2004;113(7):2156–2171
76. Agrawal K, Shrotriya R, Bachhav M. Diced cartilage under perichondrial carpet with reinforcement (DCUP) technique

Even though "otoplasty" literally means ear surgery, this term is used mainly for cosmetic surgery of external ear (pinna) aimed at correcting size, shape, position, or any congenital or acquired anomaly. Main indications for the surgery are protruding ears or prominent ears, large ears (macrotia), lop ear, constricted ears, Stahl ear, etc. More severe problems like Microtia and Anotia are grouped under ear reconstruction. A large percentage of these patients come for correction of prominent ear while other indications are relatively small in number.

Prominent Ear

Introduction

Prominent ear or protruding ear is one of the most common problems among the anomalies of the external ear. It is a congenital anomaly marked by abnormally protruding external auricle. Various terminologies like bat ear, apostasis otis, prominauris are used for this deformity. In most cases it is bilateral but can be unilateral in rare cases. It is the result of maldevelopment of ear cartilage during intrauterine life. The deformity is characterized by poorly developed antihelix and scapha either alone or with a large hypertrophied concha. The deformity can lead to emotional disorder in the child and it should be corrected early to avoid psychological distress. The aim of the surgery is to bring the ear closer to the skull while recreating all the missing ear cartilage landmarks.

History

History of surgery on prominent ear is quite old, with the earliest description in the literature by Dieffenbach (1845), who reported his technique of otoplasty in a posttraumatic ear deformity. He utilized conchomastoid suture and excised retroauricular skin in an attempt to pin back the ear.[1] Ely in 1881 used similar suture with resection of a strip of cartilage to correct bilateral prominent ears.[2] Thereafter various authors like Keen (1890), Hauck (1884), Joseph (1896) described different types of skin excisions from the back of the ear to correct this deformity.[3] However, Gersuny in the year 1903 observed that skin excision alone is not enough to achieve lasting results in otoplasty.[4]

Initial attempts of cartilage manipulation to correct the deformity were led by the work of Luckett, who created a crest by incising and folding the cartilage with sutures.[5]

The Gibson and Davis principle of cartilage warping opposite to the surgical assault is the basis of many newer techniques which rely on cartilage manipulation for correction of this deformity.[6,7] Numerous modifications of incision-scoring techniques in the area of antihelix, described by Converse, Converse and Wood-Smith, Chongchet, and Stenström are based on this principle.[8–11] Converse performed incomplete cartilage incisions in combination with fixation sutures. Chongchet and Crikelair are considered pioneers in using anterior cartilage scoring technique through posterior access to form the antihelix. Stenström used a rasp via a small posterior access to achieve similar objective.[10–12]

Roughly at the same time when cartilage scoring techniques were being developed, Mustardé used multiple nonabsorbable sutures through posterior access to create a new antihelical fold.[13]

Although it was Morestin[14] who first described conchamastoid suture to reduce the helix-mastoid distance, it is Furnas and Spira who are credited with refining this technique.[15,16]

Correction of the protruding lobule was described as early as 1969 by Spira et al who performed a wedge excision in the area of the lobule and used a deep skin-skull periosteum suture to shift the lobule into the correct position. Wood-Smith excised retrolobular skin in a fishtail-like manner with closure in V-Y fashion.[17] Unfortunately, many such techniques which rely on skin excision only do not give satisfactory long-term results because of natural elasticity of the skin. Many subsequent surgeons used different sutures by taking clue from an early article by Siegert, who used a mattress suture for fixing subcutaneous fibrofatty tissue of lobule to conchal surface, thus moving the lobule posteriorly.[18]

Anatomy of External Auricle

The auricle or external pinna is a complex three-dimensional structure. The outermost part is the helical rim. It is a smooth, curved arch. Its anterior extension is known as crus helicis. Crus helicis divides the concha into a superior cymba conchae and an inferior cavum conchae. The helix is separated from the concha by the antihelix. The antihelix in its topmost part bifurcates into superior and inferior crura. The trough between the helix and antihelix is referred to as the scaphoid fossa. The area between the two antihelical crura is known as the fossa triangularis. Lower part of the pinna has two small protrusions of cartilages which form the tragus and antitragus. Both are separated by the incisura intertragica. The cauda helicis extends posteriorly to the antitragus (**Fig. 17.1**).

The fine contour of the ear is determined by the form and shape of the elastic auricular cartilage. The lobule does not contain any cartilage, but is mainly composed of adipose and connective tissue.

The auricle is fully developed by the age of 6 years as far as the transverse growth and the depth of conchal cartilage is concerned. The auricular length might grow until the age of 11 to 12 years. There is apparent lengthening of the auricle during the natural aging process but this is because of the natural skin and soft tissue elasticity.

Neurovascular Supply

Arterial blood supply to the ear is primarily derived from branches of the external carotid artery. Superficial temporal artery supplies anterior part of pinna while occipital artery and posterior auricular artery supply posterior surface of the pinna. Venous drainage consists of veins of the same name, which ultimately drain into the external jugular vein.

The sensory innervation of the external ear is complex. Greater auricular nerve and lesser occipital nerve, both branches of cervical plexus innervate inferior surface and posterior superior surface of auricle. The auriculotemporal nerve, a branch of the mandibular component of the trigeminal nerve, innervates the anterior superior surface. The concha proper and tragus are innervated by the Arnold nerve, which is a small distal branch of the 10th cranial nerve. It is important to block this nerve by subcutaneous injection into conchal bowl in addition to blocking auriculotemporal and great auricular nerve, in order to get a complete ear block if surgery is to be performed under local anesthesia (**Fig. 17.2**).

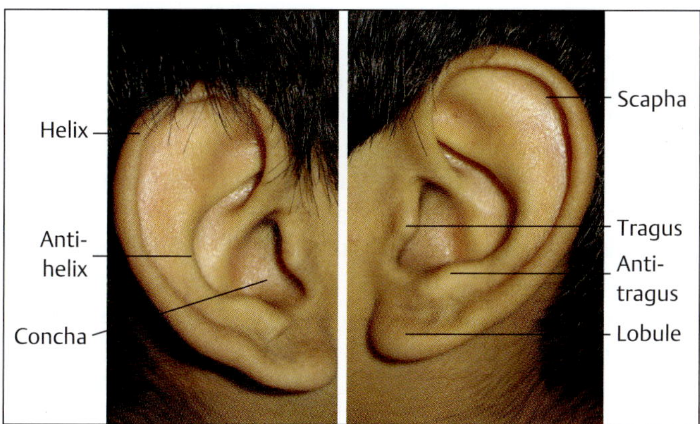

Fig. 17.1 Anatomy of a normal ear.

Anthropometry

Two important determinants to define abnormally protruding ears are cephaloauricular angle and distance. Numerous anthropometric studies were carried out to measure the distance and to calculate the angle between the ear and the head. According to Wodak, the average distance between the helical rim and the head can vary from 6 to 20 mm in adults, measured at the upper and middle measuring point, and at the level of the tail of the helix.[19] The angle between the mastoid and the helix of a normally shaped auricle should not exceed 30 degrees (**Fig. 17.3**).[20–22] Numerous other criteria for a properly shaped auricle have been suggested by various authors (**Box 17.1**).[23–25]

Applied Anatomy and Pathogenesis

The pathogenetic factors discussed in protruding ears include genetic factors, point mutations, but environmental influences during pregnancy, such as exposure to X-rays, hypoxia, as well as the intake of certain drugs like thalidomide, do play a role in the development of this anomaly.[26]

Box 17.1 Criteria of a properly shaped auricle

- The axis of the ear is almost parallel to the bridge of the nose
- The position of the auricle is approximately one auricular length behind the lateral orbital margin (55–70 mm)
- The average adult female ear is approx. 59 mm long and the average adult male ear is approx. 63 mm long
- The width of the auricle should be 50–60% of the auricular length (width: 30–45 mm, length 55–70 mm)
- The lobule should be positioned parallel to the antihelical fold in the same plane

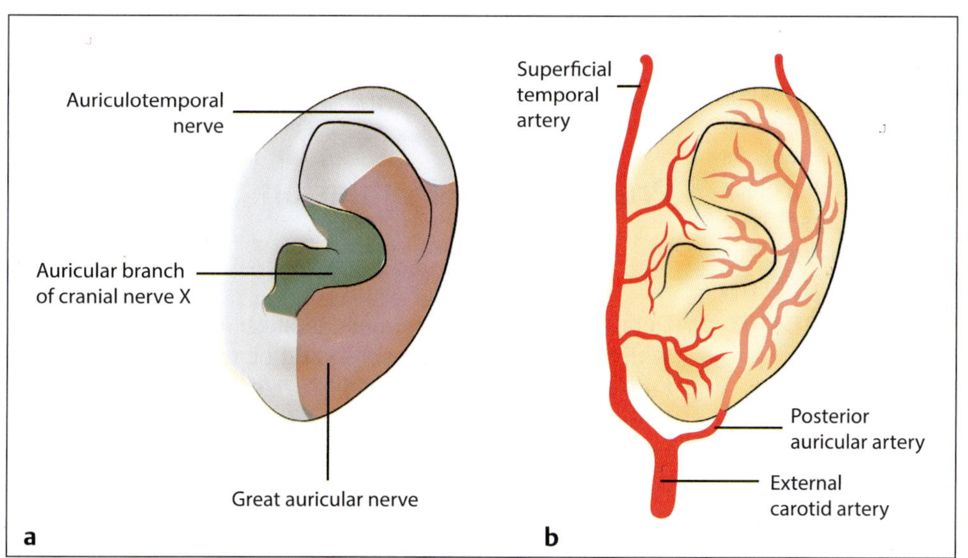

Fig. 17.2 Anatomical features of external ear. **(a)** Topography of innervations. **(b)** Blood supply.

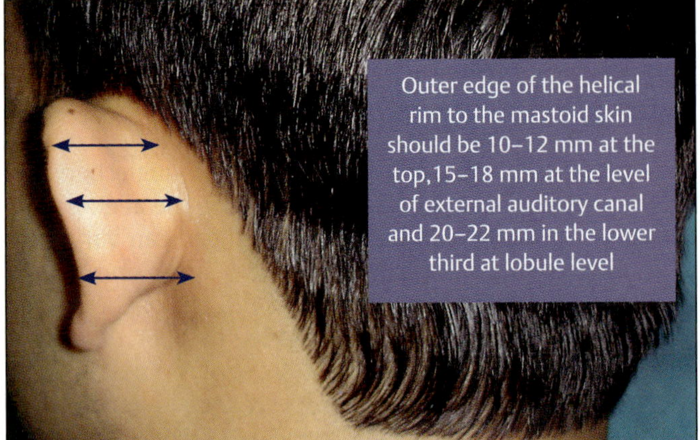

Fig. 17.3 Anthropometric features of external ear.

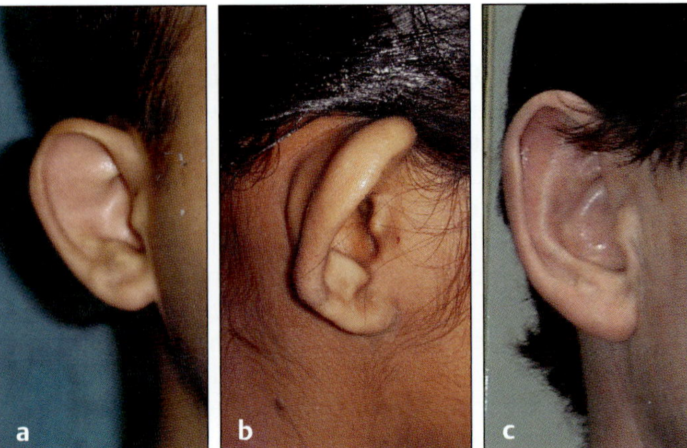

Fig. 17.4 Young dae Lee classification[30] of prominent ear. **(a)** Class I. **(b)** Class II. **(c)** Class III.

In protruding ears, deviations from the normal shape are especially apparent at the antihelix, the concha, and the lobule. The enlargement of the helix-mastoid angle especially in the mid portion is an important feature of prominent ear deformity. Another hallmark feature of this deformity is deficient antihelical fold. In addition to this, conchal hypertrophy with significantly enlarged cavum and lifted cavum conchae may also result in protruding ears. These features are found in various combinations to cause prominent ear deformity. There is apparent increase in width of the auricle as seen from an anterolateral perspective because of unfurling of antihelix and this is an important aspect of the evaluation of the effaced auricle.[27]

Incidence

Protruding ears are common in the Caucasian population, occurring with an incidence of up to 5%. About 59% of the individuals suffering from prominent ear have family history of prominent ears. The transmission is in an autosomal dominant pattern with variable penetrance. Since inner ear develops separately from external ear, hearing is normal in patients with prominent ears; however, other congenital problems, especially of urogenital tract, can be present. As per one study the prevalence of prominent ear among black African children is comparable to that of Caucasians.[28] True incidence in India is not known as many people having this deformity do not come forward for treatment because of the popular belief that large ears bring good luck and prosperity.

Classification of Auricular Anomalies

Many classifications for auricular deformities have been suggested by different authors at different times. The classification given by Weerda, which is based on severity of auricular deformity, is widely accepted and used in clinical settings.[29]

Grade I are cases with mild deformities of the auricle in which the anatomical structures of the ear is completely preserved. Examples include some milder varieties of protruding ears, cryptotias, macrotias, colobomas, as well as mild cup ear deformities.

Grade II are moderate auricular deformities. They have malformations of the basic architecture of the cartilage. These cases include severe cup ear deformities and the more severe cases of protruding ears in which the antihelix is missing and concha is hypertrophied.

Grade III are severe malformations and include microtia grade III with anotia. None of the normal structures of the pinna are recognizable. They require total reconstruction with rib cartilage framework.

Young dae Lee et al gave a simple classification specifically for prominent ear. They divided these cases into three categories depending on the severity (**Fig. 17.4**):[30]

- Class I: Absence of antihelix without conchal hypertrophy.
- Class II: Absent antihelix combined with conchal hypertrophy.
- Class III: Deep conchal bowl with well-formed antihelix.

Preoperative Evaluation

History

Detailed history of previous medical or pediatric issues which can affect anesthesia should be taken. Any concomitant anomaly which can affect surgical planning should be noted. History of previous ear surgery or otoplasty is important as the scarring of previous surgeries may affect the outcome. Family history of similar problem and psychological problems such as teasing in young patients and body dysmorphic issues in adult males should be documented.

Clinical Examination

Local physical examination should include:

- Size and depth of the concha.
- Extent of development of antihelical fold.
- Extent of protrusion of the antitragus and ear lobule.
- Assessment of the stiffness of the cartilage by palpation.
- Degree of protrusion as assessed by measuring the mastoid helical distance at three levels:
  1. Upper level: at the superior aspect of helix.
  2. Middle level: at the level of external acoustic meatus.
  3. Lower level: at the level of lobule.
- Any disparity in size and the degree of protrusion on both sides.
- A thorough ENT examination is performed. In cases of doubt, threshold audiometry with impedance testing may be required to exclude possible conductive or perceptive hearing losses.
- Additional ear abnormalities, (e.g., accessory auricles, etc.) are noted.

Photographic Documentation

Preoperative standard photographs in frontal, back, lateral, and oblique views should be done. Photographic documentation is necessary to sketch out the problematic areas. This is also recommended for follow-up and medicolegal reasons (**Fig. 17.5**).

Indications and Contraindications

Primary indication for operating on these children is psychological stress caused by teasing at school. Parents are quite aware of problems faced by these children at school so they bring them for treatment before the child starts school. Low self-esteem, general lack of self-confidence, and social isolation are some of the reasons for adults seeking surgical correction. Schwentner et al interviewed patients before and after otoplasty regarding their pre- and postoperative emotional state, using a standardized questionnaire.[31] The results of this retrospective study showed a significantly improved attitude toward life, and better self-confidence among the patients. Another study by Sirin et al showed significant psychosocial benefit in children and adult population.[32]

A child whose behavior is not cooperative, or a child with history of ear infections, persistent discharge, adult with previous failed surgery, and patients with unrealistic expectations are relative contraindications for the procedure.

Management

Nonsurgical Management

Nonsurgical therapy in the form of molding with various devices in the neonatal period offers a window of opportunity for correcting auricular deformities. While surgical therapies have to wait till the ear develops fully, these

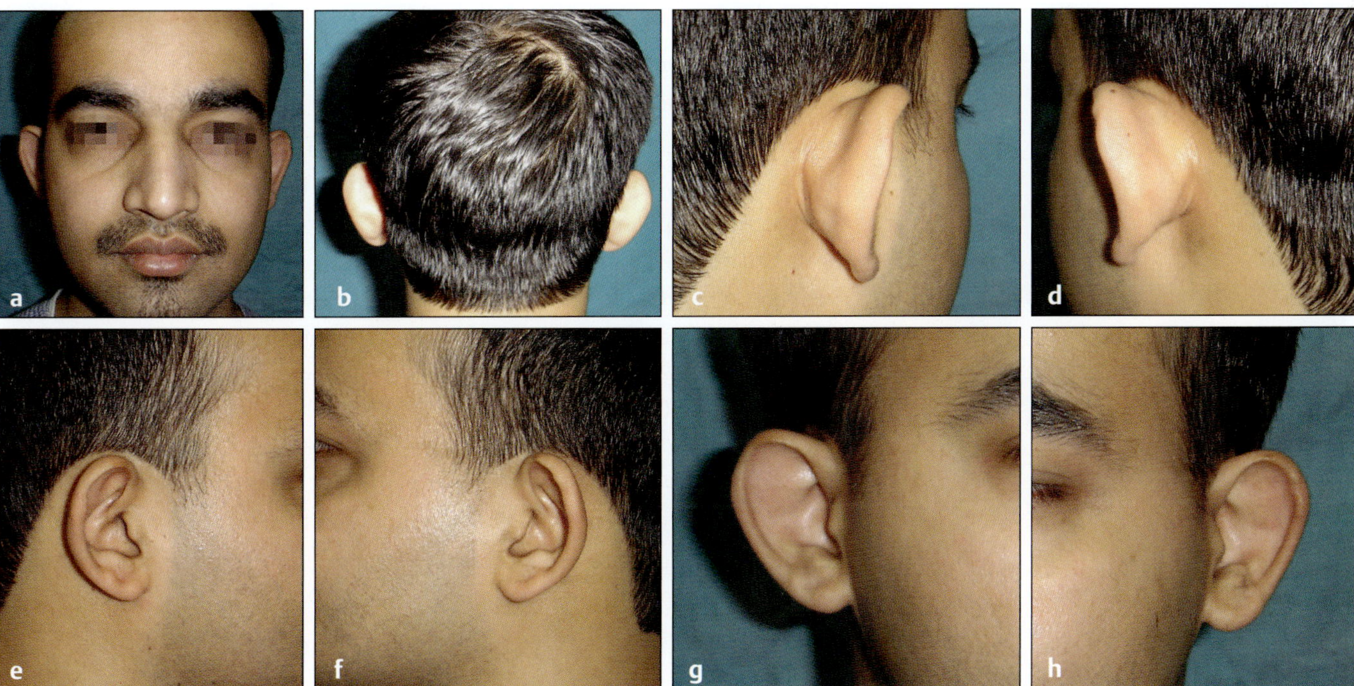

Fig. 17.5 **(a–h)** Standard views of clinical photographs. **(a)** Front, (b) From behind showing both the ears, **(c)** right oblique from behind showing medial surface of right ear, **(d)** left oblique from behind showing medial surface of left ear, **(e)** right lateral, **(f)** left lateral, **(g)** Front oblique showing lateral surface of right side, **(h)** Front oblique showing lateral surface of left ear.

techniques can be instituted long before the age of peer teasing, bullying, and loss of self-esteem.

The earliest publications on nonsurgical correction of congenital auricular deformities are in the late 1980s by Japanese plastic surgeons.[33–36] They reported successful outcome by keeping the ear into the proper position with some sort of indigenous malleable splint and maintaining it there with tape for several weeks avoiding surgery altogether in many cases.

Most articles on this subject in literature classify ear anomalies into two categories: deformations and malformations. The former anomalies have no deficiency of skin or cartilage and are suitable for splinting.

van Wijk et al published a review article in 2009 extensively covering articles published on this subject till that date. They listed different materials used for cartilage reshaping and presented them in a table form (**Table 17.1**).[37]

Many important conclusions emerge out of this review study:

- It is evident that splinting is an elegant method to correct ear deformities in the newborn, but it is unclear whether all deformed ears should be splinted.
- Splinting can be performed in many ways, provided that the ear is kept in the desired shape without distorting it.
- It is disputable until what age splinting therapy can reasonably be offered, considering the expected result, and time and effort that need to be invested. Opinions vary from "newborn only until well up to 3 or 6 months of age".
- It is unfortunate that there is no agreement about this maximum age and that their personal experiences were never clarified by patient data.
- There is no comprehensive evidence on the length of time needed for splinting.

Daniali et al recently presented their experience in a large series of patients treated with custom-made external molding device called EarWell System (Becon Medical Ltd.). They concluded that EarWell System provides consistently efficacious results in correcting lidding, conchal crus, helical rim, prominence, and Stahl deformities, with high rates of good-to-excellent qualitative outcomes.[38]

Kang et al have reported using an implantable clip made of nitinol (nickel-titanium alloy) by the name Earfold System. Long-term results will only prove usefulness and efficacy of any such system (**Fig. 17.6**).[39]

Table 17.1 Various splinting materials and methods used for correction of prominent ear

Author	Year	Splint material
Matsuo	1984	Aluwax® + tape + bandage
	1990	Cryptotia : dynamic splint
Muraoka	1985	Tape only
Brown	1986	Dental Compound(Aluwax) + tape
Bernal-Sprekelsen	1990	Dental Compound or bone wax + tape
Tan/Gault	1994	Soldering wire in 8F catheter + steri-strips + benzoin tincture.
Merlob	1995	Soft, elastic double-faced loop padding (velfoam) + foam strips
Oroz	1995	First: dental compound + Steri-strip. later Steel wire in silicon tube + steri- strip + cap
Tan	1997	Soldering wire in 8F catheter + steri-strip
Yotsuyanagi	1998	Thermoplastic material enclose ear from Posterior and anterior side
Furnas	1999	Benzoin tincture on skin + dental Compound or wire in silastic tube + tape. After few days followed by foam tape Around copper wire core + tape. When Shape is stable: tape only
Ullmann	2001	Putty soft (vinyl polysiloxane) + Steri-strips
Sorribes	2002	Specially designed clamp (night) + double adhesive tape behind ear(day)
Yotsuyanagi	2002	Thermoplastic material enclose ear from posterior + anterior side
Schonauer	2003, 2008	Wire in 6F silastic tube + steri strips
Smith	2005	Wax + Medpore tape
Lindford	2007	Wire in 6F silastic tube + adhesive skin closure strips

Source: Adapted from van Wijk et a.l[37]

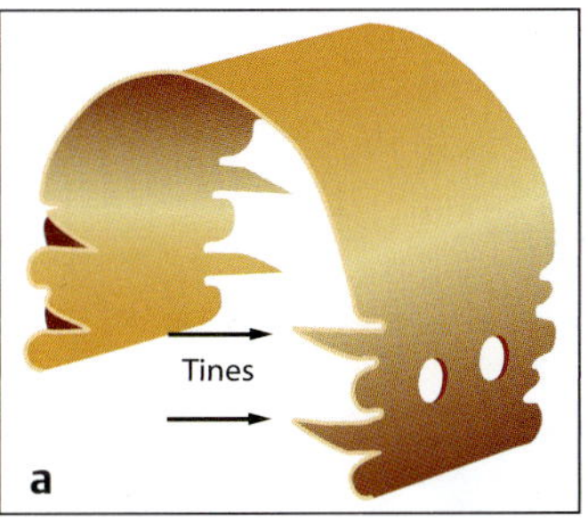

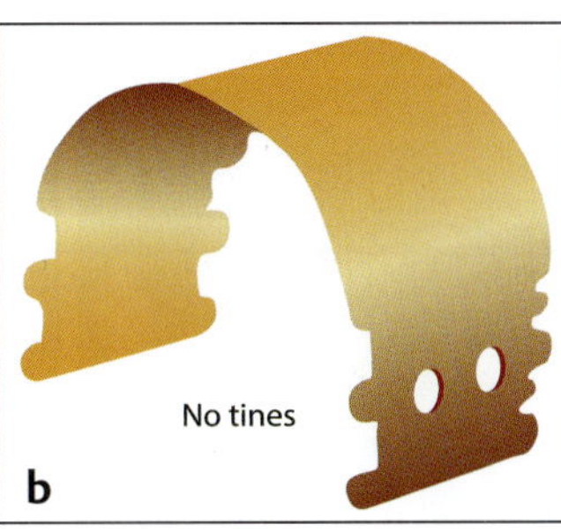

Fig. 17.6 Ear fold system.

Box 17.2 Objectives of surgery for prominent ear (Fig. 17.8)

- To reduce the cephaloauricular angle to 15–20 degrees
- To create an antihelical fold
- To achieve a smooth rim of the helix without interruption of the contours, which means no sharp edges or bends
- Reduce the prominence of conchal bowl
- Proper placement of ear lobule

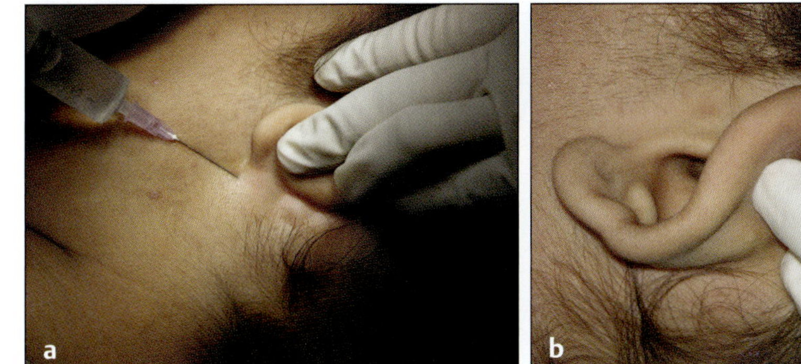

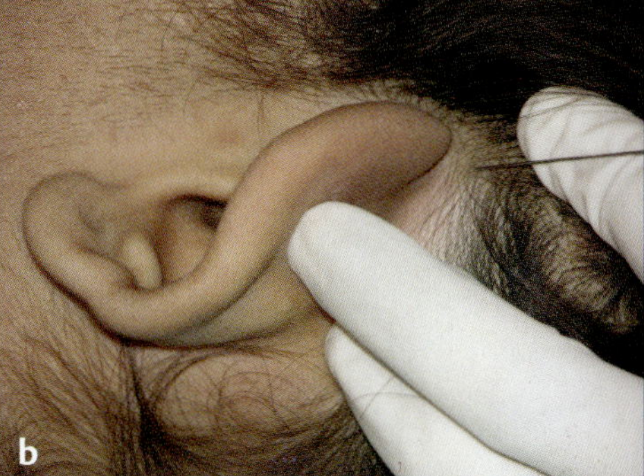

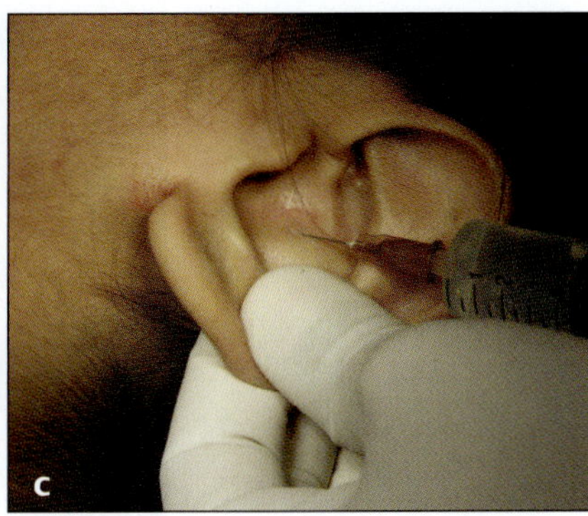

Fig. 17.7 Nerve blocks for the ear. **(a)** Greater auricular nerve block. **(b)** Auriculotemporal nerve block. **(c)** Auricular branch of X cranial nerve block.

Surgical Management

Preoperative Work-up

This includes the Haematological work-up for the fitness for surgery as per the preference of the type of anesthesia.

Timing of Surgery

The appropriate time for the correction of prominent ears depends on factors such as auricular growth, cartilage consistency, psychological strain, and the patient's wishes. The softer the auricular cartilage, the easier it is to shape the cartilage or auricle into the appropriate form and pin it back, using gentle surgical techniques.[40] By the age of 6 years, the ear completes most of its growth; therefore, an otoplasty at this time does usually not affect auricular growth to any significant extent. There is enough evidence in the literature that surgical otoplasty performed during the early years of life did not result in any significant disturbance of auricular growth.[41]

Anesthesia

The surgical correction of protruding ears is recommended to be performed under general anesthesia between the age of 5 and 6 years. However, in older children or adults with adequate compliance, the procedure can be performed under local anesthesia. Knowledge of nerve supply to pinna is essential to give effective nerve block to the ear (**Fig. 17.7**).

Position on Table

The patient's head is placed on the headrest with both the ears exposed. The endotracheal tube is fixed in the midline. Head is draped in such a way that there is access to both the ears simultaneously and the head is mobile freely during the procedure.

Surgical Principles

There are numerous techniques for otoplasty surgery and Naumann has summarized these in his review article in 2007.[42]

Many a times the choice of the surgical technique is made based on the experience of the surgeon with a particular technique. Despite individual preferences, every surgeon performing an otoplasty should have theoretical knowledge and should have practical experience with the various standard techniques (**Box 17.2**).

These objectives cannot be met by using a single technique. Out of many surgical techniques described in literature, one has to choose various combinations, depending on the type and severity of the anomaly. Most of the available techniques for correction of prominent ear can be grouped under following headings:

- Cartilage sparing techniques.
- Cartilage sculpting techniques.
- Combination techniques.
- Flap techniques.
- Lobule correction techniques.

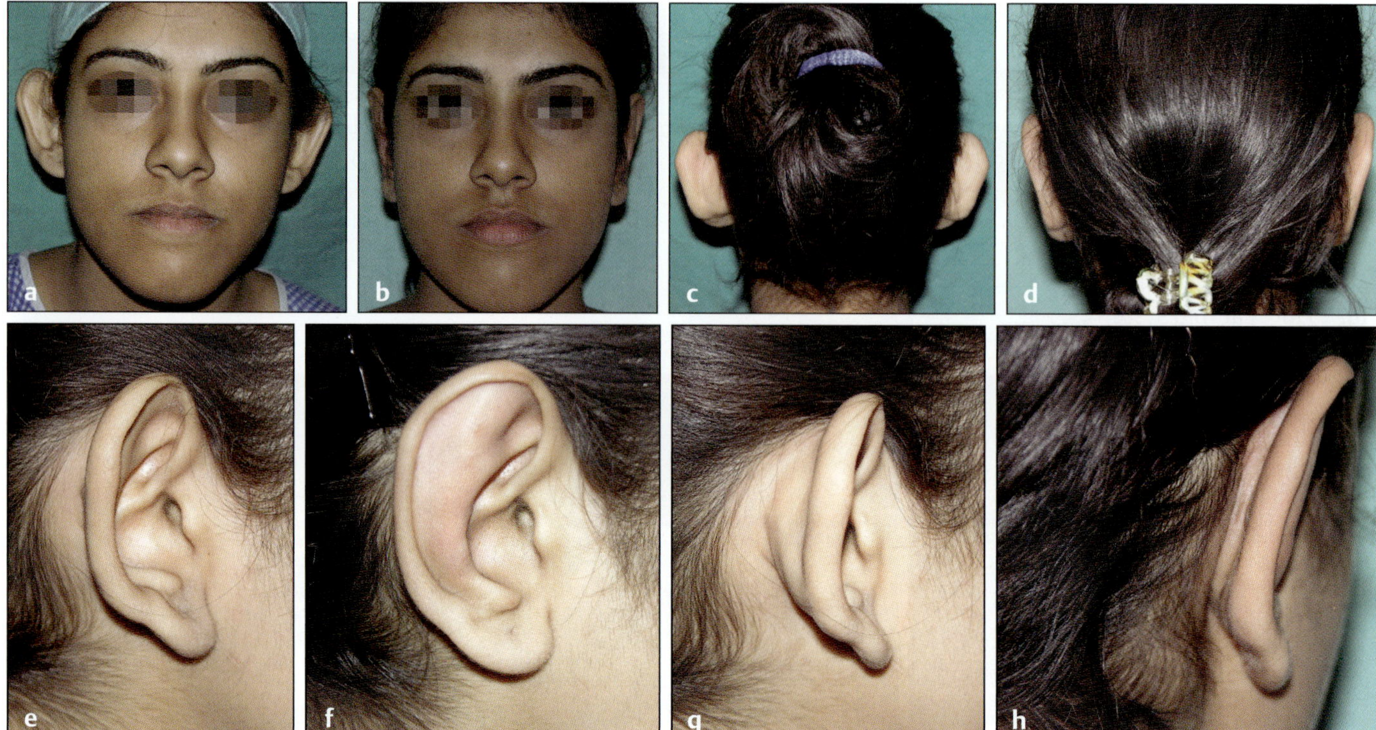

Fig. 17.8 (a–h) Achieving objectives of surgery for prominent ear. Creation of antihelix, approx 20 degree of conchofacial angle, good position of ear lobe, no break in antihelix and reduced prominence of conchal bowl.

For creation of antihelix, the cartilage sparing suture techniques are very useful if the cartilage is very thin and soft. In older children and adults, the auricular cartilage is stiff. In these cases incision techniques either alone or in combination work very well. Concha hypertrophy has to be separately addressed either by direct elliptical excision or suture fixation or a combination of both. In addition to this, the protruding lobule should be addressed by various available techniques.The ultimate goal of correction of prominent ear is highlighted in **Fig 17.8**.

Markings

Proposed antihelical fold is created by gently pressing the pinna backward and the crest of the fold is marked with a marking pen (**Fig. 17.9**). If cartilage cutting technique is planned, the proposed cut line in the cartilage (which is much beyond the proposed antihelical fold is tattooed by passing a 25/24-gauge needle dipped in ink (**Fig. 17.10**). Cartilage tattooing is also done in certain flap techniques as a guide to the extent of dissection and flap elevation. In free margin approach to the anterior surface of the cartilage, no such tattooing is necessary. Skin incision is marked in auriculocephalic sulcus or an ellipse at proper location as per the demand of the technique.

Surgical Exposure

Surgical exposure begins with infiltration of xylocaine 2% with epinephrine on the posterior and anterior surface of ear and incision line.

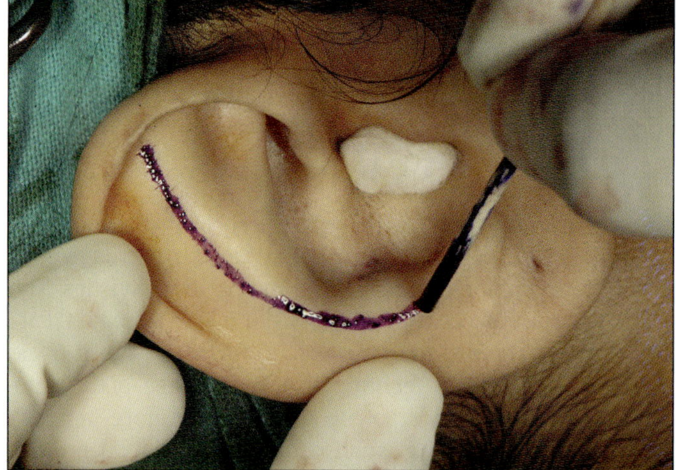

Fig. 17.9 Marking of antihelical fold.

Posterior surface of the auricular cartilage is exposed through incision long enough to give exposure needed at the upper or lower pole (**Fig. 17.11**). Bipolar diathermy is used for hemostasis and use of monopolar is avoided as it can damage the cartilage. The skin excision is not usually planned at this stage unless it is part of the particular technique to be employed. Excessive excision of ellipse of skin should be avoided at all cost as it is the main cause behind the telephone ear deformity. The dissection plane should be supraperichondrial which leaves perichondrium attached to posterior surface of the cartilage (**Fig. 17.12**). Care should be

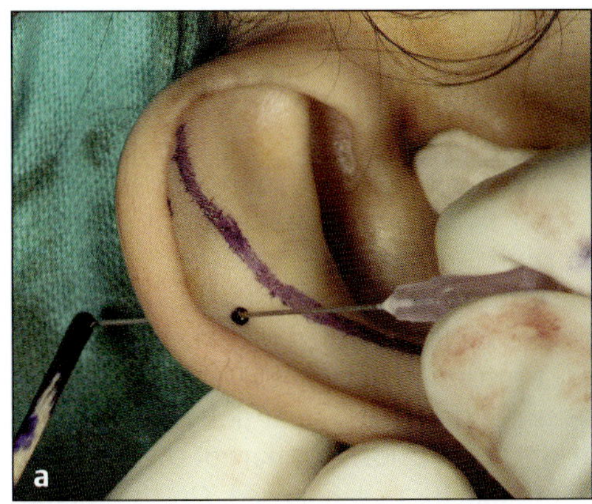

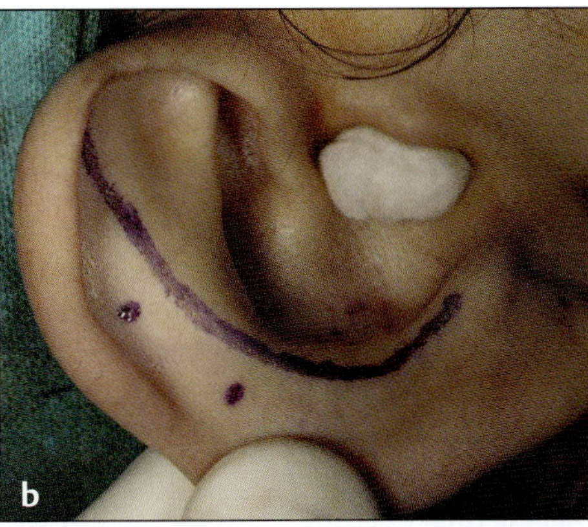

Fig. 17.10 (a, b) Tattoos in the cartilage can help in deciding incision line in anterior scoring techniques.

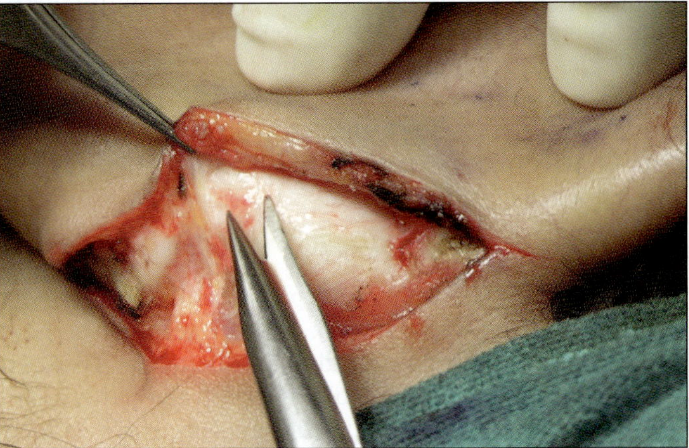

Fig. 17.11 Incision in the sulcus should be long enough to expose the whole posterior surface of cartilage.

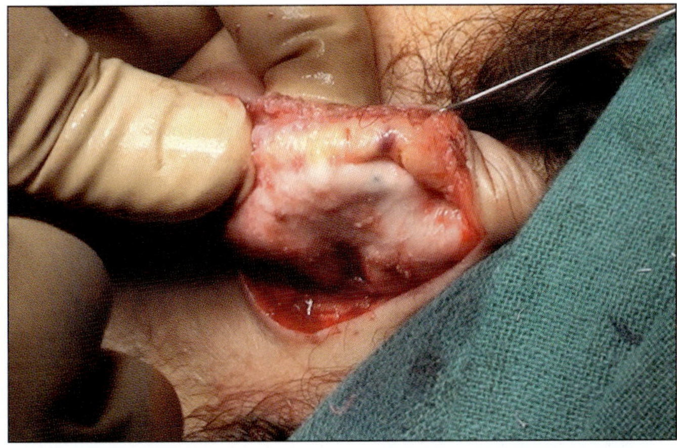

Fig. 17.12 Exposed posterior surface of the cartilage beyond tattoo marks.

taken to identify the posterior surface of the cartilaginous portion of the external auditory canal, to prevent any inadvertent injury. Extent of dissection varies as per the surgical plan.

Suture Techniques

In otoplasty, suture techniques are used for four areas as per the requirements, usually in combination or as an isolated procedure.

- To create antihelix: Conchoscaphoid suture.
- To address deep concha: Conchomastoid suture.
- To address prominent upper pole: Scaphoid fossa-temporalis fascia suture.
- To address prominent earlobe: For medial placement of the lobe, mattress sutures from the fibrofatty tissue of the lobe to the conchal cartilage or to the insertion of the sternocleidomastoid muscle.

Conchoscaphoid (C-S) Suture

In 1963, Mustardé described his otoplasty technique of using multiple conchoscaphoid sutures to create antihelical fold (**Fig. 17.13**). His technique is primarily suitable for soft and thin cartilage, which is generally present in children

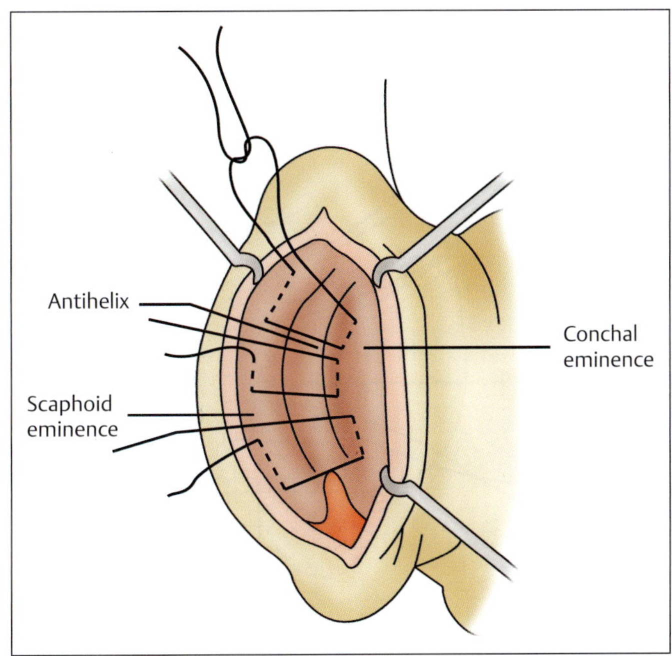

Fig. 17.13 Conchoscaphoid sutures. (Adapted from Mustardé.[43])

up to the age of 10 years. If the cartilage is firmer, there is an increased risk of recurrence with associated possibility of extrusion of mattress sutures. Recurrence rate with suture technique of antihelix plasty is reported to be as high as 25%.[43]

The first mattress suture penetrates the full thickness of the cartilage of the (potential) scaphoid fossa. The bite is wide enough for secure engagement of the cartilage but not so wide as to bend the cartilage on any axis other than the crest of the antihelix. The second bite engages a full thickness of the corresponding conchal cartilage. Mustardé sutures are pulled just tight enough to create the desired antihelix roll. After the complete series of sutures are placed, final position of the ear is checked, sutures are readjusted, knots are tied, and excess sutures are trimmed.

Kaye's modification: An alternative to the posterior approach is placement of a series of tiny incisions anteriorly, through which the mattress sutures are passed through the cartilage, and subcutaneously. The knots are cut anteriorly beneath the skin.[44]

Conchomastoid (C-M) Sutures

They were first reported by Furnas for correction of conchal hypertrophy.[15] They can be used alone or in combination with direct excision of portion of concha depending on the severity of the case. They effectively diminish the distance between the conchal rim and the mastoid area.

The dissection is extended posteriorly in supraperichondrial and submusculoareolar plane to create space to accommodate conchal cup. Mastoid fascia is identified and exposed. Few mattress sutures from posterior conchal wall to the mastoid periosteum will push the conchal bowl into the space created by dissection, effectively reducing the conchomastoid angle (**Fig. 17.14**). These sutures can be used in combination with sutures for creation of antihelix.[45]

Fossa-Fascia (F-F) Suture

Occasionally, the upper pole of a prominent ear is exaggerated in its protrusion and is difficult to correct with the usual combination of Mustardé and C-M sutures. In such situations, direct suturing of the cartilage of the triangular fossa or the scaphoid fossa to the deep temporal fascia provides excellent control over the upper auricular pole.

The ear cartilage of the anteriormost part of the scaphoid fossa and of the triangular fossa is exposed. On the medial side of the sulcus, the superficial temporal fascia is exposed. Manipulate the ear to judge the best sites for suture placement. The superficial temporal fascia then is windowed to expose the deep temporal fascia by scissors-spreading dissection in a vertical direction. One or two carefully placed sutures between cartilage and fascia are usually sufficient, since little resistance is present for the sutures to overcome (**Fig. 17.15a, b**).

Sutures for Prominent Earlobes

Prominent earlobes frequently persist after a prominent auricle has been repositioned. Several techniques have proven useful. Inferiorly extend the postauricular skin incision into the postauricular sulcus. Widen the pattern in a dumbbell shape within the posterior sulcus of the earlobe. Medial placement of the lobe can be enhanced by placing mattress sutures from the fibrofatty tissue of the lobe to the conchal cartilage or to the aponeurotic fibers of the insertion (**Fig. 17.16**).

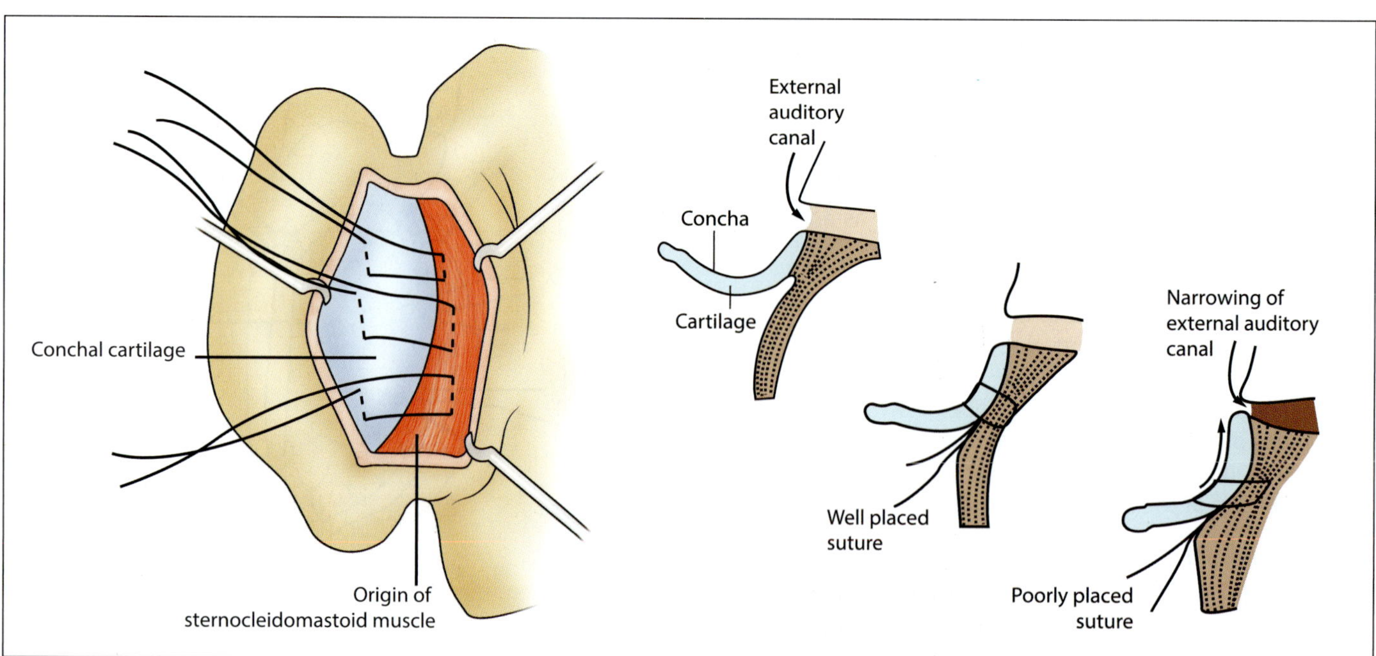

Fig. 17.14 Conchomastoid sutures.[15]

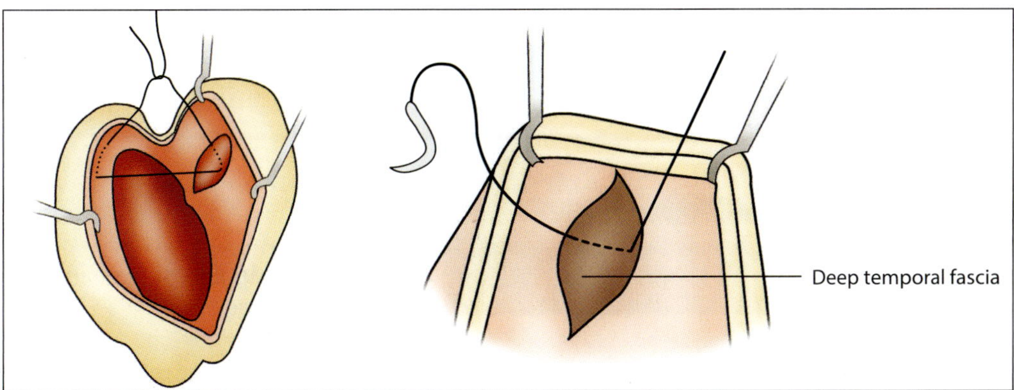

Fig. 17.15 Fossa-fascia suture.

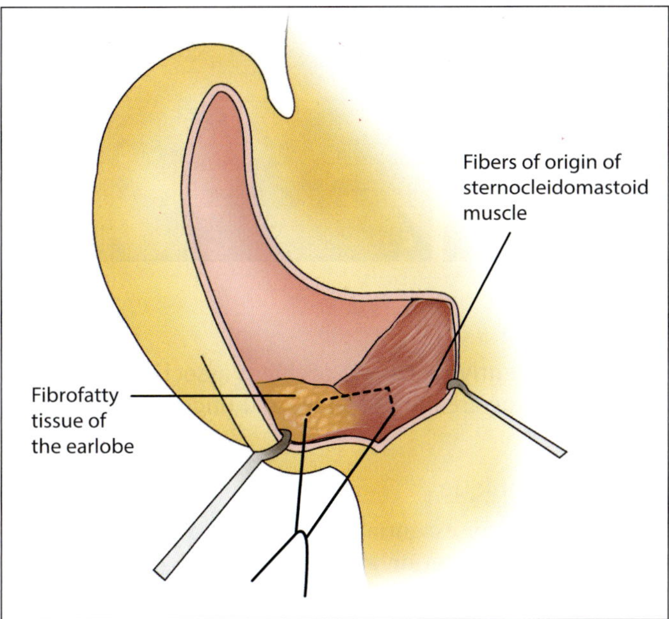

Fig. 17.16 Lobule correction sutures.

Cartilage Sculpting Techniques

In adults, in previously operated patients, in patients with heavy thick cartilages, or as a surgeon's preference, there are different types of cartilage sculpting techniques that are employed. They can be divided into following subgroups:

- Cartilage scoring, abrading techniques.
- Cartilage cutting techniques.

Cartilage Scoring, Abrading Techniques

Most of the cartilage breaking/weakening techniques are based on the studies of Gibson and Davis. The cartilage's tendency to warp to the opposite side of scoring is utilized to achieve antihelix fold. Even though the cartilage is cut in one way or other in all these techniques, they are grouped separately from cartilage cutting techniques as the cut in the cartilage in these is only for accessing the anterior surface and in no way contributing to the antihelix formation. Anterior surface of the cartilage can also be exposed by using free margin of the helix, thus eliminating the need to cut the cartilage for this purpose.[46] The anterior surface of ear cartilage is exposed and prepared to the extent required. Numerous methods and their modifications have been presented over the years which achieve the desired shape of the antihelix and conchal cartilage with scoring, incisions, grinding down with diamond drills, rasps, needles, or Adson-Brown forceps used by the authors to treat antihelix deformity.[47–50] Some of these are summarized in the following text.

Stenström Technique

In this technique, the anterior surface is accessed by creating a subcutaneous tunnel with a dissector through an opening in the cartilage between the cauda helicis and concha. The dissection continues in subperichondrial plane along the crest of the antihelix. A handheld diamond burr is used for abrading the cartilage in proposed antihelix fold area. Excessive abrasion is avoided for the fear of fracture and producing sharp edges. An ellipse of posterior skin is excised and is relied upon to maintain tubing effect. Unfortunately, there was a very high chance of recurrence with this technique.

Chongchet Technique

This technique uses a more invasive correction by degloving the entire anterior surface of cartilage. There is doubt that Chongchet was the originator of this technique.[51] An incision along a premarked tattoo line in the cartilage, approximately 6 to 7 mm away from proposed antihelix crest, gives subperichondrial access to anterior surface. The incision runs almost the entire length of the helical rim. Multiple partial thickness incisions in the cartilage in the axis of antihelix allow cartilage to fold in opposite direction. The technique is very effective since scoring is under vision and much more controlled. Once completed, the cartilage is inserted in the skin pocket and allowed to fold now along with the skin draped on both sides of cartilage. The cartilage fold is evident immediately and can be appreciated on the operation table itself. The cut in the cartilage heals in original position and does not give any telltale sign of surgery (**Fig. 17.17a, b**).

Authors' modification of Chongchet technique involves extensive anterior undermining in subperichondrial plane into conchal bowl, scoring large surface area of cartilage

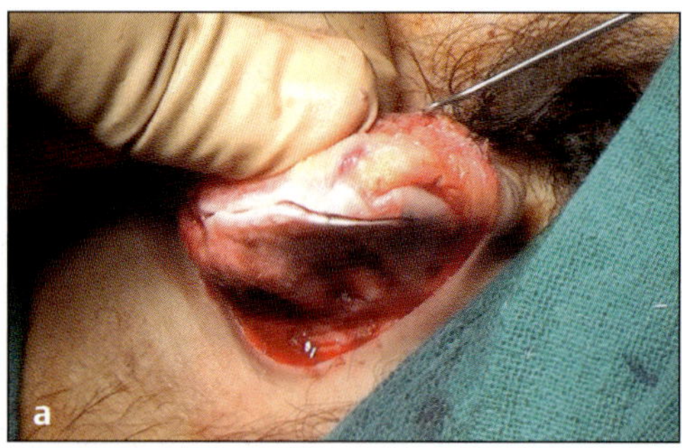

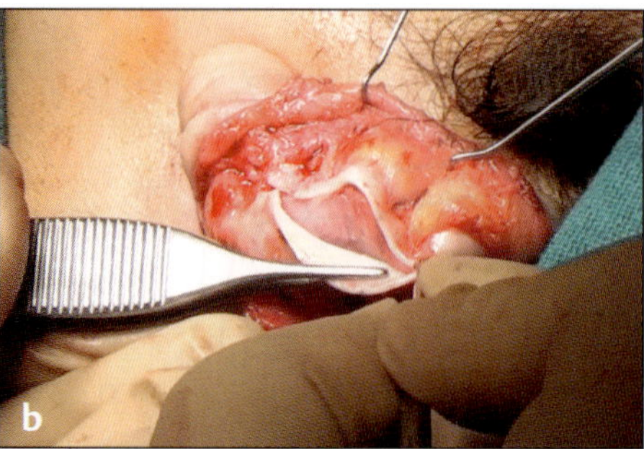

Fig. 17.17 (a, b) Exposure of anterior surface of cartilage.

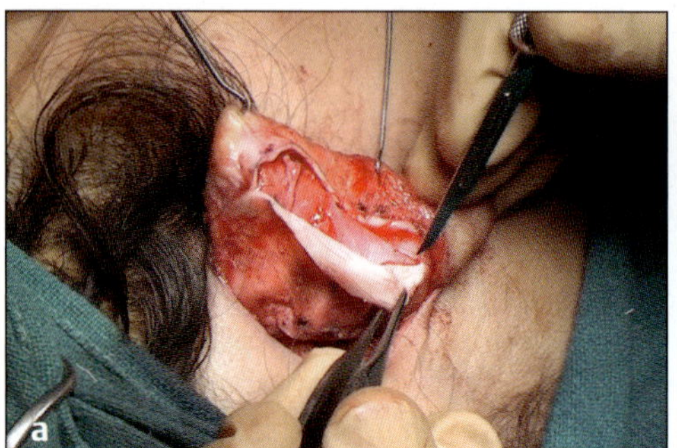

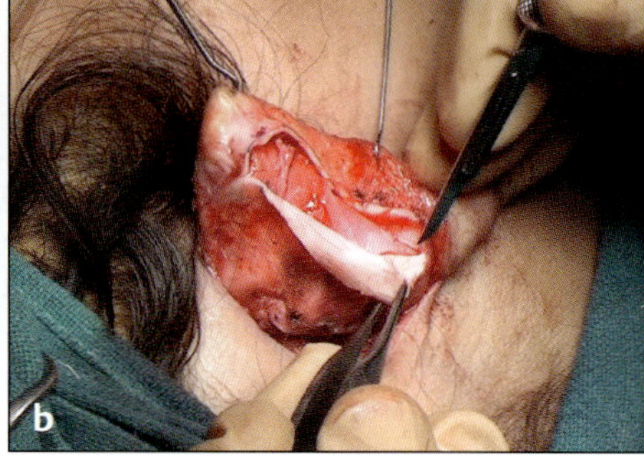

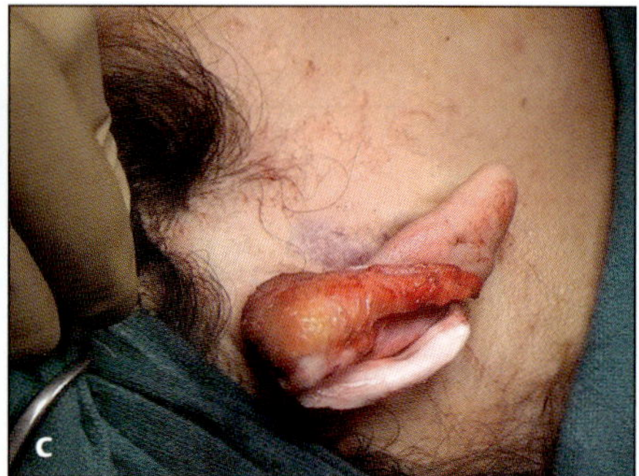

Fig. 17.18 (a–c) Anterior scoring and back cut at lower end to open conchal cup.

extending into conchal bowl, radial cuts at lower end of concha to release the cauda helix and to flatten the deep concha. These maneuvers help in creating sustainable antihelical fold without support of any suture (**Fig. 17.18a, b**).

Crikelair Technique

This is similar to Chongchet technique. Crikelair advocated extensive scoring with cross-hatching.

Cartilage Cutting Techniques

True cartilage cutting techniques re-create the prominence of the antihelix by a combination of cartilage incision, excision, and mobilization and frequently relying on sutures. They are also useful for correction of conchal hypertrophy by direct excision of cartilage. All of these techniques significantly weaken the cartilage frame and potentially lead to deformities that may be difficult to correct. If incisions of the cartilage are made too often, then these lead to an unnaturally sharp profile of the new prominences. All techniques which employ cartilage shaving, abrasion, etc., as a means of weakening the cartilage on posterior surface fall into this category.

Converse Technique

This technique uses a combination of incision and suture to make new antihelix. Using retroauricular approach, two cartilage incisions are placed parallel to the helical rim about 7 to 8 mm apart. Complete transection of the cartilage is done, including the ventral perichondrium. Sutures are used to create a tubular structure by joining two cut edges, which projects outside on the skin surface as antihelix crest. A frequently discussed problem associated with this technique is the creation of sharp and undesirable edges in antihelical area.[52]

Weerda Technique

This technique is essentially a cartilage weakening technique through posterior approach. With a diamond drill, the auricular cartilage is weakened immediately above and below the intended new antihelical fold and the antihelical crus. In addition, full-thickness mattress sutures of polydiaxanone (PDS) are placed to fix the antihelix in the intended position.[53]

Pitanguy Island Technique

This is based on an incision suture technique, in which an incised cartilage island defines the new antihelical prominence.[54–56] After exposure, cartilage island is marked in the region of the antihelix. The marked cartilage is incised all around. Free edges of the incisions are stitched together using absorbable suture material so that the cartilage island overlays the sutures cartilage and defines a new antihelix. This method is associated with various postoperative risks including sharp edges, hematoma, suture dehiscence, and asymmetry. Mayer (2018) modified Pitanguy technique by beveling cartilage island edges to 45 degrees to avoid sharp edges.[57]

Conchal Cartilage Excision Technique

This technique is used to achieve a reduction in height and/or size of the conchal bowl by direct excision of cartilage. An elliptical excision via retroauricular access, away from antihelix and suturing cut edges together, is the most acceptable way of doing it. Any excess anterior skin slowly resolves by shrinkage (**Fig. 17.19a–e**).

Combination Techniques

It is evident from the previous description that no one technique sufficiently covers all possible deformities in a given case. So many authors advocate using combination of techniques. Most favored combination technique is using cartilage sculpting similar to Chongchet together with Furnas conchomastoid suture for prominent concha. Furnas technique is without doubt the best technique to achieve conchal setback with or without direct conchal ellipse resection. Most surgeons recognize this fact and include this as an addition to whatever antihelix plasty technique they are using.[58–60] Opinions vary in use of sutures along with cartilage sculpting. In doing so one is ensuring less chances of recurrence found with pure suture technique. Although one can argue that you are also inviting complications of both techniques like suture extrusion and sharp edges for sculpting techniques.

Flap Techniques

The postauricular fascial flap is the first fascial flap utilized for prominent ear correction as described by Horlock et al in 2001.[61] Postauricular fascia is a distinct layer of intrinsic fascia in the posterior surface of the ear which extends as extrinsic postauricular fascia in the mastoid region. Horlock successfully used this flap for covering the Mustardé sutures in order to reduce the complications with these sutures. Taş has summarized all the flaps used in otoplasty in a comprehensive review article.[62] While most of the early authors used these flaps in conjunction with Mustardé technique, more recently these flaps are used as standalone procedure either as proximally based or distally based flaps.

Taş et al[63] used a proximally based dermofascioperichondrial flap technique to re-create the antihelix. Unlike previously described flap techniques, the fascial flap in this technique is used to reconstruct the antihelical fold without additional suturing or scoring methods. A crescentic shape skin excision is planned and marked on proposed antihelix. Skin is excised almost like a full-thickness skin graft. A proximally based flap is raised in subperichondrial plane by incising distal border of dermal crescent down to perichondrium. The distal dissection is carried out from the same incision in supraperichondrial plane. The proximal flap is now advanced in this pocket over the perichondrium in antihelix area and sutured to the distal margin of new antihelix. The skin now overlies the de-epithelized portion of crescent, bringing the skin margins in close approximation for suturing (**Fig. 17.20a–d**).

Cihandide et al[64] in a similar operation used distally based flap and added cartilage scoring ensuring better folding of cartilage and less chances of recurrence. The skin ellipse is marked centered over new antihelical fold. Skin excision is performed in a full-thickness skin graft fashion. The soft tissue and perichondrium is incised with the help of no. 15 blade along the proximal border of defect. The perichondrio-adipo-dermal flap is raised in subperichondrial plane. To create a natural-looking antihelical fold and scapha and to form a smooth transition between them, this flap is elevated 2 to 5 mm distal to the antihelical fold markings projected on the cartilage. Proximal dissection is in subcutaneous plane till mastoid region. Exposed cartilage in antihelix region is scored and the flap is advanced in proximal pocket and sutured to mastoid fascia, thus creating a fold of cartilage in antihelix region (**Fig. 17.21**).

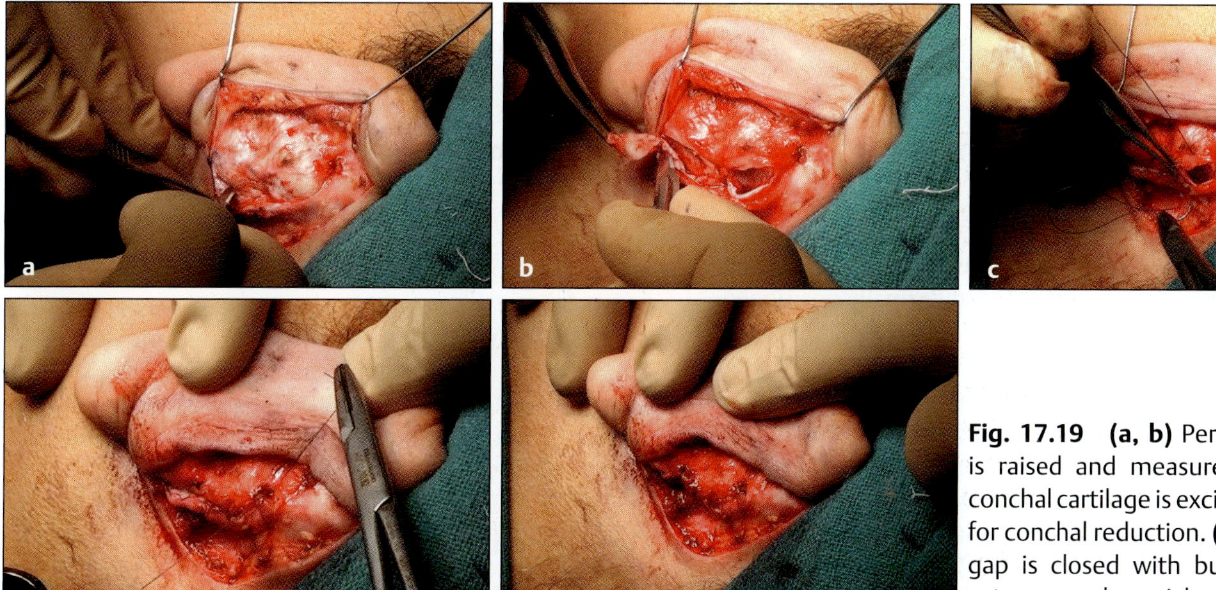

Fig. 17.19 **(a, b)** Perichondrial flap is raised and measured amount of conchal cartilage is excised from fossa for conchal reduction. **(c–e)** Cartilage gap is closed with buried mattress sutures and perichondrial flap is sutured over it.

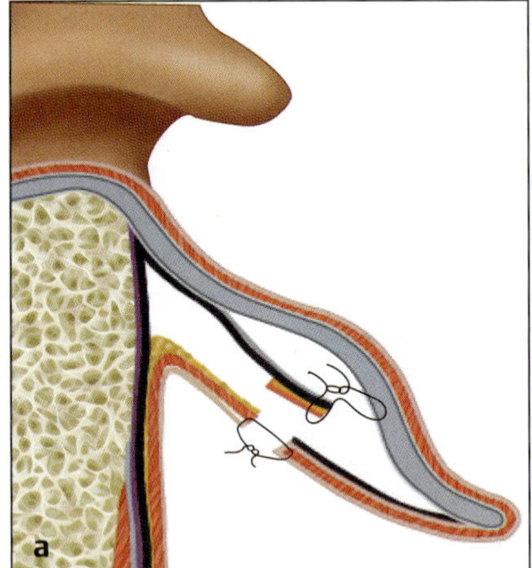

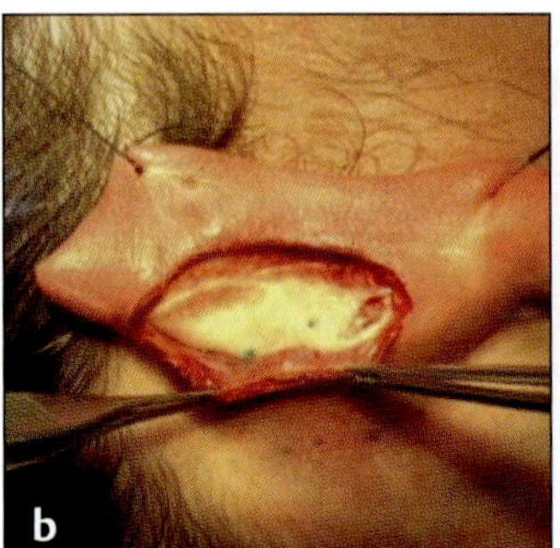

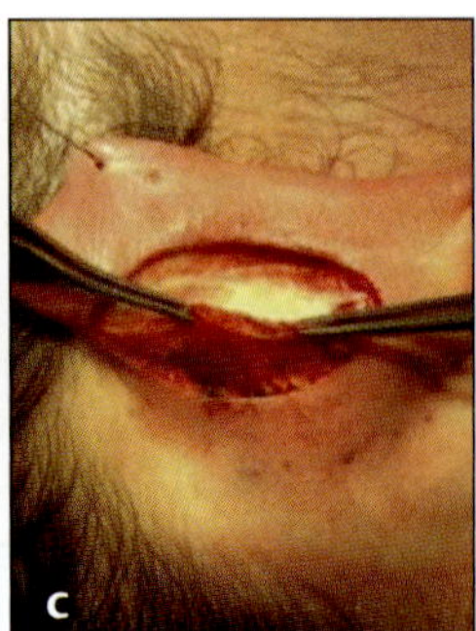

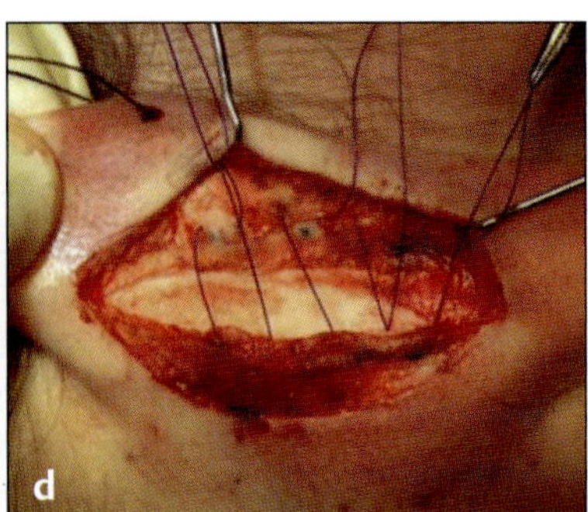

Fig. 17.20 (a–d) Proximally based dermo-fascio-perichondrial flap.

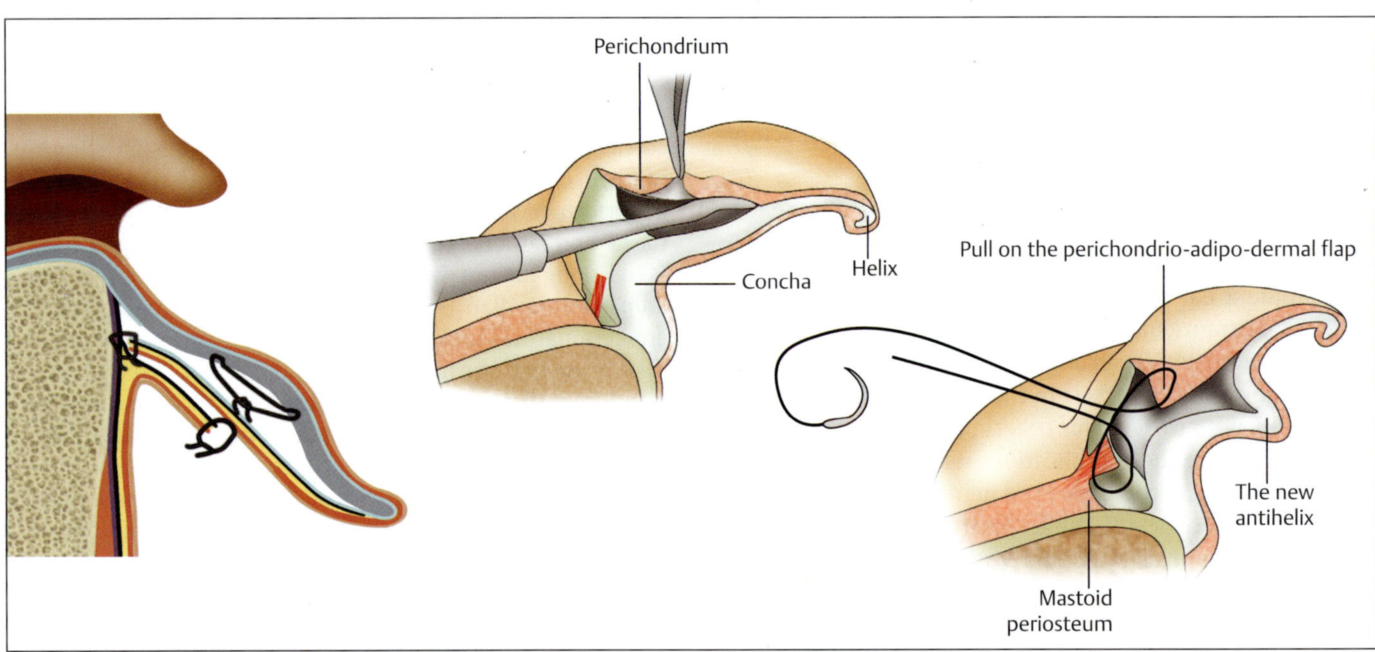

Fig. 17.21 Distally based perichondrio-adipo-dermal flap.

Techniques to Correct Protruded Lobe

A prominent lobule can be caused by medial skin excess or an abnormal caudal helicis. Correct diagnosis is essential for proper treatment. Palpation of the lobule reveals either flaccid soft tissue or a firm, long, and abnormally positioned cauda helicis. In the latter case, simple resection of the cauda helicis corrects lobule position.

For aesthetic reasons, the lobule should be adjusted parallel to plane of the upper third of the ear. To correct lobule retroauricular skin incision can easily be extended to the middle of the lobule, and subsequently skin excisions can be performed to the extent required. Many types of skin excisions, (e.g., in the shape of a fishtail, a Z-plasty, or an ellipse), in combination with fat resection in the area of the lobule have been suggested.

Skin-suture techniques alone cannot guarantee successful long-term result due to the natural elasticity of the lobular skin. Hence a suture technique described earlier should be used when applicable.

Recent Advances

Techniques will continue to be refined with an attempt to re-create the normal appearance of the ear with minimal possible incisions and the shortest recovery time.

Laser Otoplasty

Leclère et al[65] evaluated the efficacy of laser-assisted cartilage reshaping (LACR) for prominent ears using three different wavelengths: 1,064 nm (Nd:YAG), 10,600 nm (CO_2), and 1,540 nm (Er:Glass) in seven clinical studies. The success rate for ear reshaping achieved with LACR appears promising and is expected to have positive role in future. Authors are the first ones to report clinical LACR after extensive animal research. As per their experiments wavelength 1,540 nm is ideal for cartilage reshaping.

Fengfeng et al in an article published in a Chinese journal of plastic surgery in 2018 have details of parameters of various lasers which can be used for ear reshaping.[66]

Minimally Invasive Otoplasty

Over the past few years, there have been increasing calls for minimally invasive methods of otoplasty. The idea is to reduce postoperative risks, including hematoma and scarring.

Fritsch described a suture-only technique, creating a new antihelical fold with percutaneously placed and subcutaneously laid horizontal mattress sutures without an incision.[67]

Peled explained an “incision-free otoplasty,” combining a suture technique similar to that of Fritsch with blind scoring of the anterior antihelix via a small skin incision in the area of the anterior cauda helicis.[68]

Graham and Gault described a minimally invasive endoscopic-assisted method.[69] A small skin incision in the upper hairline above the auricle is made to introduce the endoscope. The cartilage in the area of the new antihelix is scored blindly from a retroauricular approach. In addition, a scapha-mastoid nonabsorbable suture is placed via small, retroauricular incisions.

Raunig did gentle weakening of the antihelical and conchal cartilage with a special diamond rasp inserted via small skin incisions at the inner side of the upper helical rim and at the caudal antihelix.[70] He relied on postoperative pressure bands to shape the ear.

Benedict and Pirwitz combined subcutaneously placed cartilage-penetrating nonabsorbable mattress sutures and blind scoring of the anterior antihelix cartilage with a scoring instrument.[71] Haytoğlu in a large series published recently compared patients with and without cartilage abrasion in incisionless otoplasty and found that there is no statistical difference in two groups of patients.[72]

Closure, Dressing, and Postoperative Care

Once the desired changes have been made to the cartilaginous contour, the skin flap is redraped. Skin is closed with interrupted sutures, which allows any collected blood to ooze out in between spaces.

Dressing needs utmost care. All the contours are filled with antibiotic impregnated paraffin gauge or antibiotic impregnated yellow wool (soft cotton made in acriflavin). With these measures, the contour of the newly formed auricle is stabilized. After soft padding a compressive double mastoid dressing is applied, preferably using a crepe bandage. Excessive pressure should be carefully avoided as it can lead to disastrous consequences.

The first dressing is usually changed on the second postoperative day to rule out a possible hematoma which if recognized early can be drained without consequences. Next dressing is changed only after about a week. Some surgeons do not like to disturb the dressing till about a week as by that time skin sticks back into the contours.

At the seventh to eighth postoperative day, the sutures are removed or trimmed if they are absorbable and the dressing is replaced with a headband. The headband should be worn for another 4 to 6 weeks, at least at night, to prevent accidental kinking of the auricle(**Fig. 17.22**). Headbands apart from maintaining the shape help in decreasing the edema as well.

Follow-up

The assessment of measurements is done in immediate postop and then at 1 month, 3 months, 6 months, and at 1 year. Measurements are done at three levels: upper, middle, and lower as described above. Follow-up photographs are taken during each visit with standard views for comparison.

Ear-to-ear symmetry is compared by measures between two sides. Symmetry is considered as excellent if the difference between two sides measure is no more than 2 mm at any of the three recorded levels, good if it is not more than 4 mm, and poor if it is more than 4 mm at any of the levels.[73]

Complications

Immediate Complications

Hematoma

Haematoma formation is more common with cartilage weakening techniques. Excessive pain soon after the surgery is the earliest indication of a developing hematoma.[74]

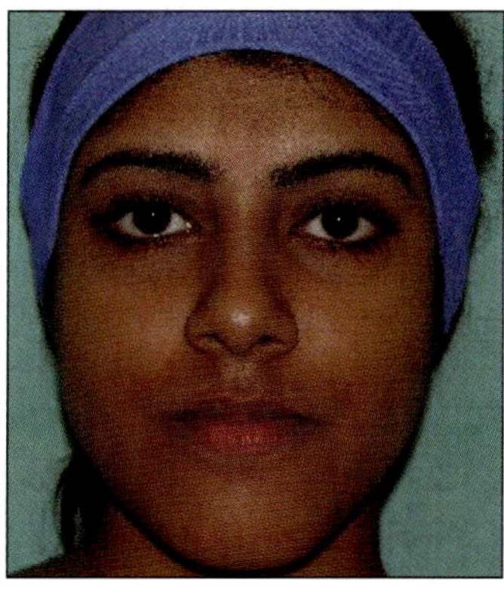

Fig. 17.22 Head band to be used for 4 to 6 weeks.

Conclusion

Prominent ear or bat ear is a congenital external auricle deformity which can be a source of great psychological distress in either sex and at any age. The most common causes of protrusion of the external ear are an underdeveloped or absent antihelix, an overdeveloped or deep concha, or a combination of both of these features.

The goal of otoplasty technique for prominent ear correction is to achieve natural appearing symmetrical auricles. Worldwide, cartilage sculpting technique is the most practiced surgical procedure. Thorough preoperative assessment of the deformity with good photographic records, precise carefully individualized surgical technique, taking care of not to create sharp edges, and meticulous hemostasis are the keys for a successful outcome. Diligent postoperative care in the initial months is the key to prevent complications and recurrence in this gratifying surgery. There are studies to indicate that patients, who had undergone otoplasty, showed an improved quality of life post surgery.

References

1. Dieffenbach JF. Die operative Chirurgie. Leipzig: FA Brockhaus; 1845
2. Ely ET. An operation for prominent auricles. Arch Otolaryngol 1881;10:97. Reprinted in Plast Reconstr Surg 1968;42:582–583
3. Keen WW. New method of operating for relief of deformity of prominent ears. Ann Surg 1890;11(1):49–51
4. Gersuny R. Über einige kosmetische Operationen. Wien Med Wochenschr 1903;53:2253
5. Luckett WH. A new operation for prominent ears based on the anatomy of the deformity. Surg Gynecol Obstet 1910;10: 635–637
6. Becker OJ. Correction of the protruding deformed ear. Br J Plast Surg 1952;5(3):187–196
7. Gibson T, Davis WB. The distortion of autogenous cartilage grafts: its cause and prevention. Br J Plast Surg 1958;10: 257–274
8. Converse JM, Nigro A, Wilson FA, Johnson N. A technique for surgical correction of lop ears. Plast Reconstr Surg (1946) 1955;15(5):411–418
9. Converse JM, Wood-Smith D. Technical details in the surgical correction of the lop ear deformity. Plast Reconstr Surg 1963;31:118–128
10. Chongchet V. A method of antihelix reconstruction. Br J Plast Surg 1963;16:268–272
11. Stenström SJ. "Natural" technique for correction of congenitally prominent ears. Plast Reconstr Surg 1963;32:509–518
12. Crikelair GF, Cosman B. Another solution for the problem of the prominent ear. Ann Surg 1964;160:314–324
13. Mustardé JC. The correction of prominent ears using simple mattress sutures. Br J Plast Surg 1963;16:170–178
14. Morestin MH. DE La Reposition et du plissementcosmetiques du pavilllion de l'orelle. Rev Orthop 1903;4:289
15. Furnas DW. Correction of prominent ears by conchamastoid sutures. Plast Reconstr Surg 1968;42(3):189–193
16. Spira M, McCrea R, Gerow FJ, Hardy SB. Correction of the principal deformities causing protruding ears. Plast Reconstr Surg 1969;44(2):150–154
17. Wood-Smith D. Otoplasty. In: Rees T, ed. Aesthetic plastic surgery. Philadelphia: Saunders; 1980:833
18. Siegert R. Correction of the lobule. Facial Plast Surg 2004;20(4): 293–298
19. Wodak E. On the position and shape of the human auricle. Arch Klin Exp Ohren Nasen Kehlkopfheilkd 1967;188(2):331–335
20. Farkas LG. Anthropometry of the normal and defective ear. Clin Plast Surg 1990;17(2):213–221
21. Farkas LG. Anthropometry of normal and anomalous ears. Clin Plast Surg 1978;5(3):401–412
22. Tolleth H. Artistic anatomy, dimensions, and proportions of the external ear. Clin Plast Surg 1978;5(3):337–345
23. Tolleth H. A hierarchy of values in the design and construction of the ear. Clin Plast Surg 1990;17(2):193–207
24. Bozkir MG, Karakaş P, Yavuz M, Dere F. Morphometry of the external ear in our adult population. Aesthetic Plast Surg 2006;30(1):81–85
25. Janis JE, Rohrich RJ, Gutowski KA. Otoplasty. Plast Reconstr Surg 2005;115(4):60e–72e
26. Takemori S, Tanaka Y, Suzuki JI. Thalidomide anomalies of the ear. Arch Otolaryngol 1976;102(7):425–427
27. Siegert R, Krappen S, Kaesemann L, Weerda H. Computer assisted anthropometry of the auricle. Face 1998;6:1–6
28. Muteweye W, Muguti GI. Prominent ears: anthropometric study of the external ear of primary school children of Harare, Zimbabwe. Ann Med Surg (Lond) 2015;4(3):287–292
29. Weerda H. Classification of congenital deformities of the auricle. Facial Plast Surg 1988;5(5):385–388
30. Lee Y, Kim YS, Lee WJ, Rha DK, Kim J. Proposal of a classification system for the assessment and treatment of prominent ear deformity. Aesthetic Plast Surg 2018;42(3):759–765
31. Schwentner I, Schmutzhard J, Deibl M, Sprinzl GM. Health-related quality of life outcome of adult patients after otoplasty. J Craniofac Surg 2006;17(4):629–635
32. Sirin S, Abaci F, Selcuk A, Findik OB, Yildirim A. Psychosocial effects of otoplasty in adult patients: a prospective cohort study. Eur Arch Otorhinolaryngol 2019;276(5):1533–1539
33. Kurozumi N, Ono S, Ishida H. Non-surgical correction of a congenital lop ear deformity by splinting with Reston foam. Br J Plast Surg 1982;35(2):181–182
34. Matsuo K, Hirose T, Tomono T, et al. Nonsurgical correction of congenital auricular deformities in the early neonate: a preliminary report. Plast Reconstr Surg 1984;73(1):38–51
35. Yotsuyanagi T, Yokoi K, Sakuraba M, Sugawara M. The use of a thermoplastic splint for treating cryptotia. Jpn J Plast Surg 1993;36:1037–1042
36. Yotsuyanagi T, Yokoi K, Urushidate S, Sawada Y. Nonsurgical correction of congenital auricular deformities in children older than early neonates. Plast Reconstr Surg 1998;101(4):907–914
37. van Wijk MP, Breugem CC, Kon M. Non-surgical correction of congenital deformities of the auricle: a systematic review of the literature. J Plast Reconstr Aesthet Surg 2009;62(6): 727–736
38. Daniali LN, Rezzadeh K, Shell C, Trovato M, Ha R, Byrd HS. Classification of newborn ear malformations and their treatment with the earwell infant ear correction system. Plast Reconstr Surg 2017;139(3):681–691
39. Kang NV, Sabbagh W, O'Toole G, Silberberg M. Earfold: a new technique for correction of the shape of the antihelix. Laryngoscope 2018;128(10):2282–2290
40. Gosain AK, Recinos RF. Otoplasty in children less than four years of age: surgical technique. J Craniofac Surg 2002;13(4): 505–509

41. Gosain AK, Kumar A, Huang G. Prominent ears in children younger than 4 years of age: what is the appropriate timing for otoplasty? Plast Reconstr Surg 2004;114(5):1042–1054
42. Naumann A. Otoplasty: techniques, characteristics and risks. GMS Curr Top Otorhinolaryngol Head Neck Surg 2007;6:Doc04
43. Mustardé JC. The treatment of prominent ears by buried mattress sutures: a ten-year survey. Plast Reconstr Surg 1967;39(4):382–386
44. Kaye BL, Kaye BL. A simplified method for correcting the prominent ear. Plast Reconstr Surg 1967;40(1):44–48
45. Furnas DW. Correction of prominent ears with multiple sutures. Clin Plast Surg 1978;5(3):491–495
46. Ahmed M, Alkhalaf H, Ibrahim E. Helix free otoplasty for correction of prominent ear. Asian J Surg 2019;42(5):621–627
47. Bulstrode NW, Huang S, Martin DL. Otoplasty by percutaneous anterior scoring. Another twist to the story: a long-term study of 114 patients. Br J Plast Surg 2003;56(2):145–149
48. Peker F, Celiköz B. Otoplasty: anterior scoring and posterior rolling technique in adults. Aesthetic Plast Surg 2002;26(4): 267–273
49. Elliott RA Jr. Otoplasty: a combined approach. Clin Plast Surg 1990;17(2):373–381
50. Keramidas EG. The use of Adson-Brown forceps to score the cartilage in otoplasty. Plast Reconstr Surg 2006;118(1):263
51. Maisels DO. Anterior scoring for bat ears; the story so far. Br J Plast Surg 1990;43(3):349
52. Staindl O. Failures and complications following otoplasty. Laryngol Rhinol Otol (Stuttg) 1986;65(11):646–651
53. Weerda H. Chirurgie der Ohrmuschel. Bd. 1 Stuttgart: Thieme; 2004
54. Pitanguy I, Cansancao A, D'Andrea S, Avelar JM. Orelhas em abano. Rev Bras Cir 1971;61:158
55. Pitanguy I, Müller P, Piccolo N, Ramalho E, Solinas R. The treatment of prominent ears: a 25-year survey of the island technique. Aesthetic Plast Surg 1987;11(2):87–93
56. Pitanguy I, Fiazza G, Calixto CA, Müller PM, Caldeira AM, Alexandrino A. Prominent ears: Pitanguy's island technique: long-term results. Head Neck Surg 1985;7(5):418–426
57. Mayer HF, Loustau HD. Modified island technique for prominent ears. Aesthet Plast Surg 2018;42:159–164
58. Bauer BS, Song DH, Aitken ME. Combined otoplasty technique: chondrocutaneous conchal resection as the cornerstone to correction of the prominent ear. Plast Reconstr Surg 2002; 110(4):1033–1040, discussion 1041
59. Andjelkov K, Sforza M, Zaccheddu R, Lazović G, Colić M. No recurrence in otoplasty: is that possible? Srp Arh Celok Lek 2010;138(9–10):546–550
60. Koul AR, Patil RK. An effective technique of helical cartilage scoring for correction of prominent ear deformity. Indian J Plast Surg 2011;44(3):505–508
61. Horlock N, Misra A, Gault DT. The postauricular fascial flap as an adjunct to Mustardé and Furnas type otoplasty. Plast Reconstr Surg 2001;108(6):1487–1490, discussion 1491
62. Taş S. Prominent ear correction: a comprehensive review of fascial flaps in otoplasty. Aesthet Surg J 2018;38(7):695–704
63. Taş S, Benlier E. A new way for antihelixplasty in prominent ear surgery: modified postauricular fascial flap. Ann Plast Surg 2016;76(6):615–621
64. Cihandide E, Kayiran O, Aydin EE, Uzunismail A. A new approach for the correction of prominent ear deformity: the distally based perichondrio-adipo-dermal flap technique. J Craniofac Surg 2016;27(4):892–897
65. Leclère FM, Vogt PM, Casoli V, Vlachos S, Mordon S. Laser-assisted cartilage reshaping for protruding ears: a review of the clinical applications. Laryngoscope 2015;125(9):2067–2071
66. Fengfeng G, Xiaobo Y, Haiyue J. Advances in clinical application of laser-assisted cartilage reshaping technique for correcting ears. Chinese J Restorative Reconstr Surg 2018;32(6):769–772
67. Fritsch MH. Incisionless otoplasty. Laryngoscope 1995; 105(5 Pt 3, Suppl 70):1–11
68. Peled IJ. Knifeless otoplasty: how simple can it be? Aesthetic Plast Surg 1995;19(3):253–255
69. Graham KE, Gault DT. Endoscopic assisted otoplasty: a preliminary report. Br J Plast Surg 1997;50(1):47–57
70. Raunig H. Antihelix plasty without modeling sutures. Arch Facial Plast Surg 2005;7(5):334–341
71. Benedict M, Pirwitz KU. Minimally invasive otoplasty. HNO 2005;53(3):230–237
72. Haytoglu S, Haytoglu TG, Yildirim I, Arikan OK. A modification of incisionless otoplasty for correcting the prominent ear deformity. Eur Arch Otorhinolaryngol 2015;272(11):3425–3430
73. Ghozlan NA. Otoplasty: a cartilage sculpting technique. Egypt J Plast Reconstr Surg 2008;32(1):145–151
74. Elliott RA Jr. Complications in the treatment of prominent ears. Clin Plast Surg 1978;5(3):479–490
75. Rajbhandari S. Repair of constricted ear. Research J Ear Nose Throat 2018;2(1):5
76. Cosman B. The constricted ear. Clin Plast Surg 1978;5(3): 389–400
77. Ferraro GA, Perrotta A, Rossano F, D'Andrea F. Stahl syndrome in clinical practice. Aesthetic Plast Surg 2006;30(3):348–349, discussion 350
78. Gleizal A, Bachelet JT. Aetiology, pathogenesis, and specific management of Stahl's ear: role of the transverse muscle insertion. Br J Oral Maxillofac Surg 2013;51(8):e230–e233
79. Yotsuyanagi T, Nihei Y, Shinmyo Y, Sawada Y. Stahl's ear caused by an abnormal intrinsic auricular muscle. Plast Reconstr Surg 1999;103(1):171–174
80. Kaplan HM, Hudson DA. A novel surgical method of repair for Stahl's ear: a case report and review of current treatment modalities. Plast Reconstr Surg 1999;103(2):566–569
81. Yotsuyanagi T, Yamashita K, Shinmyo Y, Yokoi K, Sawada Y. A new operative method of correcting cryptotia using large Z-plasty. Br J Plast Surg 2001;54(1):20–24
82. Marsh D, Sabbagh W, Gault D. Cryptotia correction: the post-auricular transposition flap. J Plast Reconstr Aesthet Surg 2011;64(11):1444–1447
83. Xu JH, Wu WH, Tan WQ. Surgical correction of cryptotia with the square flap method: a preliminary report. Scand J Plast Reconstr Surg Hand Surg 2009;43(1):29–35
84. Kajikawa A, Ueda K, Asai E, Ohkouchi H, Katsuragi Y. A new surgical correction of cryptotia: a new flap design and switched double banner flap. Plast Reconstr Surg 2009;123(3):897–901
85. Sakamoto Y, Nakajima H, Kishi K, Imanishi N. A new surgical correction of cryptotia with superior auricular myocutaneous flap. J Plast Reconstr Aesthet Surg 2010;63(12):1995–2000

18

Role of Fat Grafting in Facial Aesthetics

Satyaswarup Tripathy, Ranjit Kumar Sahu, and Subair Mohsina

Introduction

Fat grafting has become one of the most popular tools in the armamentarium of plastic surgeons to correct the congenital or acquired contour deformities of face as well as in facial rejuvenation.[1,2] There is loss of volume in congenital craniofacial syndromes and in acquired conditions such as trauma, infection, drug-related lipodystrophy, etc.[3–5] The concept of facial aging has also evolved from the traditional concept of loss of elasticity to a loss of volume support in the face.[6,7] The loss of a youthful face or contour deformities have been found to be associated with body discomfort, low self-esteem, and even depression in many patients.[8,9] These are three-dimensional deformities which require surgeons' imagination and creativity and are challenging. These have been addressed with implants or injectable fillers; however, they lacked a natural feel, had the foreign-body related risk, and were not amenable to subtle manipulations.[10] In the quest of a suitable filling material for facial defects, fat has emerged as a panacea due to its regenerative and healing properties.

Fat is autologous, found abundantly in body, safe to inject and can be repeated if required.[1] It has wider applications in different clinical scenarios. Fat contains mature adipocytes, adipose-derived stem cells (ADSC), and stromal vascular fraction (SVF) which help in filling as well as remodeling.[11–13] It provides bulk to the paralyzed atrophic muscle as well as support to the underlying scars. It brings in good capillary network and induces better healing in facial scars; hence, fat can be used to bring back a person's glorious past. For satisfactory results of fat grafting, a thorough understanding of the disease process, the basic anatomy of the facial contours, as well as reliable technique to ensure fat survival is essential. These aspects will be discussed in detail in the chapter.

History of Fat Grafting

The technique of fat grafting has undergone a sea change in its evolution since its first description in 1893 by the German surgeon Gustav Neuber.[2] He used fat from the arm for a postinfective infraorbital scar. This was followed by Vincent Czerny, in 1895, who transferred a gluteal lipoma to breast in a case of partial mastectomy.[14] These early reports transferred chunks of fat, similar to dermal graft. However, due to long-term unpredictable resorption rates, it fell out of vogue. The revolutionary change was brought in by Eugen Hollander in 1912 triggered by the complication rates following paraffin injection as fillers.[15] He suggested injection of human fat mixed with ram fat to improve survival. This was then followed by Miller in 1926, who described fat injection through hollow cannulas.[16] Although its regenerative potential was identified, attempts by Lexer and Gilles, in 1920s, demonstrated early encouraging results in patients with hemifacial microsomia and severe facial disfigurement.[17,18] However, these early results were found to be worsening over time due to resorption or formation of fibrotic masses. This led to an era of decline in fat grafting in the 1930s.[18] Because of this disrepute of fat grafting, many other types of filler cropped up in the kitty of plastic surgeons such as paraffin, silicone, gutta-percha, and rubber sponges.

The work of Illouz in the year 1980 in the field of liposuction revived the interest in fat grafting.[19] The use of a small bore cannula to remove fat from body by a minimally invasive technique was the harbinger of body contouring and fat grafting. In this way, fat was available in liquid form instead of removing en bloc fatty tissue; however, resorption rates remained high. It was Sydney R. Coleman in 1994 who standardized the approach for fat grafting, which he termed as "Liposculpture."[20,21] This process of *structural fat grafting* underscores the importance of gentle harvest, centrifugation, and injection of fat in small aliquots in different planes.[21,22] This technique still remains the gold standard with improved graft survival rates and hence pleasing aesthetic results. It further evolved with the discovery of SVF in the lipoaspirate. SVF is a potential source of ADSCs which are pluripotent and with wide regenerative potential.[11,12] This explains the role of fat in healing or replacing damaged tissues and its role in regenerative medicine. Further modifications in the harvest and delivery technique have been used for finer scars and wrinkles in the form of micro and nanofat grafting as described by Tonnard et al.[23]

Current Concepts on Graft Survival

Several theories have been described to explain the survival of fat cells. There is no consensus till date; however, a combination of these mechanisms is believed to be responsible for ensuring fat survival. The various theories are as follows.

Host Cell Replacement Theory

This was described by Neuhof and Hirschfeld in 1923.[24,25] There was an initial stage of degeneration of fat cells which was followed by regeneration at 2 to 3 months. They noticed that some wandering cells transformed into embryonal cells which developed into adult fat cells. The metaplastic fat cells were noted to have all the properties of mature fat cells.

Cell Survival Theory

This was proposed by Peer in early 1950s. He showed that adipocytes in the graft survived if re-vascularized.[26] The survival depended on the number of vital adipocytes in the graft at the time of transfer.

Niche Theory

This theory states that the microenvironment of the host bed decides the regeneration of ADSCs and hence the fat survival rate. Three zones, viz., surviving zone, regenerating zone, and necrotic zone can be identified in the grafted fat as shown in **Fig. 18.1**.[24,27] Eto et al stated that the volume of the graft survival depends on the survival of the adipocytes in the regenerating zone.[28] All the fat cells in the graft eventually die and are replaced by fat cells differentiating from ADSCs in the regenerating zone. The paracrine action of ADSCs through growth factors is also known to influence fat survival.[24]

Facial Anatomy and Relevance in the Process of Aging

A thorough understanding of the arrangement of facial soft tissue will help in planning an anatomical approach to correction of contour deformities and rejuvenation. This is important to ensure a "natural" look which lasts longer.

The facial soft tissue is arranged in five basic layers bound by retaining ligaments.[29,30] The five layers include: skin, subcutaneous tissue, musculoaponeurotic system, areola tissue, and deep fascia. Retaining ligaments attach facial soft tissue to deep fascia/bone. The various retaining ligaments are superior and inferior temporal septae, lateral orbital thickening, zygomatic ligament, masseteric ligament, and mandibular ligament.[29]

The fourth layer, i.e., areolar tissue, comprises the retaining ligaments and the deep facial spaces. In the second layer, ligaments branch out as retinacular cutis, thus dividing the subcutaneous fat into distinct compartments.[30–32]

To understand the functional anatomy better, a vertical line from lateral orbital rim can be used to divide the

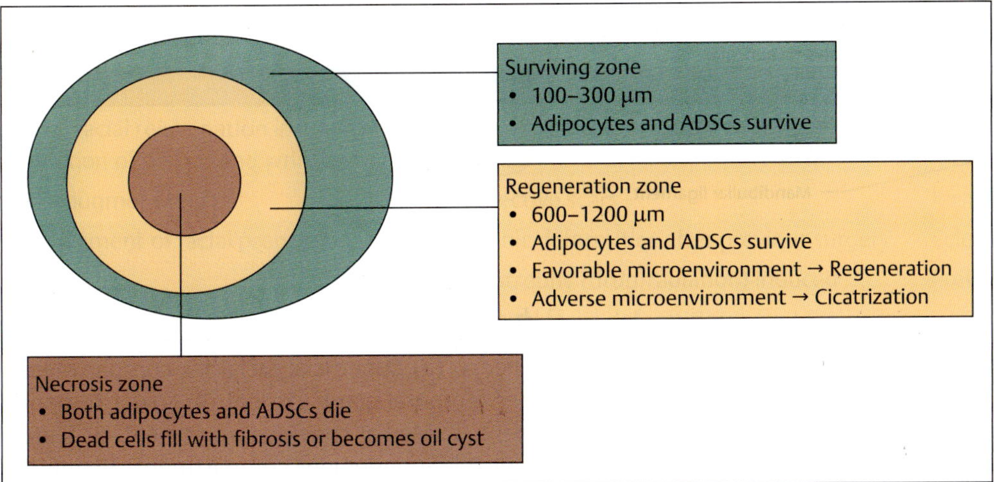

Fig. 18.1 Zones of adipocytes in the fat graft. The survival of the fat cells depends on the microenvironment resulting in four fates of the grafted fat: survival, successful regeneration, failed regeneration/cicatrization, and oil cyst formation. ADSCs, adipose-derived stem cells.

after centrifugation. This is often based on trial and error and the surgeon's expertise and hence is highly subjective. Usual volumes required for each facial area are discussed in detail later in the chapter.

Newer objective methods for assessment of facial volumes include 3D surface analysis (utilizing 3D photographs/3D computed tomography [CT] scans) and magnetic resonance imaging (MRI) volumetry.[38–42] 3D volumetric analysis requires a photograph to be captured using 3D cameras/scanners which is then digitalized by computer-aided designing (CAD) software to produce 3D digital meshes. Multiple polygons can be configured on these meshes which help in accurately configuring a mathematical representation from which volume can be calculated.[38–40] Similarly use of 3D-CT combined with volume-rendering techniques can help in assessment of volume. In MRI volumetry, the MRI images taken in prone position are first stored in DICOM (digital imaging and communications in medicine) format. A variety of software are available for carrying out volume assessment layer-by-layer by a process known as segmentation.[41,42]

High cost and radiation exposure with CT remain the limiting factors preventing wide use of these. Novel 3D scanners that help in capturing the 3D digital mesh and web-based software are now available which can pave way for reduced costs and development of alternative smartphone applications.[40]

These methods can be used not only for preoperative planning, but also for postoperative assessment of fat survival, contour, and volume changes.[38,39]

Assessment of Donor Sites

All the available donor sites for graft harvest should be noted and recorded. There is no definitive evidence correlating donor site and graft survival till date.[37] Lower abdomen and inner thigh are known to have higher concentration of ADSCs; however, they have a higher potential to wrinkle.[43,44] Posterior hip, back, love handles, and outer aspect of thigh are more forgiving and are preferred sites. Donor areas also should be marked with permanent marker in standing position.

Informed consent for the procedure and consent for photography should be taken. Patient should be counseled regarding the possible realistic outcomes, postoperative course, expected complications, and the need for repeated procedures.

Technique of Structural Fat Grafting

The technique of structural fat grafting was standardized by Sydney R. Coleman in 1994; the basic principles of this are still being adhered to.[20] Careful handling of the fat at all stages is of utmost importance as proper technique is an important factor determining the graft survival.[20,21] Care should be taken to avoid undue delay between harvest and placement of the graft. The procedure can be performed under sedation, local or general anesthesia, depending on the defect size and estimated amount of the fat to be harvested.[37] The instruments required for harvest, processing, and transfer of fat should be ensured.

Harvesting the Fat

The various techniques for harvesting fat can be classified based on mechanisms used to create pressure and the volume of tumescent solution injected into donor site. Direct excision, manual aspiration with syringe, and liposuction assisted by suction of varying pressures, ultrasound, or LASER are the various harvesting techniques described. Although there is a wide variety of techniques, it is well accepted that high pressures are traumatic for adipocytes and hence the technique standardized by Coleman for ensuring fat survival is widely practiced, which is described in detail ahead.

Fat should be harvested under low pressure as tiny parcels with intact architecture.[20,21] The size should be amenable to be injected through small cannulas in tiny aliquots to ensure a good blood supply. Access stab incisions are made in hidden areas for the donor site selected. A tumescent solution consisting of 500 mL of Ringer's lactate, 15 mL of 2% lidocaine, and 0.5 mL of 1:200,000 adrenaline is infiltrated in the donor areas in 1:1 ratio through blunt Lamis-infiltrating cannula (**Fig. 18.3**).[22,37] Unlike liposuction, superwet technique (3:1 ratio) is discouraged as the likelihood of injury to the aspirated fat cells is more.[37] The fat is harvested using blunt-tipped Coleman's cannula size ranging from 2 to 3 mm (**Fig. 18.4**). The cannula is connected to a 10 to 20 mL luer-lock syringe, thus creating a slight negative pressure. The authors use a 60-mL syringe and maintain pressure of up to 20 mL as the wide bore of the syringe makes it easier to transfer the harvested fat into smaller volume syringes. With gentle to-and-fro motion, the fat is harvested under low pressure (**Fig. 18.5**).

In cases where a large volume is required, powered low-pressure suction devices can be utilized to ease the process of harvesting.[45] However, there is a need for sterile autoclavable container between the harvesting cannula and the

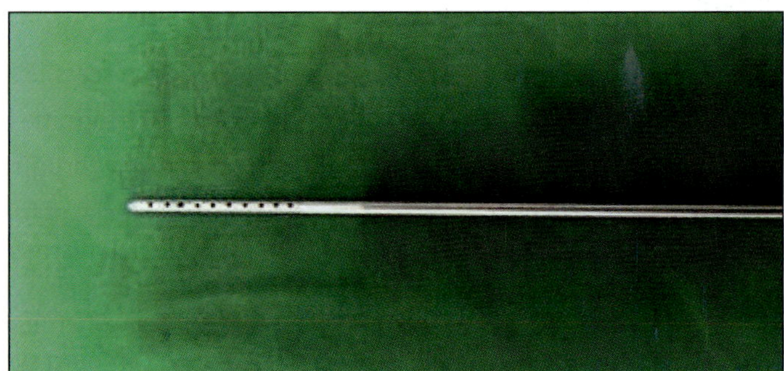

Fig. 18.3 Lamis-infiltrating cannula. Note the blunt tip and the multiple holes at the tip which help in even distribution of the infiltration solution.

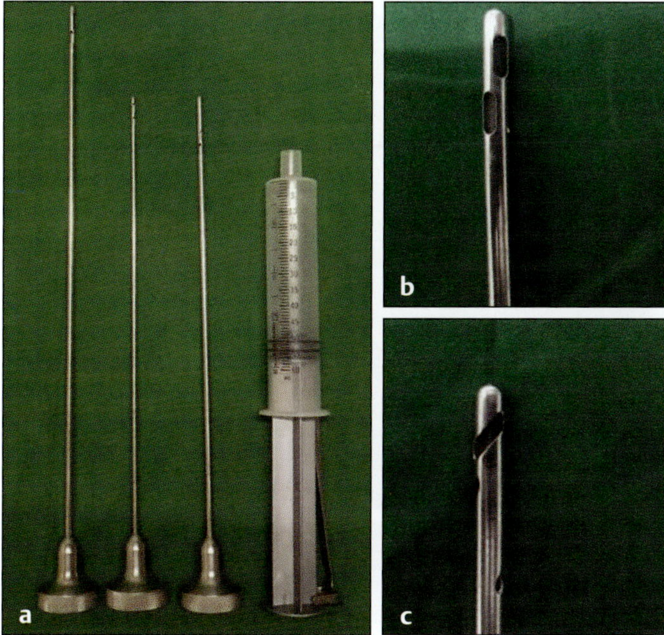

Fig. 18.4 Instruments for fat harvest. **(a)** Coleman-harvesting cannula of 2 to 3 mm size, wide-bore syringe with lock to maintain volume at 20 mL. **(b)** Coleman-harvesting cannula with blunt tip. **(c)** Tulip-harvesting cannula.

suction machine. The authors utilize a modification by interposing an infant mucous sucker as an alternative receptacle in such situations[46] (**Fig. 18.6**). Once the adequate volume has been harvested, the stab incision is closed with a 6–0 nylon suture and a transparent adhesive dressing is applied over the donor site.

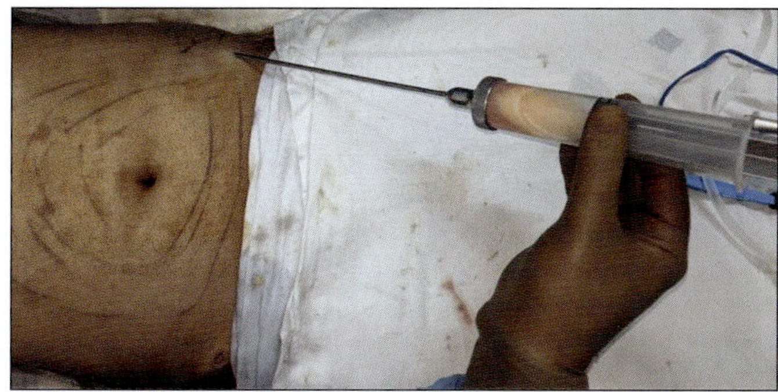

Fig. 18.5 Process of fat harvest under low pressure.

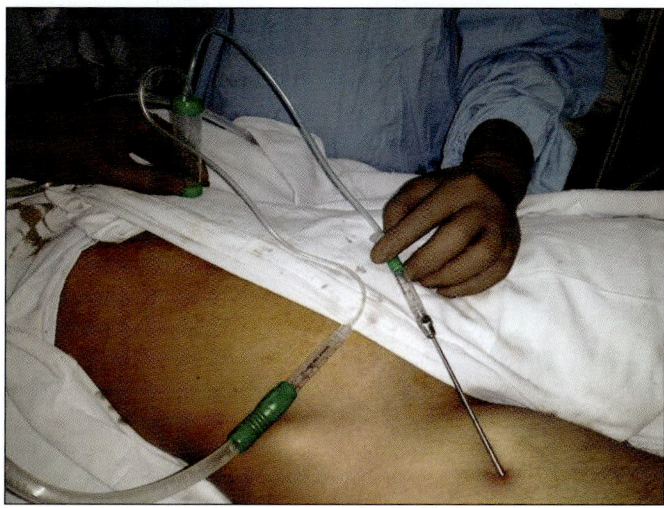

Fig. 18.6 Use of infant mucous sucker as alternative fat receptacle for large volume harvest using suction device.

Processing of Fat

The various methods of processing fat are concentration by allowing harvested fat to sediment followed by decantation, scrubbing, filtration through cotton compresses, addition of steroid hormones, and centrifugation. Many of these methods are of historical importance and have not been clinically successful. The most widely used clinically relevant methods are filtration and centrifugation. Coleman described the use of centrifugation for processing when standardizing the procedure of fat grafting. The aspirated fat in each 10-mL syringe after capping (putting the broken needle tip at the end) is then subjected to centrifugation at 3,000 rpm for 3 minutes (**Fig. 18.7a**). Values more than 3,000 rpm should be avoided as it can cause cell damage.[22,37] Centrifugation separates the viable and nonviable contents; lowermost layer is the tumescent fluid and serum, the middle layer is the pure fat-containing adipocytes, and the top layer is formed by oil and nonviable cells (**Fig. 18.7b**). In cases where the volume harvested is less and in absence of centrifuge, allowing the syringe to stand in upright position for 10 to 15 minutes will cause separation of the layers (**Fig. 18.7b, c**). The bottom layer is usually drained by uncapping the syringes gently and the top layer is decanted/soaked by gel foam (**Fig. 18.7d**). The middle layer of processed fat is then transferred to 2-mL luer-lock syringes for injection.

Placement of Graft

Based on the anatomical knowledge of fat compartments in the face, they are filled with the purified fat in a systematic manner depending on the areas to be corrected and filling from deep to superficial planes of tissues.[20-22,37] The target sites are infiltrated with adrenaline solution to induce vasoconstriction and prevent bleeding/hematoma. The stab incisions are planned in such a way so as to allow movement of the cannula in at least two directions.[22] Fat is injected using blunt tip 18 or 17 gauge Coleman cannula with an aperture proximal to the tip. The cannula is advanced into the target areas. As the tip is blunt, it tends to follow the natural planes and does not cut into new planes. The fat is not injected when the cannula is advanced to avoid clumping. As the

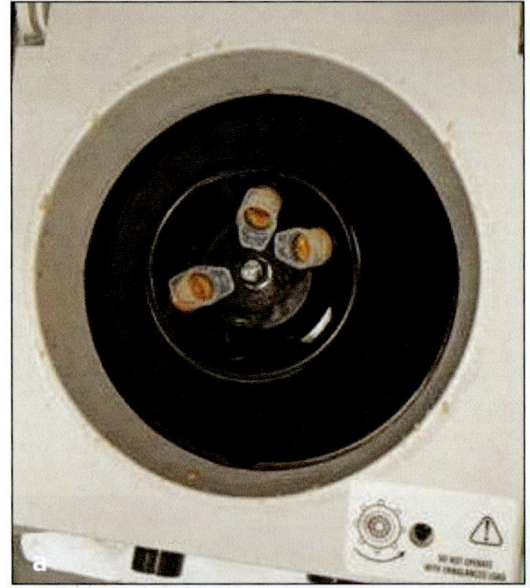

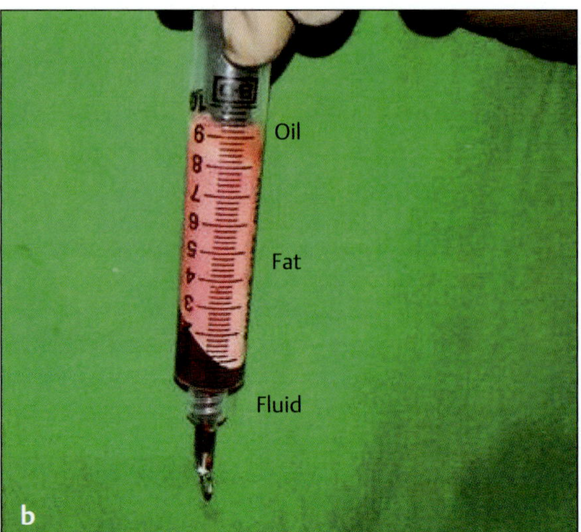

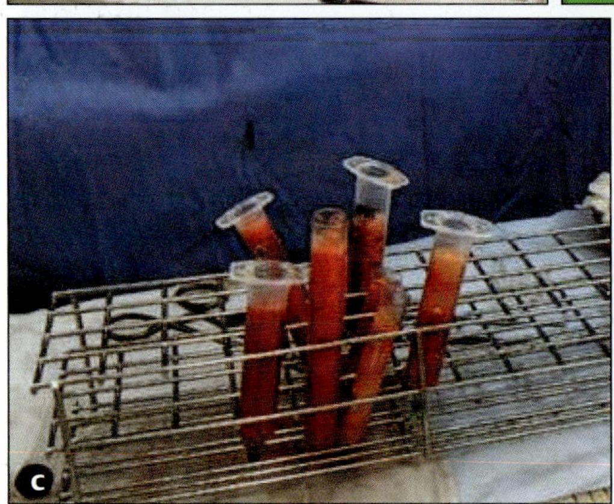

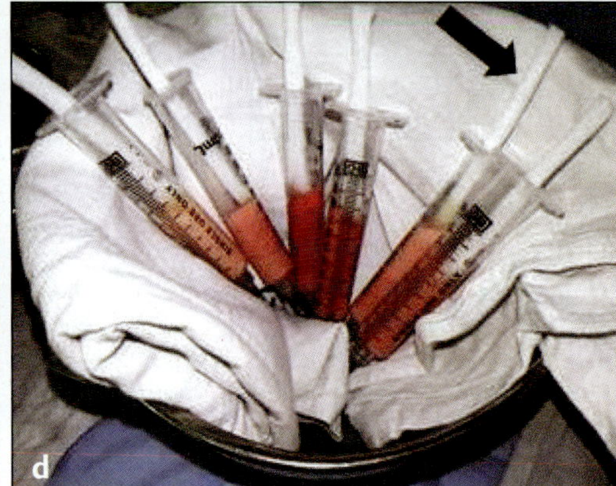

Fig. 18.7 Processing of fat. **(a)** Centrifugation of the harvested fat at 3,000 rpm for 3 minutes. **(b)** Separation of viable and nonviable cells after centrifugation. **(c)** Harvested fat allowed to separate out by keeping in upright position in situation where centrifuge is not available. **(d)** Removal of the upper oily layer by soaking with gel-foam (*arrow*).

cannula is withdrawn, fat is deposited in small aliquots, thus maximizing the contact area with the surrounding bed.[20–22] This is important to ensure fat survival as large globules can undergo central necrosis and thus resorb.[47,48] A fat-grafting gun can be used for placement of the graft as it is more precise with constant pressure and is comfortable (**Fig. 18.8**).[49] The fat should be placed in multiple planes starting from deeper to superficial planes. Placement of a large bolus and then trying to mold it by pressure should be avoided as it always leads to displacement and necrosis of some or all of the fat in the area which results in irregularity of the surface. Some gentle molding can be done during placement to make the surface smooth intraoperatively.

The structural correction begins with building up tiny aliquots. In areas of volume deficit, the placement of fat in deeper layers acts as an anchor and the subsequent placements in the superficial planes result in rejuvenation of the skin. Application of pressure should be avoided after placement of the graft as it is detrimental for its survival. The stab incisions may be left to heal on their own or may be sutured with interrupted nonabsorbable sutures.

Postoperative Care

The most common sequelae is swelling owing to the tissue edema due to the multiple passes.[22] Small strips of adhesive tapes or transparent adhesive dressing are applied over the fat-grafted areas to reduce pain and swelling. Use of ice packs, tight compressions, and deep massage is to be avoided. After the initial few days, taping is removed and gentle touch helps in lymphatic circulation.

Variations of Fat-Grafting Technique

Microfat Grafting

In this technique, the lipoaspirate size is smaller than the conventional structural fat grafting harvested using 2-mm cannulas. The fat is harvested using smaller size cannulas (<1.2 mm) and injected using cannulas as small as 0.7 mm or 23-gauge needles.[23,50] This is described for use in deep

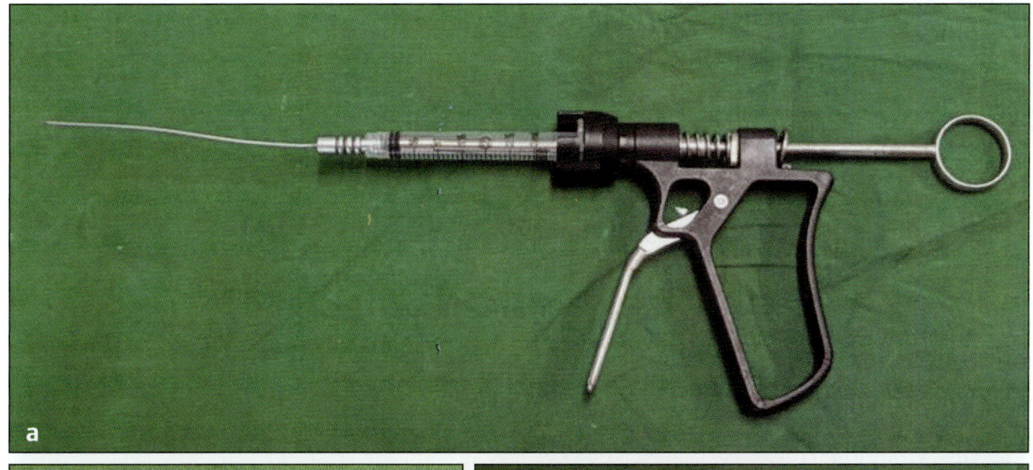

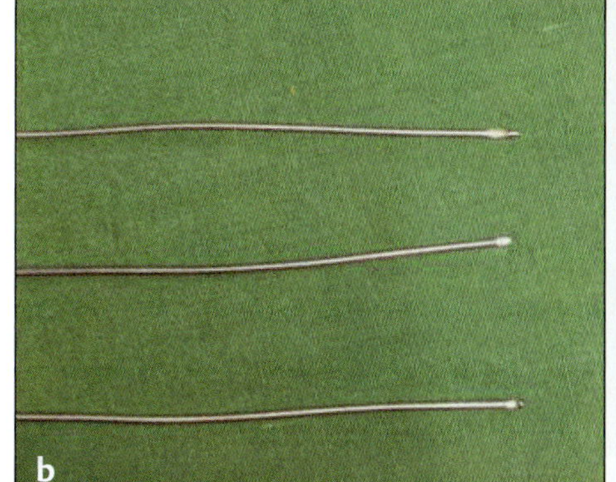

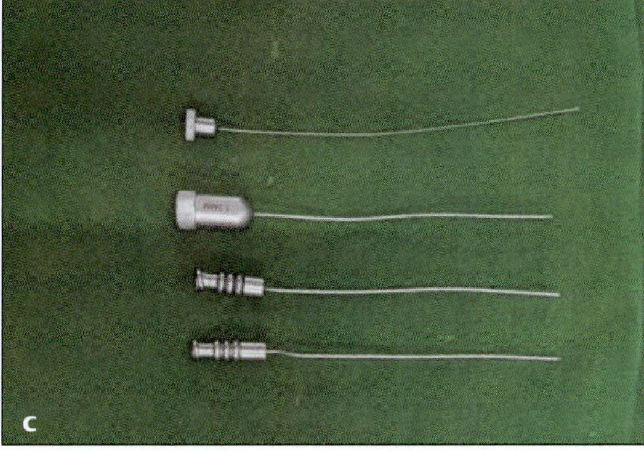

Fig. 18.8 Placement of fat. **(a)** Fat-grafting gun used for precise placement of fat. **(b)** Cannulas used for fat placement. **(c)** Note the blunt tip of the cannulas used for fat placement.

dermal layers and superficial fat compartments in the delicate areas of the face.

Nanofat Grafting

This was described for even more superficial layers or finer rhytids. The harvested fat is mechanically emulsified by passing between two luer-lock syringes. After 30 passes, a liquid suspension is obtained which is strained by a fine cloth. The resultant filtrate so obtained is known as nanofat[23] (**Fig. 18.9**). Using a 27-gauge needle it is injected to the various areas of fine wrinkles, scarring and atrophic dermis, areas of hyper pigmentation, and dark circles around the eyes in an intradermal plane till the skin blanches (**Fig. 18.9**). A novel method of delivering nanofat using microneedling devices has also been recently reported. The nanofat does not have volumizing effects, only rejuvenating effect by causing remodeling through ADSCs.[51,52] The rejuvenating effect of nanofat is brought about by an accelerated and increased production of mature collagen.[53,54]

The comparison of the three types of fat grafts is shown in **Table 18.3**.

Fat Grafting for Different Facial Regions: Practical Tips

Anatomical Fat Grafting in Face: Changing Paradigm to Delay Facial Aging

Aging is now regarded as a continuum of anatomic and physiological changes occurring in the tissues. The concept of delaying the facial decay or rather reversing the aging is now gaining popularity with the introduction of concept of injectable tissue replacement and regeneration (ITR^2) by Cohen et al.[36] This concept aims at addressing the volume loss by anatomical compartments and combines it with regenerative ingredients.

As discussed earlier, fat in the superficial compartments are tightly packed above the muscles, whereas deep compartments are loosely arranged beneath the muscles. In the ITR^2 concept, attempt is made to replace fat anatomically in the compartments in parcel sizes similar to the original arrangement. The compartments of volume loss are identified from facial topography. The deep compartments and bone losses are addressed first using structural fat grafting

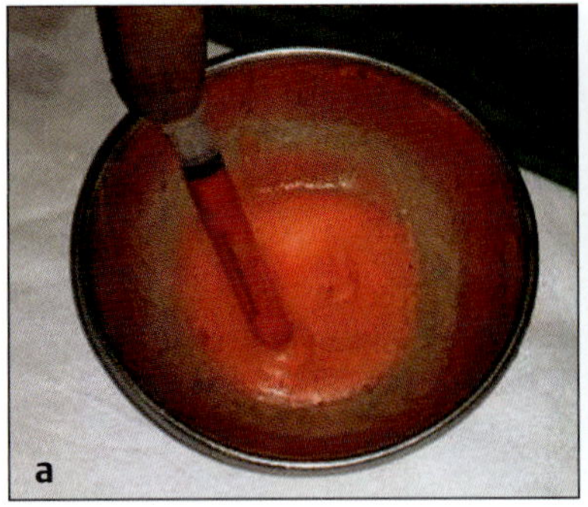

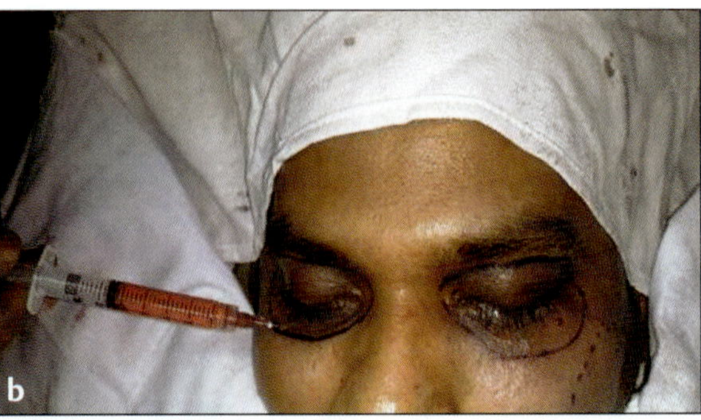

Fig. 18.9 Nanofat grafting. **(a)** Processed nanofat solution obtained by emulsifying the aspirated fat followed by filtering. **(b)** Injection of nanofat subdermally for correcting hyperpigmentation.

Table 18.3 Comparison of different types of fat grafts

Type of graft	Aliquot size	Usage
Structural fat/Macrofat	<2.4 mm	Deep fat compartments Onlay graft on bone Fat-lifts
Microfat	<1.2 mm	Superficial fat compartments
Nanofat	400–800 micron	Finer rhytids Sub/intradermal Microneedling

(macro/millifat). The superficial compartments and deeper rhytids are then addressed using microfat. Nanofat is then applied to the tear-troughs and other areas as intradermal injections to augment the regenerative effects. The authors demonstrated significant volume improvements and regenerative effects with this approach.[36]

If the patient gains weight, the fat-grafted area tends to appear as bumps or deformities if placed blindly to mask the contour irregularities. In an anatomic approach, fat is grafted within the compartments and has the potential advantage of avoiding such deformities as it will give the appearance of natural weight gain rather than irregularities.

Level of Placement of the Graft

The depth of placement of the graft depends on the facial area and the problem being treated. In areas with multiple tissue layers and with thick overlying skin, fat can be injected from periosteum to subdermal level.[22,37] Classical examples are cheek, chin, midface, pyriform aperture, and the geniomandibular groove. For other facial regions, the fat injection should be in specific anatomic planes to achieve optimum results.[37] These are as follows:

- Temporal area/Temple → Subcutaneous plane.
- Upper/lower orbit, tear trough → Preperiosteal/ Suborbicularis oculi plane.
- Lip → Submucosal plane.
- Jaw line → Preperiosteal/Submasseteric plane.

Based on the problem being treated, the level and hence the type of the graft has to be chosen appropriately. For areas of volume loss, macro/microfat should be used to attain volumizing effect. These need to be placed in deep to superficial planes. For fine scars, rhytids, hyperpigmentation, etc., both micro- and nanofat can be utilized. The rejuvenating effect can be brought about by nanofat especially in very fine rhytids and conditions requiring intradermal injections.[23,53–55]

Fat Grafting in Specific Facial Regions

The various technical aspects of fat grafting in specific facial regions are summarized in **Table 18.4**. The placement of incision and direction of injection at various regions is shown in **Fig. 18.10**.

Postoperative Outcomes

Most of the patients have satisfactory outcome because of obvious volume changes. There is improvement in the quality of skin. Rigotti demonstrated healing and normalization of affected skin in the irradiated tissue of breast following fat grafting.[56] Mojallal et al described the improvement in the adherent scars, the texture, skin suppleness, and color of the skin in burnt skin.[57] Some of the patients may need additional procedures which can be done once the inflammation subsides. The second procedure can be done after 3 to 6 months after the primary procedure.[22]

Table 18.4 Fat grafting in face: regionwise summary

Facial region	Injection site	Cannula size	Level of injection	Volume of fat injected
Geniomandibular (prejowl) groove	Mandibular border, perioral area	4 cm long, 0.7 mm (22 gauge)	Periosteum to subdermal	1–3 mL
Cheek	Midcheek, perioral area	5 cm long, 0.7 mm (22 gauge)	Periosteum to subdermal	3–7 mL
Chin	Midline of lower lip, lateral to target area	4 cm long, 0.7 mm (22 gauge)	Periosteum to subdermal	1–3 mL
Nasolabial area	Nasolabial fold, midcheek	4 cm long, 0.7 mm (22 gauge)	Subcutaneous (for nasolabial crease) Preperiosteal (for maxillary recession at pyriform aperture) Periosteum to subdermal (for both)	1–3 mL
Lip	Angle of mouth	5 cm long, 0.7 mm (22 gauge)	Submucosal beneath wet and dry lip vermilion	2–3 mL (upper lip) 3–4 mL (lower lip)
Jawline	Mandibular border, perioral area	8 cm long, 1.2 mm (18 gauge)	Preperiosteal/ submasseteric	3–6 mL
Temple	Temporal hairline	5 cm long, 0.9 mm (20 gauge)	Subcutaneous	5–7 mL
Upper orbit/upper eyelid	Eyebrow	4 cm long, 0.7 mm (22 gauge)	Preperiosteal/ suborbicularis oculi	2–3 mL
Lower orbit/lower eyelid	Midcheek, perioral	4 cm long, 0.7 mm (22 gauge)	Preperiosteal/ suborbicularis oculi	2–3 mL
Tear trough	Nasolabial area	4 cm long, 0.7 mm (22 gauge)	Preperiosteal/ suborbicularis oculi	0.5–1.5 mL

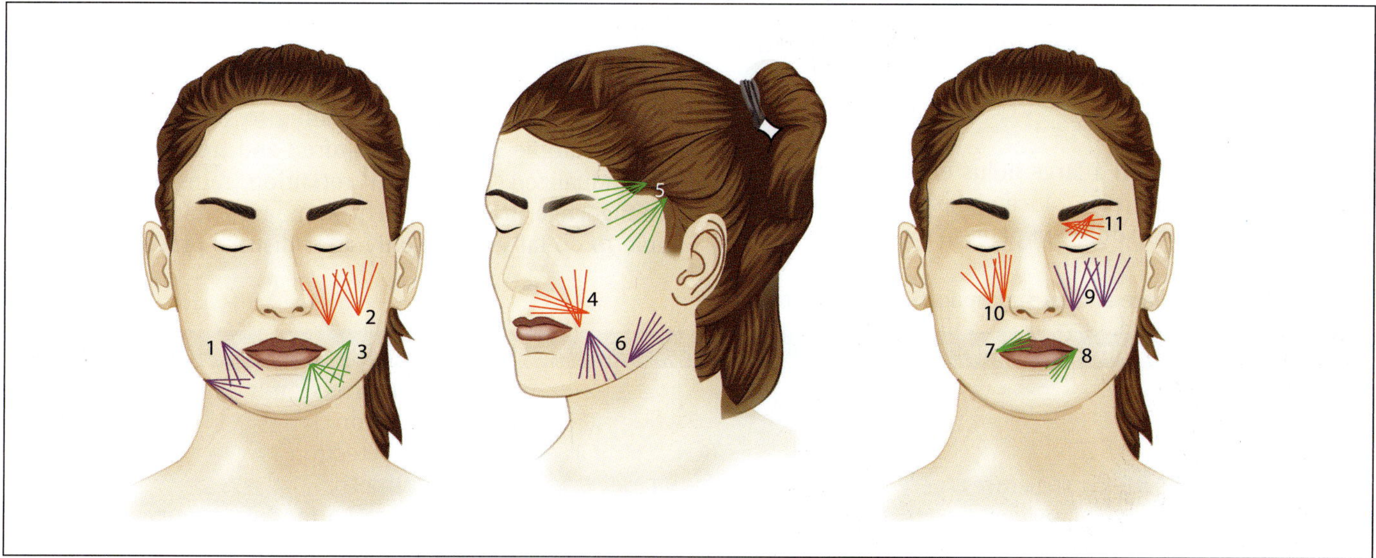

Fig. 18.10 Placement of incision and direction of injection for various facial regions; incision for fat injection for 1: geniomandibular (jowl) groove; 2: cheek; 3: chin; 4: pyriform aperture and nasolabial fold; 5: temple; 6: jawline; 7: upper lip; 8: lower lip; 9: lower orbital; 10: tear trough; and 11: upper orbital region.

Complications

Fat grafting in the face is mostly a safe procedure with a very low complication rate. Very serious complications are rarely reported.[58,59] The various complications following fat grafting are listed in **Table 18.5**.

Prevention and Management of Complications

Mastering the local anatomy and strict adherence to the basic principles can help avoid majority of the complications.[59–62]

Swelling/Bruising

Avoidance of sharp needles for fat injection will help prevent this. Treatment is conservative with light touch and will resolve spontaneously in 2 to 3 weeks.

Aesthetic Irregularity

Adherence to the anatomical principles and the standard protocol will help minimize this. If fat is placed too superficially it will be felt as a palpable lump. If a larger bolus is placed it will undergo necrosis.[63] These minor differences can be managed by liposuction/touch-up around these areas to smoothen it out before coming out of operation theater.

Infection

Infected fat tends to undergo rapid resorption. It can be prevented by maintaining strict aseptic measures starting from fat harvesting, processing, centrifugation, and placement of grafts.[59,64,65] A closed system should always be used for tumescence solution infiltration. The gloves should be always changed when injecting the fat. The oral commissure and lip areas are to be grafted at the end of facial fat grafting as it may contaminate the rest of the areas because of oral secretions.[59,66,67] Treatment requires antibiotics with or without surgical intervention.

Fat Oil Cysts

These cysts form when a large bolus of fat is injected and undergoes central necrosis.[63] It can be prevented by placing small aliquots of fat in different planes.

Injury to Neurovascular Structures

This may result in dysesthesia/headache/neurological deficit.[68–70] This can be prevented by thorough understanding of the anatomy of the danger areas such as the prezygomatic space, temporal and nasal region.[60]

Intravascular Emboli

This is a rare but devastating complication. It can lead to loss of vision, stroke, or neurological deficit.[71–73] Fat grafting of nose, eyelid, and upper cheek areas is associated with higher risk due to the retrograde communication of facial artery with ophthalmic artery.[73] Treatment includes steroids, antiplatelet agents, and hyperbaric oxygen.[59,61]

Clinical Scenarios of Restoring Facial Aesthetics Using Fat Grafting

Congenital Craniofacial Syndromes

Fat grafting plays a crucial role in replacing the volume discrepancy in the congenital deficiencies like Parry-Romberg syndrome, hemifacial microsomia, and Treacher-Collin syndrome.[3,4] The principle of specific facial fat compartment is applied in these conditions. The areas with more irregularity are addressed first. The filling of deeper areas is first performed so that they act as a support for the placement of superficial fat parcels.[74,75] It is believed that due to the pluripotent nature of the ADSCs, these cells are capable of differentiating into multilineage potentials including fat, skeletal muscle, collagen, cartilage, bone, nerves, and blood vessels in the long run, thereby achieving an acceptable outcome.[76,77] Clinical photograph of a patient of hemifacial microsomia who was managed with multiple sittings of fat grafting alone is shown in **Fig. 18.11**. The deeper layers require structural fat grafting for volumizing. Micro- and nanofat will be utilized in the stages when addressing the superficial layers, thus leading to skin rejuvenation as well. Multiple stages are required and treatment has to be individualized.[78] Although retention rates are better in younger age, in cases of Parry-Romberg syndrome, it is advisable to do fat grafting only after disease process stabilizes,

Table 18.5 Immediate and late complications of fat grafting

Immediate complications	Chronic/late complications
• Swelling • Bruises • Infection • Injury to underlying structures (nerves, vessels, muscles, gland) • Intravascular emboli: vision loss, stroke, neurologic deficit • Migration of fat • Donor site deformity	• Undercorrection • Resorption • Overcorrection • Asymmetry • Calcification/nodule/fat oil cyst • Atypical mycobacterial infection • Dysesthesia/headache • Chronic edema and fibrosis • Delayed pigmentation (tea staining)

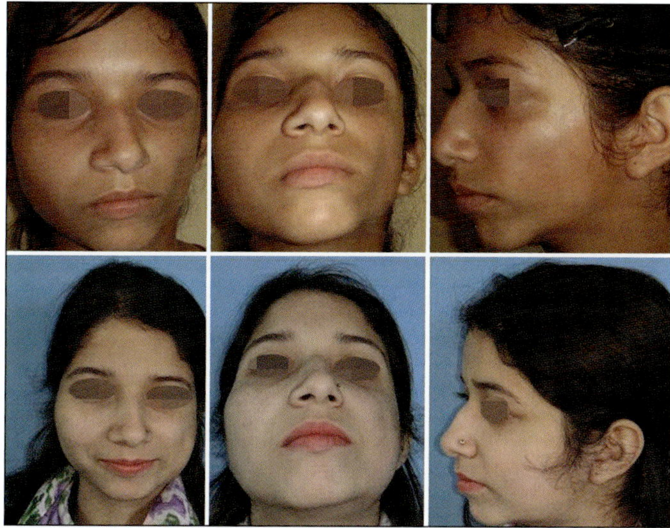

Fig. 18.11 Clinical photograph of patient of hemifacial microsomia. Upper row: preoperative. Lower row: 5 years postoperative following six sessions of fat grafting. Left to right: frontal, basal, and lateral views.

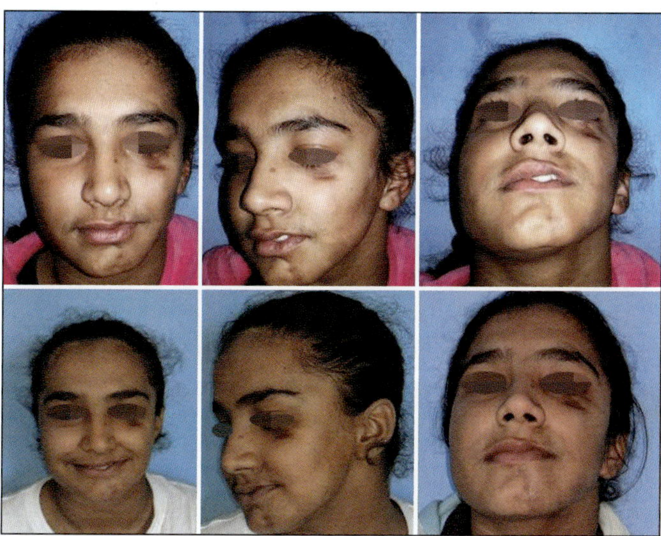

Fig. 18.12 Clinical photograph of patient of Parry-Romberg syndrome. Upper row: Preoperative. Lower row: 6 months postoperative following a session of fat grafting. Left to right: frontal, oblique, and basal views.

as during active phase fat resorption rates are higher.[79,80] Clinical photographs of a patient of Parry-Romberg syndrome treated with fat grafting are shown in **Fig. 18.12**.

Age-Related Facial Lipoatrophy

The different areas over face which need volume correction include forehead, temporal fossa, upper eyelid, lower eyelid cheek junction, cheek, nasolabial fold, upper and lower lip, marionette line, and chin areas. The volume replacement provides support to skin and helps in providing a more natural rejuvenation.[37] An anatomical approach as described earlier can provide better aesthetic outcomes. These patients often need a combination of treatments such as LASER for sun-damage or facelift for excess skin laxity.[81]

Micro- or nanofat can be used for correction of fine scars and wrinkles. The clinical photograph of a patient who underwent nanofat grafting for forehead rhytids is shown in **Fig. 18.13**. Nanofat can be used to improve the quality of the skin owing to the remodeling property and is used for treatment of hyperpigmentations, acne scars, etc.[51] The effects, however, take 3 months to be clinically evident.[23,82] The photograph of a patient who underwent nanofat grafting for correction of dark circles is shown in **Fig. 18.14**.

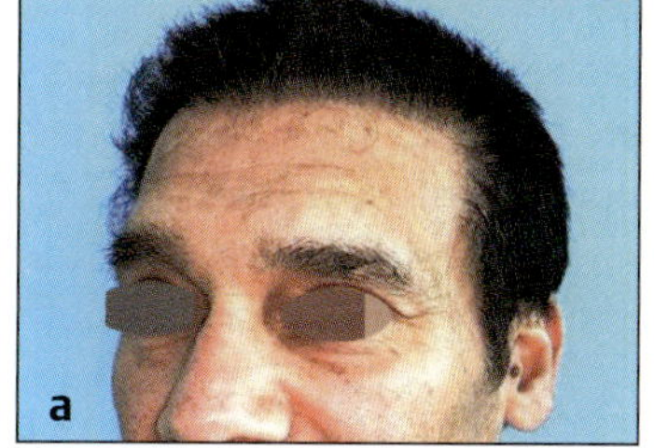

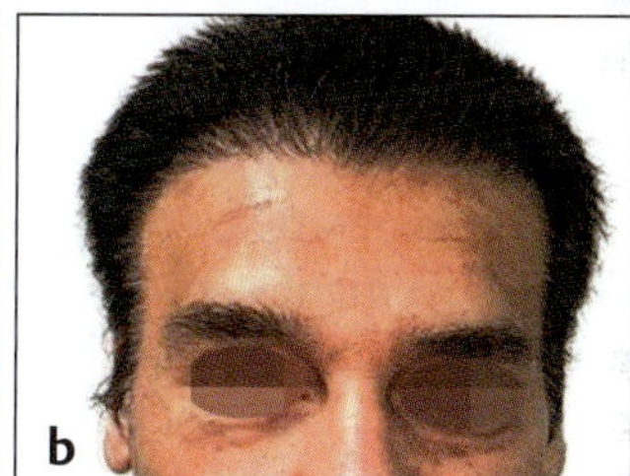

Fig. 18.13 Clinical photograph showing the effect of nanofat grafting in the treatment of forehead wrinkles. **(a)** Preoperative, **(b)** postoperative after nanofat grafting demonstrating the disappearance of the wrinkles. The patient was treated with subdermal and intradermal nanofat injections.

HIV-Associated Facial Lipoatrophy

HIV patients receive protease inhibitors and reverse transcriptase inhibitors as antiretroviral therapy which causes hypertriglyceridemia, glucose intolerance, and insulin resistance. This results in drug-associated lipodystrophy in long term with abnormal fat distribution such as buffalo hump and facial lipoatrophy.[83] The facial lipoatrophy presents as a series of defects in the form of temporal hollowing, wasting of buccal fat, atrophy of nasolabial region, and atrophy over angle of mandible region. These can be treated by aspiration of the fat for the excess humps and fat grafting for areas of volume loss.[84]

Fat Grafting for Patients with Scleroderma Affecting the Face

Scleroderma is an autoimmune chronic connective tissue disorder in which there occurs fibrosis of skin and internal organs. Fat grafting has been shown to be effective in alleviating the fibrosis in the skin to a great extent.[85] Fat results in immunomodulation and reduces the vascular inflammation.

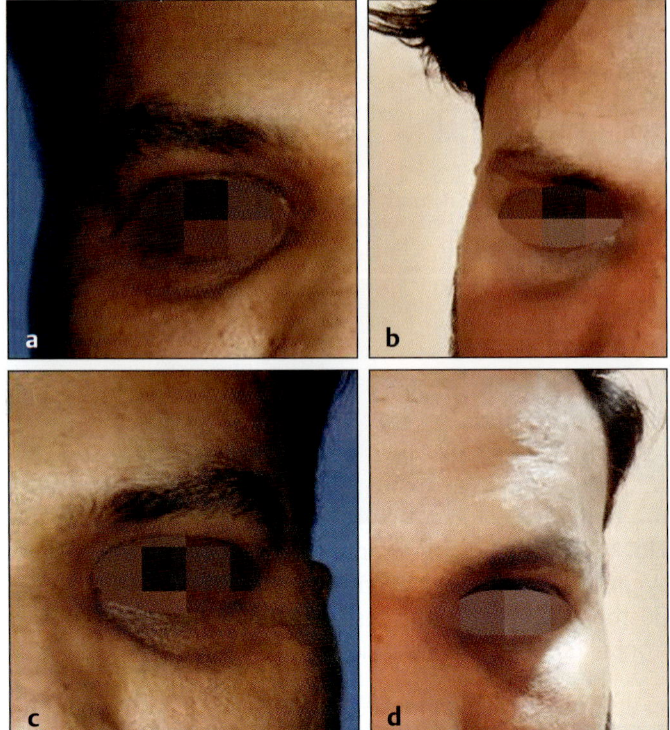

Fig. 18.14 Clinical photograph of patient who underwent one sitting of nanofat grafting for dark circles. **(a, c)** Preoperative; **(b, d)** 4 months postoperative. Though an improvement in skin quality is noted with lightening of the pigmentation, patient will need further sittings for optimum results.

It induces angiogenesis and vasculogenesis. They are essential for reducing the fibrosis by limiting the deposition of extracellular matrix proteins and increasing the collagen deposition.[85,86] The procedure effectively improves the quality of the skin and corrects the contour deformities. The photograph of a patient who underwent macro, micro, and nanofat grafting for the correction of localized scleroderma (morphea) of the face is shown in **Fig. 18.15**.

Fat Grafting in Chin and Nose Augmentation/ Postbariatric Procedures

The chin in the lower third of face plays an important role in facial aesthetics. Minor asymmetry or microgenia results in disharmony in facial proportions which hampers the beauty of the face. The double chin, bifid chin, and deep labiomental crease also result in disfigurement. These deficits can be effectively dealt with by use of liposculpture to bring in symmetry. They are filled from deep to superficial planes. Done properly, the need for other procedures adopted for chin augmentation like use of chin implants and sliding genioplasty may not be required.[87] The augmentation of chin and nose by use of fat graft is known as profiloplasty. Fat retention of up to 41% at 13 months follow-up have been reported in the literature.[88] Patients who undergo bariatric procedures may present with significant volume loss of facial compartments and skin laxity. Often these deformities can be corrected with volume replacement with fat grafting alone. Clinical photograph of a patient who presented with significant volume loss following postbariatric procedure is shown in **Fig. 18.16**.

Fat Grafting for Post-traumatic/Burn/ Iatrogenic/Radiation-Induced Scar or Contour Deformity in the Face

Scars present over the forehead, glabella, nose, nasolabial crease, temple, around the cheek, periorbital region, jowl, angle of mandible, and neck are disfiguring for the patient. The adherent depressed scars are treated by subcision, i.e., creation of space with the use of a sharp 18-gauge needle followed by fat grafting. Clinical photograph of a patient with adherent scar in the infraorbital region managed with fat grafting is shown in **Fig. 18.17**. In the deeper planes macrofat is required; however in superficial planes micro/nanofat has scar-modulating properties.[23,37,59] The early results of fat grafting on postburn scar of face is shown in **Fig. 18.18**. In posttraumatic cases with late contour deformities, fat grafting can bring about acceptable volumizing effects. The effects of fat grafting in a patient with posttraumatic contour deformity of the right zygomatic region following trauma is shown in **Fig. 18.19**.

Complementary Fat Grafting

With the better understanding of the interplay of various processes involved in facial aging, the role of autologous fat transfer in isolation and as an adjunct procedure is increasing. The aging process is now recognized as a combination of tissue laxity and volume loss as opposed to the historical concept with dominant effect of gravity.[29,31,32,36] This has led to the rise in fat grafting as an adjuvant to the various surgical and nonsurgical rejuvenation procedures.

Facelift and Fat Grafting

To obtain a more natural outcome, both the components of skin laxity and volume atrophy needs to be addressed.[31,32] To explain this concept better, an aging face can be likened to a dried raisin which has laxity and shrinkage of the outer skin as well as loss of volume. Tightening the outer shell alone to remove the wrinkles without adding volume will not help recover the original contour, but create a tailored look. Fat grafting can be combined with facelift to address areas that have fallen short after facelift.[89] The surgeon can decide based on his/her own personal results and the individual patients' topography to make a customized approach for each patient.

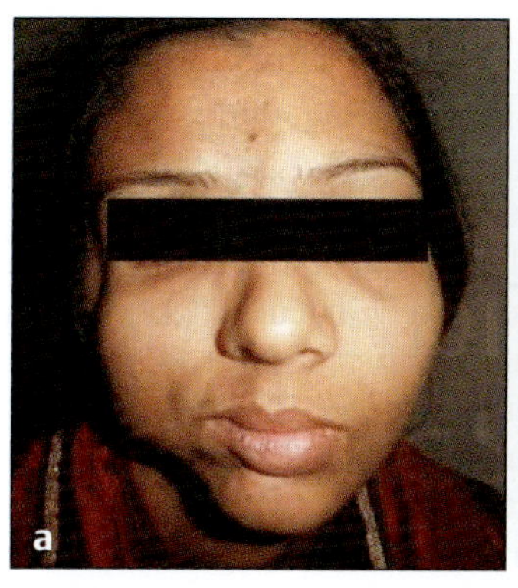
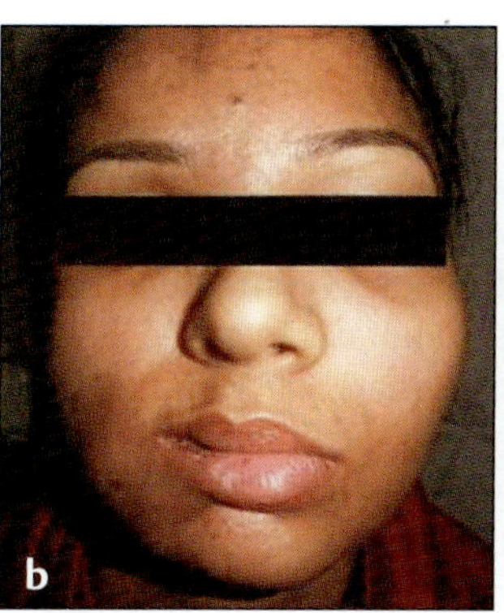
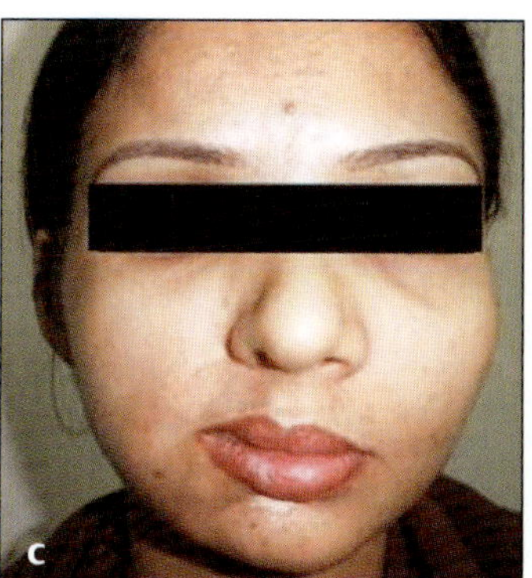

Fig. 18.15 Clinical photograph demonstrating the role of fat grafting in the treatment of patient with localized scleroderma (morphea) of face. A combination of macro, micro, and nanofat grafting techniques was utilized. **(a)** Preop, **(b)** 1 month postop, **(c)** 3-month postop. (The images are provided courtesy of Dr Ajay Hariani and Dr Lakshyajit Dhami, Mumbai, Maharashtra, India.)

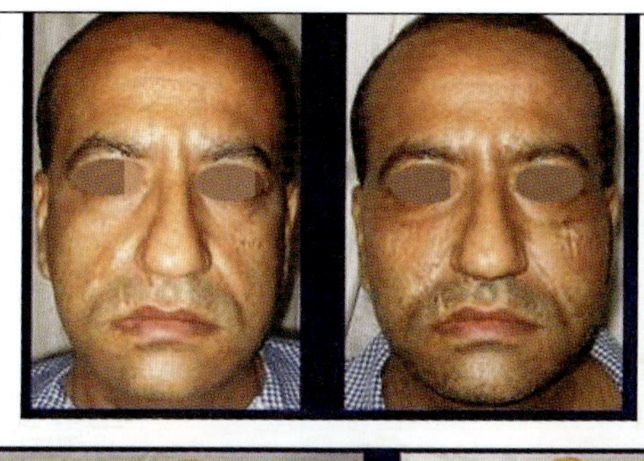
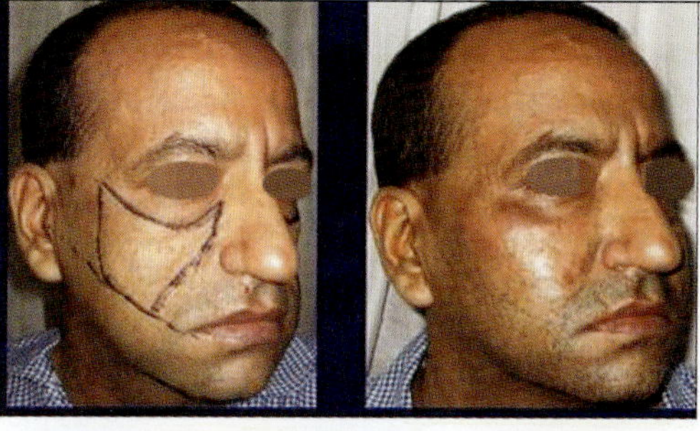
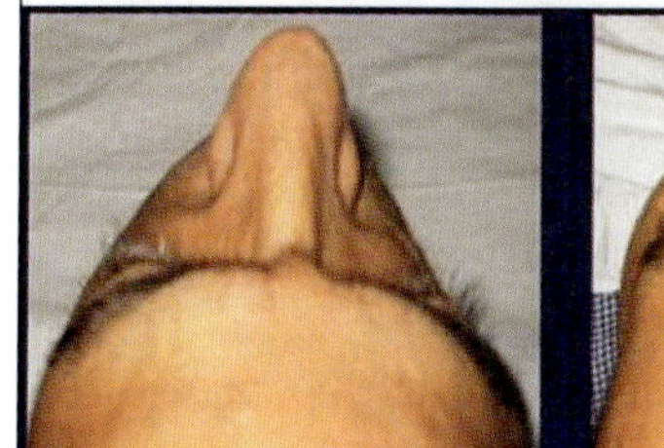
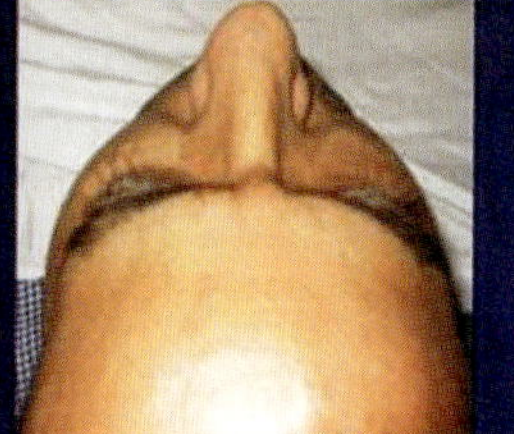
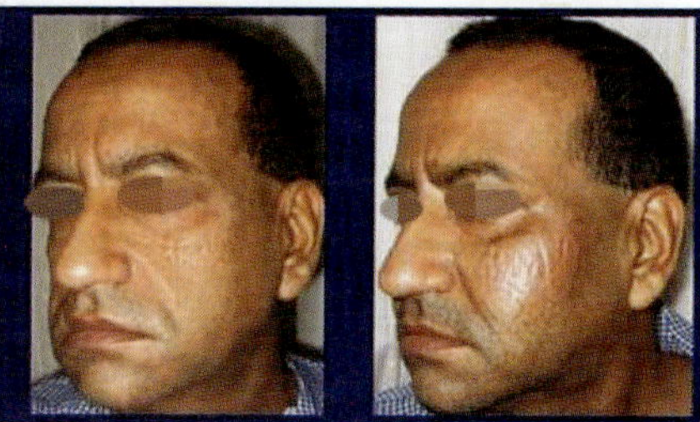

Fig. 18.16 Clinical photograph of patient postbariatric surgery with volume loss over facial compartments treated with combination of macro and microfat grafting. Upper row: frontal view (left: preop, right: postop); left oblique view (left: preop, right: postop). Lower row: Bird's eye view (left: preop, right: postop); right oblique view (left: preop, right: postop). (The images are provided courtesy of Dr Ajay Hariani and Dr Lakshyajit Dhami, Mumbai, Maharashtra, India.)

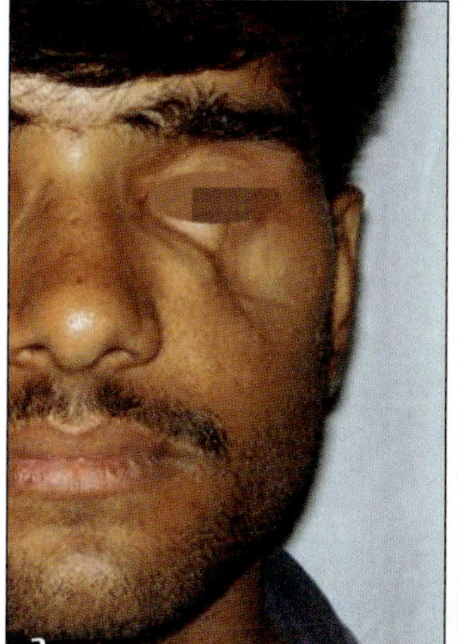
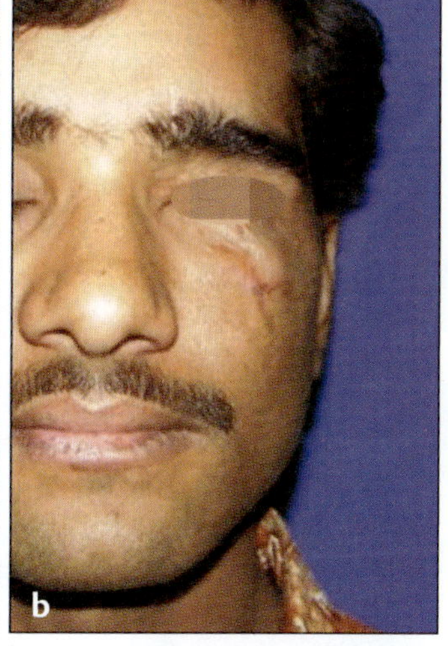

Fig. 18.17 Clinical photograph of patient with depressed scar in the left infraorbital region. The scar was treated by subcision and fat grafting. **(a)** Preoperative, **(b)** postoperative after multiple sittings of fat grafting. (The images are provided courtesy of Dr Ajay Hariani and Dr Lakshyajit Dhami, Mumbai, Maharashtra, India.)

The sequencing of the procedures has been controversial. Recent studies support fat grafting before facelift if both procedures are being performed concurrently.[89] At the beginning of the procedure, the facial landmarks are better identified and the facial planes are not opened up. However, there are few reports that suggest to use fat grafting only as ancillary procedure after all the lifts are completed either in same sitting or in a staged manner.[90] Fat grafting helps correct the deflated tissue and optimize the various surgical procedures for upper, mid, and lower face.[89,90]

Botox and Fat Grafting

Botox is one of the preferred methods for addressing deep rhytids such as glabellar grooves and marionette lines. Overcorrection with fat grafting concurrently helps address resistant creases.[90] Improved rejuvenation results have been reported when carrying out micro- or nanofat grafting 7 to 10 days after Botox injections.[91,92]

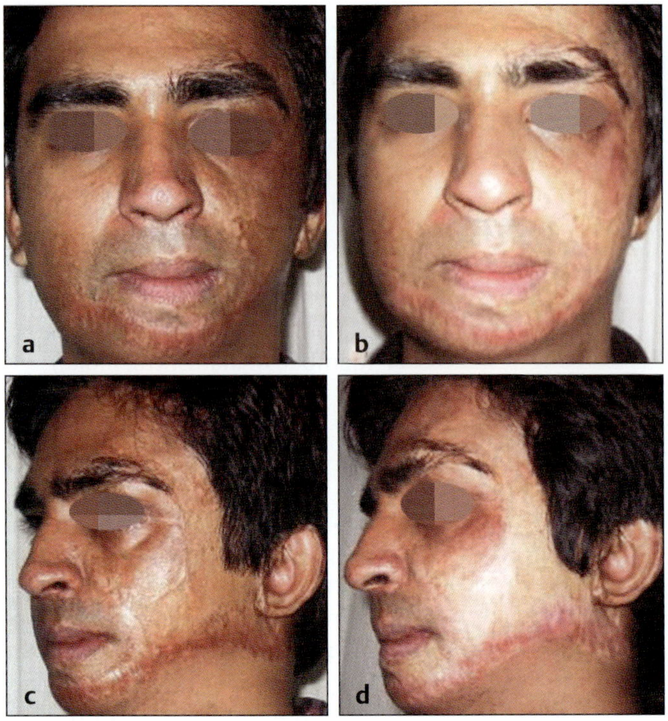

Fig. 18.18 Clinical photograph of postburn scar on face with tissue loss **(a, c)** Patient was managed with multiple sittings of fat grafting and shows improvement in scar quality and contour **(b, d)**. (The images are provided courtesy of Dr Ajay Hariani and Dr Lakshyajit Dhami, Mumbai, Maharashtra, India.)

LASER/Microneedling and Fat Grafting

Fractionated LASERs and microneedling combined with nanofat, and SVFs, have shown a significant improvement in wrinkles and tissue discolorations.[93,94] A novel topical form of nanofat (combined with a liposomal component) known as nanofat biocreme has been used in conjunction with fractionated LASER and showed significant improvement in the degree of wrinkles and skin texture.[94] The holes created by fractional LASER or needling techniques are believed to stay open for longer time and thus allowing the fat uptake in the dermis. However, further research into these is required.

Indian Scenario

The main indication for fat grafting in the Indian practice remains reconstructive procedures for post-traumatic or congenital deformities.[2,79] Regenerative property of the adipocytes is being used for radiation-induced damage and in burns.[95] However, the frequency of these procedures in our population still remains widely unexplored.

The Indian skin can be most commonly classified as Fitzpatrick type IV which is less prone to sun damage.[96] The incidence of photo damage to skin is thought to be lesser and hence the popularity of skin rejuvenating procedures is still in the early phase in our country.[97]

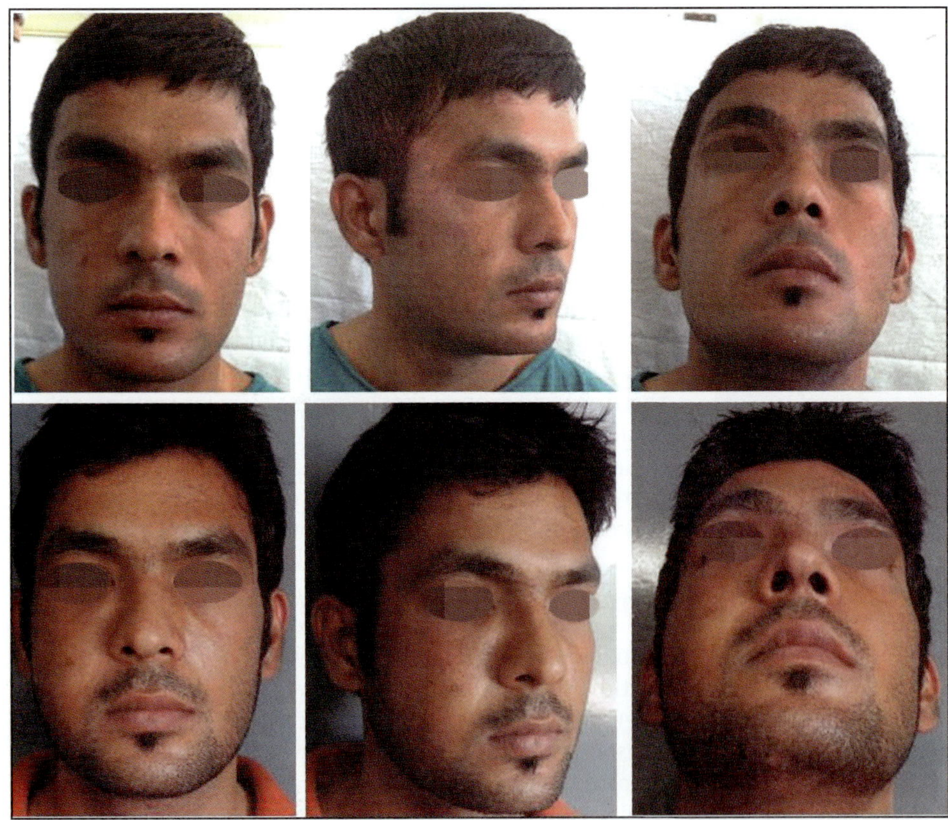

Fig. 18.19 Clinical photograph of patient of faciomaxillary trauma with contour deformity of right zygomatic region. Upper row: Preoperative. Lower row: 12-month postoperative following a session of fat grafting; left to right: frontal, oblique, and basal views.

In contrary to the general belief, a recent study on the aging process of Asian Indian faces of various ethnicity demonstrated aging changes earlier than the Caucasian skin.[98] Larger follow-up studies are required to formulate treatment protocols for Indian skin. Early use of fat grafting for volume replacement and combining it with its regenerative potential can significantly reduce the procedures required for age-related changes in the skin.

Factors Affecting Clinical Outcome

Injury to Adipocytes

Gentle handling of the fat and harvesting using low-pressure aspiration system and blunt-tip cannula are important in preventing injury to adipocytes.

Volume of the Fat

If the volume of grafted fat is more, there is increased interstitial pressure which leads to decreased tissue perfusion of the bed.[28] For this reason, significant overcorrection is preferably avoided. There is necrosis of the graft over the central region due to inadequate exposure to the source of blood supply. Also, in the transplanted fat, along with regeneration, stabilizing events such as lipid absorption (phagocytosis) and replacement with scar tissue (fibrosis) occur hand-in-hand. In smaller fat globules, if absorbed temporarily by macrophages, the space gets replaced by fibrogenesis. However, in large globules >8 mm, the necrosis of the central part forms permanent oil cysts.[99–101] Hence, the size of the aliquot should be small to ensure fat survival.

Age at Surgery

Fat retention is superior in children.[102] Elderly patients show more resorption than young patients. However, in Parry-Romberg syndrome patients, there is low retention if done at a young age. In these patients grafting should be undertaken only after disease stabilizes.[79,80] The poor blood supply of the recipient bed due to atrophic soft tissue may explain this poor retention of graft.

History of Previous Craniofacial Surgery

The fat survival rates in such cases reduce probably due to the impaired vascularity of the bed.

Nature of the Recipient Bed

In patients with scarred or avascular bed, fat survival rate is low. These cases need a staged approach with measures to optimize the bed prior to fat grafting.

Recent Advances

Novel Strategies to Improve Fat Survival

Improvement in surgical technique has led to the improvement in fat survival. Wide research is being done at various levels with the aim of improving the fat survival. Few strategies which are clinically feasible are discussed here.

Use of Combination of Fat Graft with Autologous Platelet-Rich Plasma

APRP consists of platelet concentrate of 200,000 platelets/μL, which is three to four times the concentration of a physiological clot.[103–105] It is a rich source of growth factors such as platelet-derived growth factor (PDGF), vascular endothelial growth factor (VEGF), and transforming growth factor (TGF)-β, which are known to increase fat survival in vitro.[103,104]

This promotes neovascularization, induces fibroblast activity, and stabilizes the grafted fat by polymerization of fibrin. It helps increase the concentration of adipocyte stem cells by four times and also helps in the repair of damaged adipocytes.[105,106] Clinically, it reduces skin bleeding and swelling, and improves fat survival. APRP has a good healing potential and can accentuate the effects of fat transfer. Few studies have reported results supporting the same.[107,108] APRP can be used in combination with various types of fat transfer techniques such as micro- or nanofat as well as with stem cells.

Use of Stromal Vascular Fraction

Zuk et al in 2001 demonstrated the presence of mesenchymal stem cells in human adipose tissue which led to vast research.[109] The harvested fat is enzymatically dissociated by collagenase/trypsin for 30 to 60 minutes and is then subjected to differential centrifugation. The aspirate obtained is known as SVF (**Flowchart 18.1**).[109–111] SVF is defined as the heterogeneous population of cells freshly isolated after enzymatic breakdown of adipose tissue. SVF contains a variety of cells such as blood-derived cells, endothelial cells, pericytes, lymphocytes, monocytes, and stem cells.[109–111] SVF has been used for the treatment of scars in isolation as well as in combination with autologous fat grafting.

Release of growth factors and angiogenesis improve the microenvironment and increase the graft survival by three to four times. Improved fat volume maintenance and improved skin quality have been demonstrated in studies utilizing a combination of SVF and autologous fat grafting in facial skin.[112–114]

Use of Adipocyte-Derived Stem Cells

ADSCs or stromal cells are plastic adherent culture expanded cells derived from SVF (**Flowchart 18.1**). They have the

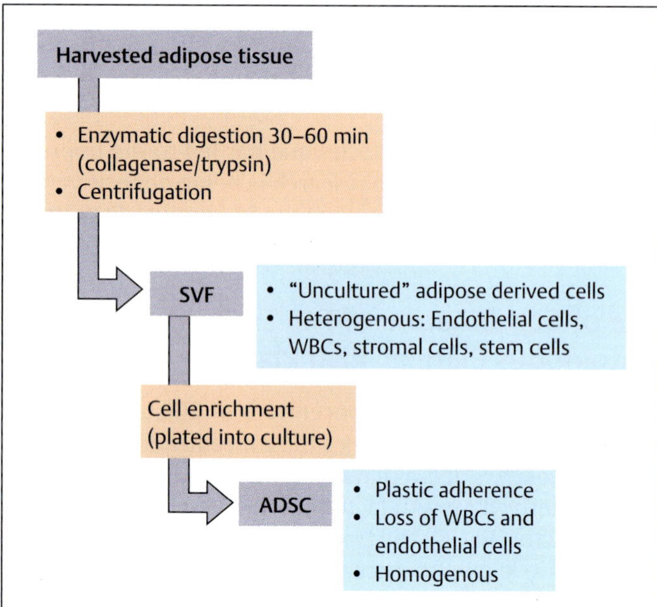

Flowchart 18.1 Steps of isolation of cell fractions from adipose tissue; SVF, stromal vascular fraction; ADSC, adipocyte-derived stem cell.

potential to differentiate into different lineages (fat, bone, cartilage, etc.) and can proliferate into large numbers in vitro.[115,116] Culture expansion of SVF after seeding in culture media for 3 to 5 weeks depletes the hematopoietic cells, thus leading to emergence of plastic adherent cells which are known as ADSCs.[117]

ADSCs produce a variety of growth factors (VEGF, PDGF, FGF, IGF-1, IL-6,7,8, TNF-α, etc.) that provide angiogenic, antioxidative, anti-inflammatory, immunosuppressive, and anti-apoptotic potential.[118–123] The immunosuppressive properties along with lack of HLA-DR expression makes allogeneic transfer possible; however, this remains to be further investigated.[122,123] The clinical application of ADSCs include their use in regenerative medicine and as a means to improve fat survival. ADSCs due to their angiogenic and antiapoptotic properties stabilize blood supply in hypoxic conditions, thus enhancing fat survival. By differentiation into adipocytes, the volume of the transplanted fat is also stabilized.[118–124]

The use of ADSCs to improve survival of fat graft is known as cell-assisted lipotransfer (CAL) first described by Yoshimura et al.[125] Although improved fat survival and volume retention with use of ADSCs has been demonstrated, there are few reports which did not show any effect of ADSCs on graft take.[126–129] However, these studies had utilized freshly obtained stem cells intraoperatively instead of cultured cells as in studies which showed significant difference.

The safety of use of ADSCs remains a concern because of its inconclusive role in tumorigenesis. Many experimental studies demonstrated its tumorigenic properties in lung, breast, and endometric cancer.[130,131] Many other reports also demonstrated a potential antitumor effect on hematopoietic, breast, and pancreatic cancer models.[132,133] RESTORE-2 trial on breast cancer patients who underwent ADSC augmented fat transfer following breast conservation therapy reported no recurrences up to 1 year follow-up.[134] However, the safety remains inconclusive and needs further research.

Recipient Site Preparation with External Volume Expansion (EVE)

Continued negative pressure to recipient bed with help of an external device promotes angiogenesis and also activates progenitor cells in the bed, thus leading to improved survival of the graft.[135–139] This has already been proven successful in large volume grafts for breast. Clinical feasibility in other areas still remains to be evaluated.

Use of Cryopreserved Fat for Facial Augmentation

Fat grafting though is a very effective and safe procedure for facial augmentation, it is associated with resorption and often requires multiple sittings. The same patient has to undergo the trauma and pain of harvesting the fat again for the procedure. To alleviate the same, researchers have contemplated in preserving the fat after the first procedure in excess of the requirement by means of cryopreservation in a liquid nitrogen tank at −196°C with a cryopreservative solution. In the subsequent procedures, the fat is rapidly thawed to 37°C for 6 to 10 minutes and used again. The safety and efficacy of the cryopreserved fat has been studied in vitro.[140–142] But it has found lesser acceptance because of the high costs associated with preserving the fat. Few recent reports demonstrated its favorable uses in clinical subjects.

Topical Nanofat

Nanofat prepared from the patient, compounded with a liposomal delivery vehicle, has been used as a topical nanofat biocreme.[94] This when used in conjunction with fractionated LASERs or microneedling techniques are thought to enter the dermis through the open pores and thus enhance the rejuvenating effect on facial skin. Further research on the mechanism of drug delivery and the efficacy remains to be studied.

Future

The future of fat grafting lies in the use of cell-based therapy and its role in regenerative medicine. The isolation, preservation, and extensive use of ADSCs and SVF will help in various clinical situations. The role of marking stem cells with tissue marker and using them in the treatment of cancer is a potential future use. Another idea being actively propagated is the banking of embryonic stem cells by prophylactic suctioning of fat for use in therapeutic emergency.[143] However, the clinical application in these directions remains unexplored. The cost of production, its processing and preservation, however, need standardization. The use of human cell-based therapies will help in predicting the survival potential of the grafted fat which tends to undergo resorption. The wound healing, regenerative, and rejuvenating potentials of these cells will help us in preventing the atrophic changes associated with aging. The extracellular matrix scaffolds and adipose tissue scaffolds will help in retaining the volume and achieving the long-term result. Biological tissues including fat when combined with many unique compounds which act as biologic or synthetic scaffold will have a potential role in the regenerative medicine.

Summary

Fat grafting has been extensively used in various clinical situations in restoring the facial aesthetics. The final results depend on its systematic harvest, processing, and placement in the tissues. It helps us in achieving the desired reproducible results in difficult situations. Earlier the use of de-epithelialized free flaps was the standard procedure of choice in patients with hemifacial microsomia which tend to sag in the long run, leading to highly unaesthetic appearance. The advent and use of fat grafts has gone a long way in treating these conditions with impunity. Its use in many difficult situations in facial scarring and antiaging properties is a boon and is a powerful tool in the kitty of plastic surgeons. The combined use of face lifts and volumization by fat grafting results in better long-term results. Use of nanofat grafting also has long-lasting results in fine facial wrinkles and hyperpigmentation. Use of fat grafting in scleroderma and HIV-associated lipodystrophy helps in changing the lives of many patients. In future, we will come across many more developments pertaining to the human cell-based therapies and use of adipose extracellular scaffolds.

References

1. Coleman SR, Saboeiro AP. Fat grafting to the breast revisited: safety and efficacy. Plast Reconstr Surg 2007;119(3):775–785, discussion 786–787
2. Neuber F. Fat transplantation. Berichtüber die Verhandlungen der deutschen Gesellschaftfür Chirurgie. Zentralbl Chir 1893;22:66
3. Rajan S, Ajayakumar K, Sasidharanpillai S, George B. Autologous fat graft for soft tissue camouflage in craniofacial microsomia. J Cutan Aesthet Surg 2019;12(4):223–226
4. Yamaguchi K, Lonic D, Ko EW, Lo LJ. An integrated surgical protocol for adult patients with hemifacial microsomia: methods and outcome. PLoS One 2017;12(8):e0177223
5. Arcuri F, Brucoli M, Baragiotta N, Stellin L, Giarda M, Benech A. The role of fat grafting in the treatment of posttraumatic maxillofacial deformities. Craniomaxillofac Trauma Reconstr 2013;6(2):121–126
6. Coleman SR, Grover R. The anatomy of the aging face: volume loss and changes in 3-dimensional topography. Aesthet Surg J 2006;26(1S):S4–S9
7. Coleman S, Saboeiro A, Sengelmann R. A comparison of lipoatrophy and aging: volume deficits in the face. Aesthetic Plast Surg 2009;33(1):14–21
8. Singhania R, Kotler DP. Lipodystrophy in HIV patients: its challenges and management approaches. HIV AIDS (Auckl) 2011;3:135–143
9. Guaraldi G, Murri R, Orlando G, et al. Severity of lipodystrophy is associated with decreased health-related quality of life. AIDS Patient Care STDS 2008;22(7):577–585
10. Funt D, Pavicic T. Dermal fillers in aesthetics: an overview of adverse events and treatment approaches. Clin Cosmet Investig Dermatol 2013;6:295–316
11. Nakagami H, Morishita R, Maeda K, Kikuchi Y, Ogihara T, Kaneda Y. Adipose tissue-derived stromal cells as a novel option for regenerative cell therapy. J Atheroscler Thromb 2006;13(2):77–81
12. Bourin P, Bunnell BA, Casteilla L, et al. Stromal cells from the adipose tissue-derived stromal vascular fraction and culture expanded adipose tissue-derived stromal/stem cells: a joint statement of the International Federation for Adipose Therapeutics and Science (IFATS) and the International Society for Cellular Therapy (ISCT). Cytotherapy 2013;15(6):641–648
13. Kapur SK, Dos-Anjos Vilaboa S, Llull R, Katz AJ. Adipose tissue and stem/progenitor cells: discovery and development. Clin Plast Surg 2015;42(2):155–167
14. Czerny V. Dreiplastische Operationen. III. Plastischer Ersatz der Brustdru¨sedurchein Lipom. Arch F Klin Chir 1895;50:544–550
15. Hollander E. Die kosmetische Chirurgie. In: Joseph M, editor. Handbuch der Kosmetik. Leipzig, Germany: von Veit; 1912: 689–690, 708
16. Miller CC. Cannula implants and review of implantation technics in esthetic surgery. Chicago: Oak Press; 1926:25–30, 66–71
17. Lexer E. Die freienTransplantationen. Stuttgart, Germany: Enke; 1919–1924
18. Gillies HD. Plastic surgery of the face. London: Frowde, Hodder, Stoughton; 1920
19. Illouz YG. The fat cell "graft": a new technique to fill depressions. Plast Reconstr Surg 1986;78(1):122–123
20. Coleman SR. The technique of periorbital lipoinfiltration. Oper Techn Plast Surg 1994;1:120–126
21. Coleman SR. Facial recontouring with lipostructure. Clin Plast Surg 1997;24(2):347–367
22. Coleman SR. Facial augmentation with structural fat grafting. Clin Plast Surg 2006;33(4):567–577
23. Tonnard P, Verpaele A, Peeters G, Hamdi M, Cornelissen M, Declercq H. Nanofat grafting: basic research and clinical applications. Plast Reconstr Surg 2013;132(4):1017–1026
24. Bellini E, Grieco MP, Raposio E. The science behind autologous fat grafting. Ann Med Surg (Lond) 2017;24:65–73
25. H. Neuhof, Hirschfeld S. The transplantation of tissues. New York: D. Appleton; 1923:1–297
26. Peer LA. Loss of weight and volume in human fat graft, with postulation of a cell survival theory. Plast Reconstr Surg 1950;217
27. Mashiko T, Yoshimura K. How does fat survive and remodel after grafting? Clin Plast Surg 2015;42(2):181–190
28. Eto H, Kato H, Suga H, et al. The fate of adipocytes after nonvascularized fat grafting: evidence of early death and replacement of adipocytes. Plast Reconstr Surg 2012;129(5): 1081–1092

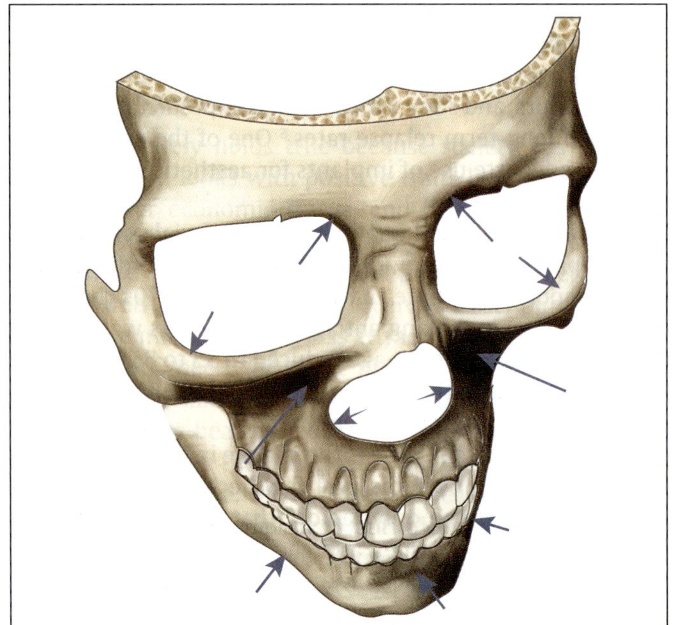

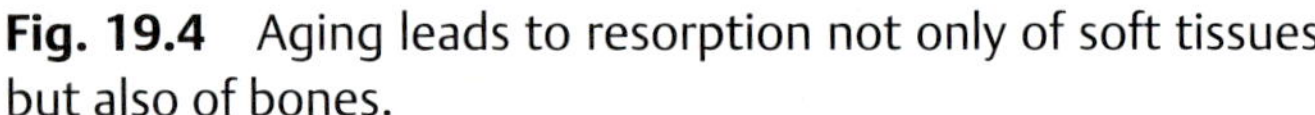

Fig. 19.4 Aging leads to resorption not only of soft tissues but also of bones.

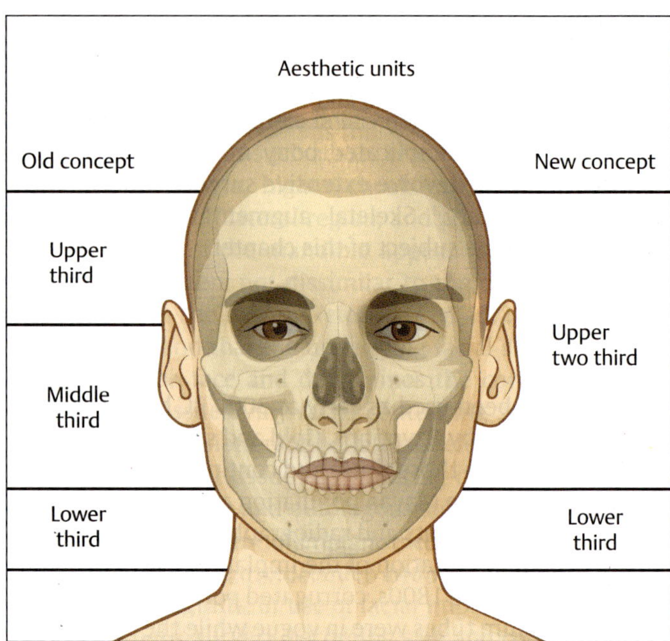

Fig. 19.5 The old and new concept of facial aesthetic units.

Table 19.1 Comparison of skeletal augmentation using implants versus autogenous augmentation

Implants	Autogenous augmentation using osteotomy/bone grafts
No donor site morbidity	Donor site morbidity
Easier and less cumbersome surgery	Difficult surgery
Lesser operating time	Longer operating times
Predictable results	Unpredictable results due to chances of bone resorption
Shorter learning curve	Longer learning curve
Greater chances of infection	Lesser chances of infection
Chances of implant rejection	No chances of rejection
Additional cost of implants	No such cost

The main advantages and disadvantages of implants over autogenous augmentation using osteotomies/bone grafts have been summarized in **Table 19.1**.

Indications and Contraindications

The major indications for facial implants are deficiencies in the facial skeleton due to aging, congenital asymmetries, trauma including accidents, asymmetry due to previous surgeries, or postcancer ablation asymmetry. Facial implants are used for:

- **Skeletal enhancement:** Enhancement refers to improvement of features of an otherwise healthy young person to give him/her more refined appearance. Facial implants can be useful in healthy, young people who have normal skeletal relationships but who have desire for a more chiseled appearance with better definition and angularity of their face.
- **Restoration:** Restoration refers to re-instatement of the appearance of an individual to his/her former youthful appearance. The term is usually applied for middle-aged individuals in whom aging has led to changes like sagging and loss of volume but these changes are not dramatic/advanced and it is possible to restore them to their youthful appearance by facial cosmetic surgery.
- **Rejuvenation:** The term "rejuvenation" is used for individuals with advanced aging. In these individuals use of facial cosmetic surgery can help in achieving a more youthful appearance but it is not possible to give them an appearance exactly similar to how they looked when young. This happens because with

advanced aging, not only the soft tissues but the skeletal structures also undergo atrophy, leading to retrusion of the midface and lower face. Use of implants will restore the facial skeleton in three dimensions to some extent and also provide support to the overlying soft tissues. The depleted volume of the soft tissues as well as tissue laxity has to be addressed using additional tools in order to rejuvenate the face to yield a more youthful appearance. In these cases, the surgeon must discuss realistic goals with the individual and suggest multimodality approach to their problem, before taking him/her up for surgery.[8] It is important to remember that more youthful results are achieved with greater ease when the goal is enhancement or restoration compared to when goal is rejuvenation.

- **Alternative/adjunct to orthognathic surgery:** Congenital skeletal hypoplasia like mandibular hypoplasia, maxillary deficiency, and malar/submalar hypoplasia benefit by the use of implants. In these patients, facial implants may be used as an alternative to orthognathic surgery if their occlusion is normal or has been corrected by orthodontic management. Implants can simulate the effect of skeletal osteotomies in such cases. Implants can also be used as an adjunct to orthognathic procedures like Le Fort I maxillary advancement, sagittal split osteotomy, or sliding genioplasty to enhance their results or to correct asymmetries occurring as a consequence of these surgeries or deficiencies left unaddressed by these procedures.[10,11]

The major contraindications to implant placement are:

- Deficiency of adequate, good quality soft tissue cover.
- Deficiencies in volumes in areas like oral or orbital apertures which do not have a stable skeletal base.
- Presence of infection.
- Inability to achieve clear margins after excision of a malignancy.[3]

Relative contraindications are uncontrolled diabetes mellitus, hypertension, or presence of psychiatric illness.

Types of Implant Materials

An **"ideal" implant** is one that is biocompatible and simulates the characteristics of the tissues for which it is intended to be used. It should be able to withstand the mechanical stresses of the forces acting over that area while retaining its form and function. It should be inert, capable of getting incorporated with the host tissues and noncarcinogenic. Besides these characteristics, an "ideal" implant should be nonallergenic, resistant to infections, and not leave any toxic products on its degradation. It should be easily available, inexpensive, and easy to sterilize. Although the implants have improved in their characteristics drastically since their inception, an ideal implant is still far from reality.

The two most common alloplastic materials used specifically for facial implants are silicone and high-density porous polyethylene (Medpor). Polymethyl methacrylate is also preferred implant material in specific areas like forehead and temporal region.

Silicone

Silicone has been extensively used in plastic surgery for over six decades and is the most common solid material used for facial implants. Medical-grade silicone is a synthetic polymer consisting of repeating chains of polydimethylsiloxane $[(CH)_{32}SiO_n]$, produced by the process of vulcanization in which oxygen, carbon, and silica are heated to achieve the polymer. The viscosity of the final product depends upon the length of the polymer chain and on the degree of cross-linkage. Hence, silicone can be found in liquid, gel, rubbery, or solid form. Liquid silicone has shorter chains and lesser degree of cross-linking while more solid forms have a greater length of chain and also more cross-linking. As facial implants, silicone has been used for augmentation of malar area, chin, and nose (**Fig. 19.6**). It has also been used for reconstruction of ear (**Fig. 19.7**) and mandibular condyle, besides being used as sheets for the reconstruction of the floor of orbit.[4]

The major advantages of silicone that have led to its widespread use are its excellent biocompatibility, pliable nature, ability to be carved easily into the desired form, ease of sterilization due to its resistance to high temperatures, and relative inertness. It is a nonporous material and has very smooth contours making its insertion simple. After insertion, the silicone implant gets encapsulated in a fibrous capsule and never gets incorporated with the underlying bone unlike porous polyethylene. Due to its smooth surface, it is more prone to seromas. It also needs to be immobilized with sutures to the surrounding soft tissue or with screws to the bone to prevent displacement. However, its smooth surface and encapsulation makes its removal, if needed, a simple procedure.

High-Density Porous Polyethylene

High-density porous polyethylene (HDPE) is another commonly used material for facial implants. It is made of repetitive carbon backbone and hydrogen side chains forming the polyethylene structure. It was developed in the 1970s. Though available both in solid and porous structure, the latter is the preferred one in medical use. Among the various densities of medical-grade polyethylene, such as low, high, and ultrahigh density, the most commonly used is the high-density variant.

HDPE is a stable biocompatible implant (**Fig. 19.8**). It is inert, causes a minimal foreign body reaction, and does not degrade over time. It is easily sterilizable and is malleable when heated but is nonpliable at room temperature. HDPE implants are commonly used for chin, malar, orbital rim, nasal, and mandibular angle augmentation. They are also used for ear reconstruction with temporoparietal fascia flap as single-stage reconstruction (**Fig. 19.9**). Its porosity allows for tissue ingrowth, thereby allowing it to get incorporated

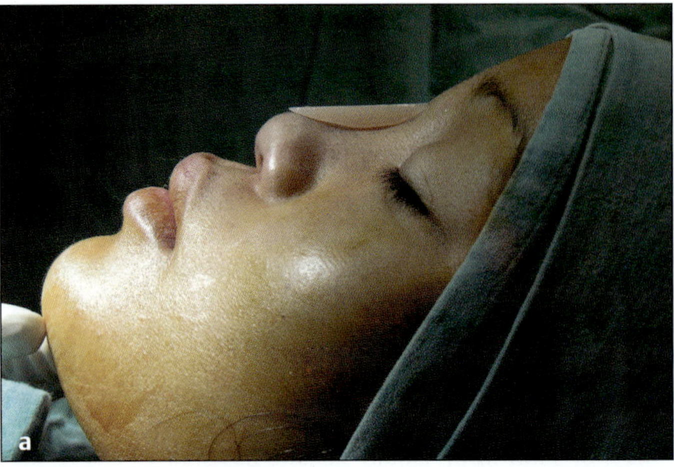

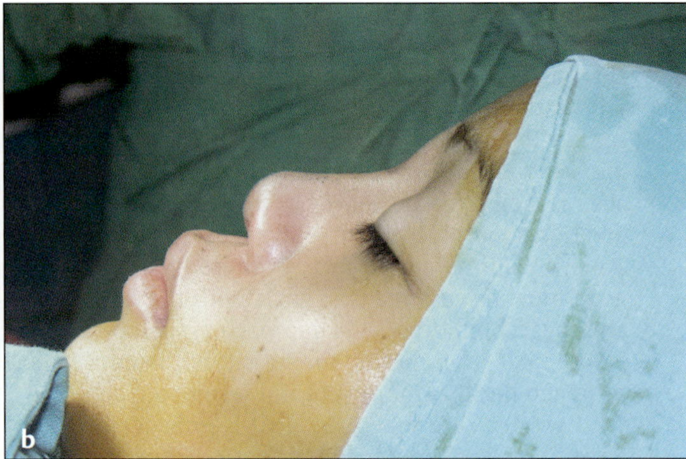

Fig. 19.6 **(a, b)** Silicone implant for augmentation of dorsum of the nose.

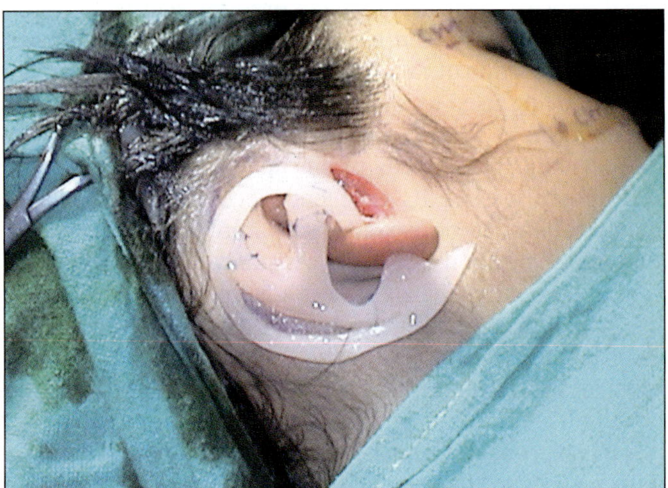

Fig. 19.7 Hand-carved silicon ear implant for microtia reconstruction.

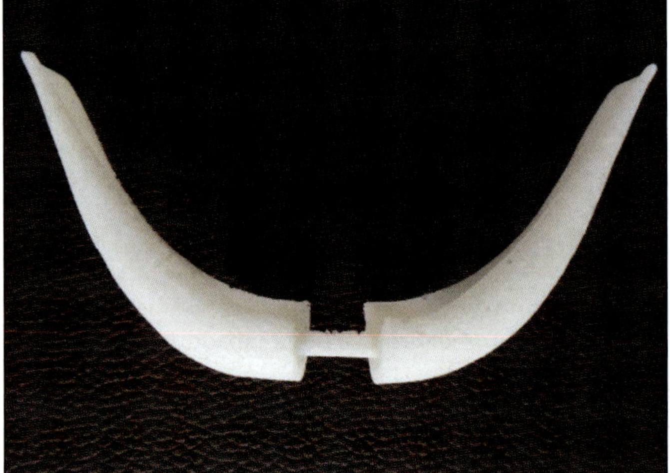

Fig. 19.8 High-density porous polyethylene implant.

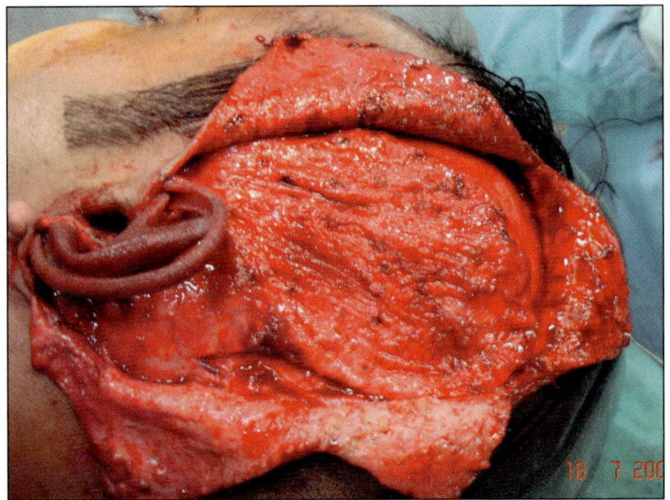

Fig. 19.9 High-density porous polyethylene ear implant being used with temporoparietal fascia flap for microtia reconstruction.

with the underlying bony structures over time. This property allows for firm attachment of the implant to surrounding structures, thereby reducing chances of implant migration. However, this property also makes it difficult to remove in the event of complications.[12] The implant is available as sheets/blocks that can be carved and also in prefabricated and customized forms. Customization can be easily done these days using computer-aided designing and three-dimensional printing, which have been discussed later.

A brief comparison of the properties of silicone versus polyethylene implants is provided in **Table 19.2**.[8]

Basic Concepts and Principles of Facial Contouring Using Implants

Facial aesthetic contouring involves achieving a balance between the soft tissue and skeletal framework to restore a youthful appearance. With age, the soft tissues and the skeleton both undergo atrophy. In many patients who have a

Table 19.2 Silicone versus polyethylene implants

Silicone	Polyethylene
Easy to carve	Difficult to carve
Flexible, hence can be easily inserted through small incision	Not flexible, requires bigger incision and implant can fracture if too much manipulation is attempted
Easily fixed using sutures	Need screw fixation
Can easily conform to underlying bony framework due to flexibility	Inflexibility results in difficult conformation; hence requires higher accuracy in designing/carving the implant
Removal easy due to capsule formation around the implant	Removal difficult as the implant gets integrated with the underlying bone
Less prone to infection	More prone to infection because of porosity
Can withstand minor infection and is salvageable	Cannot withstand infection and once infected has to be removed

good skeletal foundation, aging leading to shrinkage of soft tissues can bring out the definition of bony prominences making them look more beautiful, while in others, it can emphasize the atrophic soft tissues making them look old. The quantum of loss of both these components have to be analyzed in detail to see what elements need restoration for a good balance and harmony between these two elements.[3] An artistic ability to be able to assess and determine the exact deficiency is critical for delivering optimal results.

Use of facial implants causes three-dimensional changes in facial appearance in contrast to lifting procedures which cause only two-dimensional changes. In patients with mild or moderate changes due to aging, use of facial implants alone can sometimes restore the youthful appearance, while in those with severe changes due to aging, lifting procedures with adjuvant use of volumizing procedures like structural fat grafting can complement the results of facial implants to achieve harmony.

The six basic principles for planning facial implants as described by Terino et al are as follows:[13]

1. Purpose: The purpose of facial implants is to optimally restore the three-dimensional form and balance of the facial anatomy.
2. Practice: To achieve predictable and precise results, the surgeon must have good experience. Hence, practice is essential to understand and visualize the aesthetic changes that can be achieved by use of facial implants.
3. Precision: The implants are permanent, incompressible devices used to augment facial contours. Since face has a very delicate anatomy where even minor changes are very visible, even small errors in the size, shape, or positioning of the implants can cause major visible asymmetry postoperatively. Hence, the need for precisely designed implants cannot be over emphasized.
4. Principles of aesthetics: Implants help in improving the aesthetics of face by achieving facial balance by correcting the deficient areas by adding volume to them.
5. Predictability: Implants are made from stable, biocompatible materials and the results are predictable.
6. Permanence: Implants cause permanent changes to one's appearance and do not change due to effect of gravity or aging.

The three major promontories of nose, malar region, and the jawline along with the supraorbital rim (which is of lesser significance than the other three) define an individual's facial structure and aesthetics. By altering the volume of these promontories and carefully choosing the size, shape, and design of the implant and its positioning, one can easily cause subtle alterations and changes to a more youthful appearance. The fourth promontory of the supraorbital ridge/forehead needs alteration in very few cases but may be significant in patients who undergo gender reassignment surgery.

Applied Anatomy

The facial structures are divided into four planes from superficial to deep. The first plane is the skin, the second plane is subcutaneous tissues, the third one is the superficial musculoaponeurotic system (SMAS), and the fourth plane is the bony skeleton. Once the analysis of the face in terms of skeletal and soft tissues elements is made by analyzing each aesthetic unit and anatomic zone, the plan is made as to which areas need attention and the implant and adjuvant procedures are decided accordingly.[8] The placement of facial implants in the subperiosteal plane improves skeletal contours, which, in turn, simulate the fullness of the overlying soft tissues, thereby improving the appearance.

Analysis of facial volumes is done with respect to the following three elements in decreasing order of significance:

1. The four major bony promontories namely the nose, malar area, chin, and jawline, and supraorbital rim are of prime importance.
2. Secondary importance is given to the three minor bony promontories of premaxilla, temple, and the suborbital region.

3. Tertiary significance is given to the soft tissue areas of jowls, nasolabial region, tear-trough region, and perinasal premaxillary region to evaluate its retrusion or protrusion.

The applied anatomy of the temporal-forehead region, malar-midface region, and the premandibular jawline region is discussed in detail in the following text.[8]

Temporal and Forehead Region

The temporal fossa is a shallow concavity that lies on the lateral aspect of the skull. It is bounded by the frontal process of zygoma and zygomatic process of the frontal bone anteriorly, superior temporal lines superiorly and posteriorly, and the zygomatic arch inferiorly. Its main contents are temporalis muscle, superficial temporal artery and vein, branches of mandibular and deep temporal nerves, auriculotemporal nerve, and temporal branch of the facial nerve. When the concavity is exaggerated due to decrease in bulk of the temporalis muscle or the temporal fat pad or bony deformity, it looks aesthetically unpleasing.

Malar-Midface Region

Augmentation of the skeletal anatomy of this area leads to aesthetic changes in the contour of the cheek. The relevant anatomy is illustrated in **Fig. 19.10**. This region is divided into five well-defined anatomic zones for the purpose of augmentation using implants (**Fig. 19.11**).[3]

Zone 1

It extends from the infraorbital foramen to include *the major portion of maxilla up to the anterior one-third of the zygomatic arch.* It is the largest subspace of the malar region and its augmentation leads to maximum increase in the volume of the cheek which gives a sharp, angular appearance to the cheek. In women usually a 3-mm implant in this region is sufficient while men may require a 4- to 5-mm implant for augmentation of this area.

Zone 2

This is the second-most important zone and is formed by the *middle one-third of the zygomatic arch.* When this area is augmented along with zone 1, it accentuates the lateral cheek. This area needs augmentation in patients with narrow upper face or those having long face syndrome.

Zone 3

Comprises the *paranasal area* and *lies medial to a line drawn vertically through the infraorbital foramen.* Deficiency in this area leads to a tear-trough deformity. Augmentation of this area requires release of the origin of the orbicularis oculi muscle from the medial part of the orbit to correct the tear-trough deformity. It is important to remember that the infraorbital nerve is very sensitive to trauma; hence, the dissection to this area must proceed with utmost care to avoid injury and loss of sensations in its distribution, which may take a long time to recover. Since this area has thin skin, the implant should be very precisely designed to avoid any show through the skin.

Zone 4

Posterior one-third of the zygomatic arch forms zone 4. Intervention in this zone is likely to cause injury to the superficial temporal artery, temporomandibular joint, and zygomaticotemporal nerve. Hence, implant is avoided in this zone.

Zone 5

The *submalar zonal triangle* forms zone 5. Boundaries include zygomaticus muscle groups, their innervation, and SMAS anteriorly; masseter and its overlying tendinous fascia posteriorly; the lower bony margin of the malar eminence superiorly; gingivobuccal sulcus lateral to the oral commissure inferiorly and the nasolabial mound medially.

This region is the most significant among all the zones, and frequently requires augmentation. Augmentation of this zone leads to a full, round "apple cheek" contour by extending the midface fullness downward to the submalar region. The second-most common augmentation is the composite augmentation of zones 1 and 5. This composite augmentation is used to achieve the appearance of an accentuated malar prominence and to mimic good soft tissue volume in midface.[8]

Premandibular Jawline Region

Augmentation of the premandibular jawline is utilized to achieve a chiseled attractive and youthful appearance. Jawline region is divided into four zones as follows (**Fig. 19.12**).[3]

Zone 1

This zone constitutes the *central mentum which is the area between the two mental foramina.* The floor of the central mentum is the surface of the central mandible including the mental tubercle. In the early days of chin implants, only this zone was often augmented and led to an unattractive protuberance in the center of the chin as it made the prejowl sulcus area look more prominent. Now, the area is usually augmented using implants with lateral extensions that fit onto the mental contour snugly and give it a more natural appearance.

Zone 2

This zone is the *midlateral zone that extends from the mental foramina to the oblique ridge of the mandible.* Superiorly it is bound by the upper border of mandible and inferiorly by the lower border of mandible. The roof of this area consists of platysma, SMAS, anterior facial vein and artery, and the marginal mandibular branch of facial nerve crossing the mandible to enter the lip depressors.

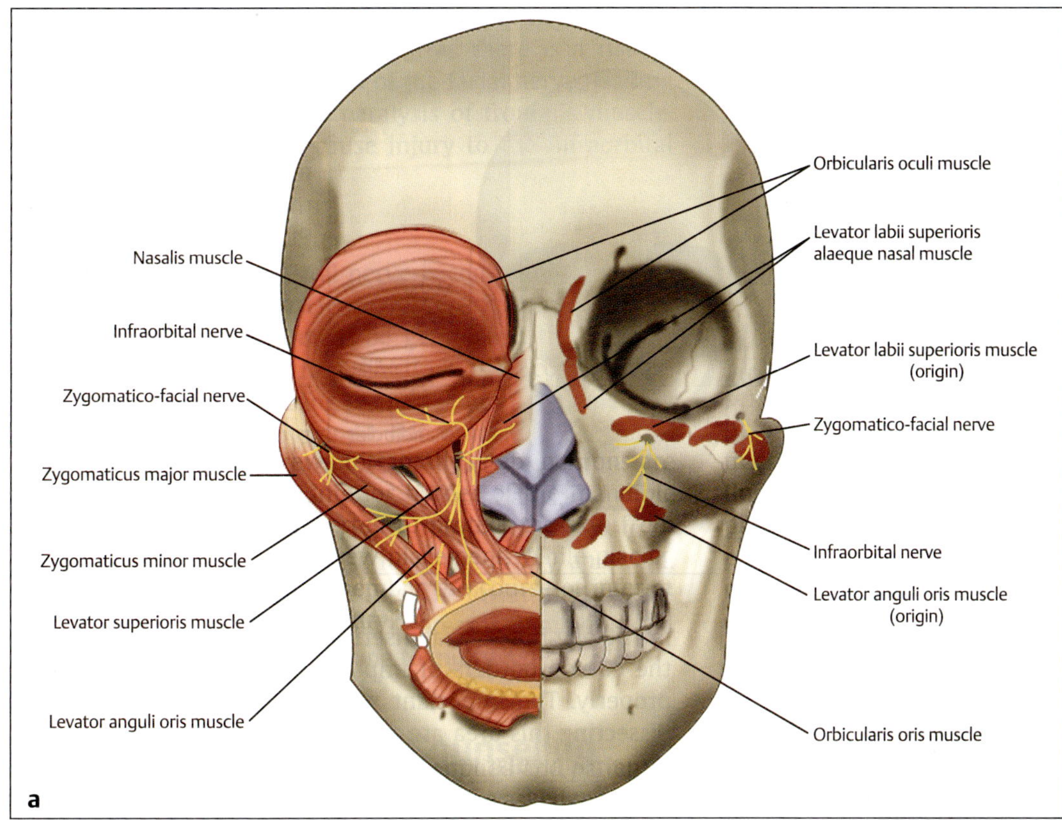

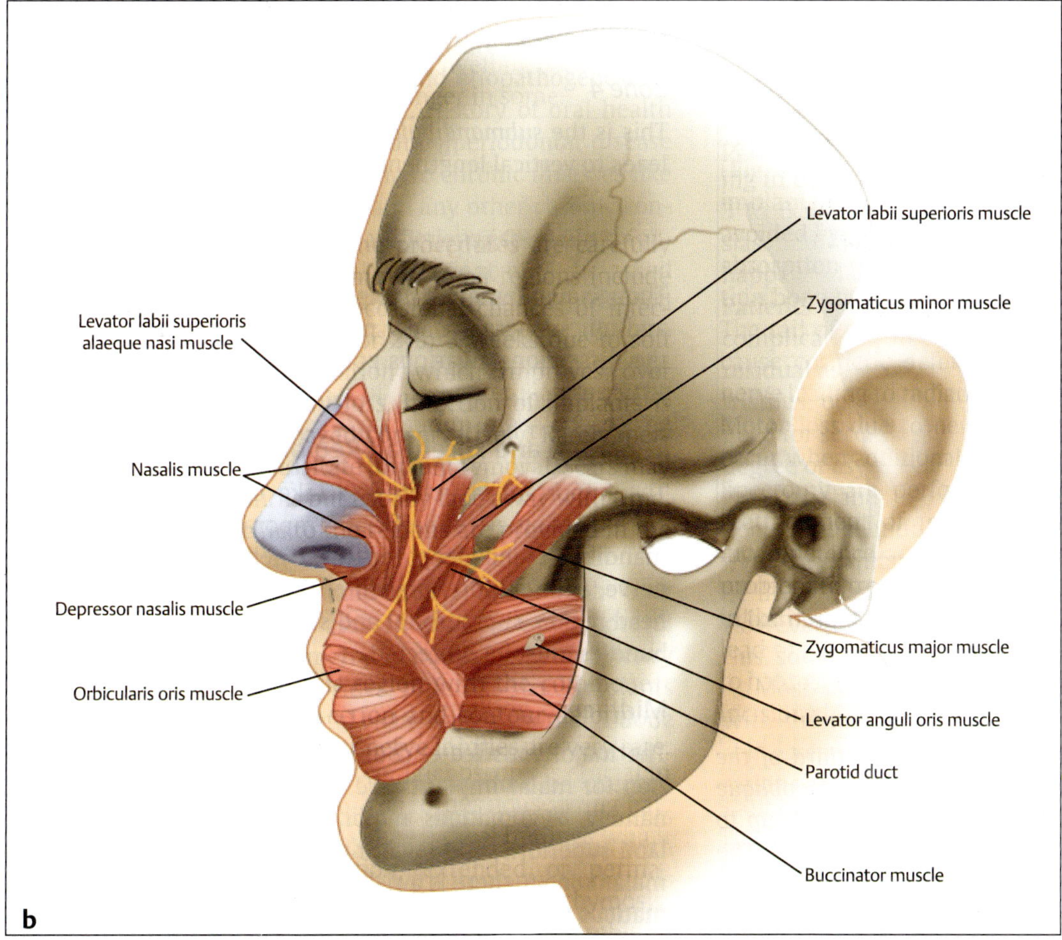

Fig. 19.10 (a, b) Musculature of the midface relevant to implants.

It is important to note here that published studies indicate that more than 47% of patients consulting for cosmetic surgery procedures meet the criteria for mental disorders. The most common mental disorders seen in patients of cosmetic surgery are body dysmorphic disorder (BDD) in 5 to 15% cases, narcissistic personality disorder in around 25% patients, and histrionic personality disorder in around 10% population.[15,16] In BDD, patients have an exaggerated preoccupation with any defect in their appearance to the point that it impairs their occupation, and social and personal relationships. These patients have an insatiable need for plastic surgery. It is recommended that plastic surgeons routinely screen their patients for BDD as a basic work-up.[17] These patients often suffer from anxiety or depression. Patients with narcissistic personality disorder have a pervasive pattern of grandiosity, constant need for admiration, and/or lack of empathy. Patients with histrionic personality have excessive emotional and attention-seeking behavior that starts in adulthood. Hence, it is important to get a psychiatric clearance before taking them up for surgery.[16,17]

Investigations

Routine Investigations

Routine investigations like complete hemogram, coagulation profile, and serology for human immunodeficiency virus and Hepatitis B and Hepatitis C virus are essential. Blood sugar profile, hormonal profile like assessment for thyroid hormone levels, chest radiographs, electrocardiogram, and echocardiogram are done whenever indicated.

Specific Investigations

Although the assessment of facial asymmetries and deficiencies is mostly clinical, radiological investigations may assist in planning implant surgery. Cephalometric radiographs and three-dimensional computerized tomography (CT) of face must be done to assess the asymmetry of the face. This information can be digitized to construct three-dimensional life-sized models that can be utilized to design customized implants with significant facial asymmetry. Use of computer-aided designing of implants is discussed below in detail. Dental X-rays, orthopantomogram, or CT scans are done to rule out any dental/bony pathology including focus of infection.

Role of Computer-Aided Designing and Computer-Aided Manufacture (CAD/CAM) and 3D Imprinting

CAD/CAM have been utilized for a long time in reconstruction of cranial defects, planning of the site of osteotomies and fixation in orthognathic surgeries, refining the contour deformities after orthognathic surgeries, besides being used in jaw reconstruction with vascularized free fibula. They have now been introduced to purely aesthetic indications as well.[18] In CAD, a CT scan of the facial skeleton is done which is then transferred to a software which analyzes the contour of the craniofacial skeleton. This can then be used to design customized implants depending on what contours are planned for enhancement. There are two techniques of designing the implants. One technique employs transmitting the CAD data to prepare wax models which are then utilized to make custom implants. The other technique is used to make streolithographic (SL) models. These models are used as a template on the basis of which virtual implants are designed. After designing these virtual implants, they are sent for approval to the plastic surgeon, who may suggest further modifications. This technique allows millimeter precision and is the preferred technique. Once the virtual implant is approved, the final implant is manufactured and is made available for use (**Fig. 19.13**).

With advent of 3D printing, the surgeon can customize the implants as an in-office procedure, bringing down the costs significantly. The main areas where CAD/CAM and 3D printing are used for purely aesthetic reasons are forehead and jaw contouring. Besides facial augmentation for aging patients and those with facial deficiencies, this can also have a role in transgender surgery when the patients request for redefinition of their facial bone structure to align with their new gender. Women have more vertical and smooth forehead contours than males who have a central prominence in lower one-third of the forehead due to development of the frontal sinus. Besides this, the prominence of supraorbital rims can make the eyes look more deep set while retrusion of the supraorbital rim makes eyes look more prominent. Men have more prominent, squarish jawline as compared to females who have more gently slanting jawlines. CAD/CAM can be used to design implants to alter the forehead and jaw to give them more feminine or masculine appearance as deemed aesthetically suitable for the individual.

The major advantage of this technique is possibility of precise refinement. Besides this, operative time is reduced due to better preoperative planning and preparedness, thereby reducing the cost of surgery.

Positioning and Anesthesia

General anesthesia with local infiltration of epinephrine mixed local anesthetic is mostly preferred for placement of implants through intraoral approach. This ensures a secure airway with endotracheal intubation. Local anesthesia with intravenous sedation can be used for forehead augmentation and external approach to chin augmentation.

After completing the preoperative markings of the area, the patient is placed. Normotensive anesthesia keeping the systolic blood pressure within range is preferred. In addition

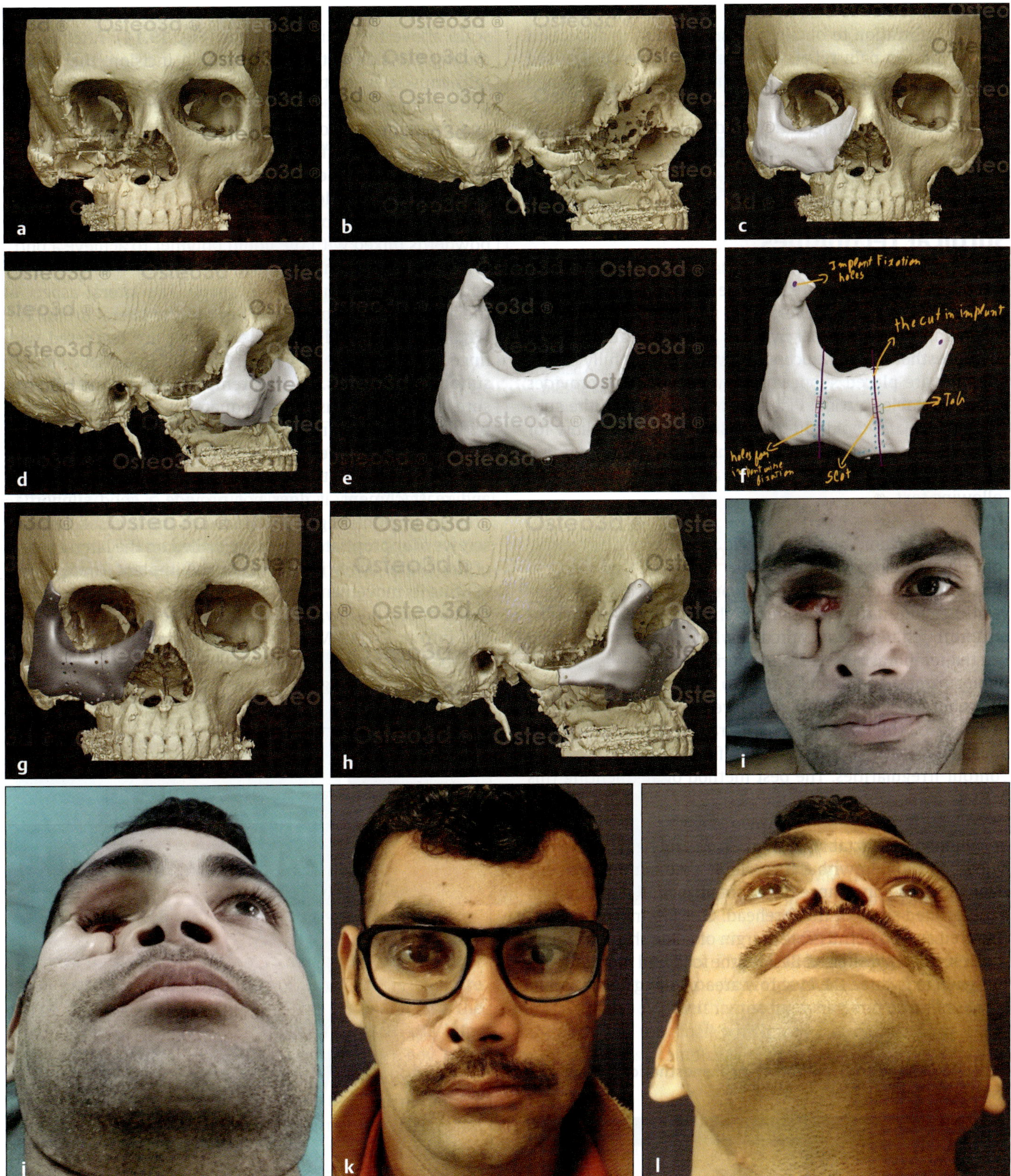

Fig. 19.13 (a) Computer-aided planning and designing for facial implants. Stereolithographic model of skull with posttrauma Rt zygomatic defect was created. Virtual implant of defect was first created and marked by the surgeon for changes. Final titanium implant was made and used during surgery. **(b–l)** Before and after pictures of the same patient operated with custom-designed implant. (These images are provided courtesy of Dr Anil Murarka, New Delhi, India.)

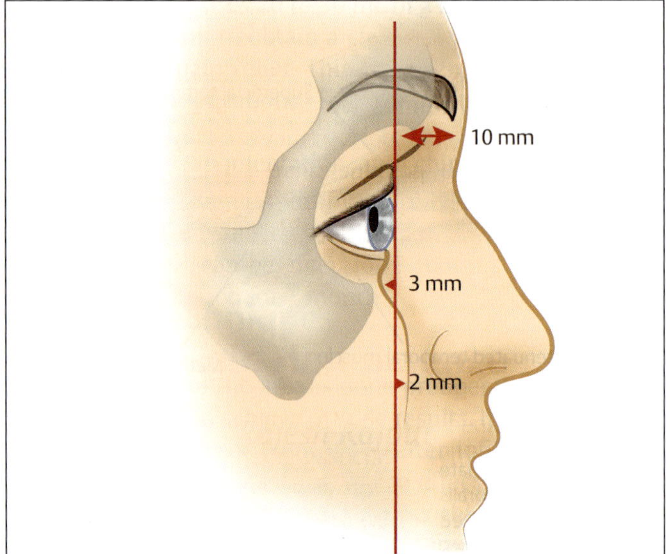

Fig. 19.17 Globe–infraorbital rim relations. In an average individual, the normal globe-infraorbital rim relationships comprise of the supraorbital rim projecting 10 mm beyond, the infraorbital rim lies 3 mm behind, and the cheek prominence 2 mm beyond the anterior surface of the cornea.

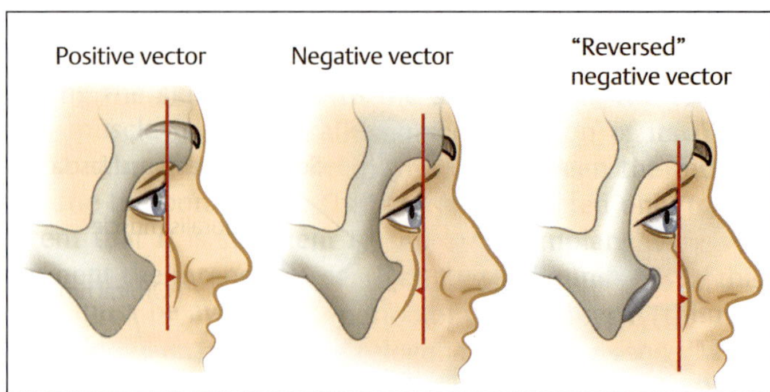

Fig. 19.18 Jelks and Jelks classification of globe–orbital rim relationships.

in **Fig. 19.18**. A negative vector is caused due to hypoplasia of the infraorbital part of maxilla. This deficiency does not usually exist alone and most of these patients also suffer from malar or submalar deficiency. Patients with negative vector are benefitted with infraorbital implants but may need implants with a malar extension when those areas are also hypoplastic. The area is approached via a subciliary/transconjunctival approach along with the intraoral incision (**Fig. 19.19**).[23]

The infraorbital nerve lies 8 mm below the infraorbital rim and in patients with hypoplastic faces it can lie anywhere 3 to 6 mm below the rim. Infraorbital nerve must be carefully preserved at all costs. The zygomaticofacial nerve is located 8 to 10 mm below the infraorbital rim on the lateral aspect of zygoma in line with the lateral orbital wall. This nerve is routinely sacrificed during the surgery. The implant is fixed with titanium screws to prevent both displacement and rotation. The malar soft tissues are sutured back in place using two figure-of-eight sutures after ensuring hemostasis. Patients who have lower eyelid retraction post blepharoplasty may in addition to implants need a lateral canthopexy.

Malar Implants

The midface consists of malar, infraorbital, and paranasal regions. Hinderer, Wilkinson, and Yaremchuk have described methods to determine the location of malar implants to give aesthetically pleasing contours (**Fig. 19.20**).[7,24,25] Multiple midface implants, if used judiciously, can mimic Le Forte III osteotomies (**Fig. 19.21**).

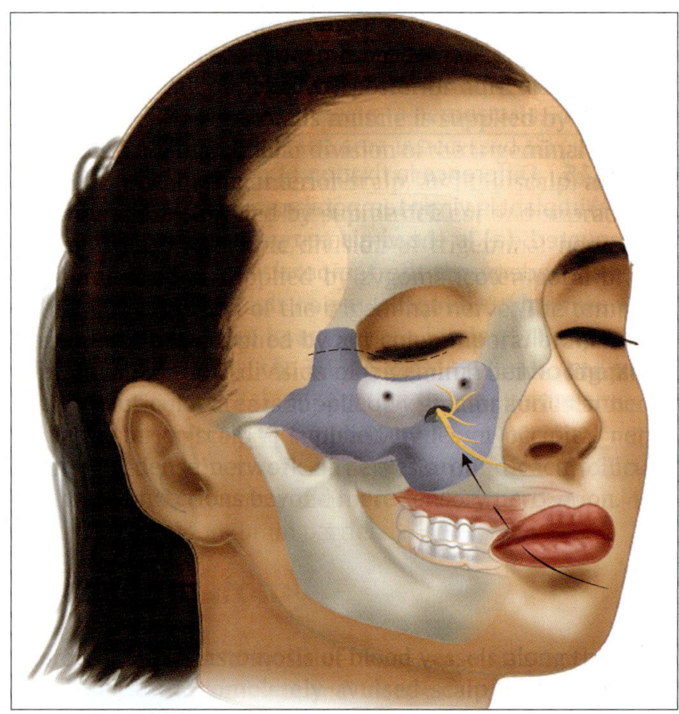

Fig. 19.19 Surgical approach to infraorbital implants.

Both silicone and porous polyethylene implants have been used for malar area; however, the author more commonly uses the latter. A rough guide to choosing these implants is that for patients with height of less than 5 feet 6 inches small or moderate implants with/without feathering are sufficient, while patients taller than this need large implants. In rare cases of extreme volume deficient or extremely tall patients, extralarge submalar implants may be required.[9]

The exposure to the malar/submalar area is best achieved by a combination of intra-oral and eyelid incisions (**Fig. 19.22**). The intraoral incision is made 1 cm above the gingivobuccal sulcus overlying the premolars on the labial aspect of the sulcus. The length of incision is around 2 to 2.5 cm (**Fig. 19.23**). While authors like Yaremchuk prefer transconjunctival retroseptal incision with lateral canthotomy, others prefer subciliary incision 1 mm below lower eyelid lash line extending to the crow-feet area, similar to

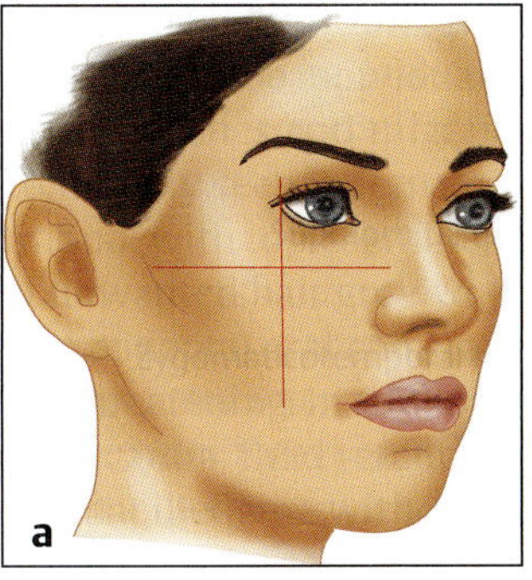

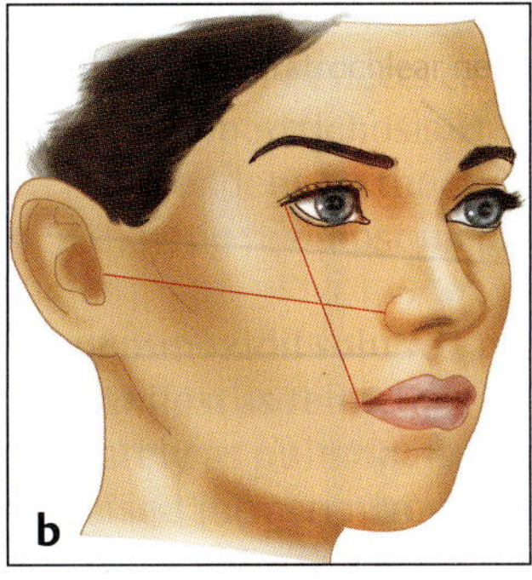

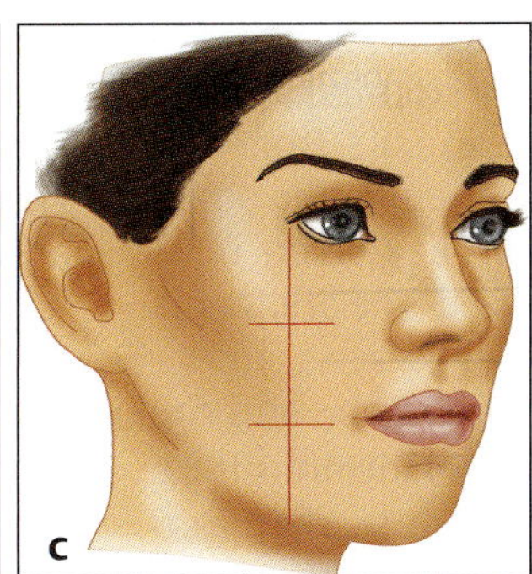

Fig. 19.20 Methods of marking for placement of malar prominence implants. **(a)** Yaremchuk method: Implant is placed slightly lateral to where a vertical line from lateral canthus of eye intersects a horizontal line through infra-orbital foramen. **(b)** Hinderer method: A line is drawn from tragus to ala and another from lateral canthus of eye to the angle of mouth. Implant is placed in the upper outer quadrant formed by intersection of these two lines. **(c)** Wilkinson method: A vertical line is dropped from the lateral canthus of eye to the border of mandible and divided into three equals. The implant is placed to achieve maximum prominence at junction of upper and middle third of this line.

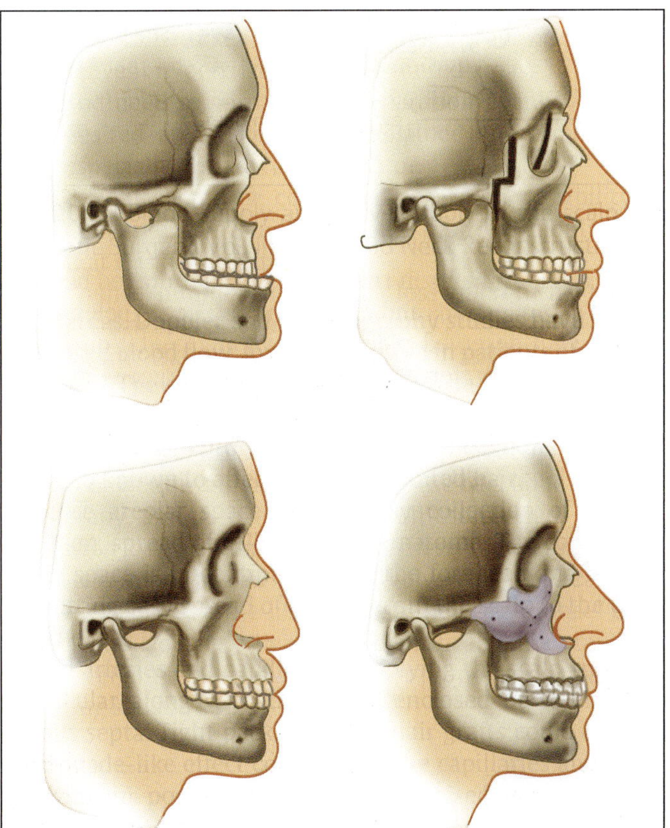

Fig. 19.21 Use of multiple midface implants mimics the effects of le Forte III osteotomy.

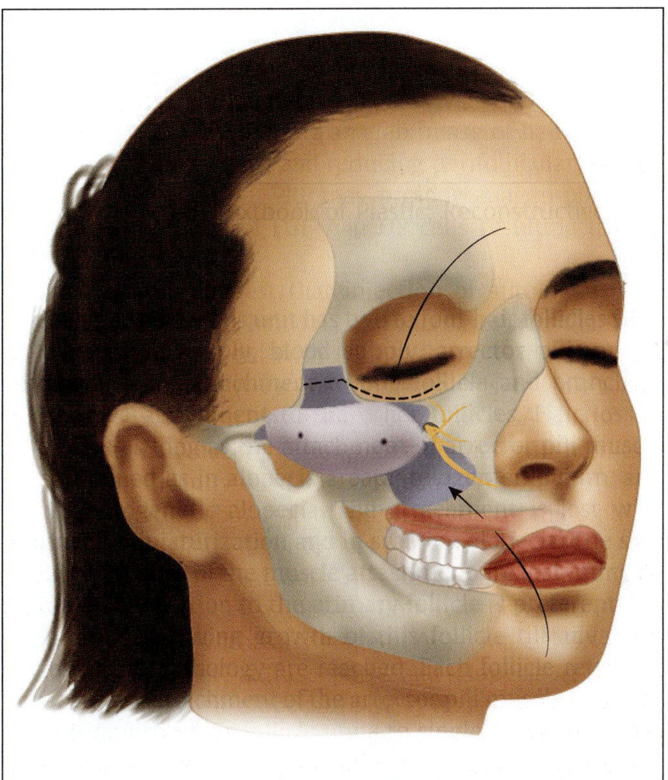

Fig. 19.22 Incisions and approach for malar implants.

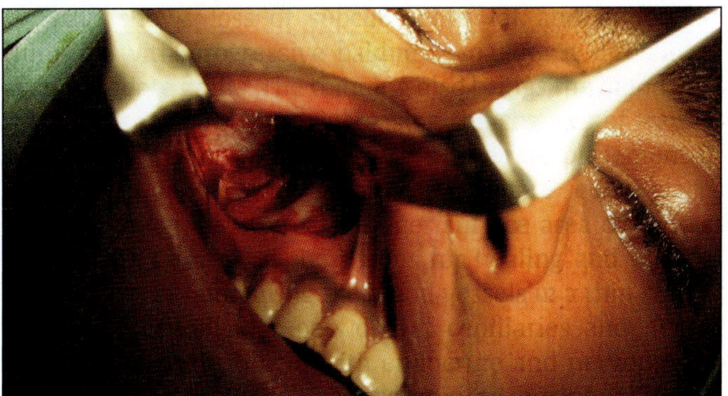

Fig. 19.23 Intraoral exposure for malar implants.

the one used for lower eyelid blepharoplasty.[25] Some authors prefer a vertical oblique incision in the region of anterior buttress at the level of first molar tooth. If implants are to be used as an adjunct procedure to rhytidectomy, then the malar region can be approached through an incision in the SMAS which can be subsequently closed. The incision in the SMAS should be transverse to avoid injury to the facial nerve branches. Zygomaticus major and zygomaticus minor muscles are transected at their origin and the zygomaticofrontal nerve is sacrificed. Then the levator anguli oris muscles are dissected from the canine fossa. The dissection proceeds subperiosteally and laterally to the zygomaticotemporal suture while medially dissection stops at the level of infraorbital foramen. Infraorbital nerve exits from the infraorbital foramen in line of the medial limbus of the pupil. Laterally, the masseter muscle or tendon may be encountered frequently but it should not be violated. The implant is placed under vision and fixed using titanium screws, ensuring that there is no dead space between the bone and the implant. While fixing the implant, one must avoid injury or traction to the infraorbital nerve. After rigid fixation, the edges of implant are feathered to ensure smooth transition and natural appearance (**Fig. 19.24**). There are many situations where malar implant is used along with other implants and aesthetic procedures (**Fig. 19.25**).

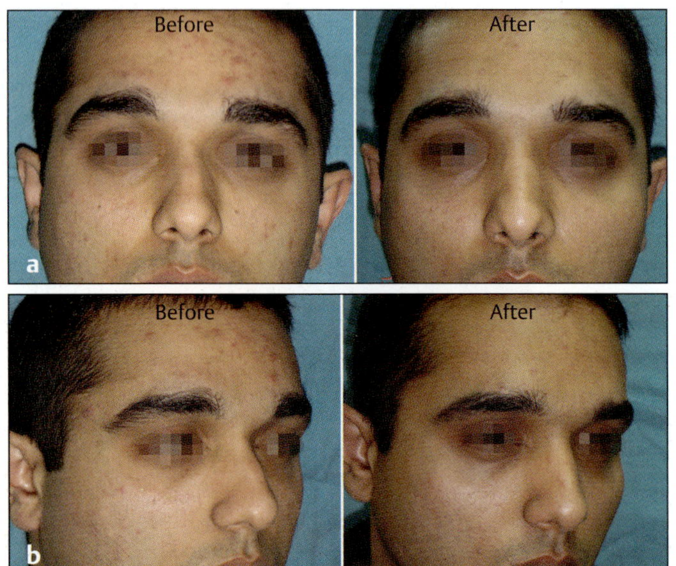

Fig. 19.24 **(a)** Malar implants—frontal view. **(b)** Malar implants—right oblique view.

Postoperatively the patient may be unable to smile, pucker the lip, and/or not speak labial words properly due to the dissection involving the muscles of lip and due to postoperative edema and paresthesias. These symptoms resolve in 2 to 3 weeks. Infection is rare unless patient is an uncontrolled diabetic or a smoker.

Some patients may need a secondary surgery due to asymmetry or after some years when the soft tissue atrophies making the implant look more visible through the scanty soft tissue envelope. When surgery is needed within a few months, it is easier to reposition or replace the implant as long as it hasn't got incorporated with the underlying bone. However, revision surgery after a few years is difficult and complicated as the porous polyethylene implant gets incorporated by tissue ingrowth and may be difficult to remove.

Nasal Implants

Use of nasal implants in rhinoplasty is discouraged because of high complications and extrusion rate. Nevertheless, they have a well-deserved place in Asian augmentation rhinoplasty and are preferred choice of many surgeons in Asian countries because of the advantage of the quick and short procedure. If judiciously used several complications associated with them can be avoided.

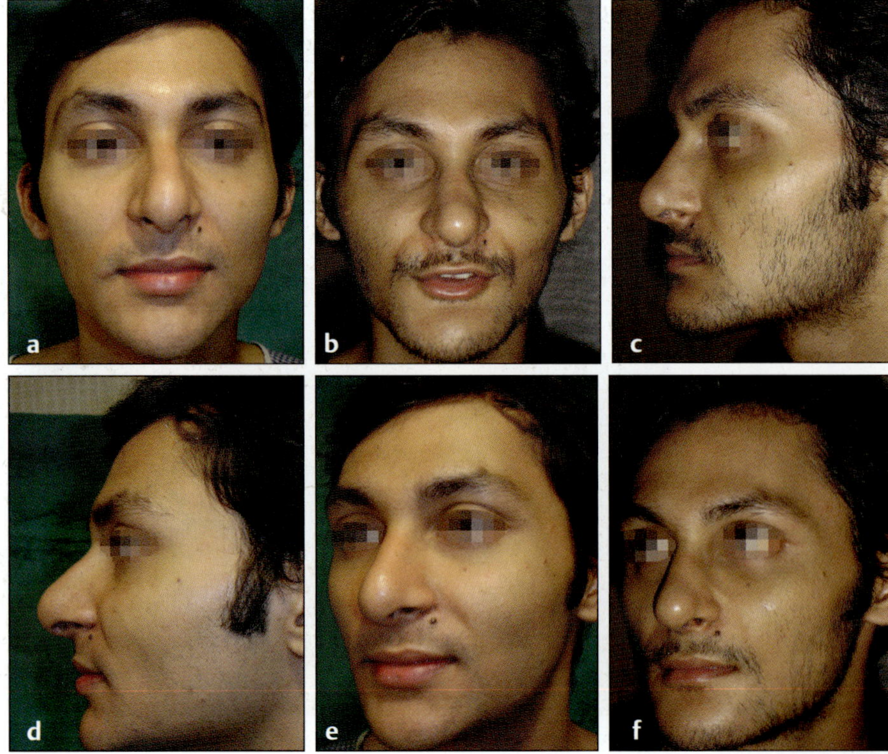

Fig. 19.25 **(a–f)** A 27-year-old male who described his face as more feminine. He underwent reduction rhinoplasty along with small submalar implant, extended chin implant, and mandibular implant to give definition to mandibular angle and more square face to achieve a more masculine appearance.

Silicone is preferred over polyethylene as the latter is associated with higher chances of infection and once infected it is difficult to remove because of soft tissue ingrowth. There are several points to be considered for successfully executing this procedure and to minimize the complications.

First and foremost is the careful selection of cases. Ideal cases are those with isolated saddle deformity with minimum or no tip issues and those who understand and accept the limitations of the procedure. They should have thick and elastic skin with abundant subcutaneous tissue, and relatively strong septum to support the implant (**Fig. 19.26**).

Second important point is selection of implant. Readymade implants are available with predesigned size and shape. Sometimes the implant does not conform to the defect and may leave a dead space between dorsum and the implant. This dead space gets filled with granulation tissue which is responsible for late infection and extrusion. For this reason the author prefers to carve the implant from a block of soft silicon as per the measurements of the defect (**Fig. 19.27**). The carved implant should have a curvature on the undersurface to fit into dorsal defect and the top of the implant should be straight with margins rounded off (**Fig. 19.28**). L-shaped implants are more prone to complications as the tip of L-segment overlies the tip cartilages and soft tissue which, apart from being unnatural, leads to constant pressure over the tip skin with movements of the upper lip (**Fig. 19.29**). This leads to thinning of the skin and ultimately culminates in exposure and extrusion of implant.

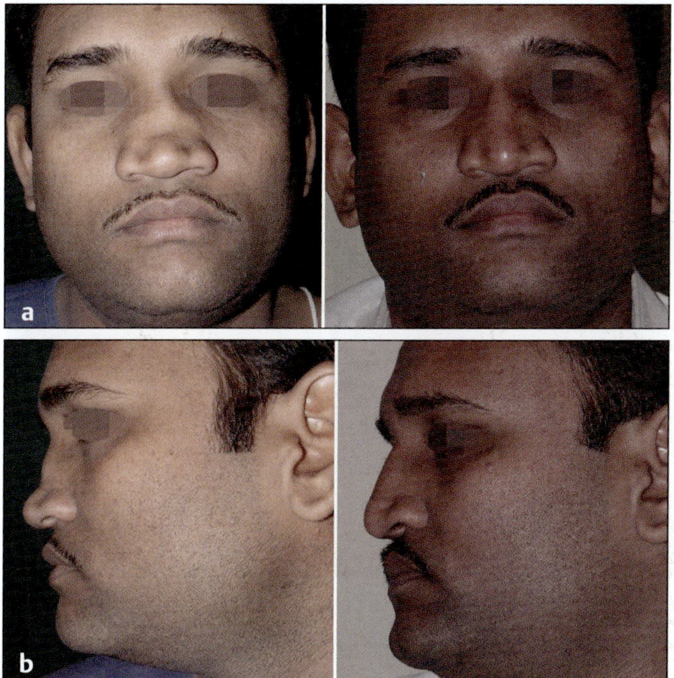

Fig. 19.26 (a, b) Nasal implant in a case with no septal support is not a good indication and prove disastrous resulting in collapse of the dorsum due to unsupported implant.

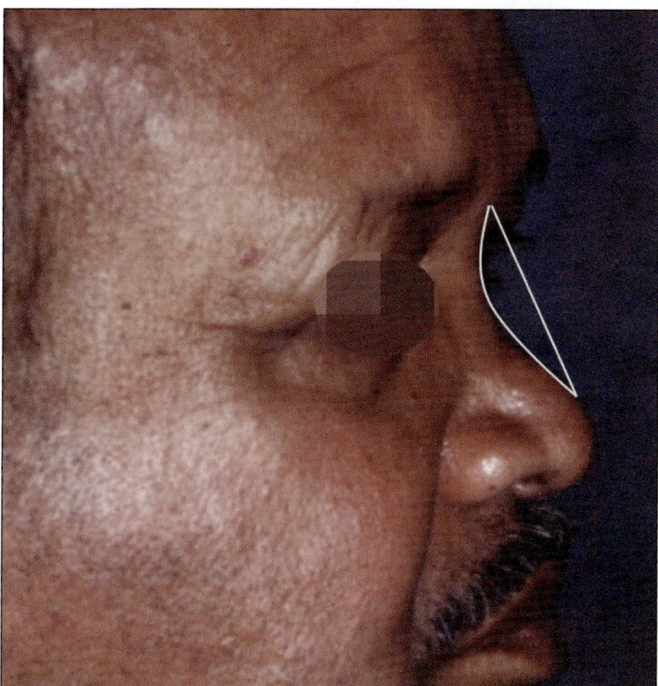

Fig. 19.27 For carving of implant measurement of length is taken from root of the nose to septal angle and depth is measured to ensure the undersurface of implant fills the defect.

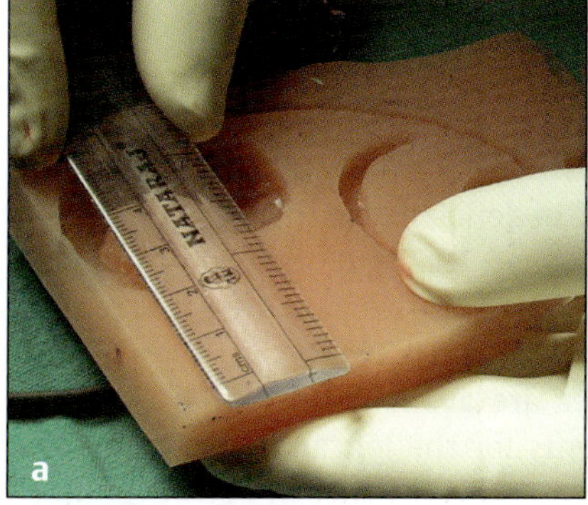

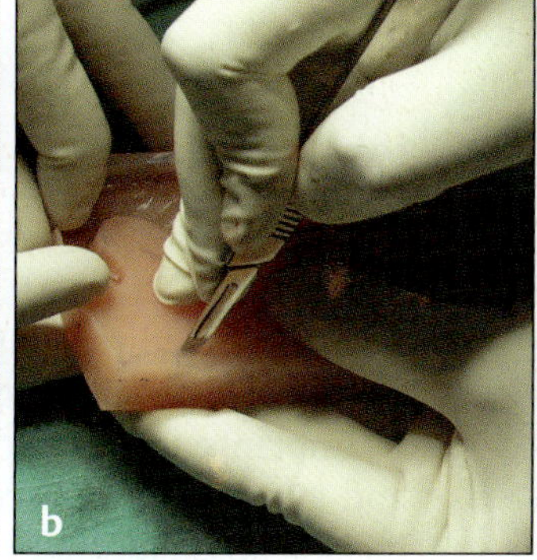

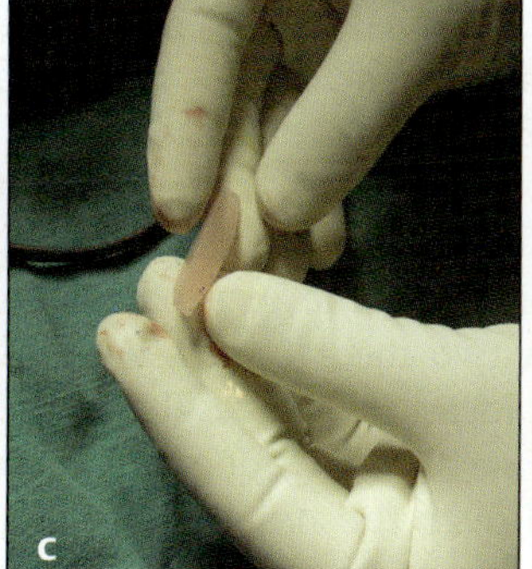

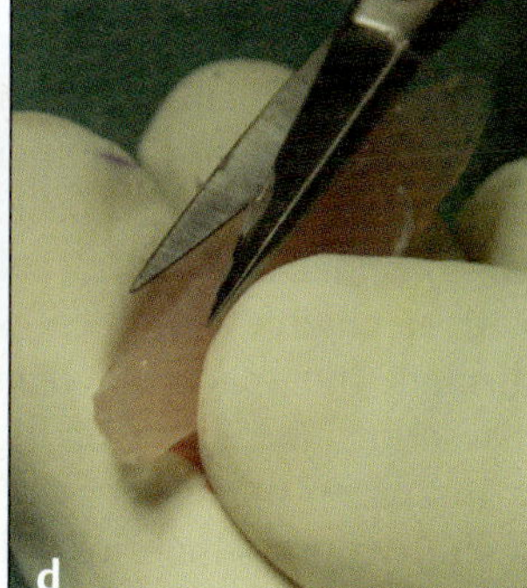

Fig. 19.28 (a–d) Implant is carved from a soft silicone block.

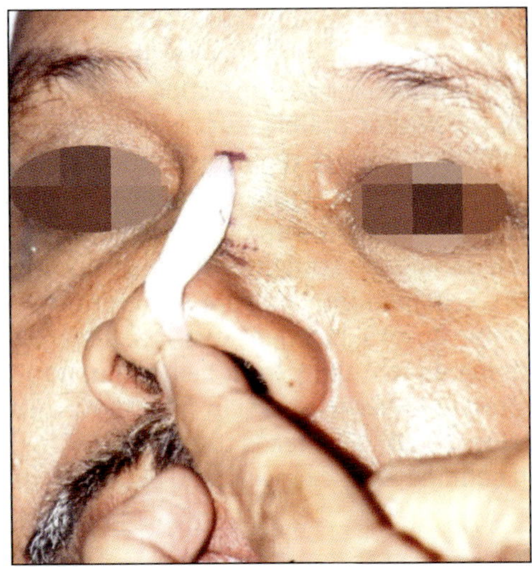

Fig. 19.29 L-shaped implant creates abnormal tip and is more prone to complications.

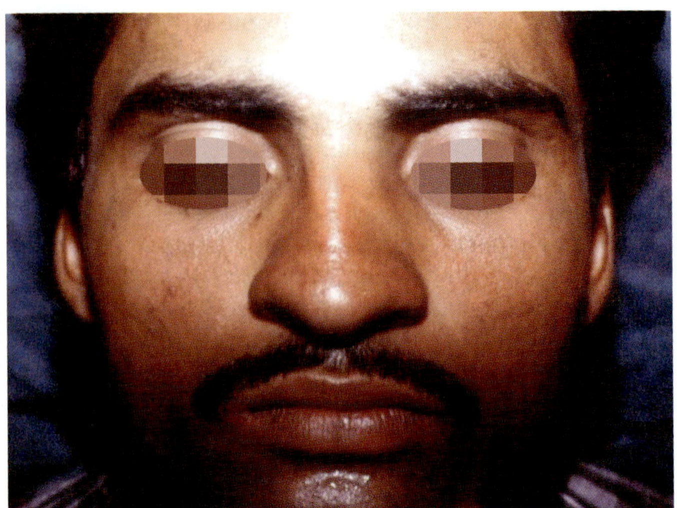

Fig. 19.30 Placement of implant through incision in one of the nostril will have a tendency to become oblique.

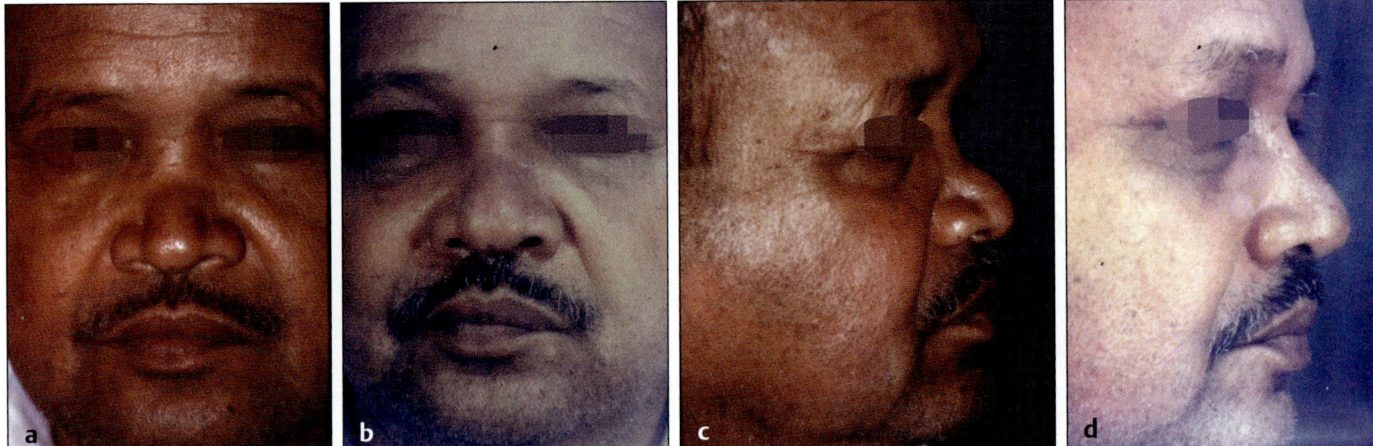

Fig. 19.31 **(a–d)** This middle-aged man approached for correction of saddle deformity of the nose. His tip was very well supported. Hand-carved silicone implant inserted through vertical columellar incision achieved a satisfactory profile.

The "I" shape implant which stops at septal angle and does not extent over the tip cartilages similar to autogenous graft is less prone to complications.

Choice of incision and creation of the pocket for implant placement are important. Unilateral intranasal incision for implant placement leads to creation of little oblique pocket; hence, the implant is likely to become oblique despite best efforts (**Fig. 19.30**). The incision also provides a weak spot for implant exposure and extrusion. Author uses a vertical midline incision in the columella for implant placement with negligible complication rate.[9] The incision is carried through the space between two medial crura with sharp dissection. By virtue of its location, the resultant pocket is in a deep plane over the cartilaginous dorsum. The dissection turns subperiosteal over the nasal bones till the nasal root. This ensures maximum thickness of subcutaneous tissue over the implant. The pocket is wide enough to snugly accommodate the implant. Carved implant as per the size and shape of the defect is pushed deep into the pocket so that distal end overlies the septal angle. The incision is closed in two layers. The procedure is quick and can be executed under local anesthesia in a day care setting (**Fig. 19.31**).

Pyriform Aperture Implants

The most common cause of deficiency in these areas are cleft lip and palate (**Figs. 19.32** and **19.33**), Binder syndrome, and maxillary fractures. Implants in this region are often used in lieu of Le forte I osteotomy (**Fig. 19.34**).

Implants for this area are available in two sizes: small and large and as crescents for the left and right sides. The incisive fossa located just above the incisors gives origin to depressor septi. Canine fossa lies lateral to the canine and

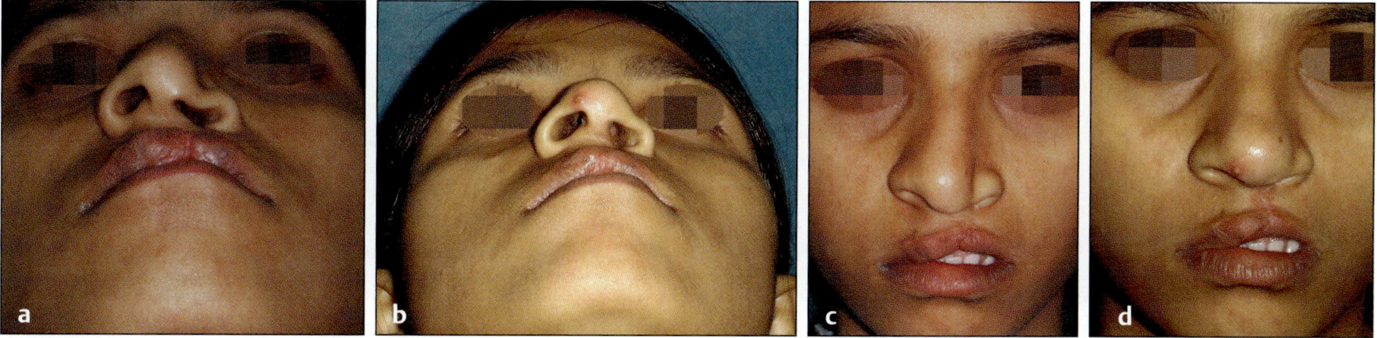

Fig. 19.32 (a–d) Impact of premaxillary implants on nose and profile. A patient of cleft lip nasal deformity with hypoplastic pyriform aperture. Managed with premaxillary implant along with rhinoplasty.

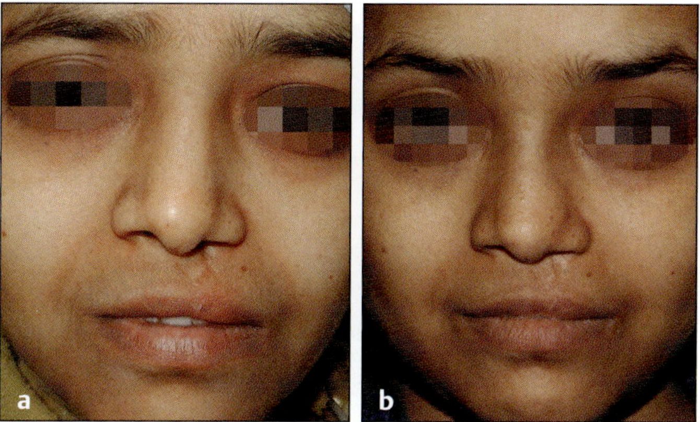

Fig. 19.33 (a, b) Long-term follow-up of a patient managed with premaxillary implant and rhinoplasty.

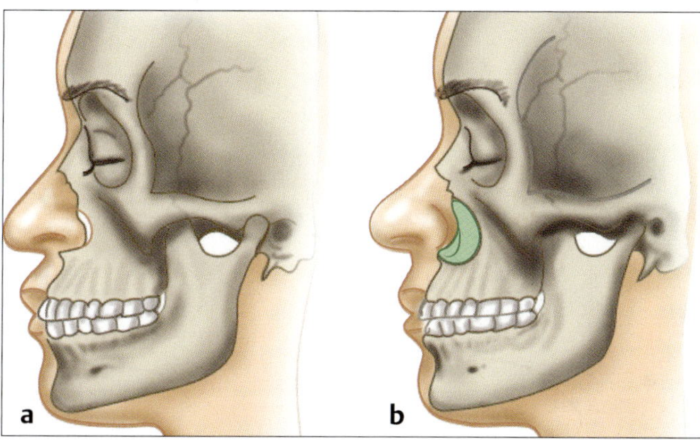

Fig. 19.34 (a, b) Diagrammatic representation of change in profile with perialar implant.

levator anguli oris originates from here. Infraorbital foramen lies superior to the canine fossa. Medial to the infraorbital foramen lies the nasal notch which is the place of origin of dilator naris which inserts into the anterior nasal spine.

The area is approached by a gingivobuccal sulcus incision located lateral to the pyriform aperture to avoid placing the final suture line over the implant. The implant is placed subperiosteally after carefully delineating the pyriform aperture while dissecting the muscles of the area and taking care not to damage the infraorbital nerve. It must be ensured that the implant does not abut into the pyriform aperture, else the patient may have breathing difficulty postoperatively. Since the lip elevators need to be dissected off to approach this area, there is temporary loss of function of these muscles which may take 2 to 3 weeks to return to normal.

Chin Implants

The chin is the most common site of facial augmentation using implants. The evolution of implants of this area has moved on from button implants and single-piece implants to the recent two-piece implants and custom-designed implants that conform better to the contours of the mandible. Augmentation of this area has an immense impact on the profile of the person and even a few millimeters of enhancement improves the appearance of these patients (**Fig. 19.35**). Chin and mandibular implants mimic the effect of sliding genioplasty and sagittal split osteotomy (**Fig. 19.36**).

Labiomental angle and lip height are two important landmarks which have bearing upon the choice of the chin implant and its placement. The implant should be appropriately augmented with additional pieces in selected cases where anterior implant placement leads to deepening of labiomental angle, giving empty toothless look to the augmented chin (**Fig. 19.37**).

Chin implants can be introduced either by a submental or an intraoral approach. The authors prefer a 1.5- to 2-cm submental incision for silicone implants which are flexible and an intraoral incision for porous polyethylene implants which are rigid and need a bigger incision. The submental incision provides a better exposure to the mandible, avoids injury to mentalis muscle and mandibular nerve, and allows for a better contouring of the implant but leaves an external scar whereas the intraoral incision avoids the scar but often leads to lower lip malfunction due to injury to mentalis muscle and frequent malpositioning of the implant.[26] Intraoral incision is usually 1 cm above the sulcus, dividing

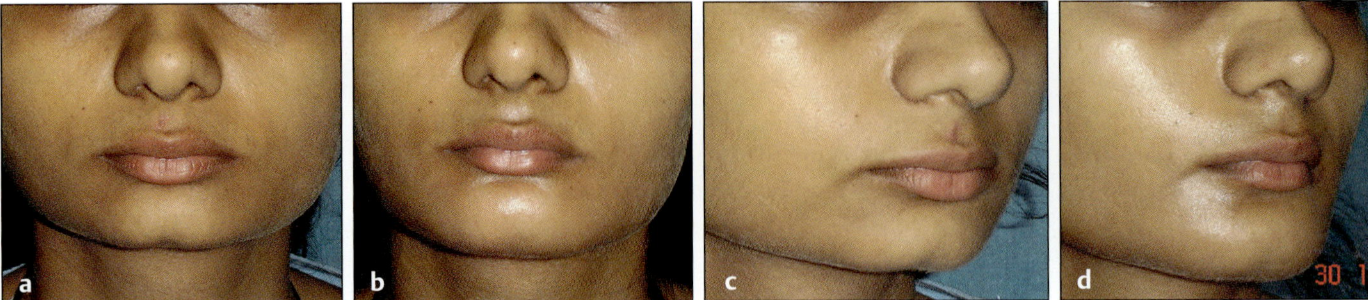

Fig. 19.35 (a–d) A 3-mm enhancement with a chin implant has made remarkable change in the profile of this young woman.

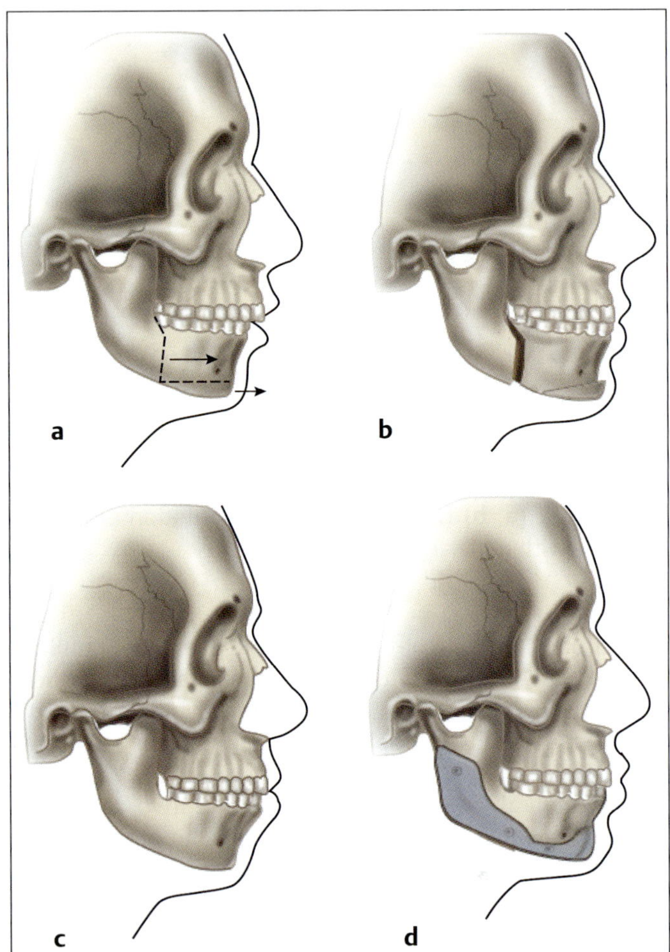

Fig. 19.36 (a–d) Chin and mandibular implants mimic the effect of sliding genioplasty and sagittal split osteotomy.

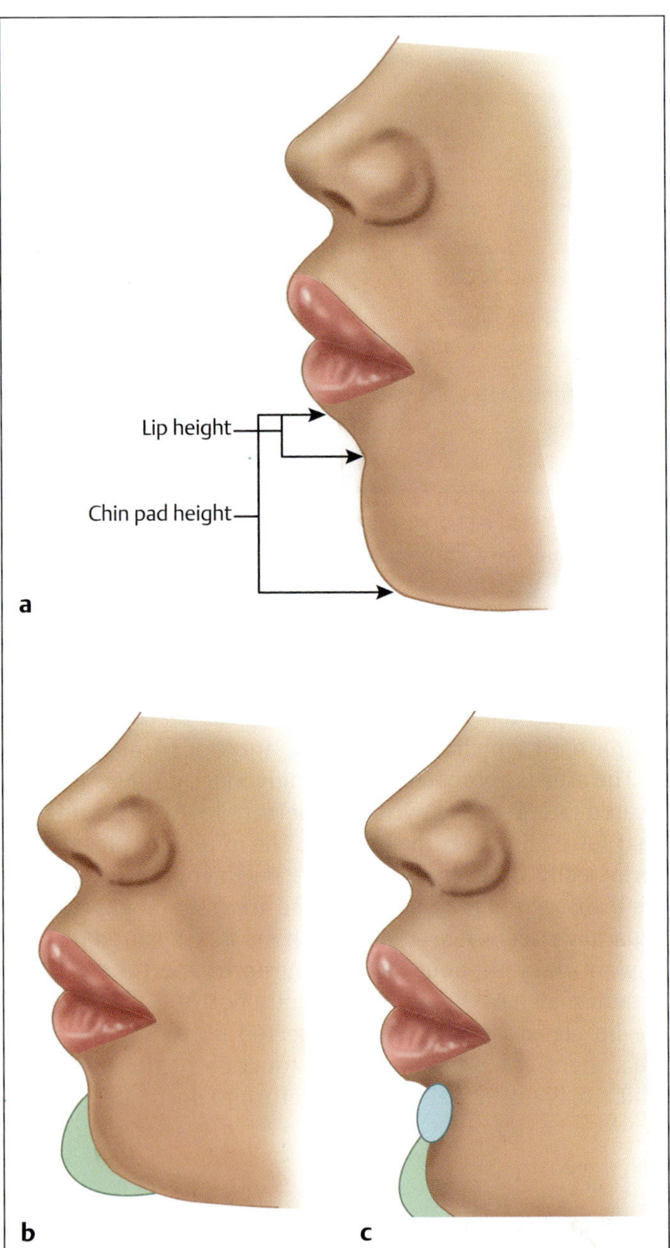

Fig. 19.37 (a) Lip height and labiomental angle should be assessed for appropriate placement of chin implant. **(b, c)** If the labiomental angle is deep, an additional strip of implant on top will prevent hollow toothless look of lower jaw.

the muscle for a short distance before a direct subperiosteal dissection to the mandibular bone (**Fig. 19.38**). Special dissectors are used to go around the lower border of mandible for wide release for natural look and to ensure better draping of soft tissue over implant (**Fig. 19.39**). The sulcus incision can be easily extended to access midlateral and posterolateral zones. There is a greater chance of injury to the mental nerve with a sulcus incision. Alternatively, a gingival approach is used. Gingival incision proceeds subperiosteally

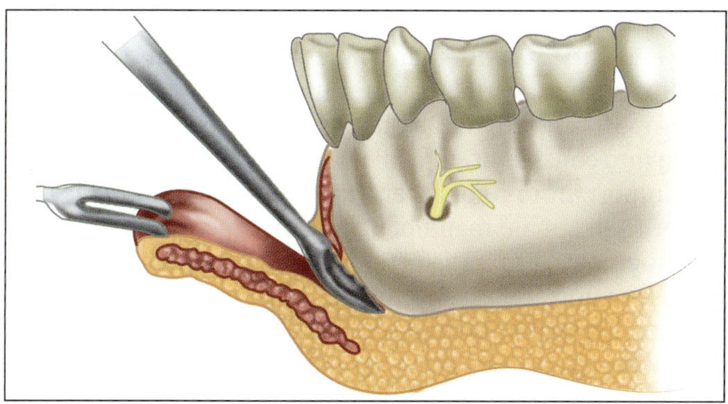

Fig. 19.38 Incision, approach, and dissection for chin implant.

right from the incision on the mucosa and avoids injury both to the mentalis muscle and mental nerve since the subperiosteal dissection from gingiva downward exposes the mental foramen, and the nerve is secured by going around it (**Fig. 19.40**).

In either approach once the bone is reached, the midline is marked with a screw or a burr to allow for correct positioning of the implant. The authors prefer the two-piece porous polyethylene implant/customized implants for the chin (**Fig. 19.41**). The connecting bar of two-piece implant allows for proper contouring of the implant over the chin and also to alter the width of the chin to suit the rest of the face. The implant is then fixed using screws and it is important that no gap is left between the implant and the bone, else the

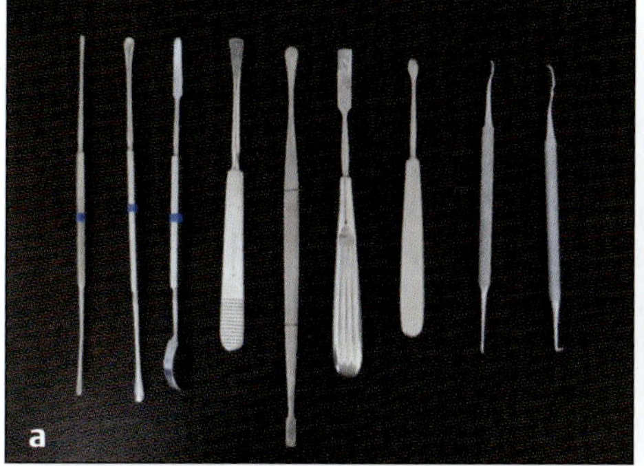

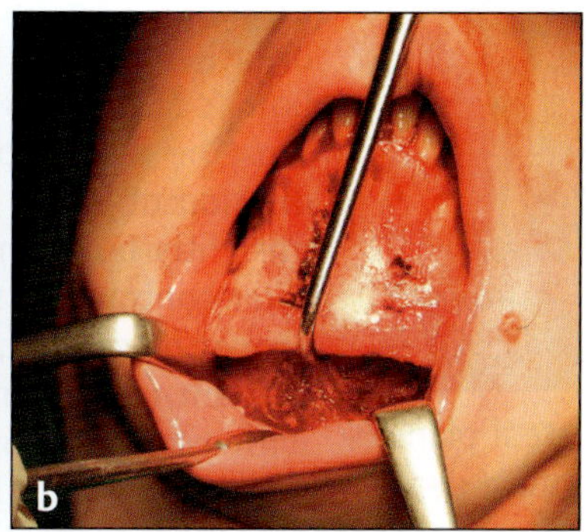

Fig. 19.39 **(a, b)** Set of special dissectors is used for wide undermining for chin implant placement.

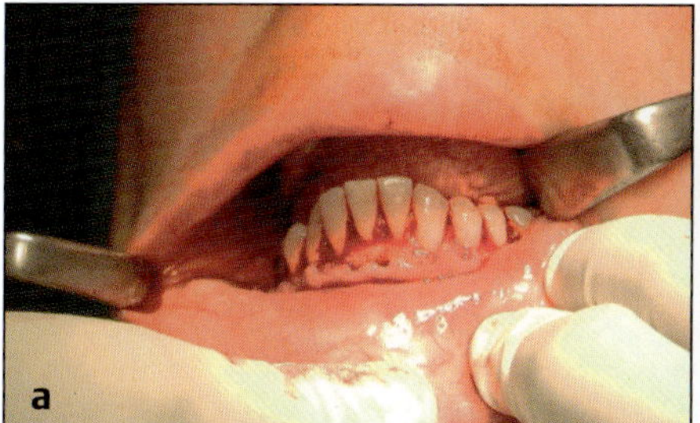

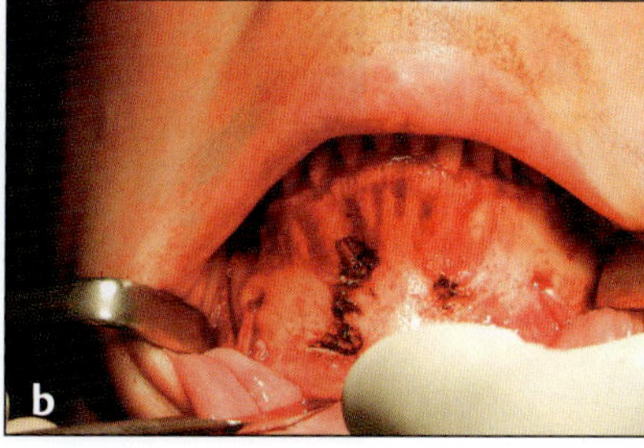

Fig. 19.40 **(a, b)** Wide dissection is done to achieve adequate exposure. Mental nerves are identified and secured out of the way while fixing the implant.

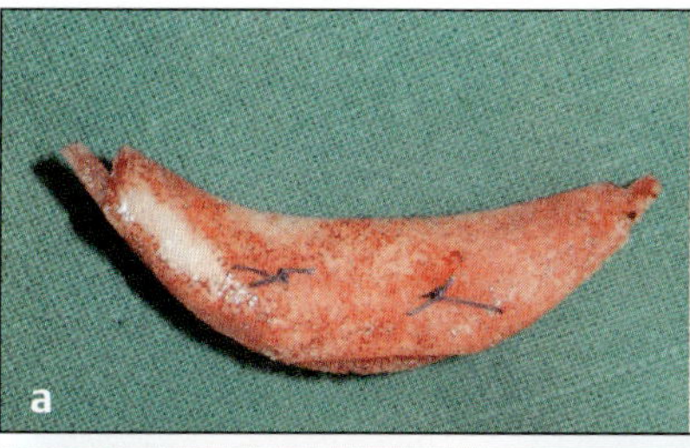

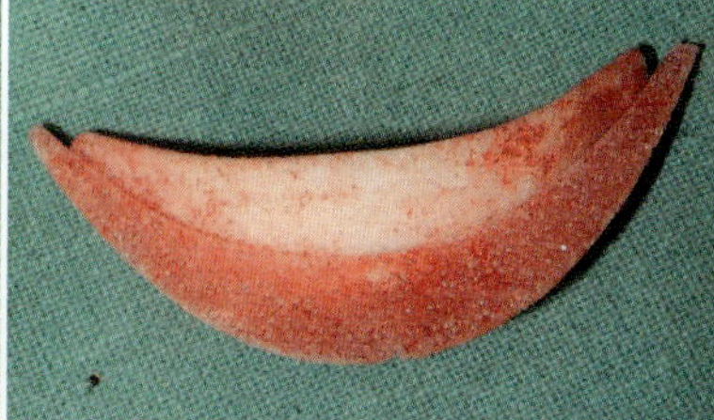

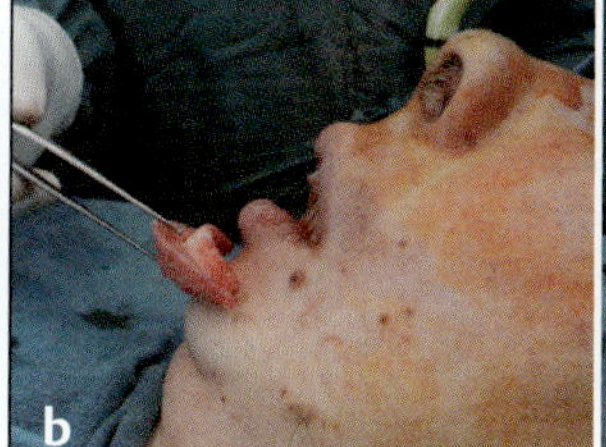

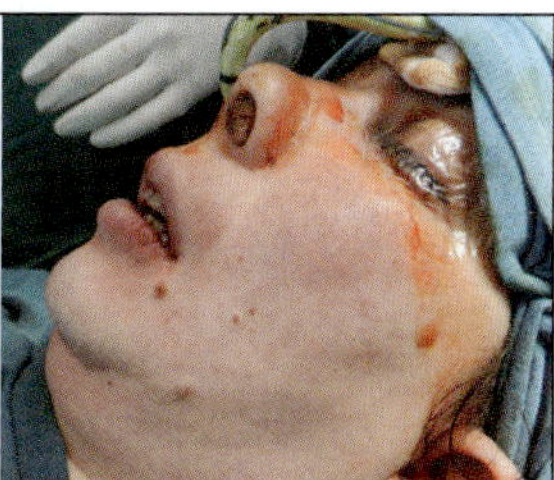

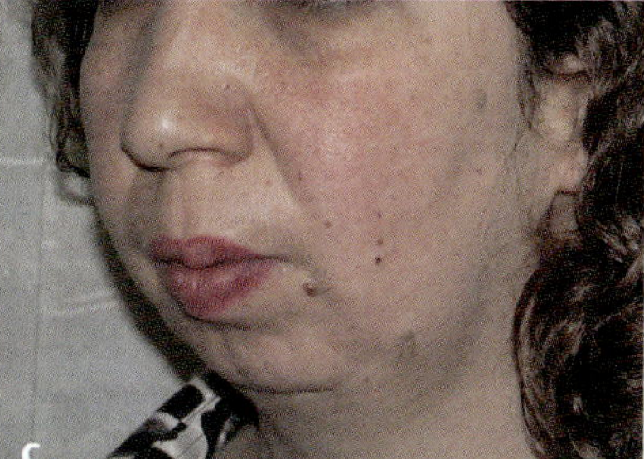

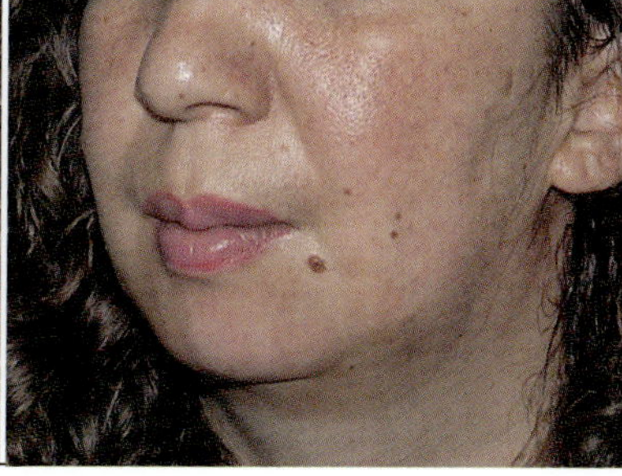

Fig. 19.41 **(a, b)** Tailor-made porous polyethylene implant for chin augmentation in a woman with retruded chin. **(c)** Postoperative results show pleasing appearance and improved balance of face.

patient may have an exaggerated augmentation (**Figs. 19.42** and **19.43**). The edges are burred to give a smooth contour (**Fig. 19.43**). Meticulous watertight closure is done including the lower lip muscle in sulcus incision. Individual papillae of gingiva are fixed in between teeth with 4–0 Vicryl in gingival incision (**Fig. 19.44**). Some of these patients may need a submental lipectomy/liposuction as an adjuvant procedure to enhance the results.

Mandibular Implants

A well-sculpted jawline is considered aesthetically appealing, hence frequently requested by both genders. The common indications for mandibular implants are individuals with a normal mandible who want a more chiseled appearance and patients with mandibular deficiency and posttraumatic deformities. The masseter muscle and the soft tissues are important parts of aesthetics of this area and must be taken into consideration while planning the size of implants. It is important to remember that a female mandible is narrower than a male mandible and care must be taken not to overaugment. The satisfaction rates of implants in mandibular region are lesser than that of chin or malar implants despite meticulous planning.[9] Hence, patients must be given a realistic picture of what is expected. Both silicone and porous polyethylene implants are available for this region.

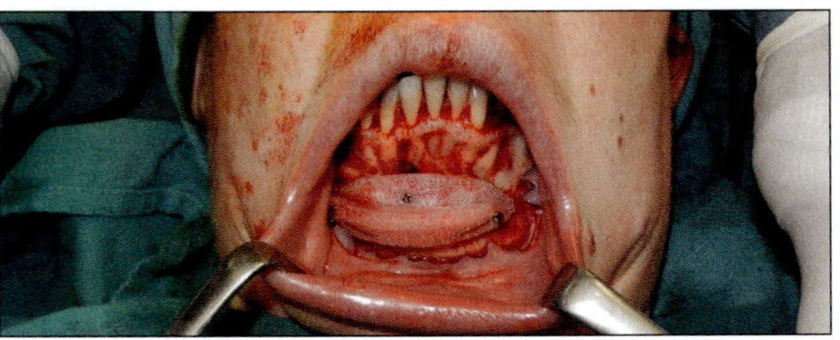

Fig. 19.42 Implants are placed in the subperiosteal plane to prevent mobility and fixed with screws to minimize dead space between implant and bone.

For mandibular implants, the authors' preferred approach is via an intraoral incision (**Fig. 19.45**). A liberal sulcus incision is preferred to expose the body and the ramus of the mandible. The anterior ramus and the body of the mandible are freed from their soft tissue attachments. The inferior border also needs to be freed of the attachments but care must be taken not to divide the pterygomasseteric sling, division of which can lead to its elevation resulting in an unsightly bulge in the midramus area whenever the masseter contracts. A set of special retractors help in exposure, proper placement, and fixation of implant (**Fig. 19.46**). The implant is then inserted, positioned accurately, and fixed with titanium screws. Any prominent bulges are burred off. While fixing the implant to the angle of the mandible, it is held in position with a clamp. In situations where it

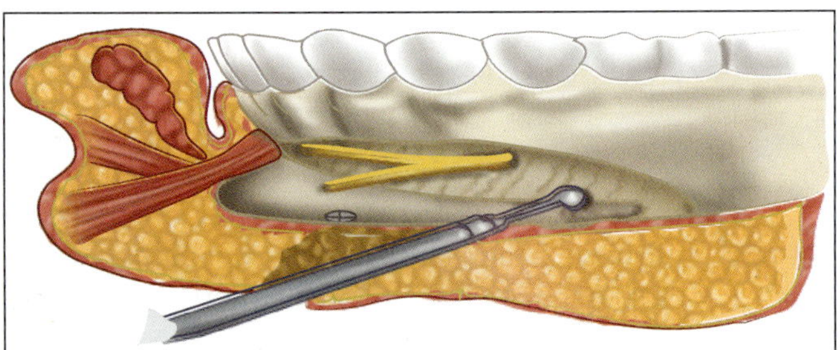

Fig. 19.43 After fixing the implant, its edges are smoothened using a burr to achieve a smooth contour.

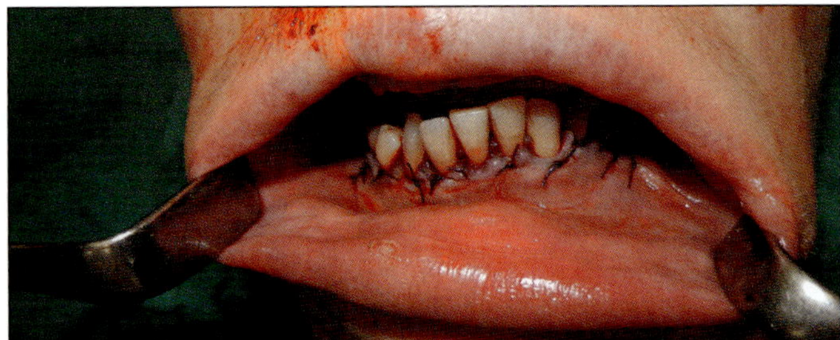

Fig. 19.44 Individual papillae are fixed in interdental space for closure of gingival incision.

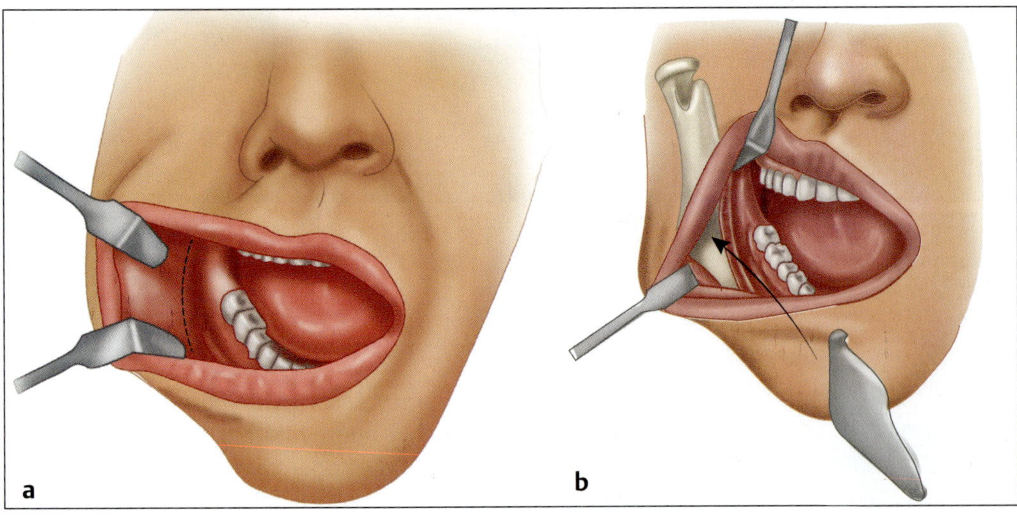

Fig. 19.45 (a, b) Incision and subperiosteal pocket dissection for mandibular implant.

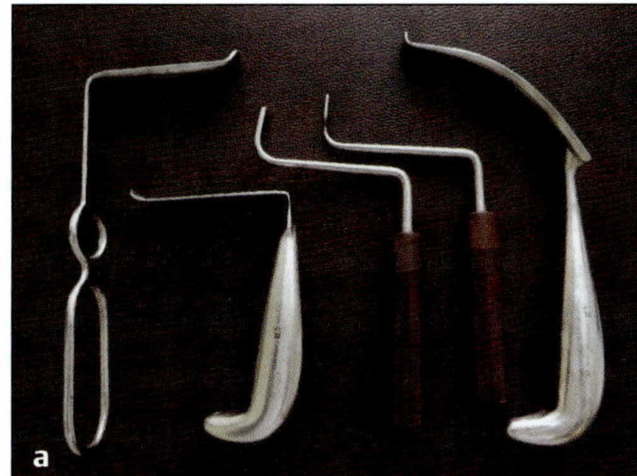

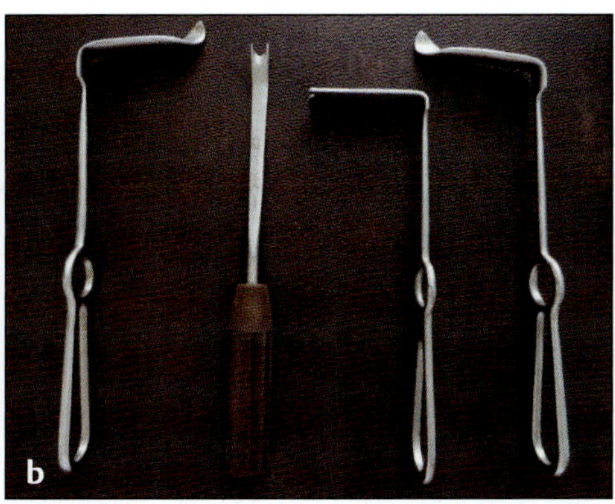

Fig. 19.46 Special retractors for angle of mandible and posterior border exposure.

is difficult to put the screws intraorally, stab incisions are made on the skin on the inferior border of the mandible and a trocar and sheath inserted to protect the skin from the trauma of drilling and screw placement. While placing screws, it is important to remember the course of inferior alveolar nerve and avoid its injury.[25]

Postoperative Care

A simple noncompressive dressing is applied and patient is nursed with head high position. Patients are asked to refrain from excessive animation or movements of the operated part for a week. As swelling is expected postoperatively, ice packs may be beneficial in most cases. Swelling usually subsides in 3 to 6 weeks but may take longer in some.

Complications

Complications are rare when the procedures are carefully planned. The complications common to all regions include hematoma/seroma collection, occasional chances of infection, compromised animation for 2 to 3 weeks due to soft tissue/nerve/muscle manipulation which improves over time and temporary sensory loss. Infection of implants is rare. It can mostly be managed conservatively. Rarely, persistent infection may necessitate implant removal. Scars may be visible for a few months but usually fade away with time.

Complications specific to the regions are provided in the following text.

Forehead/Temporal Implants

Complications are rare in this region with the commonest complication being overcorrection and contour deformity. Supraorbital and supratrochlear nerve injuries are very rare.

Cheek Implants

Asymmetry, over/undercorrection, extended or permanent paresthesia, subconjunctival/periorbital ecchymosis, implant malposition, implant mobility, hardware problem, fracture of the maxillary sinus, shooting or radiating pain due to infraorbital nerve impingement are some of the complications. Nerve impingement leading to sharp shooting pain may necessitate implant re-exploration and adjustment. In cases of maxillary sinus fracture during dissection, one must prevent the debris from falling into the antrum as that may become a source of secondary infection. However, implant placement is not contraindicated if such an eventuality happens. Major asymmetries or implant malposition may require secondary surgeries. Occasionally, few patients develop a psychological ideation of guilt in the postoperative period, are unhappy with the implant/a foreign body placement into their body, and may request their removal.[9]

Chin Implants

The most common complications are asymmetry, over (**Fig. 19.47**)/undercorrection, palpable edges, or mobility of implant. All these are iatrogenic complications which can be avoided by careful planning and execution (**Fig. 19.48**). Bone absorption may occur when an implant is placed over the thin bone of the tooth roots leading to damage of the teeth. The tail of an extended implant may project inferiorly and cause cosmetic deformity or impingement on the mental nerve leading to radiating pain that may need re-exploration. Motor loss due to nerve injury is extremely rare and may occur when additional procedures like liposuction/submental lipectomy are performed. However, improper/inadequate reattachment of mentalis muscle may lead to lower lip incompetence and exposure of the teeth. This is a difficult problem to treat and all attempts must be made to avoid this in the first place. If scar is placed too close to the sulcus, it can lead to scar contraction and formation of a food trap leading to halitosis and inability to clean the area properly. Hence the incision should be at least 1 cm away from the sulcus.[9]

Mandibular Implants

This area is more prone to wound dehiscence and implant malposition as compared to other areas. There are chances of heterotopic ossification at the region of angle of the mandible in these patients.[9]

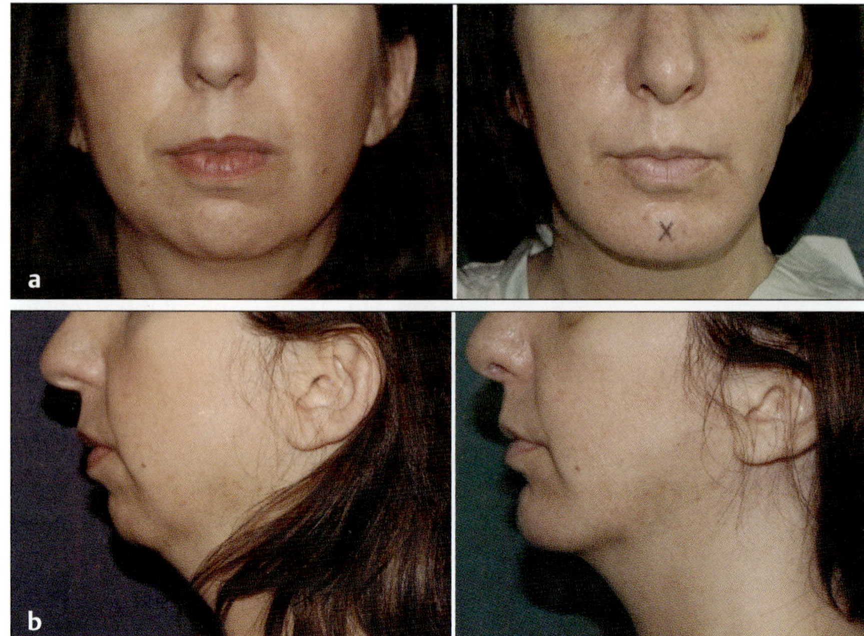

Fig. 19.47 (a, b) Chin augmentation was done in a young lady using a rather large chin implant meant for males. The result was unacceptable masculine chin.

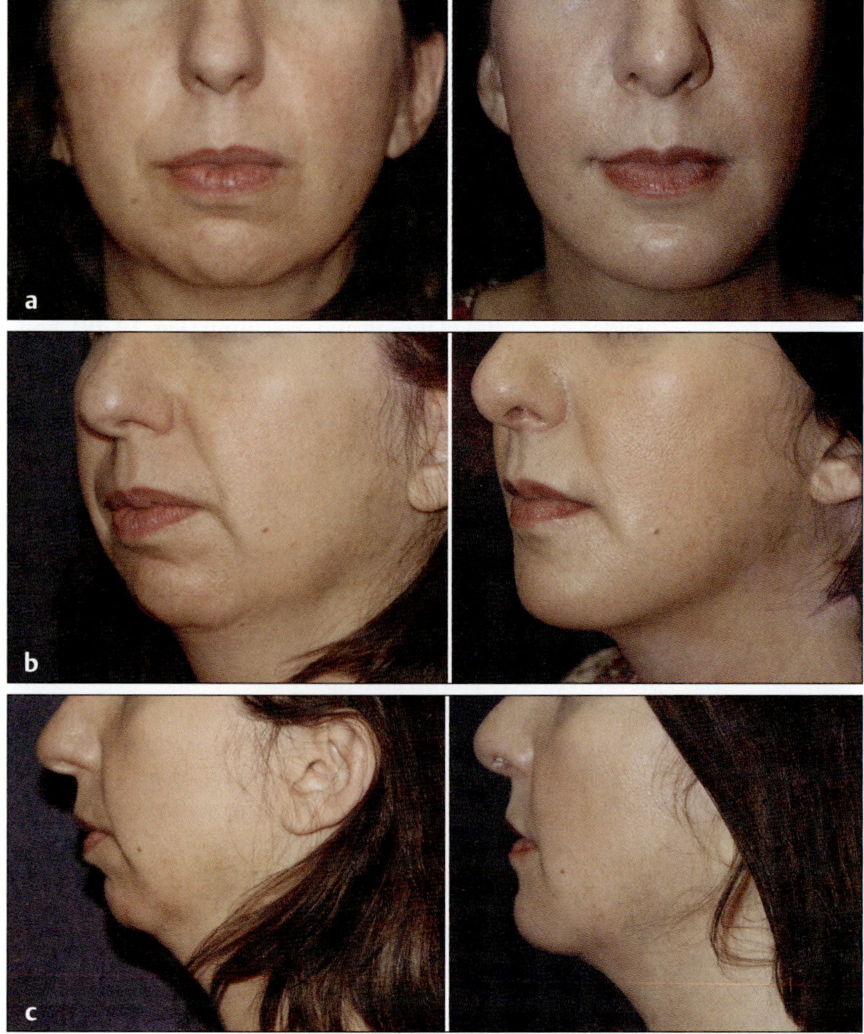

Fig. 19.48 (a–c) Revision surgery of patient in **Fig. 19.47** was performed within a fortnight to correct the error in judgment to achieve a feminine aesthetically pleasing appearance.

Conclusions

Facial implants are an important tool in the armamentarium of an aesthetic plastic surgeon. When appropriately used, it is relatively a simple surgery that can give dramatic results and is often used in lieu of osteotomies for skeletal augmentation. Facial implants will continue to form an essential part of our armamentarium in facial aesthetic surgery in the future.

References

1. Little AC, Jones BC, DeBruine LM. Facial attractiveness: evolutionary based research. Philos Trans R Soc Lond B Biol Sci 2011;366(1571):1638–1659
2. Romm S. The changing face of beauty. Aesthetic Plast Surg 1989;13(2):91–98
3. Terino EO. Alloplastic facial contouring. In: Nahai F, ed. The art of aesthetic surgery: principles and techniques. 2nd ed. Vol. 2. St Louis, MO: Quality Medical Publishing Inc.; 2011:1191–1269
4. Friji MT, Sudhakar PV. Alloplastic materials and implants. In: Agrawal K, Bhattacharya S, eds. Textbook of plastic, reconstructive, and aesthetic surgery, Vol. 1. Principles and advances in plastic surgery. New Delhi, India: Thieme; 2016:305–318
5. Quatela VC, Chow J. Synthetic facial implants. Facial Plast Surg Clin North Am 2008;16(1):1–10, v
6. Tessier P. The definitive plastic surgical treatment of the severe facial deformities of craniofacial dysostosis. Crouzon's and Apert's diseases. Plast Reconstr Surg 1971;48(5):419–442
7. Hinderer UT. Malar implants for improvement of the facial appearance. Plast Reconstr Surg 1975;56(2):157–165
8. Terino EO. Alloplastic facial contouring: surgery of the fourth plane. Aesthetic Plast Surg 1992;16(3):195–212
9. Kumar L, Sethi SS. Use of silicon implant in Asian rhinoplasty. In: Proceedings of the XII Congress of IPRAS, San Francisco, 27th July to 2 August, 1999
10. Yaremchuk MJ. Skeletal augmentation. In: Neligan PC, Warren RJ, eds. Plastic surgery. 3rd ed. Vol. 2. London: Elsevier Saunders; 2013:339–353
11. Yaremchuk MJ. Facial skeletal reconstruction using porous polyethylene implants. Plast Reconstr Surg 2003;111(6):1818–1827
12. Rubin JP, Yaremchuk MJ. Complications and toxicities of implantable biomaterials used in facial reconstructive and aesthetic surgery: a comprehensive review of the literature. Plast Reconstr Surg 1997;100(5):1336–1353
13. Terino EO, Edward M. The magic of mid-face three-dimensional contour alterations combining alloplastic and soft tissue suspension technologies. Clin Plast Surg 2008;35(3):419–450, discussion 417
14. von Soest T, Kvalem IL, Skolleborg KC, Roald HE. Psychosocial changes after cosmetic surgery: a 5-year follow-up study. Plast Reconstr Surg 2011;128(3):765–772
15. Ricci WF, Prstojevich SJ, Langley HS, Hlavacek MR. Psychological risks associated with appearance-altering procedures: issues "facing" cosmetic surgery. Oral Maxillofac Surg Clin North Am 2010;22(4):439–444
16. Hasan JS. Psychological issues in cosmetic surgery: a functional overview. Ann Plast Surg 2000;44(1):89–96
17. Dey JK, Ishii M, Phillis M, Byrne PJ, Boahene KD, Ishii LE. Body dysmorphic disorder in a facial plastic and reconstructive surgery clinic: measuring prevalence, assessing comorbidities, and validating a feasible screening instrument. JAMA Facial Plast Surg 2015;17(2):137–143
18. Chang CS, Yaremchuk MJ. Commentary on: Integrated forehead and temporal augmentation using 3D printing-assisted methyl methacrylate implants. Aesthet Surg J 2018;38(11):1169–1171
19. Ousterhout DK. Aesthetic contouring of the craniofacial skeleton. 1st ed. Boston, MA: Little, Brown; 1991
20. Gordon CR, Yaremchuk MJ. Temporal augmentation with methyl methacrylate. Aesthet Surg J 2011;31(7):827–833
21. Park YW. Frontal augmentation as an adjunct to orthognathic or facial contouring surgery. Maxillofac Plast Reconstr Surg 2016;38(1):37
22. Mulliken JB, Godwin SL, Pracharktam N, Altobelli DE. The concept of the sagittal orbital-globe relationship in craniofacial surgery. Plast Reconstr Surg 1996;97(4):700–706
23. Jelks GW, Jelks EB. The influence of orbital and eyelid anatomy on the palpebral aperture. Clin Plast Surg 1991;18(1):183–195
24. Wilkinson TS. Complications in aesthetic malar augmentation. Plast Reconstr Surg 1983;71(5):643–649
25. Yaremchuk MJ, Chang CS, Dayan E, Mrad MA, Yan A, eds. Atlas of facial implants. 2nd ed. Elsevier; 2021
26. Zide BM, McCarthy J. The mentalis muscle: an essential component of chin and lower lip position. Plast Reconstr Surg 1989;83(3):413–420

Hair Restoration

autoimmunity, and every little change or imbalance in the internal cellular environment.

Interruption in the dense network of sensory nerves during hair restoration surgery can cause altered sensation, paresthesia, hypoesthesia that sometimes continues for months. Use of tumescence can lift the nerves away from the scalp and prevent injury. Adrenaline in tumescence fluid may cause shock hair loss in the donor as well as recipient areas especially in females and in patient having thin weak follicles. It is good to strengthen the follicles with a hair care program for 2 to 4 months before planning the surgical intervention.

Different nerve supplies of the frontal and midscalp and posterior, parietal, and lateral scalp indicate the embryological difference in origin of the tissue and the hair follicles in these regions. Difference in the development may be responsible for paradoxical response of the follicles, creating a pattern where frontal and midscalp hair are lost to baldness while lateral, parietal, and occipital hair are comparatively preserved or remain less affected.

Anatomy of the Hair Follicle

Human hair follicles arise from ectoderm as well as mesoderm whereas in animals the follicles are purely ectodermal. Hence, it is easy to create or culture in animal experiments. Upregulation of Wnt signaling pathway, bone morphogenic protein (BMP), sonic hedgehog (SHh), and noggin inhibition lead to formation of evenly spaced epidermal placodes along the fetal skin at 9 weeks. Signals from the placode create an underlying dense mesenchymal condensate of dermal cells (**Fig. 20.3**). The ectodermal placodes grow down and around the dermal cluster in an oblique track forming the hair follicle and the mesenchyme contributing to the dermal papilla (DP).[4] Further proliferation of the placode cells into the dermis results in development of two bulbous cell locations. The upper cell cluster forms the sebaceous gland. The lower cellular group forms the site of insertion of arrector pili and the stem cell reservoir.[5,6]

The hair follicle has three parts. Infundibulum is the upper portion from the follicular ostium on the epidermis to the opening of the sebaceous duct. Isthmus is the midsegment (**Fig. 20.4**), between the sebaceous duct and insertion of the arrector pili or level of the stem cell bulge. Lowermost or inferior portion from insertion of arrector pili to the hair bulb consists of the hair matrix and the DP.

The infundibulum and isthmus are referred to as the permanent part of the follicle which remains constant throughout the hair cycle. The inferior segment shows periods of regression, breakdown, and regeneration according to the stages of the hair cycle. Peri-infundibular infiltration, concentric fibrosis affecting the stem cell bulge is the hallmark of androgenetic alopecia while lymphocytic infiltration around the bulb is seen in hair loss from systemic or internal causes like the swarm of bees sign, in alopecia areata.

The oval-shaped DP consists of epithelial cells with the dermal sheath attached at the lower pole and extracellular matrix of spindle-shaped fibroblasts surrounding the sides and the upper pole. Healthy, active dermal papillary cells appear large; thus, the size of the DP appears to control growth and size of the follicle. Hair matrix is the active growing portion of the hair creating layers of cells which push their way upward along the root sheaths forming the hair shaft. The innermost layer of the hair is a tough, triple cylindrical cell-compacted inner root sheath (IRS) which molds the hair. The three layers of the IRS are the cuticle, the Huxley layer, and the Henle layer. This is followed by a single-cell fat layer or companion layer of fat cells, which offers a smooth gliding movement to the hair cells. The outer root sheath (ORS) composed of glycogen-loaded cuboidal cells is in continuity with the epidermis (**Fig. 20.5**). The IRS merges

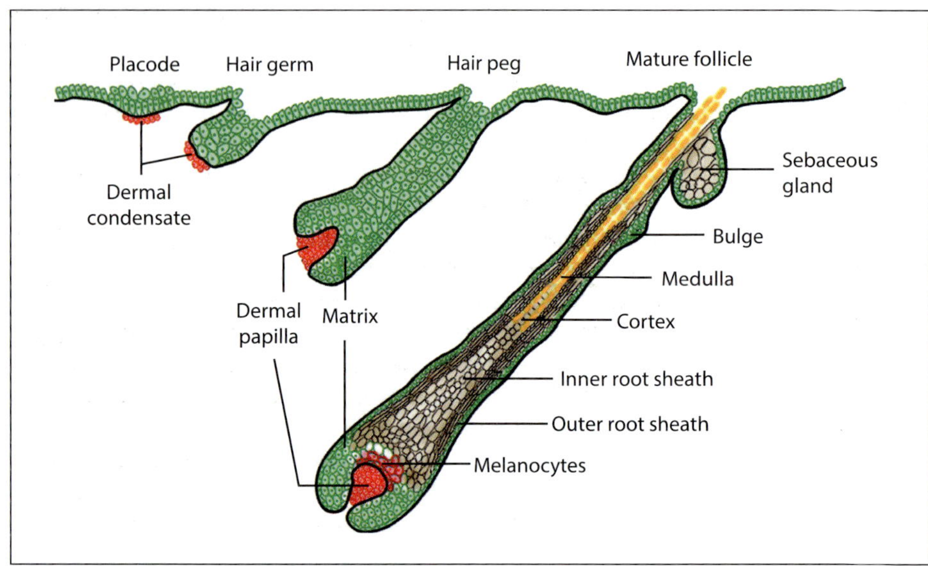

Fig. 20.3 Embryogenesis of the hair follicle.

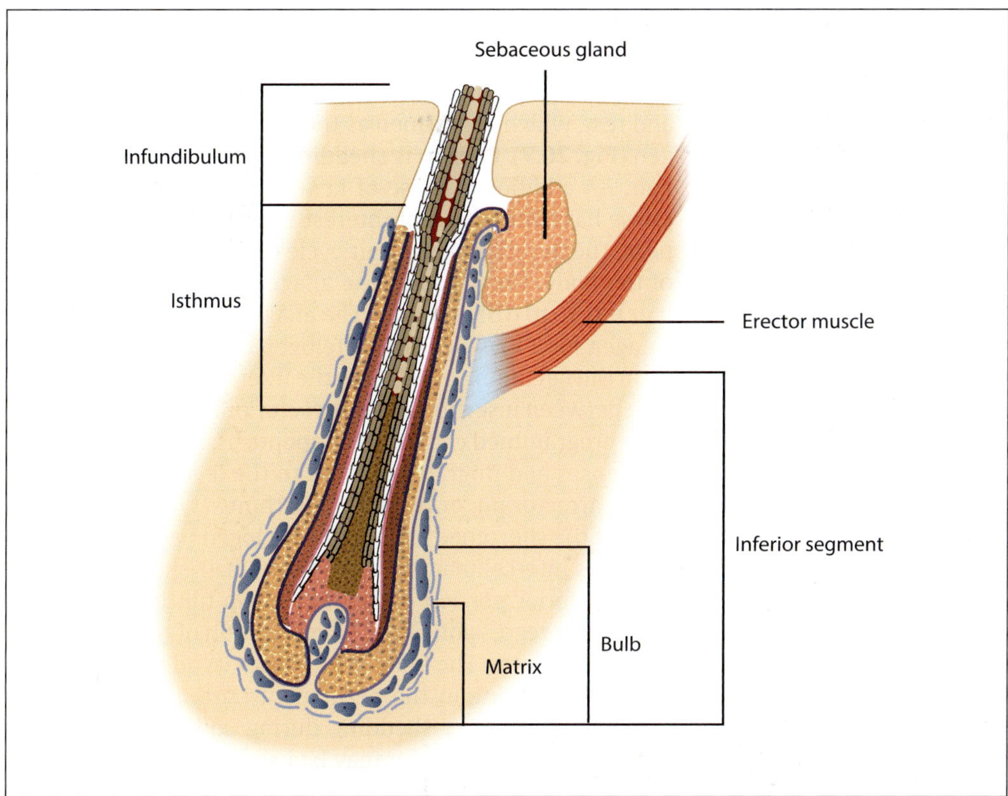

Fig. 20.4 Structure of the hair follicle.

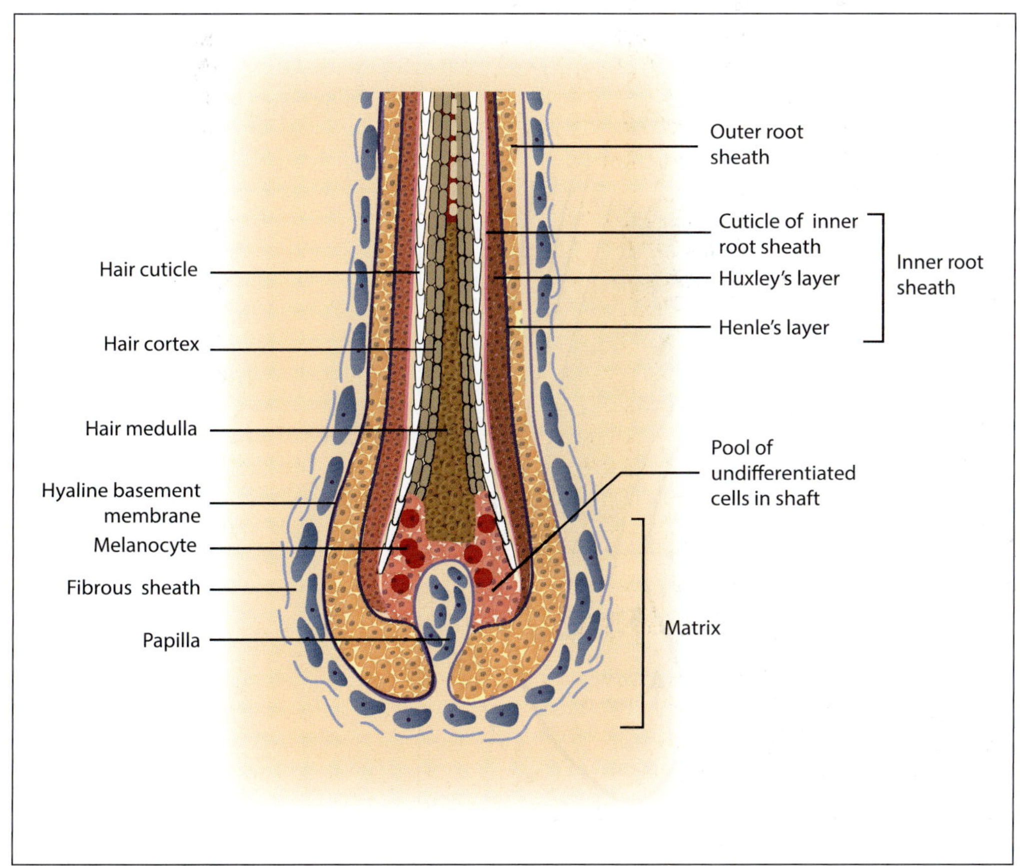

Fig. 20.5 Cellular layers of the hair follicle.

with the ORS at the isthmus. ORS at the level of the isthmus shows Langerhans cells or tissue macrophages involved in immune homeostasis, responding to microbes, antigens, and apoptotic cells. ORS also harbors sensory and light-sensitive Merkel cells. The hair shaft consists of a narrow central medulla, a thick cortex covered with a single-layered cuticle of partially overlapping keratinized cells, interlocking like scales. The hair shaft is made up of hard alpha keratin.

As the DP cells proliferate, they gradually keratinize as they move upward toward the hair shaft. The keratin deposition pushes the nucleus against the cell wall. At the level of the Auber line the nucleus is destroyed and a partially dead or zombie cell continues with more keratin deposition and functioning mitochondria, and finally it is completely dead (**Fig. 20.6**).

Follicular stem cells in the bulge area are derived from epithelial cells and mesenchymal cells and contain neural crest cells. Embryologically, neural crest cells form the nervous system, adrenal medulla, extracellular matrix of the endocrine glands, and melanocytes. Thus, indicating a close connection between follicular response to stress, nerve stimulation, neurotransmitters, neuropeptides, endocrine modulators, and hormones. The follicle is known to secrete its own prolactin and androgens. Researchers today agree that the altered response of the follicle to hormones, inflammation, and immunity is responsible for hair loss, not the androgen levels in circulation as these are often found to be normal.[7]

The Hair Cycle

The hair cycle has three main phases: growth, involution, and rest, which are termed as the anagen, catagen, and telogen (**Fig. 20.7**). Exogen is shedding or release of the telogen hair. An additional phase of kenogen or the empty follicle phase has been of recent interest in hair thinning and baldness. The duration of the hair cycle differs on different areas of the body. On the scalp the anagen growth of a terminal hair is 0.30 to 0.35 mm/day. The anagen lasts for 3 to 4 years, catagen for 3 to 4 weeks, and telogen for 3 to 4 months.

In the beginning of catagen, the inferior portion of the follicle between insertion of the arrector pili and the DP undergoes programmed cell death or apoptosis. As a result, the DP condenses and migrates upward to the level of attachment of the arrector pili or level of the isthmus, which is now the base of the shortened club-shaped telogen hair. The IRS that provides intercellular adhesion to the hair shaft exists only in the inferior portion of the follicle, up till the isthmus. In telogen on regression of the lower portion of the follicle, the IRS disintegrates. The telogen hair loses its adhesion, leaving it loosely hanging in the permanent portion of the follicle leading to excessive shedding during combing and shampoo. The club telogen hair may be held for variable duration. Unless the anagen commences immediately, the telogen hair will be shed off as exogen.

Depending on the conditions favorable for restarting the anagen and the causes precipitating a natural telogen

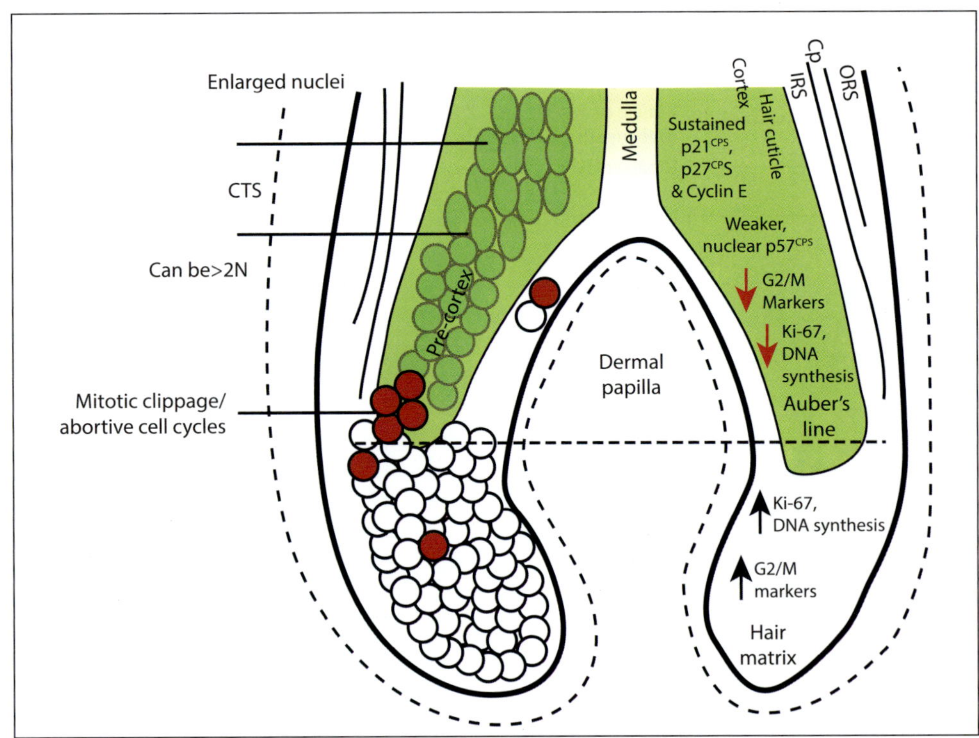

Fig. 20.6 Dermal papilla.

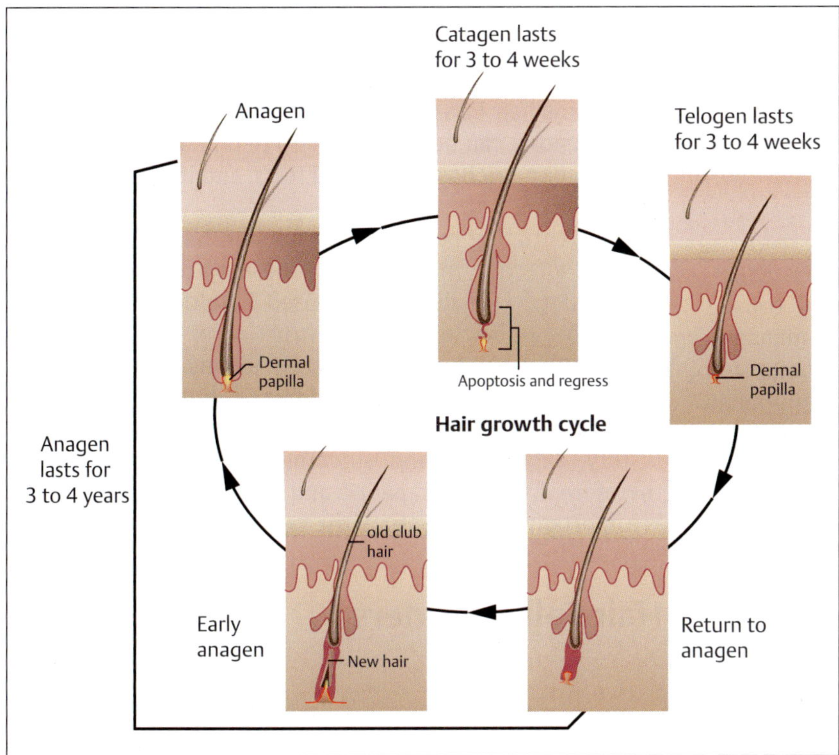

Fig. 20.7 Hair cycle.

or the telogen being a response, there is a lag phase of 2 to 5 months which may not affect all the follicles uniformly, now referred to as the kenogen or the empty follicle phase. Extended kenogen leaves empty follicles creating thinning followed by lack of hair growth or arrest of hair growth leading to progressive baldness. Sudden, rapid, cell division is required for restarting the anagen phase, which requires a favorable cellular environment, free of toxins or free radicals, reactive oxygen species (ROS), proper homeostasis, and normal internal cellular functions that are necessary for the commencement and the uninterrupted continuation of anagen. The role of nutrition is of prime importance here.

At the induction of anagen, the DP is seen to enlarge and there is a sudden burst of cell proliferation in the secondary hair germ at the lower end of the telogen hair at the level of insertion of the arrector pili. The follicle grows downward and deeper into the dermis and the subcutaneous fat. In a good healthy scalp, 80 to 90% of hair are in anagen, 2% are in catagen, while 10 to 18% are in telogen. For average count of 100,000 hair on the scalp, it is normal to lose 100 to 150 hair per day. People do not go bald because these 150 hair fall; thinning and baldness happen when these fallen hair are not replaced with new anagen hair as the hair cycle is dysregulated, slow, or arrested. In time of need, the body can not only arrest hair growth and redirect the nutrients toward more vital functions, but it can also carry out a programmed breakdown of hair cells by autophagy to retrieve essential nutrients. Timely nutritional support can repair and restore the cell cycles.[7] The telogen effluvium can be reversed back to anagen.

In animals the anagen and telogen cycles happen synchronously in a wave behaving in the same manner, together. However, in humans the hair cycles are asynchronous. Follicles in the same unit may be in different stages of the hair cycle. Hence, we have anisotrichosis where one weak, thin, or villus hair is found right next to a strong, good, growing terminal hair. Recent research shows that even areas of the scalp not showing hair loss have the same underlying pathology as the areas showing hair loss. The scalp is uniformly affected all over, but strong follicles continue to grow, while weak follicles suffer thinning and fall off. The answer lies in supporting the weak follicles and making them strong enough to stand against the cause.

Examination and Diagnosis of Hair Loss

Sandeep S. Sattur

Introduction

From time immemorial hair has played an important role in a person's body image. Well-groomed headful of hair adds to a person's confidence, be it socially or professionally. By the same token hair loss can make people self-conscious and impact their quality of life.[8] Hair loss is not life threatening but can be distressing to patients. Hair loss (alopecia) is a common problem that affects up to 50% of men and women throughout their lives.[9] Today our understanding of hair loss and its causes is better and treatments or camouflage solutions are available in most cases.

Causes of Hair Loss

An understanding of the hair follicle biology and consequently the pathogenesis of hair loss will aid in management of this condition. The hair follicle is a composite organ having dual origin from mesenchymal-epithelial interaction.[10] Healthy men and women usually have an average of 100,000 follicles on the scalp which range from 80,000 to 120,000.[11]

Hair follicles have a cyclical growth pattern having three primary phases: anagen, catagen, and telogen. The anagen or growth phase lasts 2 to 6 years, catagen symbolizes phase of involution or regression which lasts for 2 to 4 weeks, and telogen or the resting phase lasts from 2 to 4 months. The hair grows during the anagen phase and about 85 to 90% of all scalp follicles are in this phase at any given time. At the end of hair growth, the inferior portion of the follicle regresses. During the catagen phase, the lower follicle moves up to the level of the arrector pili muscle and enters the telogen phase and in some time the hair is shed. The shedding process is referred to as the "exogen" phase.[12] Approximately, 100 hair can be shed on a daily basis from the scalp by virtue of hair follicle cycling. Hair follicles that deviate from this normal physiology result in pathological conditions such as hair loss (alopecia) or hair fall (telogen effluvium).

Hair loss or hair fall can be caused if there is:

- Disturbed hair follicle cycling (telogen effluvium, alopecia areata, androgenetic alopecia, chemotherapy-induced alopecia).
- Hair follicle transformation (androgenetic alopecia/pattern hair loss).
- Damage to the hair follicle (scarring hair loss—lichen planopilaris, pseudopelade, folliculitis decalvoans, traction alopecia, deep necrotizing folliculitis, radiation-induced alopecia).
- Excessive exogen (telogen effluvium).
- Defect of the hair follicle (hair shaft disorders—monilethrix, pili torti, exogenous hair shaft damage).[13]

In many patients more than one of the above causes may be operating. The common hair complaints seen in the author's practice are hair fall, hair breakage, receding hair line, thinning, baldness, patchy hair loss, graying of hair, poor hair aesthetics (frizzy, loss of volume, limp hair, etc.). Patients usually end up mixing the complaints or sometimes more than one issue may coexist, making a clear diagnosis difficult.

Attempts have been made to classify hair loss for a more standardized approach but none have been completely accurate. From a clinical and therapeutic standpoint, it is important to discern:

- Whether we are dealing with hair fall or hair loss.
- If the hair loss is scarring or nonscarring.

The diagnosis can be reached with detailed history, proper examination, trichoscopy, blood tests, and if necessary scalp biopsy.

Differentiating between hair fall and hair loss is important for effective management—the medical term for hair loss is alopecia. Baldness is caused by either reduction in the caliber of hair or actual destruction of the hair follicle. On the other hand, hair fall merely means shedding of the hair shaft which could be caused by the alteration in the hair cycle. Although hair fall and hair loss sound similar, patient history, experience, and outcomes may be different, and therefore, from a therapeutic and prognostic perspective it is important to differentiate the two.

Hair Fall Disorders

Effluvium

Excessive hair shedding is known as effluvium. When hair fall occurs due to increase in the number of follicles in the resting phase, it is called telogen effluvium. When follicles in anagen shed, it is called anagen effluvium.

Telogen Effluvium

By definition telogen effluvium is a nonscarring, diffuse hair loss preceded by a stressful event and usually self-limiting, lasting for about 6 months.[14,15] This is the commonest hair issue seen in practice as it can also coexist with pattern hair loss. The stressors could be elements like febrile episodes, major illnesses, major surgeries, childbirth, endocrine disorders (hyper or hypothyroidism), nutritional deficiencies (iron deficiency), psychoemotional stress, etc., causing movement of a large number of follicles into resting phase (**Flowchart 20.1**). The long telogen hair are shed and replaced by the shorter new anagen hair leading to diffuse thinning seen in some patients.[15] Usually, a careful history and physical examination are sufficient to diagnose telogen effluvium. Patients will report hair shedding, usually without other symptoms, with a relatively abrupt onset. A careful history will identify a causative event like the ones mentioned above, occurring approximately 4 to 20 weeks before the onset of shedding.[16] Commonly the patient would have recovered from the illness and would not see the connection between the illness and the hair loss. On examination there would be diffuse thinning involving most of the scalp and a hair pull test would be positive. Trichoscopy would show decreased hair density with presence of empty follicles and no variation in hair shaft diameters.[17] Mostly sudden onset of hair fall is called acute telogen effluvium (ATE) and if it persists beyond 6 months it is called chronic telogen effluvium (CTE).

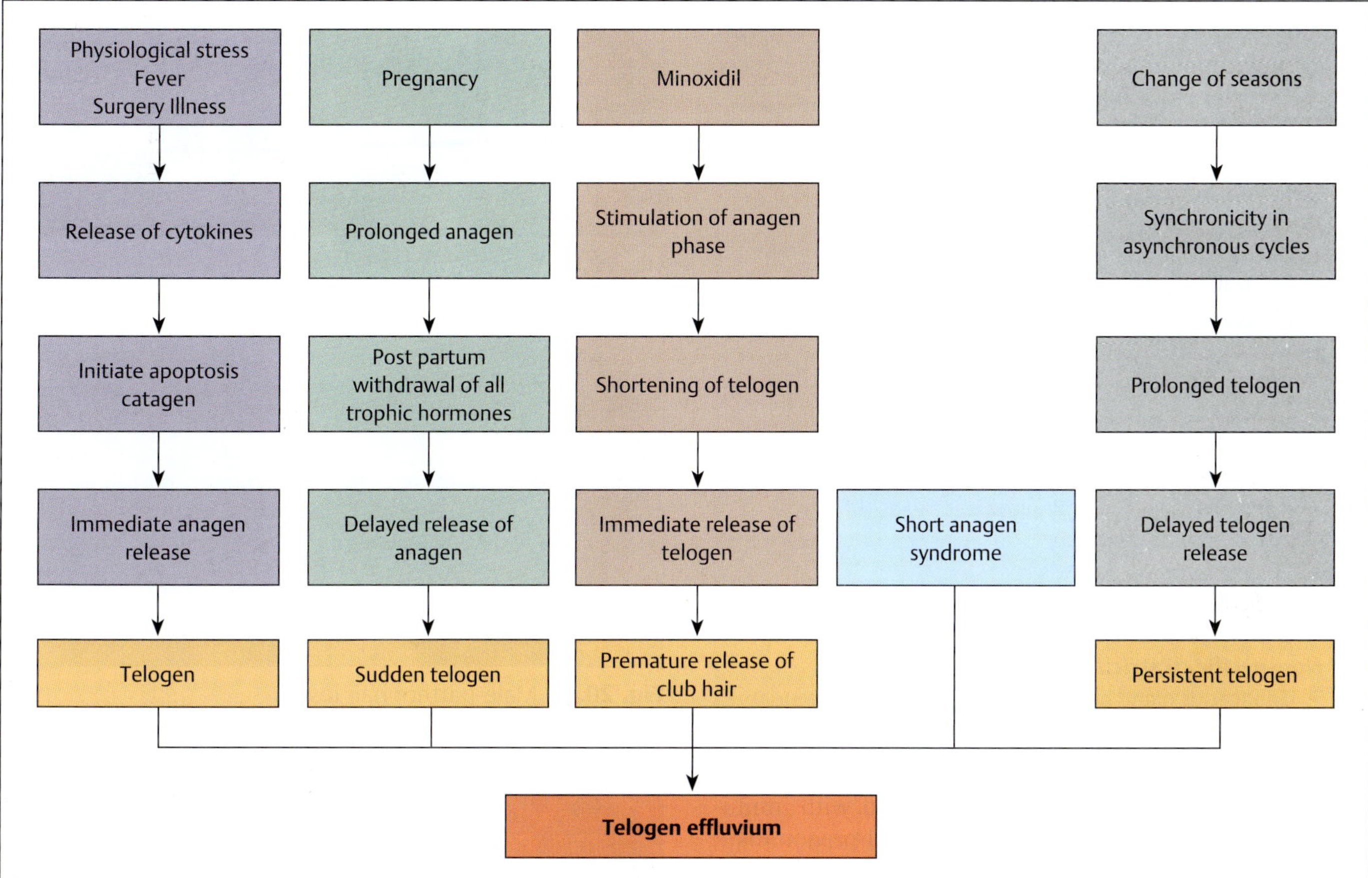

Flowchart 20.1 Pathways causing telogen effluvium.

Anagen Effluvium

Hair shafts in the growing phase are never routinely shed unless there is an impairment of the mitotic and metabolic activity of the hair follicle.[11] This is most commonly seen with chemotherapy and is almost synonymous with chemotherapy-induced hair loss. Chemotherapy targets all the rapidly dividing cells in the body and since the hair follicle has one of the highest cellular turnover rates, they are also affected along with the malignant cells. Shedding usually takes place within 14 days of administration of the offending drug, with hair regrowth upon discontinuation of the offending agent in majority of cases.[18] Other conditions where one may see anagen effluvium are alopecia areata in adults and children, heavy metal poisoning, thallium poisoning, systemic lupus erythythematosus, severe protein energy malnutrition, etc.[19] History would be obvious in these patients. On examination, the degree of hair loss varies between patients. Most hair follicles are in the anagen stage at any given time; therefore, anagen alopecia affects a large percentage of the scalp.[19] Sometimes a combination of telogen effluvium and anagen effluvium can result in complete baldness. As anagen effluvium is a nonscarring alopecia, trichoscopy shows intact follicular ostia. Usually there is no evidence of erythema, scaling, pigmentation, and scarring.[19]

Hair Loss Disorders

Hair loss can be classified into two main categories: scarring hair loss also called cicatricial hair loss and nonscarring hair loss. From a clinical perspective they could also be divided into patterned and nonpatterned or diffuse and focal. From a prognostic and treatment perspective differentiating scarring from nonscarring would be most crucial.

Scarring (Cicatricial) Hair Loss

In cicatricial alopecia, the hair follicle is irreversibly destroyed due to destruction of stem cells in the bulge area of the outer sheath, and replaced by fibrous scar tissue, leading to permanent hair loss.[20,21] From an etiological perspective, scarring alopecias are further divided into primary where the hair follicle is the sole target in a group of skin or systemic diseases and secondary where there is an injury to the hair follicle as part of general injury to the skin.[22] Histopathologically the scarring alopecias are further divided on the basis of the infiltrate around the hair follicle into lymphocyte-predominant, neutrophil-predominant, and mixed subgroups (**Box 20.1**). The treatment also varies in these two groups: principally the

Box 20.1 Classification of scarring hair loss

- **Lymphocytic cicatricial alopecia**
  - ➢ Chronic cutaneous lupus erythematosus
  - ➢ Lichen planopilaris (LPP)
  - ➢ Classic LPP
  - ➢ Frontal fibrosing alopecia
  - ➢ Graham-Little syndrome
  - ➢ Classic pseudopelade (Brocq)
  - ➢ Central centrifugal cicatricial alopecia
  - ➢ Alopecia mucinosa
  - ➢ Keratosis follicularis spinulosa decalvans
- **Neutrophilic cicatrlclal alopecia**
  - ➢ Folliculitis decalvans
  - ➢ Dessecting cellulitis/folliculities (perifoliculities abscendens et saffodiens)
  - ➢ Keratosis follicularis spinulosa decalvans (KFSD)
- **Mixed cicatricial alopecia**
  - ➢ Folliculitis (acne) keloidalis
  - ➢ Folliculitis (acne) necrotica
  - ➢ Erosive pustular dermatosis
- **Nonspecific cicatricial alopecia**
  - ➢ Sebaceous gland abnormalities (primary or secondary)

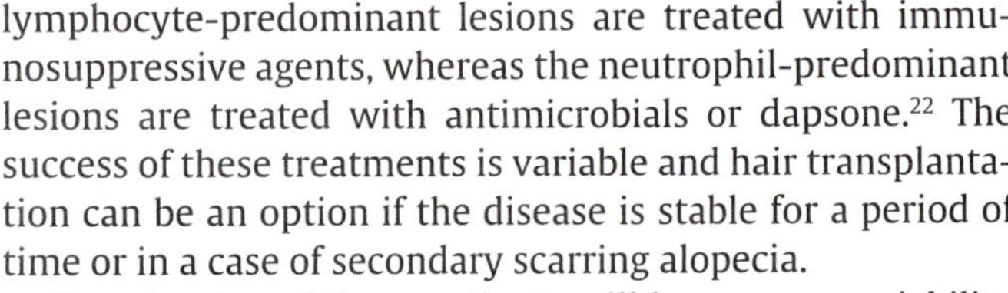

lymphocyte-predominant lesions are treated with immunosuppressive agents, whereas the neutrophil-predominant lesions are treated with antimicrobials or dapsone.[22] The success of these treatments is variable and hair transplantation can be an option if the disease is stable for a period of time or in a case of secondary scarring alopecia.

Examination of these patients will have some variability with some common features. The hair loss may be generalized, patterned, or focal. One should note the density of hair, presence of broken hairs, vellus (thin, downy premature hair) vs. terminal hairs (thick, strong mature hair), etc. (**Fig. 20.8**). Trichoscopy reveals absence of follicular ostia and scar tissue, scaling, perifollicular erythema. A scalp biopsy is usually diagnostic. One should be careful of the presentation of some of these alopecias which mimic patterned hair loss.

Nonscarring Hair Loss

Pattern Hair Loss

Androgenic alopecia is a genetically determined, patterned, progressive loss of hair from the scalp and occurs in both men and women. Both androgens and genetics play a role in its pathogenesis. The term *androgenic alopecia* is commonly used only when referring to male-pattern hair loss (**Fig. 20.9**), as the role of androgens may not be prominent in females (**Fig. 20.10**). The term *pattern hair loss* is used when referring to hair loss affecting both sexes. The proposed pathways for androgen action on the hair follicle depend on conversion of testosterone (T) to dihydrotestosterone (DHT) which is the preferred ligand for the androgen receptor in the hair follicle. 5-Alpha-reductase type 2 is the enzyme present in the hair follicles which helps to convert testosterone to DHT (**Flowchart 20.2**). In males the paradox of androgen action is seen where androgen effect on beard hair follicles helps to convert them from vellus hair to terminal hair. The reverse happens in the balding hair follicles.[23–26] A detailed pathway is explained in the accompanying figure. Male- and female-pattern hair loss are thought to represent similar clinical end points (miniaturization) of two processes that may share a few pathways, but are clearly two separate entities. Half of all men are affected by age 50, whereas 40% of women are affected by the same age.[25,27] In men symptoms can start as early as puberty and in women the onset is during the reproductive years, which is later than in men. The family history of pattern hair loss is usually present in male patients. Androgenetic alopecia or male-pattern hair loss is thought to have polygenic basis with variable penetrance and involvement of both maternal and paternal genes. There is a familial predisposition to androgenetic

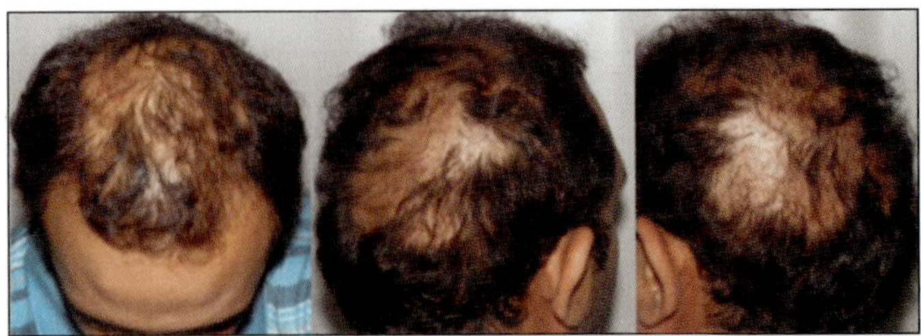

Fig. 20.8 Scarring alopecia.

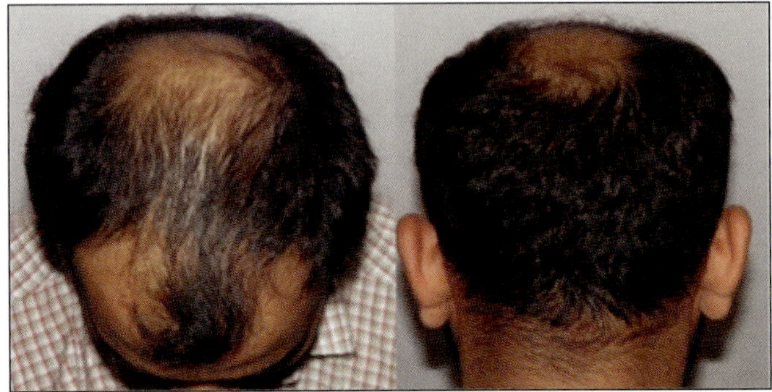

Fig. 20.9 Male-pattern hair loss.

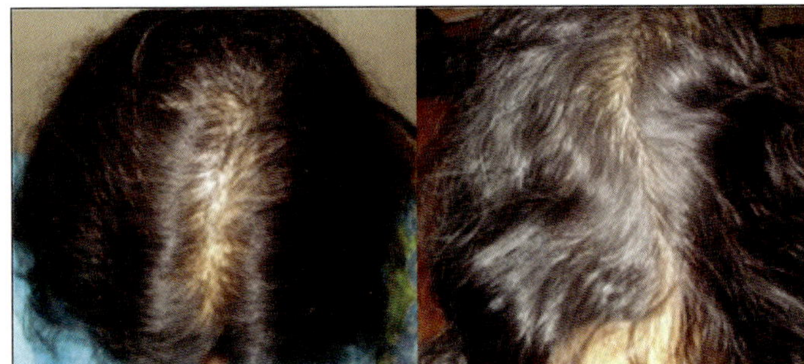

Fig. 20.10 Female-pattern hair loss.

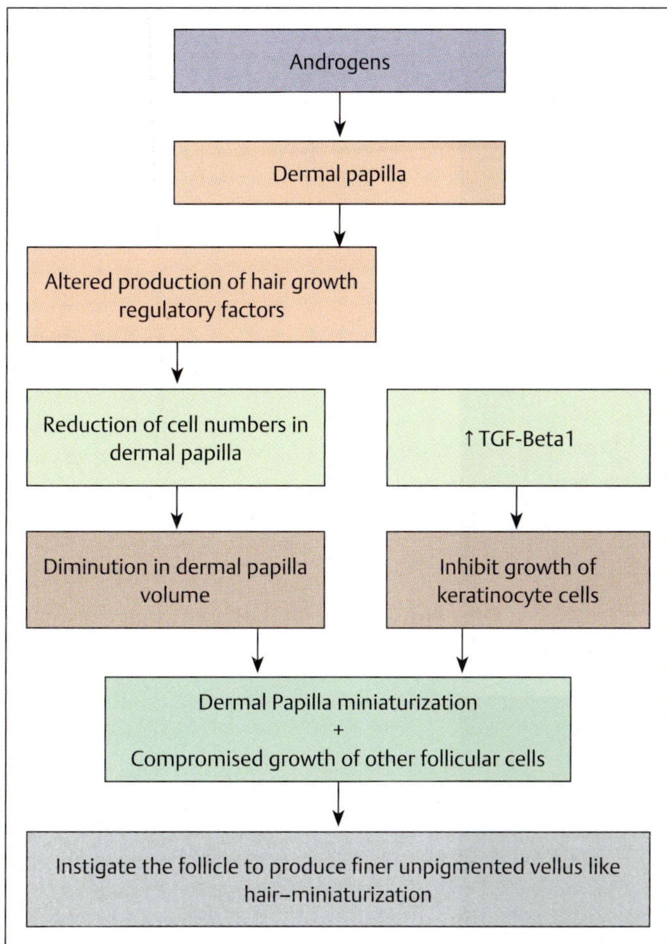

Flowchart 20.2 Pathways of androgenetic alopecia.

alopecia with sons at a five to six times higher relative risk, if their fathers were balding.[26]

In women usually an episode of telogen effluvium tends to unmask an underlying pattern hair loss issue. Pattern hair loss progresses gradually both in males and females but some patients have periods of accelerated hair loss. The examination reveals pattern distribution of hair loss. The pattern of hair loss in men starts with bitemporal recession that merges with vertex hair loss and can lead to complete baldness with sparing of the occipital fringe.

In women usually the anterior hairline is preserved but thinning occurs in the frontal and midscalp regions. Comparing the part-width between different areas of the scalp helps to confirm pattern distribution especially in women. For many men, androgenetic alopecia advances to produce complete baldness with retention of only the occipital and temporal hair regions. In contrast, total baldness at any area is rare for women. Trichoscopy is crucial in differentiating pattern hair loss from other nonscarring hair loss conditions. Pattern hair loss has typical findings which should not be missed: In the affected area there will be reduced number of follicles and significant variation in hair shaft diameter (anisotrichosis) field and predominance of single hairs. These findings should be compared with findings in the unaffected occipital area which shows normal follicular units and no hair shaft diameter variation. In advanced cases white dots may also be visible which represent hypertrophic sebaceous glands.[17] A thorough review of history, medications, and systemic findings is important to rule out other reasons for the unmasking of the androgenetic alopecia.[26]

Alopecia Areata (AA)

It is an autoimmune condition which equally affects both sexes, which may present at any age but usually has an onset before the age of 30 years. It can affect any part of the body but the scalp and beard areas are most commonly affected. It usually manifests as patchy hair loss which is accidentally discovered by the patient. There are no symptoms associated with the patch but some patients can complain of tenderness on combing hair (trichodynia has been defined as discomfort, pain, or paresthesia of the scalp related to complaint of hair loss).[28] Literature evidence suggests that AA could be caused by an autoimmune reaction involving cell-based and humoral systems, to the hair follicles due to both genetic and environmental factors.[29]

A significant percentage of patients may give history of a stressful event in the recent past such as febrile episode, severe psychoemotional stress, etc., and there could be nutritional triggers like Vitamin D deficiency.[29] Most common areas of hair loss are scalp and beard regions. Sometimes the manifestations may include multiple patches (multifocal), diffuse, total (involving the entire scalp), or universal (involving hair follicles of the whole body) (**Figs. 20.11 and 20.12**). Many patients may give history of having such patches in the past which would have recovered on their own without treatment.[29] Trichoscopic findings are diagnostic of AA. Active disease is characterized by circular areas of complete hair loss with retained follicular ostia, yellow or black dots, "exclamation mark" or tapering hairs, and broken hairs. Exclamation point hairs found at the edges of expanding areas of hair loss are a hallmark sign, being thicker at the apex and progressively thin toward the base of the hair shaft. Vellus hair is another marker of AA and may indicate late or inactive disease. In doubtful cases, a scalp biopsy would be needed to confirm the diagnosis.[17,29]

Traction Hair Loss

A form of traumatic alopecia called traction alopecia is seen in individuals due to hairdressing styles or traditional or sophisticated procedures. Males from the Sikh community who do not cut their scalp and beard hair tie them in the form of a tight knot on the head and under the beard.[30] Due to continuous traction on the hair they develop traction hair loss. Areas under greatest pressure are usually the scalp margins in the frontal and temporal regions and the submandibular regions of the beard area. Affected patches

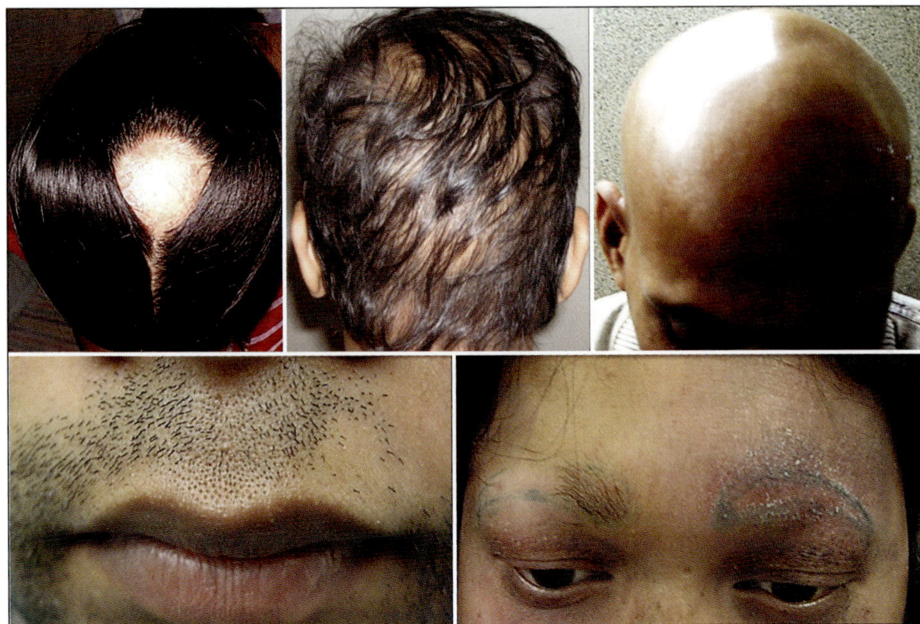

Fig. 20.11 Variation in alopecia areata.

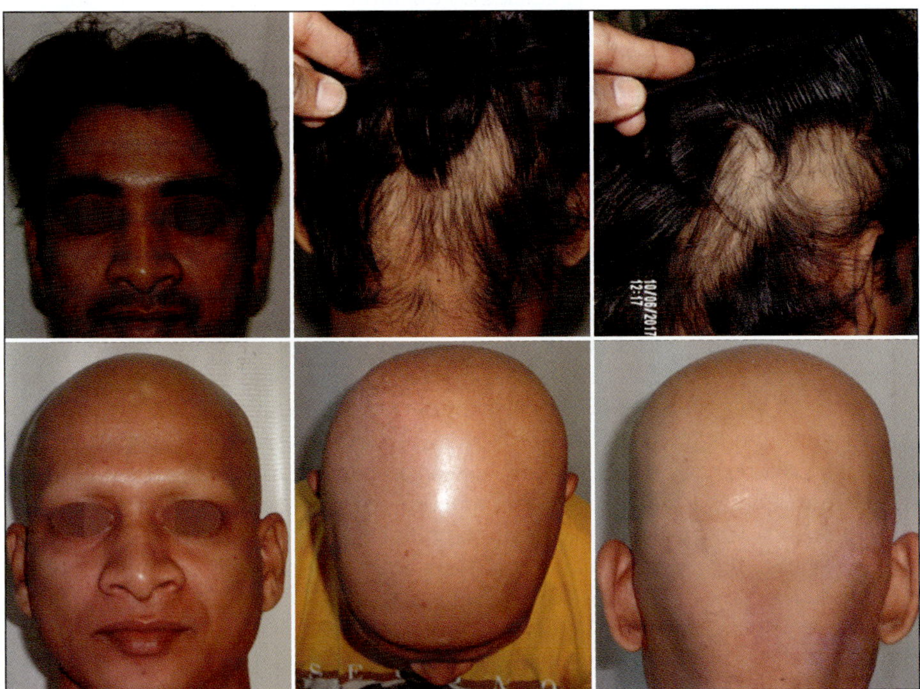

Fig. 20.12 Progression of alopecia areata from focal to totalis.

are characterized by sparse, irregularly distributed growths of short, fractured hairs. None of the areas will demonstrate complete lack of hair shafts, a distinction between trichotillomania and AA.[17] Trichoscopic findings in traction hair loss are similar to hair loss in other traumatic conditions like trichotillomania. These features include decreased hair density, broken hairs, and tulip hairs. However, flame hairs and coiled hairs are less common.[31]

Trichotillomania

Trichotillomania (TTM) is characterized by repetitive stereotypical hair-pulling from different sites. Patients experience an irresistible urge to pull out their own hair despite negative impacts to their occupational and social function. Childhood TTM affects boys more than girls and resolves spontaneously. Adult TTM affects women much more frequently than men. Patients experience an urge that they gratify by pulling out hair, engaging in this task for up to 3 hours per day. It was originally thought to be on the spectrum of obsessive compulsive disorders but now is thought to be having some differences in the psychobiology which will mandate different approaches in treatment. There is higher incidence of this condition reported in patients with psychological illness.[14] Trichoscopy findings in TTM reveal broken hair shafts of variable length with longitudinal splitting/fraying (**Fig. 20.13**). Some fractured hairs may be coiled due to the excessive traction, resembling a question mark sign.[17]

Consultation, Patient Assessment, and Diagnosis

Consultation is a critical step in the path to having a satisfied patient. When examining a patient of hair loss, it is important to understand what bothers the patient most and determining the answer to this question is most important in managing expectations and providing appropriate recommendations. It is best to have a questionnaire to be filled by the patient, which gives details and time lines of the hair complaints along with other relevant medical history.

The four tenets of consultation are (**Flowchart 20.3**):

1. Listen and Understand: Patient complaints, motivating factors, patient expectations—spoken and unspoken needs.
2. Observe and Evaluate: Degree and grade of hair loss, trichoscopy, nonscalp areas, and general examination.
3. Convey: The provisional diagnosis, need for further tests, possible treatment options.
4. Allow: The patient to take a decision on the treatment.

History Taking

In a patient with alopecia, an accurate history helps in determining the diagnosis. The important points in history are the onset of hair loss (sudden or gradual), the quantum of hair fall, any treatment taken for hair loss, family history of hair loss, dietary history (whether on any form of weight-loss diet, vegetarian/vegan, etc.), any medical comorbidities (diabetes, hypo-hyperthyroidism, hypertension, cardiac illness, psychiatric illness), drug history, smoking, lifestyle, etc. It is also important to enquire into hair care habits,

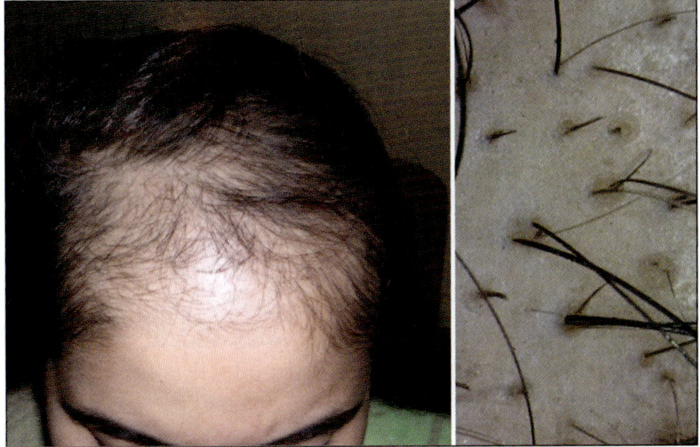

Fig. 20.13 Trichotillomania showing broken hair shaft.

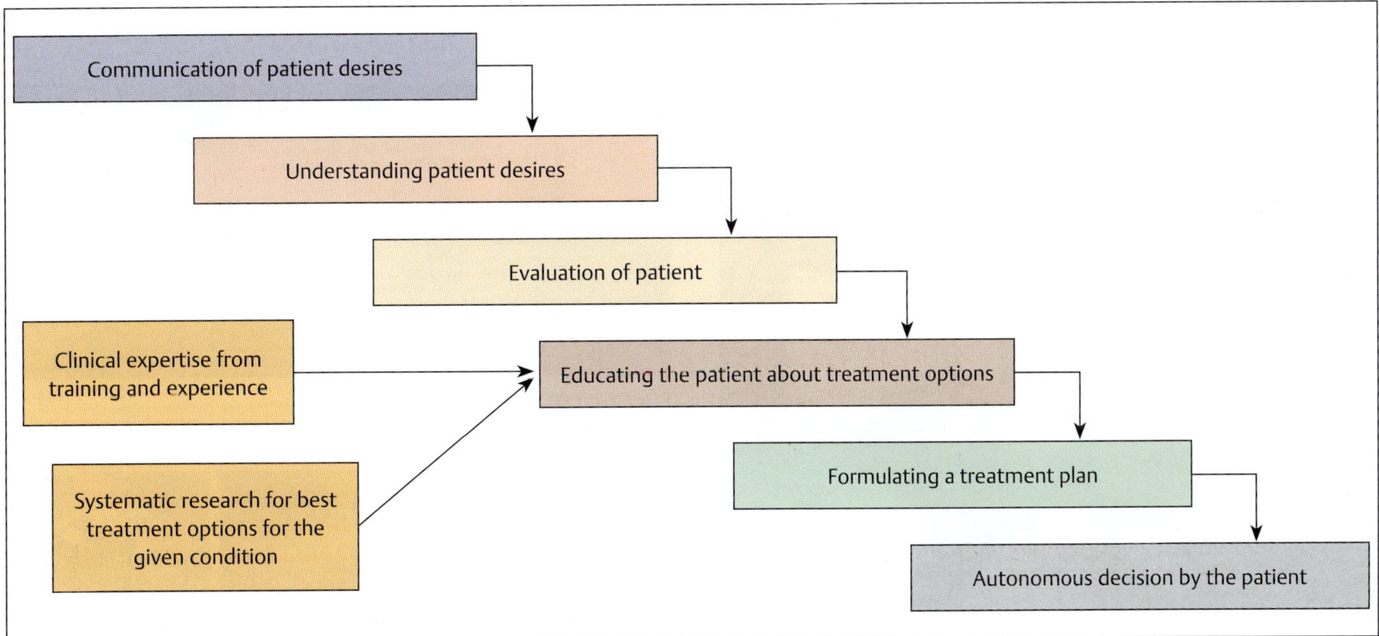

Flowchart 20.3 Pathway for formulating treatment plan of hair loss of a patient.

frequency of shampooing, use of hair color, use of procedures like straightening/perming/bleaching, etc. Many of the procedures do tend to damage the hair and cause hair breakage. In women it is important to enquire about their menstrual and obstetric history. Polycystic ovarian disease is quite common in young female patients presenting with hair loss.

Examination

The best position to examine the patient is with the surgeon standing and the patient seated on the chair for global examination (**Fig. 20.14**). The points to be examined are scalp coverage: scalp visibility, frontal hairline, temporal recession, vertex thinning, patches of hair loss, patterned or diffuse hair loss, flaking and condition of the nonscalp area.

Hair Pull Test

It is most effective when the patient has a severe condition and is in the acute phases of hair loss. A bundle hair of 4 to 6 mm diameter depending on thickness of hair (containing approximately 50 to 60 hairs) at the vertex of the scalp is held close to the root between the thumb and the fingers and firmly pulled using slow traction as the fingers slid down the hair shaft (**Fig. 20.15**). The tension should be just adequate to slightly stretch the scalp, causing mild discomfort.[32] If the hairs get removed with this action they should be counted and also observed under the trichoscope. It is important to rule out false-positives and false-negatives.

Trichoscopy

The trichoscope (**Fig. 20.16**) is as important to a hair transplant surgeon as a stethoscope is to the physician. Use of a dermoscope to examine hair and the scalp is trichoscopy. Most commonly used trichoscope is a USB-based trichoscope connected to the computer to observe, capture, and compare images of scalp and hair. One can assess the hair caliber, its density, follicular ostia, interfollicular scalp, and seborrheic activity of the scalp. With the help of a software one can measure hair thickness and calculate hair density. The first thing to observe are the hair follicle openings (ostia) also called dots. These may be normal, empty, fibrotic, or containing biological material like hyperkeratotic plugs or hair residues. The next to observe is the hair shaft: uniformity of shape and color, variability of thickness between hair shafts called anisotrichosis, number of hair shafts within a follicular unit, etc. (**Figs. 20.17–20.19**). If the anisotrichosis is more than 20% in the observed field, it is thought to be diagnostic of pattern hair loss.[17] Also the presence of broken hairs, black dots, yellow dots, white dots, and peripillar casts is helpful in diagnosing the type of hair loss.

Photography

Global photographs are helpful tools to document the state of hair loss and scalp coverage and monitor objectively the response to treatment. Photographic record should be maintained for every patient.[33] Commonly, the standard views are frontal, both side oblique views, top, and back of the scalp. In clinical studies, the photographs of vertex, midpattern, frontal, and temporal regions are standardized by using a stereotactic device assuring a constant view, magnification, and lighting for assessment.

Investigations

Patients with alopecia need to be investigated thoroughly to determine the type and cause. Complete blood count, iron

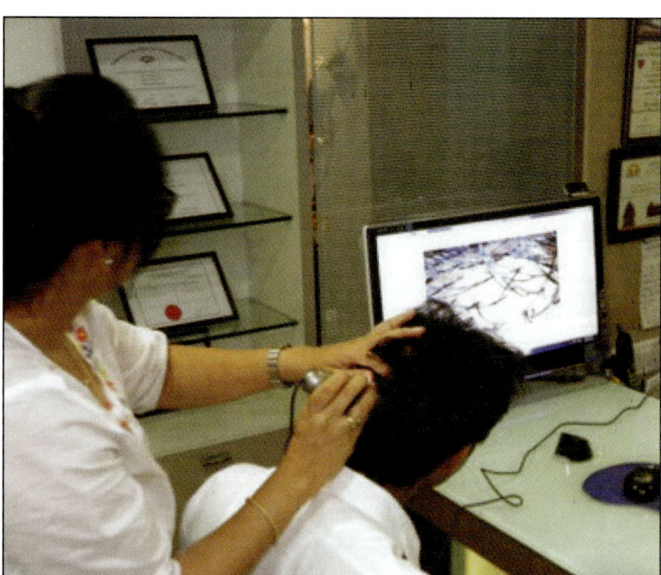

Fig. 20.14 Global examination and trichoscopy.

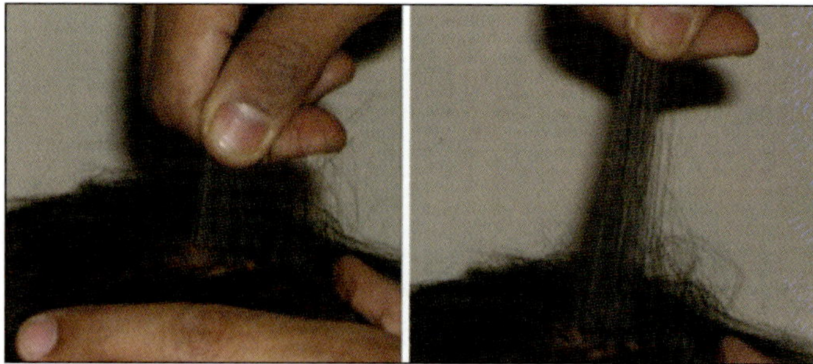

Fig. 20.15 Hair pull test.

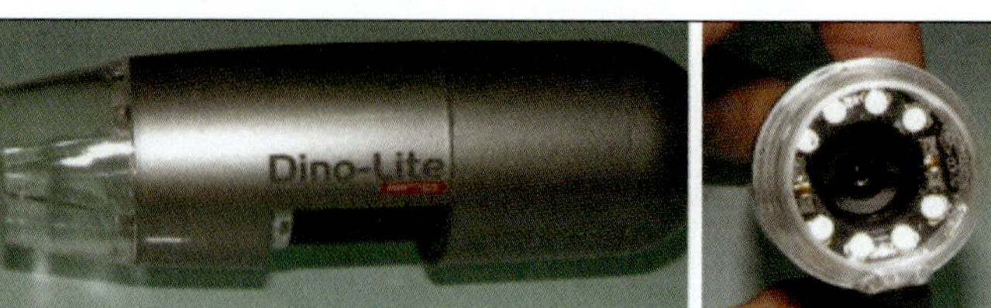

Fig. 20.16 Trichoscope.

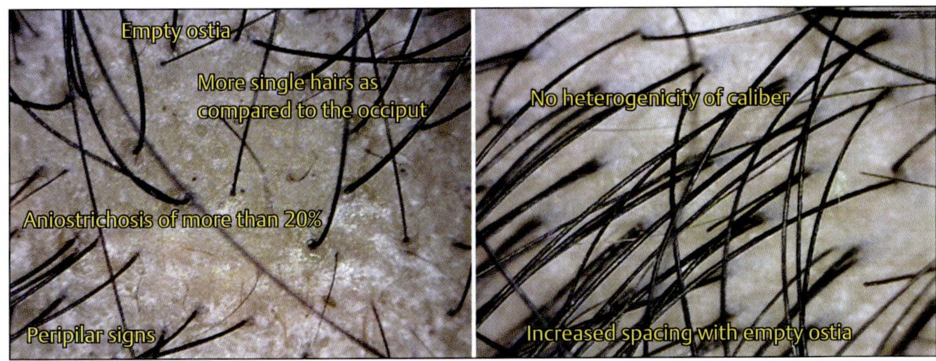

Fig. 20.17 Trichoscopy characteristics in pattern hair loss.

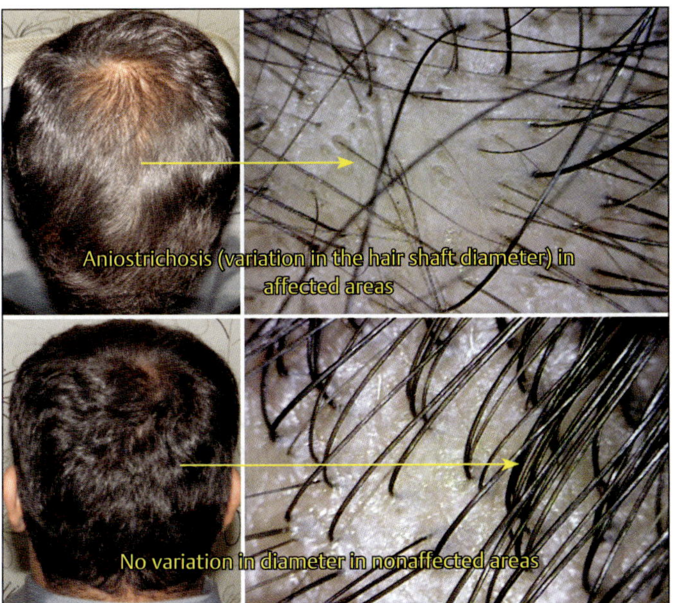

Fig. 20.18 Trichoscopic findings in pattern hair loss.

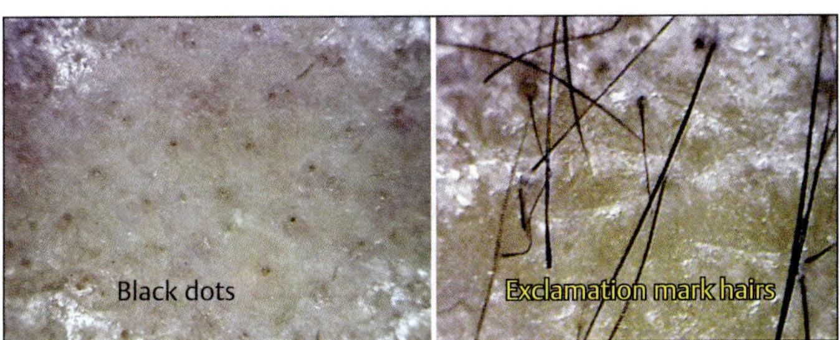

Fig. 20.19 Black dots and exclamation mark hair seen in alopecia areata.

panel, thyroid function test, autoantibodies, total testosterone, and free testosterone, ovarian hormones, luteinizing hormone, and the follicular stimulating hormone may be necessary for some patients. It is good to assess the Vitamin D and B12 levels. In men over 45 years of age, it is advisable to estimate serum prostate-specific antigen (PSA) especially if there is a plan to start finasteride therapy.[33]

Scalp Biopsy

When the diagnosis is not clear, a scalp biopsy may help to corroborate the findings and come to a conclusive diagnosis. It can also serve as an indicator of prognosis and stability of the disease.[34] Most commonly a 4 mm punch biopsy oriented in the direction of hair growth is taken from the affected area. Sometimes for reference a second sample may be taken from the normal area. The biopsy sample should be processed using vertical and transverse sections for optimum information.

Summary

Generally, hair loss is a clinical diagnosis. Depending on the patient history, clinical evaluation and trichoscopy, and additional investigations, one can arrive at a diagnosis (**Flowchart 20.4**) regarding the type and cause of hair loss. One should be able to give a rough guide to possible treatment options and prognosis. It is advisable to have questionnaire to be filled by the patient so that the surgeon does not miss out on any points in history taking and examination.

Alternate regimens have been designed to reduce the side effect profile of finasteride and improve patient compliance in practice, but evidence for these is lacking:

- The drug may be initially administered at a dose of 0.5 mg daily for a short period. This would gain patient confidence and the 1 mg per day dose may be started once the patient is comfortable.
- Alternate day dosing can be tried.
- Finasteride can be given for 3 months followed by a washout period for 1 month.

Topical Finasteride

A topical solution of finasteride has been developed to overcome the side effects associated with oral finasteride. However, this formulation is not FDA approved. A recent study comparing topical with oral finasteride showed that there was a significant decrease in the scalp DHT level, but only a 24 to 26% reduction in serum DHT.[58] However, data is still preliminary and more evidence is needed. One of the major concerns with topical formulations is contact with childbearing women, and this should be avoided.

Minoxidil

In 1979, oral minoxidil was approved for the treatment of resistant hypertension that failed to respond to standard drugs.[59] As the drug gained popularity, it was noticed that hypertrichosis was a common side effect. Every setback presents an opportunity, and the drug was tried topically to treat AGA. In 1988, topical minoxidil received FDA approval for AGA.[60]

Mechanism of Action

Minoxidil is available as 2% and 5% topical solution. 2% Minoxidil was approved for treatment of male AGA in 1988 while 5% and 2% preparations were approved in 1991 for the treatment of male and female AGA, respectively. Chemical name of minoxidil is piperidino-pyrimidine derivative. The chemical structure is 2,4-primidinediamine,6-(1-piperidinyl)-,3-oxide ($C9H15N5O$).

Minoxidil solution is by itself a prodrug, which is converted into its active form minoxidil sulfate in the ORS by the enzyme sulfotransferases. It requires a vehicle such as water, ethanol, and propylene glycol for improving the solubility of minoxidil. Propylene glycol vehicle enhances the delivery of minoxidil into hair follicles. But it is known to cause local irritation manifesting as itching and burning sensation, which led to the development of propylene glycol-free minoxidil foam. Foam preparation contains cetyl alcohol, stearyl alcohol, and butylated hydroxytoluene. It enhances the delivery and penetration of minoxidil to the hair follicle as well as causes less irritation.[61]

Minoxidil sulfation varies among individuals. Individuals with higher enzyme activity have better results compared to individuals with lower enzyme activity. It has been found that the level of follicular sulfotransferase enzyme levels remains unchanged even up to 8 weeks post therapy. This suggests that, after therapy, responders do not develop low enzyme levels nor do nonresponders convert into responders.[62] Minoxidil has the following effects on hair:

- Prolongs the latent period of the hair cycle (the time between shedding of telogen hair and the onset of the next anagen). It has been suggested that minoxidil has a key role in cell proliferation at the early stage as potassium channel activity is required for moving to the G1 phase of cell cycle.
- Opens the potassium channels leading to hyperpolarization of the cell membrane. In the presence of calcium, epidermal growth factor (EGF) inhibits the hair growth. This entry of calcium is opposed by the potassium channel openers and may lead to hair growth.
- Minoxidil also causes delay in the hydrolysis of cAMP via inhibition of phosphodiesterase, thus resulting in vasodilatory action.[63]

Pharmacokinetics

Topically used minoxidil is poorly absorbed through the skin (systemic absorption is 2% of the applied minoxidil). The absorbed minoxidil is distributed into the body and is metabolized in liver and excreted in urine as unchanged metabolite (glucuronide conjugate) within 4 days. It does not cross the blood–brain barrier.

Efficacy

Topical minoxidil is available from concentrations of 2 to 15%. A systematic review and meta-analysis of treatments in AGA showed that both 5% and 2% topical minoxidil were effective in AGA and the efficacy of 5% was more than that of 2%. Five percent topical formulation has been shown to be quite effective not only in preventing hair loss but also in hair regrowth.[64,65]

Contraindications

Though there is a paucity of literature; however, it is contraindicated in cases of hypersensitivity, pregnancy, and lactating mothers.

Side Effects

Minoxidil is generally safe, but occasionally has a few minor side effects. Irritant contact dermatitis is typically the most common adverse effects which present as itching and scaling. Paradoxical hair shedding can occur at the beginning of treatment due to stimulation of exogen as telogen follicles re-enter anagen.[57] Allergic contact dermatitis occurs uncommonly. In some individuals, the vasodilatory effects can trigger headaches and migraines. Facial hypertrichosis is more commonly seen in females and is dependent on the concentration, with topical minoxidil 5% having the most incidence of unwanted hair growth.

Accidental oral consumption of minoxidil solution can be life threatening. In adults, it can manifest as refractory shock, tachycardia, fluid retention, and rarely as pulmonary edema and papilledema without overt raised intracranial pressure. In children, it manifests with serious cardiovascular effects.

Guidelines for Use

- One mL of the minoxidil solution or half a cup of foam is applied twice daily over the scalp.
- Care to be taken to prevent run off to other areas to prevent hypertrichosis in unwanted areas.
- The need to spread the preparation evenly over the desired areas should be explained and emphasized especially with spray applicator.
- Patient should be counseled regarding possibility of increased hair shedding in the first few months and that it is only temporary.
- Counsel him/her that the hair loss will return if topical treatment is discontinued.
- Inform the need for cessation of application of the drug during pregnancy and lactation due to insufficient studies regarding its effects.

Medical treatments are an essential component of AGA treatment. Finasteride and minoxidil form the backbone of medical therapy, and their efficacy is well established. Patients may often be misinformed about these medications, and hence it is important for anyone involved in AGA treatment to be up to date on the literature so they can counsel their patients judiciously. When used scientifically, they can produce excellent results in a significant proportion of patients and bring satisfaction.

Recent Advances and Emerging Treatments for Hair Loss

Ratchathorn Panchaprateep

Introduction

Currently, the topical minoxidil, oral finasteride, and hair transplantation are the standard treatment for androgenic alopecia (AGA).[66] However, some patients get unfavorable results or experience side effects with standard treatments. There are few novel treatments which have been developed to improve clinical outcome and some of them seem to have great potential.

Physical Treatments

Platelet-Rich Plasma (PRP)

A definition of PRP is plasma with abundant platelet concentration three to seven times greater than normal. PRP contains various growth factors, including vascular endothelial growth factor (VEGF), platelet-derived growth factor (PDGF), transforming growth factor-β (TGF-β), insulin-like growth factor 1, 2 (IGF-1, 2), epidermal growth factor (EGF), hepatocyte growth factor (HGF), and fibroblast growth factor (FGF), which are secreted from the alpha granules of concentrated platelets activated by inducers.[67] These growth factors can stimulate hair growth by promoting cell proliferation and differentiation, prolonging cell survival and antiapoptotic properties, lengthening anagen phase of hair follicles, increasing angiogenesis, and reducing perifollicular inflammation.[68,69] In addition, PRP may prolong anagen phase by inducing expression of FGF-7 in DP cells resulting in hair growth stimulation.[70]

Most studies suggest that injection of autologous PRP decreases the rate of hair fall, and increases hair diameter and density in patients with AGA at 3 and 6 months after multiple sessions.[71] A recent meta-analysis revealed that 3 monthly PRP injections are effective for AGA treatment. It increases hair density[71,72] and hair diameter in men and women significantly after three injections.[73] Studies demonstrated that combination of PRP with topical minoxidil is more effective than PRP or topical minoxidil alone.[74]

PRP is used to treat both male and female AGA with satisfactory results. A significant better response to PRP is found in patients with early stage of AGA (male: Norwood-Hamilton: II-III-IVv, diffuse patterned alopecia (DPA) or diffuse unpatterned alopecia (DUPA) and female: Ludwig stages I-II, Olsen I-II).[75]

Technique

There is no standardized method to prepare PRP. PRP can be prepared by using manual or automated systems. The basic two-step centrifugation procedure is the most popular. An initial slow centrifugation at 1000 to 2500 RPM separates the erythrocytes from lighter plasma with buffy coat at the interface. Plasma and buffy coat are aspirated and then centrifuged at high speed at 2000 to 4500 RPM to pellet platelets. The automated systems are established to simplify the preparation of PRP and improve productivity and better yield of platelet and growth factors. The optimal platelet concentration to stimulate angiogenesis range from 1.5 to 3×10^6/L in most of the in vitro experiments.[76]

Platelet activation is the process to turn on the specific molecules on the surface of platelets, followed by alpha granules release of growth factors. Calcium chloride, calcium gluconate, and thrombin have been frequently used as exogenous agents to activate platelet.[77] For AGA treatment, the nonactivated PRP in liquid form is preferred, because it is easier to inject as compared to the activated PRP. 0.05–0.1 mL/cm^2 of PRP has been recommended to be used at 1 cm apart using a 27 to 30-gauge needle. Author uses it in three sessions at 1-month interval (**Fig. 20.20**). Maintenance treatment is suggested every 3 to 6 months.[78]

PRP and Hair Transplantation

The PRP is used as an adjuvant to hair transplantation to increase the graft survival, to enhance the vascular supply of scalp, and to stimulate hair growth in the area where hair thinning is observed. PRP is expected to enhance the vascular neogenesis in the scar tissue in cases of scar alopecia. PRP can be used in hair transplantation in two ways: one as a graft storage solution, and second as subcutaneous injection into the recipient and donor sites. Uebel and colleagues reported the first study in 2006 using PRP as storage solution to increase the graft survival after a transplantation.[79]

The side effects of PRP are minimal and transient. PRP injection is painful due to its acidic pH. It may also cause erythema, headache, forehead swelling, scalp dryness, and scaling.[80] PRP is a promising adjunctive treatment for AGA and can be used during hair transplantation to enhance the outcome.

Low-Level Laser (or Light) Therapy

Currently, low-level laser therapy (LLLT) has been introduced as a new treatment modality for AGA. A recent meta-analysis strongly suggests that LLLT is effective for promoting hair growth in AGA.[81] LLLT works on the principle of "photobiomodulation"; however, the exact mechanism of action is not clearly understood. It has been proposed that LLLT stimulates the growth of hair follicles, prolongs anagen phase, and promotes anagen re-entry through increased mitochondrial respiration and cell energy in the form of adenosine triphosphatase (ATP) and nitric oxide (NO). LLLT is also known to improve microvascular circulation and reduce inflammation.[82]

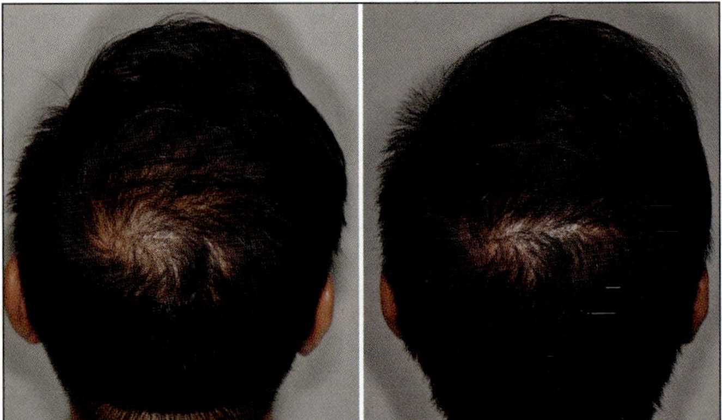

Fig. 20.20 A 46-year-old male patient with androgenetic alopecia (AGA) IV vertex at baseline and 3 months after treatment with platelet-rich plasma (PRP) for three sessions at 1-month interval.

Laser devices for the treatment of AGA are commercially available since 2007.[83] There are three types of LLLT devices: laser comb, helmet-type, and laser cap. The advantage of a comb device is that light sources can be close to the scalp because the device is required to part the hair during the usage. Helmet or laser cap devices are more user friendly. Currently, most devices use a wavelength of 630 to 660 nm and are recommended to be used daily or alternate days for 20 to 30 minutes.[81]

Majority of the studies suggest that LLLT can improve hair density, and hair thickness for both male and female AGA patients with mild-to-moderate severity (Hamilton-Norwood: IIa to V and Ludwig (savin): I to II-2).[84] It is doubtful whether the improvement seen with LLLT in various studies is long lasting.[81,84]

The office-based LED units are often used perioperatively to speed up wound healing, reduce pain and edema, and encourage hair growth.[85,86] Both donor and recipient areas are treated immediately post hair transplantation, after 24 to 48 hours, and then one to two times a week[87] (**Fig. 20.21a, b**).

Most adverse effects such as headache, skin dryness, scalp tenderness, pruritus, irritation, acne, and warm sensation are mild and transient.[84,88]

Hair Stem Cell Regeneration

Hair follicle stem cells (HFSCs) are located in the bulge region of the follicle and show characteristics of slow cycling behavior, superior clonogenicity, high proliferative capacity, multipotency, and transplant ability. The action of HFSCs in the bulge is regulated by its microenvironment called niche. Another important stem cell in hair follicle is DP cell located at the hair bulb. DP cells are special mesenchyme cells, playing a pivotal role to regulate the hair growth and renewal of neighboring tissues.[89] The interactions between epithelial, mesenchymal, and the niche are critical to hair growth and biologic process.[90]

The concept of hair cloning and hair stem cell therapy starts from extracting crucial cells from a biopsy of the healthiest scalp tissue, maturing the cells ex vivo in the laboratory, and then reinjecting into the problematic area.[91]

At present, hair follicle regeneration using chamber and patch assay has been successfully performed in mice model.[92] Tsuboi et al reported successful cell-based treatment for hair loss by using autologous dermal sheath cup (DSC) cells in human subjects. There was significant increase in hair density and cumulative hair diameter as compared

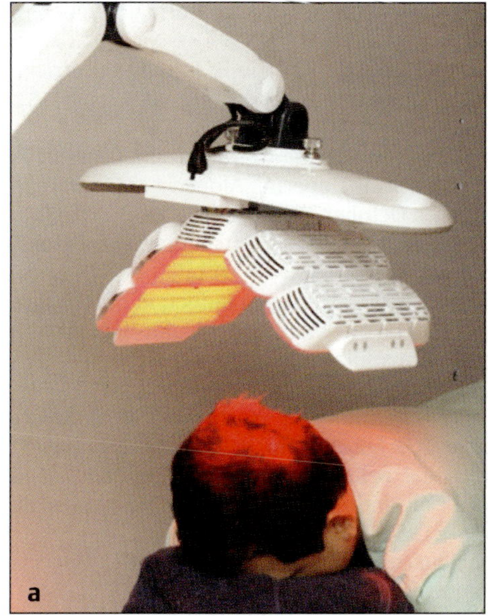

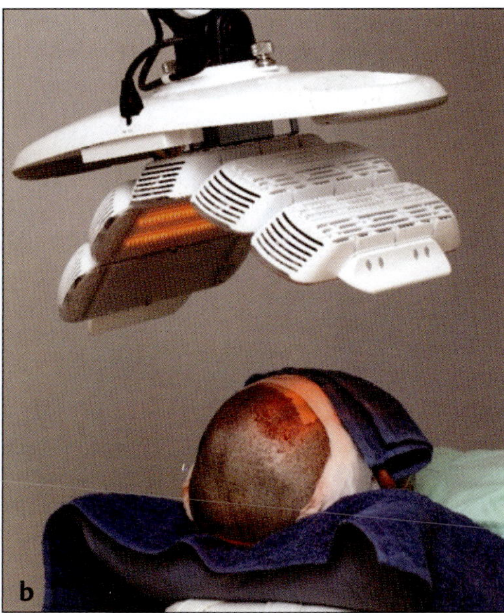

Fig. 20.21 (a) LED therapy post hair transplantation on donor area using low-power laser in wavelengths of 830 and 633 nm. **(b)** LED therapy on recipient areas using low-power laser in wavelengths of 830 and 633 nm.

with the placebo. However, the effect did not last long and turned to near baseline at 12 months.[93]

At present there is no evidence favoring clinical application of HFSC in the management of AGA. However, there seems to be potential, and stem cell–based therapy may become an alternative treatment modality of hair loss in future.

Exosomes

Exosomes are biological membrane-bound structures which are secreted from intracellular multivesicular bodies (MVBs or late endosomes) into extracellular space by a variety of cells.[94] Depending on the origin, exosomes contain many constituents of a cell, including DNA, RNAs, mRNAs, lipids, metabolites, and cytosolic and surface protein markers.[94,95] Exosome is considered as a newly identified mechanism for cell-to-cell communication.[94] It is believed to promote hair regeneration through a paracrine mechanism dependent on its source. Recent studies have reported that exosomes secreted by stem cells, including mesenchymal stem cells and DP cells, are promising for skin wound healing and hair regeneration.

The published data strongly suggest that exosomes derived from DP cells, DP-ORS cells co-culture, and 3D-spheres promote hair growth and regeneration by regulating the activity of follicular dermal and epidermal cells.[96] These in vitro findings have implications for the development of therapeutic strategies for hair loss. However, clinical application of exosomes in human is still awaited.

New Antiandrogens for Female-Pattern Hair Loss

Many new antiandrogen therapies have gained traction in recent years due to their potential efficacy in treating AGA especially in females.

Cortexolone 17α-propionate (C17P, Clascoterone)

C17P is a direct androgen receptor (AR) inhibitor with anti-inflammatory properties and weak glucocorticoid effects. C17P is found to bind the AR with high affinity in vitro and consequently inhibit AR-regulated transcription in a reporter cell line with similar efficacy to the 5α-reductase inhibitor, finasteride. When compared to another AR antagonist, C17P showed more potent antiandrogenic activity as compared to progesterone, finasteride, flutamide, and is about as effective as cyproterone acetate.[97]

For AGA, C17P is currently in a phase 2, randomized, double-blind, control study in over 400 male patients with mild-to-moderate AGA. The greatest improvement was observed in C17P 7.5% solution twice daily group. No serious adverse effects have been reported yet. It is yet to receive an FDA pregnancy safe category.

Bicalutamide

Bicalutamide is a nonsteroidal, pure antiandrogen. Very low dose of bicalutamide at 1–10 to 25 mg/day has been used to treat female-pattern hair loss. A recent study using bicalutamide in combination with other hair-enhancing therapy showed 20.2 to 27.5% reduction in Sinclair stage at 6 months.[98]

References

1. Rose Paul T, Shapiro Ron, Morgan Michael. Basic science. In: Unger, WP, Shapiro, R. Hair transplantation. 4th ed. New York: Marcel Dekker; 2004:25–48
2. Michael B. Anatomy and anatomical landmarks. In: Robert SH, Dow S. Hair transplant. 1st ed. Philadelphia, USA: Elsevier Saunders; 2006:19–25
3. Last R. Anatomy: Regional and applied. 3rd ed. London: J. & R. Churchill; 1963:2–3
4. Lindelöf B, Forslind B, Hedblad MA, Kaveus U. Human hair form: Morphology revealed by light and scanning electron microscopy and computer aided three-dimensional reconstruction. Arch Dermatol 1988;124(9):1359–1363
5. Pinkus H. Embryology of hair. In: Montagna W, Ellis RA, eds. The biology of hair growth. New York: Academic Press; 1958:1–32
6. Alonso L, Fuchs E. The hair cycle. J Cell Sci 2006;119(Pt 3): 391–393
7. Rajendra SR. A scientific hypothesis on the role of nutritional supplements for effective management of hair loss and promoting hair regrowth. J Nutrit Health Food Sci 2018;6(3): 1–11
8. Kim BK, Lee S, Jun M, Chung HC, Oh SS, Lee WS. Perception of hair loss and education increases the treatment willingness in patients with androgenetic alopecia: a population-based study. Ann Dermatol 2018;30(4):402–408
9. Price VH. Treatment of hair loss. N Engl J Med 1999;341(13): 964–973
10. Bernard BA. Advances in understanding hair growth. F1000 Res 2016;5:F1000 Faculty Rev-147. Published 2016 Feb 8
11. Murphrey MB, Agarwal S, Zito PM. Anatomy, hair. Updated 2019 Jul 14. In: StatPearls [Internet]. Treasure Island (FL): StatPearls Publishing; 2020. https://www.ncbi.nlm.nih.gov/books/NBK513312/
12. Milner Y, Sudnik J, Filippi M, Kizoulis M, Kashgarian M, Stenn K. Exogen, shedding phase of the hair growth cycle: characterization of a mouse model. J Invest Dermatol 2002;119(3):639–644
13. Paus R. Therapeutic strategies for treating hair loss. Drug Discov Today Ther Strateg 2006;3:101–110
14. Qi J, Garza LA. An overview of alopecias. Cold Spring Harb Perspect Med 2014;4(3):a013615
15. Malkud S. Telogen effluvium: a review. J Clin Diagn Res 2015; 9(9):WE01–WE03
16. Hughes EC, Saleh D. Telogen effluvium. Updated 2019 Dec 20. In: StatPearls [Internet]. Treasure Island (FL): StatPearls Publishing; 2020. https://www.ncbi.nlm.nih.gov/books/NBK430848
17. Jain N, Doshi B, Khopkar U. Trichoscopy in alopecias: diagnosis simplified. Int J Trichology 2013;5(4):170–178
18. Saleh D, Cook C. Anagen effluvium. Updated 2019 Jul 31. In: StatPearls [Internet]. Treasure Island (FL): StatPearls Publishing; 2020. https://www.ncbi.nlm.nih.gov/books/NBK482293/
19. Kanwar AJ, Narang T. Anagen effluvium. Indian J Dermatol Venereol Leprol 2013;79(5):604–612
20. Quercetani R, Rebora AE, Fedi MC, et al. Patients with profuse hair shedding may reveal anagen hair dystrophy: a diagnostic clue of alopecia areata incognita. J Eur Acad Dermatol Venereol 2011;25(7):808–810
21. Filbrandt R, Rufaut N, Jones L, Sinclair R. Primary cicatricial alopecia: diagnosis and treatment. CMAJ 2013;185(18): 1579–1585
22. Yingjun S, Qing Y, Wenjie D, Ping X, Xianjie M, Xianhui Z, Lei W, Chiyu J. Cicatricial alopecia, Alopecia, Muhammad Ahmad, IntechOpen; October 31st 2018, doi: 10.5772/intechopen.78971. https://www.intechopen.com/books/alopecia/cicatricial-alopecia
23. Itami S, Kurata S, Takayasu S. Androgen induction of follicular epithelial cell growth is mediated via insulin-like growth factor-I from dermal papilla cells. Biochem Biophys Res Commun 1995;212(3):988–994
24. Inui S, Fukuzato Y, Nakajima T, Yoshikawa K, Itami S. Androgen-inducible TGF-beta1 from balding dermal papilla cells inhibits epithelial cell growth: a clue to understand paradoxical effects of androgen on human hair growth. FASEB J 2002;16(14):1967–1969
25. Norwood OT. Incidence of female androgenetic alopecia (female pattern alopecia). Dermatol Surg 2001;27(1):53–54
26. Ho CH, Zito PM. Androgenetic alopecia. Updated 2019 Nov 19. In: Stat Pearls [Internet]. Treasure Island (FL): StatPearls Publishing; 2020. https://www.ncbi.nlm.nih.gov/books/NBK430924/
27. Norwood OT. Male pattern baldness: classification and incidence. South Med J 1975;68(11):1359–1365
28. Bukharia A, Jain N. Assessment of depression and anxiety in trichodynia patients of Telogen effluvium and Alopecia areata. Int J Med Res Health Sci 2016;5(6):61–66
29. Darwin E, Hirt PA, Fertig R, Doliner B, Delcanto G, Jimenez JJ. Alopecia areata: review of epidemiology, clinical features, pathogenesis, and new treatment options. Int J Trichology 2018;10(2):51–60
30. Kanwar AJ, Kaur S, Basak P, Sharma R. Traction alopecia in Sikh males. Arch Dermatol 1989;125(11):1587
31. Al-Refu K. Clinical significance of trichoscopy in common causes of hair loss in children: analysis of 134 cases. Int J Trichology 2018;10(4):154–161
32. McDonald KA, Shelley AJ, Colantonio S, Beecker J. Hair pull test: evidence-based update and revision of guidelines. J Am Acad Dermatol 2017;76(3):472–477
33. Blume-Peytavi U, Blumeyer A, Tosti A, et al; European Consensus Group. S1 guideline for diagnostic evaluation in androgenetic alopecia in men, women and adolescents. Br J Dermatol 2011;164(1):5–15
34. Vidal CI. Overview of alopecia: a dermatopathologist's perspective. Mo Med 2015;112(4):308–312
35. Hamilton JB. Male hormone stimulation is prerequisite and an incitement in common baldness. Am J Anat 1942;71: 451–458
36. Imperato-McGinley J, Guerrero L, Gautier T, Peterson RE. Steroid 5-alpha-reductase deficiency in man: an inherited form of male pseudohermaphroditism. Science 1974;186(4170): 1213–1215
37. Thiboutot D, Harris G, Iles V, Cimis G, Gilliland K, Hagari S. Activity of the type 1 5-alpha-reductase exhibits regional differences in isolated sebaceous glands and whole skin. J Invest Dermatol 1995;105(2):209–214
38. Azzouni F, Godoy A, Li Y, Mohler J. The 5-alpha-reductase isozyme family: a review of basic biology and their role in human diseases. Adv Urol 2012;2012:530121

39. Olsen EA, Hordinsky M, Whiting D, et al; Dutasteride Alopecia Research Team. The importance of dual 5-alpha-reductase inhibition in the treatment of male pattern hair loss: results of a randomized placebo-controlled study of dutasteride versus finasteride. J Am Acad Dermatol 2006;55(6):1014–1023
40. Finn DA, Beadles-Bohling AS, Beckley EH, et al. A new look at the 5-alpha-reductase inhibitor finasteride. CNS Drug Rev 2006;12(1):53–76
41. Zito PM, Syed K. Finasteride. Updated 2020 Feb 16. In: StatPearls [Internet]. Treasure Island (FL): StatPearls Publishing; 2020. https://www.ncbi.nlm.nih.gov/books/NBK513329/
42. Mysore V. Finasteride and sexual side effects. Indian Dermatol Online J 2012;3(1):62–65
43. Mella JM, Perret MC, Manzotti M, Catalano HN, Guyatt G. Efficacy and safety of finasteride therapy for androgenetic alopecia: a systematic review. Arch Dermatol 2010;146(10):1141–1150
44. Khandpur S, Suman M, Reddy BS. Comparative efficacy of various treatment regimens for androgenetic alopecia in men. J Dermatol 2002;29(8):489–498
45. Amory JK, Wang C, Swerdloff RS, et al. The effect of 5-alpha-reductase inhibition with dutasteride and finasteride on semen parameters and serum hormones in healthy men. J Clin Endocrinol Metab 2007;92(5):1659–1665
46. Clark RV, Hermann DJ, Cunningham GR, Wilson TH, Morrill BB, Hobbs S. Marked suppression of dihydrotestosterone in men with benign prostatic hyperplasia by dutasteride: a dual 5-alpha-reductase inhibitor. J Clin Endocrinol Metab 2004;89(5):2179–2184
47. Erdemir F, Harbin A, Hellstrom WJ. 5-alpha reductase inhibitors and erectile dysfunction: the connection. J Sex Med 2008;5(12):2917–2924
48. Hagberg KW, Divan HA, Persson R, Nickel JC, Jick SS. Risk of erectile dysfunction associated with use of 5-α reductase inhibitors for benign prostatic hyperplasia or alopecia: population based studies using the Clinical Practice Research Datalink. BMJ 2016;354:i4823
49. Haber RS, Gupta AK, Epstein E, Carviel JL, Foley KA. Finasteride for androgenetic alopecia is not associated with sexual dysfunction: a survey-based, single-centre, controlled study. J Eur Acad Dermatol Venereol 2019;33(7):1393–1397
50. Mondaini N, Gontero P, Giubilei G, et al. Finasteride 5 mg and sexual side effects: how many of these are related to a nocebo phenomenon? J Sex Med 2007;4(6):1708–1712
51. Cash TF. The psychosocial consequences of androgenetic alopecia: a review of the research literature. Br J Dermatol 1999;141(3):398–405
52. Samplaski MK, Lo K, Grober E, Jarvi K. Finasteride use in the male infertility population: effects on semen and hormone parameters. Fertil Steril 2013;100(6):1542–1546
53. Ganzer CA, Jacobs AR. Emotional consequences of finasteride: fool's gold. Am J Men Health 2018;12(1):90–95
54. Mansouri P, Farshi S, Safar F. Finasteride-induced gynecomastia. Indian J Dermatol Venereol Leprol 2009;75(3):309–310
55. Etzioni RD, Howlader N, Shaw PA, et al. Long-term effects of finasteride on prostate specific antigen levels: results from the prostate cancer prevention trial. J Urol 2005;174(3):877–881
56. Mysore V, Shashikumar BM. Guidelines on the use of finasteride in androgenetic alopecia. Indian J Dermatol Venereol Leprol 2016;82(2):128–134
57. Kanti V, Messenger A, Dobos G, et al. Evidence-based (S3) guideline for the treatment of androgenetic alopecia in women and in men - short version. J Eur Acad Dermatol Venereol 2018;32(1):11–22
58. Lee SW, Juhasz M, Mobasher P, Ekelem C, Mesinkovska NA. A systematic review of topical finasteride in the treatment of androgenetic alopecia in men and women. J Drugs Dermatol 2018;17(4):457–463
59. Zins GR; ZinsGR. The history of the development of minoxidil. Clin Dermatol 1988;6(4):132–147
60. Goren A, Naccarato T. Minoxidil in the treatment of androgenetic alopecia. Dermatol Ther (Heidelb) 2018;31(5):e12686
61. Suchonwanit P, Thammarucha S, Leerunyakul K. Minoxidil and its use in hair disorders: a review. Drug Des Devel Ther 2019;13:2777–2786
62. Goren A, Mccoy J, Kovacevic M, et al. The effect of topical minoxidil treatment on follicular sulfotransferase enzymatic activity. J Biol Regul Homeost Agents 2018;32(4):937–940
63. Goren A, Shapiro J, Roberts J, et al. Clinical utility and validity of minoxidil response testing in androgenetic alopecia. Dermatol Ther (Heidelb) 2015;28(1):13–16
64. Rundegren J. A one-year observational study with minoxidil 5% solution in Germany: results of independent efficacy evaluation by physicians and patients. J Am Acad Dermatol 2004;50(3):91
65. Rundegren J. Rapid onset of action of minoxidil 5% topical solution in a 4-month German observational study on both patients and physicians. J Am Acad Dermatol 2004;50(3):91
66. Bienová M, Kucerová R, Fiurásková M, Hajdúch M, Kolář Z. Androgenetic alopecia and current methods of treatment. Acta Dermatovenerol Alp Panonica Adriat 2005;14(1):5–8
67. Gentile P, Cole JP, Cole MA, et al. Evaluation of not-activated and activated PRP in hair loss treatment: role of growth factor and cytokine concentrations obtained by different collection systems. Int J Mol Sci 2017;18(2):408
68. Cervelli V, Palla L, Pascali M, De Angelis B, Curcio BC, Gentile P. Autologous platelet-rich plasma mixed with purified fat graft in aesthetic plastic surgery. Aesthetic Plast Surg 2009;33(5): 716–721
69. Kang JS, Zheng Z, Choi MJ, Lee SH, Kim DY, Cho SB. The effect of CD34+ cell-containing autologous platelet-rich plasma injection on pattern hair loss: a preliminary study. J Eur Acad Dermatol Venereol 2014;28(1):72–79
70. Li ZJ, Choi HI, Choi DK, et al. Autologous platelet-rich plasma: a potential therapeutic tool for promoting hair growth. Dermatol Surg 2012;38(7 Pt 1):1040–1046
71. Gupta AK, Versteeg SG, Rapaport J, Hausauer AK, Shear NH, Piguet V. The efficacy of platelet-rich plasma in the field of hair restoration and facial aesthetics: a systematic review and meta-analysis. J Cutan Med Surg 2019;23(2):185–203
72. Mapar MA, Shahriari S, Haghighizadeh MH. Efficacy of platelet-rich plasma in the treatment of androgenetic (male-patterned) alopecia: a pilot randomized controlled trial. J Cosmet Laser Ther 2016;18(8):452–455
73. Ahmad M. Effect of platelets-rich plasma on scalp hair diameter. J Cosmet Dermatol 2019;18(1):51–54
74. Singh SK, Kumar V, Rai T. Comparison of efficacy of platelet-rich plasma therapy with or without topical 5% minoxidil in male-type baldness: a randomized, double-blind placebo control trial. Indian J Dermatol Venereol Leprol 2020;86(2):150–157
75. Kachhawa D, Vats G, Sonare D, Rao P, Khuraiya S, Kataiya R. A spilt head study of efficacy of placebo versus platelet-rich plasma injections in the treatment of androgenic alopecia. J Cutan Aesthet Surg 2017;10(2):86–89

76. Giusti I, Rughetti A, D'Ascenzo S, et al. Identification of an optimal concentration of platelet gel for promoting angiogenesis in human endothelial cells. Transfusion 2009;49(4):771–778
77. Nusbaum AG, Tosti A. Commentary on a randomized placebo-controlled, double-blind, half-head study to assess the efficacy of platelet-rich plasma on the treatment of androgenetic alopecia. Dermatol Surg 2016;42(4):498–499
78. Gupta AK, Cole J, Deutsch DP, et al. Platelet-rich plasma as a treatment for androgenetic alopecia. Dermatol Surg 2019;45(10):1262–1273
79. Uebel CO, da Silva JB, Cantarelli D, Martins P. The role of platelet plasma growth factors in male pattern baldness surgery. Plast Reconstr Surg 2006;118(6):1458–1466, discussion 1467
80. Laird ME, Lo Sicco KI, Reed ML, Brinster NK. Platelet-rich plasma for the treatment of female pattern hair loss: a patient survey. Dermatol Surg 2018;44(1):130–132
81. Adil A, Godwin M. The effectiveness of treatments for androgenetic alopecia: a systematic review and meta-analysis. J Am Acad Dermatol 2017;77(1):136–141.e5
82. Gao X, Xing D. Molecular mechanisms of cell proliferation induced by low power laser irradiation. J Biomed Sci 2009;16:4
83. Dodd EM, Winter MA, Hordinsky MK, Sadick NS, Farah RS. Photobiomodulation therapy for androgenetic alopecia: a clinician's guide to home-use devices cleared by the Federal Drug Administration. J Cosmet Laser Ther 2018;20(3):159–167
84. Liu KH, Liu D, Chen YT, Chin SY. Comparative effectiveness of low-level laser therapy for adult androgenic alopecia: a system review and meta-analysis of randomized controlled trials. Lasers Med Sci 2019;34(6):1063–1069
85. Rose PT. Advances in hair restoration. Dermatol Clin 2018; 36(1):57–62
86. Kim WS, Calderhead RG. Is light-emitting diode phototherapy (LED-LLLT) really effective? Laser Ther 2011;20(3):205–215
87. Joshi R, Shokri T, Baker A, et al. Alopecia and techniques in hair restoration: an overview for the cosmetic surgeon. Oral Maxillofac Surg 2019;23(2):123–131
88. Afifi L, Maranda EL, Zarei M, et al. Low-level laser therapy as a treatment for androgenetic alopecia. Lasers Surg Med 2017;49(1):27–39
89. Ohyama M, Terunuma A, Tock CL, et al. Characterization and isolation of stem cell-enriched human hair follicle bulge cells. J Clin Invest 2006;116(1):249–260
90. Qiu W, Lei M, Zhou L, et al. Hair follicle stem cell proliferation, Akt and Wnt signaling activation in TPA-induced hair regeneration. Histochem Cell Biol 2017;147(6):749–758
91. Stenn KS, Cotsarelis G. Bioengineering the hair follicle: fringe benefits of stem cell technology. Curr Opin Biotechnol 2005;16(5):493–497
92. Zhang Q, Zu T, Zhou Q, Wen J, Leng X, Wu X. The patch assay reconstitutes mature hair follicles by culture-expanded human cells. Regen Med 2017;12(5):503–511
93. Tsuboi R, Niiyama S, Irisawa R, Harada K, Nakazawa Y, Kishimoto J. Autologous cell-based therapy for male and female pattern hair loss using dermal sheath cup cells: a randomized placebo-controlled double-blinded dose-finding clinical study. J Am Acad Dermatol 2020;83(1):109–116
94. Margolis L, Sadovsky Y. The biology of extracellular vesicles: the known unknowns. PLoS Biol 2019;17(7):e3000363
95. Kalluri R, LeBleu VS. The biology, function, and biomedical applications of exosomes. Science 2020;367(6478):eaau6977
96. Li MY, Liu DW, Mao YG. Advances in the research of effects of exosomes derived from stem cells on wound repair. Zhonghua Shao Shang Za Zhi 2017;33(3):180–184
97. Celasco G, Moro L, Bozzella R, et al. Biological profile of cortexolone 17alpha-propionate (CB-03-01): a new topical and peripherally selective androgen antagonist. Arzneimittelforschung 2004;54(12):881–886
98. Fernandez-Nieto D, Saceda-Corralo D, Jimenez-Cauhe J, et al. Bicalutamide: a potential new oral antiandrogenic drug for female pattern hair loss. J Am Acad Dermatol 2020;S0190-9622(20)30667-8

21

Hair Restoration: Planning and Surgical Management—I

Anil K. Garg and Seema Garg

Introduction

Hair transplant is a surgical procedure. Live hair follicles from one area of the body called the "donor area" are transferred to the chosen "recipient area" where the hair is needed. The goal of the hair transplant is to re-establish the aesthetic balance lost in the process of balding. The purpose of hair transplant is to restore normalcy both in the short and the long term, as the balding process is progressive.

History

The first hair transplant of intact hair follicles was performed by the Japanese physicians Okuda and Tamura.[1,2] Norman Orentreich, father of modern hair transplant surgery, gave the concept of donor dominance, stating that hair follicles taken from the occipital region and implanted in the front of the scalp will survive and continue to grow. Headington introduced the landmark concept of the "follicular unit" in 1984.[3] Each follicular unit of the adult human scalp usually consists of one to four terminal hair follicles, sebaceous glands, a neurovascular plexus, arrector pili muscle, and one or rarely two vellus follicles.[3] The above two concepts became the basic principles of hair transplant.

Bobby Limmer in 1994 gave the concept of implantation of individual follicular units (FUs) by taking a strip and dissecting FUs under a stereo microscope.[4] In 2002, Rassman and colleagues published an article about follicular unit extraction.[5] The technique of follicular unit extraction was initially known as FOX or FUSE (follicular unit extraction/follicular unit separation extraction) procedure. In 1998, Bernstein and 20 other physicians gave precise definitions of various types of graft obtained.

Principles for Hair Transplant

1. Priority of the frontal zone: Main objective of hair transplant is restoration of the anterior hairline (AHL). The frontal zone should be the highest priority. If the limited donor hair follicles are consumed to transplant areas like the vertex, transplanting in the frontal zone may be compromised. To prevent such a situation, surgeons need to plan ahead to save enough donor hair for the frontal area which may be required in the future.
2. Less is always better: Balding is a progressive process. The future bald areas may need more hairs. This rule applies especially to younger individuals whose future balding pattern is uncertain.

3. Use the "Gradient Density" technique: It is advisable to keep the density highest in the anterior and central area called "egg." Density decreases as we go posterior, near the fringe of permanent hair.
4. Do not make hair transplants "too perfect" in terms of density, location, and design of AHL. Making one area extremely dense will give a transplanted look. A straight hairline with obtuse/round off on both lateral ends of the hairline (frontotemporal angle) will look unaesthetic.
5. Transplant the future balding area: This avoids the need to repeat transplant at a short interval.

Elements of Hair Transplant

There are *four essential elements* of hair transplant. One should understand the patient's goals, should thoroughly examine the donor and recipient areas, and should have ability to meet the patient's expectations with successful execution of the procedure.

Hair transplant is a surgical procedure performed by a trained, qualified surgeon. Every bald individual is not a candidate for a hair transplant. There are a few criteria which affect the planning of hair transplant. Norwood, in 1992, categorized the factors that affect the planning of hair transplant.[6] Later on, his factors were further extended. Eight major and 11 minor factors are to be taken into consideration before planning the hair transplant (**Table 21.1**). Out of all factors, age of the patient and the donor-recipient ratio are the most important ones. However, none of these factors is a reason to defer any plan for surgery.

Red Flags for Hair Transplant

These are warning signs, indicating the increased risk of complications during or after surgery.

Medical Red Flags

Comorbidities, e.g., diabetes, hypertension, cardiac diseases, heavy smoking, alcoholism, affect the vascularity of the recipient area and affect the outcome of the hair transplant.

Objective Red Flags

If there is a significant discrepancy between the donor supply and the requirement at the recipient site, one needs to prioritize the use of harvested hair follicles. Wrong distribution of the available follicles will compromise the overall result. In any situation the frontal forelock with lateral humps get the priority.[7,8]

Subjective Red Flags

If there is discrepancy between the patient's expectations and the surgeon's capability, result may not be satisfactory. A patient with unrealistic expectations falling in the category of body dysmorphic disorder (BDD) is a contraindication to the hair transplant surgery.

Psychological Aspects of Hair Loss

Alopecia can affect women and men of all ages and has significant social and psychological impacts.[9,10] There are many young individuals who left their job or stopped going to social gatherings because of hair loss. Mental disorders such as depression, anxiety, anger, fatigue, low self-esteem, embarrassment, discomfort with appearance, lower self-regard, less sexual activity, decrease in school performance, social withdrawal, and suicidal tendency increase among alopecia patients.[10–12] We need to differentiate between the psychological trauma because of hair loss in a patient and BDD.

If a patient with BDD or any other psychological abnormality comes for treatment to a hair restoration surgeon, it

Table 21.1 Factors for consideration for hair transplant

Major factors	Minor factors
Age of the patient	Thickness of scalp
Donor recipient ratio in terms of grafts	Supporting temporal hairs
Patient preference and goal	The unique anatomy of the patient's head (size, contour, orientation, etc.)
General medical health	Tolerance of detectability during the hair transplantation process
Psychological status	Means of camouflage available
Hair characteristics	Scalp elasticity and laxity
Capabilities of Surgeon and assisting staff	Patient's potential as a candidate for alopecia reduction
Family history of baldness	Presence of "whisker hair"
	Present hair loss treatment strategy
	Hairstyling preference
	Financial capability and time constraints

is important to send him for psychological/psychiatric consultation. There is a risk of unsatisfied patient resorting to physical violence or legal issues. Hair restoration surgery shall be considered only after effective treatment of BDD.

In author's experience, there are many significant positive changes at the psychological, physical, and social levels after having a successful transplant. Such patients show increased level of confidence, feel happy, start socializing, and involve in routine activities. They feel their identity has been restored.

Counseling before Hair Restoration Surgery

Counseling before hair restoration surgery is of utmost importance. The progressive nature of hair loss, the benefits of medical treatment, and limitations of surgery should be explained to the patient. Surgeon needs to explain the mathematical facts of surgery. There is a big gap between the amount of hair loss and the supply of donor hair. Hair transplant provides coverage but not the normal density. The importance of medical treatment needs to be emphasized for retention of the existing normal hair. Such therapy needs to be used indefinitely.

The posttransplant density, the covered and uncovered bald area of the scalp, operative technique, need for shaving should be explained and should be documented. All preoperative pictures shall be taken with due consent.

Preoperative Assessment and Instructions

After the comprehensive counseling, detailed preoperative assessment and investigations are needed. A personal history, comorbidities, medications, and previous surgeries should be recorded. It is important to elicit a history of allergy, bleeding tendency, keloidal tendency, and history of convulsion(s). It is important to elicit a history of all medications ranging from herbal medicines, blood thinners, antiplatelet therapy, antiepileptics, antidepressants, acne treatment, antiallergic, antibiotics, nonselective β-blockers like propranolol and/or other medicines. History of alcohol, tobacco, opium derivatives, and smoking should also be recorded.

General physical examination, recording of vital parameters, and local examination of donor and recipient sites should be done in an organized manner. A detailed instructions sheet should be given to all the patients **(Table 21.2).**

If the hair is to be harvested from the beard, shaving of the beard should be stopped for 3 to 5 days prior to surgery. Shaving of other parts of the body like chest and abdomen shall be done 12 to 15 days prior.

Donor Area

Occipital area of the scalp is the most preferred donor site. The concept of "safe donor area" is based on a study by and experience of Walter Unger.[13] It is difficult to accurately define the safe donor area. Furthermore, there is no guarantee that all follicles within a "safe donor area" are permanent. Based on Unger study, the defined "safe donor area" will be safe in approximately 80% of patients under the age of 80 years.

Rassman and Bernstein have suggested that the "safe donor area" consists of approximately 25% of the scalp and only half of this should be used for harvesting.[14,15] They also confirmed that hair-bearing scalp is ±520 cm^2 and the average scalp contains approximately two hair/follicular unit. J. Cole advised that the total size of the safe donor area is 203 cm^2.[16] In this safe zone, Caucasians and Asians have on an average 16,649 and 15,718 FUs, respectively. If the hair follicle is harvested beyond the safe zone, there is a high risk of early hair loss.

Safe donor area has specific limits. Lowermost limit is marked using three points over the occipital region (**Fig. 21.1a**). Midpoint A in a sagittal plane over external

Table 21.2 Instructions before hair transplant as practiced by the author

Time	Instructions
1. Four weeks prior	• If scalp donor laxity is low. Scalp massage three times a day. For 15 to 20 min (for strip surgery cases)
2. Three weeks before	• Physician consultation and management of comorbidities
3. One week before	• Stop smoking and tobacco (it is better to stop three weeks before.)
4. Five days before	• Herbs, Vitamin E, and fish oil should be discontinued
5. Two days before	• Stop supplements and other nonapproved medications for hair loss
6. One day before	• Stop alcohol
7. A night before	• Stop blood thinner, aspirin, and seek fitness from a physician
8. On the day of surgery	• Stop applying minoxidil
	• Stop Ibuprofen, naproxen
	• Good sleep, if needed anxiolytic may be prescribed
	• Avoid strenuous exercise
	• Breakfast or meal as usual
	• Shampoo and regular bath

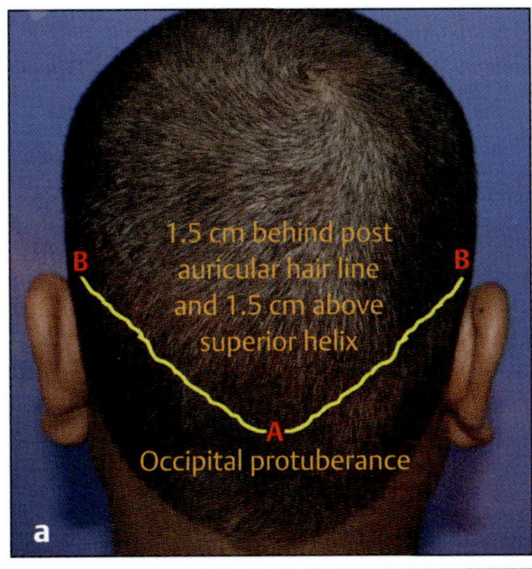

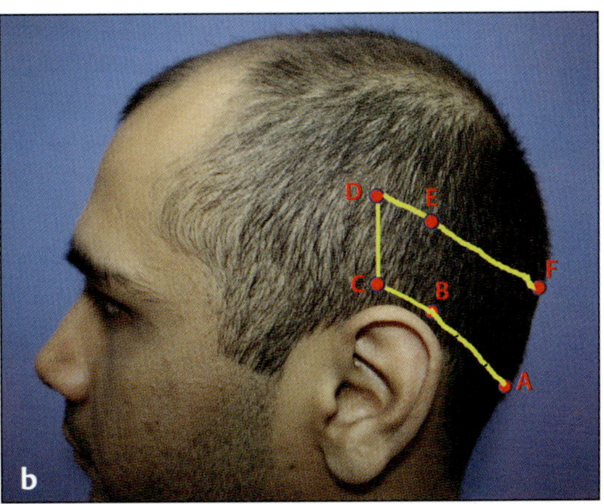

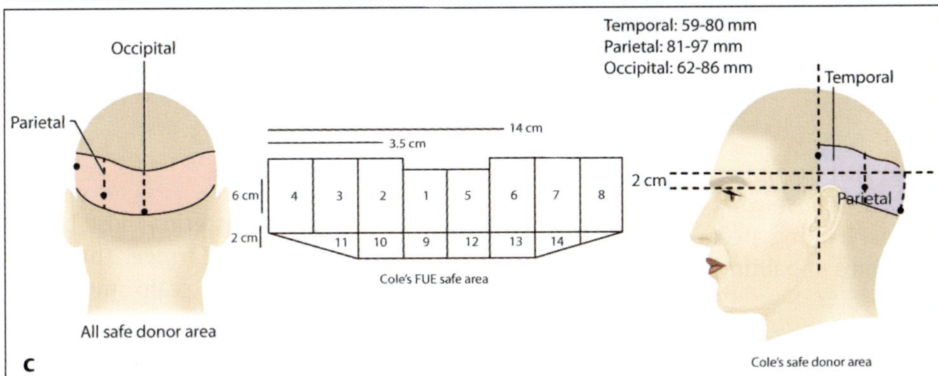

Fig. 21.1 **(a)** Scalp safe donor area. Point A marked over occipital protuberance in midline, point B is 1.5 cm behind postauricular line and 1.5 cm above helix rim. **(b)** The point C is 2 cm above the superior aspect of helix along a line drawn vertically through anterior tragus. This is the extreme lateral limit of the strip. Point D is taken 6 to 7 cm above point D. Point F is taken by drawing a horizontal line from point C across the midline, so the line joining the point D and F shows upper border of safe donor area. **(c)** Cole's safe donor area.

occipital protuberance (**Fig. 21.1a**), lateral point B is 1.5 cm behind the postauricular hairline and 1.5 cm above the superior aspect of the helix. This point is lateral most limit of a conservative length of the strip (**Fig. 21.1a**). The point C is 2 cm above the superior aspect of helix along a line drawn vertically through anterior tragus (**Fig. 21.1b**). This is the extreme lateral limit of the strip.

The line joining these three points A, B, C is the lower and lateral limits of the safe hair zone (**Fig. 21.1a, b**). The area below occipital protuberance is the neck region. Hair harvested from neck region is susceptible to early fall. Also, strong neck muscles in the area may increase the tension on suture line resulting in widening of scar. While planning for strip, one should look for existing miniaturization in this region.

Upper limit of safe area is marked in relation to the line of lower limit. Width of the safe donor area at its anterior limit is 6 to 7 cm. The width in center is decided by a horizontal line drawn from point "C" (**Fig. 21.1b**) across the midline. This will be the superior limit of the safe donor area in the midline. While planning for the strip, the area 1 cm below and 2 cm above permanent hair-bearing zone should be left so as to camouflage the donor scar.

Assessment of Donor Area

The donor area should be examined for progressive pattern of hair loss in the crown, retrograde hair loss, and thinning or miniaturization of the hair in the donor area. In scalp donor area, approximately 90% of hair remain in the anagen phase and 10% in the telogen phase. If telogen hair is more than 30%, the surgery should be deferred and the cause should be treated.

The success of hair transplant depends on the quality of the donor area. The donor area is to be evaluated for skin elasticity and glidability (for follicular unit transplantation [FUT] cases), number of available FUs, and number of hair in FUs. The thickness, curvature, and color of hair are as important as the number of follicles.

Methods for Calculation of Donor Density

Subjective assessment based on the experience of the physician is important. The density, thickness, and anagen:telogen ratio can be objectively assessed by digital dermoscope or folliscope.

Using a rubber stamp one square centimeter area is marked (**Fig. 21.2**). Hair follicles within the marked area are counted using a densitometer which is an illuminated magnifying lens (**Fig. 21.3**). Alternatively, self-illuminated trichoscope can be used.

Recipient Area

The success of hair transplant depends on proper planning. There is a need to restore natural-looking hair in the AHL and various scalp zones. While doing hair transplantation

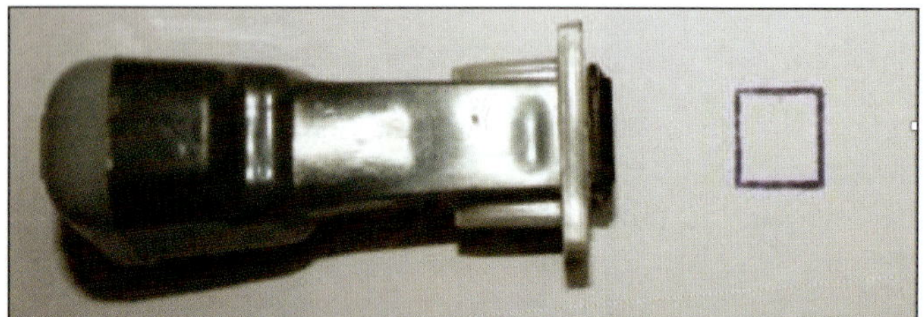

Fig. 21.2 A simple rubber stamp having one square centimeter area. The rubber stamp mark is created over the scalp to calculate the density of hair follicles.

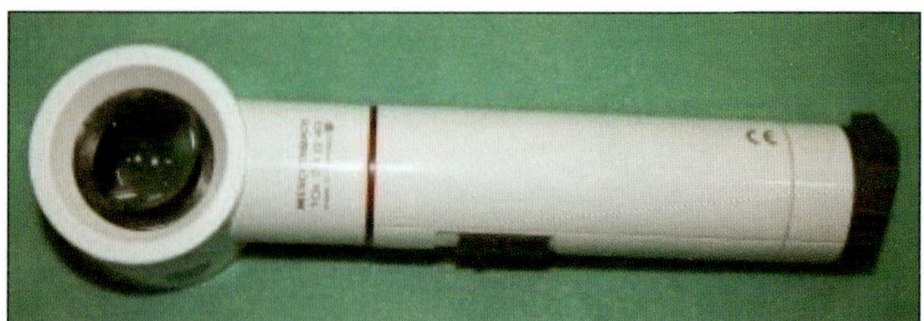

Fig. 21.3 Self-Illuminated trichoscope for counting hair in a 10×10 mm area.

there shall be a balance between total donor supply and present bald as well as future balding area. Hence, a detailed account of various zones of balding scalp is essential.

Topical Zones of Balding Scalp

The balding area of the scalp extends from AHL to upper border of occipital fringe. It is divided into three zones: frontal area, midscalp area, and the posterior-most balding area that is vertex or crown. There are different zones of balding scalp (**Fig. 21.4a–d**).[17]

Frontal Region

This is the most frontal balding area of the scalp which extends from AHL to an imaginary line joining the apex of frontotemporal angles. The posterior border is a little curved.

Frontal Hairline Zone

This is the anterior border of the frontal area, usually 2 centimeter in width, commonly called anterior hairline. This zone is further subdivided into irregular zones including macro and micro irregularities, transition zone, and defined zone.

Midfrontal Point (Trichion)

This is the anterior midpoint of the hairline. This important aesthetic landmark plays an important role in designing of the AHL.

Frontal Tuft (Forelock)

This is a small circular area, located centrally in the frontal zone, just behind the defined zone of the AHL. This is a high-density zone which is aesthetically important.

Midscalp

This is the top and horizontal area of the scalp. The anterior border is a curved line joining apex of both frontotemporal areas; the posterior border is anterior border of the vertex which includes vertex transition point. The lateral border on both sides is limited by temporal and parietal fringes.

Vertex (Crown)

This is a posterior-most area of the balding scalp of male pattern hair loss. This is usually oval, round, or oblong as per whorl pattern of the crown. It starts from the vertex transition point.

Vertex Transition Point

This point is situated between the posterior-most border of midscalp and upper border of occipital fringe. This is the point where the horizontal portion of the scalp starts sloping down.

Anterior Temporal Point

These are sharp angles at the anterior-most point of the occipital fringe on the forehead. It plays an important role in the framing of the face.

Frontotemporal Triangle

This develops as a part of male pattern baldness. These are alopecic areas situated anterolaterally between the lateral aspect of the frontal area (hairline zone) and temporal fringe. The posterior apex of the triangle is aligned to the lateral canthus of the eye.

Anterior Temporal Fringe

Anterior-most vertical portion of temporal fringe is commonly known as temporal triangle. This also has an important contribution to the framing of the face.

Superior Temporal Fringe

This is the small, anterior, superior border of temporal fringe, which starts from the apex of the frontotemporal triangle to an imaginary line aligned to the tragus of the ear.

Parietal Fringe

The superior border of the parietal fringe starts from the posterior border of superior temporal fringe (an imaginary line aligned to the tragus of the ear) to the start of occipital fringe.

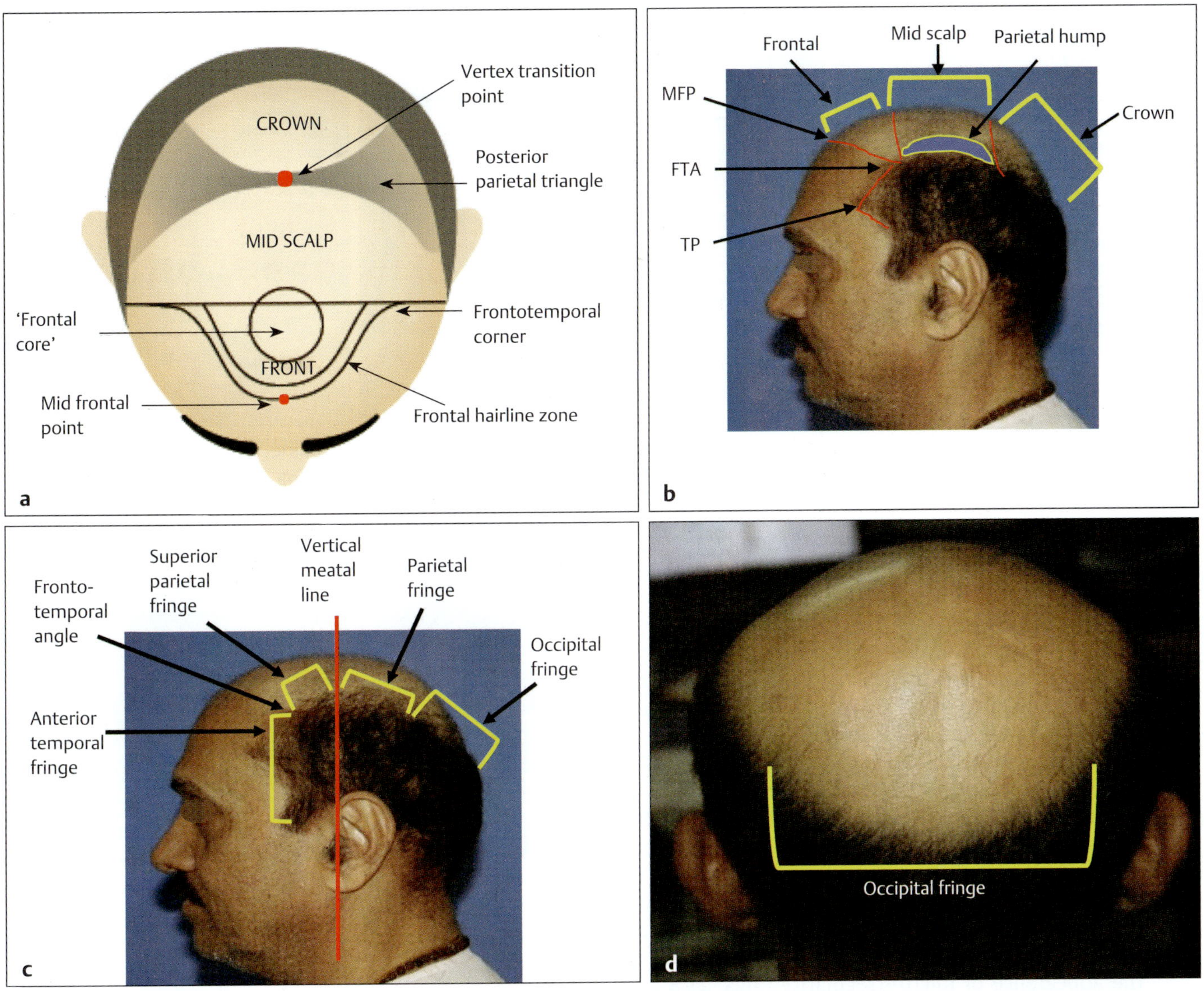

Fig. 21.4 **(a–d)** Topical zones of balding scalp. FTA, frontotemporal angle; MFP, mid frontal point; TP; temporal point.

Occipital Fringe

It is the superior border of occipital hair which makes the inferolateral border of alopecic vertex area.

Planning of Hair Transplant in Various Zones

Frontal Area and Anterior Hairline

The reconstructed hairline should be natural looking with enough density. It should have futuristic outlook and should not have the footprint of grafting.[18,19] The aesthetic curvature of the forehead should be designed in the natural shape of hairline. In males, the hairline is usually triangular or oval in shape (**Fig. 21.5**).

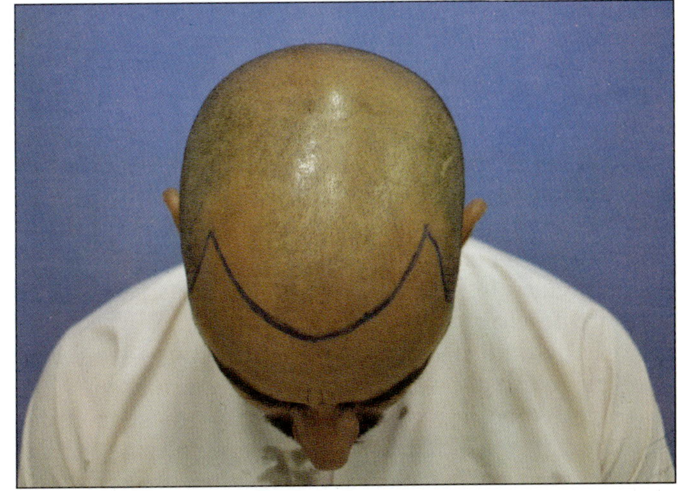

Fig. 21.5 Oval hairline in Indian Asian.

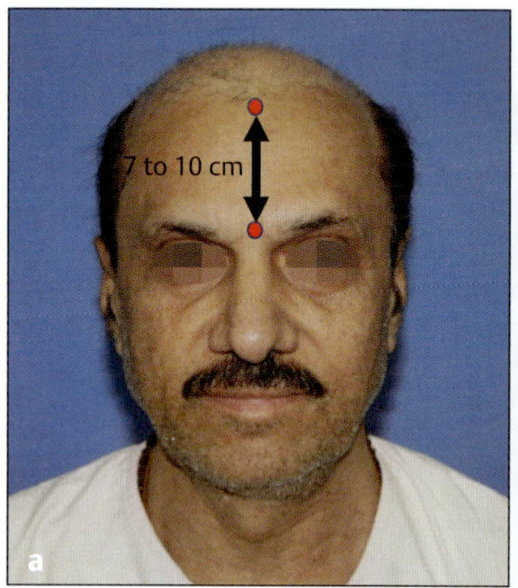

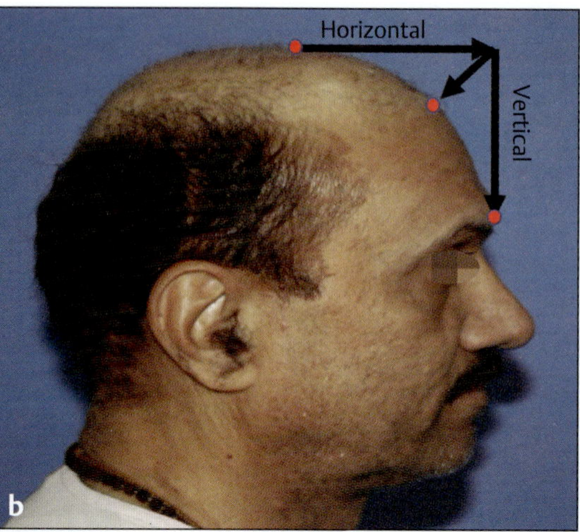

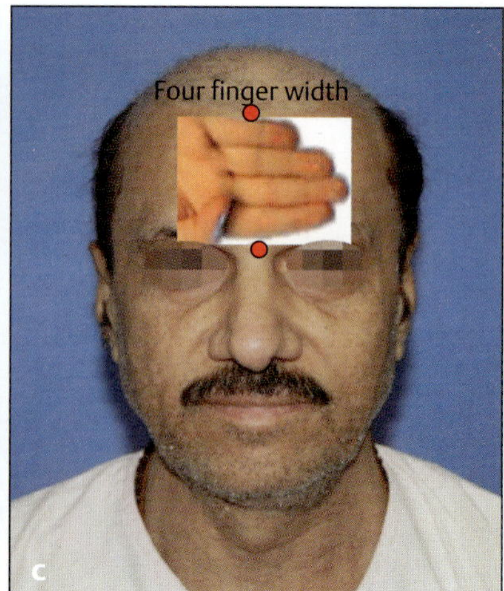

Fig. 21.6 Placement of the midfrontal point. **(a)** A point 7 to 10 cm from glabella in the midline. **(b)** Point at the junction of the vertical and horizontal plane. **(c)** Approximately four fingers from glabella is midfrontal point.

Placement of AHL is aesthetically very important. It is better to place it at a higher level than lower. A high-placed hairline can be shifted lower but the reverse is not possible. The hairline is marked four fingers or 7 to 10 cm above the glabella or at a point on the forehead where the vertical plane of forehead and horizontal plane of scalp meet (**Fig. 21.6a–c**). Final placement of AHL should be individualized depending on the size and shape of the head, degree of alopecia, and patient's wish. Patient's desire for low hairline can be addressed by constructing "widow's peak."

The male AHL consists of three subzones (**Figs. 21.7–21.9**):

1. *The anterior-most "transition zone" (TZ)* is approximately 0.5 to 1 cm wide. It is an irregularly irregular zone which merges in a defined zone. On close observation, normal hairlines have small intermittent triangular areas of higher density which contribute to the appearance of micro-irregularity (**Figs. 21.8** and **21.9**). Parsley has called these areas of intermittent density "clusters" and the area between them "gap." Hairline without "gap" and "clusters" makes it unnatural straight line.

   While observing the hairline from a distance, the line looks serpentine or curvaceous. This irregularity is called "macro irregularity." Martinick has used the term "snail tracking" to describe it.[20] Parsley has attributed this macro irregularity to the existence of a central mound (the widow's peak) and a lateral mound on either side (**Fig. 21.9**).[21] Micro and macro irregularities work together in the transition zone to create a natural-looking hairline.[22]

   The width and density of the transition zone should be adjusted based on the severity of hair loss. The greater the degree of hair loss, the wider and more diffuse the transition zone should be, mimicking the pattern found when more severe hair loss occurs.
2. *Posterior portion called "the defined zone" (DZ)* is 2 to 3 cm wide area immediately posterior to the transition

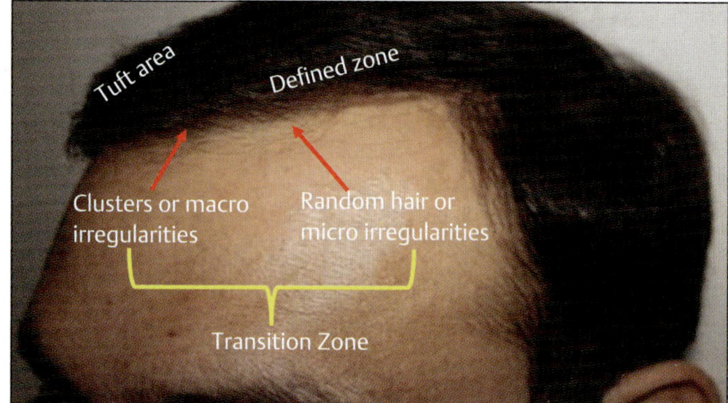

Fig. 21.7 Zones of anterior hairline and frontal tuft area.

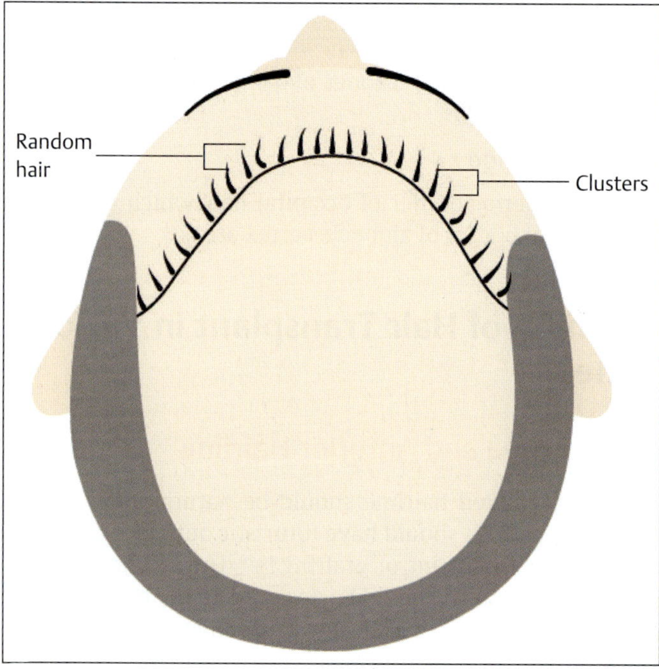

Fig. 21.8 Clusters and sentinel hair.

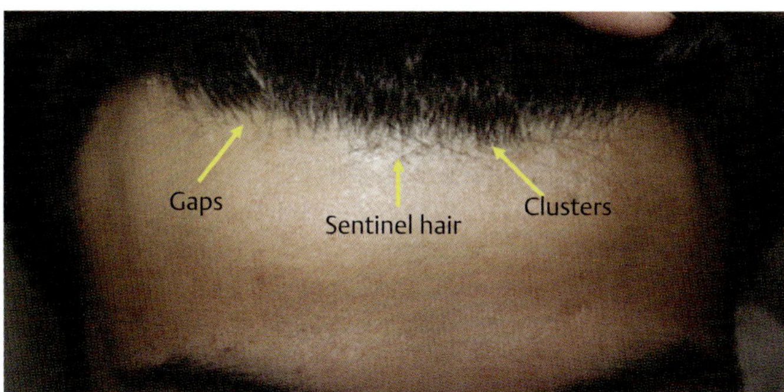

Fig. 21.9 Sentinel hair, gaps, and clusters.

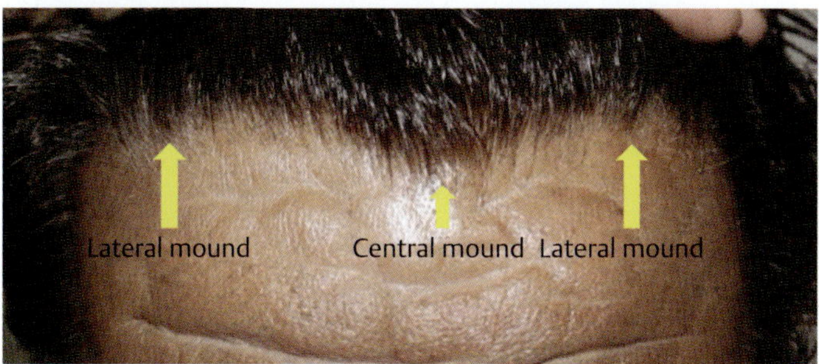

Fig. 21.10 Photograph showing the central mound (the widow's peak) and two lateral mounds on either side of the central mound.

zone. In this area, the hairline should develop a higher degree of definition and density (**Fig. 21.7**). Density in this zone creates a fuller-looking hairline by limiting the distance that can be seen past the transition zone.

3. Frontal "tuft area" is a small but aesthetically significant oval area that overlies the central portion of the defined zone directly behind the transition zone in the midline (**Fig. 21.7**). This area has higher degree of density than the rest of the defined zone.

Collectively, all three zones contribute to the overall appearance of the AHL (**Figs. 21.7–21.10**). **Box 21.1** shows the tips for designing the AHL.

It is not uncommon to have patients desiring to have hairline lower than recommended. There are two methods to accomplish their desire. A widow's peak may be created in the midline to give an illusion of a low hairline. If the patient desires to fill the temporal recession, the frontotemporal angle may be shifted anteriorly. This maintains the aesthetic look with less graft.

Frontotemporal Angle

The frontotemporal (FT) angle is formed by frontal and temporal lines, which is characteristic of male pattern baldness (**Fig. 21.11a, b**).[23] Recreating a soft frontotemporal angle is

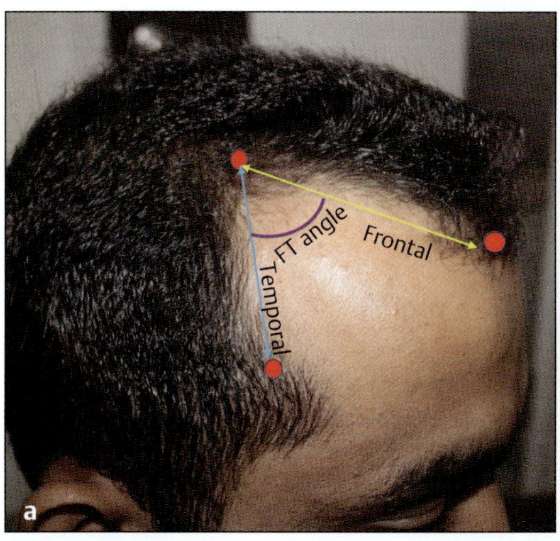

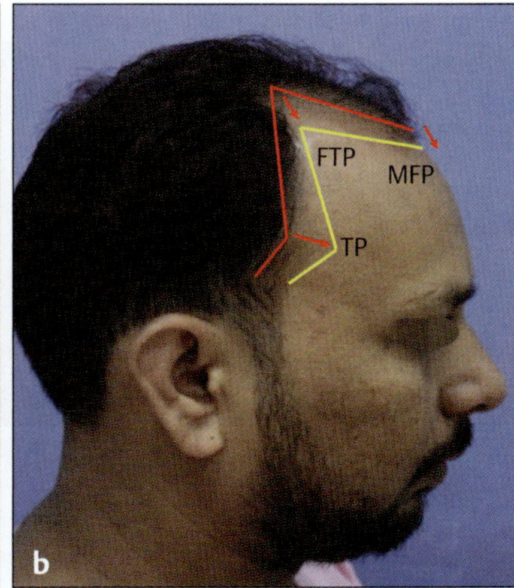

Fig. 21.11 **(a)** The frontotemporal angle is formed by the frontal and temporal hairline. **(b)** In male pattern baldness anterior hairline recedes, and frontotemporal angle deepens. All the points, midfrontal point (MFP), frontotemporal point, and also temporal peak point recede in proportion. The yellow line shows the original frontotemporal line while the red line shows receded line because of androgenetic alopecia.

Box 21.1 Tips for anterior hairline

- Avoid hair transplant before 23 years of age, but if required make a conservative hairline, avoid transplant in temporal and vertex area in younger age group. Medical treatment is strongly recommended postoperatively.
- Placement of hairline at a higher level is preferred.
- Create micro- and macro-irregularities using single follicular unit (FU). Two FUs and three FUs should be used in defined and forelock zone.
- Midfrontal point shall be lower or at the level of frontotemporal point but should not be higher.
- The distance between midfrontal point and temporal peak point in the lateral profile shall be less than 3 cm.
- Both frontotemporal points shall be aligned to lateral canthus of the eye.
- If parietal hump has receded down to the extent that the lateral end cannot meet the temporoparietal fringe, parietal hump should be rebuilt.

one of the most difficult and important aspects of hairline creation. Blunting this angle or placing it too low gives an unnatural look.

Estimation of Frontotemporal Points

In mild-to-moderate hair loss, where there is only a little loss of temporal hair, the existing temporal hair becomes the inferior border of the frontotemporal triangle while the future AHL becomes the superior border of the triangle. The apex of the frontotemporal triangle is aligned to the lateral canthus of the eye (**Figs. 21.12a–c and 21.13a–c**).

In a severe degree of hair loss when temporal hair has receded and lateral fringe has dropped, recreating "lateral hump" helps. The lateral hump is located superior to the ear and is a semicircular area of hair that bridges the lateral fringe to the midscalp region (**Fig. 21.14a–c**). Recreating such a lateral hump gives the lateral epicanthal line a target

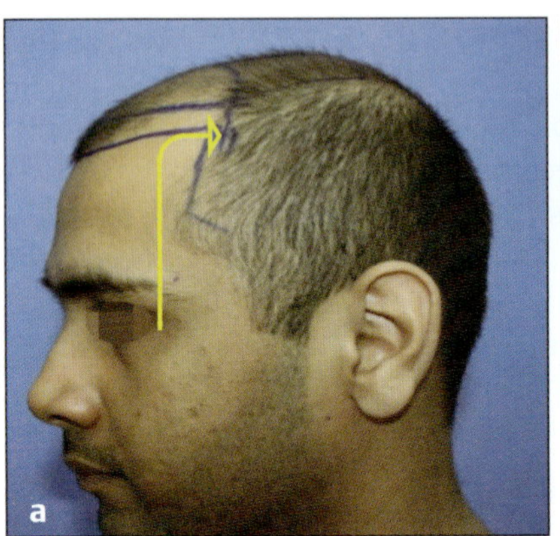

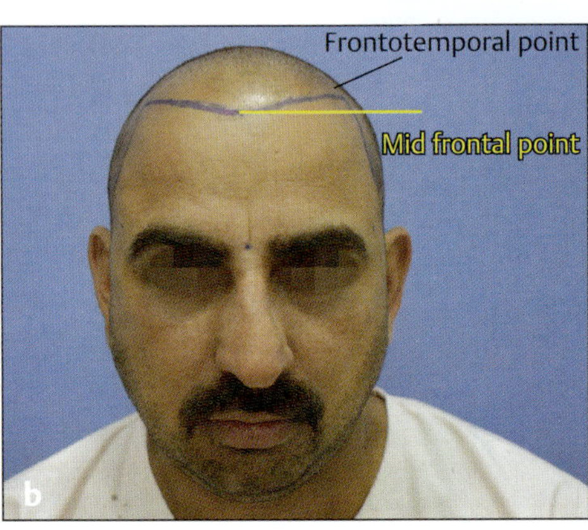

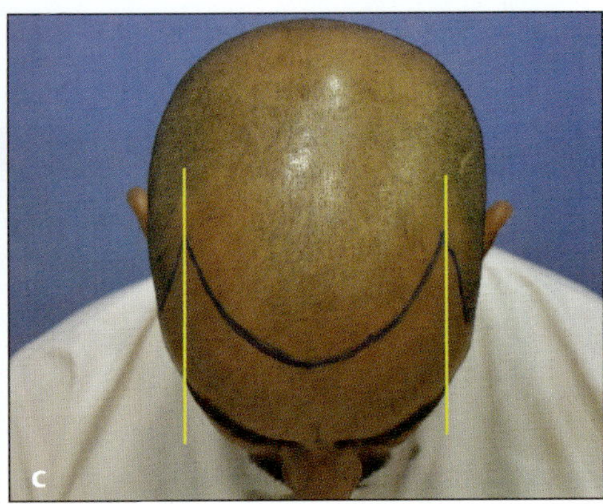

Fig. 21.12 **(a)** Drawing a line from lateral epicanthus of the eye posteriorly toward a point where it meets the remaining temporal hair. **(b)** Make sure the hairline created by this point does not slope downward toward the ear but looks parallel or slopes upward when viewed from the side, meaning the level of the frontotemporal point is higher or at the same level to the midfrontal point. **(c)** Frontotemporal points shall be placed in the line of the lateral epicanthus.

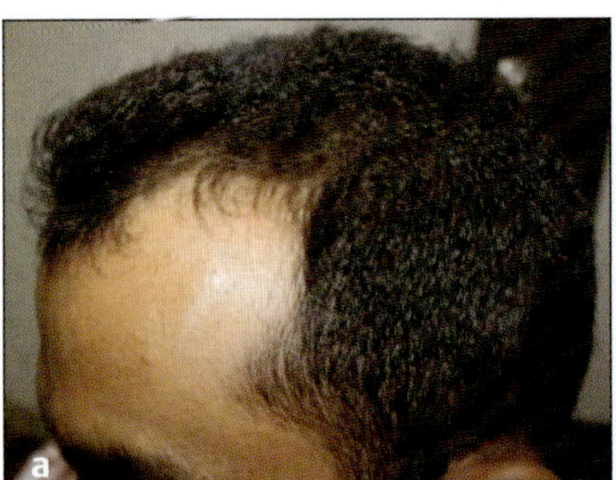

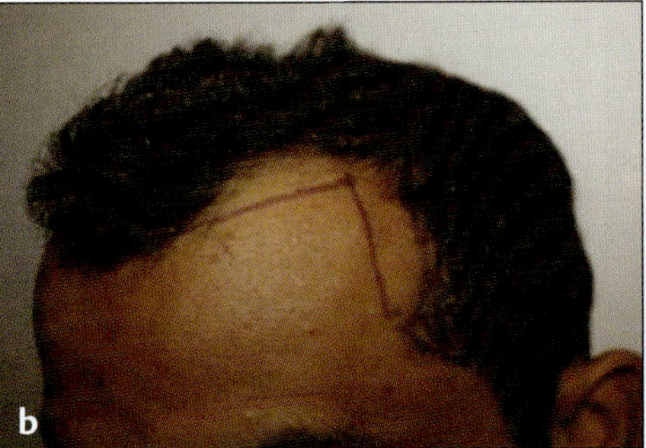

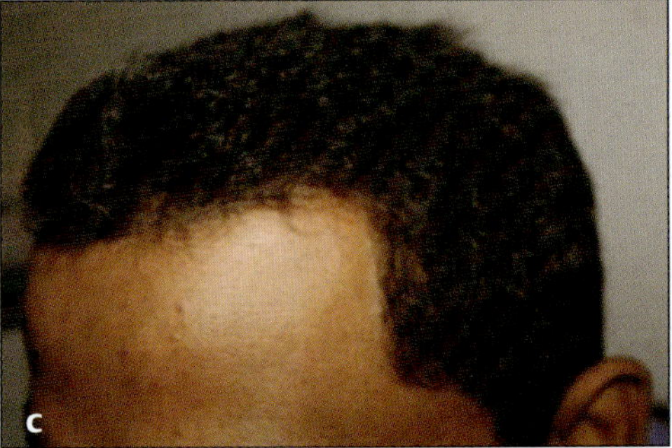

Fig. 21.13 **(a)** The minimal loss in the temporal region. **(b)** Planning of frontotemporal triangle. **(c)** Postoperative picture after temporal area reconstruction.

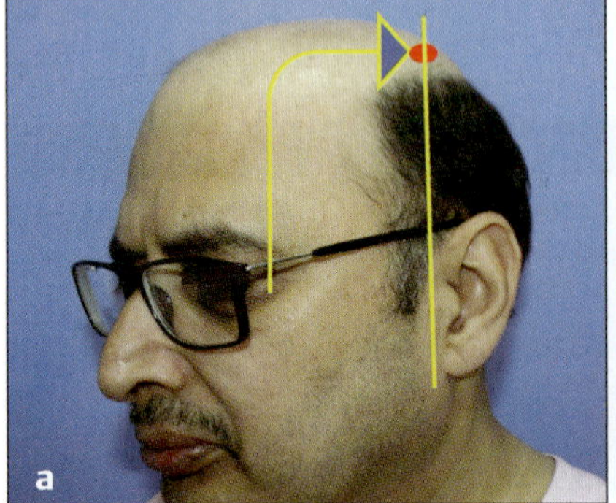

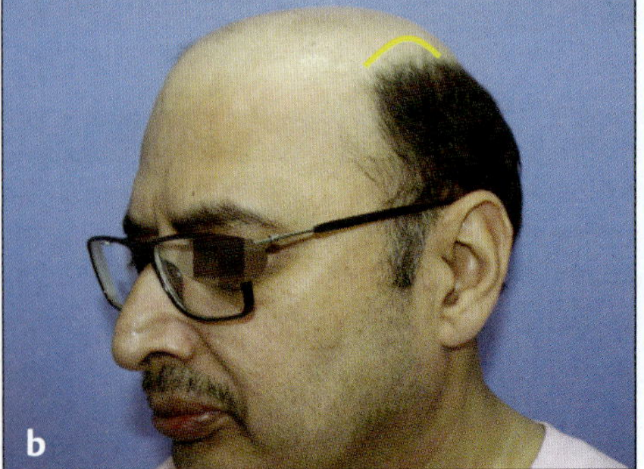

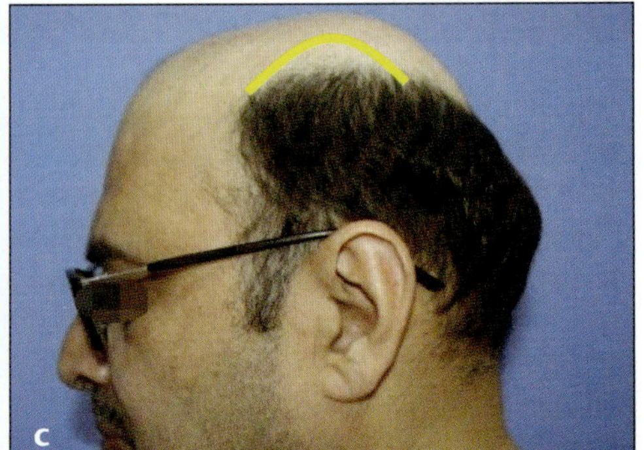

Fig. 21.14 **(a)** In the more severe degree of hair loss when temporal hair has receded and lateral fringe has dropped—visualizing and recreating "lateral hump" helps. **(b, c)** The lateral hump is located superior to the ear and is a semicircular area of hair that bridges the lateral fringe to the midscalp region.

to intersect. They usually meet near the top of a hump or approximately 1 cm anterior to a line drawn vertically from the auditory meatus. The temporal line usually becomes the inferior border of the frontotemporal angle.

Temporal Fringe (Triangle)

Hair loss in the temporal area causes loss of temporal point and recession of anterior temporal line resulting in a larger forehead, which significantly affects the aesthetic appearance of the face. When temporal point lies in the line of sideburn or the temporal fringe becomes concave hair transplant is indicated.

The temporal point is placed above the lateral end of the eyebrow over the forehead. Mayer has described the placement of temporal points.[24] The temporal point is a point of intersection of two imaginary lines; one is drawn from the tip of the ear lobe to mid-frontal point and the second line is drawn from the base of the nose to the center of the pupil extending up to the scalp (**Fig. 21.15**). The angle of hair in the temporal area should be kept as flat as possible. Usual graft implantation density is kept around 20 to 25 grafts per square centimeters.

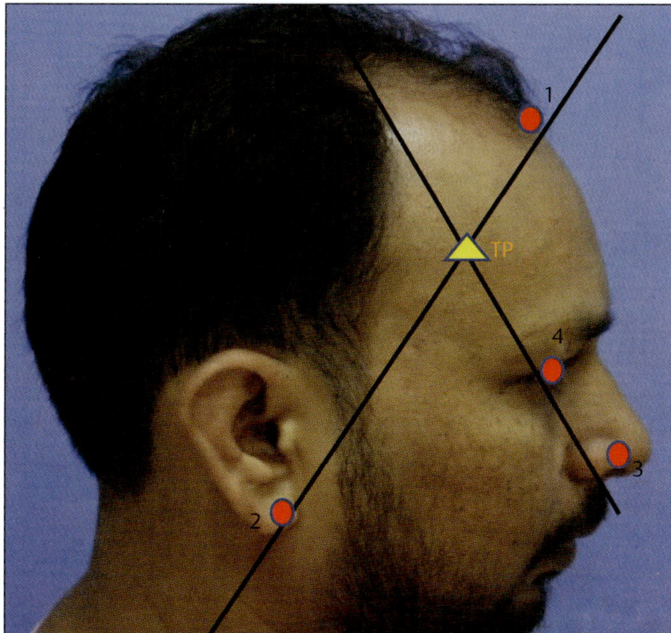

Fig. 21.15 Mayer's method of temporal peak point—red dots are landmark points. Point 1 is midfrontal point, point 2 is the tip of ear lobule, point 3 is base of the nose, point 4 is midpupil point, and TP is the temporal peak point.

Midscalp

This is a horizontal, slightly curved area of the scalp. Hair is facing forward in the central area and on the lateral side, it turns laterally. One should follow the angle and direction of existing hair. Usually the hair angle is 25 to 35 degrees. Multifollicular unit grafts are preferred in the midscalp area.

In the advanced grade of baldness, the lateral fringe drops to a point where the frontal hairline cannot connect it. In such a case, there is a need to restore lateral (parietal) fringe. The anterior portion of the parietal hump blends with the upper temporal line (**Fig. 21.16a–c**). The existing hair always helps in deciding the angle of implantation. Density is 20 to 30 grafts per square centimeter.[25]

Vertex

Vertex is not a very important aesthetic unit of the scalp. However, hair restoration of the scalp is incomplete if the crown is left unattended even if the donor site is limited. There are multiple approaches to hair restoration in vertex, which are summarized in **Box 21.2**. Vertex is divided into upper, middle, and lower subzones (**Fig. 21.17**). The whorl is part of the middle and lower zones.

The best guide for implantation is existing thin hair, which is known as vellus hair (ghost hair). Existence of vellus hair helps in determining hair patterns in vertex. If a patient does not have any whorl left, it is better to place a single whorl off center, precisely on the side of the part with the arc matching the part line (**Fig. 21.18**). If the patient parts his hair from left to right, the whorl should be designed clockwise on the left side of the head so that the upper limb of the vertex arc matches with the hair part. Also matching the same direction of the hair part, facilitates hairstyling.[26]

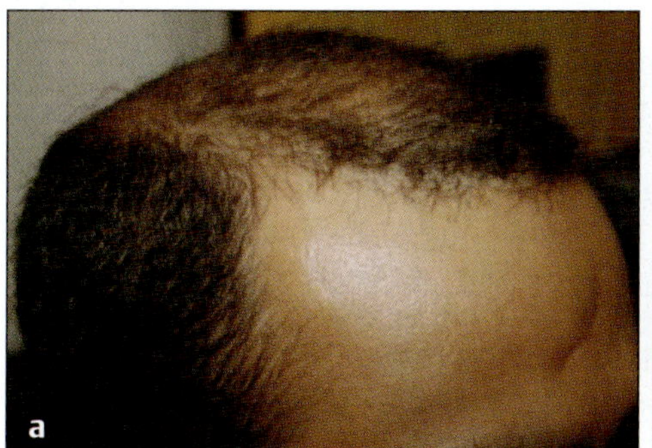

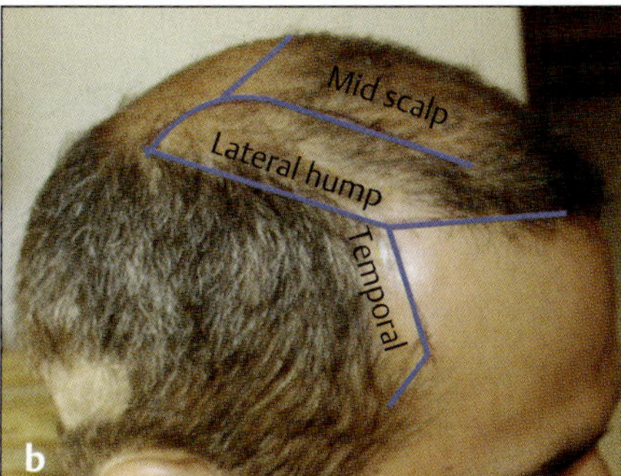

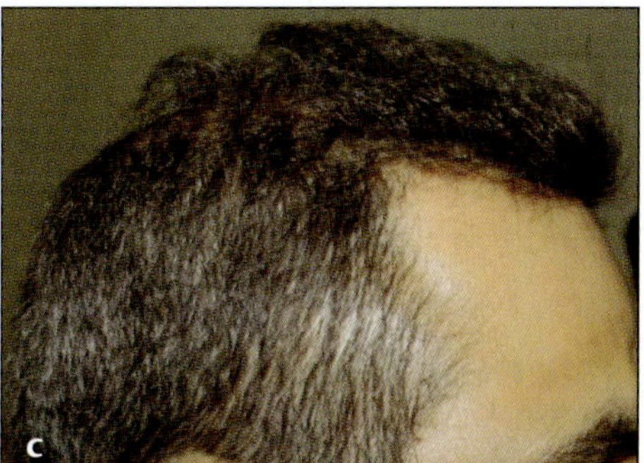

Fig. 21.16 **(a)** Loss of hair in parietal hump and midscalp. **(b)** Marking for the restoration of the parietal hump with temporal fringe and midscalp area. **(c)** Postoperative picture after the restoration of midscalp, parietal hump, and temporal fringe.

Box 21.2 Options for vertex transplant

- Do not transplant at all.
- Transplant entire vertex with uniform density.
- Transplant entire vertex with graded density. Less in center and more at the periphery.
- Transplant only at the periphery.
- Transplant in the uppermost zone of vertex, hair in a downward direction.
- Creating an anterior-lateral border of vertex only.
- Augment the visual density by scalp micro-pigmentation.
- Use body hair donor follicles with scalp as "combination grafting."

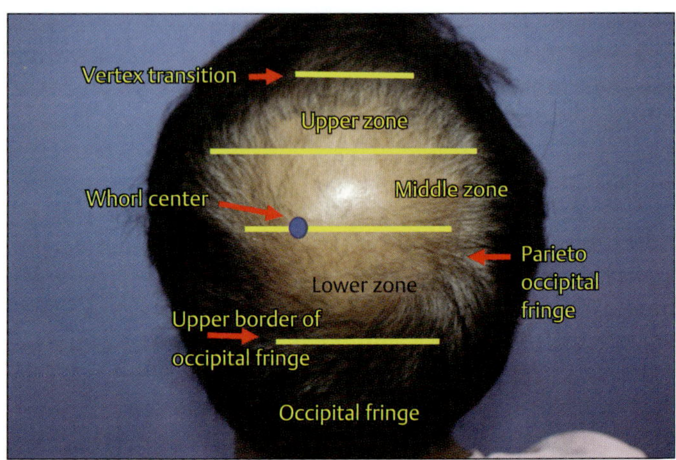

Fig. 21.17 Zones of vertex.

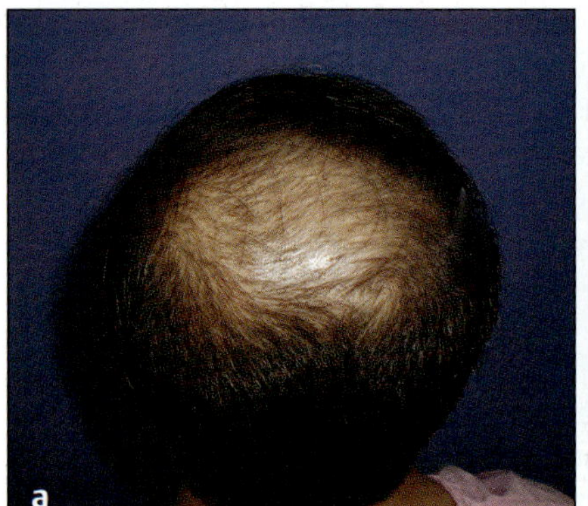

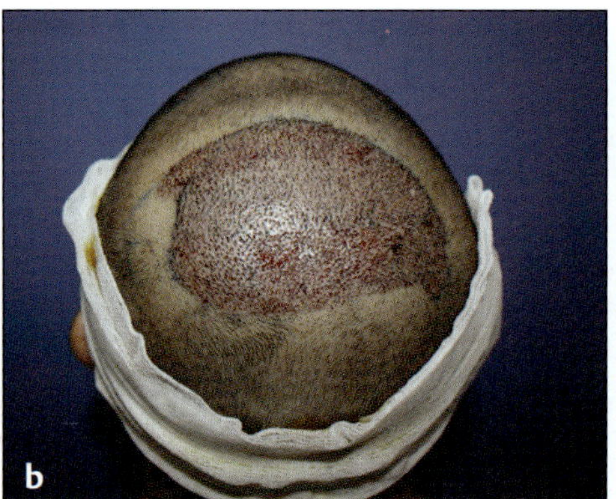

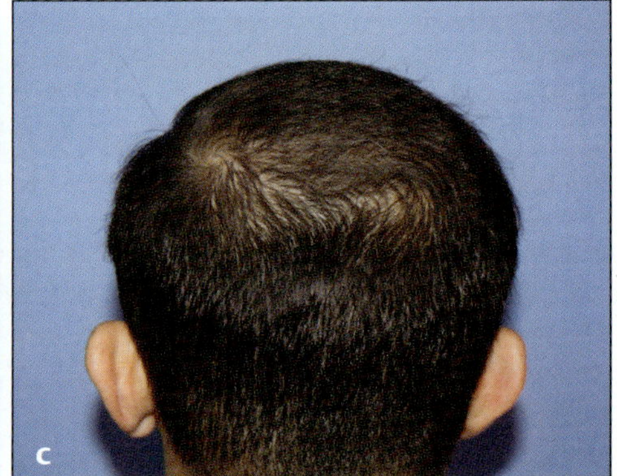

Fig. 21.18 **(a)** A 35-year-old man, before hair transplant. **(b)** After implantation of 2,306 FUE grafts over the vertex. **(c)** Early results of hair transplant.

Angulation of hair is important in vertex. The natural angle of hair increases from the nape of the neck and is highest in the anterior-most area of the upper zone of the vertex which further goes down in the midscalp to AHL. There should be a gradual transition of the angle of implantation for its natural appearance. The preferred angulation in the lower zone is 10 to 20 degrees and near the vertex transition zone, it may go up to 35 to 45 degrees. It is always advisable to start implanting from the center of the whorl. Mostly smaller FUs (1 FU, 2 FUs) should be implanted in the center of the whorl and the lower half of the crown. Larger FUs are used for the upper arc of vertex, while 3 hair FU grafts are placed lateral to the whorl to create the sweep of hair. Higher density in the upper arc of the vertex gives a look of higher density to the lower vertex and posterior midscalp region as well.[26]

Hair Restoration for Female Hair Loss

The pattern of hair loss and AHL differs in the female.[27] The female hair loss is usually diffuse with an intact AHL which may eventually be thinned out or may recede.[28] The loss of hair does not lead to complete baldness because all the hair from the hair FUs are not lost.[29]

While transplanting in females,[30,31] few cautions are important. Usually, women have very high expectations and desire to have a normal density of hair over the whole scalp. Female patients also demand to have a low AHL. Careful evaluation is essential to exclude frontal fibrosing alopecia and conditions mimicking the female pattern hair loss. Females with unrealistic expectations and generalized thinning including occipital fringe are contraindications for hair transplant.[32]

The creation of the female hairline is more complex as compared to men. This needs more density as well as coverage of a larger area of the scalp with limited donor supply. One needs to evaluate the availability and the requirement of FUs correctly. Most often the AHL remains intact, which may recede only in advance stages of hair loss. Very rarely women may have hair loss akin to male patterns.[33,34]

The characteristic features of the AHL of the female are cowlicks, widows' peaks, undulations, temporal mounds, and low positioning. As per Nusbaum,[35] the average distance from midbrow to the lowest central hairline point was 5.5 cm. The average distance from the central midpoint of the hairline to the lateral mounds was 4 cm, and the temporal points on average were located 1 cm above and behind the lateral canthus. Successful aesthetic restoration of a female hairline is dependent on accurately reproducing these features (**Figs. 21.19 and 21.20**).

The midfrontal point or central point of the hairline is kept almost 5 to 6 cm from the midpoint of eyebrow. The implantation angle of hair follicles is at an acute angle, almost parallel to the skin. The temporal mounds are convex. The temporal peak point is designed almost 1 to 2 cm above and behind the lateral canthus.

While transplanting, one layer of single-hair FUs is placed anteriorly followed by two to four hair FUs to restore the hairline area. The strong multi-FUs are placed in more aesthetically important areas away from the AHL.

Anesthesia

The detail of the anatomy of the scalp nerves is mentioned in the anatomy section. The scalp donor involves the occipital, parietal, and a part of the temporal area. The recipient area

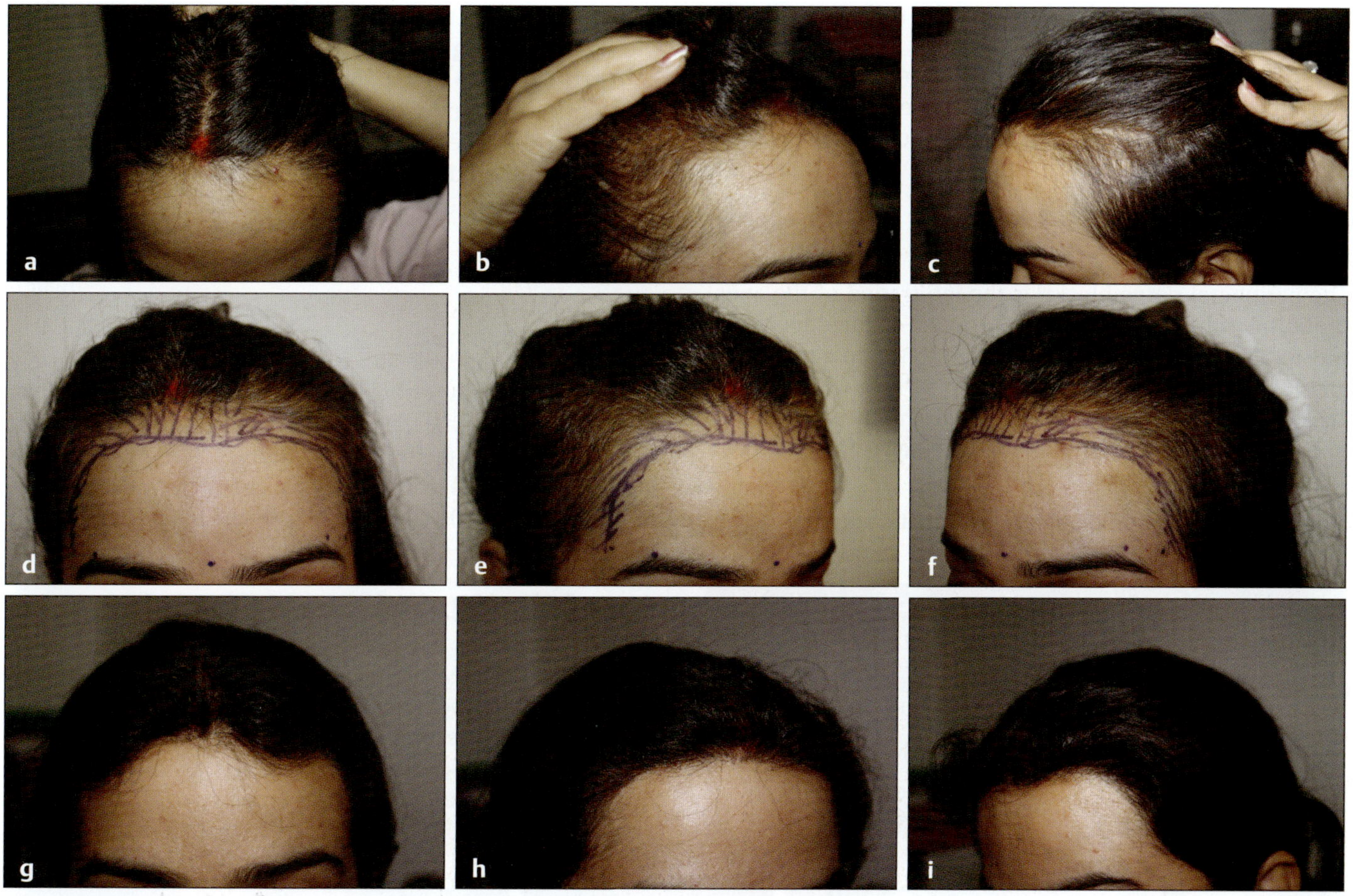

Fig. 21.19 **(a–c)** Preoperative pictures showing the posteriorly placed anterior hairline and thinning in the frontotemporal area. The patient wanted to have lower anterior hairline (AHL). **(d–f)** The hairline was designed and finalized. **(g–i)** 11 months follow-up result of 2,231 grafts by strip method.

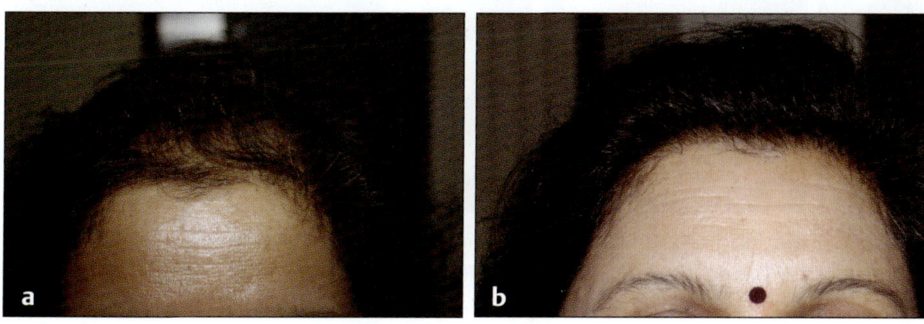

Fig. 21.20 **(a)** Female pattern hair loss with intact anterior hairline and low density. **(b)** Results after 12 months of hair transplant.

is usually the frontal and midscalp region, extending to the vertex. The field block, peripheral nerve block, and tumescence anesthesia are used for anesthetizing the scalp in the hair transplant procedure.[36,37]

Every surgeon uses different combinations of local anesthetic solution. The common constituents are local anesthetic agents, adrenaline, and normal saline. The author uses the different combinations for peripheral nerve blocks and tumescent anesthesia (**Table 21.3**).[38]

The Field Blocks

The field block is the infiltration of anesthetic solutions in the periphery of the operative field.[39] In the recipient area, the nerves travel from anterior to posterior, so the infiltration of the anesthetic solution should be anterior to the anterior hairline. In the occipital donor area, the nerve supply is from inferior to superior, so the anesthetic solution is injected inferior to the donor area.

The Peripheral Nerve Blocks

The peripheral nerve block[40] is the infiltration of the anesthetic solution around the nerve trunk. For the donor area, the local anesthetic agent is injected around the greater and lesser occipital nerve. An insulin syringe or 3 mL Luer Lock syringe with a 30-gauge hypodermic needle is used. The area is ice-cooled to minimize the pain of needle prick (**Fig. 21.21a**). The injection sites for greater occipital nerve and lesser occipital nerves are marked by keeping the three fingers, index, middle, and ring finger together vertically at the level of superior nuchal line in the prone position. Vibrator tip is kept near needle prick site for pain alleviation (**Fig. 21.21b**). The local anesthetic is infiltrated after raising wheel lateral to index and ring fingers to block lesser and greater occipital nerves on both sides (**Fig. 21.21c**).

Table 21.3 Combination of local anesthetic agents for blocks and tumescence

For nerve and field block	For tumescent anesthesia
Lidocaine 2% × 20 mL	Lidocaine 2% × 5 mL
Ropivacaine/Bupivacaine 0.5% × 20 mL	Ropivacaine/Bupivacaine 0.5% × 5 mL
Normal saline × 40 mL	Normal saline × 90 mL
Epinephrine (1:1,000) × 0.5 mL	Epinephrine (1:1,000) × 0.5 mL

For the recipient area, the solution is injected around supratrochlear, supraorbital, and zygomaticotemporal nerves. These nerves innervate the majority of the scalp recipient area. Block is given in the supine position. Index, middle, and ring fingers are placed over the forehead pointing down, keeping the middle finger in the midline between the eyebrows (**Fig. 21.22a, b**). The supraorbital notch is palpated lateral to index and ring fingers. One mL of local anesthetic solution is injected around the supratrochlear and supraorbital nerves on both the sides. If the supraorbital nerve, block should be given carefully. Trauma to the nerves may lead to anesthesia and or hypoesthesia, swelling, ptosis, or bruising.

The Tumescence Anesthesia

The tumescent anesthesia[37] is the infiltration of a relatively large volume of dilute anesthetic solution in the entire operative area. The tumescence infiltration reduces the quantity of anesthetic agents used and gives a longer period of local analgesia. Maximum of 30 mL of the tumescent fluid (**Table 21.3**) per 100 cm^2 is used over the scalp.

Art of Slit (Site) Making in Recipient Area

The "slit (site)" means puncture wounds or tunnels created in the skin and subcutaneous tissue in the recipient area for the purpose of insertion of the hair follicles. Creation of the slit is an art and science both. The slits should be created in a way that guest follicles fit in properly without jeopardizing the circulation.[39] The art is to create natural-looking

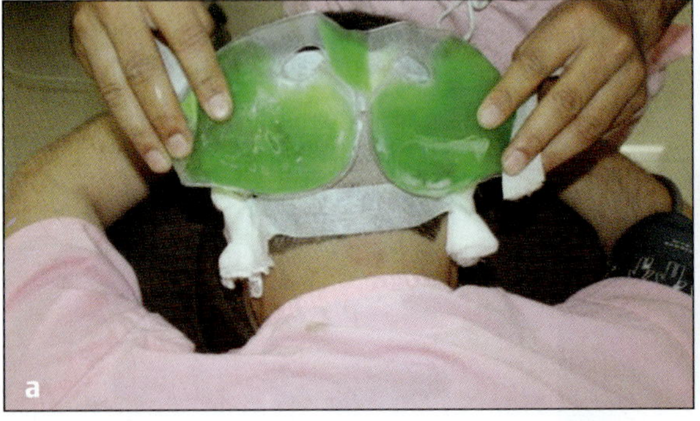
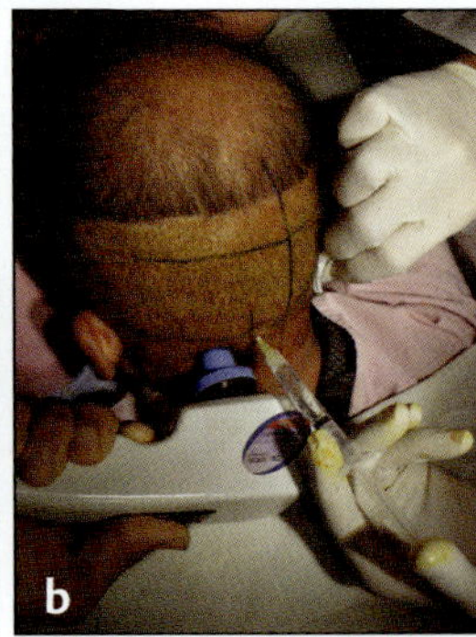
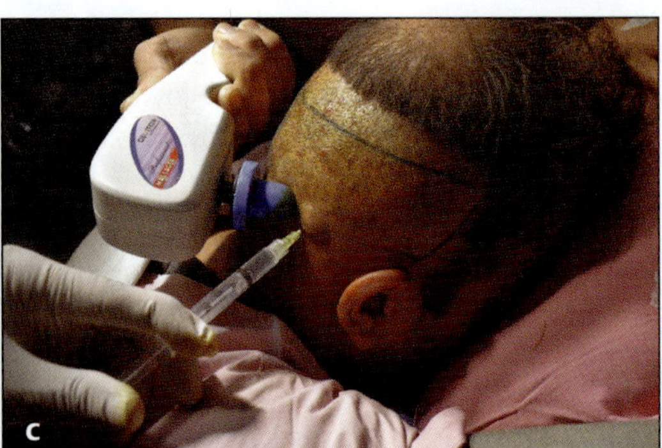

Fig. 21.21 **(a)** Ice pack over the occipital area. **(b)** Marking of greater occipital nerve. **(c)** Wheel created by infiltration of solution. Use of vibrator near the injection site, ice pack, and fine bore needle decrease the pain during the infiltration of anesthetic solution.

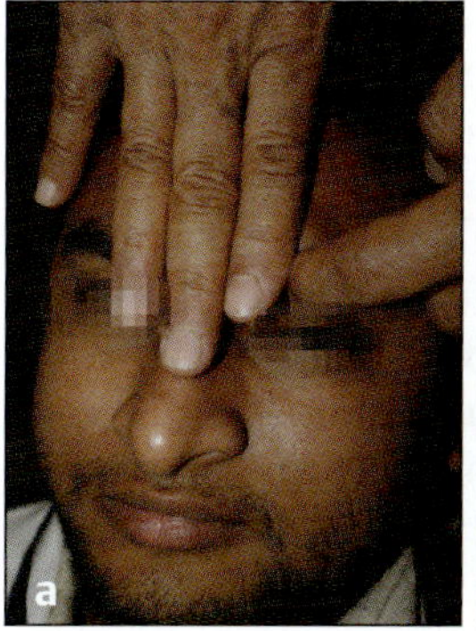

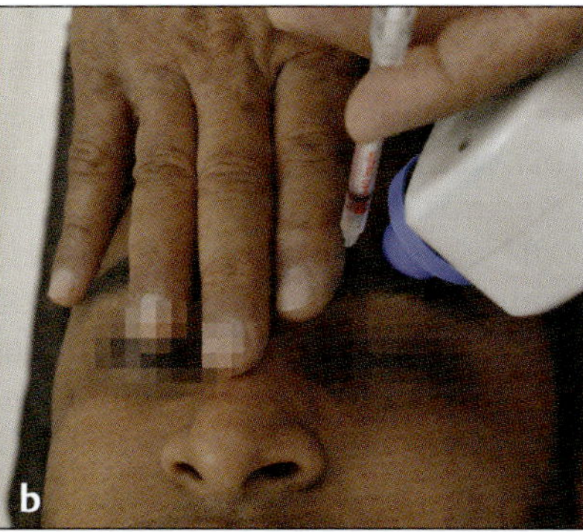

Fig. 21.22 **(a)** Supraorbital nerve block by keeping three fingers over the forehead, positioning the middle finger over the nose. Supraorbital notch is felt lateral to index and ring fingers. **(b)** Anesthetic solution is injected keeping the vibrator near the injection site.

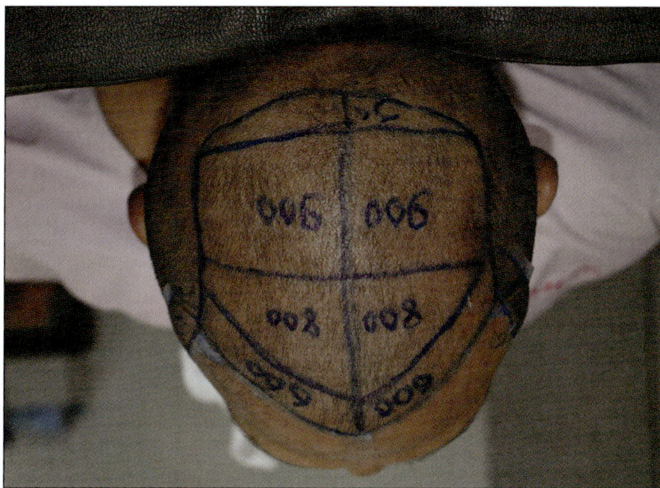

Fig. 21.23 Planning of grafts in scalp zones.

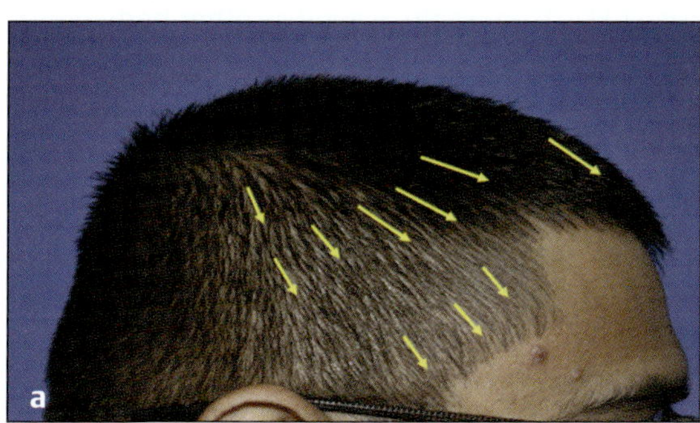

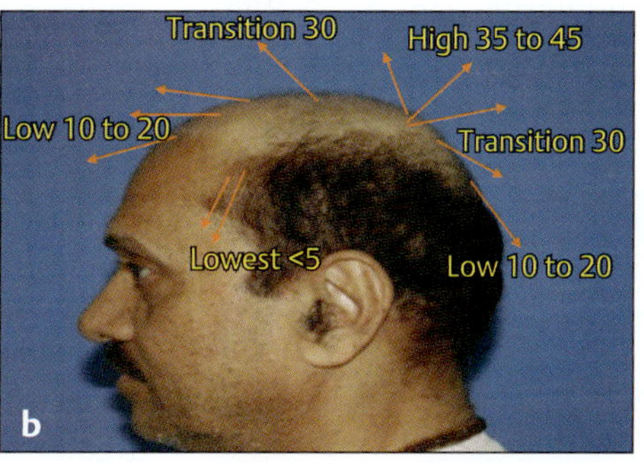

Fig. 21.24 **(a)** Figure showing the direction of hair in a different region. **(b)** Different angles of hair in different directions.

scalp. If the slits created are not proper in terms of size, width, depth, direction, and angle, the aesthetic outcome is compromised.[41]

The distribution of grafts in various zones should be planned and noted on a sheet as shown in the **Fig. 21.23**. Accordingly, the slits should be created over the recipient area.

The depth and width of slits should match the dimension of the follicular grafts. If the slit is larger than graft, it will pop out. Large linear slits may cause vascular trauma, which may, in turn, affect graft survival. If slits are smaller than graft size, there will be difficulty in implanting them. The forceful insertion will cause trauma to the graft, which will affect the hair growth. So, the slit depth and size should match the graft size. It is prudent to create different sizes of the slit for 1 FU, 2 FU, and 3 FU grafts.

The direction of the slit will decide the angle and direction of the growing hair. The angle of hair means the angle between the hair shaft and the scalp surface. The hair angle varies in different zones of the scalp (**Fig. 21.24b**). If the direction of hair does not match with the existing hair, the natural look will be compromised. If existing hair is absent then the direction and angle are decided as per the scalp zones as shown in **Fig. 21.24a**.

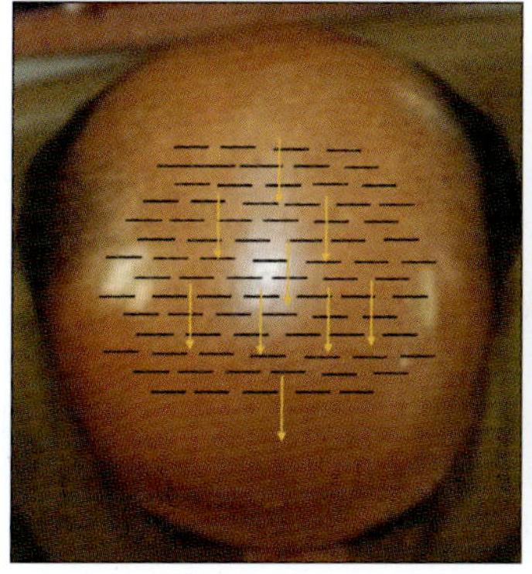

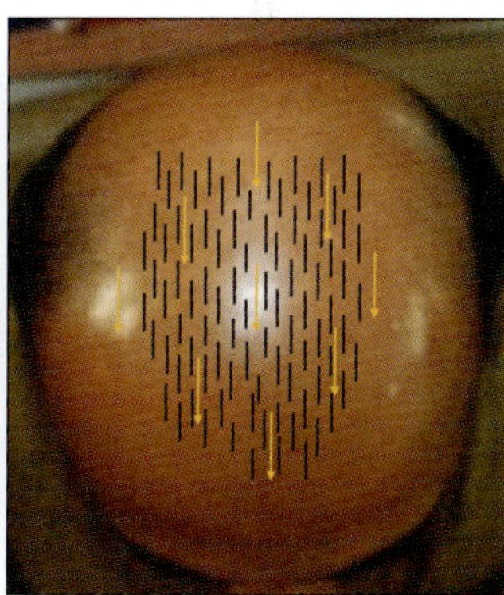

Fig. 21.25 **(a)** Coronal slits, which are perpendicular to the direction of the hair. Black lines show slits and yellow arrows show the direction of hair. **(b)** Sagittal slits which are parallel to the direction of hair growth.

The orientation of the slit is designated in relation to the direction of the hair. The slits could be coronal or sagittal. Both types of slits are created with blades, and have their own advantages and drawbacks. The orientation of the slit affects the visual density and amount of vascular trauma (**Fig. 21.25a, b**).

Instruments for Slit Creation

There are many slit- or site-making instruments in the market. There are many published and unpublished innovations done by many surgeons. Slit-making instruments have a handle (**Fig. 21.26a**), and the cutting edge is in the form of a blade or a needle. The hypodermic needles of size No. 18, 19, 20, and 21G are used (**Fig. 21.27a, b**). The cutting edge of the blades could be straight (rectangular shape) or angled. The blades commonly used are available in different sizes from 0.7 to 1.2 mm (**Fig. 21.26b, c**) (**Table 21.4**). Some surgeons use cut-to-size shaving blades.

Procedure of Slit Creation

The slit creation is done either by hypodermic needle, blade, or both, depending on the choice of the surgeon. Most of the surgeons prefer to start from back to front. Many surgeons divide the entire recipient area in multiple zones.[42] A good planner allots specific number of grafts for AHL, front tuft area, temporal triangle, frontal area behind the hairline, midscalp area including parietal fringe and vertex (**Fig. 21.28a**). This will help in proper distribution of the grafts and will avoid mismatch.

The angle and direction of slits for every recipient zone are listed in **Table 21.5** (**Fig. 21.28b**). The table also shows the different densities for individual zones, but the final estimation of density of graft depends on the supply of the grafts and surgeon's and patient's decisions.

Table 21.4 Size of the needle and blade as per the number of FU in graft

FU	Needle size	Blade size
1 FU	20 gauge	0.7 mm
2 FU	19 gauge	0.8–0.9 mm
3 FU	18 gauge	1.1 mm
4 FU	18 gauge	1.1–1.2 mm

Abbreviation: FU, follicular unit.

Follicular Unit Excision

FUE or follicular unit extraction, now called excision, is the most popular method for follicle harvesting.[43,44] FUE involves harvesting of donor hair follicles from the safe donor area using a circular knife called "punch." This is a versatile technique to harvest FUs from scalp as well as other body donor sites such as the beard, chest, and rest of the body.[45] The procedure has achieved increasing popularity, as compared to the strip method (FUT) of follicle harvesting.

In 2017, a nomenclature committee of ISHRS concluded that the term "follicular unit extraction" is inappropriate and misleading because it is a histological term rather than an anatomical and surgical term.[46] The committee recommended "follicular unit excision" as it explains the two steps of the process: incision and extraction. The term also carries greater surgical implication that this is a surgical domain.[46]

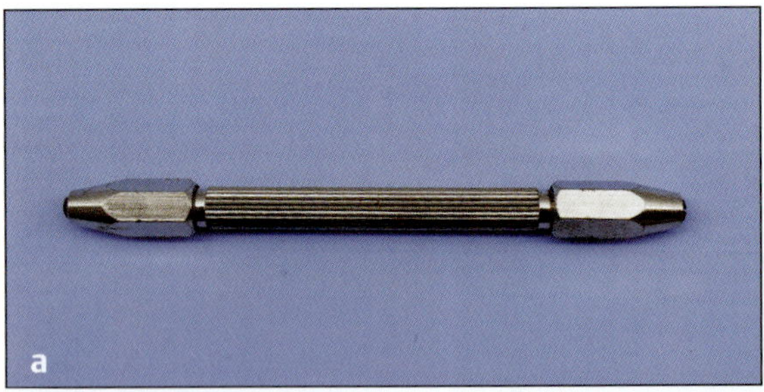
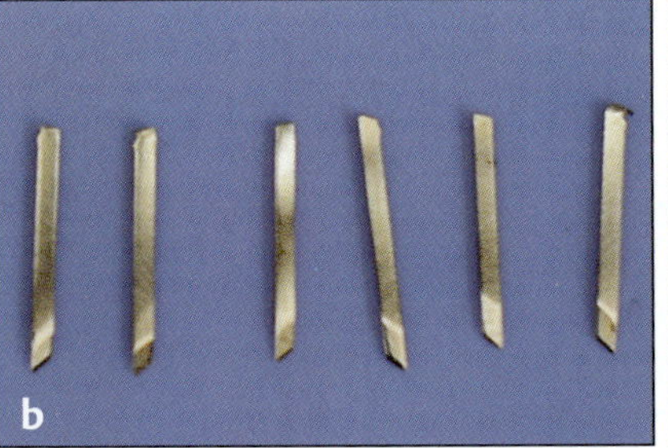
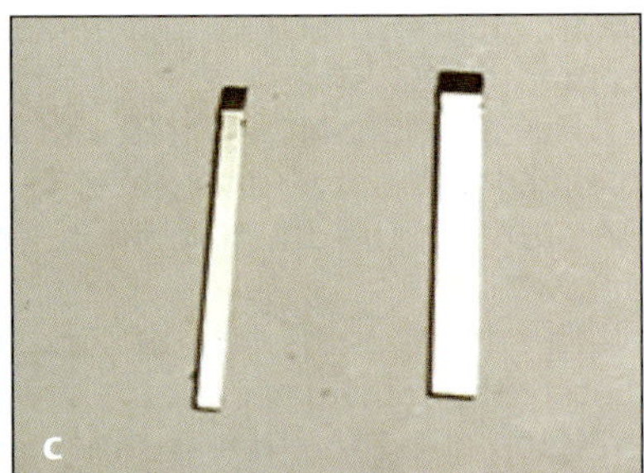

Fig. 21.26 **(a)** Chisel blade handle, both blade/needles can be loaded on the handle. **(b)** Different sizes of angled blades. **(c)** Rectangle blades.

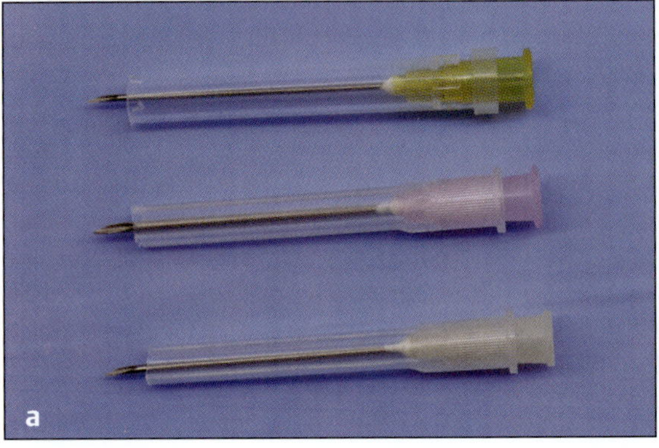
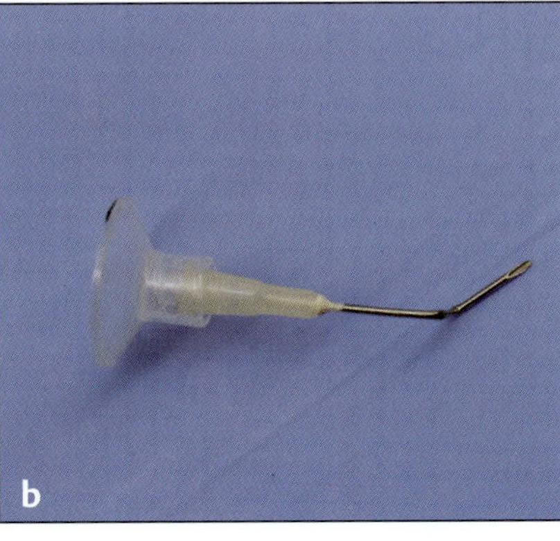

Fig. 21.27 **(a)** Hypodermic needles with guard for depth control. **(b)** Bent needle to facilitate the angle of the slit for the temporal area.

Table 21.5 Specification of slits in different zones of scalp

Scalp zone	Angle (degree)	FUs	Average density (G/sq. cm)	Direction	Special features
Anterior hairline zone	10–15	1 FUs 2 FUs	35–45	Centre-forward, lateral side-laterally	Micro- and macro-irregularities should be created
Forelock, rest of frontal zone	10–20	2 FUs 3,4 FUs	Forelock 45 Remaining 25–30	Forward	Follow existing hair
Temporal zone	3–5	1 FU	15–20	Upper-downward anteriorly Lower-downward posteriorly	Follow existing hair, when using a needle, bend it If using a blade, keep handle close to skin
Parietal fringe	10–15	1 FU, 2 FUs	20–25	Downward anteriorly	Follow existing hair
Midscalp	25–35	2, 3, 4 FUs	20–30	Central anteriorly Lateral side-slightly laterally	Follow existing hair
Vertex transition	25–35	2, 3, 4 FUs	20–30	Central-anteriorly Lateral side—slightly radially	Follow existing hair
Vertex whorl	10–15	1 FU, 2FUs	15–20	Make whorl	Follow existing whorl Draw whorl and perform
Occipital fringe	5–10	2 FUs, 3 FUs	20–25	Downward	Follow existing hair

Abbreviations: FUs, follicular units; G/sq. cm, grafts/square centimeter.

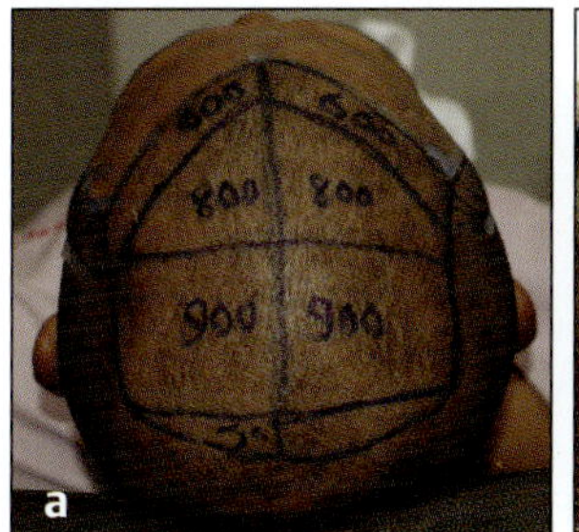

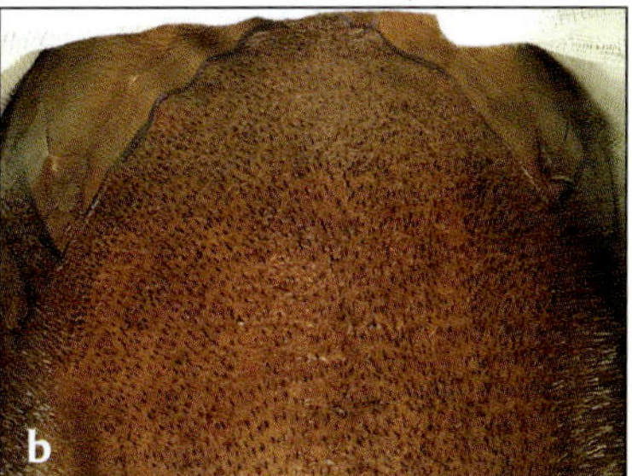

Fig. 21.28 **(a)** Planning of slits. **(b)** Slits after gentian violet staining.

Follicular unit excision is defined as the surgical technique that refers to circumferential incision of the skin around the follicular unit bundle or group of hair follicles to extract a full-thickness skin graft containing hair follicle(s), intradermal fat, dermis, and epidermis.[46]

Indications of FUE

A few conditions where FUE is the preferred choice over the strip method of hair transplant are:

- A person wishing to keep short hair.
- Tight scalp.
- Tendency of hypertrophic scar or keloid.
- Wanting to go back to work early.
- Low pain threshold.
- Secondary case where strip has already been harvested.
- For FU harvest from body donor sites.
- As part of the combination procedure.

Surgical Steps

While performing FUE, first the epidermis is *scored* to enter the deeper tissue and thereafter follicular unit is *dissected* from surrounding dermal tissue (**Fig. 21.29a–c**). Scoring of epidermis and dissection of follicles together constitutes "follicular unit excision."

The FUE is performed in four steps:

1. *Alignment*: The long axis of the punch is kept along or parallel to the hair shaft (**Figs. 21.30a** and **21.31a**).
2. *Engagement*: The cutting edge of the punch is fixed over the skin surface for scoring the epidermis. The punch is centered on the exit point of hair or preferably the epidermal blush (**Fig. 21.30b**).
3. *Advancement*: Using the rotational and/or oscillatory and axial force the punch is advanced deeper in the dermis to separate follicle from all surrounding attachments, which is the dissection of the follicle unit (**Fig. 21.30c**).
4. *Extraction*: The dissected FU is removed from the skin (**Fig. 21.31a–d**).

The precise depth of the insertion of punch is the key to harvesting an intact FU. The follicle is firmly attached to the surrounding tissues called "tethering." The tethering is linked to the existence of various lateral connections between the dermal sheath, pilosebaceous elements, and connective tissue of the hypodermis. There is also a deep tethering between the hair follicle and the subcutaneous fat at the bottom of the FU neurovascular attachments.[47]

One of the challenges in FUE donor harvesting is the variability in the viscoelastic properties of donor areas.

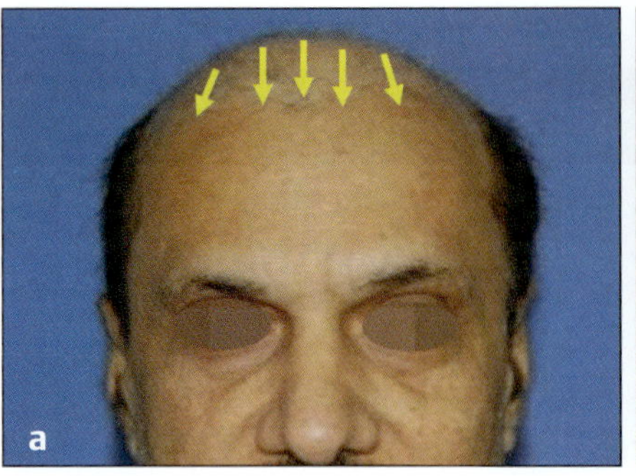

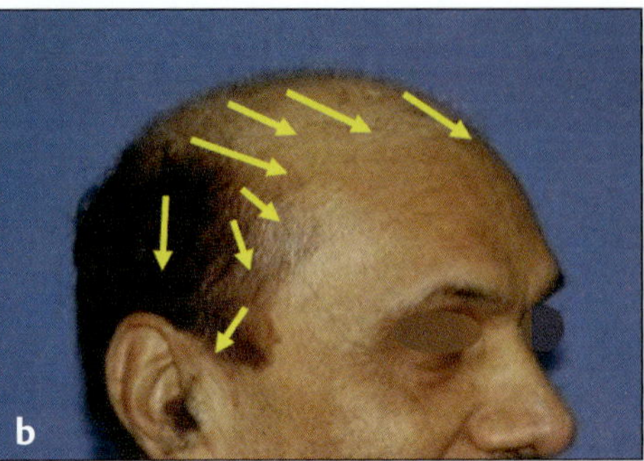

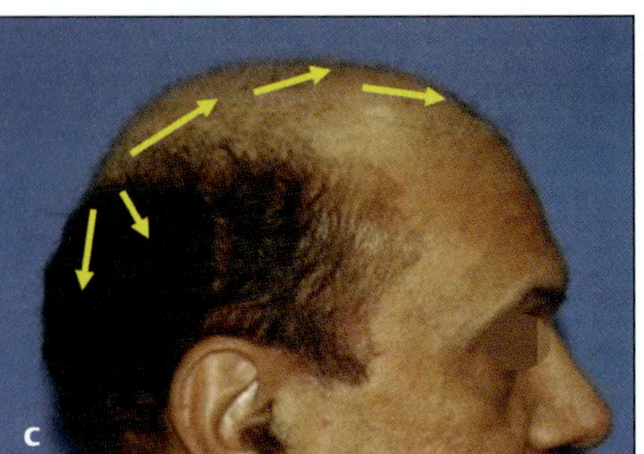

Fig. 21.29 **(a–c)** Direction of hairs in different region.

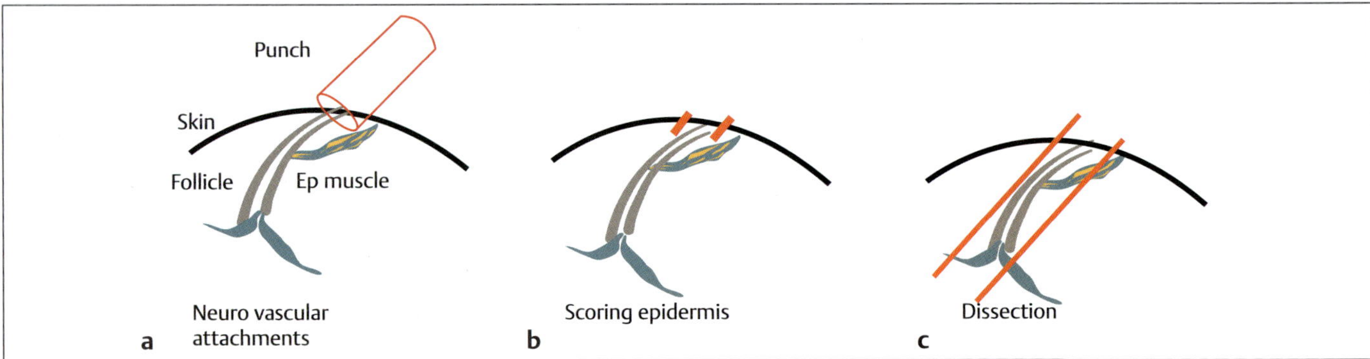

Fig. 21.30 Surgical events. **(a)** Follicle with its attachments. **(b)** Scoring of the epidermis by the punch. **(c)** Dissection of the follicle from its attachments.

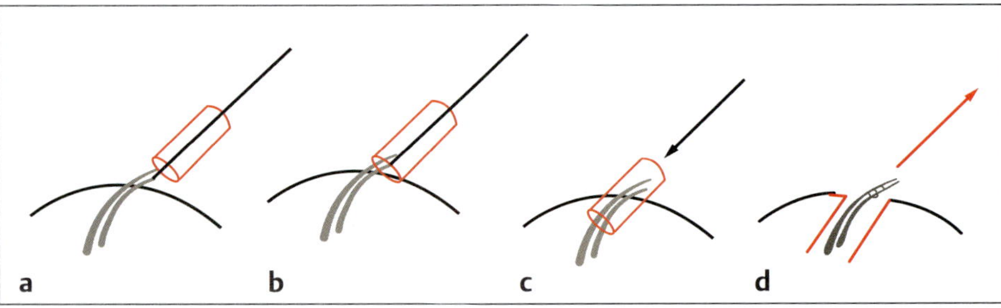

Fig. 21.31 Steps of follicular unit excision (FUE). **(a)** Step I: alignment. **(b)** Step II: engagement. **(c)** Step III: advancement. **(d)** Step IV: extraction of dissected follicle.

The patient-to-patient variation of tissue quality contributes to the challenges of donor harvesting.

Instruments

FUE instruments have punch and a handle. A wide range of such instruments are available.[48] The handle could be manual or it may be motorized (**Box 21.3**).

Punch

The punch is a circular knife to dissect the follicle or follicular unit. The diameter of the punch is variable, ranging from 0.7 to 1.2 mm. The punch size of less than 0.8 mm is called a small punch, between 0.8 mm and 1.0 mm is medium, and punch bigger than 1.0 mm is labeled as large punch. The good quality punch should have a thin and strong wall with a smooth surface. The larger punch has less transection rate but results in more scar and greater vascular compromise. Small diameter punches cause more root transection, and will harvest thinner grafts bearing fewer follicles per FUs, but cause less donor scarring. Most of the surgeons use 0.9- to 1.00 mm-diameter punches for scalp and 0.7 to 0.8 mm for harvesting body hair follicles.

Box 21.3 Instruments used for follicular unit extraction (FUE)

- Punches of 0.7 mm to 1.0 mm in diameter (sharp or dull).
- Handle: Manual or motorized.
- Magnifying glass 3× to 4.5×.
- Chair for the patient.
- Forceps for extraction of grafts.
- Implantation instruments: Forceps, implanters.

Depending on the cutting edge of the punch, the punch can be sharp (**Fig. 21.32a**) or dull (**Fig. 21.32f**). The dull punch

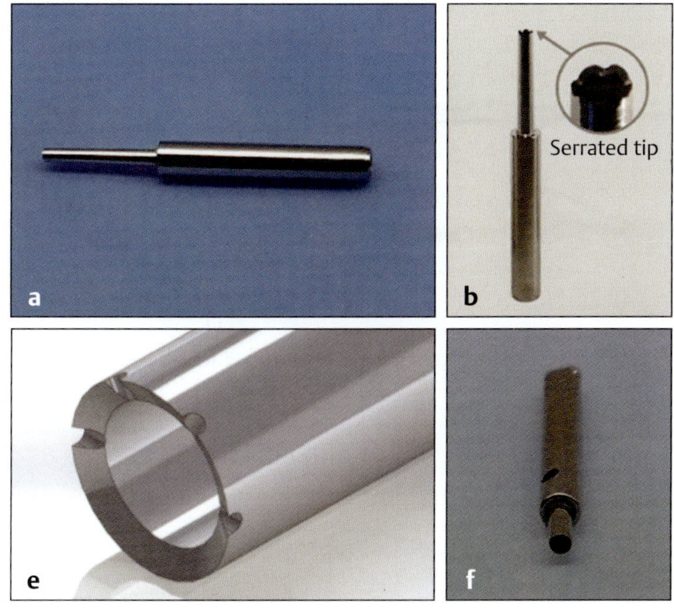

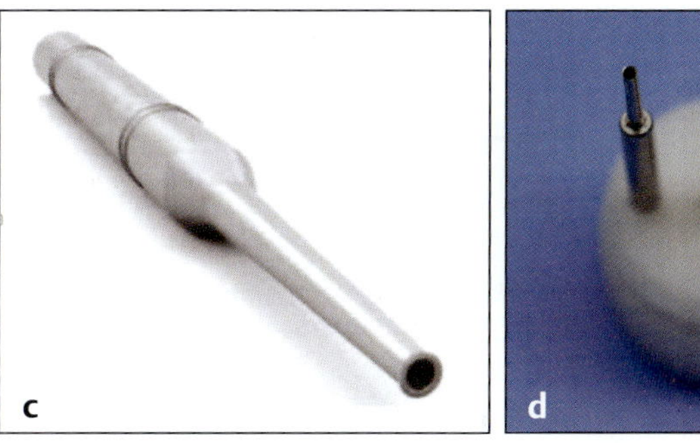
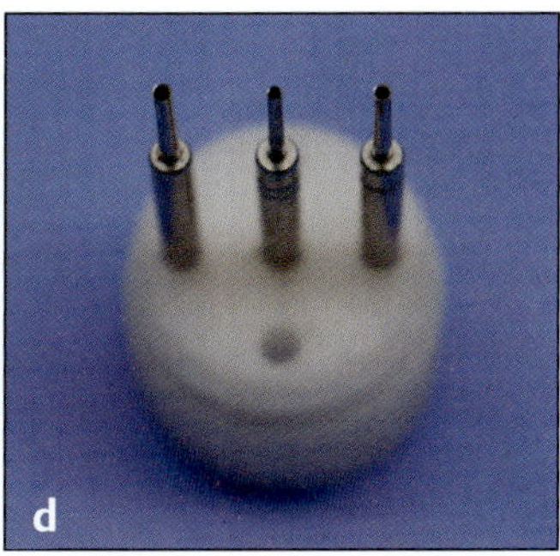

Fig. 21.32 **(a)** Cole sharp punch. **(b)** Cole sharp serrated thin wall punch. **(c)** Devroye hybrid punch with an outer edge for scoring and inner edge for dissection. **(d)** Trivellini flared punch. **(e)** Trivellini punch for long hair. **(f)** Dull punch.

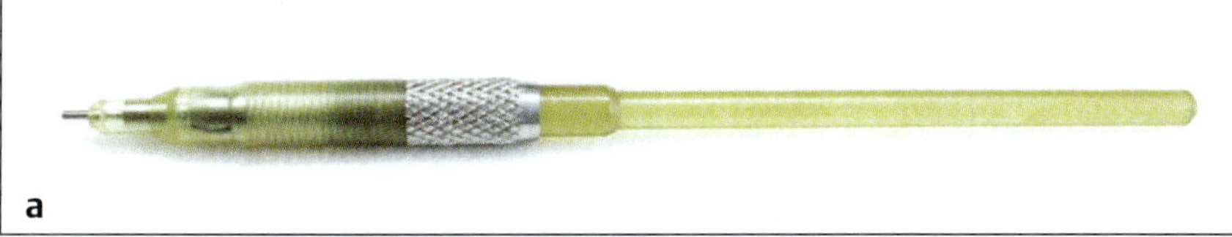
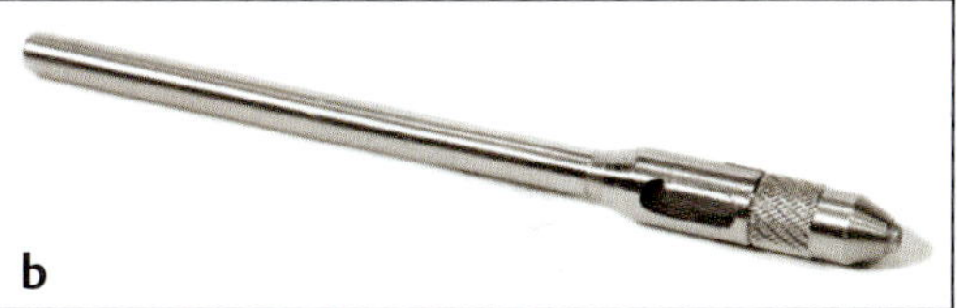

Fig. 21.33 **(a)** CIT manual punch handle. **(b)** Versi manual handle for follicular unit excision (FUE).

needs more pressure to cut as compared to the sharp punch. The cutting edge of punch can be outside bevel, inside bevel, or middle bevel. There are different types of punch edges in different instruments (**Fig. 21.32a–f**). Overall, the objective is to harvest a good quality graft with more perifollicular tissue at a good speed.

John Cole has been promoting sharp punches and he has simplified the biomechanics of extraction to support his theory.[49] When force is applied over the skin, there is compression of the skin and follicle underneath. The dull punch needs more force to cut the skin, which leads to more distortion, thereby increasing the transection rate and risk of buried grafts. If the sharp punch is used, less force will be required to cut the skin, so there will be minimal distortion and better graft quality. He further devised an ultrasharp serrated punch to reduce the friction injury. The potential problem with a sharp punch is high-transection rate, which is a matter of concern. It can be minimized with practice.

The hybrid punch is flared (trumpet-shaped, **Fig. 21.32d**) at the end with a sharp outer edge for scoring and dull inner edge for dissection.[48] This design helps in reducing the transection of hair follicles (**Fig. 21.32c**). The selection of sharp or dull punch is as per the choice of surgeon.

Handle

These punches are mounted over the handles. The handle is used for creating axial, rotational, and/or oscillatory force to score the epidermis and finally dissect the follicle. The handles are manual or motorized.

Most of the manual FUE handles are made of stainless steel and autoclavable. There are different varieties of handles, with most commonly used being CIT manual punch handle (**Fig. 21.33a**) and Versi handle (**Fig. 21.33b**).

To improve the speed of follicles harvesting, the punch is mounted on a battery operated or electrically powered motorized handle.[50,51] The motor revolves at a speed of 100 to 20,000 RPM (**Fig. 21.34a, b**). Initially, the revolutions were unidirectional, but in the advanced systems, the oscillatory movements have been added. The punch is mounted over the motorized handle and placed around a follicle unit. The rapid axial rotation of the punch allows for fast scoring and easy separation of the follicle.

During the initial phase of the motorized method of FUE, the graft yield was less due to the strain put on the follicular unit through rapid rotation, tension, heat, and friction. Later, these problems were resolved by reducing the speed of rotation and the addition of the oscillatory movement.

Harris developed the *SAFE system*[47,52] which utilizes "blunt" instrumentation to dissect the FUs with minimal risk of follicle transection. Harris introduced the dull Hex punch on a motor (**Fig. 21.35a, b**). The potential problem with dull punch was the increased incidence of buried grafts and slow speed of extraction in comparison to the sharp punch.

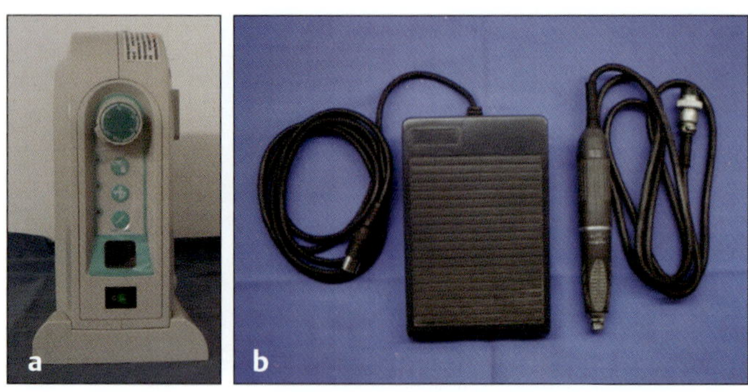

Fig. 21.34 Basic motorized system for follicular unit excision (FUE). **(a)** Basic console for control of the speed of motor. **(b)** A motor and handle for holding the punch and foot paddle for control.

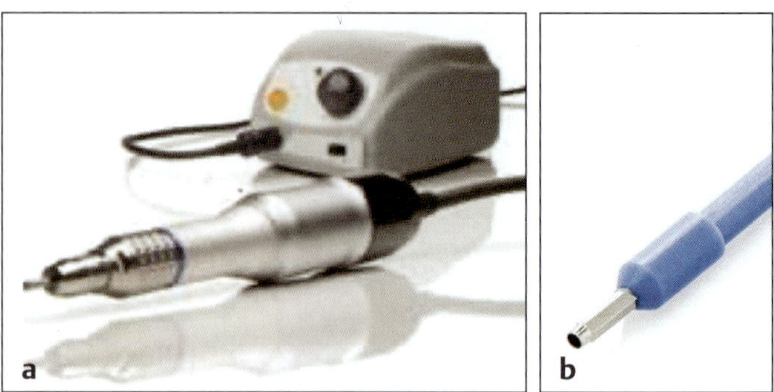

Fig. 21.35 **(a)** Harris SAFE system. **(b)** Harris hex dull punch.

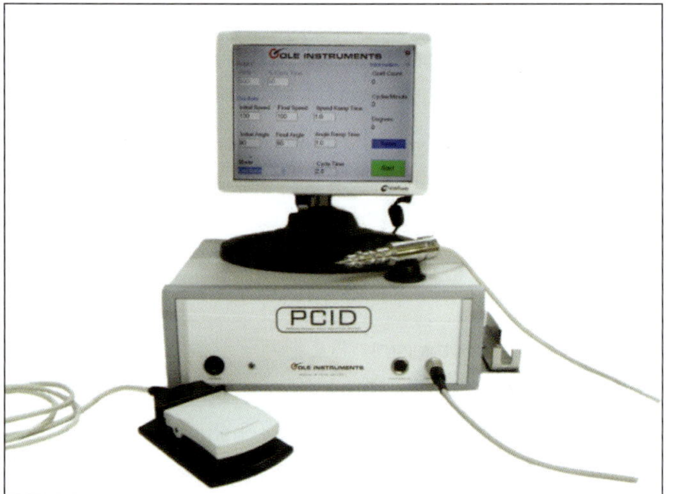

Fig. 21.36 Cole PCID system.

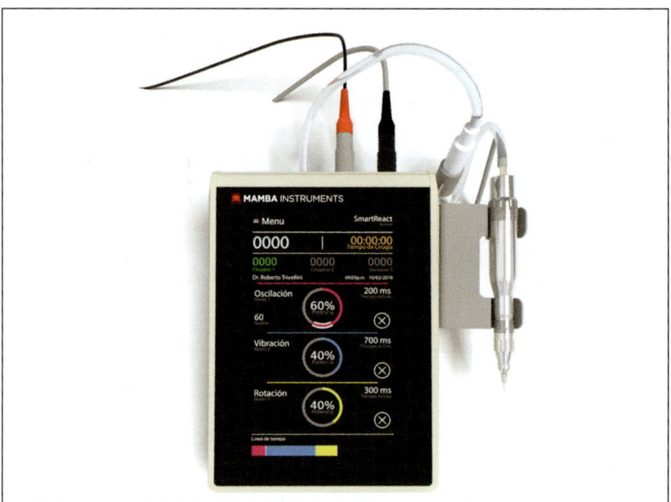

Fig. 21.37 Trivellini Mamba system.

Powered Cole isolation device is a programmable device developed by J. Cole. This advance system[48,49] allows for more precise control of rotation, oscillation, arc of rotation, and the depth control (**Fig. 21.36**).

Trivellini Device developed by Dr. Roberto Trivellini, the Mamba FUE Device is a multifunction programmable motor that incorporates in-line suction, rotation, oscillation, and vibration.[47,48] The device also uses a unique flat punch design called the "Edge-Out" punch (**Fig. 21.37**).

Devroye system—developed by Dr. Jean Devroye—is a battery-powered device using an oscillating flat punch controlled by a foot pedal.[47,48] This precision device works with very short arc punch oscillation (**Fig. 21.38**).

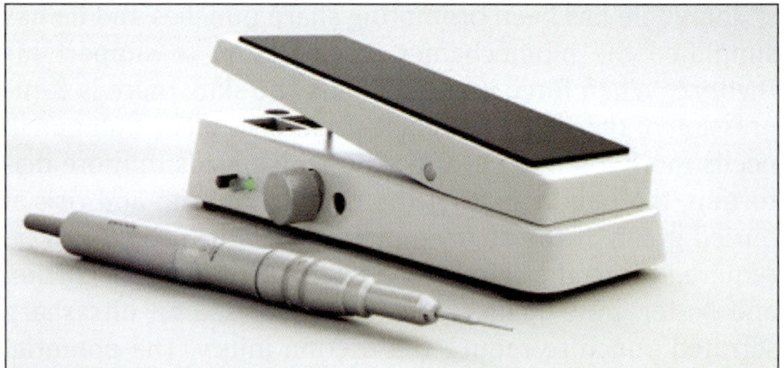

Fig. 21.38 Devroye system with a hybrid punch.

Suction-Assisted Motorized Device/Neograft

This is a motorized device with a sharp punch and both negative and positive pressure mounted on a right-angled hand piece (**Fig. 21.39**). The negative pressure sucks the graft after dissection and are collected in a chamber.[47,48] The grafts can be implanted in premade slit by another device attached to the machine using pneumatic positive pressure. The system did not gain popularity because of technical problems. The grafts were collected in a dry chamber, risking desiccation.

Image-Guided Robotic Device

Restoration Robotics developed a digital image-guided robotics system in 2011 capable of scoring FUs with an image-guided motorized punch (**Fig. 21.40**).[47,48] The robotic system is composed of a computer, a mechanical arm, a

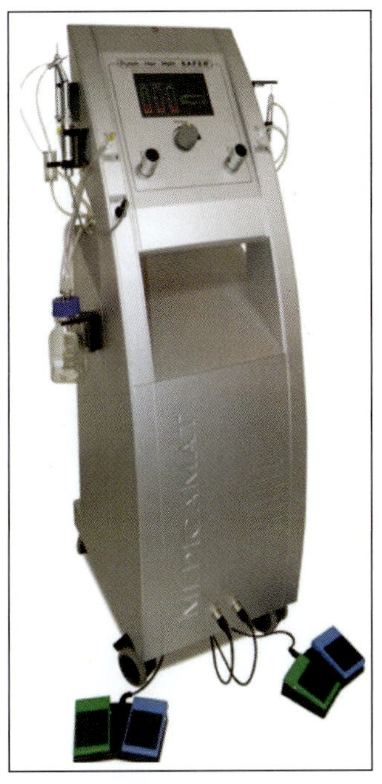

Fig. 21.39 Neograft suction-assisted system.

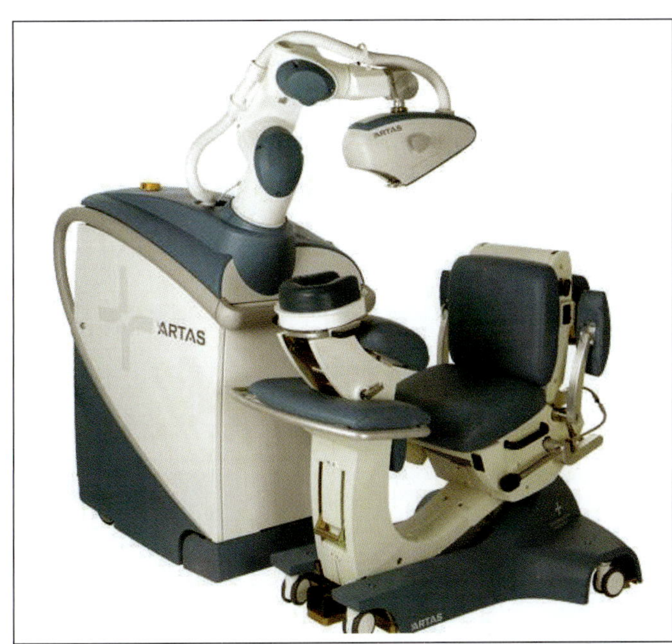

Fig. 21.40 ARTAS robotic device.

punch mechanism, a video-imaging system, and a user interface. Its dissection technique is enabled by two punches that are concentrically arranged. The small diameter inner punch has sharp-cutting capabilities to score the uppermost part of the skin, and the outer dull punch has a blunt edge that dissects the FUs from the surrounding tissue, minimizing injury to the grafts. The device can suggest the target unit; align the punch for precise scoring, and deeper dissection. The robotic system utilizes the Harris SAFE methodology. The dissected follicle is removed manually. To stretch the skin surface, a skin tensioner is used.

The robot is an expensive device and uses multiple disposable materials, which increases the cost of the procedure. The use of robots will undoubtedly overcome human error, shorten the learning curve, and reduce the surgeon's time. Still, it cannot bypass the surgeon, as evaluation of donor area and recipient area planning needs an experienced specialist.

Operative Procedure

Operation Theater Setting

One should perform hair transplantation in a well-equipped operation theater setting. There should be a facility for general anesthesia as well as resuscitation equipment. The atmosphere of the theater should be patient-friendly. There should be an operating table or chair as per the preference of the surgeon. One should consider the requirement of specific positioning of the patient as well as the surgeon for a long period of time. The comfort of the patient as well as the surgeon should be kept in mind. Thai massage chair (**Fig. 21.41a**) or modified dental chair (**Fig. 21.41b**), or surgical operating table with some modifications (**Fig. 21.41c**) can be used for the comfort of the patient. Comfortable prone and lateral position will facilitate cooperation from the patient.[53] A simple DVD player can be used for patients' entertainment (**Fig. 21.41d**). To avoid claustrophobia, a hole can be made (**Fig. 21.41e**) on the head-end side of the operating table with a silicone ring. There should be good cold light. Surgery should be performed preferably using 3.5 or 4.5× magnification.

Technique of FUE Harvesting

The punch is mounted on the handle, first epidermal scoring and then dissection of the FU is performed by advancing deeper in the dermis. Manual harvesting can be performed using two steps or one-step technique.[47,54]

Manual FUE

Two-Step Manual FUE Technique

A sharp punch is mounted on a handle, aligned to the hair shaft, engaged at the exit point or epidermal blush, and epidermal scoring is performed using oscillating force. In the second step, the sharp punch is replaced with a dull punch. This punch is inserted through the same incision. Maintaining the same angle, the punch is advanced deeper by oscillating movement and axial force. Once the arrector pili muscle is cut, there is a feeling of giving way which is the end point. The punch is removed and the FU is picked up using a forceps. The initial few follicles should be examined for transection, angulation, and depth of hair follicles as further guide.

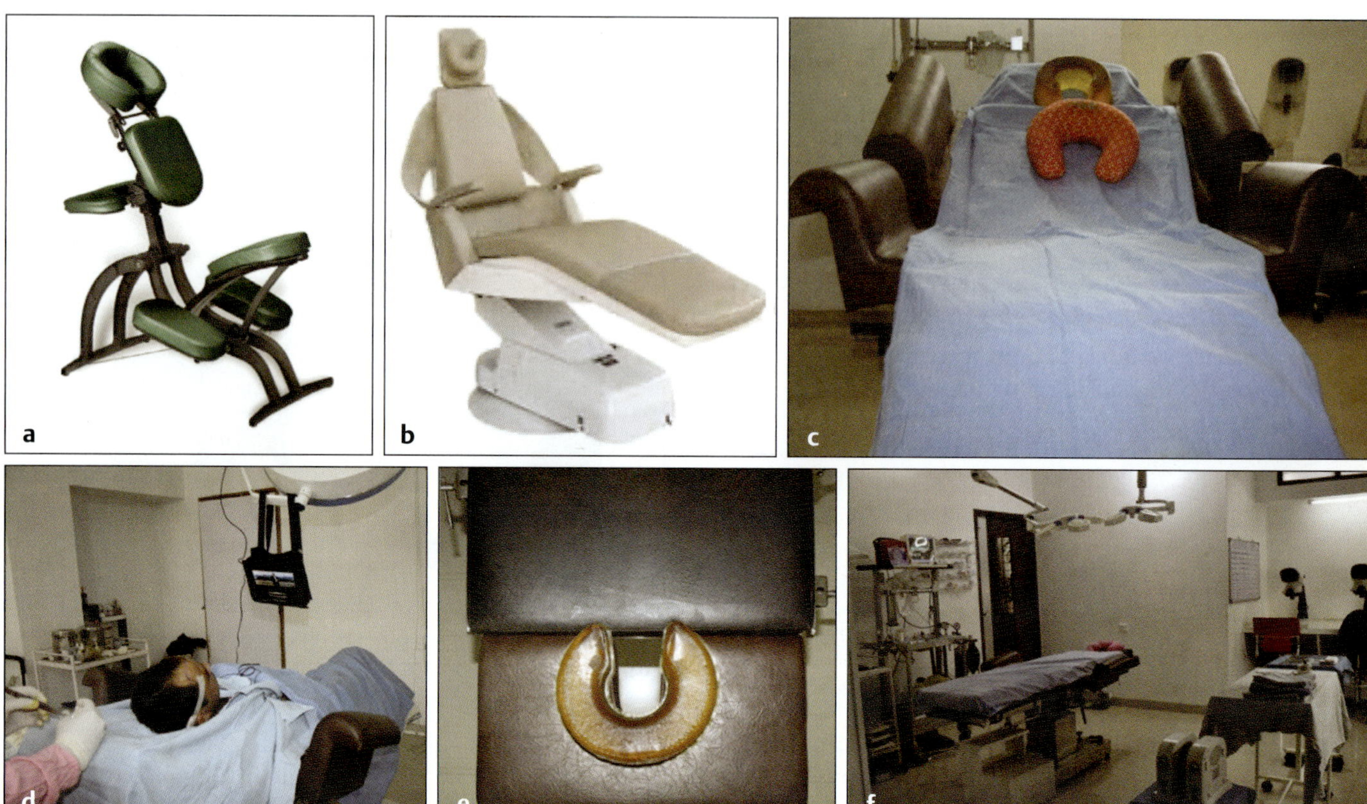

Fig. 21.41 **(a)** Thai massage chair. **(b)** Modified dental chair. **(c)** Operating table with extra cushion, attached cushioned handle, and neck pillow. **(d)** Car DVD player hanging from the light. **(e)** Horseshoe-shaped hole on the head end of the operation table. **(f)** Operation room equipped with all emergency equipments including an automated defibrillator.

Single-Step Manual FUE

The scoring of epidermis and dissection of the follicle unit is performed using the same punch in one step. The depth is chosen depending upon the length of the hair follicle which is usually 3 to 4 mm. The CIT handle has a depth control; otherwise, a guard can be used to control the depth of penetration of punch. After completing the precise depth dissection, the punch is removed. The graft is harvested and examined for any injury, direction, and length.

Motorized FUE Method

The punch is mounted on the motorized handle. One should hold the motor handle in a pen-holding position, stabilize the grip, adjust the RPM of the motor, and target the follicle. The exit point of the follicle is targeted at the center of the punch. The author advises centering the punch over epidermal blush. Epidermal blush is identifiable under magnification (**Fig. 21.42e**). In slow-motion, the punch is engaged in the epidermis, and scoring of the epidermis is done. The punch is advanced further deep with steady pressure to dissect the follicle to its full depth. The speed of the motor is adjusted during the procedure as per tissue resistance (**Fig. 21.42a–j**).

The depth of punch is controlled by using a depth guard over the punch. The depth of punch is decided as per the length of the follicle. Initial few follicles are examined after extraction for decision making (**Fig. 21.42a–c**).

Manual versus Motorized Harvesting

It is suggested that beginners should start with the manual harvesting method. The slow oscillatory movement in the manual method reduces the risk of damage to the follicles. In motorized extraction, the movement is rotatory and/or oscillatory. The deeper the punch goes, the more it releases the follicle from its ties. If dissection is too deep, the follicle may twist on itself, ending in as a "buried graft," commonly seen with a motorized punch in an inexperienced hand. The significant advantage of oscillation of a manual punch is the avoidance of complete twisting of the follicle. Another advantage of manual extraction is that the surgeon is able to recognize the variation in the tissue resistance at different levels; accordingly, the force and movements can be adjusted. Slow speed is the limitation of the manual method. The motorization has significantly increased the speed of FU harvesting.

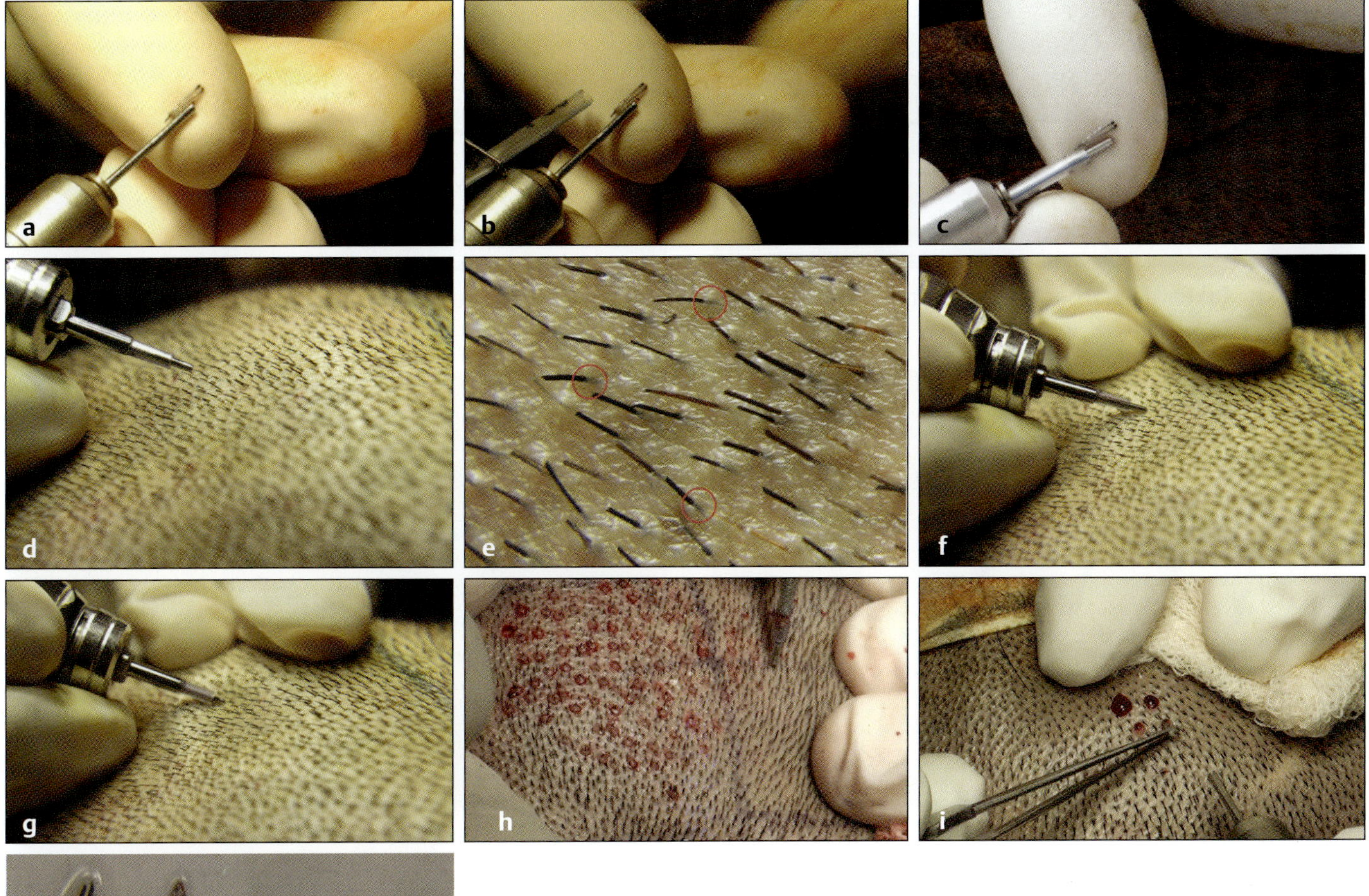

Fig. 21.42 **(a–c)** How to apply depth guard. **(a)** The first few test grafts are harvested, and the length of graft is assessed. **(b)** Infant feeding tube or other silicone tube is taken. **(c)** The silicone tube guard is mounted over the punch, so the punch reaches just above the level of bulb of the hair follicle. **(d–j)** Steps of follicular unit excision (FUE). **(d)** (Step I) alignment. **(e)** Centering the center of the punch to epidermal blush. **(f)** (Step II) engagement. **(g)** (Step III) Advancement. **(h)** Dissected follicle in its place. **(i)** (Step IV) Removal or extraction of the dissected follicle. **(j)** Extracted FUs.

Grafts Injury

Follicular graft may sustain various types of injuries during harvesting. It is crucial to examine the harvested grafts to identify various types of injuries and modify the procedure.

Transection is division of a follicle along its entire length. A graft is considered completely transected when all of the follicles are cut transversely. The partial transection is when some follicles are cut, leaving one or more intact follicles (**Fig. 21.43a**, **b**).

Capping or Topping is a small segment of epidermis and dermis without a hair follicle (**Fig. 21.44**). In most cases, this is due to not having achieved sufficient depth with the punch before liberating the graft.

Pluck is naked follicles devoid of all or part of surrounding connective tissue sheath (CTS), outer root sheath (ORS), inner root sheath (IRS), and the dermal papilla (DP). In some instances only the IRS may remain (**Fig. 21.45**).

Broken or Fractured Follicle(s): The follicles are broken into two or more pieces. Such trauma typically results from an excessive force applied with forceps during the extraction of FUE (**Fig. 21.46**).

Safe Excision Density[55–57]

How many follicles can be extracted? One should consider donor area limitations and avoid excising from areas likely to be affected by androgenetic alopecia (AGA). This usually means excluding the nape of the neck, superior lateral

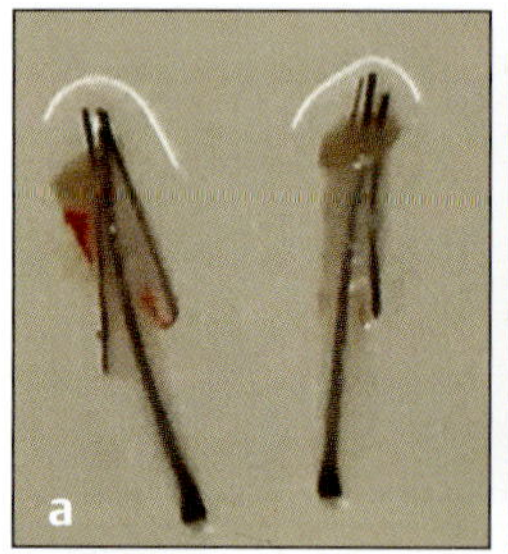

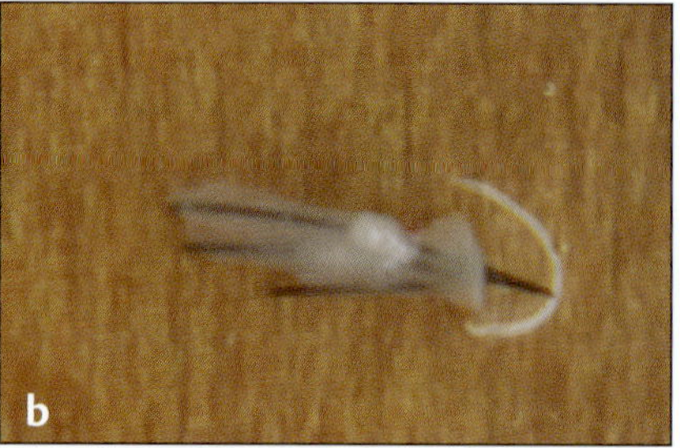

Fig. 21.43 **(a)** Partial transection. **(b)** Complete transection.

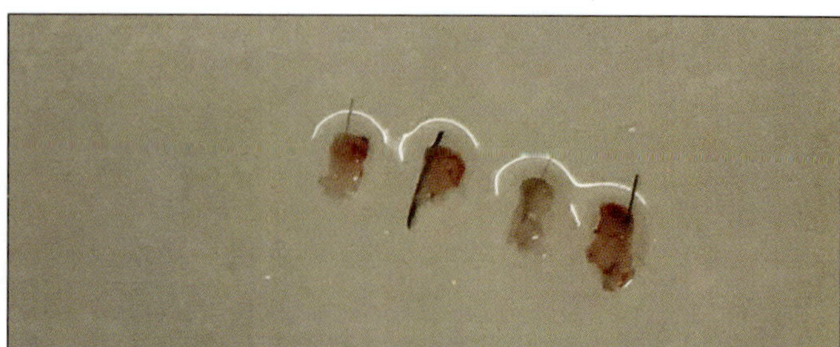

Fig. 21.44 Capping of the follicle.

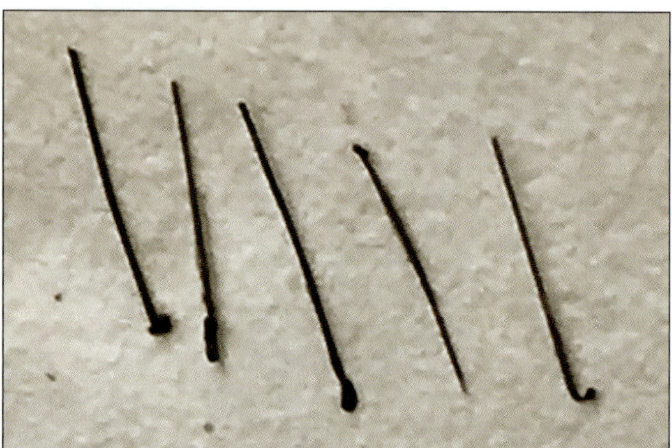

Fig. 21.45 Plucks.

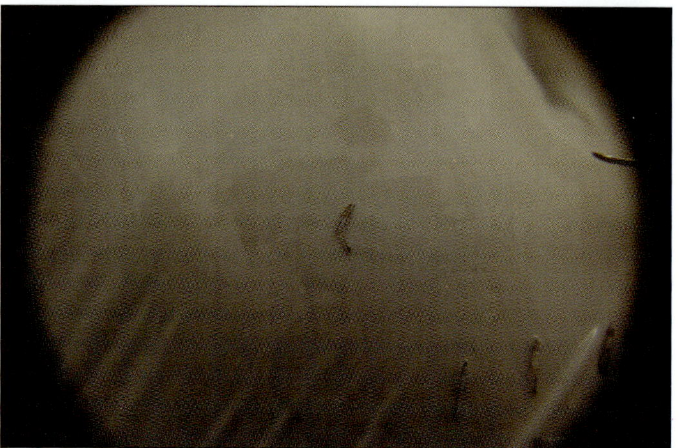

Fig. 21.46 Fracture of the hair shaft in follicle.

fringes, and the superior aspect of the occiput near the region of the balding crown.

Most FUE experts recommend 10 to 15 grafts excision/ cm^2 as a safe single-pass density[56] in a person with a baseline average density of 65 to 75 grafts/cm^2. James Harris[52] reported routine use of higher excision density in the range of 20 to 25 grafts/cm^2. In the case of a patient with an average baseline density of 70 grafts/cm^2, an excision density of 10 to 15 grafts/cm^2 leaves a residual FU donor density of 55 to 60 grafts/cm^2. FUE harvesting with the same excision density would further reduce residual density to 40 to 45 grafts/cm^2. Visible thinning may be expected when the residual density is between 40 and 50 grafts/cm^2, especially in short hairstyle with straight and thin hair. The extraction shall be uniform, to avoid "moth-eaten appearance" (**Fig. 21.47**).

Mega Session

With more and more experience of FUE, sharp punches, and more sophisticated motorized devices, a large number of follicles can be harvested in one session. When grafts extracted are more than 2,000 to 2,500 grafts in one session, then it is called *mega session*.[55] When the grafts are more than 4,000 grafts in one session, it is called a *giga session*. From scalp donor area, extraction of more than 3,000 grafts in one session is not advisable. Author considers approximately 2,500 grafts in one session from the scalp donor area is the safe limit; of course, it depends on the donor density too.

Contraindications for FUE Surgery

The FUE procedure is not preferred in the following situations:

- Patient with extensive scarring of the donor area.
- Patients having a high curl of hair where there is risk of high transection of follicles.
- The surgeon does not have adequate training and skill.
- The patient not willing to shave the head; unshaven FUE is an option.
- Female patients where the shaving of the donor area is not feasible, the strip method is the choice, or unshaven FUE is an option.

Graft-Holding Solution

During the interval between the graft extraction and implantation, hair follicles are devoid of circulation, supply of oxygen, and nutrition. This period is called "graft out of body time" or "ischemia time." The graft during this period is kept or stored in a "graft-holding solution." This prevents desiccation of graft and minimizes ischemic injury to hair follicles.

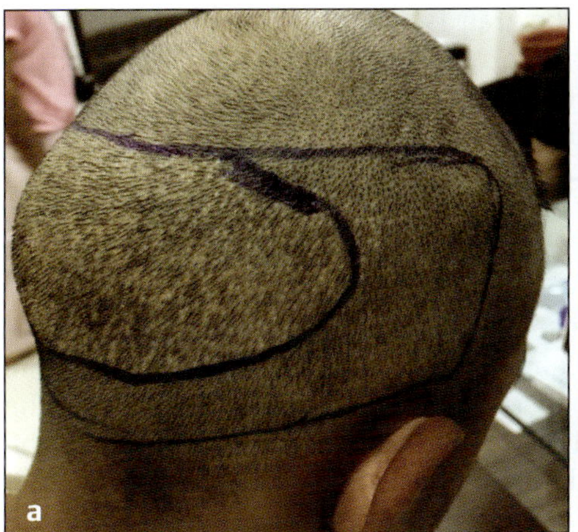

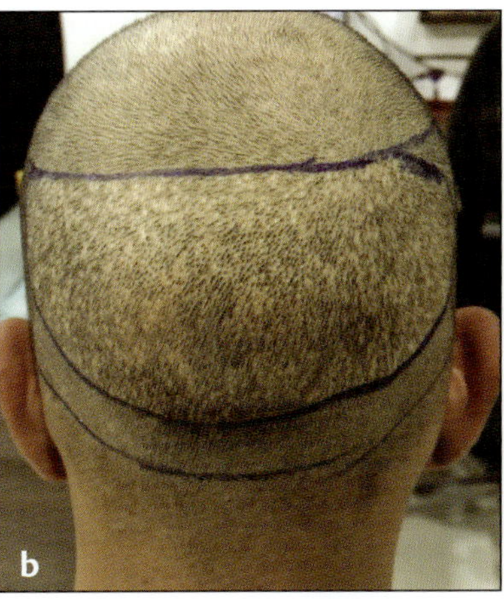

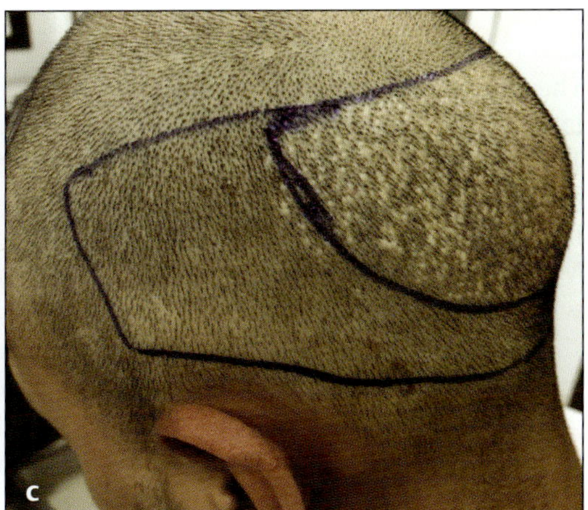

Fig. 21.47 (a–c) Overharvested donor area. The grafts were extracted from the central occipital area, using a large size punch with overharvesting, leading to extensive scarring and moth-eaten appearance. The second harvesting was planned to leave the central occipital area, and grafts were harvested from both lateral and inferior areas only.

Graft Injuries

The out-of-body time and the temperature of the graft might affect the survival of hair follicles. Ischemia causes injury to rapidly dividing cells of hair follicles, called "*ischemic injury*" or "storage injury."[58–60] If the supply of oxygen is not restored quickly, the rapidly dividing cells may undergo apoptosis resulting in loss of graft.

The temperature also affects the metabolism of cells. By lowering the temperature, oxygen demand of a cell can be lowered. The oxygen consumption at 5°C is about 6% of the requirement at 37°C.[58–61] Too low temperature disrupts the membrane ATP, sodium, and potassium pump. The influx of sodium attracts water into cells leading to cell swelling and increases the calcium which activates degenerative enzymes. The resulting injury is called "*cold injury*." Hence, the graft should be preserved at an optimum temperature.

Kim[62] and Limmer[63] concluded that storage of hair follicles in chilled saline decreases the survival of grafts. The cold injury can be controlled by maintaining the oncotic pressure of the graft-holding solution. The chilled Hypothermosol solution is one of the graft storage solutions which prevents cell swelling even at low temperature.[58,59]

Common extracellular graft-holding solutions have the composition similar to plasma. Commonly used are normal saline, lactated ringer, autologous plasma, platelet-rich plasma (PRP), balance salt solution (BSS). Ringer lactate and normal saline are popular graft-holding solutions for approximately 2 hours of ischemia time.[60] The autologous plasma and PRP have shown beneficial results in terms of early growth and thickness of hair.[63–65]

Alternatively, intracellular-holding solutions with composition of intracellular fluids with high potassium and low sodium levels are used. The higher osmotic pressure prevents the influx of sodium and water, and prevents swelling at lower temperature. Examples are Hypothermosol, Viaspan (University of Wisconsin solution), CryoStor, Unisol, and KPS1. The grafts stored in these fluids should be maintained between 2 and 8°C.[66]

In general, normal saline or ringer lactate are used for approximately 2 hours.[67] If one expects longer ischemia time then chilled Hypothermosol with or without ATP or autologous plasma as a graft-holding solution without chilling should be used.

Box 21.4 Advices for good outcome of transplant

- Magnification >3.5×.
- Good cool operative light.
- Adequate surgeon's time.
- Comfortable positioning of patient and surgeon.
- Good operation theater ambience.
- Good tumescence and analgesia.
- Minimum "graft out of body time" or "ischemia time."
- Precise depth control of slit.
- Slit dimensions in accordance to graft size.
- Control of bleeding.
- Good harvesting and implantation technique.
- Trained assistants/technicians.

Implantation of Hair Follicles

The implantation of hair follicle is the process of inserting the dissected or harvested FUs into the recipient area. Implantation is one of the critical steps in the process of hair transplant. No matter how safely a surgeon has harvested and stored the grafts, but the final step of implantation, if not done efficiently, the outcome of the transplant may be compromised. All measures shall be taken to get best outcome of the transplant (**Box 21.4**). This implantation can be done in many ways, depending on the surgeon's choice. The outcome depends not on the technique but depends on how efficiently the technique is executed.

Slit Making and Implantation

The slits (sites) could be premade and implantation is done later or slit and implantation are done simultaneously. This is surgeon's preference. In the former technique, slits are made throughout the recipient area and then FUs are implanted later. This is the most commonly used method. Many surgeons feel that the graft ischemia time is shorter with this technique.

Slit making and implantation may be done simultaneously. This is usually performed using implanters or by using a needle by stick-and-place method. With this procedure the slit size can be monitored and discrepancy between the slit size and graft size can be avoided.

Procedure of Implantation

The graft can be grasped either at the lower end (near bulb) or at epidermal end (hair shaft) for implantation.

While implanting the graft the lower end of the graft (root end) is grasped. The fat below the bulb or perifollicular tissue near the bulb is used to grasp the graft (**Fig. 21.48a**). This is not advisable, especially for FUE grafts, as they have relatively less perifollicular tissue as compared to the FUT grafts. Authors feel it is better to avoid this technique as the technicians may not be efficient enough to understand the severity of this microtrauma to the matrix cell, which may affect the quality and thickness of the hair.

Alternatively, the graft is grasped at the epidermal level or the hair shaft. In this technique, the entire length of the follicular graft remains untouched. This is called "No-touch to root" technique and is the author's preferred technique (**Fig. 21.49a, b**).

Instruments used for Implantation

The instruments used for implantation depends on the technique used. Implanters were devised for ease, precision, automation, and to reduce the time of implantation. The grafts are loaded in the channel of the implanter, and the plunger pushes the grafts in a slit. There are many types of implanters with little difference, but all of them work on the similar principle.

The Choi implanter[68,69] has been used widely across the world. The other implanters are Lion, KNU,[70] Lead M implanters, and Indian Sava implanters.[71] The use of implanter is a useful armamentarium in practice as it minimizes the dependence on the assistant. Once the team becomes more adept, the speed of implantation increases with minimum trauma to the grafts.

The Choi implanter has a needle with a bevel (**Fig. 21.50**). The needle is attached to the main body, with an attached plunger that works through a spring located in the body of the implanter.[69,70] It is a two-step process. First, the graft is loaded by the assistant into the bevel part of the needle. The graft is grasped at the epidermal end, loaded through

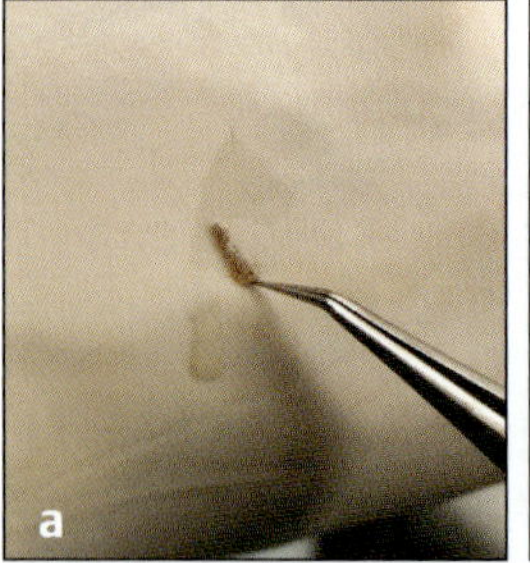

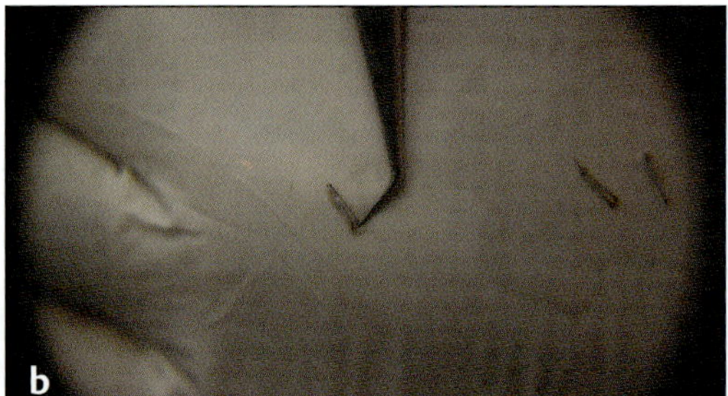

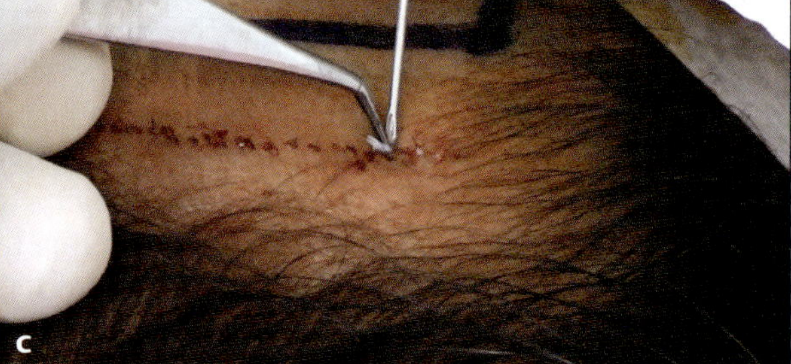

Fig. 21.48 **(a)** Grafts grasped at root level. **(b)** Chances of injury to bulb. **(c)** Implantation by touching the root of graft/hair follicles using stick-and-place technique.

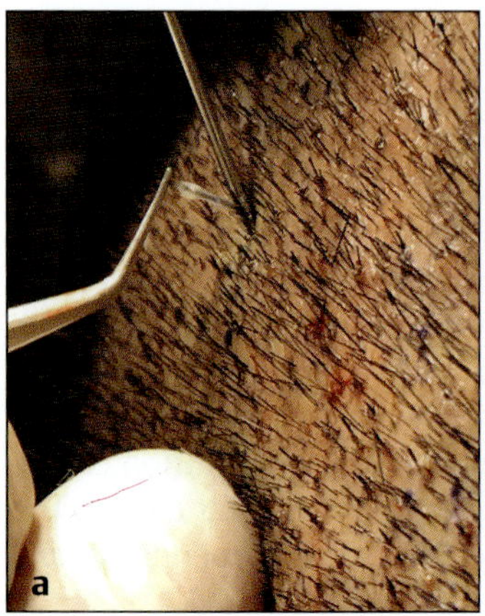

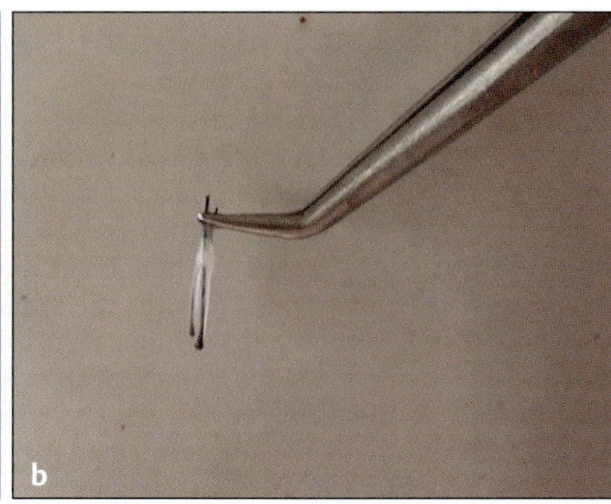

Fig. 21.49 **(a)** No-touch to root technique of holding the graft. **(b)** Stick-and-place technique by no-touch to root technique.

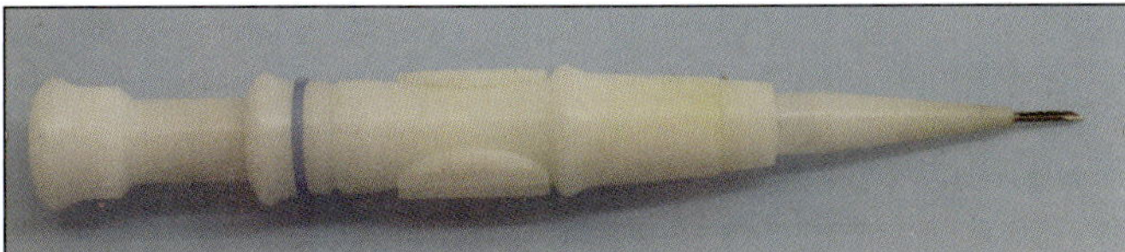

Fig. 21.50 Choi implanter.

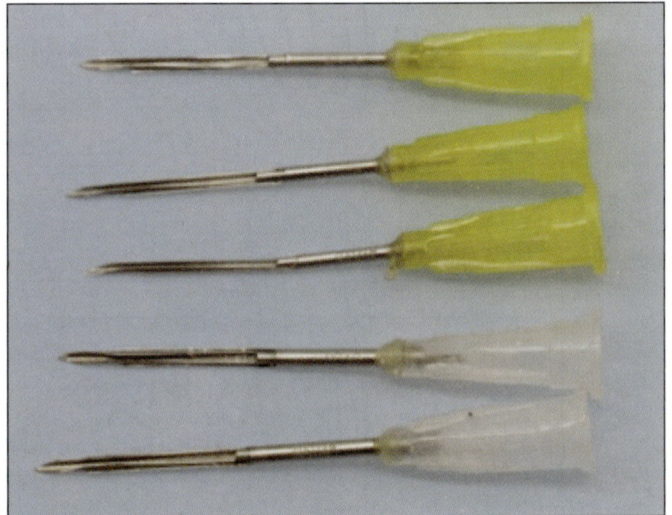

Fig. 21.51 Sava implanter.

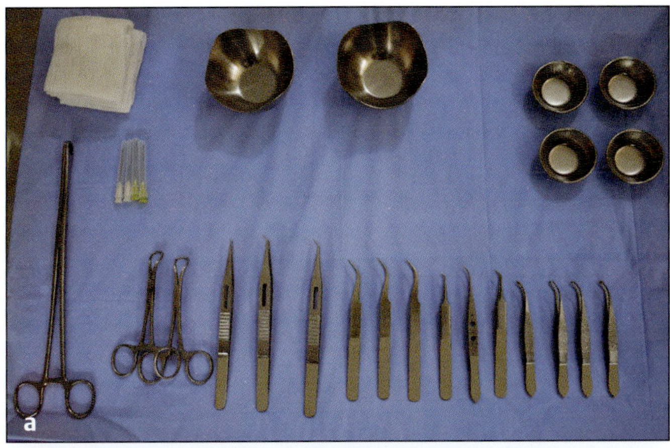

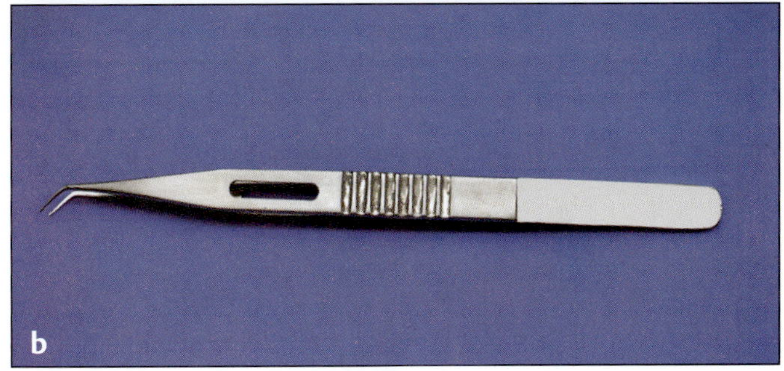

Fig. 21.52 **(a)** Instrument trolley for implantation. **(b)** Jeweler's forceps for implantation.

bevel end and slid up in the channel of the needle. The entire length of the graft remains in the channel except the epidermal part or hair which is kept outside the channel. In the second step, the implanter is inserted into the slit at the desired angle and direction. The needle is inserted facing the bevel toward the skin; the graft is delivered into the slit by pushing the plunger. This has learning curve. It requires readjustment of the grafts in the initial phase, but once surgeons and technicians become familiar, the process becomes fast and smooth.

The Sava implanter (**Fig. 21.51**) was invented by Dr. Sanjiv Vasa.[71] These implanters come in three sizes. The graft is loaded in the bevel of the transplanter needle which is then used to make a slit; the graft is then pushed into the cavity using a forceps.

Most of the surgeons are comfortable with implantation using fine-tip nontooth jewelers' forceps without any implanter (**Fig. 21.52a, b**). A combination of a forceps and the hypodermic needle is commonly practiced. The forceps are used for grasping and manipulating the graft and the needle is used for making slit and insertion at the same time. Alternatively, if slits are premade, then needle acts as a dilator and the bevel of the needle is used to deliver the graft in the slit (**Figs. 21.47 and 21.48**). Some surgeons use two forceps, one for dilating the slit and the other one for implanting the graft. The author prefers to use hypodermic needle number 19 and 20-gauge for stick-and-place technique in premade slits (**Fig. 21.52a, b**).

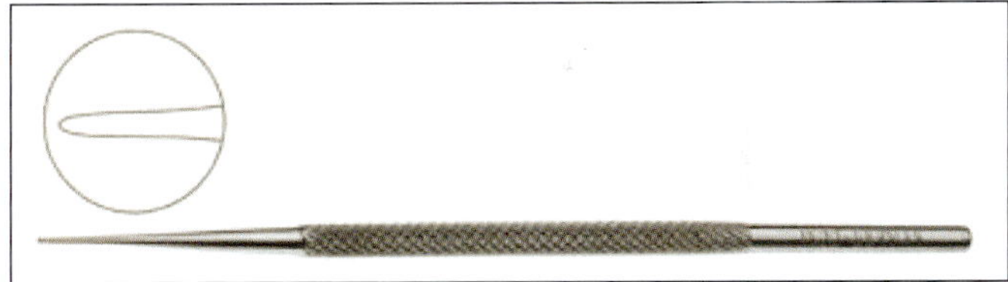

Fig. 21.53 Slit dilator (the lacrimal punctum dilator which comes in different sizes can be used, or custom-made dilators are available).

Occasionally one needs to use a slit dilator for dilating the premade slits. These are metallic-pointed reusable devices which facilitate the implantation of the follicular unit (**Fig. 21.53**).

Technical Errors during Implantation

There are few technical errors which are commonly encountered during implantation.

The ejection /popping out of previously implanted graft during implantation of the adjacent graft is called popping (**Fig. 21.54a**). The force of implantation pushes the adjacent graft. This usually occurs when large size graft is implanted in a relatively smaller or a shallow slit. Active oozing from the slits and rough handling of the graft may also cause popping of grafts. The surgeon should supervise and watch over the assistant's work to avoid such errors.

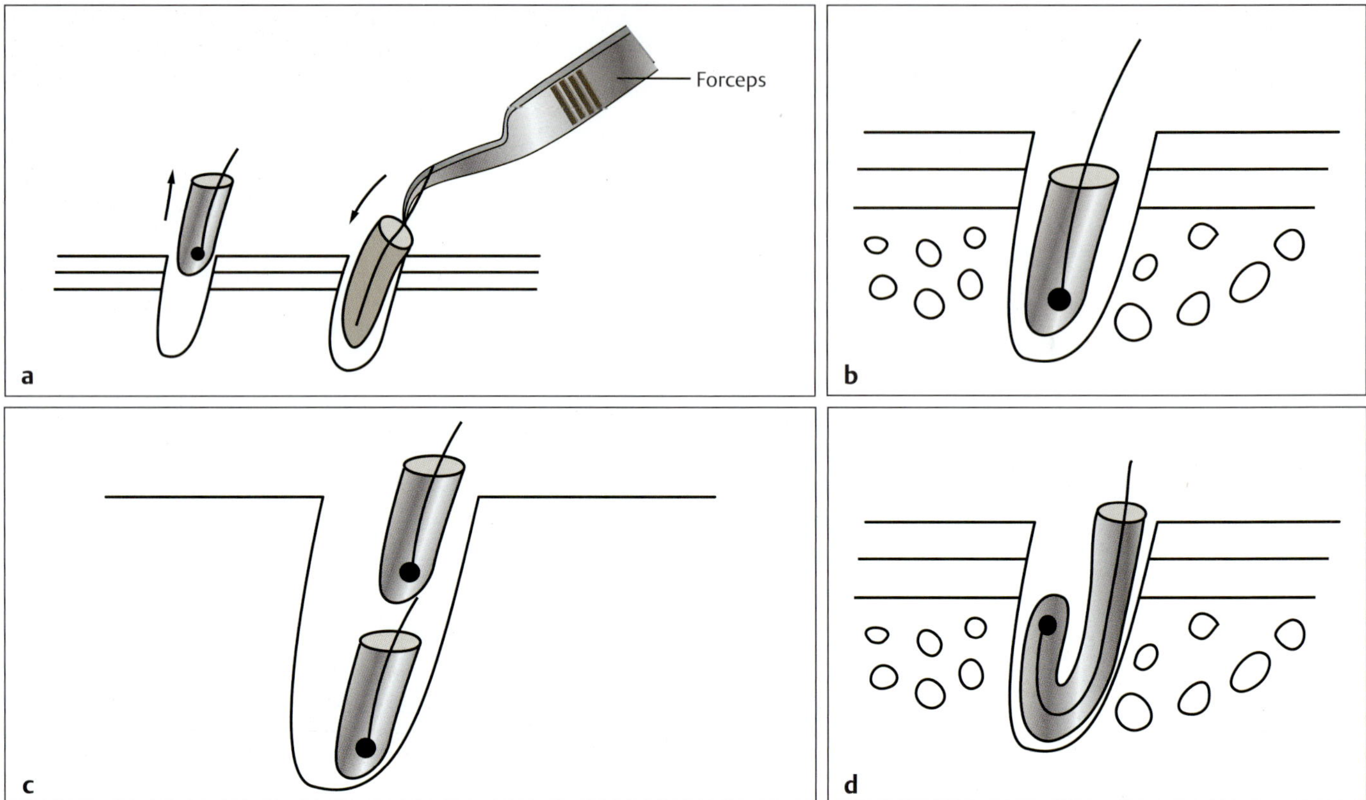

Fig. 21.54 **(a)** Popping-ejection of previously implanted grafts while implanting graft nearby. **(b)** Deep insertion of the graft. **(c)** Piggy backing-grafts implanted one over another. **(d)** Bent graft.

Deep insertion of graft means the graft is implanted below the epidermal surface (**Fig. 21.54b**). This can happen if the slit is deeper than the length of the graft and excessive pressure is applied for insertion of graft or to control the bleeding. The deep insertion of the graft may lead to the formation of inclusion cyst and ingrowing hair. The correct dimension of the slit, good control of bleeding, and magnification can prevent such errors.

Piggy backing is implantation of second graft in the same slit (**Fig. 21.54c**). It happens because of the deep insertion of the first graft and poor visibility. It will lead to an inclusion cyst and ingrowing hair.

Bent graft happens when a large graft is forcibly inserted in a shallow slit; the graft may bend over itself and bend in a shape of "J" (**Fig. 21.54d**). This may lead to kinky hair growth.

Postoperative Care and Instructions

After completion of implantation, the recipient and donor areas are cleaned with normal saline. The debris and blood shall be removed gently.

Care of Recipient Area

No antibiotic ointment or dressing is applied on the recipient area. The author advises not to use any cap or cloth over the recipient area (**Fig. 21.55a**). The grafts may stick to the cap and may get explanted while removing the cap. A cap can be used after 48 to 72 hours. The common advice is to irrigate the recipient area with saline 4 to 6 hourly for 3 to 4 days to prevent drying. Head wash with plain water is advised on the fourth postoperative day. One should avoid rubbing the scalp for 8 to 10 days. After tenth postoperative day, povidone iodine scrub or shampoo head wash is given, which is continued for 4 to 5 days.

Donor Area Care

The FUE donor area after cleaning with saline is dressed with an antibiotic ointment (**Fig. 21.55b, c**). The dressing can be removed after 24 hours and the donor area is left open and topical antibiotic is applied twice a day for 10 days.

Medication

Author prefers to give oral antibiotics for 5 days with analgesics and anti-inflammatory. As per the preference of the surgeon, topical minoxidil and other medical treatment are advised to prevent the loss of existing hair after 10 to 12 days postoperatively.

Positioning

Patient shall sleep in supine position for first 2 days and can use soft pillow.

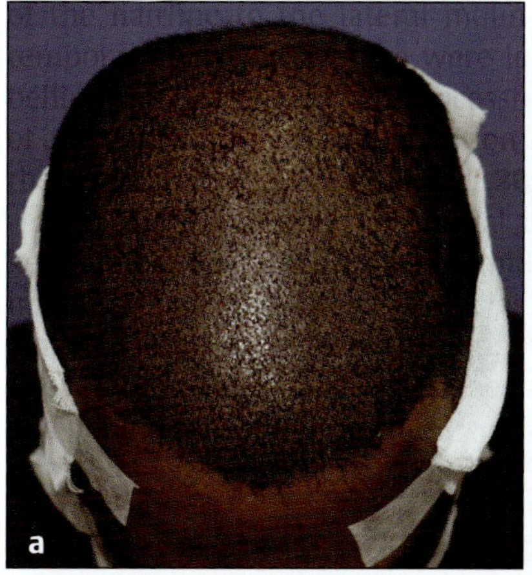
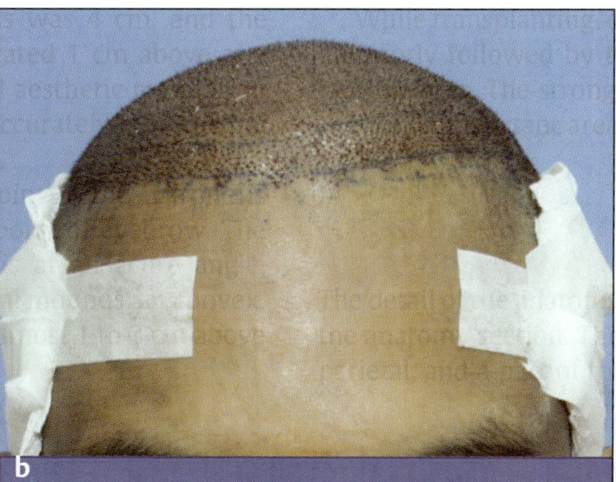
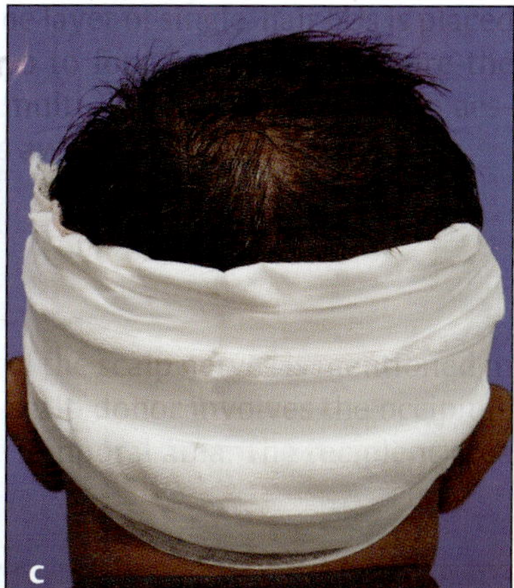

Fig. 21.55 (a) Recipient area. **(b, c)** Dressing follicular unit excision (FUE) donor area.

Postoperative Complaints and Complications

Postoperative pain is usually within tolerable limit and is relieved with oral analgesics. Itching is a common complaint especially in the recipient area because of dryness. Keeping the area moist may reduce itching. Postoperative periorbital edema may appear on the second or third day of the procedure and may take a week to subside. It can be avoided if the patient lies in a supine/semisupine position for the first 2 days. Systemic corticosteroid and cold compresses may be given to reduce the edema.

Temporary loss of existing hair known as "shock loss" may occur in 10 to 20% of men and 40 to 50% of women. Chances of shock loss increase if more grafts are implanted per session, especially in women. Proper counseling of the females before hair transplant is mandatory. The temporary nature of hair loss must be explained to the patients. Topical 5% minoxidil application 1 week before and 5 weeks after surgery reduces the chances of shock loss. Effluvium of the hair is the temporary loss of the implanted grafts which may be noticed in the first 2 to 3 months after the procedure.

Final Outcome

Result of hair transplant is appreciable after 4 months of the procedure and full growth of hair may take 8 to 12 months (**Fig. 21.56**). Rarely there may be poor growth of hair and may take longer to grow.

Body Hair Transplant

The occiput is the universal donor area for hair follicles. However, there are situations when occipital area is not adequate to fulfill the requirement. The other areas like beard, torso, extremities, axilla, and pubic area can be used as donor area, with an added advantage that the growth of hair in these areas is androgen dependent.[72–74]

There are 5 million hair follicles on the human body. Except for the scalp hair, most of the other body hairs are vellus. However, a proportion of these hairs have androgen sensitivity, and they become terminal hair (androgen hair) around puberty.[75] The density and quality are variable in different individuals.

The body hair has different physiology from region to region. It is essential to know the hair characteristics and hair cycle before harvesting (**Table 21.6**). The scalp hair follicles are 85% in anagen, while in body it varies from 20 to 70%. The anagen phase of facial hair follicles is much longer as compared to other body regions.[75–77]

All body hairs are not suitable for transplant. Thick, long, having a proportion of multi-FUs similar to scalp hair are suitable. True has given five criteria for the selection of torso hair for implantation. These are based on the hair density, similarity with the scalp hair, proportion of multi-FUs, hair-bearing area, and length of hair.[78]

Indications and Planning

The body hair can be used during first hair transplant procedures.[79] The indications are the patients wanting to have maximum coverage and density in a single procedure.

- Patients with advanced grade baldness (Norwood type VI and VII), where more than 5,000 grafts are needed in a single procedure.
- Young patients with the genetic history of developing Norwood grade VII, to preserve the scalp hair follicles for the future.
- Young candidates refusing to take finasteride and medications to control ongoing hair loss. There are high chances of early miniaturization and the need for large hair restoration.

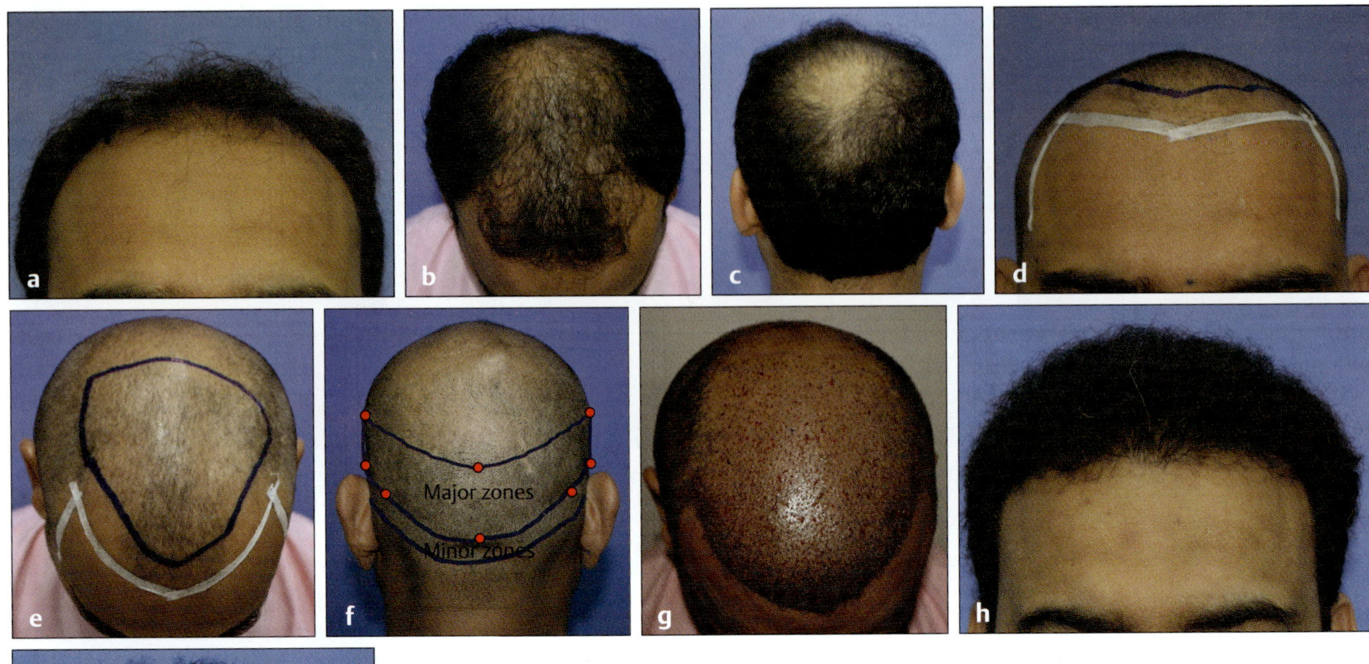

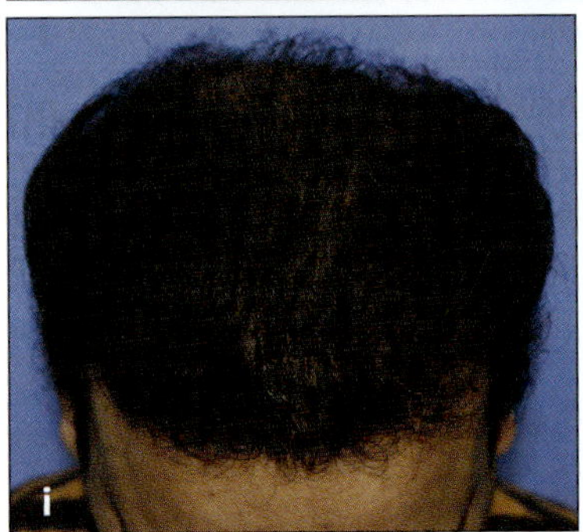

Fig. 21.56 **(a)** Young bald man. **(a, b)** Preoperative pictures. **(d, e)** Planning for front and midscalp coverage using 5,000 grafts on two consecutive days. **(c)** Donor area before shaving. **(d)** Hairline and recipient area marking. **(f)** Markings of safe donor area. Based on scalp donor area density a total of 11,670 mostly multi-follicular units are available. **(g)** On two consecutive days 2,890 from scalp donor area and 2,110 grafts from beard donor area (total 5,000 grafts) were harvested and implanted. **(h,i)** Follow-up results after 11 months.

Table 21.6 Hair cycles in different body regions[76,77]

Body site	Anagen (%)	Telogen (%)	Anagen duration	Telogen duration	Follicle depth
Scalp	85	15	2–6 y	3–4 mo	5–7 mm
Beard	70	30	1 y	10 wk	2–4 mm
Upper lip	65	35	16 wk	6 wk	1–2.5 mm
Armpit	30	70	4 mo	3 mo	4–5 mm
Chest/back	30	70	1–2 y	3–6 mo	2–5 mm
Arms	20	80	13 wk	5 mo	2–4 mm
Legs	20	80	16 wk	6 mo	2–4.5 mm
Pubic area	30	70	4 mo	3 mo	4–5 mm
Eyebrows	10	90	4–8 wk	3 mo	2–2.5 mm

- The thick and curly beard hair, along with scalp hair increases the visual density and gives a bounce to the implanted hair.[80–83]

Patients who have undergone hair transplant and want to have more fullness, and have visible bare scalp, inadequate coverage of bald area, and visible donor scar are the candidates for revision hair transplant, and body hair may be used for the purpose.[72,79,81,84] It is always preferable to use the scalp hair follicles for reconstruction of AHL irrespective of the stage of surgery. If body hair is to be used to augment the AHL, hair follicles from chest and abdomen are used along with scalp hair. To augment or cover forelock and midscalp area, beard hair along with hair follicles from torso can be used. For coverage of vertex, to avoid unnatural look, beard hair should be used in combination with hair from torso and scalp (**Figs. 21.57a, b and 21.58**).

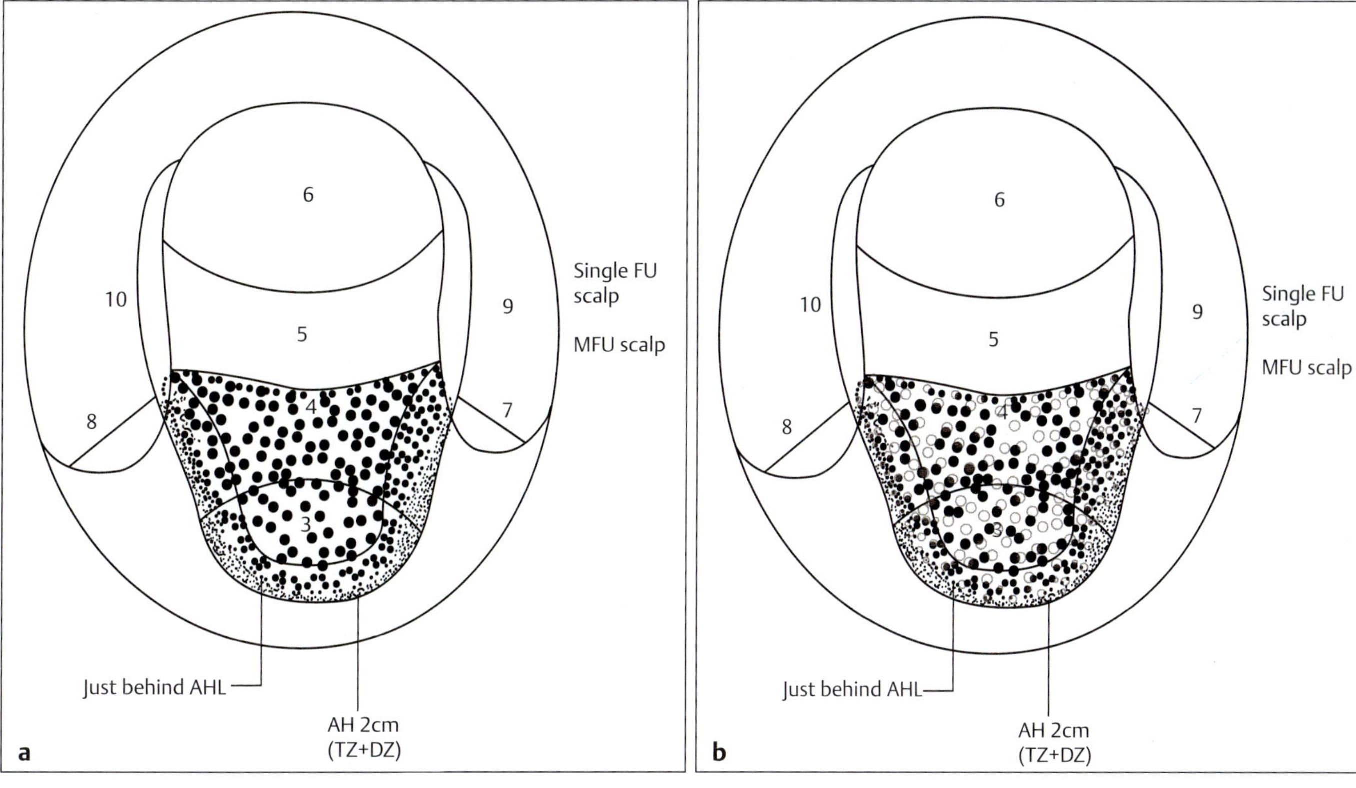

Fig. 21.57 Planning for a combination of scalp and body (beard) hair follicles in Norwood type IV male pattern baldness. **(a)** First, all scalp hair follicles are implanted in the recipient area, leaving spaces for body (beard) hair follicles. **(b)** The body hair follicles are implanted in spaces left in between scalp hair follicles. Abbreviations: FU, follicular unit; MFU, multifollicular unit; AHL, anterior hairline; TZ, transition zone; DZ, defined zone.

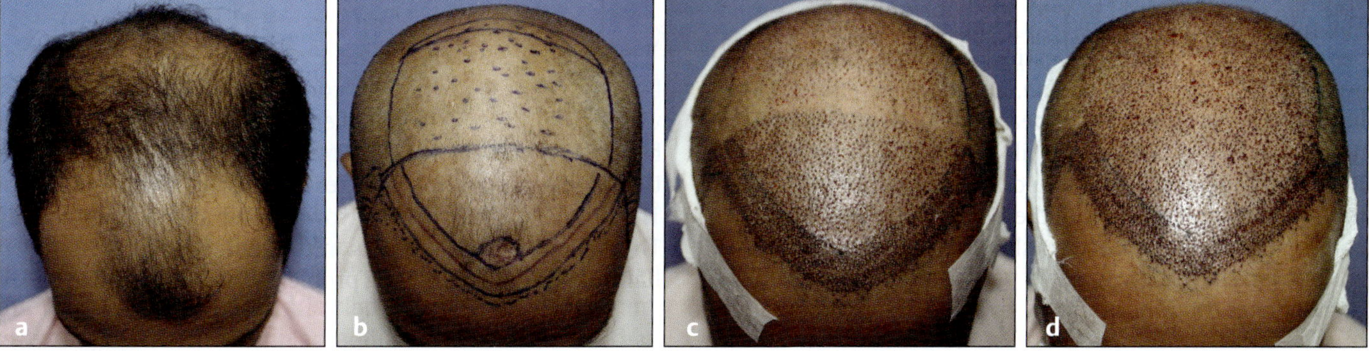

Fig. 21.58 **(a–d)** The master plan of combination grafting of scalp hair follicles and body hair follicles. The first 2 cm of the anterior hairline reconstruction is done using only scalp hair follicles. The remaining area of the scalp is covered in a ratio of 2:1 scalp and body hair. The combination ratio depends on available scalp hair follicles and body hair follicles.

Technique

The patient should be explained in detail regarding the procedure, approximate time of the procedure, the technique of anesthesia, and positional changes required during extraction.

It is advised to shave the beard hair 3 to 5 days preoperatively. Other body parts should be shaved 10 to 15 days before, because of the slow growth rate of torso hair.[85] The desired length of body hair on the day of hair transplant is 2 mm. If the hair has grown longer, it can be shortened using hair clipper leaving 2 mm shaft (**Fig. 21.59**). Gray hair needs dyeing to improve visibility during surgery.

Some physicians advocate the preoperative application of minoxidil 6 to 8 weeks before harvesting. Prior application of minoxidil increases the number of anagen hair.[84] The minoxidil is stopped 2 to 3 days prior to surgery.

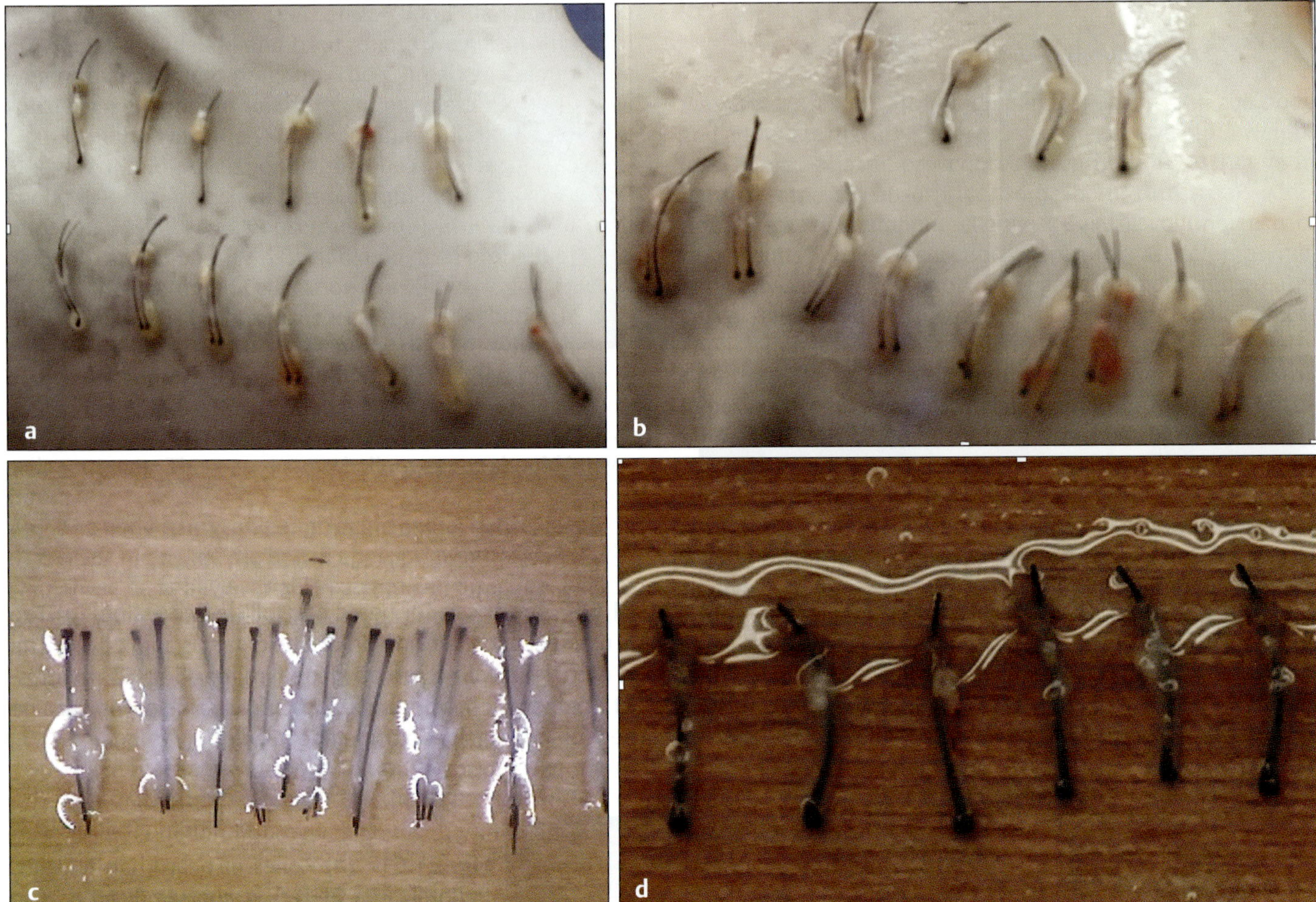

Fig. 21.63 **(a)** Chest hair follicles, **(b)** abdominal hair follicle, **(c)** scalp hair follicle, and **(d)** beard hair follicles.

The design of the AHL is one of the most crucial aspects of natural-looking hair restoration. The limitation of hair transplant is the discrepancy between the donor supply and demand of recipient area. The body hair follicles are additional donor hair to cover the deficit. Beard and torso are commonly used body donor area.

The results of successful hair transplant are seen after 4 months, and it takes around 8 to 12 months to have the final outcome.

References

Overview of Hair Transplant

1. Okuda S. Clinical and experimental studies on hair transplanting of living hair. Jpn J Dermatol Urol 1939;46:537–587 (in Japanese)
2. Tamura H. Pubic hair transplantation. Jpn J Dermatol 1943; 53:76
3. Headington JT. Transverse microscopic anatomy of the human scalp: a basis for a morphometric approach to disorders of the hair follicle. Arch Dermatol 1984;120(4):449–456
4. Limmer BL. Elliptical donor stereoscopically assisted micrografting as an approach to further refinement in hair transplantation. J Dermatol Surg Oncol 1994;20(12):789–793
5. Rassman WR, Bernstein RM, McClellan R, Jones R, Worton E, Uyttendaele H. Follicular unit extraction: minimally invasive surgery for hair transplantation. Dermatol Surg 2002;28(8): 720–728
6. Unger WP. Surgical planning and organization. In: Hair transplantation. 5th ed. London: Informa Health Care; 2011: 114–134
7. Limmer B. Isolated frontal forelock. Hair Transplant Forum 1993;3(5):17–19
8. Nusbaum BP. Frontal forelock: overall design. Hair Transplant Forum 1995;5(1):1-5
9. Springer K, Brown M, Stulberg DL. Common hair loss disorders. Am Fam Physician 2003;68(1):93–102
10. Cash TF. The psychology of hair loss and its implications for patient care. Clin Dermatol 2001;19(2):161–166
11. Yazıcı E, Erol A. Psychiatric approach to alopecia. Turkiye Klinikleri J Cosm Dermatol Special Topics 2015;8:73–78
12. Aghaei S, Saki N, Daneshmand E, Kardeh B. Prevalence of psychological disorders in patients with alopecia areata in

comparison with normal subjects. ISRN Dermatol 2014;2014: 304370
13. Unger W, Scolish N, Giguere D, et al. Delineating the "safe" donor area for hair transplanting. Am J Cosmet Surg 1994;11: 239–243
14. Bernstein RM, Rassman WR. Follicular transplantation: patient evaluation and surgical planning. Dermatol Surg 1997;23(9): 771–784, discussion 801–805
15. Rassman WR, Carson S. Micrografting in extensive quantities: the ideal hair restoration procedure. Dermatol Surg 1995;21(4): 306–311
16. Cole J, Devroye J. A calculated look at the donor area. Hair Transplant Forum Int 2001;11:150–154
17. Unger WP. Surgical planning and organization. In: Hair transplantation. 5th ed. New York: Informa Health Care; 2011: 109–112
18. Shapiro R. Principles and techniques used to create a natural hairline in surgical hair restoration. Facial Plast Surg Clin North Am 2004;12(2):201–217
19. Rose PT, Parsley WM. Science of hairline design. In: Haber RS, Stough DB, eds. Procedures in dermatology: hair transplantation. 1st ed. New York: Elsevier; 2006;55–71
20. Martinick J. Advent of the trainer placer board. Hair Transplant Forum Int 2009;19(1):8–10
21. Parsley B. Hair transplant goals based upon natural hair patterns. In: Unger W, Shapiro R, eds. Hair transplantation. 4th ed. New York: Marcel Dekker, Inc.; 2004,5C:151–161
22. Rose PT. Considerations in establishing the hairline. Int J Aesth Restorative Surg 1998;1:24–26
23. Simmons C. Five old lines and three new lines that can help when designing a male temporal hairline or when transplanting the frontotemporal apex. Hair Transplant Forum Int 2004;14(6):201–203
24. Mayer ML, Perez-Meza D. Temporal points: classification and surgical techniques for aesthetic results. Hair Transplant Forum Int 2002;12:147–158
25. Limmer BL. The density issue in hair transplantation. Dermatol Surg 1997;23(9):747–750
26. Ziering C, Krenitsky G. The Ziering whorl classification of scalp hair. Dermatol Surg 2003;29(8):817–821, discussion 821
27. Shapiro J. Clinical practice: hair loss in women. N Engl J Med 2007;357(16):1620–1630
28. Olsen EA. The midline part: an important physical clue to the clinical diagnosis of androgenetic alopecia in women. J Am Acad Dermatol 1999;40(1):106–109
29. Friedman DO. Hair transplantation for female androgenetic alopecia. Hair Loss J 1992;7(3):1–7
30. Unger WP. Hair transplantation in females. In: Unger WP, Nordstrom RE, eds. Hair transplantation. 2nd ed. New York: Marcel Dekker; 1988:295–300
31. Unger WP, Unger RH. Hair transplanting: an important but often forgotten treatment for female pattern hair loss. J Am Acad Dermatol 2003;49(5):853–860
32. Unger R. Planning in female hairline. In: Unger W, Shapiro R, eds. Hair transplantation. 5th ed. New York: Informa Health Care; 2011:182
33. Ludwig E. Classification of the types of androgenetic alopecia (common baldness) occurring in the female sex. Br J Dermatol 1977;97(3):247–254
34. Hamilton JB. Patterned loss of hair in man: types and incidence. Ann N Y Acad Sci 1951;53(3):708–728
35. Nusbaum BP, Fuentefria S. Naturally occurring female hairline patterns. Dermatol Surg 2009;35(6):907–913
36. Wolf BR. Overview of anesthesia. In: Unger W, ed. Hair transplantation. 5th ed. New York: Informa Health Care; 2005:227–37
37. Canfield DW, Gage TW. A guideline to local anesthetic allergy testing. Anesth Prog 1987;34(5):157–163
38. Shipton EA. Review article new formulations of local anaesthetics: part I. Anesth Res Prac 2012;546409:1–11
39. Farjo B, Farjo N. Dense packing: surgical indications and technical considerations. Facial Plast Surg Clin North Am 2013;21(3):431–436
40. Khan S. Nerve block and local anesthesia. In: Unger W, ed. Hair transplantation. Philadelphia: Elsevier Saunders; 2006
41. Alhaddab M, Kohn T, Sidloi M. Effect of graft size, angle, and intergraft distance on dense packing in hair transplant. Dermatol Surg 2005;31(6):650–653, discussion 654
42. Lam SM. Basic principles of slit creation. In: Lam SM, ed. Hair transplant 360 for physician Vol. I. 1st ed. New Delhi: Jaypee Brothers Medical Publishers; 2014:89–91
43. Bernstein RM, Rassman WR, Szaniawski W, Halperin A. Follicular transplantation. Int J Aesthetic Restorative Surg 1995;3:119–132
44. Bernstein RM, Rassman WR. The aesthetics of follicular transplantation. Dermatol Surg 1997;23(9):785–799
45. Garg AK, Garg S. The use of body hair with scalp hair for "combination grafting" to enhance visual density of hair transplantation and increase coverage in advanced alopecia. Hair Transplant Forum Int 2018;28(6):217–223
46. Mejia R. Redefining the "E" in FUE: Excision = Incision + Extraction. Hair Transplant Forum Int 2018;28(1):5–6
47. Garg AK, Garg S. Donor harvesting: follicular unit excision. J Cutan Aesthet Surg 2018;11(4):195–201 http://www.jcasonline.com/text.asp?2018/11/4/195/251407
48. True RH. The terminology used in follicular unit excision: recommendation of FUE committee ISHRS. Hair Transplant Forum Int 2019;29(3):98–106
49. Cole J. Commentary: Donor area harvesting. In: Unger W, ed. Hair transplantation. 5th ed. London (UK), New York: Informa Health Care; 2011;296–298
50. Onda M, Igawa HH, Inoue K, Tanino R. Novel technique of follicular unit extraction hair transplantation with a powered punching device. Dermatol Surg 2008;34(12):1683–1688
51. Ors S, Ozkose M, Ors S. Follicular unit extraction hair transplantation with micromotor: eight years experience. Aesthetic Plast Surg 2015;39(4):589–596
52. Harris JA. Follicular unit extraction: the SAFE system. Hair Transplant Forum Int 2004;14: 157, 163–164
53. Miao Y, Fan ZX, Jiang W, Hu ZQ. Patient in the sitting position to improve comfort in follicular unit extraction. Plast Reconstr Surg Glob Open 2016;4(11):e1141
54. Harris JA. Conventional FUE. In: Unger W, ed. Hair transplantation. 5th ed. London (UK): Informa Health Care; 2011:291–292
55. Bernstein RM, Rassman WR, Anderson KW. Follicular unit extraction mega sessions: evolution of a technique. Hair Transplant Forum Int 2004;14:97–99
56. Keen SA, Rassman WR. Determining safe excision limits in FUE. Hair Transplant Forum Int 2018;28(7):8–10
57. Devroye J. Donor area harvesting. In: Unger W, ed. Hair transplantation. 5th ed. London (UK): Informa Health Care; 2011:247–248

58. Cooley J. Ischemia reperfusion injury and graft storage solutions. Hair Transplant Forum Int 2004;13(4):121–127
59. Cooley J. Holding solutions. In: Unger WP, Shapiro R, eds. Hair transplantation, 5th ed. New York: Informa Health Care; 2011:321
60. Cole JP, Reed WM. The optimal holding solution and temperature for hair follicle grafts. Hair Transplant Forum Int 2012;22: 17–22
61. Beehner M. 96 hrs study of FU grafts out of body survival comparing saline to hypothermal/ATP solution. Hair Transplant Forum Int 2001;21(2):33
62. Kim JC, Hwang S. The effects of dehydration, preservation temperature and time, and hydrogen peroxide on hair grafts. In: Unger WP, Shapiro R, eds. Hair transplantation. 4th ed. New York: Marcel Dekker; 2004:285–286
63. Limmer R. Micrograft survival. In: Stough D, ed. Hair replacement. St. Louis, MO: Mosby Press; 1996:147–149
64. Uebel CO, da Silva JB, Cantarelli D, Martins P. The role of platelet plasma growth factors in male pattern baldness surgery. Plast Reconstr Surg 2006;118(6):1458–1466, discussion 1467
65. Greco J. Preliminary experience and extended applications for the use of autologous platelet-rich plasma in hair transplantation surgery. Hair Transplant Forum Int 2007;17(4):131–132
66. Garg AK, Garg S. A histological and clinical evaluation of plasma as a graft holding solution and its efficacy in terms of hair growth and graft survival. Indian J Plast Surg 2019;52(2): 209–215
67. Mathew AJ, Baust JM, Van Buskirk RG, Baust JGG. Cell preservation in reparative and regenerative medicine: evolution of individualized solution composition. Tissue Eng 2004; 10(11-12):1662–1671
68. Choi YC, Kim JC. Single hair and bundle hair transplantation using the Choi transplanter. In: Stough D, ed. Hair replacement. St Louis, MO: Mosby Year-Book; 1996:125–127
69. Choi YC, Kim JC. Single hair transplantation using the Choi hair transplanter. J Dermatol Surg Oncol 1992;18(11):945–948
70. Lee SJ, Lee HJ, Hwang SJ, et al. Evaluation of survival rate after follicular unit transplantation using the KNU implanter. Dermatol Surg 2001;27(8):716–720
71. Vasa S. The implanters. In: Mysore V, ed. Hair transplantation. New Delhi: Jaypee Brothers; 2016:262–265
72. Jones R. Body hair transplant into wide donor scar. Dermatol Surg 2008;34(6):857
73. Mahadevia B. Donors other than scalp: beard and chest. In: Mysore V, ed. Hair transplantation. New Delhi: Jaypee Brothers; 2016:307–312
74. Poswal A. Use of body and beard donor hair in surgical treatment of androgenic alopecia. Indian J Plast Surg 2013;46(1):117–120
75. Bleyl SB, Braver PR, Francis-West PH. Development of skin and its derivatives. In: Schoewolf GC, ed. Larsen's textbook of embryology. 4th ed. Philadelphia: Churchill Livingstone, Elsevier; 2009:202–205
76. Schneider MR, Schmidt-Ullrich R, Paus R. The hair follicle as a dynamic miniorgan. Curr Biol 2009;19(3):R132–R142
77. Paus R, Cotsarelis G. The biology of hair follicles. N Engl J Med 1999;341(7):491–497
78. True R. FUE from the beard and body. In: Lam S, Williams K, eds. Hair transplant: follicular unit extraction. 11th ed. Vol. 4. New Delhi: Jaypee Brothers; 2016:417–434
79. Umar S. Use of body hair and beard hair in hair restoration. Facial Plast Surg Clin North Am 2013;21(3):469–477
80. Umar S. Hair transplantation in patients with inadequate head donor supply using nonhead hair: report of 3 cases. Ann Plast Surg 2011;67(4):332–335
81. Brandy DA. Chest hair used as donor material in hair restoration surgery. Dermatol Surg 1997;23(9):841–844
82. Saxena K, Savant SS. Body to scalp: evolving trends in body hair transplantation. Indian Dermatol Online J 2017;8(3):167–175
83. Umar S. Body hair transplant by follicular unit extraction: my experience with 122 patients. Aesthet Surg J 2016;36(10):1101–1110
84. Umar S. Use of beard hair as a donor source to camouflage the linear scars of follicular unit hair transplant. J Plast Reconstr Aesthet Surg 2012;65(9):1279–1280
85. Poswal A. The preshaving protocol in body hair-to-scalp transplant to identify hair in anagen phase. Indian J Dermatol 2010;55(1):50–52

22

Hair Restoration: Surgical Management of Alopecia—II

Anil K. Garg and Manoj Khanna

FUT (Strip Technique) of Hair Transplant

Introduction

Hair restoration surgery began in the 1950s with Norman Orentreich, the famous New York dermatologist, who discovered the principle of donor dominance. He used 4-mm round punch grafts from the occipital scalp to be transplanted to the frontal and midscalp regions of baldness. This concept of donor dominance still is the basis of all modern hair restoration procedures. In the early 1980s, the large 4-mm round punch containing 16 to 20 hairs was replaced by smaller punches and smaller grafts. These minigrafts were of 5 to 10 hairs and micrografts of 1 to 2 hairs. However in the late 1980s, following Headington's histological thesis of hair growing in natural clusters on the scalp of 1 to 4 hairs called "follicular units,"[1] Limmer[2] began to transplant grafts that were dissected along this natural plane. This was the birth of follicular unit transplant (FUT).

Strip harvesting for FUT began in the 1990s, and remains the golden standard of hair restoration surgery till date. In spite of numerous advertisements and intrusion by numerous faculties into this sphere, the best hair transplant surgeons still maintain that even now, "strip surgery" consists of more than 60% of their practice.

Safe Donor Area for FUT

The advantage of FUT is that maximal area of permanent hair could be harvested within safe limits[3] from the permanent hair-bearing zone and dissected into grafts, which would give a natural appearance to the transplanted scalp. It was essential to remain within the safe limits of the donor zone. For further details, refer to Chapter 21 on "Hair Restoration: Planning and Surgical Management—I" in Volume VI. The lower limit of the donor zone is the bony occipital protuberance. Hair below this bony landmark is not scalp hair but neck hair. Also, below the bony protuberance, the neck muscles will cause a pull on the suture line leading to eventual widening of the scar. To achieve a good horizontal scar, the author uses a scale to draw a transverse line passing through the occipital protuberance to limit the lower end of the incision and get a straight-line scar. If miniaturization is present in this area, which is termed as "retrograde hair loss," it is better to move the incision a little higher. Also, if more than one sitting is anticipated, it is advisable to start a little higher to be able to include the scar of the earlier surgery in the subsequent strip.

Design of Strip

The horizontal incision should end 2 cm from the postauricular hairline. For further details, refer to Chapter 21 on "Hair Restoration: Planning and Surgical Management—I" in Volume VI. The lateral extent of the donor harvest can safely reach a line drawn vertically upwards from the anterior aspect of the tragus about two finger breadth or 2 cm above the top of the ear. This is an advanced area for harvesting. It is advisable that the beginner should limit himself to the more conservative lateral limit which is 2 cm posterior to the postauricular hairline and 2 cm above the superior aspect of the ear. It is better to mark out the entire lower border of the incision from above the ear to the lateral limit on the opposite side for this helps in better delineation of the eventual stitch line and therefore gives a more aesthetic and symmetrically placed scar.

The width of the scalp to be harvested can vary from 8 to 10 mm, and if scalp laxity permits it can go up to 1.5 cm or more. But this needs experience and expertise. The scalp is maximally tense in the bony mastoid region and it is better to reduce the width in this area rather than encounter difficult closure and a wider scar. The length of the donor strip can vary from 15 to 30 cm depending on the size of the skull but is usually shorter in females. If lesser grafts are required, it is better to only use one-half of the scalp and the other virgin half can be used in the subsequent session. Hair loss is an ongoing process and is better to harvest limited hair within comfortable limits.

Strip Harvest Procedure

The donor area is usually trimmed using a guarded trimmer leaving 1 to 2 mm or a little longer hair in the area to be harvested. It is better to trim 2 to 3 mm beyond the donor area on both sides to prevent the hair entering into the incision line during closure. The upper edge is secured by transparent adhesive tape to hold the hair away from the harvest zone.

Local anesthesia as described in Chapter 21 on "Hair Restoration: Planning and Surgical Management—I" in volume VI is injected below the incision line. The author uses a multibladed knife with two blades at two ends to score the incision. This is done before normal saline or the local anesthetic solution is injected into the donor area. The author does not inject adrenaline solution into the donor area or the recipient area, although some surgeons do so to have a cleaner field of surgery. Scoring is done before infiltration and avoid the donor area becoming broader which will lead to harvesting of lesser number of grafts. Scoring can be done using a single blade or a multibladed knife.

The multiple-bladed knife, with numerous blades, causes extensive damage to the hair roots, and is obsolete. Scoring is done only into the epidermis and superficial dermis. The double-bladed knife produces two parallel cuts which will create a nice straight scar during closure (**Fig. 22.1**). The ends of the incision are joined to the lateral limits using single no. 15 blade. The trichophytic incision, which is 1 to 2 mm beyond the incision line (usually the lower one) is now marked (**Fig. 22.2**). The area is then infiltrated well with normal saline by the author in the supragaleal plane to minimize bleeding and to create a proper dissection plane. It is prudent to wait for 15 to 20 minutes before starting the procedure to allow the hydrostatic effect. The author deepens the incision on all sides into the deep dermis, but short of the hair follicles. It is extremely important to see the direction of the hair where the incision is made, and follow the angulation to avoid inadvertent damage. The entire strip is divided into three sections with the central area usually having the best quality and density of hair. The two lateral sections are further subdivided into two zones with the lateralmost temporal zones having the finest hair which are used for the hairline and especially for the temporal triangles.

The procedure can start from any one side, usually the right. The incision is deepened only into the superficial fat and then double hooks are placed on both sides and retracted to separate the incision. The donor strip to be excised is pulled firmly by double hooks (**Fig. 22.3**), while the hooks on the side of the incision which will remain is held firmly against the scalp to prevent the remnant margin separating from the depth and the galea at the base. The strip to be harvested is ripped apart from the base in the subcutaneous connective tissue plane with the help of the double hook by this "traction technique" (**Fig. 22.4**). Any fibrous adhesions creating resistance is divided with a surgical blade. The procedure is used to separate the floating island of donor strip from its base along the subcutaneous connective tissue plane. Interestingly because this opens in a natural plane on its own, most blood vessels and nerves are left undamaged in the depth and there is minimal bleeding. This also minimizes the postoperative paresthesia or anesthesia in the scalp which is a common problem encountered in many patients and can last up to 6 months or more.

Once the strip from this zone has been harvested and proper hemostasis achieved, the trichophytic incision along the zone of removed strip is excised but not deeper than 1 to 2 mm to avoid injury to the pilosebaceous elements below. The area is closed using a running 2–0 Nylon suture to oppose the incision lines. Subsequently the central zone is harvested the same way and then the lateral zone of the other side and the entire area is stitched using 2–0 Nylon temporarily, only to be reopened and closed in layers after the slits have been made (**Fig. 22.5**).

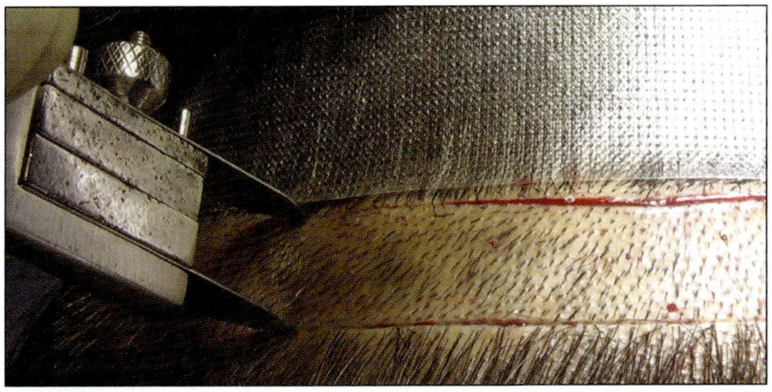

Fig. 22.1 Double-bladed knife with two no. 10 blades to give parallel incision.

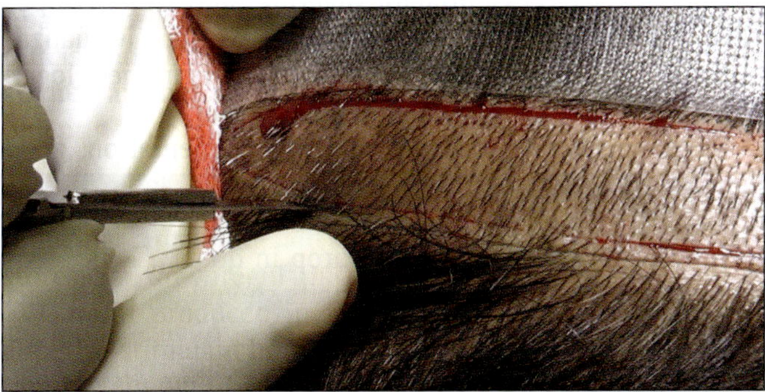

Fig. 22.2 Trichophytic incision at lower border of incision.

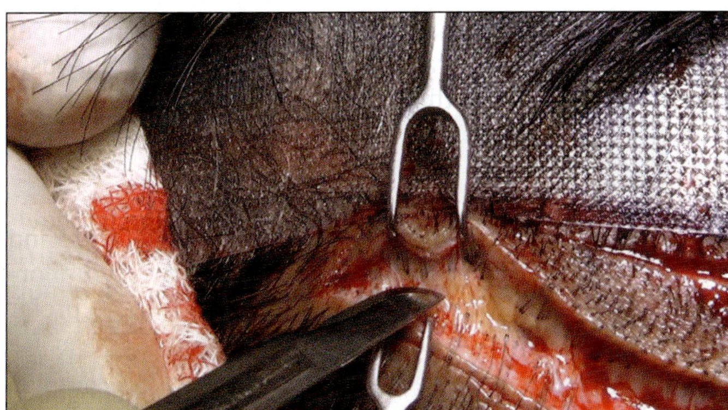

Fig. 22.3 Intact follicles along incision line deepened by retraction using double hooks.

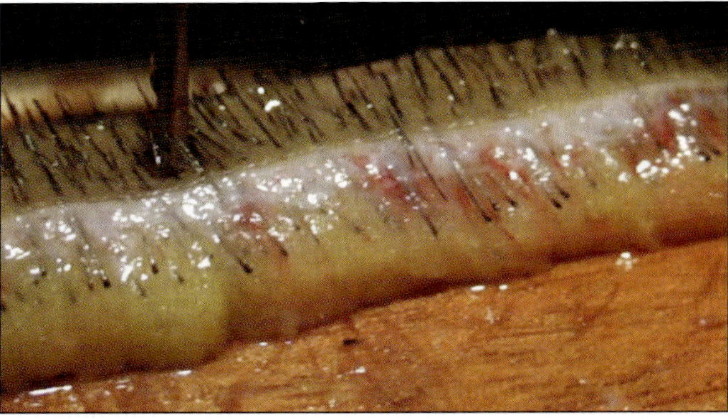

Fig. 22.4 Harvested strip by traction technique with all follicles intact.

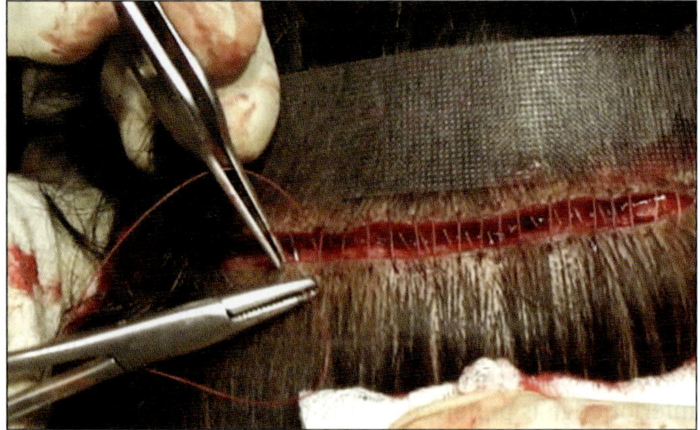

Fig. 22.12 Multiple bites of 4–0 Vicryl Rapide placed symmetrically across suture line.

The sutures are cut, if required, 10 to 14 days from the date of surgery. **Figs. 22.13 and 22.14** show long-term results of single session of FUT for hair restoration.

Harvesting Second Strip Graft

In cases where a second strip has to be taken, it is advisable to include the previous scar in the excised strip. This reduces the tension in the stitch line, making it easier to close due to removal of the scar and the scar tissue in the base. The second hair transplant should be undertaken at a gap of at least 9 months or preferably 1 year after the previous surgery. Proper head massage for 10 minutes twice daily or more for a month before the procedure increases scalp laxity. The yield of any subsequent procedure is usually less than the previous one. Sometimes the patient wants maximum harvest and is not bothered about the scar it may be better to take a strip a few mm away from the previous incision. Later, the two scars can be excised as a single strip to get a single scar in the donor zone if the patient desires.

FUT and FUE Combination

Introduction

The "combination of FUE and strip" means performing both FUE and strip graft procedures simultaneously on the scalp to harvest more hair follicles. The combined procedure is performed within the safe graft harvesting limit. If the graft is harvested beyond the safe donor area limit while attempting to harvest more graft, the transplanted hair may fall much earlier.[7] Similarly, if one intends to harvest more graft by FUT, a wider strip will be required.[8] This is likely to cause excessive postoperative pain, widening of scar or a hypertrophic scar. A careful balance needs to be struck to take advantage of both procedures, without causing

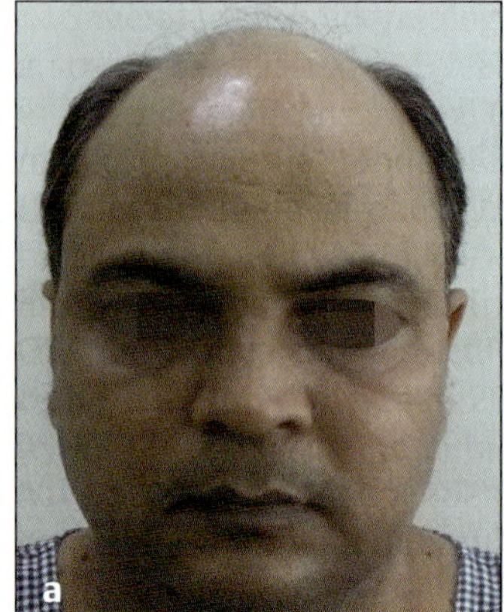

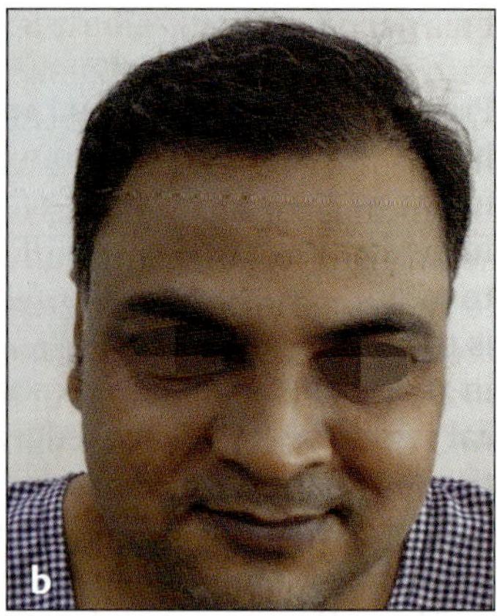

Fig. 22.13 **(a, b)** Grade 7 baldness after one session of Strip with 6,400 grafts.

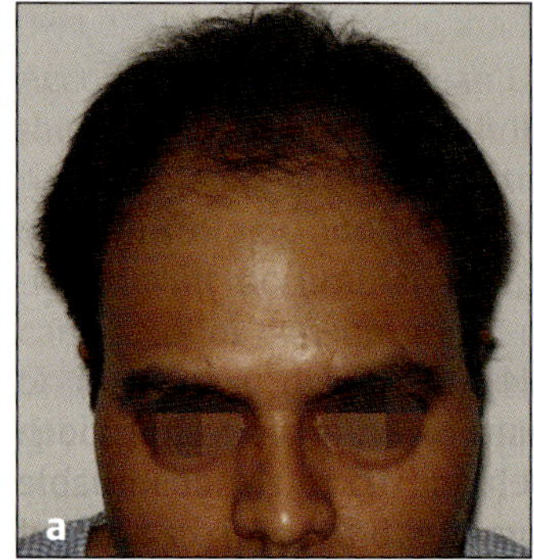

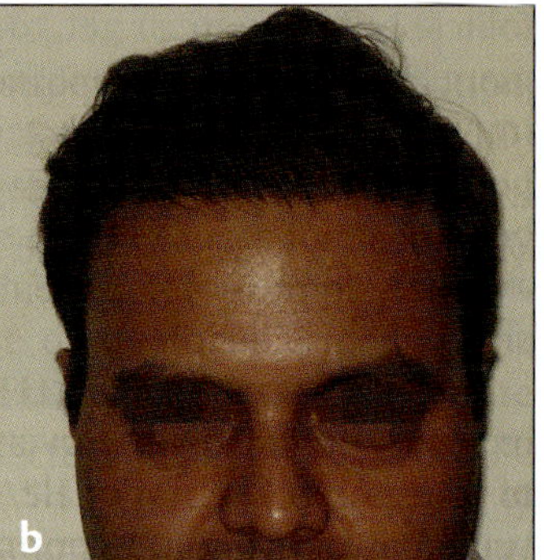

Fig. 22.14 **(a, b)** Grade 3 baldness after one session by follicular unit transplant (FUT) with 3,100 grafts.

complications of either technique. In higher grade baldness, the combination technique gives larger number of grafts. It is indicated in the patients who want to avoid multiple procedures and intend to have maximum coverage and high density in minimum sessions.[9–11]

The combination technique could be primary in which both techniques are used in the same sitting or in two different sessions.[12] This requires good planning, counseling, and discussion with patient.

Marking for strip harvest is done in relation to occipital protuberance. An additional 1 cm wide area is marked above the strip area for additional strip, in case there is need to harvest more. Rest of the safe donor area is marked for FUE harvest (**Fig. 22.15a, b**). If there is no retrograde alopecia, graft can be extracted even from the area below the planned FUT strip (**Fig. 22.15a–d**).

Procedure

Maximum utilization of donor area within a safe limit should be the ultimate aim of the hair transplantation. For this, a hair restoration surgeon must have expertise in both the techniques of strip surgery and FUE.

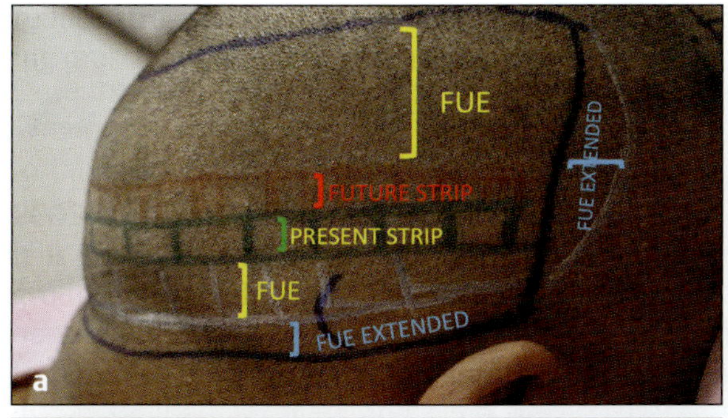

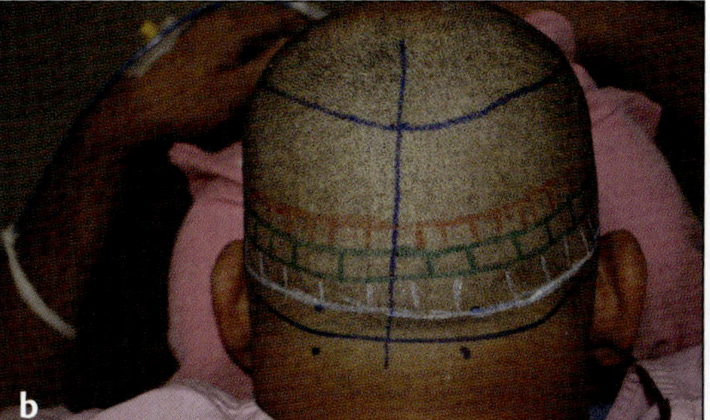

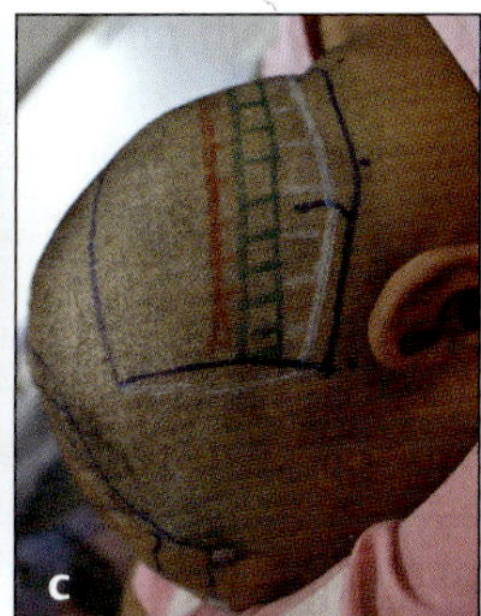

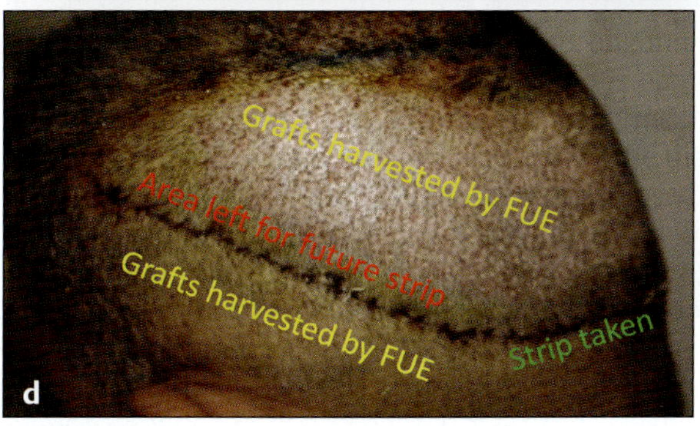

Fig. 22.15 (a–c) Donor area planning in a case of a combination method of strip and follicular unit extraction (FUE). The blue outline defines the total safe donor area. Green mark indicates the strip harvest area. Red outline marks the area of additional strip if needed. Rest of the area within the safe zone is used for FUE harvest, provided there is no sign of retrograde hair loss. **(d)** Graft harvesting by FUE and strip method. The area just above the strip suture line is left intact for future strip removal.

Primary Combination Technique

After donor anesthesia and tumescence, FUT and FUE are performed one after the another. The sequence varies from surgeon to surgeon. Many surgeons prefer to extract follicular unit from the marked area with FUE before harvesting the strip. To reduce the ischemia time, the FUE units are implanted till the slivering is done and then FUT grafts are implanted. This is the sequence followed if both the harvesting techniques are done on the same day.

Some surgeons harvest FUT strip first and close the donor wound. Slivering is done and FUT grafts are implanted. Following day FUEs are harvested and implanted. This reduces the ischemia time and avoids surgical team fatigue.

Secondary Combination Technique

This is performed in two different sittings at an interval of 9 to 12 months. If primary surgery is performed with strip, then depending upon the elasticity of scalp, strip and/or FUE are done. This again must be planned in consultation with the patient (**Fig. 22.16**).

Reconstructive Hair Transplant for Face and Scalp

Introduction

The hair follicular transplant is commonly done to treat androgenic scalp alopecia; but there are a very wide range of indications for hair transplant other than male pattern baldness. Other indications include scalp and facial scars, secondary to burn, trauma, and cancer reconstruction,[13,14] congenital conditions like facial hypotrichosis or atrichia, lowering of hairline for transgenders, cleft lip scars, alopecia following facelift, and forehead lift procedures, etc.

Beard and Moustache Reconstruction

The beard and moustache are the signs of masculinity. The trend for facial hair restoration is increasing day by day. The recent survey conducted by International Society of Hair Reconstruction Surgery (ISHRS) shows increase in demand for beard and moustache restoration from 1.5% in 2013 to 4% in 2017 and eyebrows from 4.5 to 15%, respectively.[15]

Planning for Beard and Moustache Restoration

The template of beard and moustache restoration is designed as per the requirement of the patient. Usually, such patients present with specific pattern in their mind. A final template is made, and the number of grafts is designated to cover the desired area.

The number of grafts required depends on the area to be restored and the availability of the donor area. Caution needs to be exercised while harvesting scalp hair in the first attempt as these patients may demand scalp hair transplant in future. It may be worthwhile to look for available donor hair follicles in the submandibular and neck region. The author usually uses 1,800 to 2,500 grafts for beard and

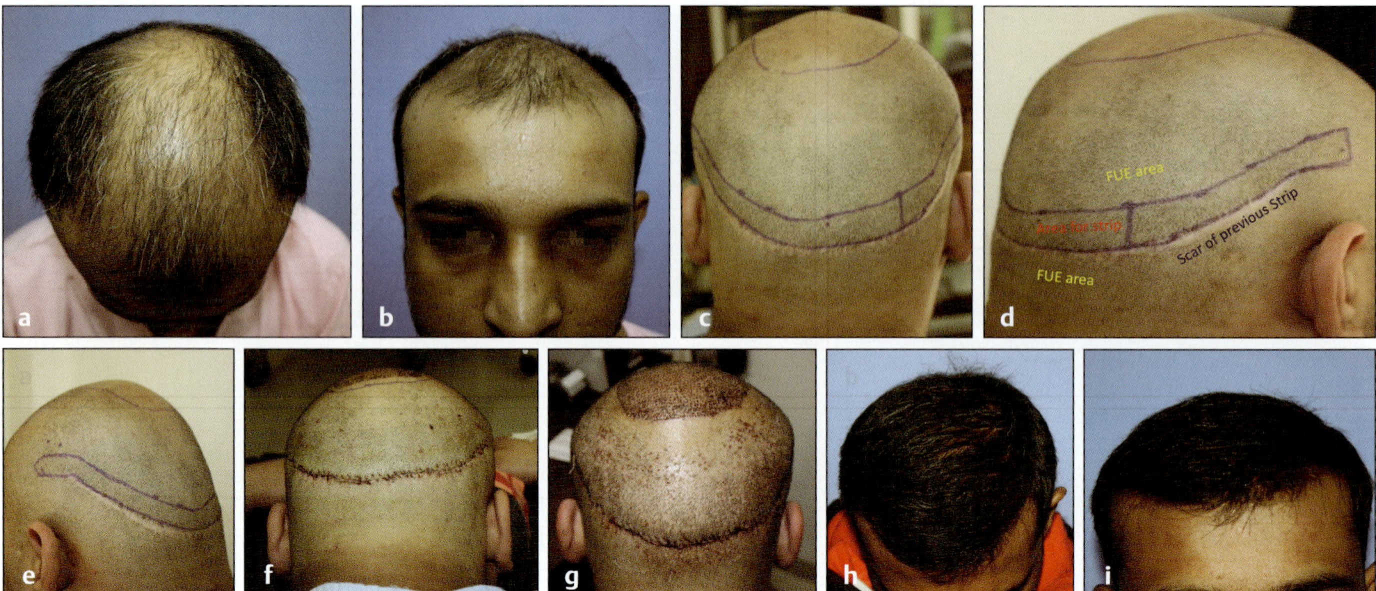

Fig. 22.16 (a, b) A 26-year-old having grade VI androgenic alopecia. Had undergone strip harvesting one-and-half years back. Presented for coverage of remaining midscalp and crown. **(c–e)** Second strip of 8 mm width and 28 cm length along with follicular unit extraction (FUE) from rest of the safe donor area has been planned. **(f, g)** Total 2,044 follicular unit transplant (FUT) grafts were harvested and at the same sitting 1,562 FU were extracted by FUE. Total 3,606 grafts were implanted over midscalp, crown, and anterior hairline. **(h, i)** Result after 1 year of follow-up.

moustache restoration. Complete moustache requires 200 to 400 grafts, goatee 300 to 500 grafts, cheek 500 to 600 grafts, and sideburn requires 300 to 400 grafts on each side. A secondary touch-up may be required in the future.

A higher density is kept in the central moustache and central area of the cheek, where two hair follicles are implanted. The author uses only single and two hair FUs to have more coverage and for naturalness. The superior border of the cheek with bumps looks more natural and attractive. Single-hair FUs are used on borders, and if available, follicles from the neck are preferred for moustache and border of the beard area.

Anesthesia

Infiltration of local anesthetic is painful over the face. It is preferable to apply prilox gel 1 hour before surgery. Anesthesia is started with facial nerve blocks, (i.e., infraorbital, mental, and auriculotemporal nerve blocks). The anesthetic solution is prepared using 1% lidocaine, 0.5% ropivacaine, with 1:100,000 adrenaline. It is advisable to use tumescence infiltration for tissue turgor, uniform long-lasting anesthesia, and hemostasis.[16]

Slits Creation and Implantation

Apart from the density, the direction, angle, and curl of hair are to be considered to give a natural look. The angle of hair is almost parallel to the skin. The hair in the central area of moustache faces downward, while in the lateral area it goes downward and laterally.

In the cheek, the direction may vary from person to person. There may be a natural whorl near the angle of the mandible. It is safer to follow the direction of existing hair in the region. If there is no hair in the region, it is better to keep the direction downwards. In the lower area of the cheek especially over the angle of the mandible, direction of the hair is usually downward and backward. In the central area of the goatee, the direction of the hair is downward and on the lateral side downward and laterally.

Facial implantation is performed using coronal slits with 19- and 20-gauge hypodermic needles or blade made in a brick pattern. The needles are bent to facilitate the flat angulation of implantation.

Postoperative Care and Instructions

Patients are instructed to avoid hot liquids and solid food on day 1. Using a straw to drink is preferred. A semiliquid diet for 2 days and face wash after 5 days of restoration is recommended. Any antibiotic cream can be applied. After 12 days of surgery, the patient is allowed to use moisturizing lotion and gentle pressure over the implanted hair to keep the angle of hair flat. It has been observed that there is a natural tendency of straightening of hair during healing; hence, gentle pressure is recommended for 4 to 6 months postprocedure. The hair is expected to grow after 4 months of surgery (**Figs. 22.17–22.20**).

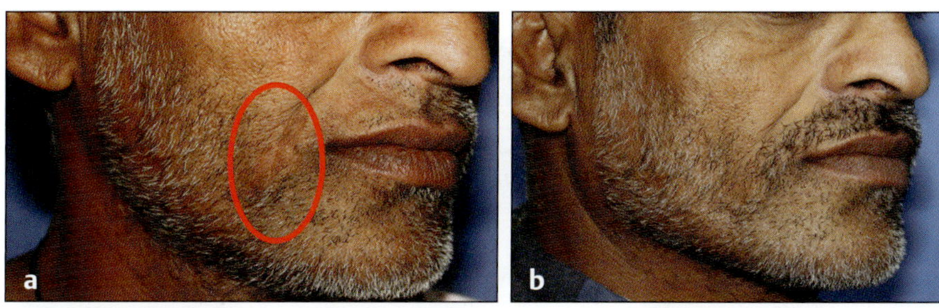

Fig. 22.17 A 34-year-old man with hypotrichosis on the right side of moustache and beard. **(a)** Preoperative, and **(b)** after implantation of 350 follicular unit (FU) grafts.

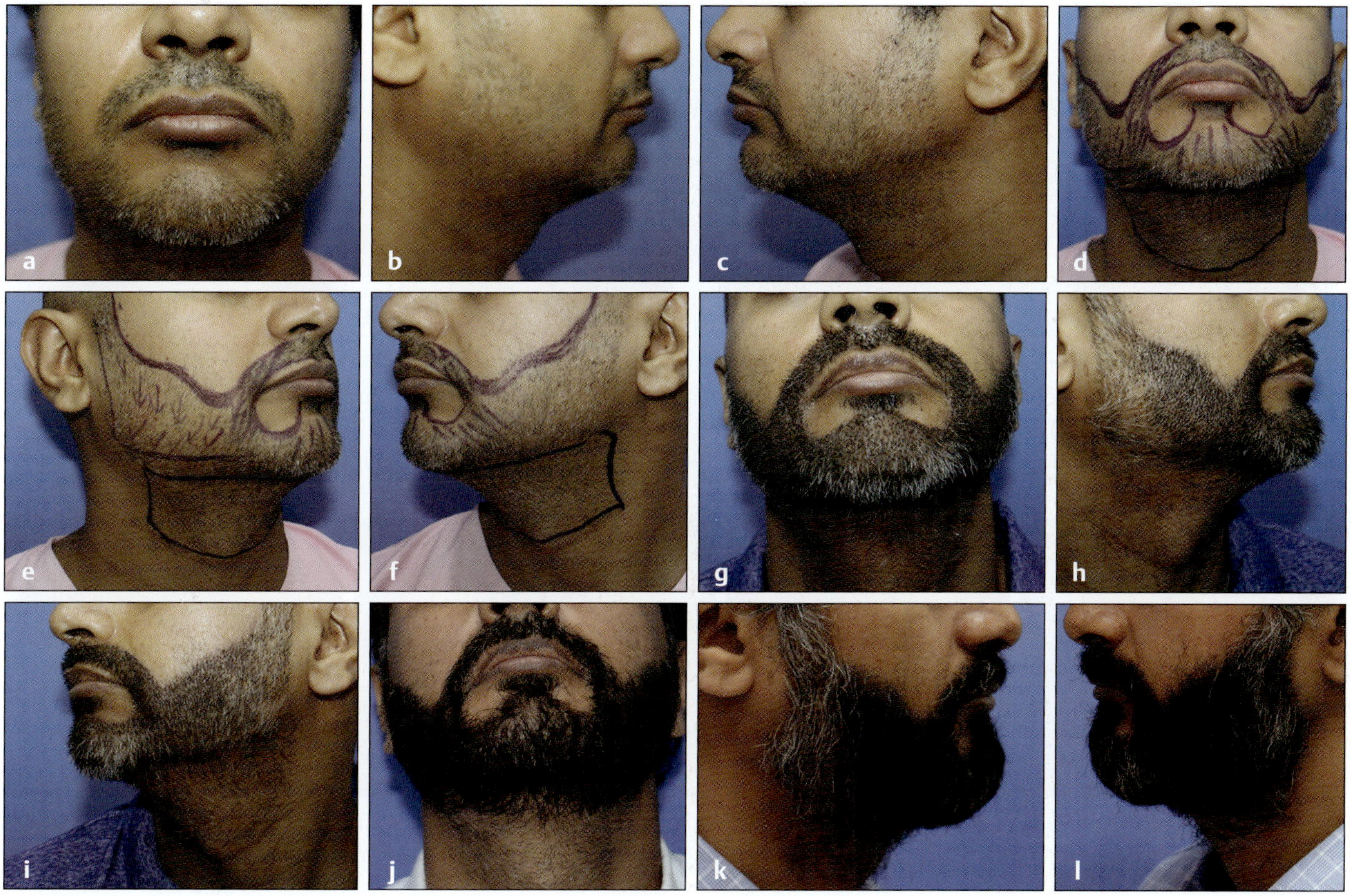

Fig. 22.18 Augmentation of beard and moustache. **(a–c)** Preoperative pictures of a young man desiring to have thick moustache, goatee area, and augmentation of superior border of cheek with bumps. **(d–f)** Planning of hair transplant. Total 2,000 follicular unit (FU) grafts were extracted from the scalp and 665 from the neck. **(g–i)** Postoperative result after implantation of 2,665 grafts. **(j–l)** Long-term follow-up result after 12 months.

Eyebrows Reconstruction

The eyebrow reconstruction is the commonest facial hair transplant procedure. The reconstruction of eyebrows has evolved from the use of full-thickness graft of strip from the scalp[17,18] to a hair-bearing flap, and finally, the use of microhair follicles transfer from the scalp.[19–21]

The shape of eyebrow varies in men and women. The women have high-arched eyebrows while male eyebrows are flat, nonarched, and masculine. Patients who come for eyebrow augmentation or reconstruction usually draw the template themselves.

The length of the eyebrow ranges from 4.0 to 5.5 cm. The eyebrows have three parts, the head (medial one-fifth), the tail (outer one-third), and body connecting the head and tail. The head is usually square or oval, 5 to 10 mm long, and its medial border corresponds with the vertical line drawn from the medial canthus of the eye. The distance between medial borders of two eyebrows is wider in females as compared

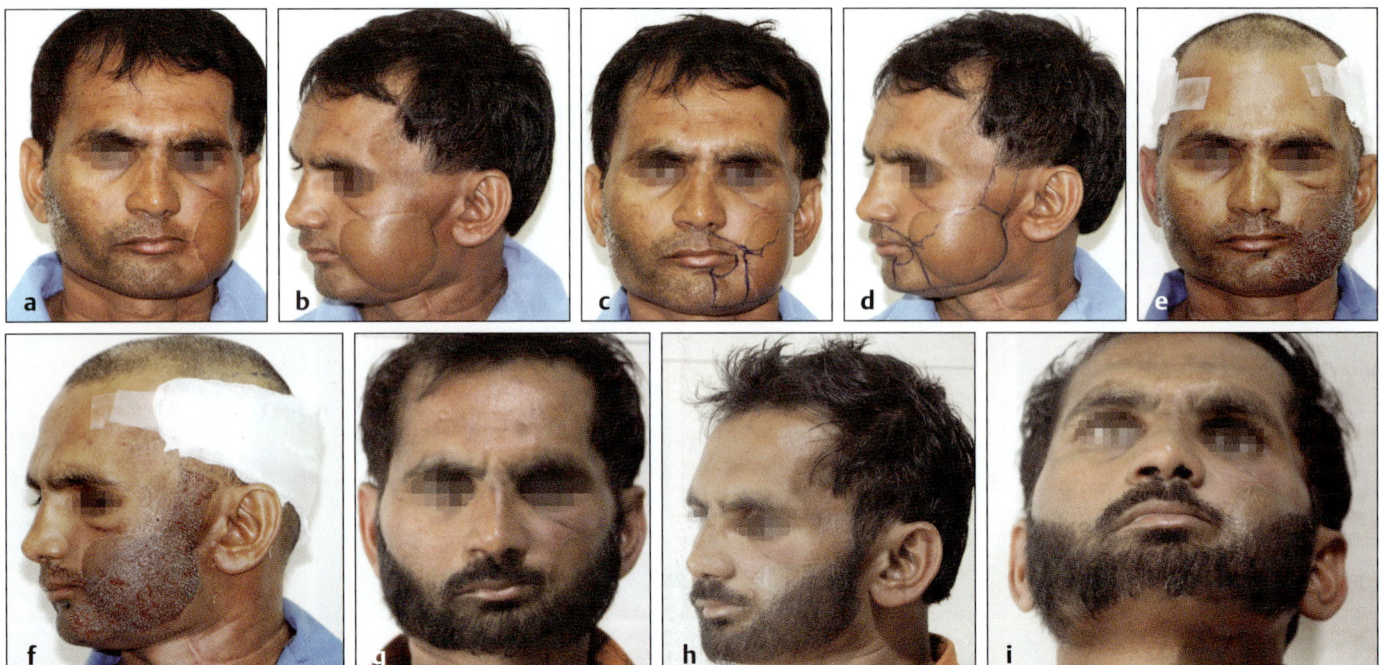

Fig. 22.19 Beard hair transplant over anterolateral thigh (ALT) flap in a 38-year-old man treated for carcinoma of buccal mucosa. **(a, b)** Left cheek reconstructed with ALT followed by radiotherapy. **(c, d)** Details of zones of beard reconstruction after 1 year of radiotherapy. **(e, f)** Total 2,100 scalp graft harvested by follicular unit extraction (FUE) and implanted. **(g–i)** One year follow-up result. (These images are providedcourtesy of Dr. Kinnar Kapadia, Ahmedabad, Gujarat, India.)

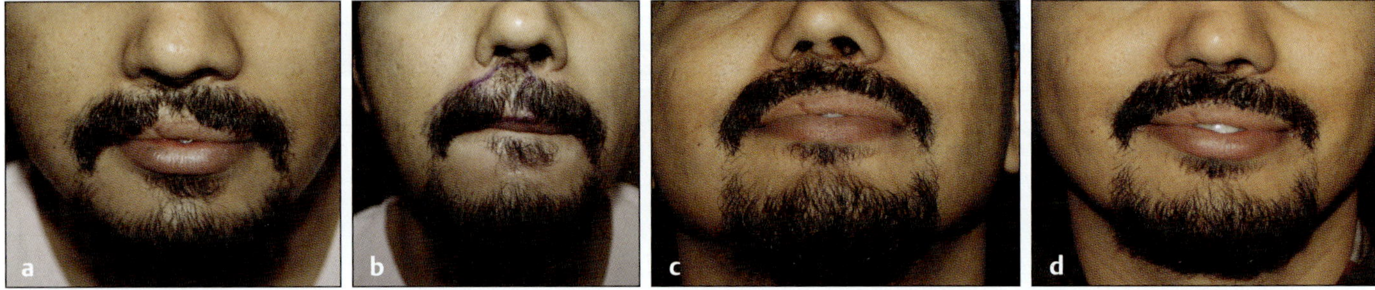

Fig. 22.20 A young boy with a cleft lip scar treated with follicular unit extraction (FUE) grafts. **(a)** Cleft lip scar. **(b)** Making of area for hair transplant. **(c)** Results, coronal view after hair transplant. **(d)** Results after hair transplant.

to their male counterparts. The body is dense, wide, 25 to 30 mm long, and the most prominent part of the eyebrows. The hair is more vertical in the head, and starts curving gradually as they move laterally.

The hair in the body of the eyebrow in its upper part is directed slightly downward, while in lower part it is slightly upward, making a crisscross pattern (**Fig. 22.21**). The tail is usually 10 mm long, having the lowest density, and descends from the peak of the arch laterally. Some women like the tail to be horizontal, and some may desire to have slightly down.

The FUs are harvested by taking a small strip from midoccipital area[22] or by FUE. The grafts are dissected under a microscope to prepare single and two follicular unit grafts. Two hair follicle grafts are needed for the body. While harvesting the hair follicles, the hair shaft shall be kept 10 to 15 mm long to know the curvature of hair. One should always keep the concavity of the hair toward the skin. The author prefers coronal slits using 20-gauge hypodermic needles. The use of implanter is a good alternative. The angle of the slits or implantation angle of hair is almost parallel to the skin (**Fig. 22.22**).

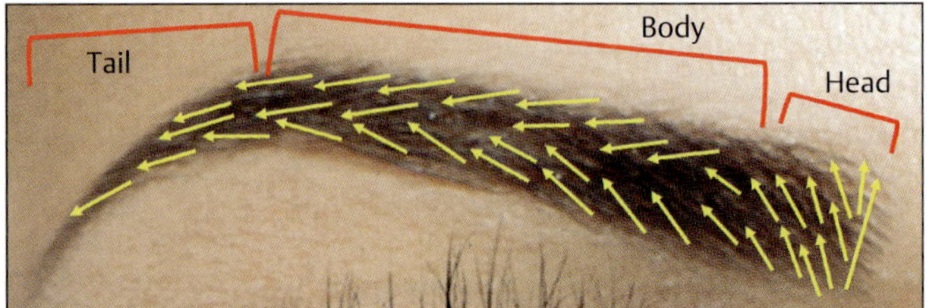

Fig. 22.21 Parts of eyebrows with hair directions in different parts.

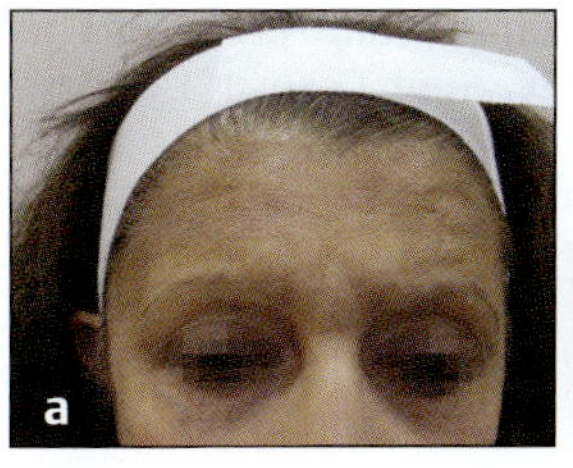
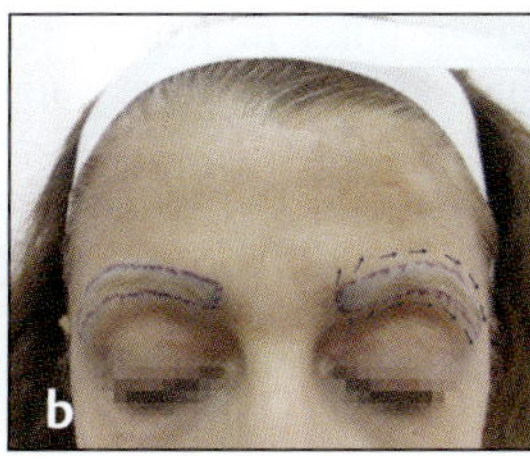
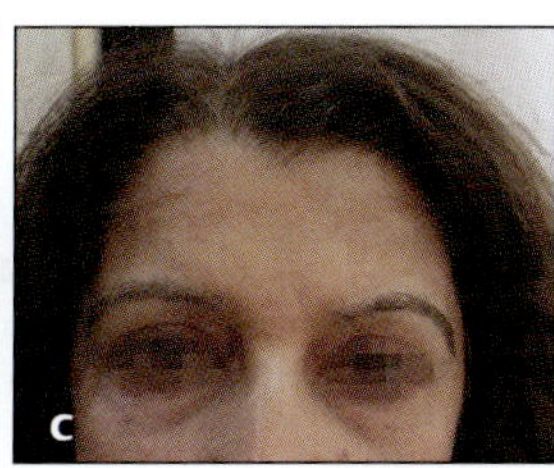

Fig. 22.22 **(a)** Senile eyebrow loss in 62-year-old female. **(b)** Planning of slits for eyebrow hair transplant. **(c)** One-year postoperative result after implanting 460 grafts (approx. 230 grafts on each side) by follicular unit extraction (FUE). (These images are provided courtesy of Dr. Sumit Agrawal, Mumbai, Maharashtra, India.)

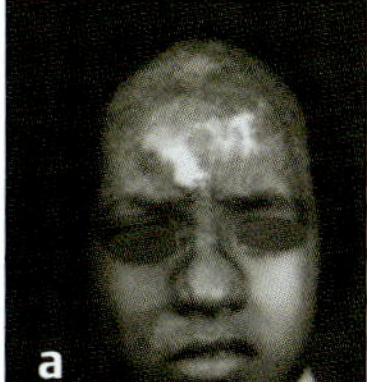
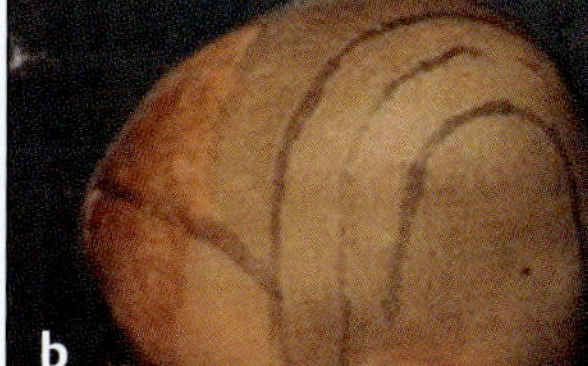
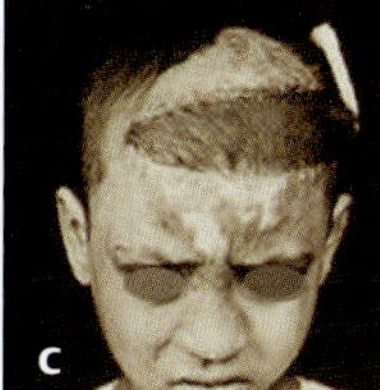
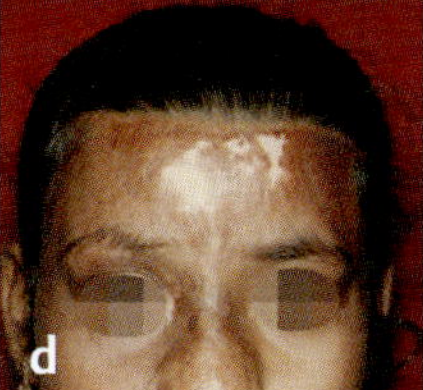
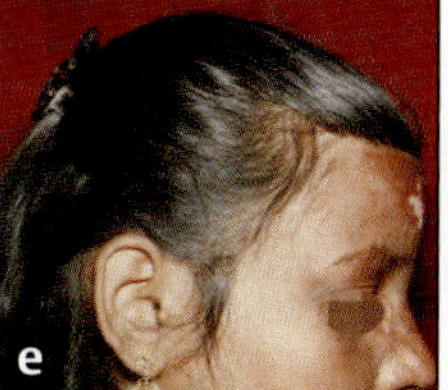
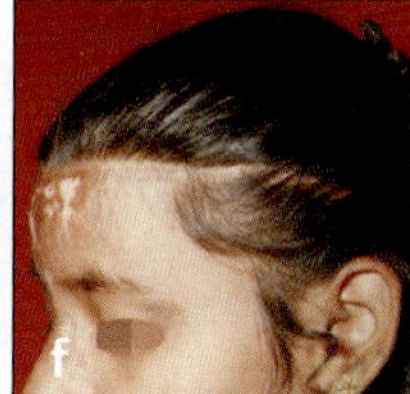

Fig. 22.23 Postburn scar alopecia managed using Juri flap. **(a)** Alopecia involving frontal area and anterior hairline with postburn hypopigmented scar. **(b)** Left-side temporoparietal Juri flap has been planned to cover the bald frontal area. **(c)** reconstructed frontal hairline after transfer of the flap. **(d–f)** Follow-up result after 3 years. The leftover bald area is well covered with long hair. Comment: Junctional scar and flat hairline are the hallmark of Juri flap. This can be corrected by transplanting few hairs to make an aesthetically pleasing female anterior hairline. A tissue expander could be used to cover the remaining scar. (These images are provided courtesy of Dr. Karoon Agrawal, New Delhi, India.)

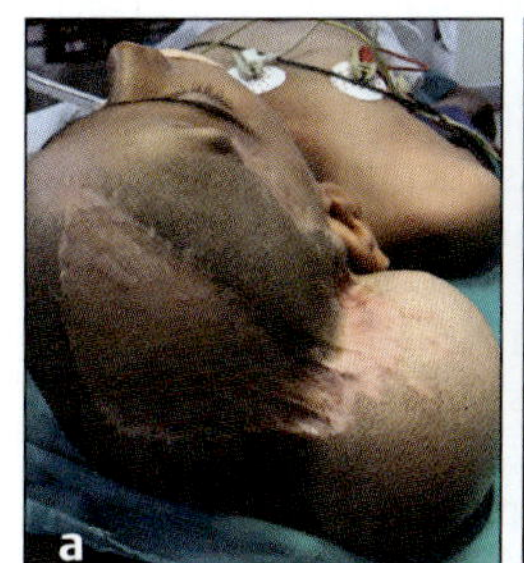
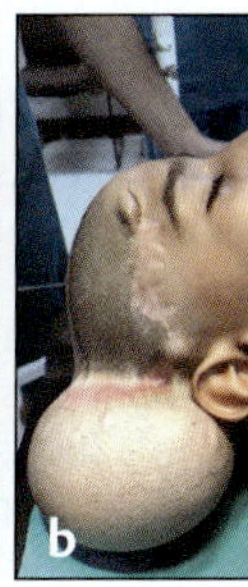
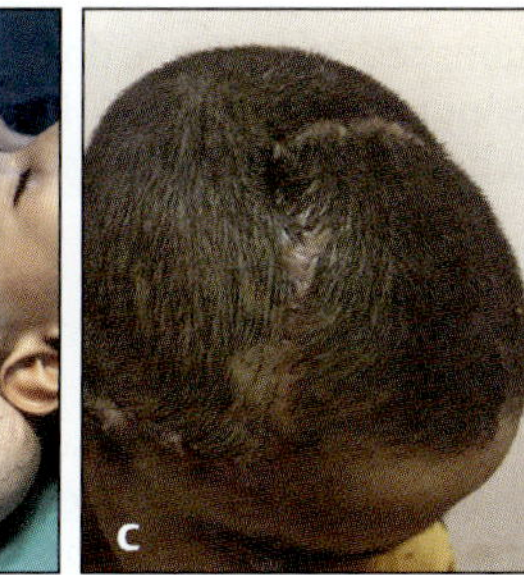
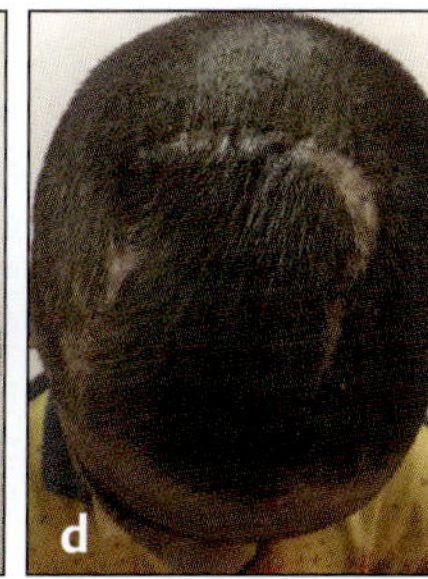

Fig. 22.24 A case of postelectric burn scar alopecia of scalp treated with tissue expansion. **(a, b)** Right frontoparietal scar of scalp with 250-mL tissue expander in situ. The expander was inflated over a period of 2 months. **(c, d)** The skin graft was excised, the tissue expander removed, and the flap has been used to cover the defect. (These images are provided courtesy of Prof. Pradeep Goil, SMS Medical College, Jaipur, Rajasthan, India.)

Postoperatively the recipient area is left open. Postoperative swelling is a common feature. Water wash is advised fifth postoperative day. After 10 days, cleaning with soap and water is permitted. Antibiotic cream or moisturizing lotion is applied gently. Hair starts growing after 3 to 4 months of implantation. The patient must be informed during preoperative consultation that the character and growth pattern of the implanted hair will be different than the original eyebrow and will have the character of donor hair. The grafts from scalp needs regular trimming.

Nonhair Transplant Methods of Surgical Hair Restoration

The hair restoration of the scalp as a surgical procedure was started way back in 1926 by Hunt,[23] as surgical excision of an alopecic patch and advancing hair-bearing scalp flap close to the alopecic patch. Passot in 1931,[24] Taabor in 1939,[25] and Lamont in 1957[26] described lateral scalp flaps for treatment of frontotemporal baldness. The publication by Juri[27] in 1975, introducing pedicle flap for frontal hairline reconstruction was a breakthrough. Initially small temporal flap was used, and later long temporo-parieto-occipital flap with two delay procedures was used. The Juri flap did not gain popularity because of the high failure rate, unnatural hair orientation, and its high density.

The detail of nonhair transplant procedures is beyond the scope of this chapter. However the options are as follows.

Full-Thickness Hair-Bearing Skin Grafts

Flap procedures:

- Local flaps: Transposition, rotation, advancement.
- Temporo-occipito-parietal pedicle/Juri flap (**Fig. 22.23**).
- Lateral scalp flap.
- Temporal vertical flap.

Alopecia Reduction Procedures

- Alopecia reduction (AR) alone and primary closure.
- Alopecia reduction with prior use of tissue expansion (**Fig. 22.24**).
- Alopecia reduction with intraoperative stretching.

Summary

The hair restoration surgery has come a long way. With time the procedure has achieved very high level of aesthetic outcome. The hair transplant is a wholesome science and art. Every surgeon has his or her preference in choosing the instruments, anesthesia, and surgical technique depending upon the experience and exposure. Overall result at the end remains the same. There is no doubt that for successful outcome every hair transplant surgeon should learn both FUT and FUE techniques and practice whatever they are comfortable with. What is ultimately required is achieving the result which makes the patient happy and the surgeon satisfied. The hair transplant surgery has a learning curve; however, it is practice that makes a surgeon perfect.

References—FUT

1. Headington JT. Transverse microscopic anatomy of the human scalp: a basis for a morphometric approach to disorders of the hair follicle. Arch Dermatol 1984;120(4):449–456
2. Limmer BL. Elliptical donor stereoscopically assisted micrografting as an approach to further refinement in hair transplantation. J Dermatol Surg Oncol 1994;20(12):789–793
3. Unger W, Solish N, Giguere D, et al. Delineating the "safe" donor area for hair transplanting. Am J Cosmet Surg 1994;11: 239–243
4. Pathomvanich D, Amonpattana K. Slivering of the donor strip in normal saline to avoid graft desiccation. Hair Transpl Forum Internat 2011;21(1):12–13
5. Garg AK, Garg S. A histological and clinical evaluation of plasma as a graft holding solution and its efficacy in terms of hair growth and graft survival. Indian J Plast Surg 2019;52(2): 209–215
6. Kim D. Planning off inferior in the Frechet and Rose trichophytic closures. Hair Transplant Forum Int 2008;18(6):211–214

References—Combination

7. Bernstein RM, Rassman WR, Anderson KW. Follicular unit extraction mega sessions: evolution of a technique. Hair Transplant Forum Int 2004;14(3):97–99
8. Garg S, Garg A. Study of ropivacaine block to reduce postoperative pain after strip harvesting, and the relationship of strip width to post-operative pain. Hair Transplant Forum Int 2019;29(5):186–189
9. Crisostomo MR. Combined strip, and FUE technique. In: Lam SM, Williams Jr K, eds. Book hair transplant 360. 1st ed. New Delhi: Published by Jaypee Brothers; 2016:383–415
10. Unger WP. My approach to the consultation. In: Unger WP, Shapiro R, Unger R, Unger M, eds. Hair transplantation. 5th ed. New York: Informa Healthcare; 2011:63–90
11. Crisostomo MR, Crisostomo MGR, Tomaz DCC, Crisóstomo MCC. Untouched strip: a technique to increase the number of follicular units in hair transplants while preserving an untouched area for future surgery. Surg Cosmet Dermatol 2011;3(4):361–364
12. Garg AK, Garg S. The use of body hair with scalp hair for "combination grafting" to enhance visual density of hair transplantation and increase coverage in advanced alopecia. Hair Transplant Forum Int 2018;28(6):217–223 10.33589/28.6.0217

References—Beard

13. Epstein J. Hair restoration to eyebrows, beard, sideburns, and eyelashes. Facial Plast Surg Clin North Am 2013;21:457–467
14. Barrera A. The use of micrografts and minigrafts for the treatment of burn alopecia. Plast Reconstr Surg 1999;103(2): 581–584
15. ISHRS. 2013 Practice census results. https://ishrs.org/media/statistics-research/
16. Kulahci M. Moustache and beard hair transplanting. In: Unger W, Shapiro R, eds. Hair transplantation. 5th ed. New York: Informa Healthcare; 2011:465

References—Eyebrows

17. Matsuda K, Shibata M, Kanazawa S, Kubo T, Hosokawa K. Eyebrow reconstruction using a composite skin graft from sideburns. Plast Reconstr Surg Glob Open 2015;3(1):e290. Published 2015 Feb 6. doi:10.1097
18. Silapunt S, Goldberg LH, Peterson SR, Gardner ES. Eyebrow reconstruction: options for reconstruction of cutaneous defects of the eyebrow. Dermatol Surg 2004;30(4 Pt 1):530–535, discussion 535
19. Scevola S, Nicoletti G, Randisi F, Faga A. Refinements in brow reconstruction: synergy between plastic surgery and aesthetic medicine. Photomed Laser Surg 2014;32(2):113–116
20. Epstein J. Eyebrow, and eyelash transplantation. In: Unger WP, ed. 5th ed. Hair transplantation. New York: Informs Healthcare; 2011:460
21. Gandelman M, Epstein JS. Hair transplantation to the eyebrow, eyelashes, and other parts of the body. Facial Plast Surg Clin North Am 2004;12(2):253–261
22. Farjo B, Farjo N, Williams G. Hair transplantation in burn scar alopecia. Scars Burn Heal 2015;1:2059513115607764

References—Nonhair Transplant Methods of Surgical Hair Restoration

23. Hunt HL. Plastic surgery of the head, face and neck. Philadelphia: Lea & Febiger; 1926
24. Passot R. Cirurgie Esthetique Pure: Techniques et Resultats. Paris, G. Doin et Cie; 1931
25. Taabor HT. The problem of premature alopecia: its surgical treatment. Minerva Dermatol 1961;36:214–217
26. Lamont ES. A plastic surgical transformation: report of a case. West J Surg, Obstet Gynecol 1957;65(3):164–165
27. Juri J. Use of parieto-occipital flaps in the surgical treatment of baldness. Plast Reconstr Surg 1975;55(4):456–460

Body Contouring

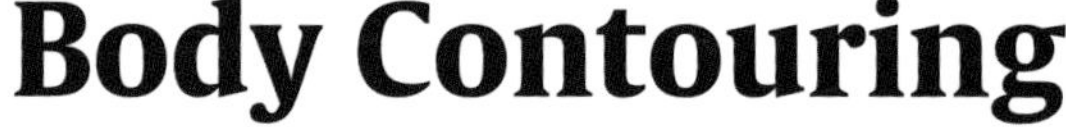

23

Obesity and Its Management

Vikas Singhal and Adarsh Chaudhary

intervention, BMI criteria be lowered by 2.5 points. Even at a BMI less than 25 a significantly higher percentage of Asian populations is diabetic and suffers from MetS.[12,13]

The Metabolic Syndrome

Several international societies such as WHO and International Diabetes Federation (IDF) recognize obesity as a part of a cluster of abnormalities called the MetS, the basic underlying cause being insulin resistance. Insulin resistance in various tissues leads to hyperglycemia, hypertriglyceridemia, and low levels of high-density lipoprotein (HDL) cholesterol. Most patients with type 2 diabetes mellitus have these features of insulin resistance and, in addition, are often hypertensive and abdominally obese. The definition of MetS initially given by WHO in 1998 considered insulin resistance as an essential component associated with metabolic problems. This has subsequently been modified by other societies, and a commonly used definition given by the IDF which considers central obesity as an essential factor is detailed in **Table 23.2**. Whether obesity is the cause or the effect of MetS remains open to debate. However, identification of this cluster of abnormalities in an individual confers a substantial additional cardiovascular risk over and above the risk associated with each individual abnormality.[14]

Causes of Obesity

While lifestyle changes due to a change in environmental factors have globally led to rise in prevalence of obesity, it has also been recognized that they are just one of the several reasons. Particularly in those suffering from severe obesity at an early age, genetic factors may be more important. Apart from the major interplay of genetic and lifestyle factors which account for most obese patients, it is imperative to exclude hormone disorders and exogenous factors such as some commonly used medicines that may cause weight gain.

Genetic Causes

It has been shown that genes influence several mechanisms that contribute to obesity such as dietary intake, metabolism, and physical activity (**Fig. 23.2**).[15] Whitaker et al showed that the odds ratio for obesity in adulthood associated with having one obese parent was 2.2 at 15 to 17 years of age.[16] If both the parents are obese, the risk of the child being obese is three to four times. Studies of adopted children have shown their BMI is much more likely to be similar to the biological parents than the adoptive parents, hence emphasizing genetics over lifestyle.[17]

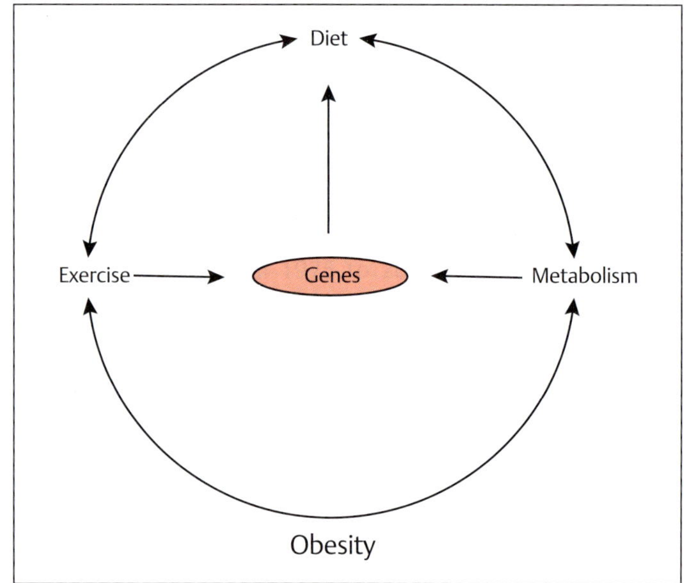

Fig. 23.2 Genetics, environment, and obesity causation.

Table 23.2 WHO and IDF definitions of the metabolic syndrome

Metabolic syndrome	WHO (1998)	IDF (2005)
Essential	Insulin resistance or type 2 diabetes plus any two of five below	Central obesity (waist circumference criteria specific to population) plus any two of four below
Obesity	BMI >30 kg/m^2 or waist: hip ratio (WHR) >0.90 (male) or >0.85 (female)	Central obesity as above
Hyperglycemia	As above, either impaired fasting glucose or impaired glucose tolerance	Fasting glucose >100 mg/dL
Dyslipidemia	Triglyceride >150 or HDL <35 (male) or <39 (female)	Triglyceride >150 or on Rx
Dyslipidemia second criteria		HDL <40 mg/dL (male) or <50 mg/dL (female) or on Rx
Hypertension	>140/90 mm Hg	>130 mm Hg systolic or >85 mm Hg diastolic or on Rx
Other criteria	Microalbuminuria	

Abbreviations: BMI, body mass index; HDL, high-density lipoprotein; IDF, International Diabetes Federation; WHO, World Health Organization.

Several mutations in the satiety hormone leptin gene (obesity gene) have been implicated in obesity development. Leptin acts as an adipocytokine that regulates food intake and energy expenditure. When adipose tissue stores are high, leptin is stimulated. Leptin binds to its receptor in the hypothalamus and in turn stimulates the pro-opiomelanocortin (POMC)/cocaine- and amphetamine-regulated transcript (CART) neurons which produce the anorexigenic peptides (primarily melanocyte-stimulating hormone) and inhibit the orexigenic neuropeptides. The net effect of leptin is to reduce food intake and promote energy expenditure. Mutations of the melanocortin 4 receptor (MC4R) also lead to loss of satiety sense which causes obesity.

Syndromic Obesity

Obesity may be part of a syndrome due to one or several genetic mutations. Most of these syndromes are associated with developmental disorders and mental retardation. Prader-Willi syndrome is the most common polygenic syndrome characterized by obesity onset in early childhood, and it is associated with hyperphagia, short stature, and small hands and feet.[18] Other syndromes, such as Bardet-Biedl (Laurence-Moon syndrome) and Wilson-Turner syndrome, also typically present in early childhood, and super obesity is a feature of these. Children and adolescents presenting with super obesity should be evaluated by a pediatrician for genetic and hormonal causes of obesity as some of them are quite treatable.

Hormonal Causes

Several endocrine disorders account for secondary causes of obesity in children and adolescents.[19] These causes may be central due to disorders of the hypothalamus or secondary hypopituitarism. The common ones being disorders of thyroid, pancreas, adrenals, and sex hormones. Morbid obesity in children and adolescents requires evaluation and exclusion of hormonal disorders.

Women tend to gain weight after menopause due to change in the estrogen-to-progesterone ratios. Several neurohumoral pathways are regulated by the gut and adipocyte hormones such as ghrelin, leptin, and adiponectin which play a major role in obesity homeostasis.

Hypothalamic Obesity

Hypothalamic obesity is due to damage to the hypothalamic structures by various causes such as tumors (craniopharyngioma), trauma, radiotherapy, and genetic disorders such as Prader-Willi syndrome. Some causes of secondary hypopituitarism are growth hormone deficiency, diabetes insipidus, hypogonadotropic hypogonadism, and central hypothyroidism. Children typically have reduced muscle mass, central obesity, puffy face, reduced sexual development, and sometimes are of short stature with low-energy levels. The treatment strategy is based on the primary underlying cause and may include somatostatin analogues, sympathomimetics, triiodothyronine, sibutramine, surgery, etc.

Cushing Disease

An adenoma of the pituitary gland can lead to large amounts of adreno-cortico-tropic hormone (ACTH) secretion which in turn leads to hypercortisolism and hence weight gain. Typically, patients have moon-like facies, buffalo hump, and central obesity associated with diabetes. Preliminary evaluation is done by testing the morning 8 am cortisol level and dexamethasone suppression test.

Thyroid Disorders

Thyroid hormones control the metabolism. Hypothyroidism can lead to fluid retention, slower than normal metabolism and weight gain. Low T3, T4, and high thyroid-stimulating hormone (TSH) are present. However, obesity in itself can be a stress factor leading to mild TSH elevation, so generally mild elevation of TSH up to 8 in obese patients with normal T3 and T4 does not require treatment as it is the effect of obesity rather than the cause.

Gut Hormone Disorders

Apart from leptin, two other neurohumoral hormones adiponectin and ghrelin have been found to be the key in obesity pathogenesis. We have already discussed the major role of leptin in obesity regulation.

Adiponectin is produced mainly by the adipocytes. It stimulates oxidation of fatty acids in the muscle, hence reducing circulating fatty acids, reducing adipose tissue stores, and downregulating obesity.

Ghrelin produced in the stomach is an orexigenic or appetite-stimulant hormone. Diets that are based on starvation are shown to increase the ghrelin levels which is why they may not work. Several therapies for obesity are based on ghrelin inhibition. Bariatric surgeries such as sleeve gastrectomy and gastric bypass have been shown to reduce ghrelin levels, and this is thought to be one of the major mechanisms of weight loss and metabolic improvements after the surgery.

Other gut hormones such as glucagon-like peptide-1 (GLP-1) behave in a manner similar to insulin and hence are also known as incretins. They improve the insulin sensitivity and inhibit glucagon, which metabolizes sugars and induces lipolysis. GLP-1 agonists such as liraglutide not only are used as a treatment for type 2 diabetes but also are used as antiobesity drugs in higher doses. Bariatric surgeries where the proximal foregut is bypassed have been shown to increase the incretins and reduce anti-incretins (peptide YY, etc.) which is believed to be the major mechanism that confers metabolic benefits immediately after the surgery although the weight loss takes time.

Drug-Induced Obesity

Several commonly prescribed drugs lead to weight gain. Not only can obesity be due to eating disorders and mental health problems but the treatment can further lead to weight gain. Most antipsychotic drugs and common antidepressants lead to weight gain as summarized in **Table 23.3**. Glucocorticoids in high doses also lead to obesity. With improved glycemic control after patients are started on insulin or oral hypoglycemic agents such as sulfonylureas, they often gain weight, sometimes making it further difficult to control the glucose. If patients are on drugs with the potential for weight gain, an attempt should be made to substitute these with drugs that are weight neutral or promote weight reduction.

Dietary Causes

An unhealthy diet has a major implication in obesity causation. It is known to be the predominant factor when compared to lack of physical activity and metabolism in causation of obesity. It is extremely difficult to compensate a poor diet with exercise. An unhealthy diet may be due to several reasons, both genetic and environmental. Changes in diet pattern due to easy access to energy-rich processed foods have been felt to be a major factor contributing to the exponential rise in obesity world over in the past two decades. Diet is seen to have lot of variation with ethnicity, geography, and socioeconomic patterns. Even within India, different patterns of diet have been identified. Some North Indian diets may have a high proportion of cereals and oils while staple South Indian diets on the other hand tend to be rice based with a varying proportion of meats.[20]

High-energy processed foods and beverages, which are rich in fats and carbohydrates, are implicated in most obesogenic diets. Sweets, baked items, snacks, and carbonated beverages have been found to be disproportionately high in typical diets of obese individuals.[21] The portion size may be another factor when food availability is not a problem. Diet assessment when treating obesity hence requires a detailed food diary and thorough assessment by a nutritionist.

Table 23.3 Drugs causing weight gain

Antipsychotics	Most subgroups
Antidepressants	Tricyclic antidepressants, MAO inhibitors
Anticonvulsants	Valproate, carbamazepine
Antihistaminergic	Cyproheptadine, flunarizine
Antidiabetics	Sulfonylureas, insulin preparations
Glucocorticoids	High doses
Beta-blockers	Nonselective, (e.g., propranolol)
Sex hormones	Estrogens, megestrol acetate, tamoxifen
Others	Some antineoplastic drugs, oral contraceptives

Abbreviation: MAO, monoamine oxidase.

Weight gain is common after cessation of smoking. This may be due to nicotine withdrawal that leads to increased appetite. It is common to gain 4 to 5 kg weight in few months after stopping smoking, although the weight gain tends to plateau within a year of stopping, and using nicotine replacement has been shown to reduce weight gain.[22]

Heavy alcohol intake especially beer and whiskey can over time lead to weight gain. While mild-to-moderate amount of alcohol intake usually does not cause weight gain and has even been shown to have a protective effect in some studies, heavy intake is associated with obesity due to added calories from the alcohol, associated consumption of fatty snacks, etc.[23]

Eating Disorders

Almost 30% of obesity is associated with some eating disorder. Hence a psychological evaluation is an essential component of managing obesity. Bulimia, depression, anxiety disorder, or stress-related eating due to various stressors such as work stress and sexual abuse need to be screened. Several questionnaires have been developed to screen for eating disorders. One of these is the SCOFF questionnaire, where if two or more questions are answered as yes, the sensitivity for identifying an eating disorder such as anorexia and bulimia is high.[24]

The SCOFF questions:

- Do you make yourself **S**ick because you feel uncomfortably full?
- Do you worry that you have lost **C**ontrol over how much you eat?
- Have you recently lost more than **O**ne stone (14 lb) in a 3-month period?
- Do you believe yourself to be **F**at when others say you are too thin?
- Would you say that **F**ood dominates your life?

Physical Activity

A sedentary lifestyle lowers energy expenditure and promotes weight gain. Physically passive behavior or inactivity such as sitting for prolonged time, watching television, etc., promotes obesity. A large cross-sectional survey by Indian Council for Medical Research from different zones of India showed that a vast majority of responders were physically inactive and less than 10% were performing any recreational physical activity.[25] This may be due to several factors including cultural and socioeconomic reasons. Gross differences have emerged due to urbanization in India, with studies showing urban men may be five times less physically active than rural men, and urban women seven times less physically active than rural women.[26] Physical inactivity has compounded the twin epidemics of obesity and diabetes in India.

Daily energy expenditure has several components apart from exercise-related physical activity, including the basal metabolic rate (BMR), thermic effect of food (TEF), and nonexercise activity thermogenesis (NEAT). Sitting for prolonged periods over 8 hours daily has been shown to confer similar risk of cardiovascular problems as smoking one pack of cigarettes. NEAT is shown to have wide variation in calorie consumption among individuals.[27] NEAT typically includes the energy consumed in all activities other than exercise, sleeping, and food digestion. While BMR and TEF are largely nonmodifiable, NEAT can be modified. Walking is a major influence on NEAT. Increasing NEAT by walking has been shown to make a substantial difference in energy consumption.[28,29]

Pathogenesis of Obesity

As we can tell from the various possible causes of obesity, it is a complex multifactorial disease. The basic underlying physiology is an imbalance between energy production and energy consumption. There are several mechanisms that control the energy balance. Afferent pathways from the stomach, intestines, pancreas, and other glands act via gut hormones, leptin, etc. to stimulate the central system primarily in the hypothalamus. This then acts via efferent pathways to control and balance the food intake with energy consumption (**Fig. 23.3**). There are several points of potential disruption of this pathway that can lead to obesity.

Clinical Effects of Obesity

Obesity is similar to cancer, in that it can affect every organ of the body. The common comorbid conditions are as shown in **Fig. 23.4**. We have already discussed how visceral obesity increases the chances of MetS, which typically includes high blood pressure, dyslipidemia, and type 2 diabetes apart from obesity. We have also discussed how MetS predisposes to an additional risk of cardiovascular complications. We will review some common obesity-associated conditions.

Diabetes Mellitus

It is estimated that almost 85% of type 2 diabetics are overweight, and approximately 30% of obese patients have type 2 diabetes due to several common factors.[30] With as little as 5 to 10 kg weight loss, the glycemic control is seen to improve irrespective of the BMI. The coexistence of diabetes and obesity in epidemic proportions has been referred to as the diabesity epidemic with measures suggested to intervene early.[31]

Obstructive Sleep Apnea (OSA)

OSA patients suffer from periodic cessation of breathing during sleep. It is usually due to the disruption of airflow in the upper respiratory system due to increased neck girth and poor compensation of the pharyngeal anatomy. Patients with OSA usually present to clinic with day time somnolence,

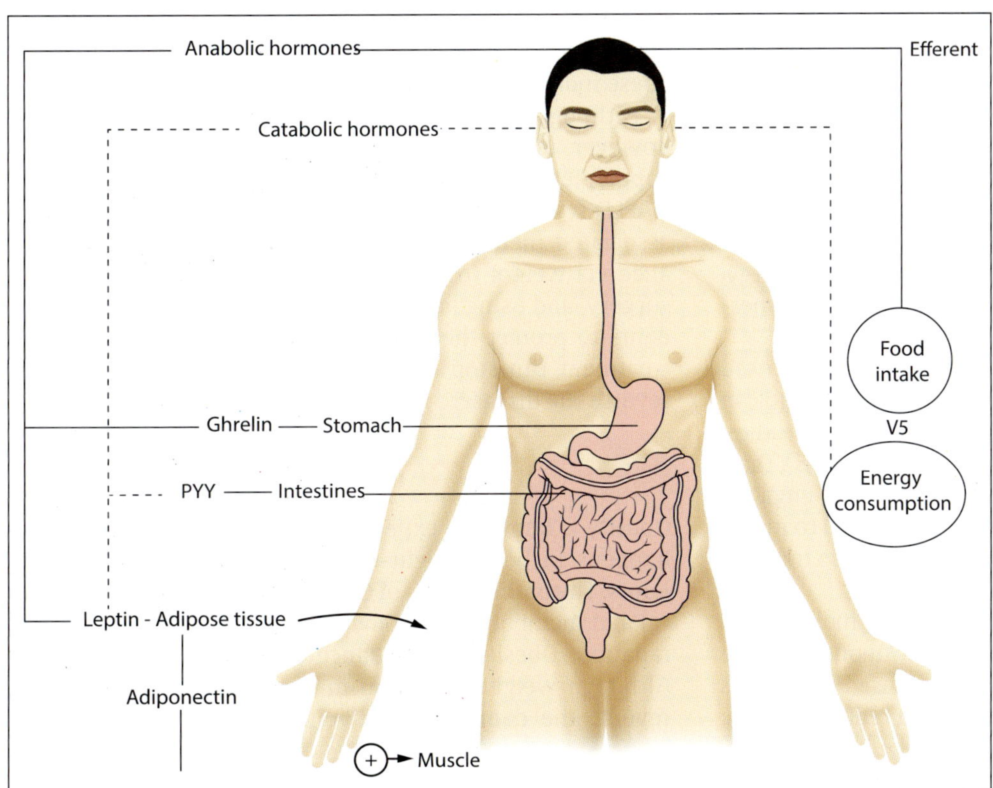

Fig. 23.3 The energy regulation pathways whose dysregulation leads to obesity.

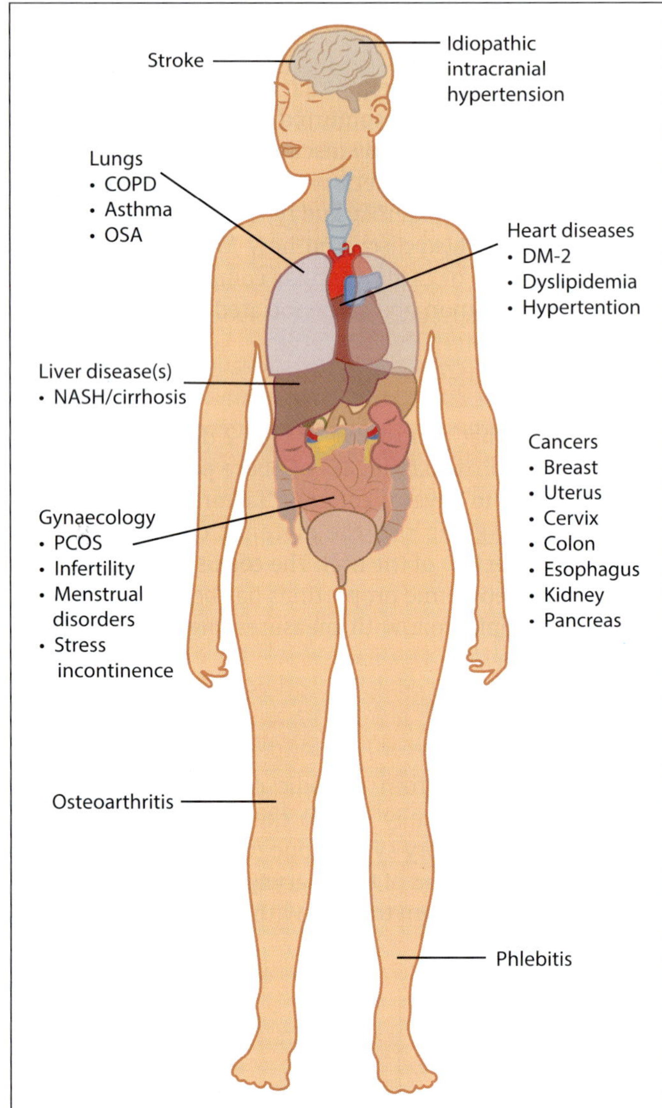

Fig. 23.4 Common obesity-associated comorbid conditions.

snoring, waking up not feeling refreshed, increased lethargy, and weight gain. OSA over time leads to pulmonary hypertension that can progress to right heart failure.

The Epworth sleep scale is a scoring system that is used to risk-stratify patients for likelihood of sleep apnea and can be used for screening purposes in clinic for sleep studies. Respondents are asked to rate, on a 4-point scale (0–3), their usual chances of dozing off or falling asleep while engaged in eight different activities.[32] Sleep studies are used to measure the oxygen levels of patients at night; they also monitor activity levels and wakefulness.

Management of OSA includes weight loss, smoking cessation, reduced alcohol intake, and continuous positive airway pressure (CPAP). CPAP machines are used in patients to effectively keep airways open in a bid to reduce hypoxic episodes.

Several large epidemiological studies have demonstrated a strong association between weight gain and an increase in the odds of developing OSA. In one study it was estimated that 58% of moderate-to-severe OSA was a result of the development of obesity.[33] Hamilton and Joosten found that patients with mild OSA who gained 10% of their baseline weight had a sixfold-increased risk of progression of OSA and conversely argued that an equivalent weight loss could result in more than 20% improvement in OSA severity. Additionally, cardiometabolic risks associated with OSA have been found independent of weight. Sleep duration and consistency are vital in regulating leptin and ghrelin levels, suggesting that OSA patients will likely find weight management challenging, leading to a vicious cycle of metabolic problems.[34]

Nonalcoholic Steatohepatitis (NASH)

According to the American Gastroenterological Association, the diagnosis of nonalcoholic fatty liver disease (NAFLD) requires evidence of hepatic steatosis, either by imaging or by histology, and that there are no causes for secondary hepatic fat accumulation including, for example, significant alcohol consumption, use of steatogenic medication, or hereditary disorders.[35] NAFLD encompasses the entire spectrum of fatty liver diseases, ranging from fatty liver to steatohepatitis to cirrhosis. NASH requires the presence of hepatic steatosis and inflammation with hepatocyte injury/ballooning with or without fibrosis. Notably, this can progress to cirrhosis, liver failure, and, on occasion, liver cancer. NAFLD is currently the most common form of liver disease in developed countries with an estimated prevalence of 20 to 30%, which increases to 50% in diabetics and to 70% in obese individuals.[36]

Although the gold standard for diagnosis is a liver biopsy; however, ultrasound can be indicative and can be further supplemented by a fibroscan. Treatment strategies for NAFLD revolves around the identification and treatment of associated metabolic conditions, improving insulin resistance via weight loss, exercise, pharmacotherapy, bariatric surgery, and using hepatoprotective agents such as antioxidants to protect the liver from secondary insults.[37] Timely treatment can stop the progression to cirrhosis and even reverse the disease.

Osteoarthritis (OA)

Obesity is known to expedite joint damage due to OA. This happens in both weight-bearing and non-weight-bearing joints. The pathogenesis of OA is mediated by both mechanical and metabolic factors including cytokine-mediated degradation. Obesity can enhance both these mechanisms.[38] Although weight reduction in obese individuals does not reverse the damage to the joint but has been shown to reduce stress on the joint, reducing pain, gradually improving muscle tone, and can greatly improve mobility.

Polycystic Ovarian Syndrome (PCOS)

PCOS is the most common endocrine disorder in women. It is present in 12 to 21% of women of reproductive age group and largely goes undetected. It is associated with obesity and MetS. The prevalence of PCOS has been found to be more than 30% in women with BMI >30. It is a condition typified by hyperandrogenism. Its presenting features can range from subtle hirsutism to oligomenorrhea and infertility. Polycystic ovarian syndrome is named such due to the fact that it is a syndrome that requires the presence of a number of clinical features to meet the diagnostic criteria. The most common diagnostic criteria used are the Rotterdam criteria. The Rotterdam criteria require the presence of two of the following: oligo/anovulation, hyperandrogenism (clinical hirsutism or biochemical), or polycystic ovaries on ultrasound.[39]

The condition is thought to stem from both environmental and genetic factors. Initially there is an increase in the release of gonadotropin-releasing hormone (GnRH) from the hypothalamus which increases the levels of luteinizing hormone (LH). The increase in LH leads to increase in androgen production by the theca cells. The testosterone/androgen is converted into estrone in the adipose tissues which suppresses follicle-stimulating hormone (FSH) production. The result of this imbalance is that follicular maturation is arrested due to low FSH and low estradiol which leads to the accumulation of immature follicles in the ovaries.[40] Increased central obesity and insulin resistance are commonly seen in females with PCOS and are contributing factors to infertility.[41]

Treatment is multipronged and depends on the symptoms that the patient finds most distressing. The aim of weight reduction is to improve fertility. Reduction in weight leads to lower testosterone levels, lower insulin resistance, and lower diabetes risk. Women are advised to maintain a healthy weight with a BMI between 19 and 25. This can be achieved through following a diet-and-exercise routine. Losing as little as 5% weight has been shown to restore menstrual cycle regularity and ovulation, thus improving fertility, and significantly reducing the risk of diabetes and cardiometabolic complications. Metformin at a dose of 500 mg twice daily can aid in weight loss and improve fertility. Clomiphene citrate is a medication used to increase ovulation, in conjunction with advised weight loss.[42]

Obesity and Cancers

Obesity has been determined to have a causal role in several cancers, particularly breast, uterus, colon, kidney, pancreas, esophagus. In nonsmokers, obesity has been shown to be the single largest preventable cause of cancer. Several mechanisms have been proposed to explain the increased incidence of several cancers in obese patients including DNA damage due to the chronic inflammatory state, high levels of insulin and insulin-like growth factors, and high levels of estrogens produced from adipocytes.[43,44]

Not only are these cancers seen more often in obese patients but the overall risk of dying from the cancer is much higher. In a study Calle et al demonstrated that all-cause mortality in cancer patients with BMI more than 40 was 52% higher in males and 62% higher in females compared to those with a BMI less than 40.[45]

Mental and Physical Disability

Irrespective of the comorbidities, obesity can cause a lot of mental and physical disabilities. The stigma of obesity can lead to obese individuals getting secluded with less social support and fewer social networks. Such factors can put obese individuals at greater risk of developing psychological distress, and consequently, anxiety disorders.[46] The anxiety disorders may also conversely lead to weight gain and obesity. Severe stress can disrupt the hypothalamic-pituitary-adrenal axis which can lead to appetite dysregulation, with increased cravings for high-sugar and high-fat foods.

Scott et al used the World Mental Health Survey Initiative to analyze the association between anxiety and obesity in more than 62,000 participants worldwide. The results showed a pooled odds ratio of 1.5 for severe obesity with anxiety disorders. As also noted in other studies, the association was stronger in women and younger people.[47]

Obesity limits physical activity and patients enter a vicious cycle of weight gain and limitation of activity which ultimately impairs the quality of life (QOL). The impairment in QOL has been shown to get worse with increasing class of obesity.[48]

Evaluation

Body Mass Index (BMI)

Although BMI categorization is widely used, it has several limitations due to its reliance on only weight and height of an individual. Other factors of importance such as abdominal adiposity, age, ethnicity, muscle mass, or gender are not considered.[49,50] BMI is unable to differentiate between lean mass and adipose tissue. For example, athletes and bodybuilders, by BMI criteria usually get classified as overweight or even obese.[51]

As BMI does not include any measurement of the waist, it cannot assess central obesity, which is a recognized risk factor in the development of cardiovascular diseases. This is a major limitation in certain ethnicities such as the Asian population as even at a lower weight (less BMI) due to high body fat ratio, particularly visceral fat, they are at a much higher risk of cardiometabolic complications. Particularly in the overweight category by BMI it becomes more important to use additional measures of obesity such as the waist circumference to make the evaluation more sensitive to detect metabolic risk.

Waist Circumference

A waist circumference ≥40 inches (102 cm) for men and ³35 inches (88 cm) for women is considered elevated and indicative of increased cardiometabolic risk.[52] However, these figures vary according to the ethnicity. The International Diabetes Federation consensus defined central obesity (also called as visceral, android, apple-shaped, or upper body obesity) in Europe as a waist circumference ≥94 cm in men and ≥80 cm in women.[53] Even lower cut-off points for central obesity have been proposed to be ≥90 cm in South Asian men and ≥80 cm in South Asian women.

Waist circumference is used with BMI for identifying adults at increased risk for morbidity and mortality, particularly in the BMI range 25 to 35 kg/m^2. Waist circumference measurements in patients with BMI ≥35 kg/m^2 may be unnecessary, as they usually do not add additional risk information.

The Waist-to-Hip Circumference Ratio (WHR)

WHR is another commonly reported anthropometric index. WHR is an index of relative fat distribution (i.e., trunk vs. extremity), and epidemiological studies have reported that it is related to the risk of cardiovascular diseases (CVD) and premature mortality. WHR >0.90 for men and >0.85 for women has been shown to confer substantially increased metabolic risk.[54] However, WHR does not confer additional advantage in evaluation of obesity than BMI or waist circumference, so it is infrequently used by clinicians, and is not currently recommended as part of the routine obesity evaluation by the American Heart Association (AHA) or The Obesity Society (TOS).[52]

Skin-Fold Measurement

Carried out using special skin calipers, skinfolds are pinched and elevated and the diameter of the fold is measured. This measures SAT and specific sites are used, (e.g., triceps). It is simple and low cost, but it is less reliable in very obese individuals.[55]

Body Fat Percentage

Body fat percentage is total body fat expressed as a percentage of total body weight. There is no uniform definition of obesity based on total body fat. Most researchers have used >25% in men, and >30% in women, as cut-off points to define obesity.[56]

Several formulas are available for body fat percentage estimation. They generally take into account the fact that body fat percentage tends to be ten percentage points higher in women than in men for a given BMI. A person's percentage body fat tends to increase as they age, even if their weight and BMI remain constant. Body fat percent is correlated with the risk of cardiovascular disease and its risk factors (diabetes mellitus, hypertension, dyslipidemia). Body fat percentage has been shown to be more sensitive in detecting individuals with early cardiovascular risk than BMI.[57] It can be estimated with greater accuracy by body composition analysis (BCA) by different methods.

Body Composition Analysis

The human body is made up of water, proteins, fats, and minerals. BCA is a physical test that measures the proportion of these components in an individual. Most of the tests, in general, measure the fat-to-lean mass ratio. Traditionally, the two-compartment model was used for BCA that divided body weight into fat mass (FM) and fat-free mass (FFM). This involves underwater weighing or densitometry (hydrostatic weighing) for measuring the total body density and deuterium isotope dilution (hydrometry) for total body water. Both are then used to calculate body composition.[58]

A more accurate measurement of body composition can be achieved by the multicompartment model that includes direct measurement of total body water (TBW), bone minerals, proteins, fats, and other body components. This utilizes a range of high-tech options to simple and low-cost anthropometric methods that we will briefly discuss.

CT/MRI

Computed tomography (CT) and magnetic resonance imaging (MRI) are accurate methods for assessing body composition and regional fat distribution at tissue-organ level. They can accurately quantify body fat percentage and visceral and subcutaneous fat. MRI poses less risk of radiation exposure. However, these are expensive and lack portability, so not useful in field studies.

Dual Energy X-Ray Absorptiometry (DXA)

It estimates the fat-free mass, fat mass, and bone mineral density for specific regions like the arms, legs, and trunk. It provides highly accurate and reproducible results for body fat and lean body mass with extremely limited exposure to X-ray. Hence it is safe for all except pregnant women and is regarded as the gold standard for BCA. One downside is that it cannot differentiate between visceral and subcutaneous fat, limiting its applicability for that purpose.

Anthropometric Methods

These methods are most widely used for epidemiological purposes because of ease of performance and low cost. Anthropometric measures include a broad range from simple weight, height, waist circumference, skin fold thickness, to the more advanced bioelectrical impedance analysis (BIA) used for BCA. BIA is the method of choice in fitness centers and requires minimal expertise.

Bioelectrical Impedance Analysis (BIA)

It is based on the principle that fat is a poor conductor of current. A very low-voltage imperceptible current is used for the test. The current conductive abilities of the body are a result of the electrolytes contained in body water, and using the electrical impedance the different proportions of body components such as fat mass, muscle mass, etc., are estimated. The machines are portable, easy to use, and widely available. The cost varies widely based on accuracy parameters and additional functions. However, there are some factors which can affect accuracy including body hydration, age, and ethnicity.[59] Let us review the BCA chart of a 38-year-old female patient with BMI 37 (**Fig. 23.5**). What is striking is that her body fat is 55%, which puts her at a very high cardiometabolic risk even though she has class 2 obesity based on BMI alone. What the BCA also tells us is that she has a high visceral fat and low muscle mass, with excess weight estimated at 39.7 kg all due to excess fat.

Edmonton Clinical Obesity Staging System

All the above methods to evaluate obesity do not take into account the existing comorbidities and degree of functional impairment of a person. While they act as surrogate

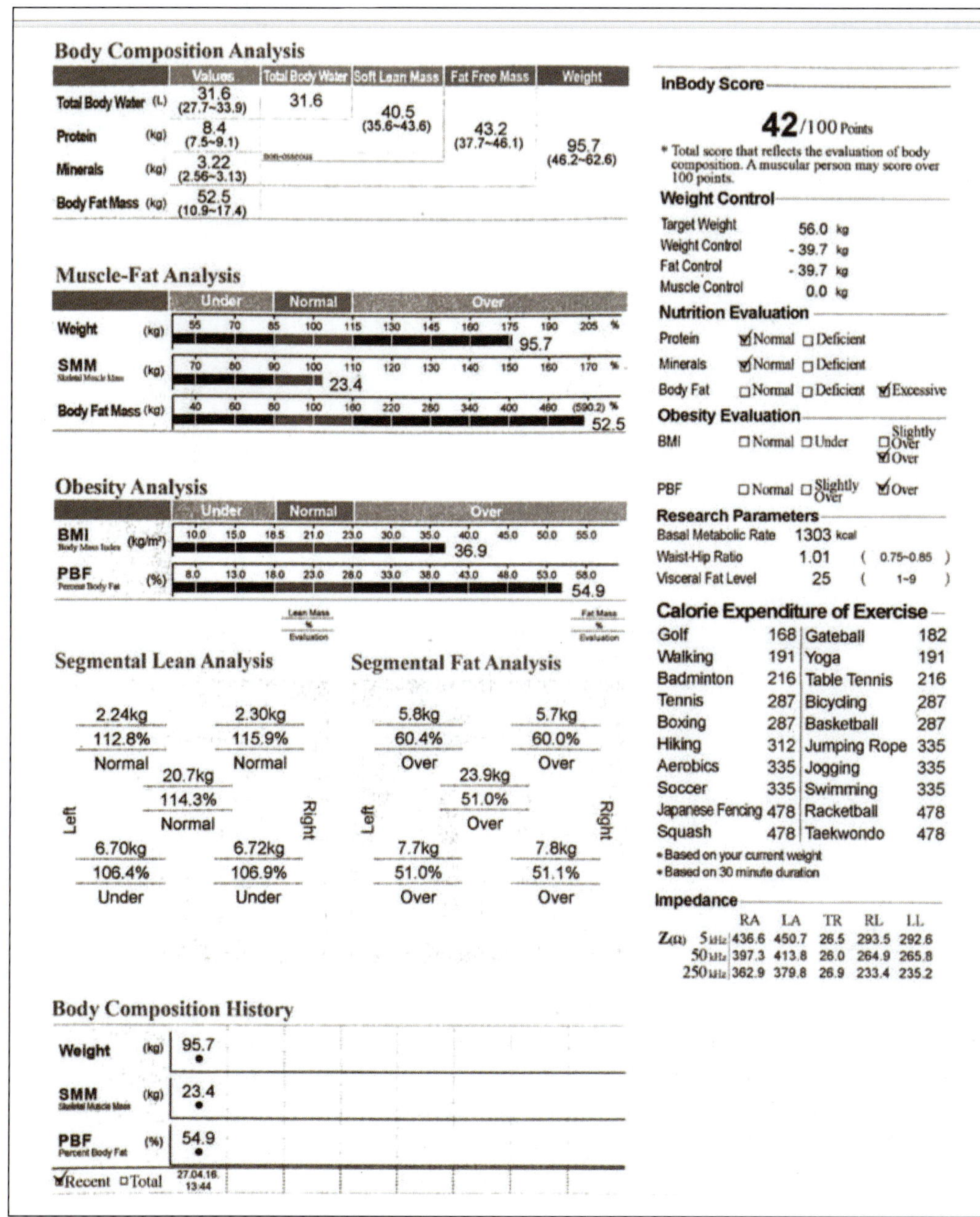

Fig. 23.5 Body composition analysis chart of a 38-year-old patient.

measures, complementing the obesity parameters with a simple disease-related and functional staging system would provide additional clinical information to guide and evaluate treatment. The rationale for a clinical staging system is also based on the notion that patients with existing health problems related to obesity should be treated more aggressively than those without them.[60]

It is toward this objective that obesity researchers in Edmonton, Canada devised a five-stage clinical staging system called the Edmonton Obesity Staging System (EOSS) that considers the metabolic, physical, and psychological parameters in order to determine the optimal obesity treatment (**Table 23.4**). EOSS has been reported to be a better predictor of mortality than BMI or MetS.[61]

Dietary Management of Obesity

Whichever method of weight loss an individual pursues whether medical or surgical, diet management is at the core of treatment. If the diet is not right most methods are destined to fail. Various large studies such as the "look AHEAD trial" have shown that interventions based primarily on dietary management generally help lose 5 to 10% of total weight with peak weight loss within 1 year of the intervention often followed by some degree of weight regain.[62,63] However even a 5 to 10% weight loss has been shown to confer metabolic benefits with improvement in the quality of life.

The "My plate" concept of a balanced diet was given by US Department of Agriculture (USDA) Centre for Nutrition policy and promotion in 2011 (**Fig. 23.6**). It is a good visual representation of the recommended proportion of grains, fruits, vegetables, and protein in an ideal plate along with a serving of dairy.[64]

The caloric requirement per day for an individual varies widely based on several factors, the most important of which is the level of baseline physical activity. In practical terms, one good way to start a diet plan is to assess the baseline daily caloric intake (by recording the past 24-hr food recall) and deducting 500 calories from that. This is also what for most people would constitute a "low-calorie diet" (LCD). The usual target LCD for women is 1,000 to 1,500 calories per day and for men 1,500 to 2,000 calories per day. As such, LCD is not a particular type of diet but calorie restriction based on low-carbohydrate or low-fat content or both.[65] The calorie limit or target is set to encourage weight loss as the calorie intake is lower than what the body requires for metabolic needs and physical activity, resulting in breakdown of energy stored in the fat cells.

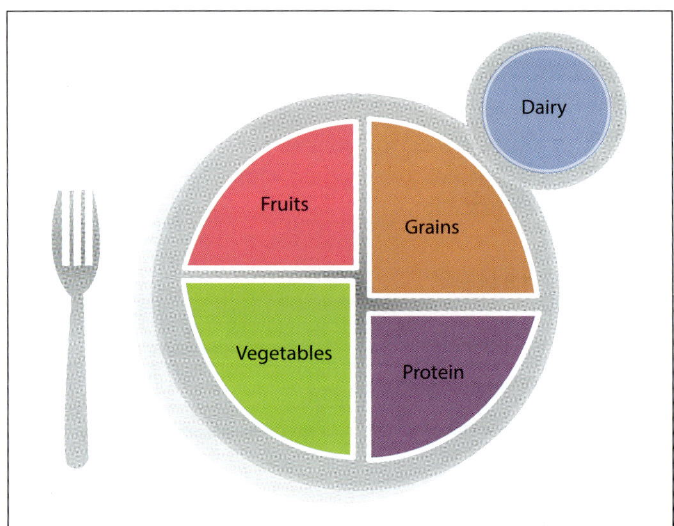

Fig. 23.6 My Plate concept (USDA).

Table 23.4 Edmonton obesity staging system (EOSS)

Stage	Parameters	Intervention recommended
0	• No comorbidities or risk factors • No physical or psychological problems • No functional limitation	• Healthy diet and physical activity counseling
1	• Early risk factors, (e.g., borderline diabetes, fatty liver) • Mild functional limitation, (e.g., dyspnea on moderate exertion)	• Intense diet and exercise • Monitor risk factors
2	• Established comorbid disease, (e.g., diabetes, hypertension, osteoarthritis, etc.) • Moderate limitation of ADL	• Diet, exercise, and psychological counseling • Consider pharmacotherapy and metabolic surgery • Treat and monitor comorbidities aggressively
3	• Significant end-organ damage, (e.g., heart failure, complications from diabetes, etc.) • Severe functional limitations	• Intense obesity management including metabolic surgery • Aggressive management of comorbidities and their complications
4	• Severe chronic disabilities due to obesity and associated conditions with severe functional or psychological limitations	• Individualized management as feasible with occupational and psychological support

Abbreviation: ADL, activities of daily living.
Source: Adapted from Sharma and Kushner 2009.[60]

"Very low-calorie diet" (VLCD) is based on a diet plan of 800 calories a day or less. These are only administered under medical supervision and the duration is generally limited to 12 weeks at a time, or sometimes in combination with a low-calorie diet. Their use is restricted to obese adults with BMI over 30. The usual daily limit of 800 kcal is approximately one-third the average caloric needs of a man (2,500 kcal) and about half that of a woman (2,000 kcal).[66] VLCDs are recommended only in certain circumstances, such as preparation for bariatric surgery, part of an infertility treatment, etc. They are not recommended for long-term weight management due to side effects, and although they may lead to good short-term weight loss, but majority regain weight after stopping them.

Some special types of diet have been in vogue such as Keto diet, Vegan diet, Mediterranean diet, Paleo diet, Atkins, etc. These diets are based on exclusion of specific nutrients and food groups. The Keto diet for example is based on high fat, adequate protein, and very low carbohydrates. This was initially popularized for treatment of pediatric epilepsy and then for weight loss.[67] There have been a lot of studies about low fat versus low carbohydrate diets as well and what has been found is that ultimately it is the calorie content of the diet which drives the weight loss, although some balance must be maintained between the carbohydrates and fats.[68] High protein maintains the muscle mass and adds to satiety keeping the calorie content relatively low so generally it is part of diet regimens. Most special diets are difficult to follow long-term and are associated with side effects. Each individual has a different dietary preference; therefore, it is important to understand that the kind of "diet" being advised should be individualized based on not just their needs but also their likings, to be effective.

Exercise for Obesity Treatment

Exercise in isolation of other interventions has a limited role in weight reduction, but, on the other hand, it is an important component of an obesity management program. Exercise, in particular, refers to a planned, repetitive activity done for physical fitness. This distinguishes exercise from physical activity which is a broader term that apart from exercise includes NEAT, TEF, and BMR, as discussed previously. While even small amounts of exercise has cardiometabolic benefits, increasing NEAT consistently, promotes energy expenditure and helps with maintaining weight. A number of obese patients may not be able to exercise due to physical disability but still can increase NEAT by simple activities such as intermittent walks that can even be done at the workplace.[69]

Exercise prescription for a patient should include recommendations about aerobic activity, strengthening and toning exercises, and breathing exercises. In addition, there need to be recommendations based on the baseline capacity of the individual for exercise frequency, intensity, time, and type (FITT).[70]

In order to achieve health benefits and "maintain" weight, moderate-intensity aerobic physical activity for a minimum of 30 minutes a day, five days a week (150 minutes per week) has been recommended by the US Department of Health and Human Services.[71] However, in order to lose weight, studies by the American College of Sports Medicine (ACSM) have shown that typically 250 to 420 minutes per week (average 60 min 6 d/wk) of moderate-intensity exercise is required long-term, although in conjunction with a diet program 150 to 250 minutes per week may be sufficient.[72] Muscle-strengthening exercises of moderate or higher intensity which involve all the major muscle groups should be performed twice or more often per week.

Apart from the exercise duration, the intensity is also important but is more subjective based on the physical ability of the individual. In case of specific musculoskeletal problems, consultation of a physiotherapist or exercise physiologist should be sought.

Behavioral Modification

Psychological assessment and counseling are important aspects of an obesity management program. Patients need to be screened for eating disorders and other psychological problems. Some patients may have an underlying psychiatric illness which is undiagnosed such as depression or bipolar disorder which needs management by a psychiatrist. The commonest cause of weight regain is an inability to undergo the behavioral change and lifestyle modification required to fight the lifelong disease of obesity.

Behavioral modification requires a multidisciplinary effort. The diet part addresses food choices. Several studies in children and adolescents show that behavioral interventions early in life can make a substantial difference in understanding right food choices and adapting them.[73] Exercise provides a major positive reinforcement not just by imparting a feeling of well-being, but it is shown that release of endorphins normalizes serotonin and other neuromodulators, improving cardiovascular health. Cognitive behavioral therapies need a sustained effort by the patient. The "Change model" given by Prochaska et al works through five stages of Precontemplation, Contemplation, Preparation, Action, and Maintenance, where gradually the patient recognizes the problem, makes the change, and makes it last.[74–76]

Drugs for Obesity Treatment

Before administering medicines for treatment of obesity, the first step is to exclude treatable medical causes of obesity such as hormonal disorders. All the comorbidities need to be evaluated and treated. If the patient is on medication causing weight gain, then the medication needs to be changed to

diabetes, hypertension, OSA, etc.[88,89] Patients should have previously enrolled in and tried to lose weight in a medical weight management program. These broad guidelines have since been adapted to suit different populations.

In keeping with the WHO recommendation to intervene at lower BMI for Asian population due to the increased metabolic risk, bariatric surgery is recommended at a lower BMI in Asians (Asia Pacific Consensus 2005), at BMI >37 or BMI >32 with any of obesity-associated medical problems.[90]

The International Federation for Surgery for Obesity (IFSO)—APC 2011 consensus recommends bariatric surgery in Asians at BMI >35, or more than 30 with obesity-associated comorbidities, or BMI ≥27.7 if diabetes cannot be controlled with best medical management.[91]

Metabolic Benefits of Surgery

Almost all obesity-associated comorbidities have been seen to significantly improve and even get cured in a large percentage of patients after bariatric surgery. Some of the given percentages from different studies, varying with different procedures are as follows:[87,92,93]

- Type 2 diabetes cured in 60 to 80% patients.
- Dyslipidemia cured in over 60% patients.
- Hypertension cured in 50 to 65% patients.
- Obstructive sleep apnea improved in over 80% with cure in most.
- Heart function improved significantly in heart failure patients.
- Asthma improved in 60 to 70% patients.
- Osteoarthritis (joint pains) significantly improved in over 40% patients.
- Nonalcoholic fatty liver disease improved in 70 to 90% patients.
- Stress urine incontinence—40% resolved.
- Polycystic ovarian syndrome—cured in over 60% patients.

Pories et al as early as 1995 published cure rates of 83% for type 2 diabetes after Roux-En-Y gastric bypass (RYGB).[94] Metabolic benefits of surgery for diabetes, dyslipidemia, OSA, etc. have been shown even in patients with mild obesity (BMI <35).[95,96] To emphasize that the primary objective of bariatric surgery in some patients is treatment of metabolic problems and not weight reduction, the term "metabolic surgery" was coined by Rubino.[97] Metabolic surgery has been compared with best medical treatment in various studies so far.[98,99] Schauer et al in a publication of their 5-year follow-up results comparing 150 obese patients with type 2 diabetes and poor glycemic control showed that after 5 years glycemic control with HbA1c less than 6 persisted in 29% of 50 patients having undergone RYGB versus 23% of 50 patients having undergone sleeve gastrectomy, versus only 5% of 50 patients who continued on best medical management.[100]

Mechanisms of Weight Loss and Metabolic Improvement after Surgery

Surgery causes physical and chemical changes in the body and alters the digestive process so as to achieve rapid weight loss. Some bariatric procedures are primarily restrictive in nature, some malabsorptive, some both. Almost all additionally cause metabolic changes. Gastric volume restriction results in diet restriction, increased gastric emptying, and early satiety. Resection of the gastric fundus and greater curve as in sleeve gastrectomy has been shown to have metabolic changes such as reduction of ghrelin causing early satiety.[101] Bypass of the foregut as in the Roux-En-Y gastric bypass procedure causes malabsorption of food and nutrients as the digestive enzymes from the biliary-pancreatic bowel limb are not able to mix with the food being carried down the alimentary limb (Roux limb) till the distal bowel (common channel). Other hormonal changes occur due to bypass of the proximal small intestine (foregut theory) or undigested food reaching the jejunum (hindgut theory) resulting in increased level of incretins (insulin-like hormones), (e.g., GLP-1), and reduced anti-incretins, (e.g., PYY, GIP), resulting in reduced insulin resistance and metabolic benefits such as immediate cure of diabetes after surgery in majority of patients.[102]

Common Bariatric Procedures

Bariatric procedures have undergone several modifications and newer procedures have been devised over time in quest for the ideal procedure that causes weight reduction with metabolic benefits but minimizes nutritional deficiencies. The procedure should also not impair the quality of life in itself due to severe restriction or malabsorption.

Most procedures that are primarily restrictive such as the laparoscopic adjustable gastric band or primarily malabsorptive such as bilio-pancreatic diversion with duodenal switch (BPD-DS) are done very selectively now. The IFSO 2016 worldwide survey of bariatric procedures showed that 685,874 procedures were performed in 2016 of which 92.6% were primary procedures and 7.4% revisional procedures for weight regain. As per the survey laparoscopic sleeve gastrectomy was the most performed primary bariatric/metabolic procedure (53.6%), followed by laparoscopic Roux-en-Y gastric bypass (30.1%), and laparoscopic one-anastomosis/mini-gastric bypass (4.8%).[103] We will discuss the key points of some procedures.

Laparoscopic Adjustable Gastric Banding (Also Known as the Lap Band)

A hollow, inflatable band made of silicone rubber is placed around the proximal stomach, creating a small pouch and a narrow passage into the rest of the stomach. The band can be tightened or loosened over time to change the size of the passage by adjusting the amount of saline in the inflatable band that is connected via a tubing to a port placed subcutaneously in an easily accessible location on the abdominal wall. This is a restrictive procedure and patients can lose on average 30 to 40% of excess weight. Although it has the lowest short-term procedure-related complications, there is a high percentage of weight regain and long-term complications such as band erosion in almost one of three patients, requiring removal of a large number of bands (**Fig. 23.8**).[104] However, they are still useful in very motivated patients who understand and implement the lifestyle changes required.

Laparoscopic Vertical Sleeve Gastrectomy

It involves removal of the greater curve side of the stomach by use of laparoscopic staplers after placing a bougie along the lesser curve (**Figs. 23.9 and 23.10**). It works by restriction with metabolic changes including ghrelin reduction. Expected weight loss is average 50 to 70% of the excess weight. The main complication is gastric staple line leak as it is a high-pressure system. The leak rate is 1 to 2% mostly within a week of surgery.[105] There is a slightly higher weight regain after 5 years follow-up than RYGB and other malabsorptive procedures as this is a primarily restrictive procedure so patients need to be particularly compliant with healthy diet and exercise.[106] Due to an overall favorable profile of weight loss, metabolic benefits, technical simplicity, and very low long-term side effects, sleeve gastrectomy has now become the most commonly done bariatric procedure worldwide.

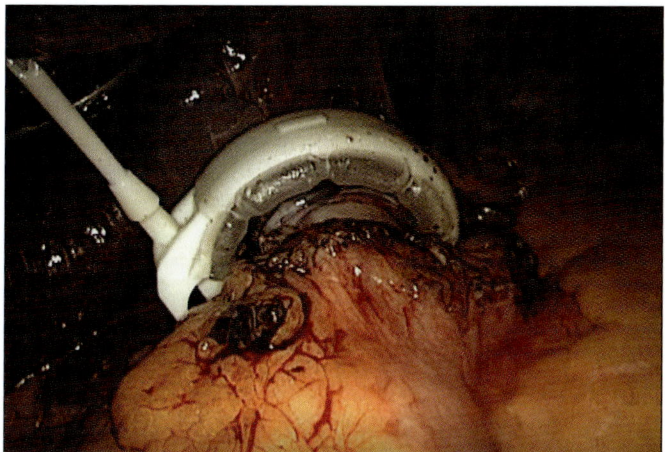

Fig. 23.8 Laparoscopic view of an eroded gastric band during removal surgery.

Laparoscopic Roux-en-Y Gastric Bypass (RYGB)

In this method a small gastric pouch is made. The jejunum is transected at 50 to 100 cm from the duodenojejunal junction. The jejunum is measured to make a 100 to 150 cm Roux/alimentary limb at which point a side-to-side jejunojejunostomy is done. The Roux limb is taken up either antecolic or retrocolic, and gastrojejunostomy is done connecting it to the gastric pouch, keeping the gastrojejunal anastomoses narrow (**Figs. 23.11 and 23.12**). The surgery works by a combination of restriction, malabsorption, and metabolic changes. If patients eat food high in carbohydrates, they may also experience dumping syndrome. The procedure leads to average weight loss of about 60 to 75% of excess weight, extensive metabolic benefits, and significant improvement in reflux disease, and it is a time-tested procedure still considered as the gold standard by most bariatric surgeons.[107] Apart from nutritional deficiencies, some complications in the long term specific to this procedure are risk of internal hernias, gallstone disease, and reoperations.

Laparoscopic One-Anastomoses Gastric Bypass (OAGB)/Minigastric Bypass (MGB)

This is a primarily malabsorptive procedure. A long gastric pouch is made to minimize biliary reflux and then a

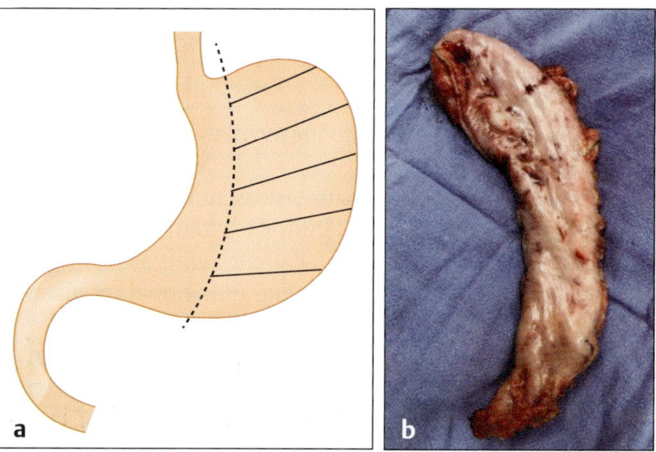

Fig. 23.9 (a, b) Line diagram of sleeve gastrectomy and the resected specimen.

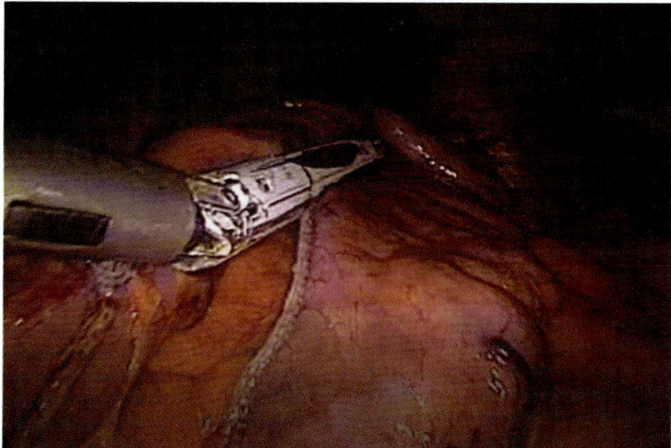

Fig. 23.10 Laparoscopic stapler applied along the bougie placed along lesser curve.

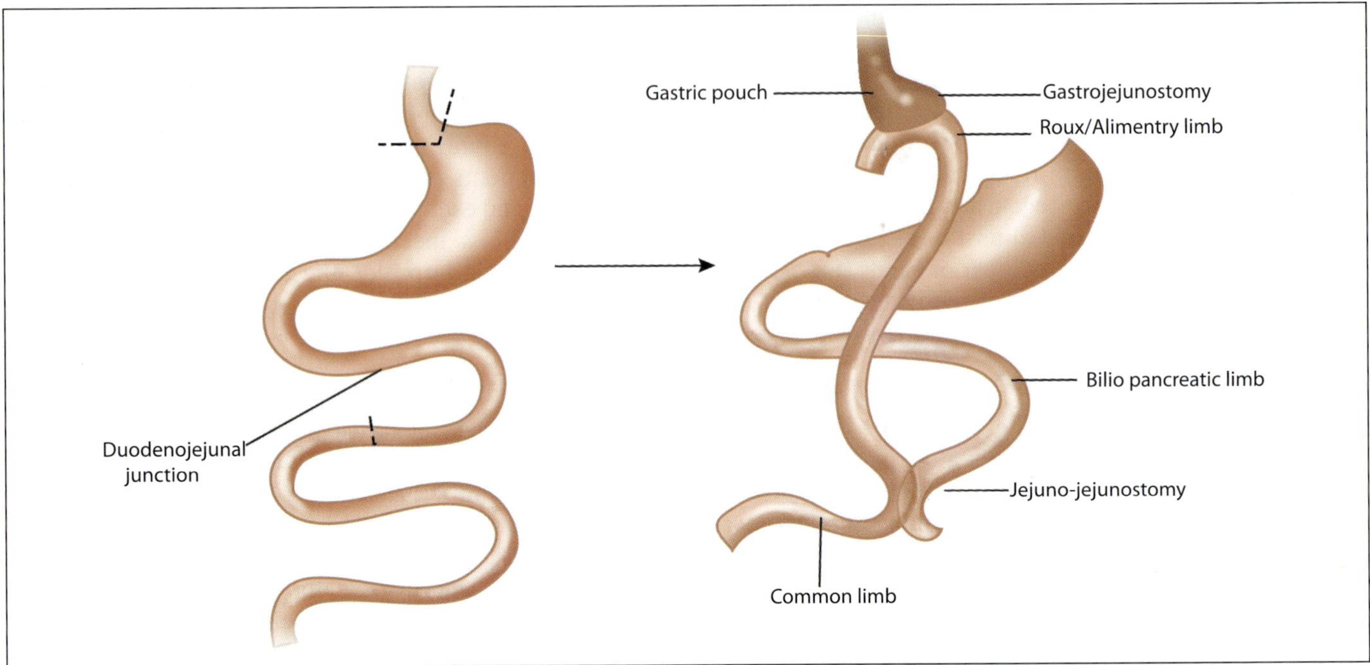

Fig. 23.11 Line diagram of the Roux-En-Y gastric bypass procedure.

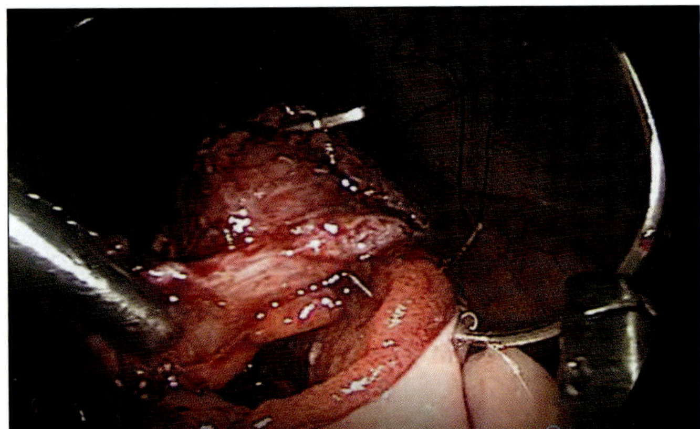

Fig. 23.12 Closure of the gastrojejunostomy (Roux-En-Y gastric bypass [RYGB]).

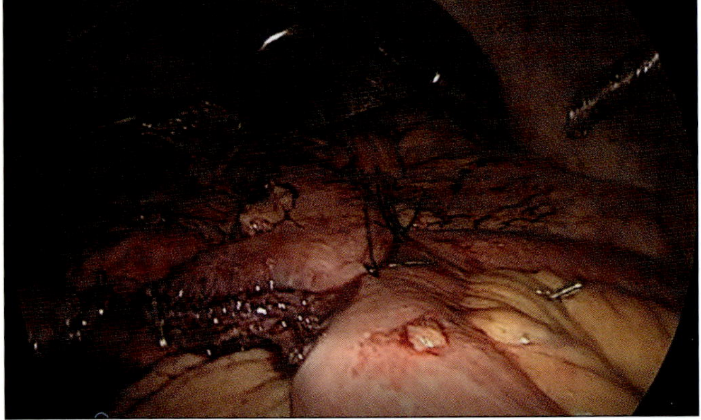

Fig. 23.13 Loop gastrojejunostomy (one-anastomoses gastric bypass [OAGB]/minigastric bypass [MGB]).

loop gastrojejunostomy is done at 150 to 200 cm from the duodenojejunal junction (**Fig. 23.13**). This procedure has been shown to have excellent weight loss and resolution of comorbidities. It is technically simpler than RYGB with less risk of internal hernias. However, there is 1 to 2% risk of symptomatic bile reflux apart from increased risk of nutritional deficiencies.[108]

Complications of Surgery

Complication rate for laparoscopic technique is now far less than that for open surgeries.[109] The risk of 30-day mortality has been reported as 0.1 to 0.2%.[110] The overall incidence of serious perioperative complications in large studies has been reported at 1.6 to 3.5% including bleeding, anastomotic leak, infections, thromboembolic events, anesthesia-related complications, etc.[111]

In the long term, the main risk is nutritional deficiencies such as deficiency of vitamin B1, vitamin B12, vitamin D, iron, and micronutrients.[112] Patients who are compliant with multivitamin supplements and nutritional monitoring usually do not suffer from nutrient deficiencies.

The success of a bariatric procedure has been arbitrarily defined by the American Society for Metabolic and Bariatric Surgery (ASMBS) as reduction of minimum 50% of excess weight. Weight recidivism after bariatric surgery has various definitions: one being regain of more than 10 kg from the nadir weight loss. While most patients are able to maintain the weight reduction in the long term after bariatric surgery, various studies have reported that 10 to 30% of patients may regain a significant portion of the lost weight. The causes are multifactorial including lack of compliance with a healthy diet, physical activity, psychological factors, sometimes related to the surgery.[113] The assessment for weight regain needs to be multidisciplinary and compliance with lifestyle measures needs to be monitored before considering any patient for revision bariatric surgery.[114]

Multidisciplinary Approach to Bariatric Surgery

With bariatric surgery the key to success is choosing the right surgery along with the patient, extensive perioperative counseling and follow-up. Patients need to understand the surgical process and the lifelong changes they need to make after surgery. The hospital stay after surgery is on average 2 to 3 days. Patients get discharged on a liquid diet for 2 weeks. They do not require special diets but are able to eat regular healthy diet with wide variety of foods, just in smaller amounts. They need to be compliant with lifelong multivitamin supplements. They should show commitment to follow a healthy high protein diet, regular exercise, and follow-up regularly. Extensive guidelines have been given by the American Society for Metabolic and Bariatric Surgery (ASMBS) for preoperative assessment, dietary and psychological assessment, postoperative nutritional monitoring, etc.[115] This requires a multidisciplinary approach. Some patients may have extensive comorbidities that also need to be managed by a bariatric physician before and after surgery, with close monitoring and adjustment of medication once they improve.

Special Considerations for Running a Bariatric Program

The essential components of a bariatric surgery program, apart from the surgeon of course, include a trained dietician, psychologist, and a coordinator to help out patients. Lot of morbidly obese patients suffer from physical and mental disabilities and accordingly need help. Besides special equipment such as bariatric table in the operating room, long operating instruments, bariatric beds and furniture, clothing, large blood pressure cuffs, intensive care facility, etc., are needed.[116]

Bariatric Surgeon's Perspective: Aesthetic Surgery in Postbariatric Surgery Patients

Massive weight loss after a bariatric procedure leads to reduction of subcutaneous and visceral fat which may leave the skin loose and redundant. As a consequence, the overhang skin can lead to functional problems apart from being a cosmetic problem. This can be over the entire body, but particularly affects the abdomen, thighs, chest, buttocks, and upper arms (**Fig. 23.14a, b**). Skin overhang can lead to recurrent and severe intertriginous rashes, dermatitis, ulceration, and wounds that are often unresponsive to medical therapy.[117,118]

The problem in some patients may be so severe that redundant breasts and abdominal wall skin could exacerbate back pain. Patients usually suffer from odor, have difficulty in maintaining personal hygiene, and may have difficulty with ambulation and other functional problems. They usually try to hide and manage the loose skin with the clothing worn and may have several psychological problems.[119]

The desire for aesthetic surgery after bariatric surgery has been shown to vary but is generally more in females, younger patients, and after massive weight loss.[120] Studies have shown that although most patients desire body contouring surgeries but few undergo them. Kitzinger et al in their survey of 252 patients postgastric bypass with massive weight loss showed that while 74% of the patients desired undergoing aesthetic surgery, only 21% received it. The most common surgery was abdominoplasty (59%) followed by lower body lifts (20%). The common reason for this discrepancy is financial problems mostly due to insurance constraints.[118,121] The utilization of aesthetic surgery is even lower in Indian patients due to several reasons such as financial and cultural differences, lack of a multidisciplinary approach, etc.

The goal of the surgery is to help regain the form and function of the affected body parts. This may require a staged approach to improve outcomes and for reducing complications. The risk of complications has been seen to be higher when patients have undergone aesthetic surgery after a bariatric surgery compared to patients who undergo it for other reasons, likely due to the massive weight loss and nutritional deficiencies in these patients. The risk of complications was lower when the weight loss had stabilized for a minimum of 3 months before the aesthetic procedure.[122] Most physicians and surgeons agree that both aesthetic and reconstructive operations are best performed at least 6 months after weight stabilization has occurred, and no earlier than 18 to 24 months after bariatric surgery. Before the aesthetic procedure it is imperative to exclude nutritional deficiencies. The patient is assessed for protein malnutrition by clinical evaluation and assessing serum albumin level. If patients are compliant with complete bariatric vitamin supplements, deficiencies are rare. Some vitamin and mineral deficiencies in bariatric patients to screen for are summarized in **Table 23.6**.

Metabolic Benefits of Liposuction

Overweight patients typically without metabolic problems may be candidates for liposuction. Some studies have shown that there may be an improvement in metabolic

Table 23.6 Common nutritional deficiencies after bariatric surgery

Nutrient	Sources	Symptoms	Test	Treatment
Vitamin B12	Egg, meats, fortified cereals	Pernicious anemia, vertigo, peripheral neuropathy, angina or heart failure, psychosis if severe	Vit B12	B12 orally disintegrating/ nasal/sublingual/ intramuscular 1000 mg every 2 wk
Folic acid	Fruits and vegetables, egg, meats	Overlap with Vit B12 deficiency Fetal neural tube defects in pregnancy	Folic acid	Multivitamin tablets In pregnancy specific oral folate supplementation
Vitamin B1 (thiamine)	Eggs, nuts, whole grains	Dry Beri Beri: peripheral neuropathy, convulsions Wernicke encephalopathy: Korsakoff psychosis	Thiamine	Multivitamin twice daily If severe: oral thiamine 100 mg thrice daily, intravenous if severe
Vitamins A, E, K (fat soluble)	Dairy, nuts, green vegetables	Vit A: night blindness Vit E: peripheral neuropathy, anemia Vit K: bleeding	Vitamin levels not routinely tested	Multivitamin twice daily Specific vitamin if required
Vitamin D and calcium	Milk, eggs, fish	Cramps, muscle weakness, osteoporosis	Vit D Calcium	Calcium-D3, if severe oral Vit D3 60,000 units weekly
Iron	Egg yolk, green leafy vegetables, red meats	Pallor, weakness, fainting, brittle nails, muscle cramps, depression	Iron Ferritin	Oral ferrous bis-glycinate, if not responsive then intravenous iron therapy
Minerals: Zinc Selenium Copper	Dairy, eggs, whole grains, fruits, and vegetables	Hair loss, neuropathy, cramps, delayed wound healing, anemia	Levels though not routinely tested	Multivitamins containing trace minerals

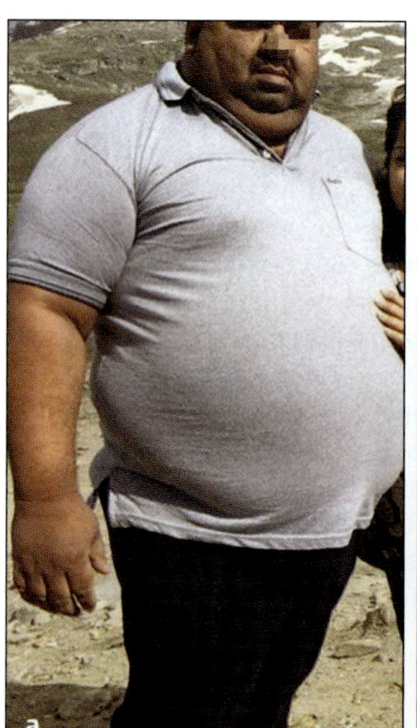

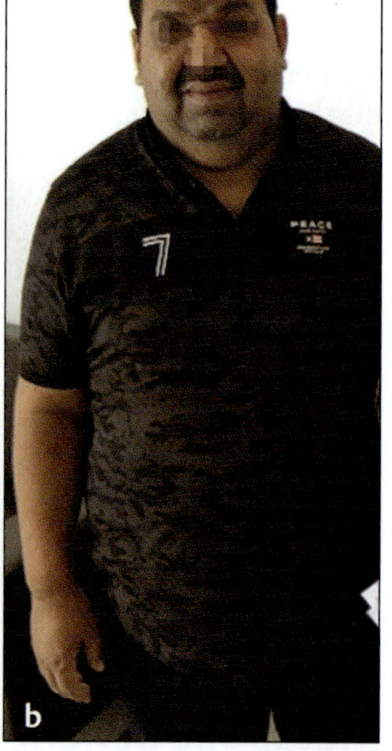

Fig. 23.14 A 35-year-old patient **(a)** presurgery and **(b)** 6 months postsurgery with weight reduction from 160 to 105 kg with resolution of obstructive sleep apnea (OSA).

parameters after decrease in subcutaneous fat in overweight individuals.[123] However this has been refuted in larger studies where removing even large volume of subcutaneous fat average 9 to 10 kg did not confer metabolic benefits in the long-term.[124,125] Nonetheless, liposuction and other body contouring procedures have benefits such as improvement in body image which can help the patient increase physical activity and improve their quality of life.

References

1. De Lorenzo A, Soldati L, Sarlo F, Calvani M, Di Lorenzo N, Di Renzo L. New obesity classification criteria as a tool for bariatric surgery indication. World J Gastroenterol 2016;22(2):681–703
2. Bays H. Central obesity as a clinical marker of adiposopathy; increased visceral adiposity as a surrogate marker for global fat dysfunction. Curr Opin Endocrinol Diabetes Obes 2014;21(5):345–351
3. World Health Organization. Controlling the global obesity epidemic. World Health Organization. 2015;7(1):1–2. http://www.who.int/nutrition/topics/obesity/en/. Accessed May 28, 2020
4. World Health Organization. Fact sheet obesity and overweight. World Health Organization 2011;1–5. https://www.who.int/health-topics/obesity#tab=tab_1. Accessed May 28, 2020

5. Vos T, Allen C, Arora M, et al; GBD 2015 Disease and Injury Incidence and Prevalence Collaborators. Global, regional, and national incidence, prevalence, and years lived with disability for 310 diseases and injuries, 1990-2015: a systematic analysis for the Global Burden of Disease Study 2015. Lancet 2016;388(10053):1545–1602
6. Ahirwar R, Mondal PR. Prevalence of obesity in India: a systematic review. Diabetes Metab Syndr 2019;13(1):318–321
7. Tripathy JP, Thakur JS, Jeet G, Chawla S, Jain S, Prasad R. Urban rural differences in diet, physical activity and obesity in India: are we witnessing the great Indian equalisation? Results from a cross-sectional STEPS survey. BMC Public Health 2016;16(1):816
8. Kopelman P. Health risks associated with overweight and obesity. Obes Rev 2007;8(Suppl 1):13–17
9. World Health Organization. WHO Global Database on Body Mass Index (BMI): an interactive surveillance tool for monitoring nutrition transition. Public Health Nutr 2006; 9(5):658–660. http://www.journals.cambridge.org/abstract_S1368980006001078. Accessed May 30, 2020
10. de Onis M, Onyango AW, Borghi E, Siyam A, Nishida C, Siekmann J. Development of a WHO growth reference for school-aged children and adolescents. Bull World Health Organ 2007;85(9):660–667
11. Tchernof A, Després JP. Pathophysiology of human visceral obesity: an update. Physiol Rev 2013;93(1):359–404
12. Misra A, Chowbey P, Makkar BM, et al; Consensus Group. Consensus statement for diagnosis of obesity, abdominal obesity and the metabolic syndrome for Asian Indians and recommendations for physical activity, medical and surgical management. J Assoc Physicians India 2009;57(2):163–170
13. Nishida C, Barba C, Cavalli-Sforza T, et al; WHO Expert Consultation. Appropriate body-mass index for Asian populations and its implications for policy and intervention strategies. Lancet 2004;363(9403):157–163
14. International Diabetes Federation. The IDF consensus worldwide definition of the metabolic syndrome. Obes Metab 2005;2(3):47–49. https://www.idf.org/component/attachments/attachments.html?id=705&task=download. Accessed May 29, 2020
15. Yang W, Kelly T, He J. Genetic epidemiology of obesity. Epidemiol Rev 2007;29(1):49–61
16. Whitaker RC, Wright JA, Pepe MS, Seidel KD, Dietz WH. Predicting obesity in young adulthood from childhood and parental obesity. N Engl J Med 1997;337(13):869–873
17. Silventoinen K, Rokholm B, Kaprio J, Sørensen TIA. The genetic and environmental influences on childhood obesity: a systematic review of twin and adoption studies. Int J Obes 2010;34(1):29–40
18. Khan MJ, Gerasimidis K, Edwards CA, Shaikh MG. Mechanisms of obesity in Prader-Willi syndrome. Pediatr Obes 2018;13(1): 3–13
19. Stipančić G, Šepec MP. Secondary causes of obesity in children and adolescents. Cent Eur J Paediatr 2018;14(1):1–11
20. Kehoe SH, Krishnaveni GV, Veena SR, et al. Diet patterns are associated with demographic factors and nutritional status in South Indian children. Matern Child Nutr 2014;10(1):145–158
21. Baker P, Friel S. Processed foods and the nutrition transition: evidence from Asia. Obes Rev 2014;15(7):564–577
22. Pankova A, Kralikova E, Zvolska K, et al. Early weight gain after stopping smoking: a predictor of overall large weight gain? A single-site retrospective cohort study. BMJ Open 2018;8(12):e023987
23. Traversy G, Chaput JP. Alcohol consumption and obesity: an update. Curr Obes Rep 2015;4(1):122–130
24. Hill LS, Reid F, Morgan JF, Lacey JH. SCOFF: the development of an eating disorder screening questionnaire. Int J Eat Disord 2010;43(4):344–351
25. Anjana RM, Pradeepa R, Das AK, et al; ICMR-INDIAB Collaborative Study Group. Physical activity and inactivity patterns in India: results from the ICMR-INDIAB study (Phase-1) [ICMR-INDIAB-5]. Int J Behav Nutr Phys Act 2014;11(1):26
26. Yadav K, Krishnan A. Changing patterns of diet, physical activity and obesity among urban, rural and slum populations in north India. Obes Rev 2008;9(5):400–408
27. Steelman GM, Westman EC. Obesity: evaluation and treatment essentials. Boca Raton: CRC Press; 2016:1–216
28. Villablanca PA, Alegria JR, Mookadam F, Holmes DR Jr, Wright RS, Levine JA. Nonexercise activity thermogenesis in obesity management. Mayo Clin Proc 2015;90(4):509–519
29. Levine JA. Nonexercise activity thermogenesis (NEAT): environment and biology. Am J Physiol Endocrinol Metab 2004;286(5): E675–E685
30. Kalin MF, Goncalves M, John-Kalarickal J, Fonseca V. Pathogenesis of type 2 diabetes mellitus. In: Principles of Diabetes Mellitus. 3rd ed. New York: Springer International; 2017:267–277
31. Verma RK, Kaur B, Mishra R, Himanshu D. Recent trends of diabesity and its non-clinical management among urban pts. Res J Recent Sci 2015;4((ISC-2014)):261–264. http://www.isca.in/rjrs/archive/special-ISC-2014/44.ISCA-ISC-2014-Oral-9FMS-02.pdf
32. Johns MW. Sleepiness in different situations measured by the Epworth Sleepiness Scale. Sleep 1994;17(8):703–710
33. Joosten SA, Hamilton GS, Naughton MT. Impact of weight loss management in OSA. Chest 2017;152(1):194–203
34. Romero-Corral A, Caples SM, Lopez-Jimenez F, Somers VK. Interactions between obesity and obstructive sleep apnea: implications for treatment. Chest 2010;137(3):711–719
35. Chalasani N, Younossi Z, Lavine JE, et al. The diagnosis and management of non-alcoholic fatty liver disease: practice guideline by the American Association for the Study of Liver Diseases, American College of Gastroenterology, and the American Gastroenterological Association. Hepatology 2012;55(6):2005–2023
36. Hannah WN Jr, Harrison SA. Effect of weight loss, diet, exercise, and bariatric surgery on nonalcoholic fatty liver disease. Clin Liver Dis 2016;20(2):339–350
37. Adams LA, Angulo P. Treatment of non-alcoholic fatty liver disease. Postgrad Med J 2006;82(967):315–322
38. King LK, March L, Anandacoomarasamy A. Obesity & osteoarthritis. Indian J Med Res 2013;138:185–193
39. Fauser BCJM; Rotterdam ESHRE/ASRM-Sponsored PCOS consensus workshop group. Revised 2003 consensus on diagnostic criteria and long-term health risks related to polycystic ovary syndrome (PCOS). Hum Reprod 2004;19(1):41–47
40. Escobar-Morreale HF. Polycystic ovary syndrome: definition, aetiology, diagnosis and treatment. Nat Rev Endocrinol 2018;14(5):270–284
41. Deng D, Gao W, Liao M, Suzuki T, Ohishi Y. Supercontinuum generation from a multi-ring holes tellurite microstructured fiber pumped by a 2 micron high power mode-locked fiber laser. Opt Components Mater 2013;X:8621
42. Homburg R. Polycystic ovary syndrome. Best Pract Res Clin Obstet Gynaecol 2008;22(2):261–274

43. Gregor MF, Hotamisligil GS. Inflammatory mechanisms in obesity. Annu Rev Immunol 2011;29(1):415–445
44. Roberts DL, Dive C, Renehan AG. Biological mechanisms linking obesity and cancer risk: new perspectives. Annu Rev Med 2010;61(1):301–316
45. Calle EE, Rodriguez C, Walker-Thurmond K, Thun MJ. Overweight, obesity, and mortality from cancer in a prospectively studied cohort of U.S. adults. N Engl J Med 2003;348(17): 1625–1638
46. Gariepy G, Nitka D, Schmitz N. The association between obesity and anxiety disorders in the population: a systematic review and meta-analysis. Int J Obes 2010;34(3):407–419
47. Scott KM, Bruffaerts R, Simon GE, et al. Obesity and mental disorders in the general population: results from the world mental health surveys. Int J Obes 2008;32(1):192–200
48. Kolotkin RL, Crosby RD, Williams GR. Health-related quality of life varies among obese subgroups. Obes Res 2002;10(8): 748–756
49. Gómez-Ambrosi J, Silva C, Galofré JC, et al. Body mass index classification misses subjects with increased cardiometabolic risk factors related to elevated adiposity. Int J Obes 2012;36(2): 286–294
50. Bray GA, Bouchard C. Handbook of obesity: epidemiology, etiology, and physiopathology. 3rd ed. New York, NY: Taylor & Francis, Inc.; 2014
51. Burkhauser RV, Cawley J. Beyond BMI: the value of more accurate measures of fatness and obesity in social science research. J Health Econ 2008;27(2):519–529
52. Jensen MD, Ryan DH, Apovian CM, et al. American College of Cardiology/American Heart Association Task Force on Practice Guidelines; Obesity Society. 2013 AHA/ACC/TOS guideline for the management of overweight and obesity in adults: a report of the American College of cardiology/American Heart Association task force on practice guidelines and the obesity society. Circulation 2014; 129(25, Suppl 2):S102–S138
53. Alberti SG, Zimmet P. The IDF consensus definition of the metabolic syndrome in children and adolescents. Int Diabetes Fed 2007;1–24
54. World Health Organization. Waist circumference and waist-hip ratio. WHO Expert 2011;8–11. 10.1038/ejcn.2009.139. Accessed May 28, 2020
55. Madden AM, Smith S. Body composition and morphological assessment of nutritional status in adults: a review of anthropometric variables. J Hum Nutr Diet 2016;29(1):7–25
56. Okorodudu DO, Jumean MF, Montori VM, et al. Diagnostic performance of body mass index to identify obesity as defined by body adiposity: a systematic review and meta-analysis. Int J Obes 2010;34(5):791–799
57. Yamashita K, Kondo T, Osugi S, et al. The significance of measuring body fat percentage determined by bioelectrical impedance analysis for detecting subjects with cardiovascular disease risk factors. Circ J 2012;76(10):2435–2442
58. Hu F. Obesity epidemiology. 1st ed. New York: Oxford University Press; 2008:1–512
59. Sergi G, De Rui M, Stubbs B, Veronese N, Manzato E. Measurement of lean body mass using bioelectrical impedance analysis: a consideration of the pros and cons. Aging Clin Exp Res 2017;29(4):591–597
60. Sharma AM, Kushner RF. A proposed clinical staging system for obesity. Int J Obes 2009;33(3):289–295
61. Kuk JL, Ardern CI, Church TS, et al. Edmonton Obesity Staging System: association with weight history and mortality risk. Appl Physiol Nutr Metab 2011;36(4):570–576
62. Look AHEAD Research Group. Eight-year weight losses with an intensive lifestyle intervention: the look AHEAD study. Obesity (Silver Spring) 2014;22(1):5–13
63. Wadden TA, West DS, Delahanty L, et al; Look AHEAD Research Group. The Look AHEAD study: a description of the lifestyle intervention and the evidence supporting it. Obesity (Silver Spring) 2006;14(5):737–752
64. Agriculture USD of H and HS and USD of 2015–2020 Dietary Guidelines for Americans. 8th ed. 2015;47:245–251 http://health.gov/dietaryguidelines/2015/guidelines/. Accessed June 1, 2020
65. Hession M, Rolland C, Kulkarni U, Wise A, Broom J. Systematic review of randomized controlled trials of low-carbohydrate vs. low-fat/low-calorie diets in the management of obesity and its comorbidities. Obes Rev 2009;10(1):36–50
66. Strychar I. Diet in the management of weight loss. CMAJ 2006;174(1):56–63
67. O'Neill B, Raggi P. The ketogenic diet: pros and cons. Atherosclerosis 2020;292:119–126
68. Gardner CD, Trepanowski JF, Del Gobbo LC, et al. Effect of low-fat VS low-carbohydrate diet on 12-month weight loss in overweight adults and the association with genotype pattern or insulin secretion the DIETFITS randomized clinical trial. JAMA 2018;319(7):667–679
69. Malaeb S, Perez-Leighton CE, Noble EE, Billington C. A "NEAT" approach to obesity prevention in the modern work environment. Workplace Health Saf 2019;67(3):102–110
70. Burnet K, Kelsch E, Zieff G, Moore JB, Stoner L. How fitting is F.I.T.T.?: a perspective on a transition from the sole use of frequency, intensity, time, and type in exercise prescription. Physiol Behav 2019;199:33–34
71. Piercy KL, Troiano RP, Ballard RM, et al. The physical activity guidelines for Americans. JAMA 2018;320(19):2020–2028
72. Donnelly JE, Blair SN, Jakicic JM, Manore MM, Rankin JW, Smith BK; American College of Sports Medicine. Appropriate physical activity intervention strategies for weight loss and prevention of weight regain for adults. Med Sci Sports Exerc 2009;41(2):459–471
73. Habib-Mourad C, Ghandour LA, Moore HJ, et al. Promoting healthy eating and physical activity among school children: findings from Health-E-PALS, the first pilot intervention from Lebanon. BMC Public Health 2014;14(1):940
74. Prochaska JO, Diclemente CC, Norcross JC. In search of how people change: applications to addictive behaviors. J Addict Nurs 1993;5(1):2–16
75. Yoo S, Kim H, Cho HI. Improvements in the metabolic syndrome and stages of change for lifestyle behaviors in Korean older adults. Osong Public Health Res Perspect 2012;3(2):85–93
76. Mastellos N, Gunn LH, Felix LM, Car J, Majeed A. Transtheoretical model stages of change for dietary and physical exercise modification in weight loss management for overweight and obese adults. Cochrane Database Syst Rev 2014; (2):CD008066
77. Scerbo MH, Felinski MM, Bajwa KS, Wilson EB, Shah SK. Endoscopic primary bariatric procedures. In: Nguyen NT, et al., eds. The ASMBS textbook of bariatric surgery. New York, NY: Springer International; 2020:391–402
78. Kumar N. Endoscopic therapy for weight loss: gastroplasty, duodenal sleeves, intragastric balloons, and aspiration. World J Gastrointest Endosc 2015;7(9):847–859
79. Abu Dayyeh BK, Kumar N, Edmundowicz SA, et al; ASGE Bariatric Endoscopy Task Force and ASGE Technology Committee. ASGE Bariatric Endoscopy Task Force systematic review and meta-analysis assessing the ASGE PIVI thresholds

for adopting endoscopic bariatric therapies. Gastrointest Endosc 2015;82(3):425–38.e5
80. Courcoulas A, Abu Dayyeh BK, Eaton L, et al. Intragastric balloon as an adjunct to lifestyle intervention: a randomized controlled trial. Int J Obes 2017;41(3):427–433
81. Vicente C, Rábago LR, Ortega A, Arias M, Vázquez Echarri J. Usefulness of an intra-gastric balloon before bariatric surgery. Rev Esp Enferm Dig 2017;109(4):256–264
82. Yorke E, Switzer NJ, Reso A, et al. Intragastric balloon for management of severe obesity: a systematic review. Obes Surg 2016;26(9):2248–2254
83. Barrichello S, Hourneaux de Moura DT, Hourneaux de Moura EG, et al. Endoscopic sleeve gastroplasty in the management of overweight and obesity: an international multicenter study. Gastrointest Endosc 2019;90(5):770–780
84. Hedjoudje A, Abu Dayyeh BK, Cheskin LJ, et al. Efficacy and safety of endoscopic sleeve gastroplasty: a systematic review and meta-analysis. Clin Gastroenterol Hepatol 2020;18(5): 1043–1053.e4
85. Buchwald H, Estok R, Fahrbach K, Banel D, Sledge I. Trends in mortality in bariatric surgery: a systematic review and meta-analysis. Surgery 2007;142(4):621–632, discussion 632–635
86. Sjöström L, Narbro K, Sjöström CD, et al; Swedish Obese Subjects Study. Effects of bariatric surgery on mortality in Swedish obese subjects. N Engl J Med 2007;357(8):741–752
87. Buchwald H, Avidor Y, Braunwald E, et al. Bariatric surgery: a systematic review and meta-analysis. JAMA 2004;292(14): 1724–1737
88. Gastrointestinal surgery for severe obesity: National Institutes of Health Consensus Development Conference Statement. Am J Clin Nutr 1992; 55(2, Suppl)615S–619S
89. NIH. North American Association for the Study of Obesity and the National Heart, Lung, and Blood Institute. The practical guide: identification, evaluation, and treatment of overweight and obesity in adults. NIH;2000: 26–27. https://www.nhlbi.nih.gov/files/docs/guidelines/prctgd_c.pdf
90. Lee WJ, Wang W. Bariatric surgery: Asia-Pacific perspective. Obes Surg 2005;15(6):751–757
91. Kasama K, Mui W, Lee WJ, et al. IFSO-APC consensus statements 2011. Obes Surg 2012;22(5):677–684
92. Sjöström L. Review of the key results from the Swedish Obese Subjects (SOS) trial: a prospective controlled intervention study of bariatric surger y. J Intern Med 2013;273(3):219–234
93. Sjöström L, Lindroos AK, Peltonen M, et al; Swedish Obese Subjects Study Scientific Group. Lifestyle, diabetes, and cardiovascular risk factors 10 years after bariatric surgery. N Engl J Med 2004;351(26):2683–2693
94. Pories WJ, Swanson MS, MacDonald KG, et al. Who would have thought it? An operation proves to be the most effective therapy for adult-onset diabetes mellitus. Ann Surg 1995;222(3): 339–350, discussion 350–352
95. Cohen RV, Pinheiro JC, Schiavon CA, Salles JE, Wajchenberg BL, Cummings DE. Effects of gastric bypass surgery in patients with type 2 diabetes and only mild obesity. Diabetes Care 2012;35(7):1420–1428
96. Proczko-Markuszewska M, Stefaniak T, Kaska Ł, Sledziński Z. Early results of Roux-en-Y gastric by-pass on regulation of diabetes type 2 in patients with BMI above and below 35 kg/m². Pol Przegl Chir 2011;83(2):81–86
97. Rubino F. From bariatric to metabolic surgery: definition of a new discipline and implications for clinical practice. Curr Atheroscler Rep 2013;15(12):369
98. Schauer PR, Kashyap SR, Wolski K, et al. Bariatric surgery versus intensive medical therapy in obese patients with diabetes. N Engl J Med 2012;366(17):1567–1576
99. Xie XF, Zhang WL, Li Q, Li N, Wang C. Bariatric surgery versus conventional medical therapy for obese patients with type 2 diabetes: a meta-analysis. Chinese J Evidence-Based Med 2013;13(6):728–734
100. Schauer PR, Bhatt DL, Kirwan JP, et al; STAMPEDE Investigators. Bariatric surgery versus intensive medical therapy for diabetes: 5-year outcomes. N Engl J Med 2017;376(7):641–651
101. Langer FB, Reza Hoda MA, Bohdjalian A, et al. Sleeve gastrectomy and gastric banding: effects on plasma ghrelin levels. Obes Surg 2005;15(7):1024–1029
102. Spector D, Shikora S. Neuro-modulation and bariatric surgery for type 2 diabetes mellitus. Int J Clin Pract Suppl 2010;64(166):53–58
103. Angrisani L, Santonicola A, Iovino P, et al. IFSO Worldwide Survey 2016: primary, endoluminal, and revisional procedures. Obes Surg 2018;28(12):3783–3794
104. Himpens J, Cadière GB, Bazi M, Vouche M, Cadière B, Dapri G. Long-term outcomes of laparoscopic adjustable gastric banding. Arch Surg 2011;146(7):802–807
105. Sakran N, Goitein D, Raziel A, et al. Gastric leaks after sleeve gastrectomy: a multicenter experience with 2,834 patients. Surg Endosc 2013;27(1):240–245
106. Salminen P, Helmiö M, Ovaska J, et al. Effect of laparoscopic sleeve gastrectomy vs laparoscopic roux-en-y gastric bypass on weight loss at 5 years among patients with morbid obesity the SLEEVEPASS randomized clinical trial. JAMA 2018;319(3):241–254
107. Adams TD, Davidson LE, Litwin SE, et al. Weight and metabolic outcomes 12 years after gastric bypass. N Engl J Med 2017;377(12):1143–1155
108. Mahawar KK, Jennings N, Brown J, Gupta A, Balupuri S, Small PK. "Mini" gastric bypass: systematic review of a controversial procedure. Obes Surg 2013;23(11):1890–1898
109. Nguyen NT, Goldman C, Rosenquist CJ, et al. Laparoscopic versus open gastric bypass: a randomized study of outcomes, quality of life, and costs. Ann Surg 2001;234(3):279–289, discussion 289–291
110. Chang SH, Stoll CRT, Song J, Varela JE, Eagon CJ, Colditz GA. The effectiveness and risks of bariatric surgery: an updated systematic review and meta-analysis, 2003–2012. JAMA Surg 2014;149(3):275–287
111. Birkmeyer NJO, Dimick JB, Share D, et al; Michigan Bariatric Surgery Collaborative. Hospital complication rates with bariatric surgery in Michigan. JAMA 2010;304(4):435–442
112. Toh SY, Zarshenas N, Jorgensen J. Prevalence of nutrient deficiencies in bariatric patients. Nutrition 2009;25(11-12): 1150–1156
113. Karmali S, Brar B, Shi X, Sharma AM, de Gara C, Birch DW. Weight recidivism post-bariatric surgery: a systematic review. Obes Surg 2013;23(11):1922–1933
114. Mahawar KK, Himpens JM, Shikora SA, et al. The first consensus statement on revisional bariatric surgery using a modified Delphi approach. Surg Endosc 2020;34(4):1648–1657
115. Mechanick JI, Apovian C, Brethauer S, et al. Clinical practice guidelines for the perioperative nutrition, metabolic, and nonsurgical support of patients undergoing bariatric procedures—2019 update: cosponsored by American Association of Clinical Endocrinologists/American College of Endocrinology, the Obesity Society, American Society for

Metabolic & Bariatric Surgery, Obesity Medicine Association, and American Society of Anesthesiologists. Executive summary. Endocr Pract 2019;25(12):1346–1359

116. Ide P, Fitzgerald-O'Shea C, Lautz DB. Implementing a bariatric surgery program. AORN J 2013;97(2):195–206, quiz 207–209
117. McMahon MM, Sarr MG, Clark MM, et al. Clinical management after bariatric surgery: value of a multidisciplinary approach. Mayo Clin Proc 2006;81(10, Suppl):S34–S45
118. Abela C, Stevens T, Reddy M, Soldin M. A multidisciplinary approach to post-bariatric plastic surgery. Int J Surg 2011; 9(1):29–35
119. Sarwer DB, Thompson JK, Mitchell JE, Rubin JP. Psychological considerations of the bariatric surgery patient undergoing body contouring surgery. Plast Reconstr Surg 2008;121(6):423e–434e
120. Giordano S, Victorzon M, Stormi T, Suominen E. Desire for body contouring surgery after bariatric surgery: do body mass index and weight loss matter? Aesthet Surg J 2014;34(1): 96–105
121. Kitzinger HB, Abayev S, Pittermann A, et al. The prevalence of body contouring surgery after gastric bypass surgery. Obes Surg 2012;22(1):8–12
122. van der Beek ESJ, van der Molen AM, van Ramshorst B. Complications after body contouring surgery in post-bariatric patients: the importance of a stable weight close to normal. Obes Facts 2011;4(1):61–66
123. Ybarra J, Blanco-Vaca F, Fernández S, et al. The effects of liposuction removal of subcutaneous abdominal fat on lipid metabolism are independent of insulin sensitivity in normal-overweight individuals. Obes Surg 2008;18(4):408–414
124. Mohammed BS, Cohen S, Reeds D, Young VL, Klein S. Long-term effects of large-volume liposuction on metabolic risk factors for coronary heart disease. Obesity (Silver Spring) 2008;16(12):2648–2651
125. Klein S, Fontana L, Young VL, et al. Absence of an effect of liposuction on insulin action and risk factors for coronary heart disease. N Engl J Med 2004;350(25):2549–2557

24

Liposuction and Liposculpture

Lakshyajit Dhami and Shrirang Pandit

Introduction

The popularity of liposuction over the past four decades has revolutionized the technique of body contouring. It has transformed the way we look at shaping the body. The prospect of modifying the form with a tiny incision was an unbelievable idea. The possibilities were mind boggling. The added benefit of losing few kilos and getting lighter on the weighing scale was the clincher. Liposculpture now has evolved as the most reliable method of manipulating fatty tissue. Addition of fat to enhance contours, with lipofilling or fat grafting, has a very sound scientific backing in contemporary plastic surgery literature.

With this popularity, liposuction has been in the top three, for several years running, of all the aesthetic surgeries being performed. Liposuction requires thoughtful planning and an artistic eye to achieve aesthetically pleasing results. The goal is to remove target fat, leaving the desired uniform body contour and smooth transition between treated and untreated areas.

Anatomy of Fat Distribution

Adipose tissue is a loose connective tissue composed mostly of adipocytes. In addition it contains stromal vascular fraction (SVF) including preadipocytes, fibroblasts, vascular endothelial cells, and immune cells like macrophages. The types of adipocytes are white, brown, or beige cells (**Fig. 24.1**). These can be stored as essential, subcutaneous, or visceral fat. Essential fat is found in brain, bone marrow, nerve sheath, and membranes of various organs, and it is essential for good health.

White fat is made up of large white adipocytes and is used as energy reservoir. It also plays a major role in the function of various hormones including Leptin and Insulin. Brown fat is primarily found in babies but adults may retain a very small amount in the neck and shoulder. This fat burns fatty acids to keep us warm. Beige fat is somewhere in between white and brown fats. If the activity of the brown and beige fat is somehow stimulated, it may prevent obesity.

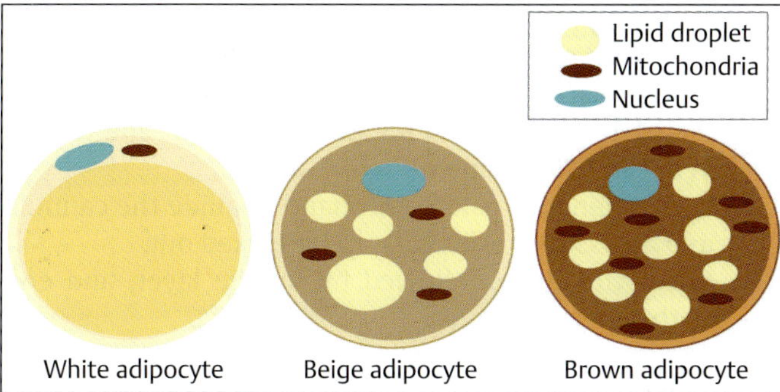

Fig. 24.1 Morphological anatomy of three different types of fat cells. White adipocytes store energy as fat droplets, while brown adipocytes are packed with powerhouses called mitochondria, which contains iron, giving them brown colour.

In an obese patient seeking liposuction, an increase in fat content may be either hypertrophic, hyperplastic, or both. Hyperplastic obesity predominates as body fat levels exceed 40% over body mass index (BMI), where there is an increase in the presence of total number of adipocytes. This obesity is also more resistant to diet and exercise regimes. In hypertrophic obesity, which is most commonly seen in clinical practice, the number of fat cells remains constant, while only the size of the fat cells varies with change in weight.[1]

History and Scientific Perspective

The concept of removing excess fat from localized body sites to achieve body contouring is credited to Charles Dujarrier.[2–4] This dates far back to 1921, when he attempted to remove subcutaneous fat using a uterine curette on calves and knees of a ballerina. An inadvertent injury to the femoral artery led to gangrene and an eventual amputation of the leg. This unfortunate complication arrested further progress in this field, but nevertheless, it was a valiant attempt at that time.[5]

Schrudde, in 1964,[6] revived interest in this procedure and extracted fat from the leg, gaining access through a small incision with a curette, but was faced with a daunting task of managing the resultant hematoma. Subsequently, Pitanguy[7] in 1964 favored en-bloc removal of both fat and skin to remove excess thigh adiposities, but the extensively noticeable incisions did not allow the technique to become popular.

Modern Liposuction, in technique and instruments, began with the gynecologists Giorgio Fisher and his father Arpad Fisher from Rome in 1974.[4] They developed the instruments and their early cannula contained a cutting blade within. They eventually developed a blunt hollow cannula connected to a suction apparatus and published their results in 1976. They developed the technique of crisscross tunneling from multiple access sites with their improved cannula and demonstrated good results with fewer complications. In 1978, Kesselring and Meyer[8] published results of a sharp curettage aided by suction. The technique did not gain much acceptance in view of the significant complications.

Pierre Fournier[9] of Paris, in 1983, improvised on the Fischer's liposculpture technique and was the initial advocate of the "dry technique" of liposuction. He went on to become an authority in liposuction and fat transplantation and later promoted the benefits of tumescent anesthesia with the use of lidocaine.

Liposuction procedure became popular in 1982, when a French surgeon Yves-Gerard Illouz presented his method, which demonstrated a suction-assisted method for removing fat cells. Illouz used fine infiltration cannulas to inject fluid into the tissues to break up the fat deposits.[3,10,11] This technique was called a "wet technique" in which a solution of hypotonic, vasoconstrictor saline, and hyaluronidase were infiltrated into the adipose tissue prior to aspiration. He termed this as a "dissecting hydrotomy" which facilitated removal of fat and reduced trauma with less bleeding.

In early 1980s, several interspecialty courses were held and Julius Newman, an otolaryngologist, was the first to use the term "LipoSuction."[4] He went on to establish the American Society of Liposuction Surgery. The first article on liposuction appeared in literature in July 1984.

Jeffery Klein, now at San Juan Capistrano, California, initially described the tumescent technique for lipoaspiration in June of 1986 and the first article describing this technique was published in January 1987.[12] Since then, lipoaspiration and fluid management have added a greater safety dimensions. Ultrasonic liposuction was developed by Italian surgeon, Michael Zocchi in 1996.[13] In India, the wet technique of liposuction gained much popularity in 1990 after Illouz conducted a live operative workshop at Hyderabad.

The procedure has evolved over the last 30 years with greater understanding of the biochemical and physiological properties of liposuction as well as biomedical and technological advancement. Suction-assisted lipoplasty (SAL) has undergone an enormous evolution, leading to tremendous improvement in the technique, patient safety, and surgical outcome, which we practice today.

These advances have also made possible removal of larger volumes of fat with rewarding results, accompanied by negligible blood loss and relatively trifle complications.

General Considerations

Mechanism of Fat Removal

- **Avulsion of fat:** When liposuction is done using large caliber cannula using a powerful suction, the fat globules are avulsed from the stromal network and neurovascular structures with a severe tearing force.
- **Emulsification:** With finer cannula liposuction using a wet technique, the targeted fat globules are gently separated from each other and the surrounding structures. This process allows these globules and fat cells to become loose and get emulsified.

Basic Principles

It is worthwhile reiterating Illouz's principle as surprisingly little has changed over time **(Boxes 24.1 and 24.2)**.

Author's Basic Principles of Liposuction

- Patient evaluation with history, thorough examination, counseling, and informed individualized consent.
- Preoperative assessment of the skin and fat, topographic marking, documentation, and photography of the area for liposuction.
- Regional anesthesia preference over general or local anesthesia.
- Intraoperative calf massage and/or stockinette support.
- Use smooth, even, and adequate infiltration with tumescent/wet technique. Allow sufficient time before suction.
- Use appropriate assisted liposuction device and noncollapsible suction tubing with powerful suction machine.
- Use blunt-tip cannula with optimum number of holes, directed away from the skin and proper diameter of the cannula for the area to be treated (medium for deep and fine caliber for superficial liposuction).

Box 24.1 Illouz's technical principles of liposuction

- Use blunt cannula
- Create many tunnels
- Dissecting hydrotomy is useful
- Operate deeply
- Use the retraction of the skin

Source: Adapted from Illouz 1989.[14]

Box 24.2 Illouz's ten commandments of adipoaspiration

- Create only tunnels:
  - ➢ Never create a cavity
  - ➢ Never undercut
- Be as gentle as possible:
  - ➢ Only use small, blunt instruments
  - ➢ Use the least possible number of passages
- Respect the superficial layer of fat
- It is not so much what is removed that is important, but what is left behind
- Use, anticipate, and estimate skin retraction instead of fighting against it
- Do not undertake an "important" resection that is locally and generally dangerous
- Indications should be restrictive. Adipoaspiration is not a panacea
- All fat resection is final
- Results in the operating room approximate the final result
- This technique demands "blind" surgery

Source: Adapted from Illouz 1989.[15]

- Tunnel liposuction in fan shape with only forward and backward movements.
- Multiple access incisions for crisscross suctioning and feathering the margin for smooth contour and to prevent "end-hits" injury.
- Use of nondominant smart hand to guide the cannula and assess the residual fat to be sucked out.
- Start with deep, followed by middle layer, and end with superficial layer.
- When in doubt—undercorrect rather than overcorrect.
- Leave the access port/incision site open, or apply loose sutures, for free seepage of the residual fluid especially after large-volume liposuction.
- Adequate hydration and early assisted mobilization in immediate postoperative period.
- Judicious use of compression garment for 3 months to achieve final contouring "in vivo sculpture."

Preoperative Assessment

Successful liposuction surgery necessitates that only an appropriate patient with realistic expectation is selected for the procedure. It is of paramount importance that the operating surgeon consults and examines the patient thoroughly and then counsels and discusses to assess suitability for the desired and planned procedure. Patients with a history of frequent and significant weight fluctuations, and no set diet or exercise regime, have a high probability of weight gain post liposuction.

Evaluation also covers the usual risk of the surgical procedure and any specific risk factors pertaining to patient's general well-being and metabolic comorbidity.

Skin Elasticity

Large adiposity of the abdomen, buttocks, medial arms, or inner thighs tends to have excess volume of fat. The weight of fat overstretches the panniculus and results in ptosis of the skin overlying the area. In these cases, it is required to reduce the large fat volume so as to permit effective skin retraction. Massive all layers liposuction (MALL) effectively addresses the issue better. The amount of skin shrinkage after this procedure is remarkable and the clinical results are appreciable.

If there is any need for an additional excisional procedure to achieve expected results, it too should be discussed in detail with its pros and cons.

The **informed consent** for liposuction is like for any other cosmetic/aesthetic surgery but a special emphasis must be made on the following points:

- Liposuction is not the first choice for the treatment of obesity. After surgery, there is fat and weight loss, but primary aim is to reshape.
- There is a limitation to the number of areas or amount of fat that can be suctioned in one session.
- The skin may not have enough elasticity to recoil after the fat is removed and may lead to recurrence of skin fold and irregularity.

- Pre-existing asymmetry will be addressed during the surgery but some asymmetry may still persist.
- After large-volume liposuction there is a possibility of skin devascularization and skin loss with delayed healing and/or scarring.
- Postsurgery, there is a phase of edema/swelling which needs judicious use of compression garment. Failing to comply with this may result in delayed recovery and healing with unsatisfactory results.
- It may be necessary to carry out an additional surgery for residual correction.

Indications

Aesthetic Indications

The types of patients who seek liposuction are classified as follows:

- **Ideal patient** is slim and has isolated, unwanted pockets of fat with good skin elasticity (**Fig. 24.2**).
- Patient with **localized fatty deposits** which refuses to reduce in spite of strict diet and exercise (**Fig. 24.3**).
- **Localized cellulite:** These patients have "orange peel skin" which is unsightly and is due to the fat globules protruding between the subcutaneous tissue septa (retinacula cutis). Liposuction benefits by deflating the deep subcutaneous fat to reduce the pressure on the septa and correct the cellulite deformity (**Fig. 24.4**).
- **Obese patient:** Young patients with good skin elasticity, who are unable to reduce weight, seek surgical intervention to help them get rid of fat from a given area. Liposuction may not achieve perfect results, but it can lead to a permanent fat and weight loss which may help inspire the patient to bring about lifestyle changes (**Fig. 24.5**).
- **Obese patient with skin laxity:** The liposuction procedure is not ideally suited for these patients. But some who have physical incapacity due to excessive fat (**Fig. 24.6**) would benefit with large-volume liposuction. These patients may even plan to have an excisional surgery at same session or later (**Fig. 24.7**).

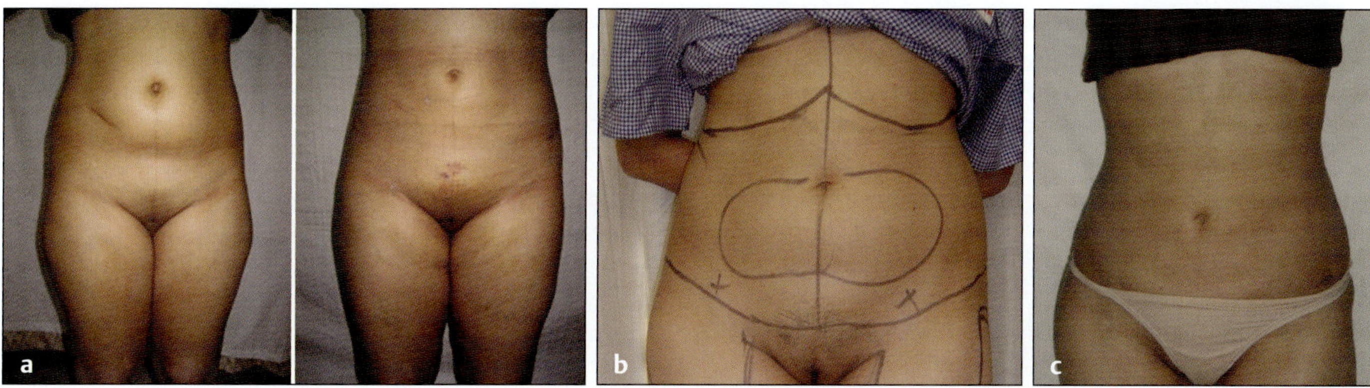

Fig. 24.2 Ideal patient for SAL. **(a)** Pre- and postoperative pictures of the result of liposuction of abdomen, medial thigh and trochanter. Good reshaping and redraping of skin after lipo-aspiration of 4 liters. Appendectomy scar has also resolved with subcision effect of liposuction cannula. **(b)** Ideal patient with no skin laxity. **(c)** Excellent result with only SAL of 5 liters for reshaping of abdomen. Abbreviation: SAL, suction-assisted liposuction.

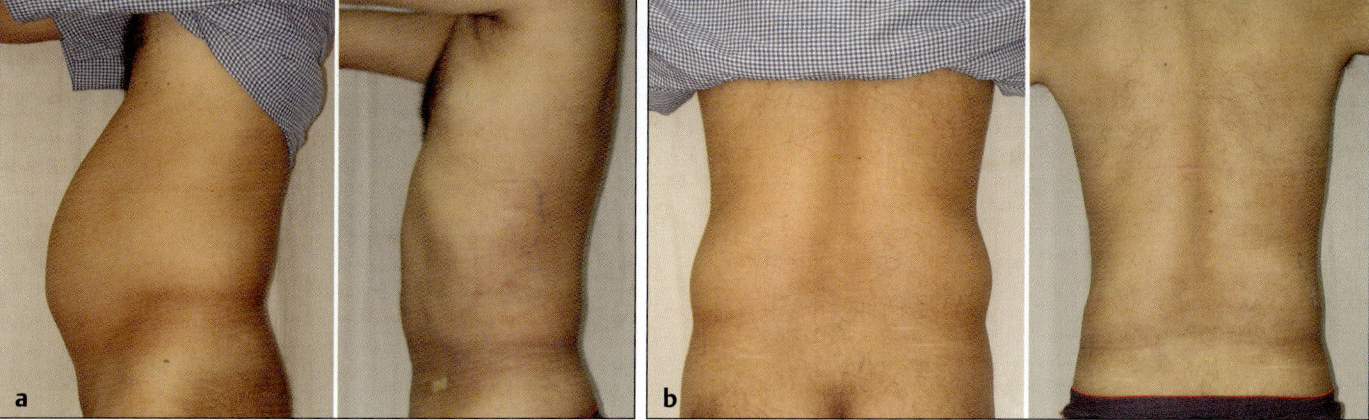

Fig. 24.3 Localized fatty deposit treated with SAL. **(a)** Abdomen and flanks pre- and postoperative—lateral views. **(b)** Pre- and postop—posterior views. Abbreviation: SAL, suction-assisted liposuction.

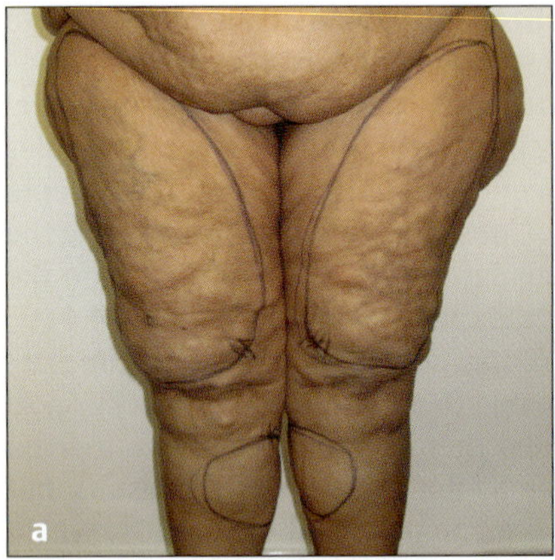
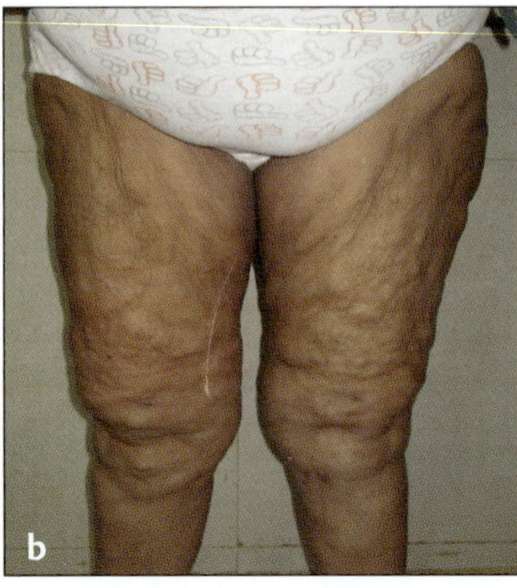

Fig. 24.4 Lipodystrophy anterior thigh with multiple lipomatosis. **(a)** Preoperative. **(b)** After PAL showing good reduction of deep seated fat on trochanter and knee roll, but only partial reduction of superficial subcutaneous fat in anterior thigh. Abbreviation: PAL, power-assisted liposuction.

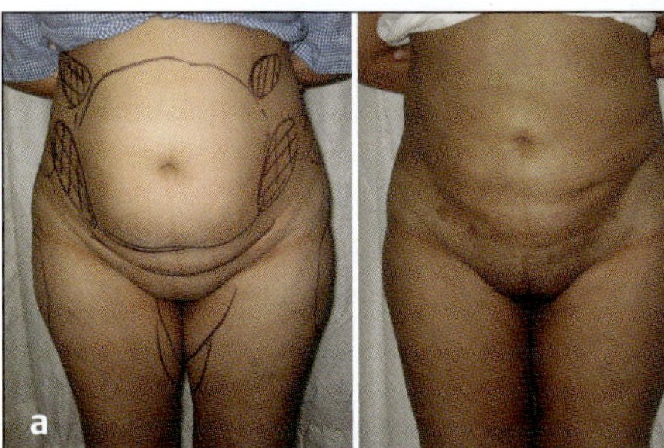
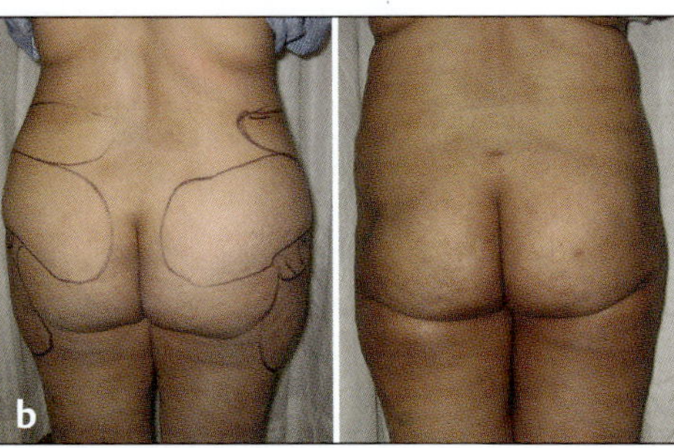
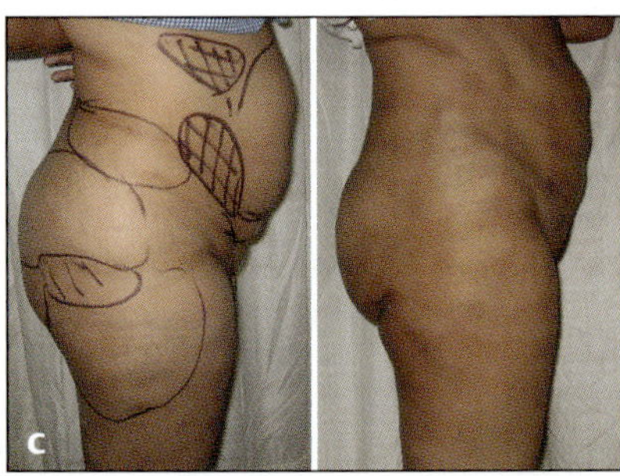

Fig. 24.5 Generalized obesity—liposuction of abdomen, trochanter, and medial thigh. (total Infiltration 11 liters and lipo-aspiration 12 liters) **(a)** Pre- and immediate postoperative picture with marking. Liposuction is avoided in cross-hatch marked area. **(b)** Marked area for liposuction of part of buttocks, flanks, and trochanter—preop and postop. **(c)** Lateral views—pre- and immediate postoperation.

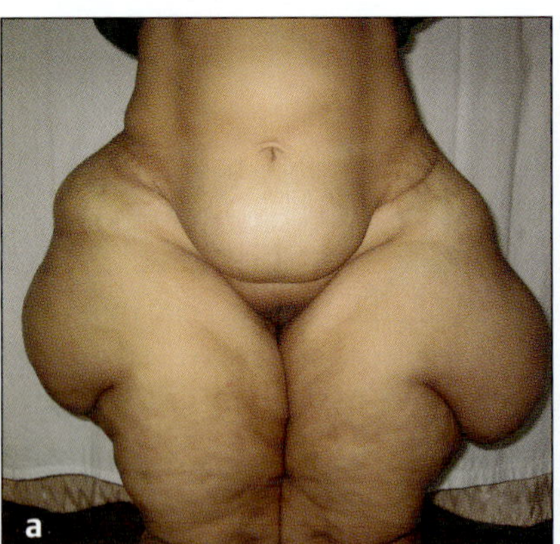
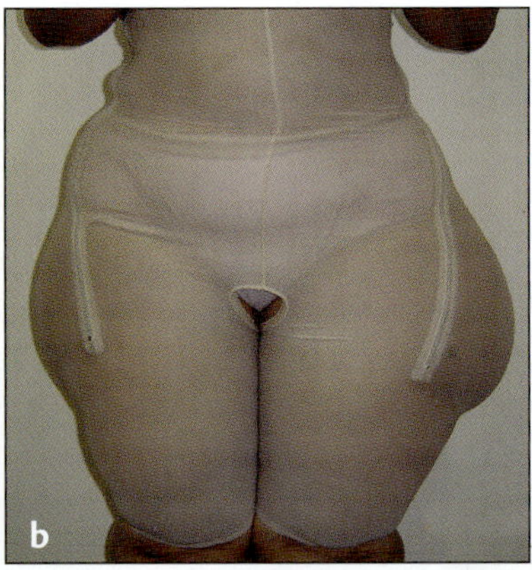

Fig. 24.6 Lipodystrophy in trochanteric region. Unable to sit in a chair. **(a)** Preop and **(b)** Immediate postoperative image with pressure garment.

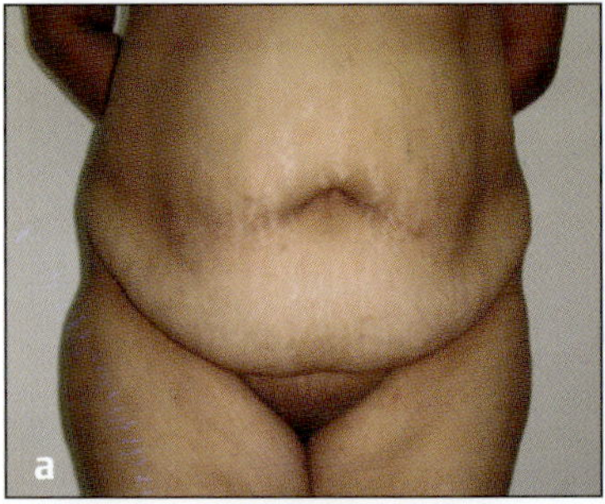
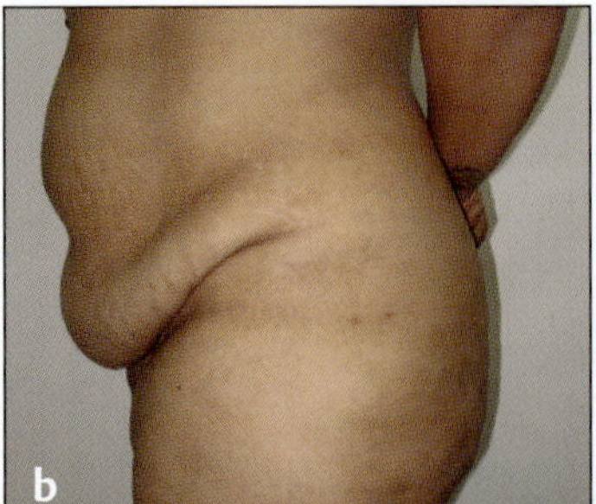
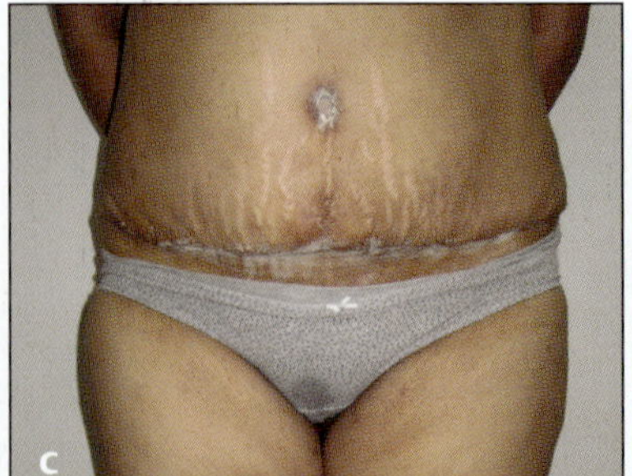
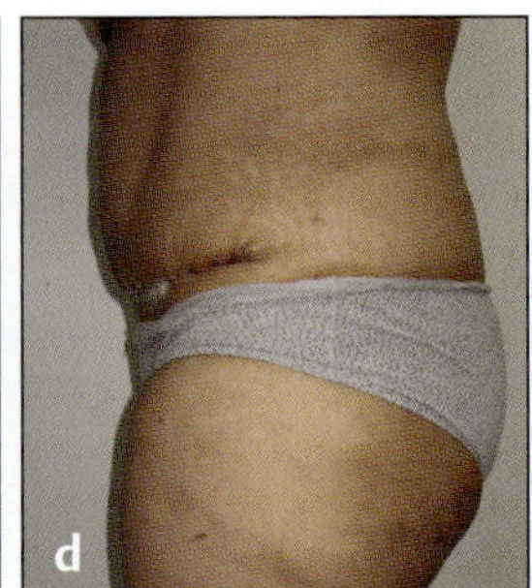

Fig. 24.7 A 47-year-old 93-kg female patient with obesity. **(a)** Preoperative image front. **(b)** Preoperative left lateral view. **(c, d)** Postoperative front and lateral image after PAL of medial and lateral thighs with lipo-abdominoplasty. Infiltration 13 liters, lipoaspiration 14.5 liters. Resected skin flap weighed 1.2 kg. Abbreviation: PAL, power-assisted liposuction.

- **Postbariatric surgery patient:** These patients too can benefit from liposuction, which leads to permanent fat cells loss from a given area. They invariably have loose excessive skin and are best suited for an adjuvant dermolipectomy procedure (**Figs. 24.8 and 24.9**).

Nonaesthetic Indications

Lipodystrophy Syndromes

There are areas of hyper and hypotrophic fat which may require a combined procedure of liposuction with fat filling to achieve symmetry (**Fig. 24.10**). Adipose tissue disorders, Dercum disease (adiposis dolorosa), benign symmetrical lipomatosis (Madelung disease), large lipomas (**Fig. 24.11**), familial multiple lipomatosis (**Fig. 24.12**), etc., are managed with liposuction.

Axillary Hyperhidrosis

A small cannula of 2.5 to 3 mm is used for suction very close to the dermis. UAL or LAL technique provides better result.

Skin Flap Thinning

In a bulky myocutaneous or fasciocutaneous flaps, liposuction helps achieve aesthetically acceptable contour by debulking the fatty subcutaneous layer. The procedure is usually performed 4 to 6 months after flap cover (**Fig. 24.13**).

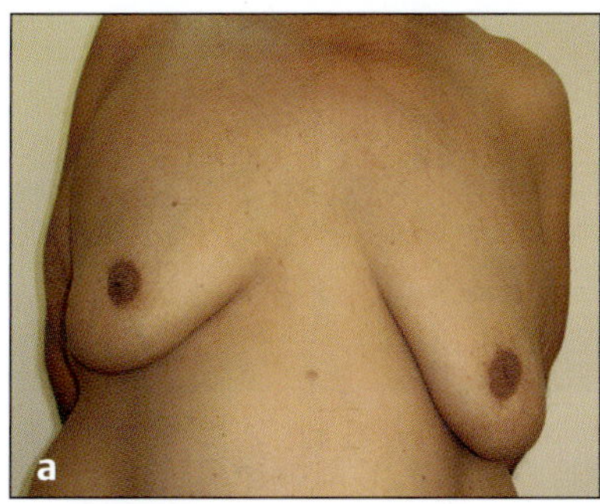

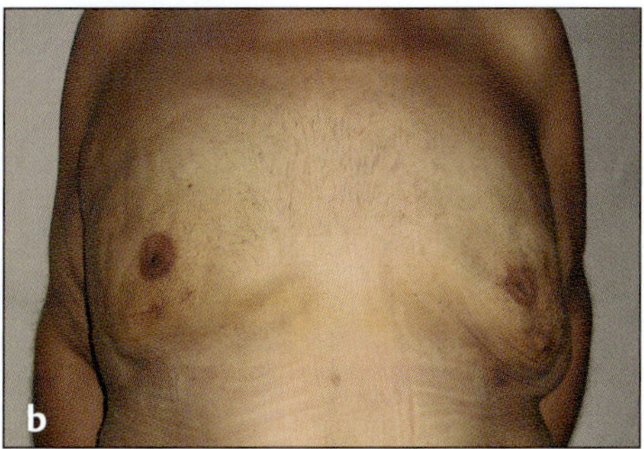

Fig. 24.8 Postbariatric surgery residual Gynecomastia: **(a)** Preliposuction. **(b)** Immediate postliposuction.

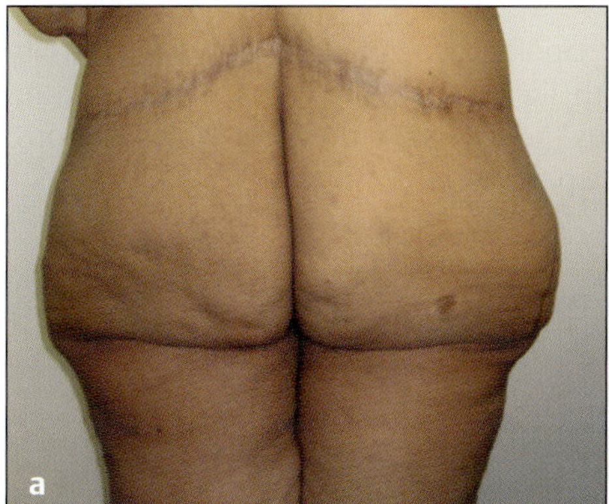

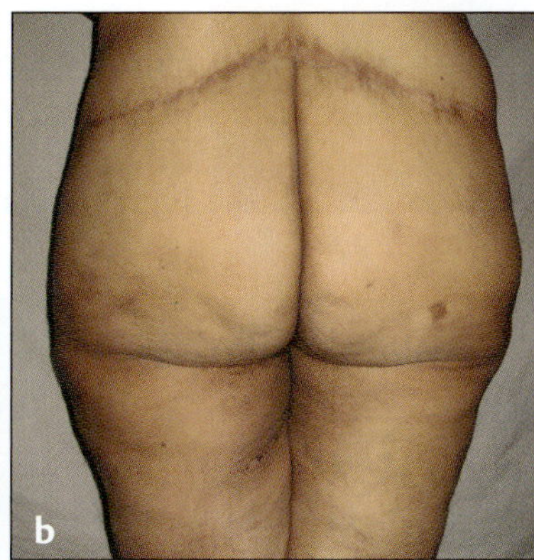

Fig. 24.9 Post bariatric surgery residual fat in buttocks: **(a)** preliposuction. **(b)** Immediate postliposuction.

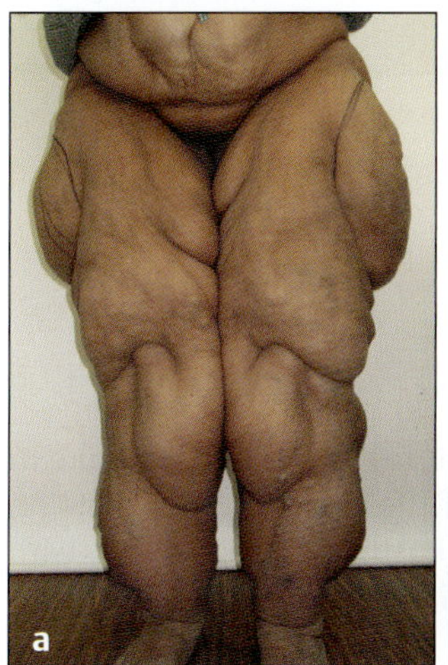

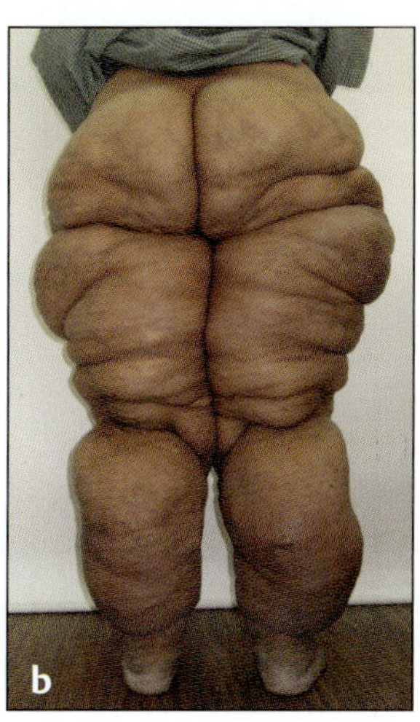

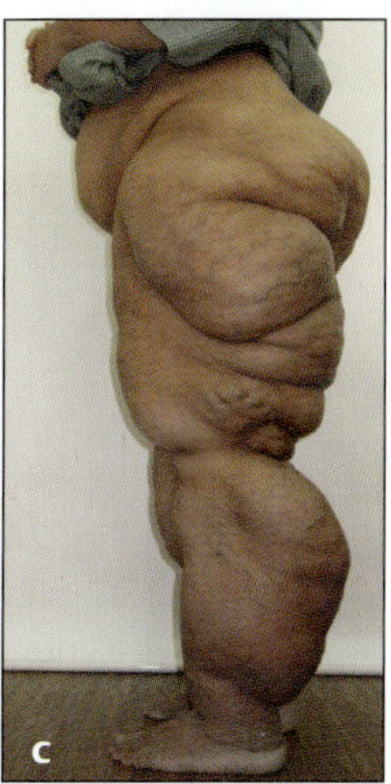

Fig. 24.10 Lipodystrophy of the lower part of body. **(a)** Front view. **(b)** Posterior view. **(c)** Lateral view.

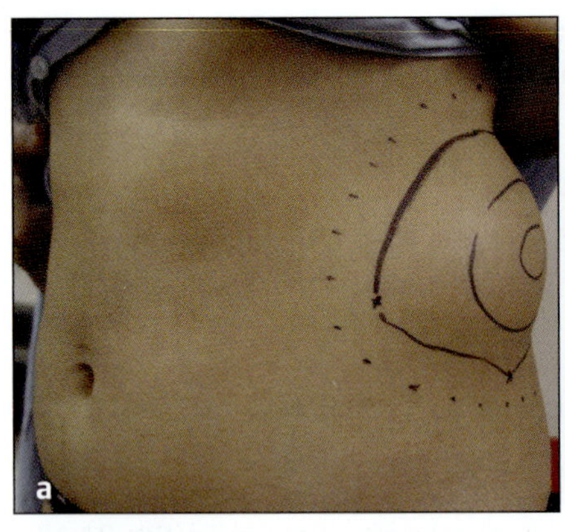
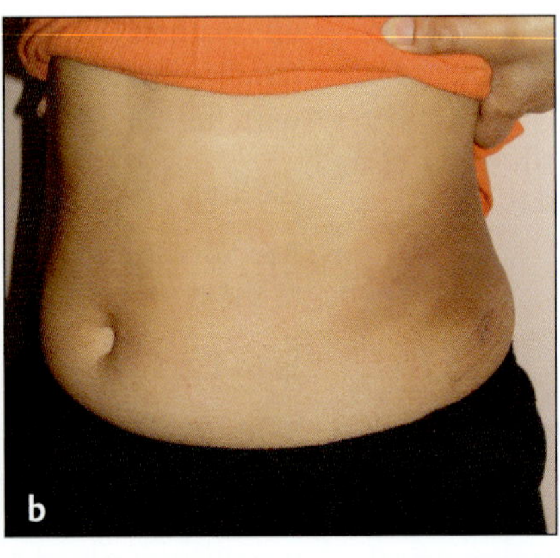

Fig. 24.11 Lipoma in flank managed with liposuction. **(a)** Preoperative picture with marking. **(b)** Postoperative result after liposuction.

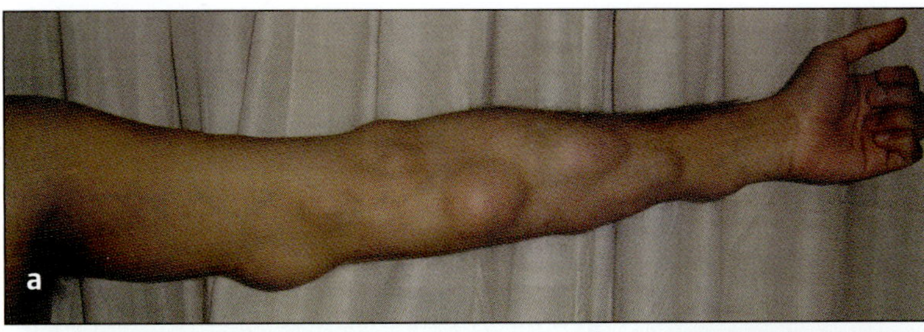
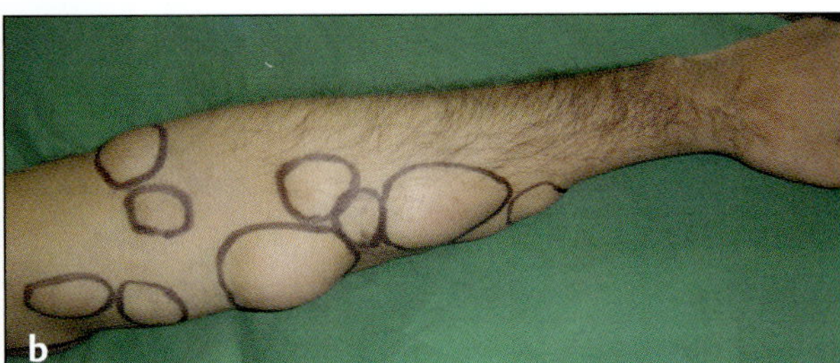
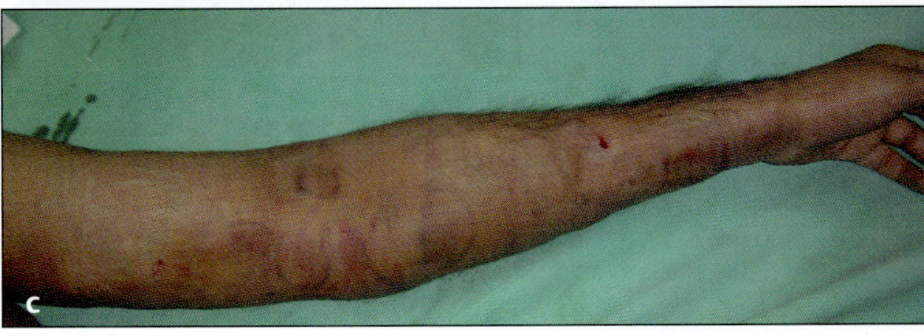

Fig. 24.12 Lipomatosis of left upper extremity managed with liposuction. **(a)** Preoperative picture. **(b)** Markings delineate the multiple lesions. **(c)** Immediate postliposuction.

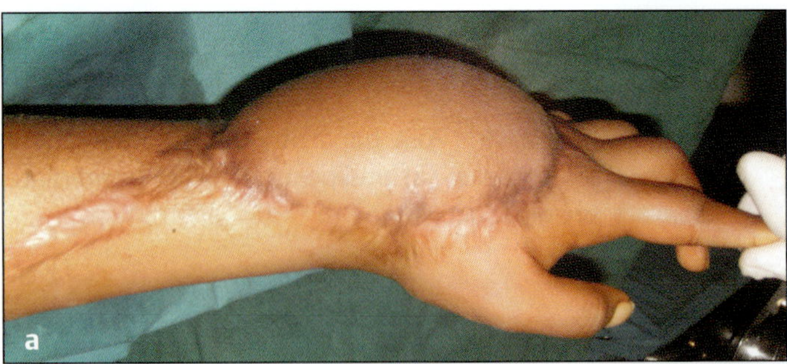
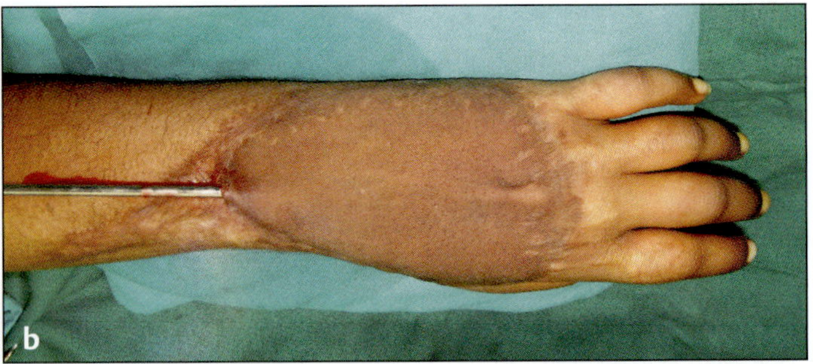
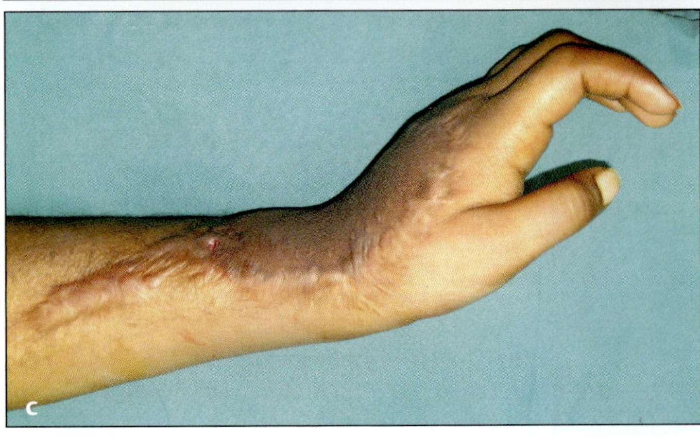

Fig. 24.13 Flap thinning with SAL. **(a)** Preoperative picture of a bulky groin flap over dorsum of the wrist. **(b)** Flap thinning using liposuction cannula. **(c)** Postliposuction result with dorsiflexion of the wrist. Abbreviation: SAL, suction-assisted liposuction.

Lipoedema

After ruling out lymphedema, liposuction is carried out along longitudinal axis, with fine and long cannula, so as not to damage the lymphatics.

Lymphedema of Extremities

The accumulated lymph may stimulate adipose tissue deposits and marked fat cell hypertrophy may be seen in patients with chronic lymphedema. Liposuction is indicated when the edema fails to respond to conservative treatment.

HIV-Induced Fat Deposits

Lipodystrophy, with redistribution and accumulation of fat, and hyperlipidemia are seen in HIV-infected individuals **(Fig. 24.14)** who are managed with liposuction.

Investigations

There are very few specific investigations required before liposuction procedure. Routine investigations are carried out from the point of view of anesthesia. Specific investigations for liposuction are bleeding profile (prothrombin time and partial thromboplastin time), abdominal and breast sonography when indicated.

Marking and Photography

Preoperative marking in standing position with indelible waterproof marking pen is an essential step. In lying down position, the anatomy changes significantly and errors can occur in judgment. Patient is made to stand, preferably in front of a mirror. This helps patient to assess, contribute, and confirm the area that will be treated. This marking provides "topographic map" which allows the surgeon to visualize the targeted convexities of fat deposits. The areas for liposuction are marked in circles from the center to periphery (**Figs. 24.5 and 24.15**). Areas to be avoided and zone of adherence are marked with cross hatching. Pre-existing asymmetry, scars, unevenness, and dimpling are marked and shown to the patient. The area to be treated is recorded with a rough estimate of infiltration and expected lipoaspiration quantity.

Photographs are taken, once the marking is complete, in various postures and at different angles. These pictures are

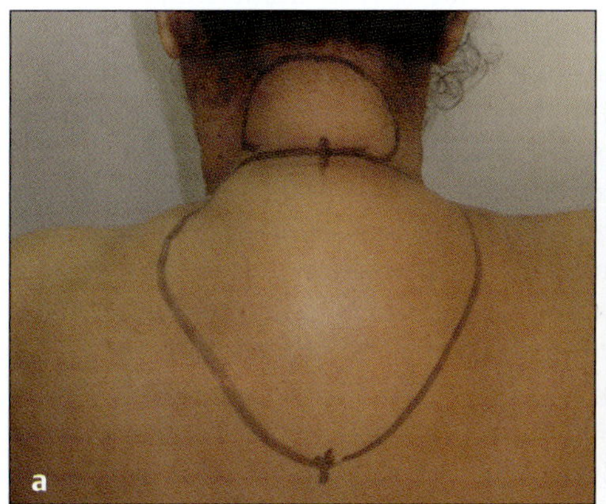
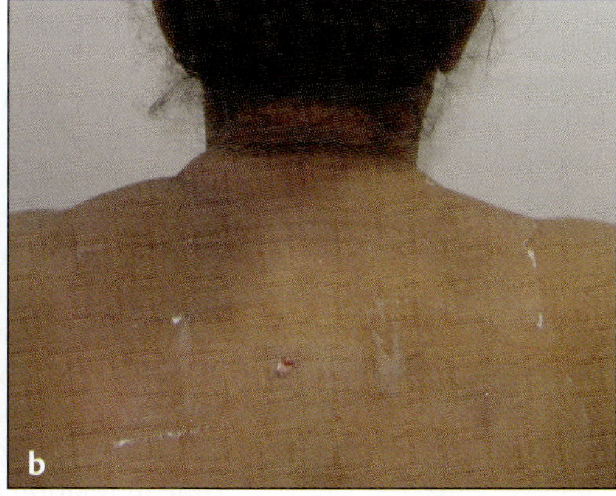

Fig. 24.14 Lipodystrophy over back (buffalo hump) in a patient on retroviral medicine for human immunodeficiency virus (HIV). **(a)** Preoperative image with marking, **(b)** 3 days postoperative.

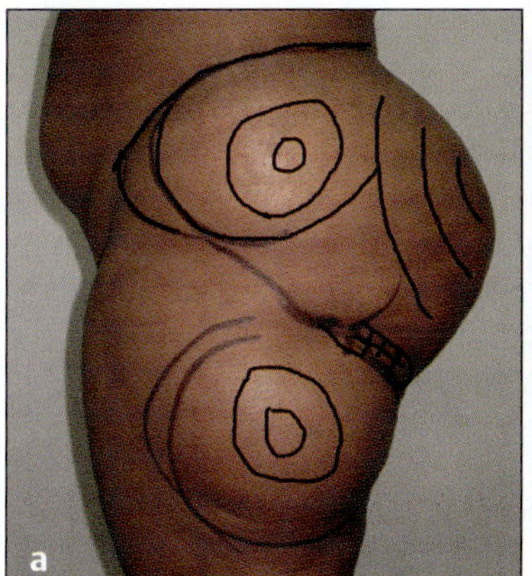
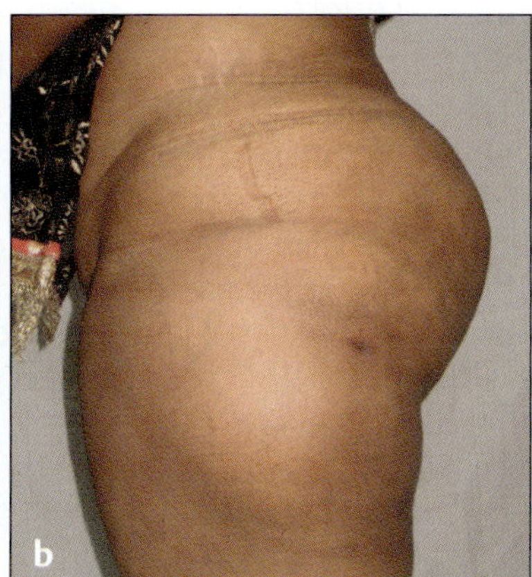
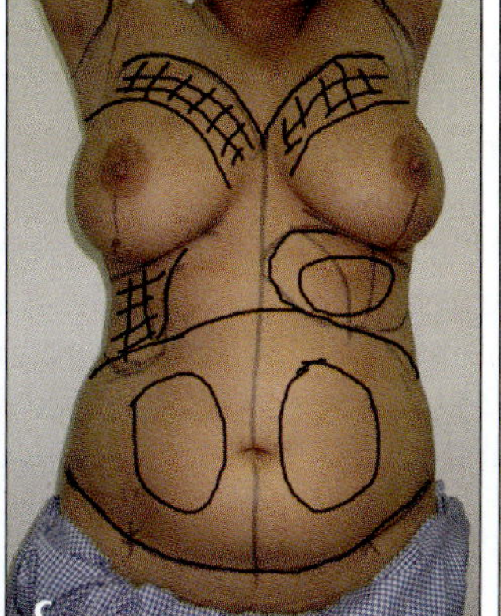
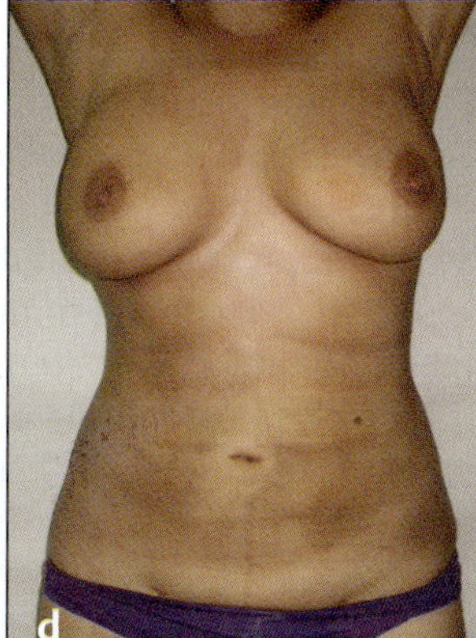

Fig. 24.15 Topographic marking for liposuction. **(a)** Preoperative marking in buttocks and trochanter. **(b)** 3 weeks post liposuction image. **(c)** Preoperative marking in abdomen and breast in another patient. **(d)** Two months post liposuction image after 10 liters infiltration and 10 liters of aspiration.

shown to the patient for one final confirmation and are kept for digital display in the operating room for a quick reference during surgery.

Anesthesia

The anesthesia technique is based on multiple factors like duration, area, and extent of procedure, volume of expected lipoaspirate, patient's positioning during liposuction, and general health of the patient. The surgery can be performed under general anesthesia, regional or under local anesthesia with or without sedation. No single anesthesia technique has proven to be superior over another.

The anesthesia is kept as simple as feasible with the operative time not exceeding 4 hours. This is best achieved with surgery being done by a team of two to three plastic surgeons. Author prefers to use spinal or epidural anesthesia, supplemented with tumescent anesthesia. Many times a combination of anesthetic techniques are used to minimize the use of anesthetic drugs and keeping the safety of the patient in mind.

Tumescent Anesthesia

The concept of tumescent anesthesia has revolutionized the technique of liposuction. Tumescence is the state of being "swollen and firm." The tumescent anesthesia may be defined as "subcutaneous, periadipose, hyperhydrostatic pressurized, megadosed, ultradilute, epinephrinized, local anesthetic field block."[16]

A dose of lidocaine 35 mg/kg of body weight is considered safe optimal therapeutic threshold, with doses up to 55 mg/kg, approaching the margin of safe therapeutic window.[17] It is safe to infiltrate up to 3.5 to 4.5 liters of tumescent solution with 800 mg of lidocaine in 1-liter fluid, when used in a patient of 80 to 100 kg body weight.

Pre-existing liver disease slows lidocaine breakdown. Lidocaine should be avoided in patients on β-blocker or tricyclic antidepressant. A combination of lidocaine with bupivacaine in the infiltration solution leads to synergetic analgesic/local anesthetic effects allowing reduced concentration, while the side effects of both are different. The total dose of bupivacaine should not exceed 8 mg/kg body weight.

After infiltration of tumescent solution, the optimal anesthesia occurs in 15 to 30 minutes. The peak plasma concentration occurs at around 12 hours; the local analgesic effect may last up to 18 hours, and total elimination of lidocaine may take up to 48 hours.[18]

Adrenaline

Author's infiltration formula has 2 mg of 1:1000 adrenaline in each 1000 mL Ringer lactate. The vasoconstriction with this concentration reduces blood loss significantly for most procedures.[19]

Even with 31 ampoules of adrenaline added into infiltration of 15,500 mL, side effects like tachycardia and/or hypertension attributing to the large dose of adrenaline have not been noticed. Halothane as a general anesthetic gas is avoided while using high dose of adrenaline.

Instrumentation

Cannulas

One of the most important and variable equipment required for a liposuction is the cannula. One has to choose from innumerable variety and designs depending upon various situations (**Fig. 24.16**).

Diameter

Initially when SAL was the only modality, the belief was to use large diameter (8–10 mm) cannula because of its ability to remove large quantity of fat rapidly with minimum effort and time. The use of such large cannula resulted in surface irregularities, unevenness, ridges, and increased postoperative pain. It also led to wide spread tissue traumatization, and widespread bruising due to damage to the neurovascular structures and sometimes resulted in skin necrosis.

Improvement in the result was achieved with the use of finer cannula as small as 2.5 mm diameter or smaller. It also reduced the traumatization of subcutaneous fibrous septae and accompanying neurovascular bundles and facilitated better and faster healing. This allows multiple entrance ports even in exposed parts of the body and hence more suited for aesthetic sculpturing and refinements.

The operating surgeon needs to select optimum size of the cannula to balance between better results and the duration of the surgery. **Table 24.1** indicates the efficiency in time in relation to the diameter of the cannula.

Length

The length determines the reach of the cannula tip for extraction of the fat. The shaft of the cannula also needs to be sufficiently thin to get the best internal diameter without losing the strength to prevent bending. Besides, the inside of the shaft of the cannula should be ultrasmooth, as roughness causes increased resistance at liposuction, and also tends to harbor tissue and blood because of difficulty in cleaning the internal surface after every surgery.

Shape

Most of the cannulas used for liposuction have a straight shaft. However in certain areas for better access, there is a need to use curved cannula to prevent end hits. The surgeon also needs to be extra careful and control the direction of the tip to prevent any inadvertent internal or external injury.

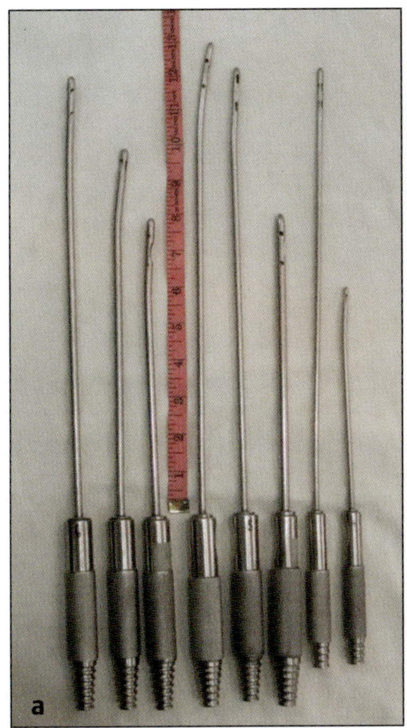
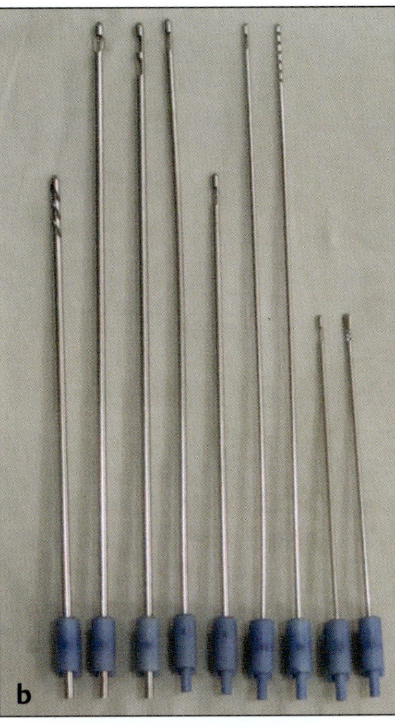
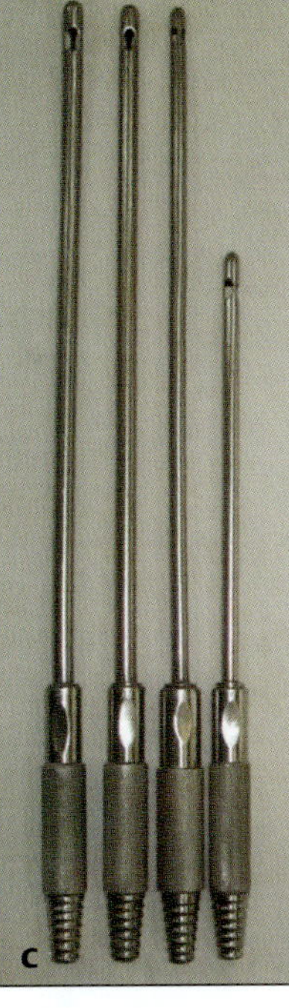

Fig. 24.16 Liposuction cannulas. **(a)** Cannula for SAL 4 to 6 mm diameter, 8 to 14 inches length. **(b)** PAL cannula 2.4 to 5 mm with assorted length. **(c)** Large-size cannula—not used in clinical practice any more. Abbreviations: PAL, power-assisted liposuction; SAL, suction-assisted liposuction.

Table 24.1 Relationship of cannula diameter with rate of aspiration

Comparison of cannula diameter (mm)	Change in the surface area and suction efficiency (surface area = πr^2)
5 mm compared to 6 mm	(3.14×3.0^2) vs. (3.14×2.5^2) = 31.4% more efficient
4 mm compared to 5 mm	(3.14×2.5^2) vs. (3.14×2.0^2) = 35.1% more efficient
3 mm compared to 4 mm	(3.14×2.0^2) vs. $(3.14 \times 1.5.0^2)$ = 43.7% more efficient

Note: Using 6 mm compared to 3 mm cannula is four times more efficient and faster.
Surface area: 3.14×3^2= 28.26 compared to 3.14×1.5^2 = 7.065.
Abbreviations: r = radius, π = pie = 3.14.

Handle

Unlike the shaft of the cannula, the handle needs to be strong, nonslippery, and comfortable. There should be a mark for thumb placement which determines the position of the opening of the cannula and curve of the cannula tip in the opposite direction. The diameter of the tube end of the cannula handle should match the diameter of the suction tube. Interchangeable cannula shaft mounted on the single handle is an interesting modification.

Tip

Primarily there are three main types of cannula tips. These are round, atraumatic with side aperture, tapered or bullet shaped with side aperture, and cannula with aperture at the tip (**Fig. 24.17**). As adipose tissue offers very little resistance, blunt-tip cannula causes minimum bleeding and bruising. More resistance is experienced while passing through the compact fibrotic tissue and needs extra effort to push through.

A tapered or bullet-shaped cannula will meet with reduced resistance but is more likely to traumatize the septa and connective tissue. Hence, this does not find favor with majority of the surgeons.

The aperture tip cannula with an opening at the end of the cannula has a direct access to the fatty tissue when it is pushed through. The fat extraction is efficient with reduced resistance, but with a high incidence of injury to the neurovascular structures. Invariably when this cannula is withdrawn from the incision site, strands of traumatized fibrous tissue stuck at the tip are seen. These cannulas have become almost obsolete in clinical practice.

Aperture

The opening or aperture of liposuction cannula is located on the side of the shaft at some distance from the tip. A single aperture on the shaft has relatively limited cutting edge. Multiple inline apertures can significantly increase the total cutting edge which can be reduced by offsetting the

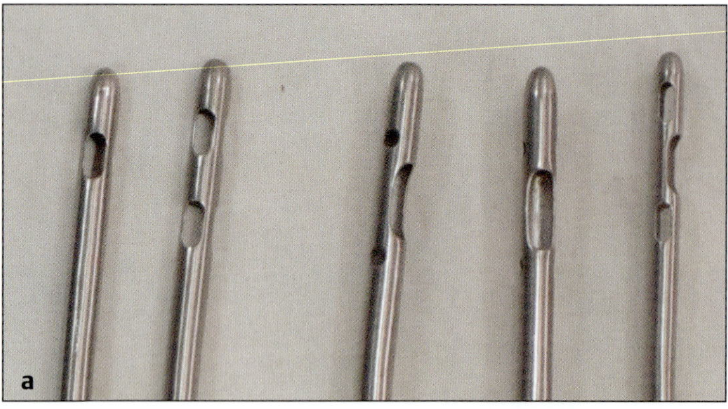

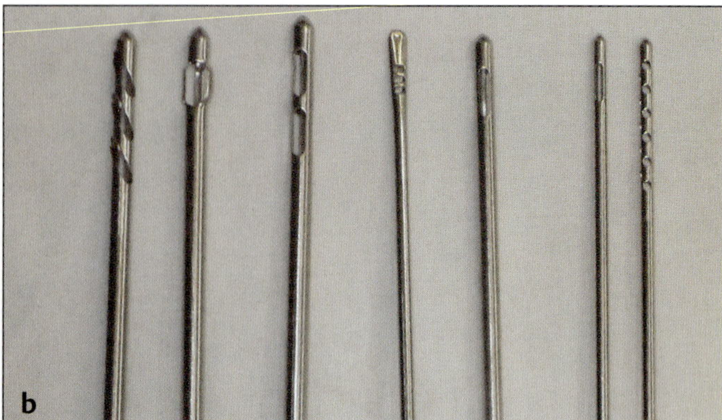

Fig. 24.17 Cannula assorted sets. **(a)** Assorted SAL cannula tips, Single and Double Mercedes types for deep liposuction with quick evacuation. Single large hole with 4 small holes for superficial liposuction. **(b)** PAL cannula assorted tips—cutting, flower-shaped Mercedes, double Mercedes, and with single or multiple holes. Flat tip for facial liposuction and 1 mm multiple holes tip to harvest the fat for use as transplant. Abbreviations: PAL, power-assisted liposuction; SAL, suction- assisted liposuction.

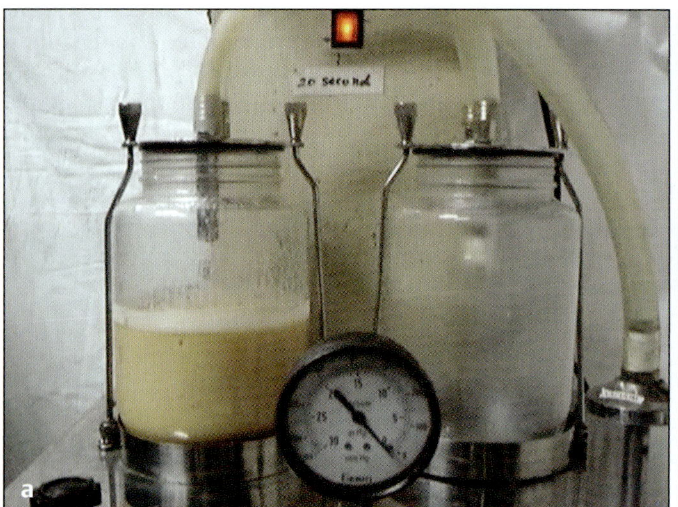

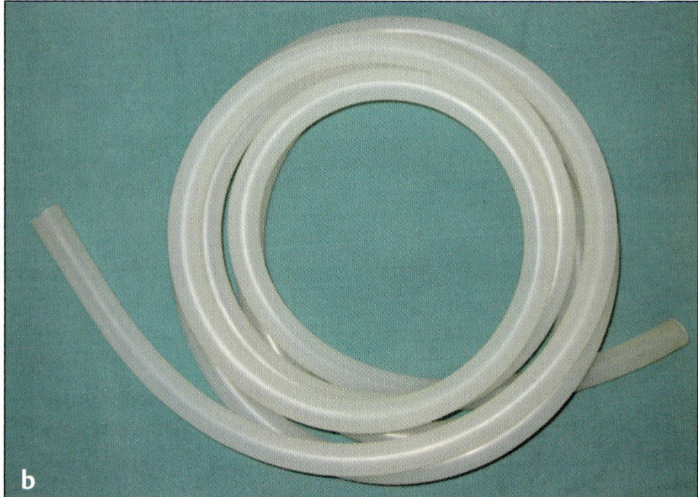

Fig. 24.18 Machine. **(a)** Liposuction machine with fat-filled bottle and suction power minus 1 atm in 20 seconds. **(b)** Silicone noncollapsible suction tube.

apertures. It will continue to provide an increased advantage of uniform fat harvesting without excessive cutting. These are most efficient in harvesting fat, producing minimal tissue damage. Mercedes or double Mercedes apertures help in a very fast and efficient large-volume liposuction.

In summary, 4- to 6-mm-diameter cannulas with single or double Mercedes apertures are used for deep large-volume liposuction, 3 to 4 mm diameter for superficial or small volume liposuction, and 2.5- to 3-mm-diameter cannulas are used for face-and-neck area, and skin etching during high-definition liposculpture.

Suction Machine and Tubes

The liposuction machine should be powerful enough to produce minus 1 atm. (760 mm Hg) in about 15 to 20 seconds, else there will not be enough suction power transmitted at the aperture of the cannula and the liposuction will not be efficient (**Fig. 24.18**).

Another school of thought recommends lower negative pressure suction, apparently more efficient while causing less bleeding.[20] However, the authors have not seen any particular benefit with this theory, except when a very fine cannula is used to extract miniscule amount of fat as in the face or submandibular region.

The suction tubes should be single-use, noncollapsible, flexible, transparent, or autoclavable and made of silicon with an inner diameter of 10 mm and wall thickness of 3 mm. The length should not ideally exceed 2 meters so as not to lose out on the suction power at the tip of the cannula.

Newer Modalities

Ultrasonic-Assisted Lipoplasty (UAL)

The effect of the ultrasound waves in the subcutaneous tissue is to emulsify the adipose tissue and at the same time preserve the vessels and the nerves. The application of ultrasonic energy to more selectively target adipose tissue is attributed to Zocchi.[21]

The microbubble formed due to this energy eventually implodes, leading to fat globule fragmentation and emulsification. With high ultrasonic energy, the cell wall may also fragment with the release of intracellular contents. There is tissue specificity and selectivity of this energy for adipose tissue so the other structures remain unaffected. For the sound energy to transmit and dissipate the heat produced, a wetting solution infiltration is a must before UAL.

The first-generation ultrasonic devices were with solid probes. The second-generation probes were with hollow cannula for simultaneous liquefaction and aspiration (SONOCA).[22] This aspiration of the fluid reduced the cooling effect of solution and hence they were replaced by the third-generation ultrasonic device—VASER (Vibration Amplification of Sound Energy at Resonance; Sound Surgical Technologies, Louisville, CO) (**Fig. 24.19**).[23] This system could deliver energy in a pulsed or continuous mode. There were concentric rings near the probe tip increasing fragmentation efficiency at lower and safer power settings. UAL also reduces the blood loss and ecchymosis.

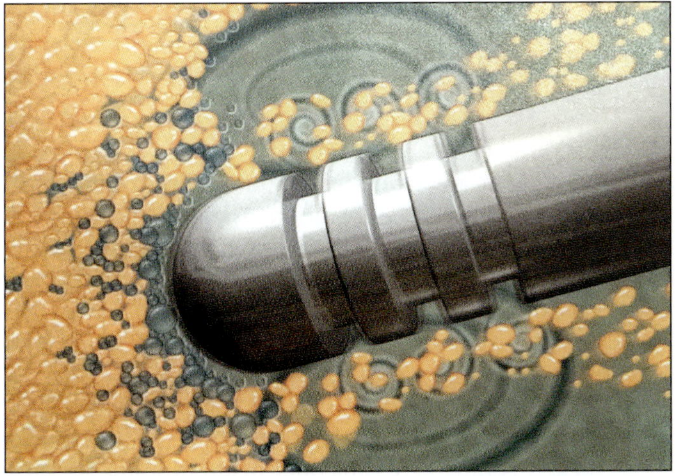

Fig. 24.19 Ultrasonic-assisted liposuction (UAL) emulsification of fat.

On the negative side, the UAL has a learning curve and requires larger incisions to accommodate the probe protector. There is a risk of skin burns, if the infiltration fluid is inadequate, probe is very close to the skin, or the probe is not in continuous harmonious movement. Another drawback is that UAL requires an additional surgical step of liquefaction prior to the process of lipoaspiration with either SAL or power-assisted lipoplasty (PAL), increasing the operative time.

UAL is indicated while treating a fibrous area, (e.g., gynecomastia, back of trunk, in redo-liposuction or when a better skin contraction is desired to tackle skin laxity) (**Fig. 24.20**). This is the technique of choice for high-definition body contouring.

Power-Assisted Lipoplasty (PAL)

The technique of PAL was initiated by Angelo Rebelo In, December 1997.[24] Flynn suggested that the electrically operated devices were less noisy compared to the air-driven ones. The weight of the hand piece was comfortable and the vibrations produced were acceptable.[25]

Coleman evaluated the efficacy of PAL devices. There was an overall 30% increase in the fat extraction speed and 45% increase in the quantity of fat extracted.[26] Katz et al observed that the time taken for same volume of liposuction was 35% less, pain, ecchymosis, and edema reduced by 32 to 38%, and surgeon fatigue reduced by 49% which are important specially while performing large-volume liposuction.[27] The senior author has been using power-assisted device (**Fig. 24.21**) since 2002 and has been able to perform large-volume liposuction to the tune of 15 to 25 liters in around 3 to 4 hours comfortably.

Laser-Assisted Lipoplasty (LAL)

With laser the fat is destroyed in situ before it is evacuated. The technique has been in use since 1998.[28] The Nd-YAG 1064-nm or Diode 1320/1470-nm energy is delivered through a fiberoptic device. Once the tip of the fiber is in the adipose tissue, a forward and backward movement is performed in a fan-shaped manner. The procedure is repeated

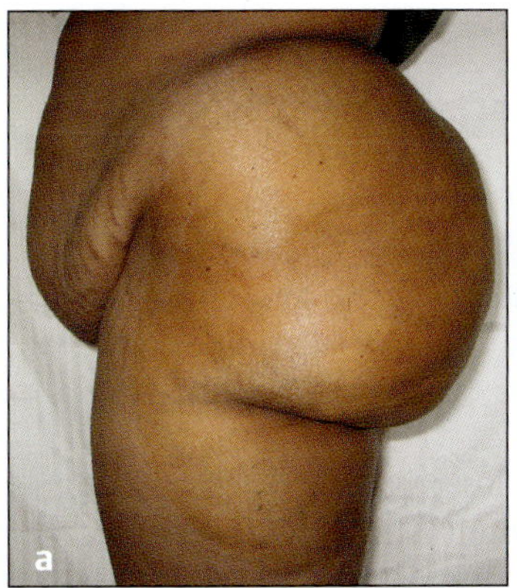

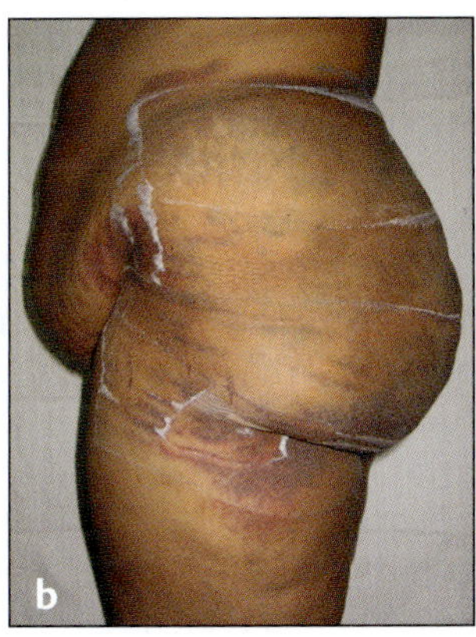

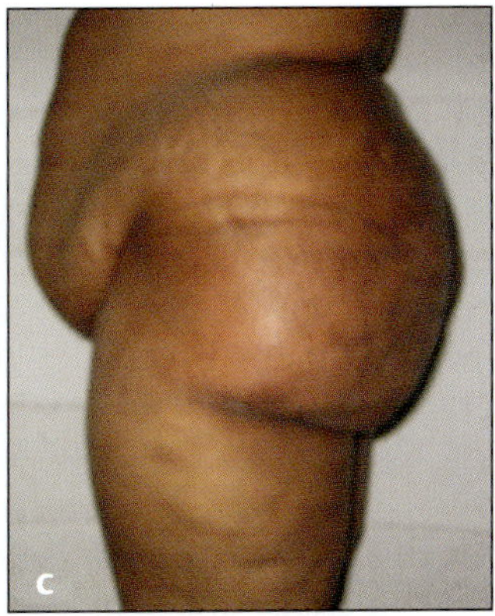

Fig. 24.20 UAL for LFD buttocks with gluteal ptosis. **(a)** Preoperative. **(b)** Immediate post UAL of 5.5 litres. **(c)** Skin tightening, skin lift and correction of ptosis after 3 months. Abbreviation: LFD, Localised fatty deposits. UAL, Ultrasonic-assisted liposuction.

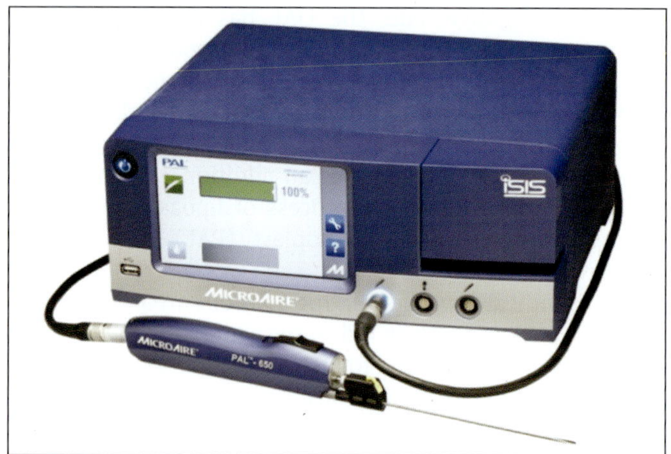

Fig. 24.21 MicroAire power-assisted liposuction device. Console, cable, and a hand piece.

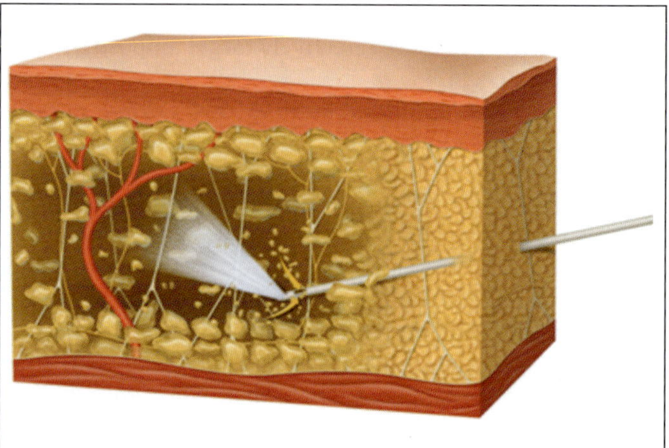

Fig. 24.22 Mechanism of water jet–assisted liposuction.

at different depths, starting with deep layer and moving superficially. Occasionally, a popping sound may be heard due to bursting of the fat cells when the laser energy is delivered. Once there is a loss of resistance to the moving fiber, the emulsified fatty fluid with fat cells is either drained or aspirated with suction cannula. The laser lipolysis is beneficial for a small pocket of fat and has shown to produce skin contraction with adequate heat being generated under the dermis.[28]

Water Jet-Assisted Liposuction (WAL)

This method of liposuction allows a controlled and selective fragmentation of fat globules. A fan-shaped liquid jet fragments the fatty tissue. The process of infiltration, detachment, and suction is happening simultaneously. The cannula can be inserted and moved very smoothly into the fatty tissue, owing to the continuous water jet spray.

Taufig[29] has noted that the surgery time can be reduced by more than 40% and the complications reported are miniscule. This technique is useful for harvesting fat which can be used as a live fat graft (**Fig. 24.22**).

Radiofrequency-Assisted Liposuction (RFAL)

RFAL technique harnesses bipolar radiofrequency energy to disrupt the adipose cell membrane and cause lipolysis. RF causes thermal injury at the subdermal level leading to skin contraction.[30] The external electrode channels the energy predominantly within the fat and is focused upward toward the subdermal fibrous septal network. The internal electrode also acts as a suction cannula (Bodytite). The device is safe with continuous impedance and temperature monitoring.

Plasma-Assisted Liposuction

The use of helium-driven plasma energy is a new and promising technique for nonexcisional soft tissue and skin tightening. The technology uses a gentle RF waveform to convert an inert Helium gas into a cold plasma using very little energy involving excited states of helium ions existing between a liquid and a gas phase. The energy is applied at subcutaneous level as an additional procedure, after liposuction is complete.[31]

Operative Technique

Skin Preparation and Draping

Patient is given povidone-iodine or chlorhexidine bath preoperatively. In the operation theater, painting is done with warm 5% povidone-iodine from neck to ankle, circumferentially. Patient is then made to lie on the OT table, covered with sterile sheets.

Positioning and Incisions

The position of the patient is kept such that the area that is to be sucked is fully accessible and made prominent. Most of the liposuctions can be carried out in either supine or prone posture with minor alterations. Access incisions are marked taking into consideration the reach to the areas to be addressed and keeping them well-concealed in shadow, hair-bearing area or natural crease lines. Multiple incisions may be needed to address an area for good contouring.

Modalities

The nomenclature given for a variety and amount of infiltration fluid, when compared to the estimated lipoaspiration, is quite often confusing. It may be broadly classified as dry or wet technique.

In *dry technique*, no fluid is injected in to the tissues. It has limitation as the suction amount is limited and causes significant blood loss, frequently requiring blood transfusion.[32]

Currently the dry technique is used only when a very small amount of fat is to be harvested.

In *wet technique*, which is currently the most commonly used procedure, the amount of infiltration equals to the amount of expected aspiration. In *super wet technique*, the infiltration is almost three times the amount of presumed aspiration.

In *tumescent anesthetic technique*, the liposuction is carried out purely under local anesthesia with tumescent fluid. The term is sometimes interchanged with wet technique.

Infiltration Fluid

Infiltration of tumescent solution (**Table 24.2**) is done with a fine 1-mm-diameter, blunt-tip, 10- to 30-cm-long cannula, so as to reach all the areas. The cannula has multiple holes near the tip in spiral fashion to permit smooth and uniform diffusion. It is advisable to use motorized pump, when large amount of fluid is to be infiltrated. Infiltration ports used are mostly the same as for liposuction.

The author has experienced an appreciable reduction in tissue swelling postoperatively with Ringer lactated (RL), instead of normal saline. RL solution also prolongs the stability of epinephrine secondary to a more acidic pH of 6.3.[33]

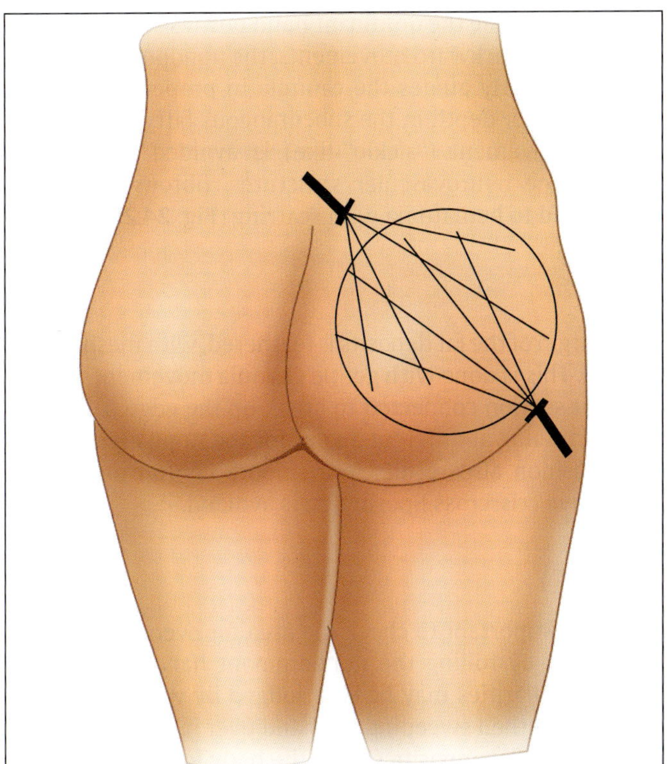

Fig. 24.23 Pretunneling with only radial to-and-fro cannula movements.

Pretunneling

Once sufficient time has passed after the infiltration, the pretunneling (**Fig. 24.23**), is carried out using a blunt-tip cannula, which is to be used for suction, keeping the machine off. The cannula is moved "to and fro" in radiating fashion in multiple layers from deep to superficial. This is done with the suction tube attached to allow drainage of fluid in the tube. The deep layer will have smoother passage of the cannula, while the superficial layer has somewhat gritty feeling. The tactile feedback during pretunneling helps in establishing a pseudoplane, where lipoaspiration will be done.

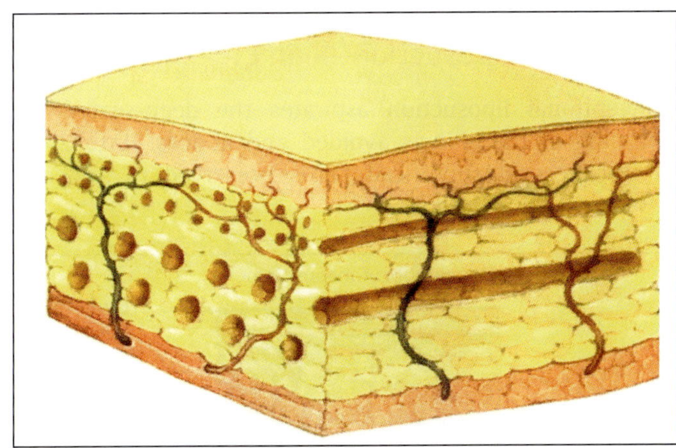

Fig. 24.24 Tunnels liposuction—larger diameter cannula for deeper fat and finer ones for superficial fat.

Deep Debulking

The fat extraction with deep debulking begins in radial fashion (**Fig. 24.24**) as guided by the preoperative marking with long, even and gentle strokes, as many as required, so as to empty the tunnel or till blood-tinged fluid appears in

Table 24.2 Composition of tumescent solutions used by the author in wet technique

Drug	Tumescent fluid	Tumescent anesthetic solution
Ringer lactate (RL)	1000 mL	1000 mL
Inj. Adrenaline	2 mg	2 mg
Inj. Triamcinolone	10 mg	10 mg
Inj. Lidocaine 2%	200 mg (10 mL)	600–800 mg (30–40 mL) (maximum 35 mg/kg body weight)
Inj. Bupivacaine 0.5%	25 mg (5 mL)	100 mg (20 mL)

the tubing. While the dominant hand pushes and carries out forward and backward movements, the nondominant, smart hand constantly guides the cannula in proper direction as well as proper depth in the subcutaneous fatty layers. Side-to-side movement ("sickle"-like) is avoided, which may damage the neurovascular structures, fibrous septa, and would lead to hematoma with scarring (**Fig. 24.25**).

Undermining

The margin of the fat deposits is feathered, with mesh undermining. This is done with gentle cannula movement, with or without suction connected to break up the edge. Tunneling and suctioning at different angles for the same area in crisscross fashion also results in a smooth contouring. But an aggressive crisscross liposuction is avoided.

Defining

It is very important to check the area for evenness, visually as well as by rolling the nondominant hand over treated area. Irregularities may be well judged by wetting the skin surface and then sweeping the hand over it. Also keep comparing with the opposite side of the body for symmetry. The end point is when all possible deep and middle layer fat is evacuated, leaving behind a pinch thickness of approximately 2 to 2.5 cm.

Superficial Liposuction—Skin Etching

Conventional liposuction aspirates the deep-seated fat. Thinning of the skin is avoided and at least 1 to 2 cm of thickness of superficial fat is preserved to save the dermal-subdermal vascular plexus. Superficial liposuction is carried out only when the skin retraction is desired or while doing high-definition (HD) body contouring. The cannula used is 2- to 2.5-mm-diameter blunt-tip. The holes are always directed away from the skin, except when skin etching is done.

Beware of over aspiration. Knowing when to stop is the hardest lesson. What is left behind determines the result. If the skin appears lax after deep suction, it may be helped with controlled superficial suction, to stimulate skin contraction. This is done with skill, based on the expertise and experience.

> "Aesthetic sense is hard to describe, and is more innate than learnt."

Closure

The entry site through which the liposuction is performed are sutured loosely or left open. These serve as drainage points for the residual fluid. The drainage may continue for up to 2 to 5 days and usually seals off on its own (**Fig. 24.26**).

Postoperative Management

There should be controlled temperature in recovery room. Good oxygenation and adequate IV fluid should be given. Deep vein thrombosis (DVT) prophylaxis using calf pump or stockinet is essential in most of the patients and early mobilization under supervision is encouraged. In selected patients, low-molecular heparin may be given. Patients are encouraged to start their normal routine activities at the earliest.

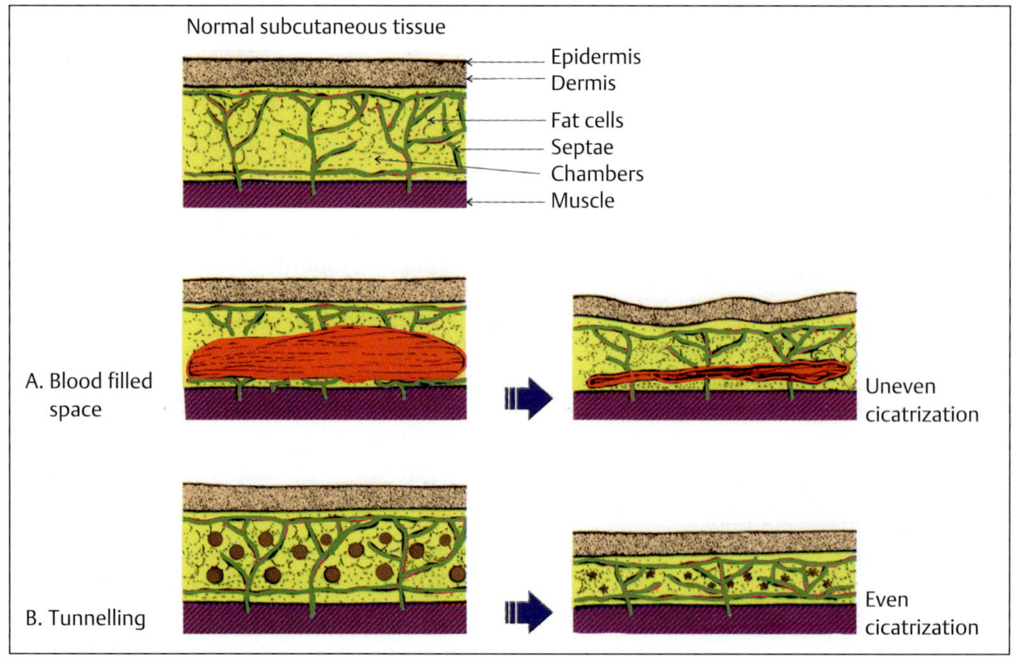

Fig. 24.25 Avoid side-to-side sickle-like movements to prevent blood filled cavity and cicatrization.

Pressure Garments

Patients start using pressure garments (**Fig. 24.27a–c**) within 48 hours of surgery. The garment should be comfortable, should provide moderate pressure, and should be used round the clock. This promotes reabsorption of fluid and most importantly allows skin to contract smoothly with reduced chance of skin fold formation. The compression garment also provides comfort to the patient during mobilization.

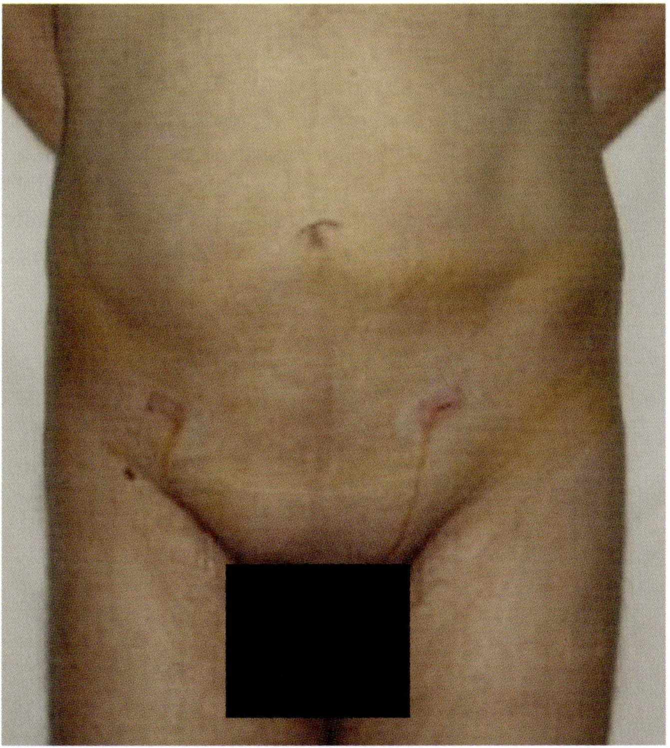

Fig. 24.26 Allow free drainage by keeping access port open postoperatively.

Liposuction in Specific Anatomical Area

Face and Neck

An ideal patient is young, nonobese with good skin elasticity, and has fat restricted in the isolated pockets of submandibular, cheeks, or nasolabial area. Patients with hypoplastic bony contour are not suitable candidates.

Patient who has submandibular fat/double chin with hypoplastic chin benefit from liposuction combined with chin augmentation. The presence of platysma band is a relative contraindication and may need surgical correction. Presence of ptotic submandibular gland may give a pseudoappearance of excessive fat and needs to be addressed separately.

Most of the facial recontouring procedures are done under tumescent anesthesia using 2.5- to 3-mm-diameter fine cannulas at 80% of minus 1 atmosphere pressure. Incisions for the approach are as shown in **Fig. 24.28a–e**. Postoperatively, patients are immediately put on a pressure dressing with a chin strap to prevent any collection.

A word of caution, in infrahyoid region, deep infiltration of local anesthetic should be avoided, as it may temporarily paralyze and affect the function of the strap muscles, leading to difficulty in deglutition. There is also a possibility of damage to the mandibular branch of facial nerve. Hence, it is important to mark and avoid any deep suction in these specific areas of concern.

Upper Extremity

The arm and forearm are easily amenable to liposuction. Upper extremity liposuction is feasible under either general or tumescent anesthesia. The anteromedial arm is the most common area desired by the patient, but must be respected due to the thin subcutaneous fatty layer.

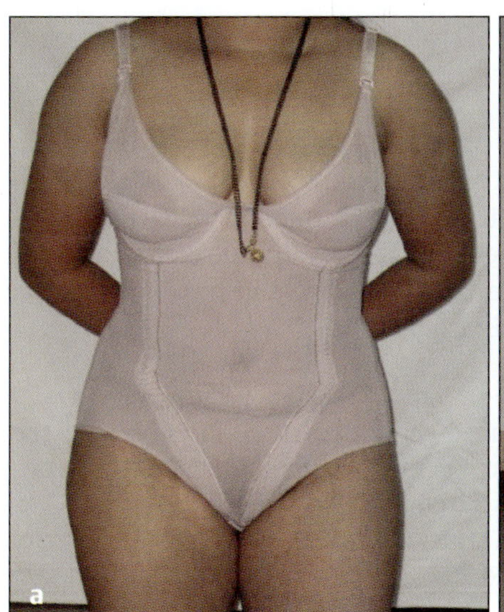

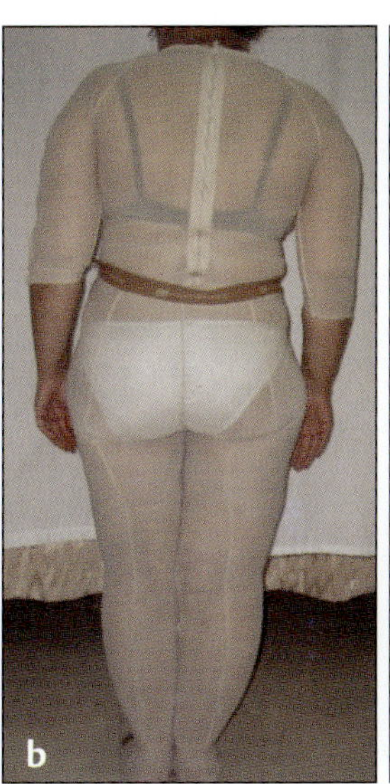

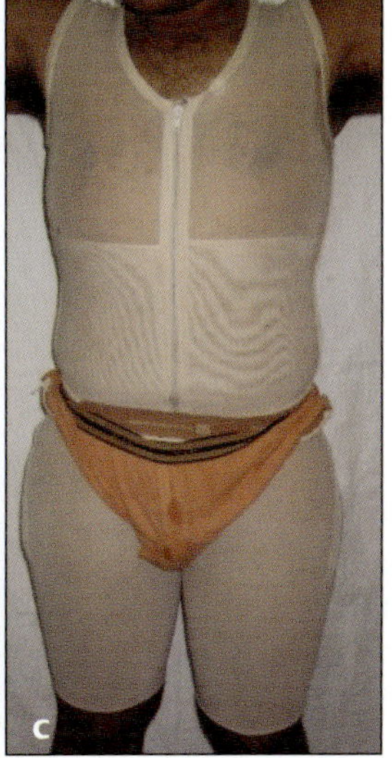

Fig. 24.27 Pressure garment. **(a)** Pressure garment for abdomen and breast support with shoulder strap to prevent folding while seating. **(b)** Two piece pressure garment covering all area, worn over undergarments. **(c)** One piece pressure garment with open crotch and undergarments worn over.

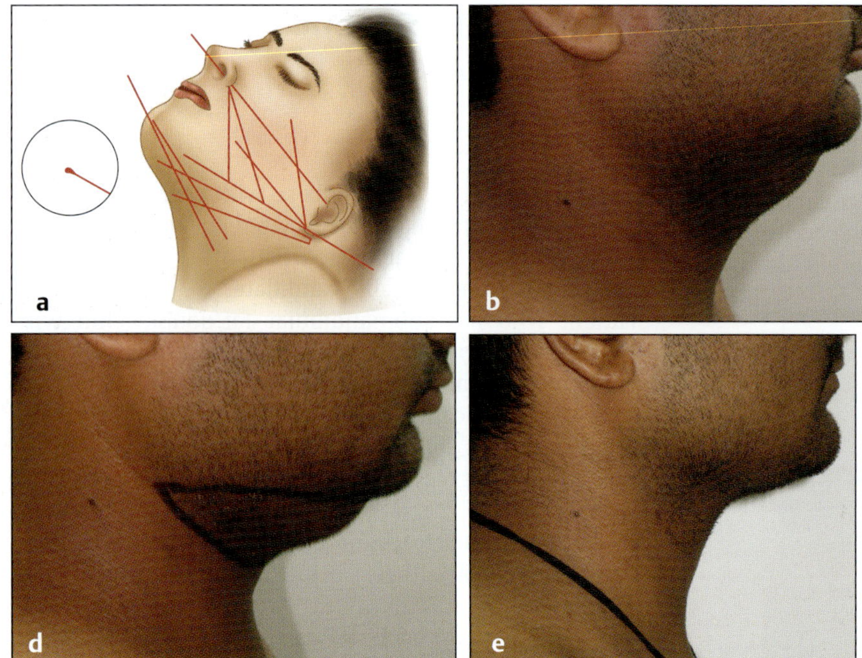

Fig. 24.28 Inconspicuous access incisions for liposuction of face, chin, and neck. **(a)** Diagrammatic representations of hidden access incisions. **(b, c)** Young man with double chin side view in straight gaze and deformity accentuated with neck flexion. **(d)** Marking, **(e)** Five months postliposuction.

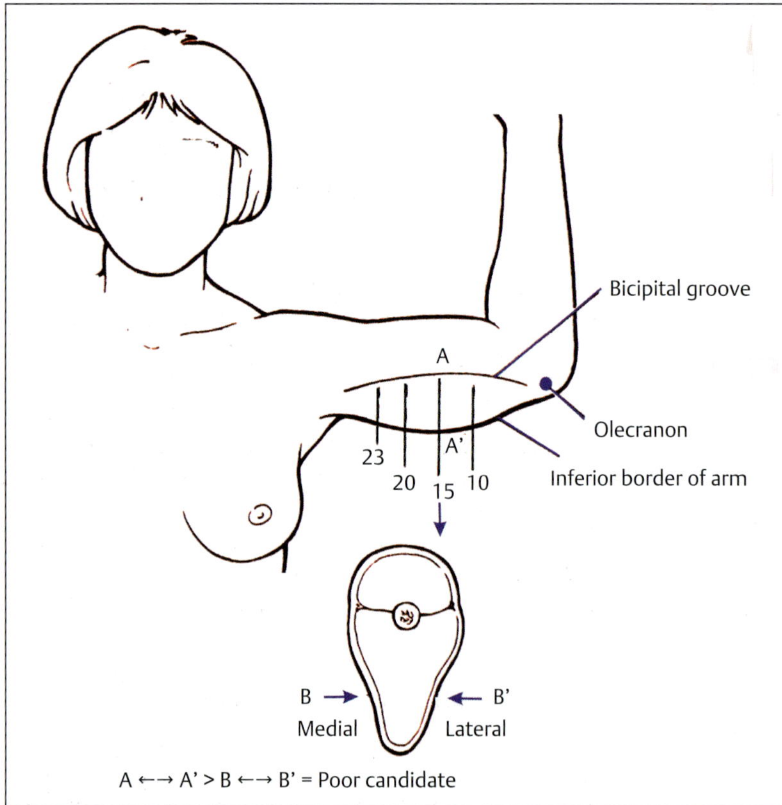

Fig. 24.29 Local fat deposit (LFD) in arm. Planning and feasibility to treat with liposuction. If the pinch thickness B to B' is more than height A to A'. It is feasible to get good result with Liposuction alone. If the ratio is reverse, it is preferable to plan excisional surgery like Brachioplasty.

The access incision for liposuction of medial arm is near medial epicondyle keeping the patient in supine position with arms 80 to 90 degrees abducted. For lateral and proximal arm, the access incision is in the posterior axillary fold with the patient in prone position and arms abducted. The forearm is managed through a small incision near the elbow crease, one each on medial and lateral sides. The cannula size preferred is 3 to 4 mm in diameter.

When the pinch thickness is more than the laxity of the skin (**Fig. 24.29**), the results of liposuction are rewarding (**Fig. 24.30a, b**). When the medial arm skin is hanging due to excessive fat and loose skin, with the overhanging skin more than the pinch thickness, it is best treated with brachioplasty in combination with liposuction. Aggressive liposuction can be done in the areas to be excised, but in the adjacent area and margins of excision, only deep liposuction should be done to maintain vascularity, while achieving smooth contour.

Trunk/Back Contouring

The back of the trunk is a large area with thick skin. After the liposuction, this skin contracts very well and hence provides excellent results. Patients with skin folds around the bra strap area demand this procedure the most (**Figs. 24.30a, b and 24.31a, b**). Patients are operated in prone position and the approach incisions are posterior axilla–arm junction and in lower back area. In author's experience, the quantity of infiltration here always exceeds the amount of lipoaspirate. Use of powered device is preferred as the fat is more fibrotic. Postoperatively the patients can comfortably lie on their back, which obliterates the dead space reducing the possibility of seroma formation.

Breast Reduction and Reshaping

Breast reduction of 30 to 50% of their preoperative size can be carried out with liposuction alone, especially in young patients having good skin elasticity. The lifting effect of the residual breast is achieved as a result of reduced weight and volume leading to retraction of collagen fibers (**Fig. 24.32a–d**). The nipple-areola complex also shrinks with reduction of breast volume and following superficial periareolar suctioning. These results should not be compared with the classic surgical reduction mammaplasty, but the procedure of liposuction does provide appreciable results without transection of lactiferous ducts or unsightly scars. Young unmarried girls are the best candidates for breast reduction with only liposuction. Liposuction could be additional contouring procedure in lateral and axillary tail region during breast reduction surgery. It is also used to address the left-over asymmetry at the end of the procedure.

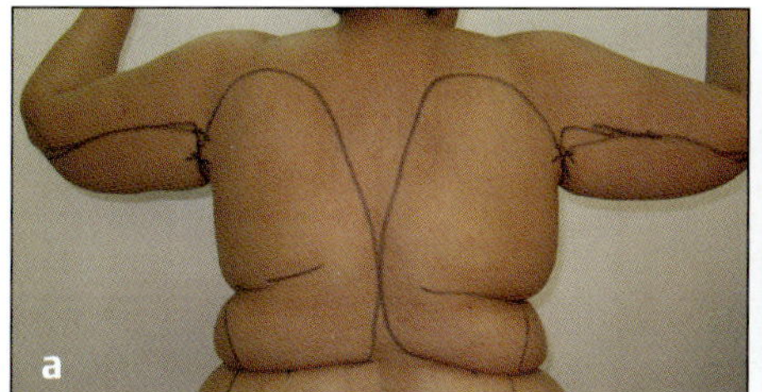
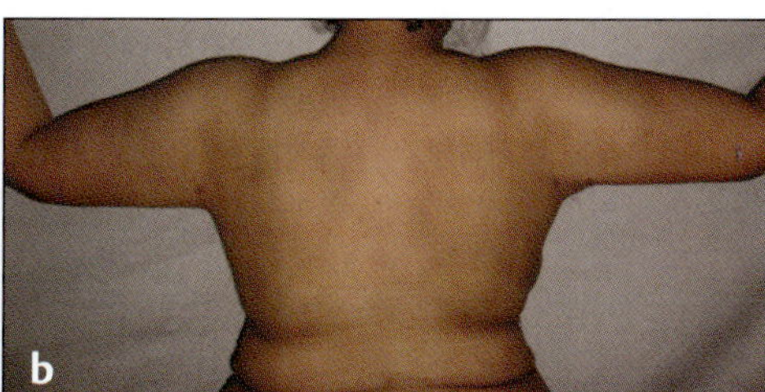

Fig. 24.30 **(a)** Fat deposits in arms and upper back with marking, preoperative view, **(b)** postliposuction after PAL. Abbreviation: PAL, power-assisted liposuction.

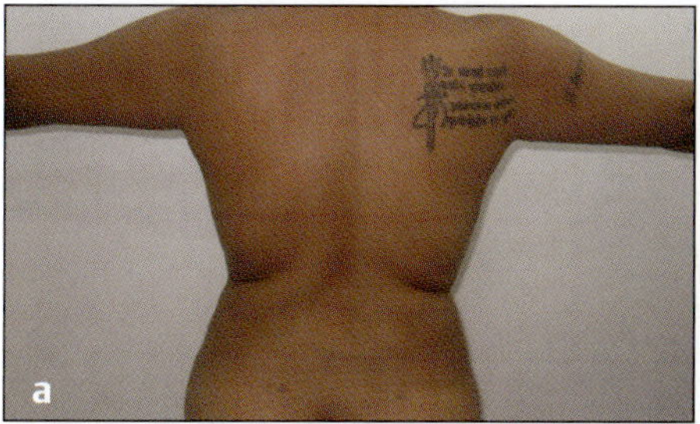
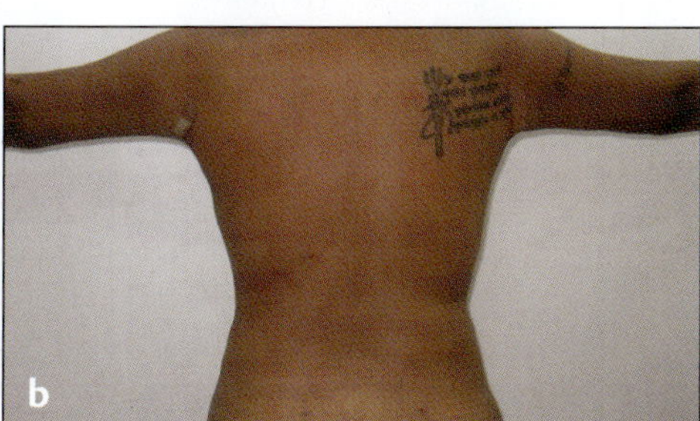

Fig. 24.31 Liposculpture of arm and back using PAL. **(a)** Preoperative, **(b)** postoperative view. Abbreviation: PAL, power-assisted liposuction.

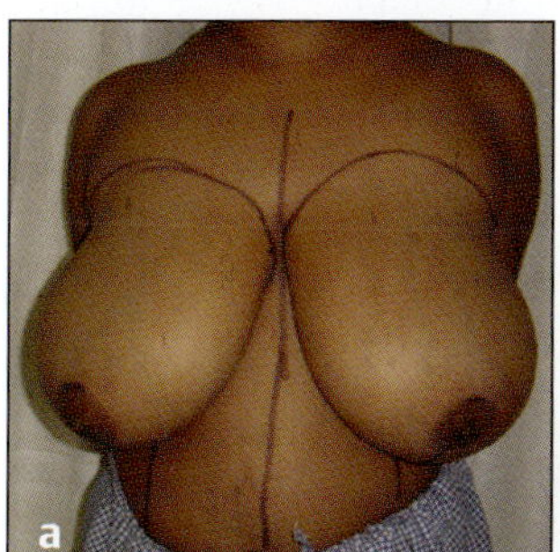
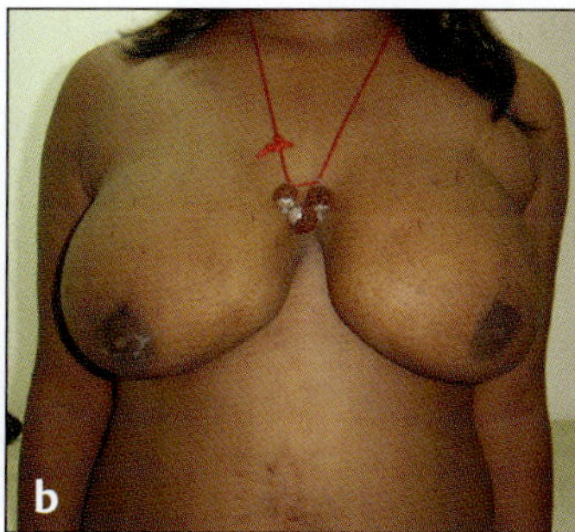
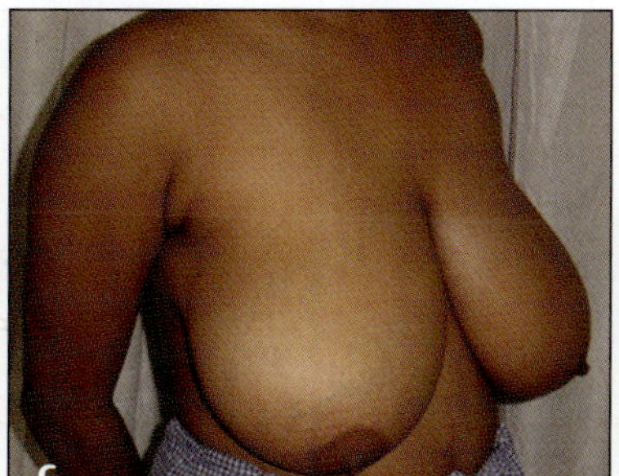
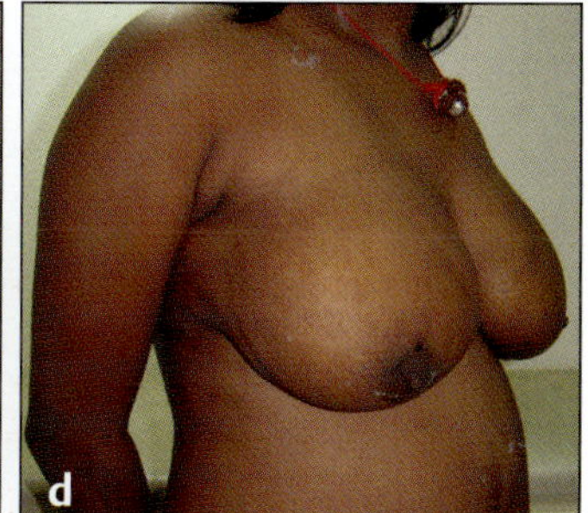

Fig. 24.32 Breast primary fatty hypertrophy. **(a, c)** Preoperative front and right oblique views. **(b, d)** Six weeks after UAL showing reduction with breast lift and areola shrinking. Abbreviation: UAL, ultrasonic-assisted liposuction.

Gynecomastia

Gynecomastia is one of the most requested surgical corrections in men as it causes embarrassment by their feminine appearance. Liposuction followed by gland excision is the treatment of choice even in true gynecomastia. Suctioning under the areola and periphery together with limited gland excision would prevent any deformity (**Fig. 24.33a–f**).

UAL and PAL have the advantage of fragmenting the gland and partly removing it along with the fat. In SAL technique a cutting cannula may be used to help remove part of the fibrotic tissue.

Abdomen and Flanks Contouring

Liposuction for the abdomen is demanded by more than 75% of the patients, amongst all undergoing liposuction. Liposculpture of the abdomen usually gives an excellent result but may also be unforgiving. Sometimes it is difficult to predict skin retraction. Presence of stria indicates poor dermal quality. A simple test to determine the fat quantity is by pinch test and the abdominal muscle integrity is by straight raising the legs (**Fig. 24.34a–e**).

Men have an "apple" shape with "spare tyre" "love handles" distribution of fat in the flanks. In men the dermis also tends to be thick and fat is more fibrous, so the results with only liposuction are more gratifying. Another large population of men (almost 50%) with "pot belly" who seek liposuction may have bulk of their fat intra-abdominal. These patients may be helped only partially with liposuction.

Fat distribution in women is "pear shaped" and the fat is usually found extra-abdominal with presence of striae commonly seen in postpartum abdomen. There could be an excess skin either below or above the umbilicus or global, associated with poor elasticity demonstrated by delayed recoil of stretched skin. Results with liposuction alone may not be very rewarding and patients are better advised to go for additional skin excision procedures.

Patients with primary lipodystrophy may be managed with liposuction alone, but more severe types with flaccid skin and/or muscle diastasis would need additional skin excision along with rectus muscle repair. Current concept of managing this group of patients is to carry out block lipoabdominoplasty, where an aggressive but judicious discontinuous undermining liposuction of the abdomen and flanks is incorporated. This allows thinning and easy caudal advancement of flap while preserving the perforators and intercostal vessels. For details refer to Chapter 25 on "Abdominoplasty and Lipoabdominoplasty" in Volume VI.

Occasionally in patients with huge panniculus, it is advisable to stage the procedure, when either liposuction or abdominoplasty is done first, depending on primary concerns of the patient. The second procedure is deferred for at least 3 months.

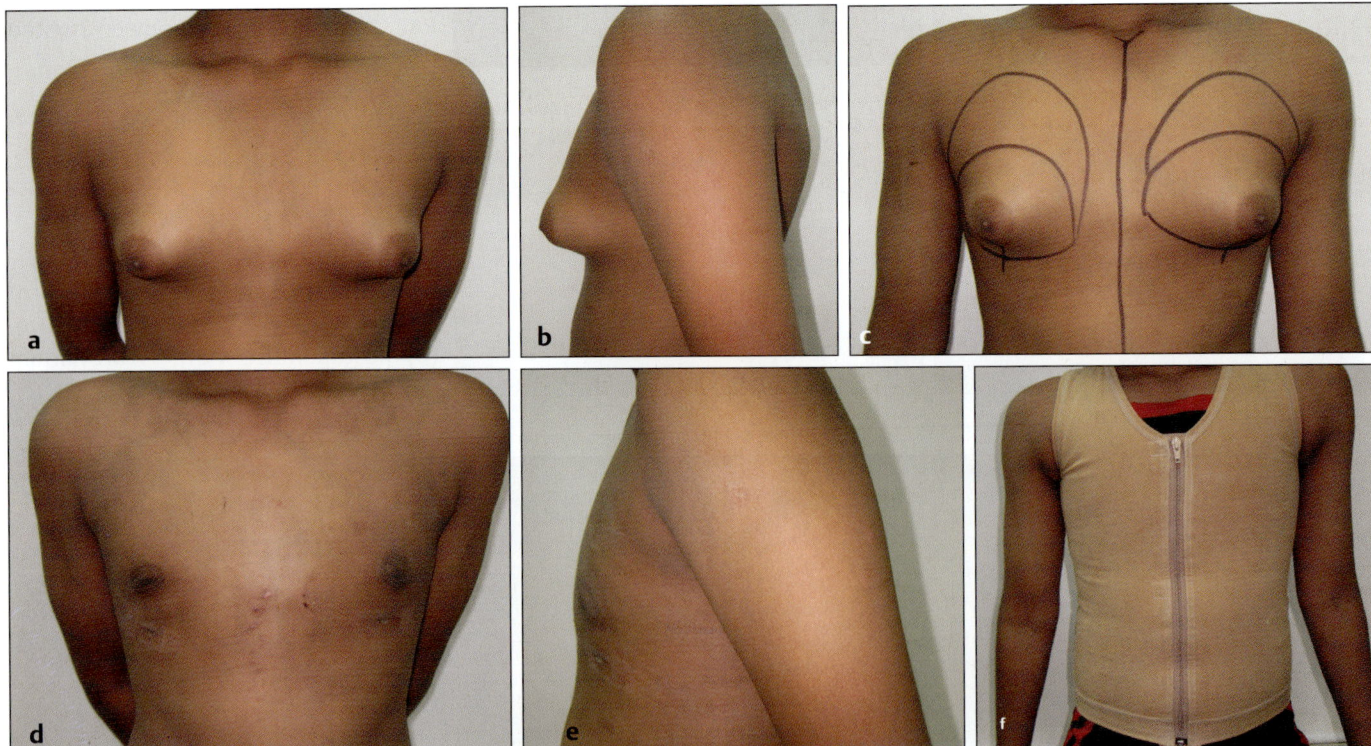

Fig. 24.33 Liposuction for true gynecomastia with glandular tissue. **(a, b)** Preoperative front and lateral views. **(c)** Marking for liposuction. **(d, e)** Removal of fat and gland using ultrasonic-assisted liposuction (UAL). Postoperative front and lateral views. **(f)** Postoperative pressure garment was prescribed for 3 months.

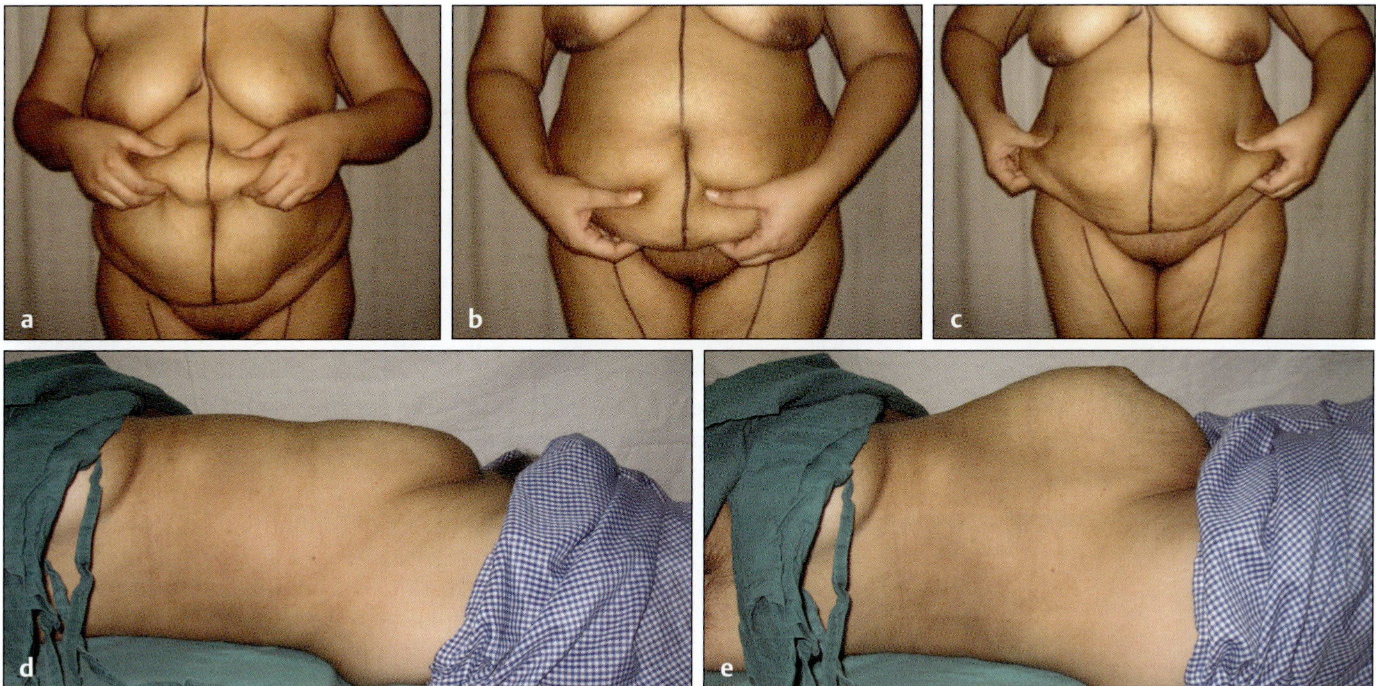

Fig. 24.34 Pinch test method. **(a)** Supraumbilical. **(b)** Infraumbilical. **(c)** Flanks. **(d)** Abdomen in supine position. **(e)** Anterior abdominal muscle laxity demonstrated by leg raising.

The procedure of liposuction of abdomen may be carried out comfortably under spinal/epidural anesthesia. Sometimes it is necessary to additionally infiltrate tumescent anesthetic in the submammary region. The surgery is carried out in supine position with the table in a jack knife (head low–leg low) position to bring the abdominal wall into hyper extension. Also an incision in the submammary fold to access the fat in costal and subcostal region prevents inadvertent injury to the anterior abdominal wall. Incisions are placed in the groin medial to the anterior superior iliac spine. An additional incision is taken hidden in the umbilicus for good contouring and to get an aesthetically pleasing midline groove. The surgeon should lift the skin and fat of the lower abdomen with the nondominant hand and the infiltration starts from deep and continues in to the superficial layer.

UAL or LAL helps in better skin contraction and contouring. There is significantly more fat in the layer deep to scarpa fascia than in the superficial layer. The surgeon should leave at least 0.5 to 1 cm of subdermal fat intact.

To access the flanks through groin incision, use a curved cannula with nondominant hand guiding the cannula. A special effort should be made to remove the fat from periumbilical region by crisscross technique in a manner that the aperture of cannula faces toward the umbilicus. Postoperatively patients are advised to wear pressure garments continuously through the day and are also asked not to sit for longer than 10 to 15 minutes at a stretch in a chair at right-angled position. They may sit for longer hours in an easy reclining posture.

Buttocks Reshaping

Buttocks and trochanteric liposuction is the second most commonly desired area, especially in Indian woman. This is performed under regional anesthesia, while the patient is in a prone position with the table in a jack knife position with a soft pillow support under the pelvic bone, making the area more prominent and easily approachable for liposuction. The area of buttocks touching each other in standing position should be marked and liposuction medial to this line should be restricted (**Fig. 24.35**) and (**Fig. 24.15**). Incisions taken at three places usually suffice to access the entire gluteal and trochanteric area. UAL is preferred to achieve good skin contraction and prevent buttocks ptosis (**Fig. 24.20a–c**). Postoperatively patients can be made to lie on their back with pressure on the gluteal area. When properly executed, this procedure can bring about gratifying results. The contour continues to improve over a period of 6 to 12 months (**Fig. 24.36a, b**).

Thigh and Calf

The fat distribution in thigh and calf varies in men and women. Excessive fat is mainly found in women and gynecoid men. A trochanteric fat (saddle bag) primarily needs deep liposuction to recontour and a controlled judicious superficial liposuction for skin contraction. The infragluteal fat folds (banana roll) are best tackled with superficial liposuction alone. A deep liposuction in this area may lead to secondary gluteal ptosis of the buttocks, which is difficult to correct.

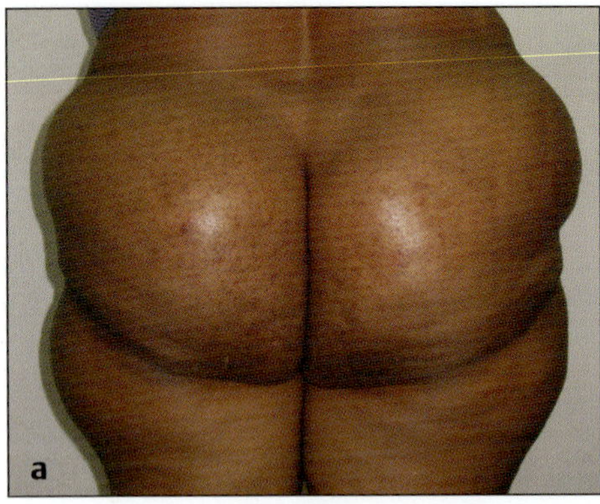
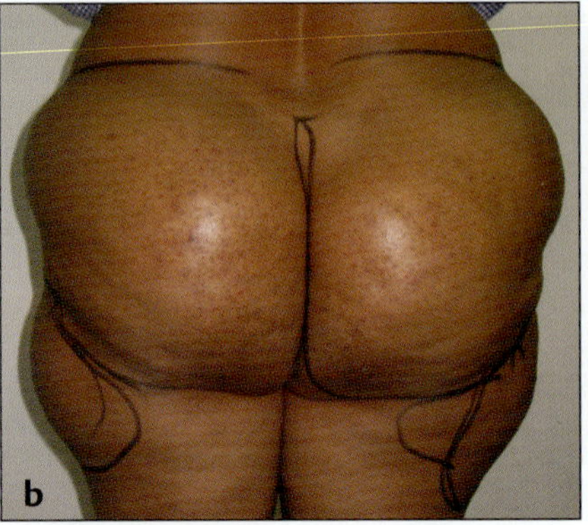
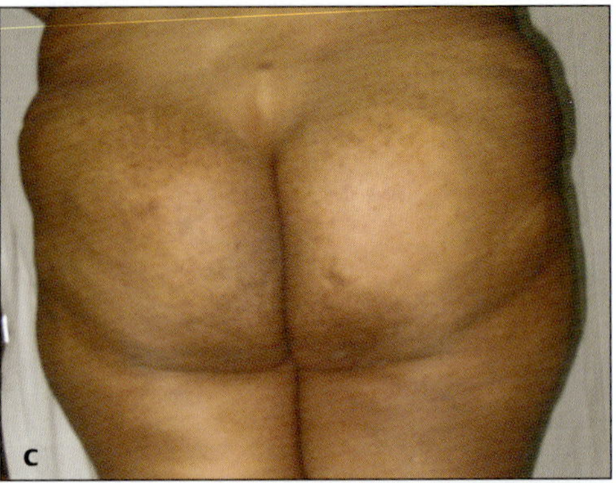

Fig. 24.35 LFD buttocks addressed using SAL. **(a)** Preoperative view of LFD buttocks and trochanter. **(b)** With marking. **(c)** After SAL. Abbreviations: LFD, local fat deposits; SAL, suction-assisted liposuction.

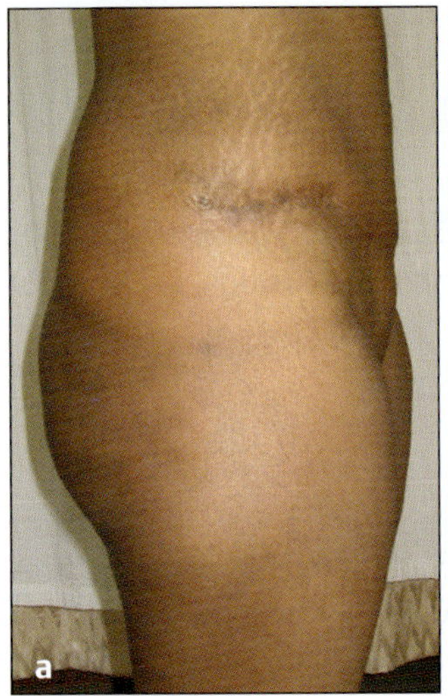
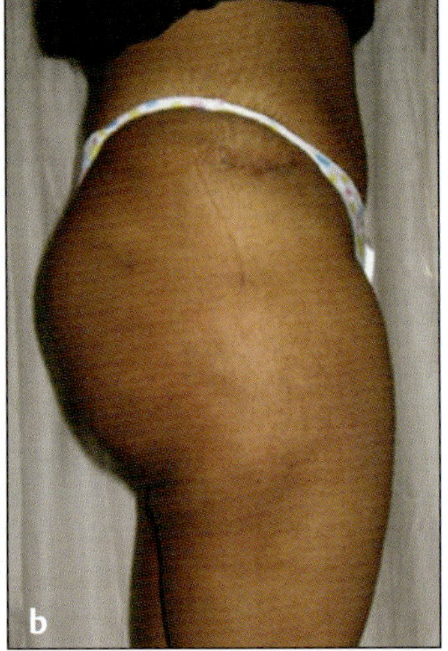

Fig. 24.36 Reshaping of buttocks with PAL thigh and gluteal fold. **(a)** Preoperative view. **(b)** Reshaping by PAL in surrounding area. No augmentation procedure has been used. Abbreviation: PAL, power-assisted liposuction.

Patients are operated in prone position with approach incision in the lateral gluteal crease.

Patients with a history of bulky medial thigh, kissing, or rubbing against each other desire to have fat removed from this area. The suction is mainly done in the superficial layer in supine position with thighs abducted and externally rotated. The liposuction is easy in this area, so much so that it is likely to be oversucked. Hence, the surgeon should exercise caution to prevent overzealous suction. The medial knee roll fat may also be suctioned while doing a medial thigh liposuction.

Liposuction may be combined with medial thigh plasty, but care should be taken to restrict aggressive liposuction only under the skin marked for excision. Surrounding area may also be liposuctioned for better advancement of the skin edges and for smooth uniform contour.

Even though routine anterior thigh liposuction is considered unadvisable, it may be tackled to some extent while doing circumferential thigh contouring. Only deep liposuction should be done, else there is a high probability of suprapatellar ptosis of the skin which is difficult to correct.

The calves and ankle area are suctioned in prone position with fine 3-mm–long cannula with small approach incisions near the popliteal crease on medial and lateral sides. An additional incision may be placed closer to ankle for better access (**Fig. 24.37a–d**).

Large-Volume/Mega Liposuction

Evaluation of the skin quality is the key to decision-making in body contouring. When the body contour deformity involves multiple anatomical areas with abundant skin excess, patient has to choose one of the following:

- Complex and combined excision procedures done in multiple sessions with resultant long scars, which could be unsightly especially in dark Indian skin.
- Tradeoff with a simple single-session procedure of large-volume suction-assisted lipoplasty (megaliposuction), with minimal access incision scars, quick wound healing, and fast recovery, but with visible skin excess and folds, which may be hidden under normal clothing.

A simple question to be answered is, "Would you like to look better with your clothes, or even without your clothes?" Younger and not so obese women and men wish to look good in and out of their clothes, while older and obese women and men desire to get rid of their bulges, to look good and in shape with their normal clothes on. They consider unfavorable "the risk-benefit ratio" of an option of multiple lengthy excisional procedures, with increased morbidity, compared to the option of less expensive, less time-consuming procedure of deflating the deformed contour bulges, with large-volume liposuction, making them look healthy and fit under the normal clothing.

Some of the unmarried boys and girls also desire not to have large surgical scars, which may be a deterrent to finding a suitable matrimonial match.

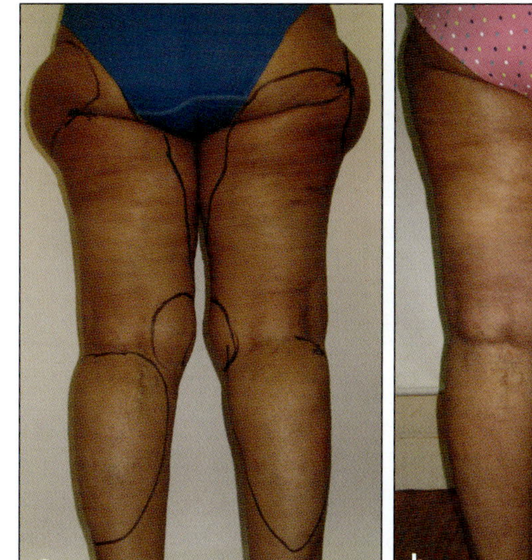
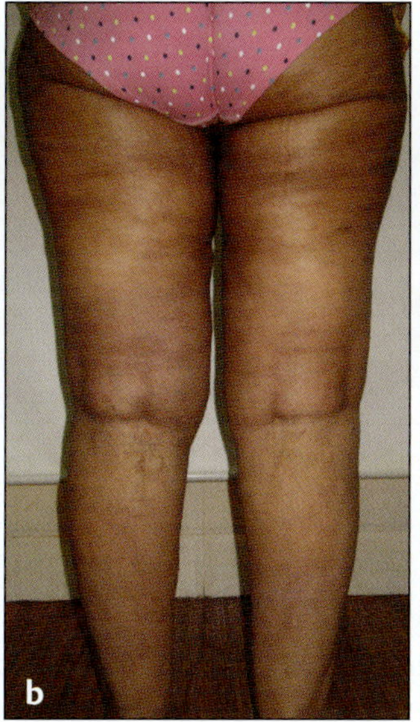
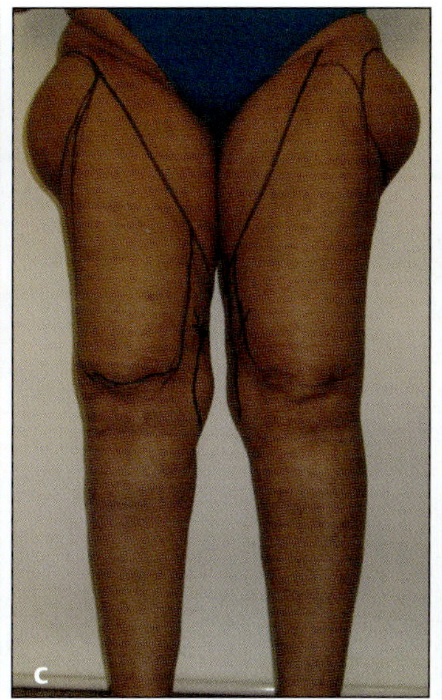
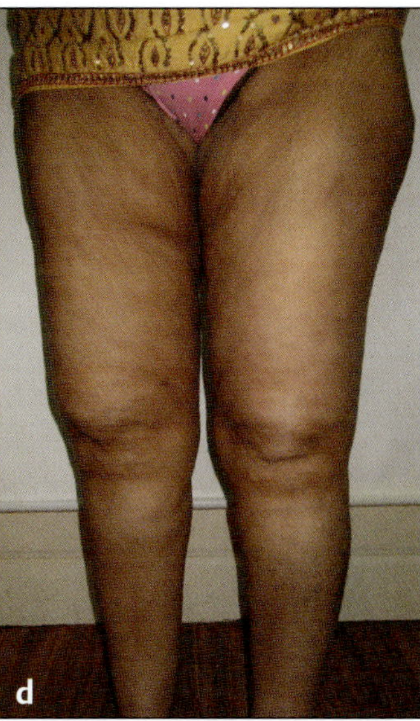

Fig. 24.37 LFD trochanter, medial thigh, medial knee roll, and calf. **(a, c)** Preoperative back and front views with marking. **(b, d)** Postoperative result after PAL of marked area. Abbreviations: LFD, local fat deposits; SAL, suction-assisted liposuction.

The term "megaliposuction" was coined by Pierre F. Fournier in 1996[34] during which 10 liters or more of a mixture of adipose tissue, infiltration fluid, and the patient's blood is extracted in one session. The American Association of Plastic Surgeon defines large-volume liposuction as removal of more than 5 liters of total lipoaspirate in a single session.[35–37]

Through the years, liposuction has advanced, now allowing megaliposculpture to be performed such that more than 10 liters of supernatant fat can be extracted without posing any greater risk to the patient, when compared to a conventional aesthetic liposculpture[38] (**Fig. 24.38a–f**).

Over the years, with gain in experience since 1986, the senior author, with a team of two or more plastic surgeon operating simultaneously, could routinely extract an average of 10 to 12 liters reaching to a maximum of 25 liters, in patients weighing an average of 78 kg and maximum up to 178 kg, in a single session[32] (**Fig. 24.39a–e**).

The goal of large-volume liposuction is to extract maximum possible subcutaneous fat in a single session. It provokes beneficial biological, metabolic, physiological, and psychological modification by losing almost an average of 10% of preoperative body weight.[32,38]

The important points to be taken into consideration are as follows:

- Avoid in chronic smokers and advise to abstain from smoking at least 3 weeks before surgery.
- Plan to complete the surgery in less than 4 hours.
- Use of regional anesthesia with supplemental tumescent or shorter duration general anesthesia.
- Massive all layer liposuction "MALL"[39] is the method of choice using 5- to 6-mm-size cannula.
- The access incisions are left open to allow free drainage of residual fluid or any serous exudate.
- Compression garments are avoided in the immediate postoperative period and not until the patient is ambulatory and the sensation has returned. The fluid seepage usually reduces in about 24 to 48 hours, after which the garment can be safely worn.

Large-volume liposuction is just one instance in the overall management of obesity. After megaliposuction, patients are better motivated to carry out dieting, exercise, and life style changes. This will bring further weight reduction and an improved overall health.

High-Definition Body Contouring

Moving on from pure debulking liposuction procedure, the concept of selective debulking has evolved. This has developed into a specialty of high-definition (HD) body contouring. Creating contour lines that will define body areas in an aesthetic manner is HD body contouring. The contour also depends on the volume encompassed under the surface. Adding or subtracting volume will enhance and highlight the body surface.

The concept of HD contouring is of positive and negative areas, also called as light and shadow effect on the body. The convex surface reflects the light, while concavities or hollow area creates shadow. Alfredo Hoyos, a Colombian plastic surgeon, has studied, developed, and evolved this concept of HD, 3D, and 4D body sculpting surgery.[40]

Thousands of exercise regimen and innumerable diets have been described to achieve the perfect "six pack abs" or a "washboard" stomach. Very few succeed in achieving and maintain it for long. Many people do succeed in getting a muscular body, but the shape is not amply evident over the surface. It is for this group of people, liposuction

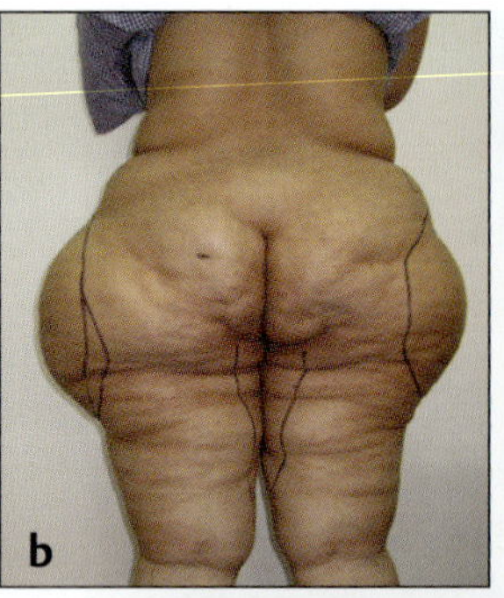

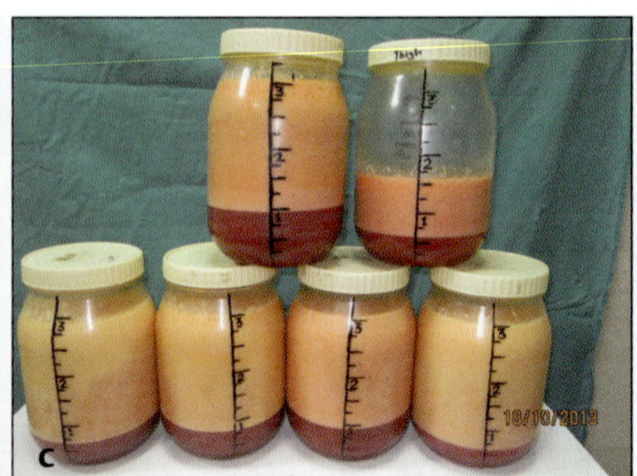

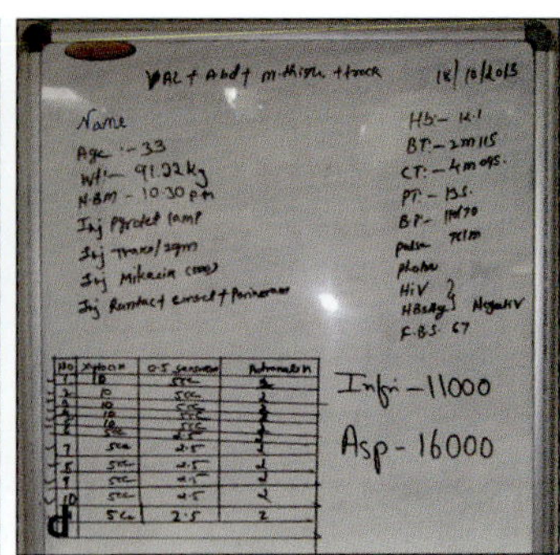

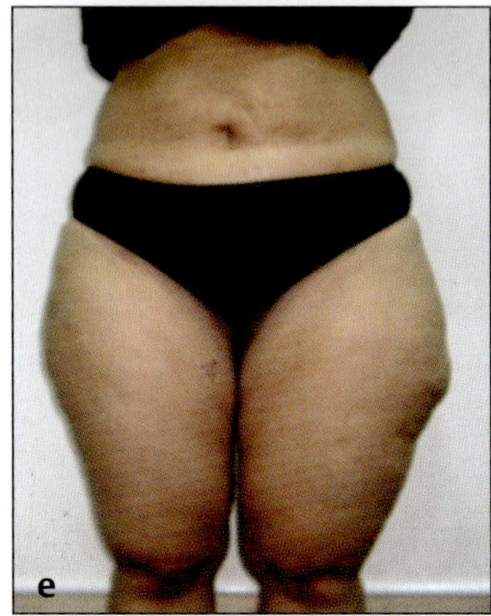

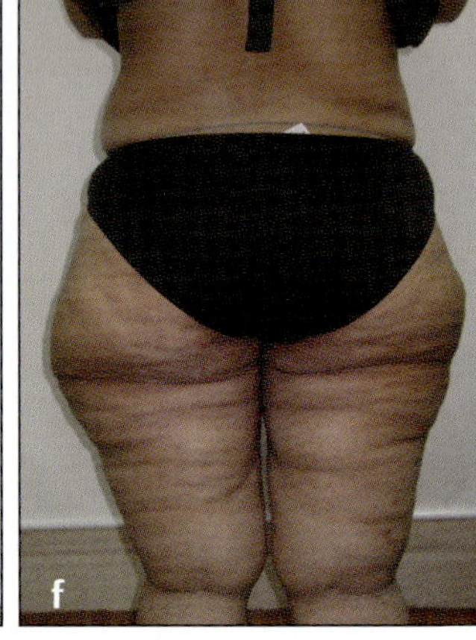

Fig. 24.38 Large-volume liposuction. **(a, b)** Preoperative anterior and posterior views with marking of the abdomen, medial thigh, and trochanteric area of LFD. **(c)** 16.5 liters of lipoaspirates. **(d)** Patient's data on display during surgery. **(e, f)** 8 months follow-up, anterior and posterior views after UAL combined with PAL. Abbreviations: LFD, local fat deposits; UAL, Ultrasonic assisted liposuction; PAL, power-assisted liposuction.

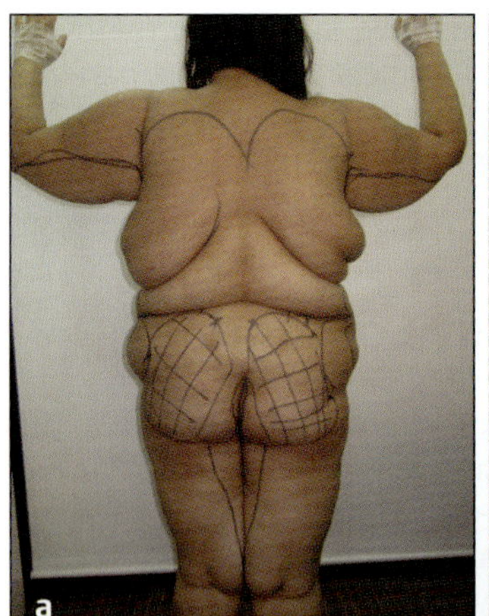

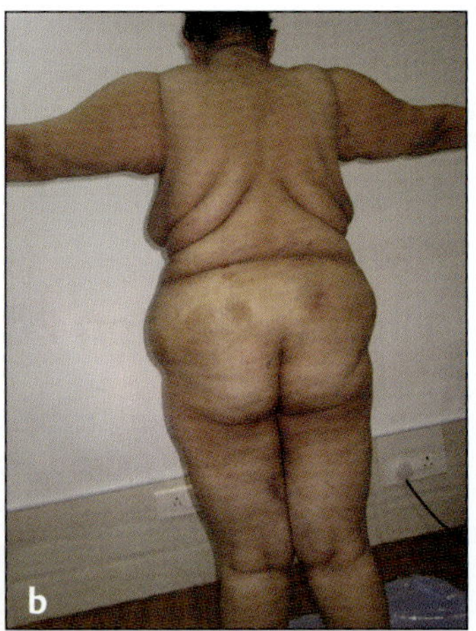

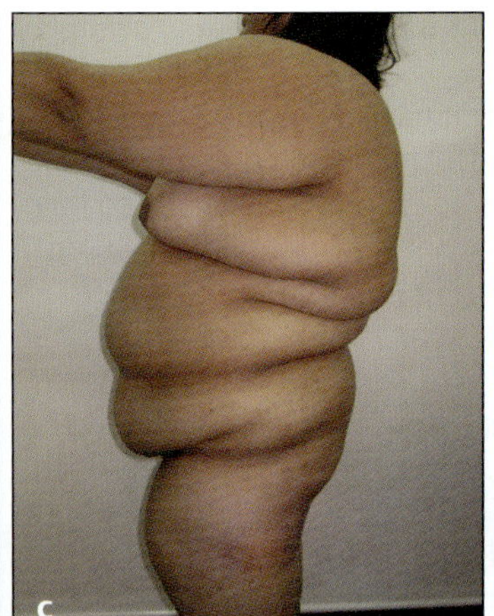

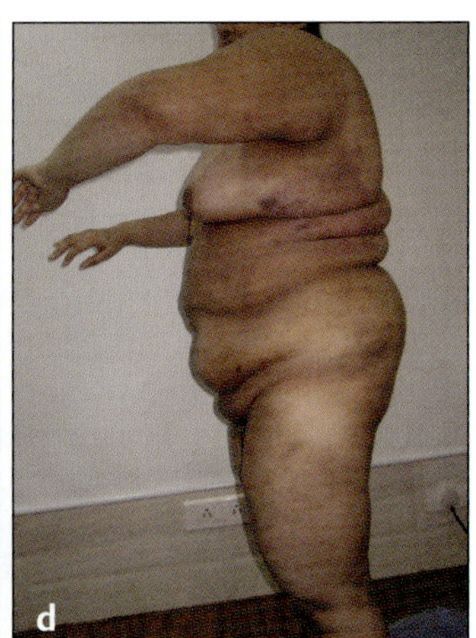

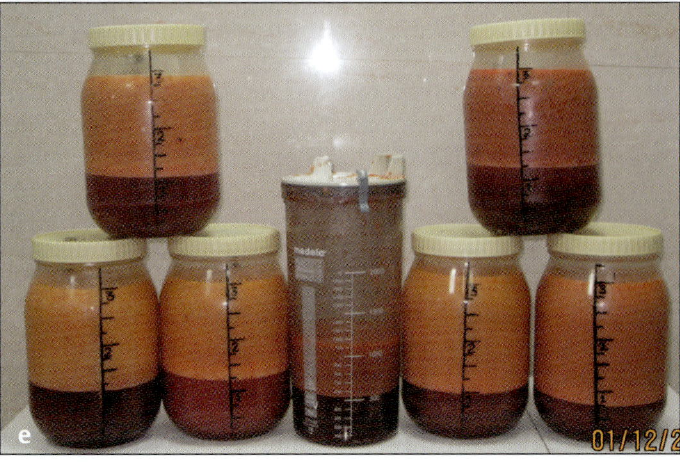

Fig. 24.39 Megaliposuction back, medial arms, medial thigh and abdomen and fat transplant both buttocks. **(a, c)** Preoperative pictures with marking. (cross marked gluteal area for fat filling) **(b, d)** Postoperative pictures. **(e)** Lipoaspiration bottles (3 liters each) showing >19.5 liters of aspirate. (total liposuction 21 liters—fat transplantation of 660 ml in left and 720 ml in right buttock).

can be a great tool to bring out the desired definition of the underlying musculature. Enhancing the definition of these muscles will convert the torso into a well-defined structure (**Fig. 24.40a–c**). Fat transplant may also be added to enhance the volume of a muscle.

Marking

The muscles are put through range of motion and under strain to study their contour, assess their bulk, and identify the borders and then surface marked (**Box 24.3**). Different color pencils are used to highlight areas that are to be deflated with liposuction or enhanced with fat transplant to create the light and shadow effect. This is a fairly exhaustive exercise, but must be carried out painstakingly (**Fig. 24.41a–c**).

Ideal Patient for High-Definition Body Contouring

- Age and sex no bar. Younger people with good skin tone, elasticity with minimal or no stretch marks or striae are the best suited.
- Should not be obese. Exercising regularly with decent amount of muscle bulk and fit to undergo long anesthesia and surgery.
- Well-motivated and without any body dysmorphic disorder.
- Should have good quantum of firm subcutaneous fat which can be suctioned.

Box 24.3 HD body contouring area for preoperative marking

- The clavicle and the sternum
- The deltopectoral muscle groove
- The insertion and three segments of deltoid muscle
- Hollow between the triceps and posterior belly of deltoid
- The groove between the deltoid and biceps muscle
- The inferior border of pectoralis major muscle
- The tendinous intersections of rectus abdominis
- The supraumbilical midline groove
- The lateral border of rectus abdominis
- The location of external oblique and serratus anterior
- The lateral border of the latissimus dorsii muscle
- The paraspinal muscles

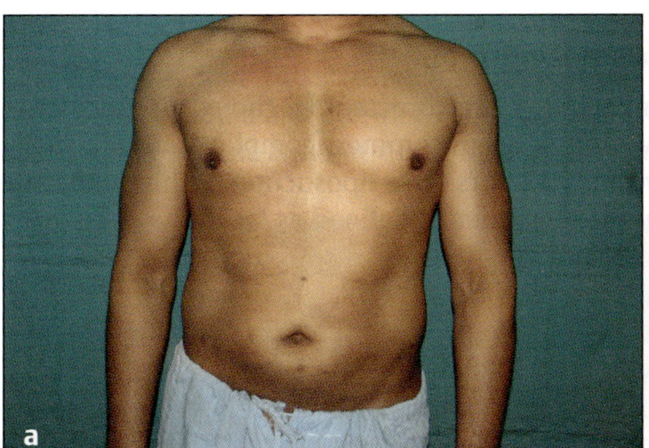
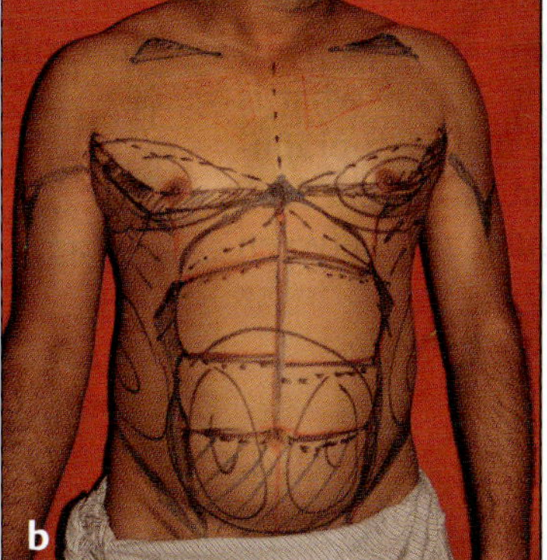
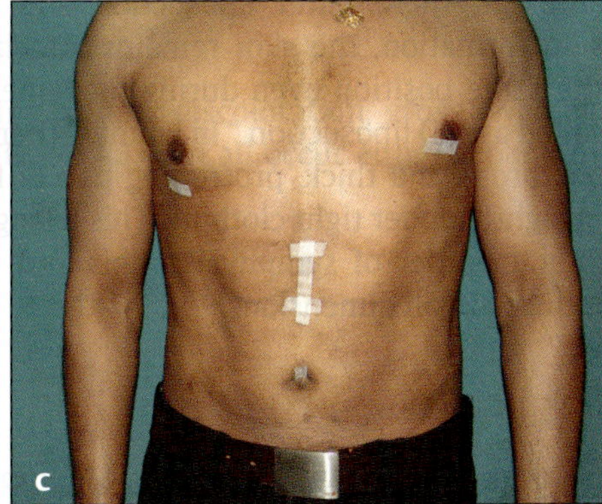

Fig. 24.40 High-definition (HD) liposuction chest and abdomen. **(a)** Preoperative appearance of abdomen and chest, **(b)** marking for HD liposuction. **(c)** HD UAL postoperative result. Abbreviation: UAL, ultrasonic-assisted liposuction.

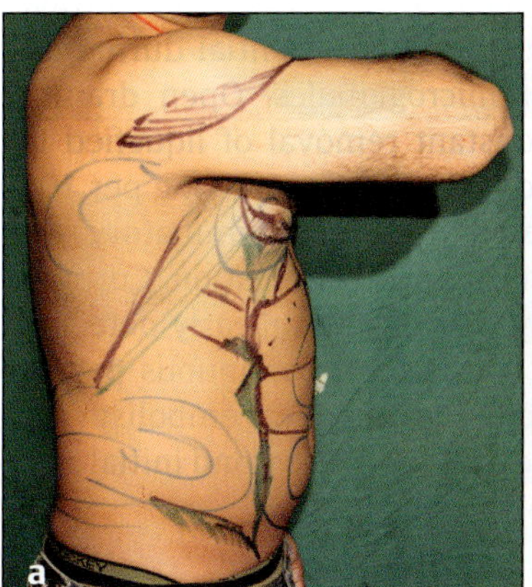
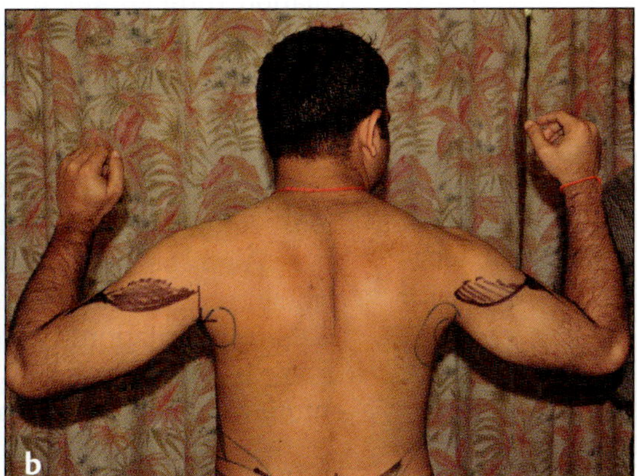
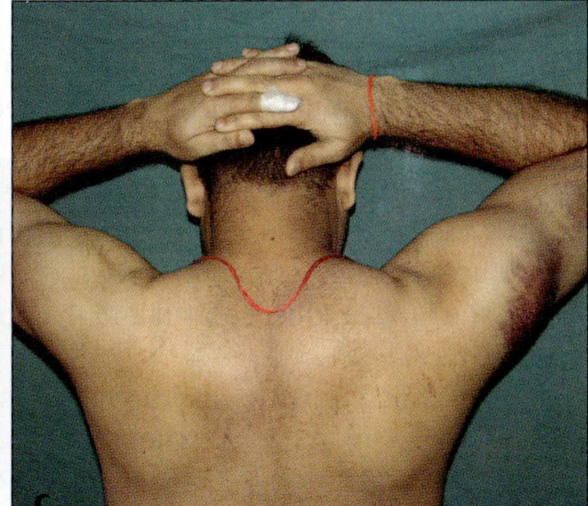

Fig. 24.41 High-definition (HD) liposuction deltoid region and arm. **(a, b)** Marking for HD liposuction lateral view, **(c)** HD UAL postoperative result. Abbreviation: UAL, ultrasonic-assisted liposuction.

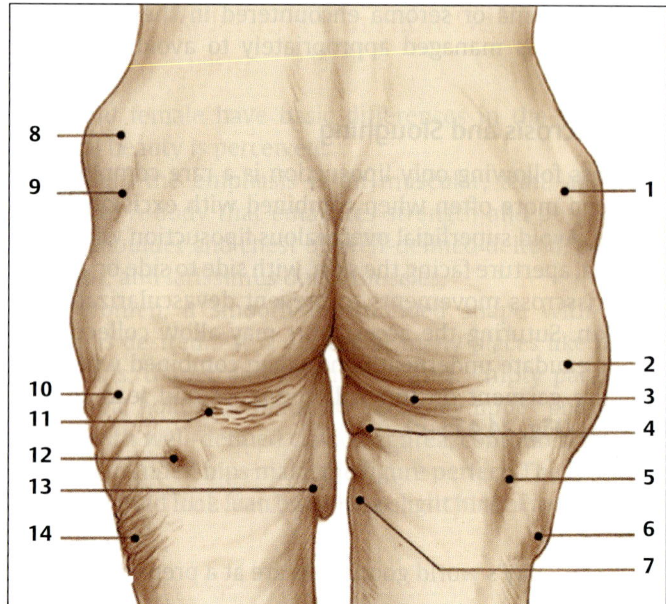

Fig. 24.44 Postliposuction sequelae and aesthetic complications. All types of possible sequelae: 1 and 8, Residual bumps; 2, Insufficient suction; 3, Postoperative banana; 4, Internal waviness; 5, 7 and 12, Grooves; 6, Step deformity; 9, Depression; 10, Waviness; 11, Bunch of little bananas; 13, Ptosis; 14, Wrinkles.

or together and affect patient's postsurgical social schedule. These should be anticipated and the patients are forewarned, more so, while treating the face, as any visually disturbing occurrences can seriously upset them.

Hematomas/Seromas

Small hematomas or seromas are unsightly and do generally resolve on their own. Some hematomas can be treated conservatively with aspiration. Any hematoma that becomes persistent and remains untreated may turn into a chronic pseudocyst. This pseudocyst can be treated with needle aspiration followed by an injection of sodium tetradecyl sulfate into the cavity, followed by local pressure to obliterate the space (**Fig. 24.46a, b**).

Swelling

Swelling is almost inevitable and is seen between the third and the fifth postoperative day. It can restrict physical and social mobility. Anti-inflammatory medication may be of some value. Swelling can mask some irregularities that will manifest over the next few weeks. Dermal edema may be apparent as orange peel skin. The lymphatics in the surgical area may go into a lymphatic shock. Gentle massage improves the lymphatic drainage (**Fig. 24.47**).

Sensory Changes/Paresthesia

Patients invariably experience reduced sensation in the area treated till there is subcutaneous edema. This may last for initial 2 to 3 weeks and resolves on its own. Some patients may experience hypersensitivity of the skin and would benefit by frequent gentle massage.

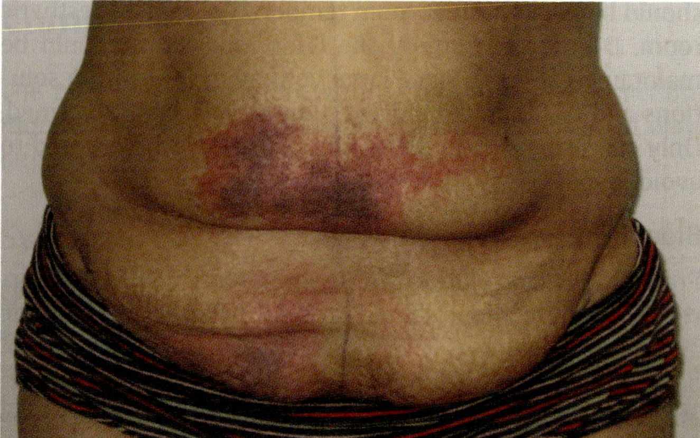

Fig. 24.45 Complication: Postliposuction contusion and edema.

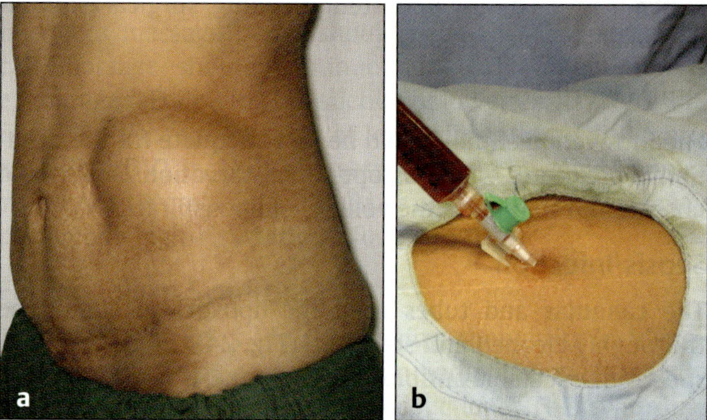

Fig. 24.46 Complication. **(a)** Post-PAL seroma left flank. **(b)** Aspiration of serosanguinous fluid followed by injection of a sclerosant: sodium tetradecyl. Abbreviation: PAL, power-assisted liposuction.

Late Aesthetic Complications

Surface Irregularities

After aggressive superficial liposuction, surface irregularities, rippling, or indentations are not uncommon. Strong vacuum force can lead to uncontrolled aspiration and may result in over-resection. One should avoid pinching of skin fold against the cannula tip, barring some exceptions, to prevent uncontrolled suction. The pressure exerted by the nondominant assisting hand can at times cause rippling and waves. Keeping the suction cannula at one place for too long can lead to unsightly depression. Repeat liposuction, subcision, lipofilling, liposhifting, or skin excision may be needed for harmonization and smoothening of the surface (**Fig. 24.48a, b**).

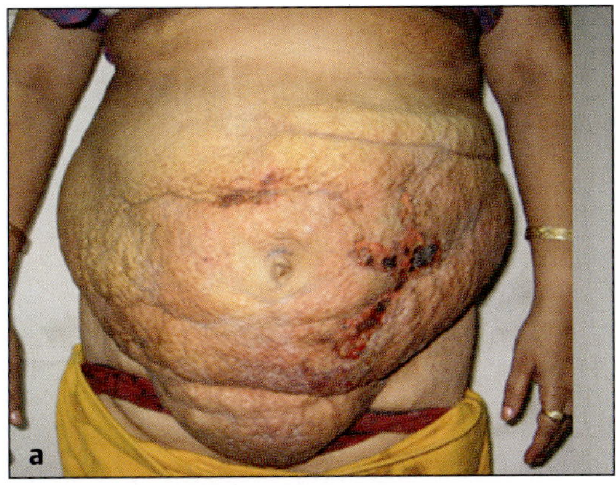
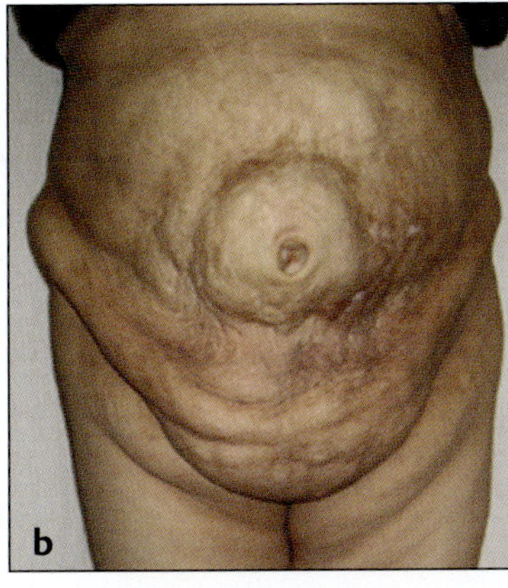

Fig. 24.47 Complication. **(a)** Immediate Post-SAL erythema, edema and skin excoriation. **(b)** Late post liposuction occult hernia and excess skin resulting in folds. Abbreviation: SAL, suction- assisted liposuction.

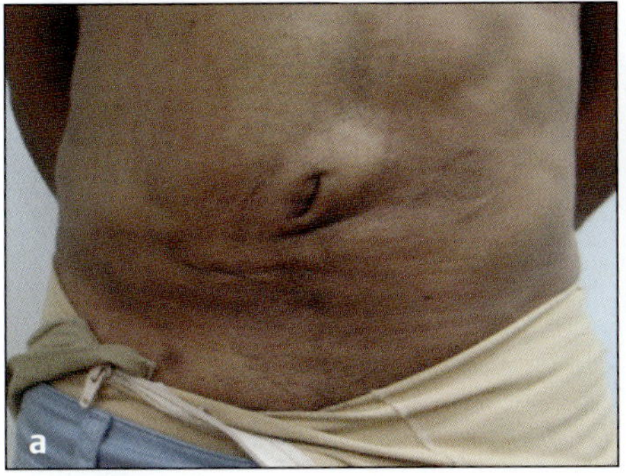
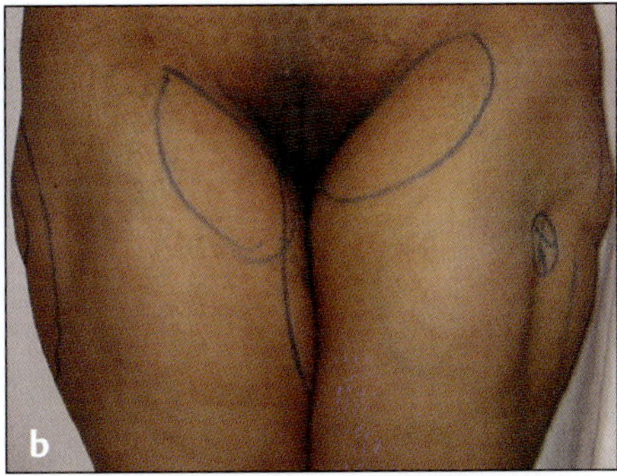

Fig. 24.48 Surface irregularities, rippling, and indentations after aggressive superficial liposuction. **(a)** Abdomen. **(b)** Thighs and groin.

Asymmetry

Absolute symmetry on two sides of the body is difficult. Some margin of error is acceptable as a normal variation. Good preoperative photographs should be used as a reference during surgery to manage any existing asymmetry.

Unnatural and artificial appearance is a disturbing complication. It is a result of lack of artistic outlook and planning on the part of the surgeon. A six-pack abdomen designed on a man having visceral (intra-abdominal) fat looks very ugly. Indiscriminate use of fat graft can also contribute to this problem.

Liposuction Port Scars

Unsightly scars at puncture sites may occur in some cases, especially when large cannula or an ultrasonic cannula is used. These may become hypertrophic and painful. Topical applications of steroid, silicone gel, and pressure can help.

Skin Adherence and Retraction

The skin and soft tissue does remain hard, and feels unnatural and unyielding for several weeks. Indiscriminate superficial and subdermal suctioning may result in skin adherence to deep structures. This can give rise to intense fibrosis and distortion. Skin adherent to the muscle below may manifest as abnormal skin movement.

Long-Lasting Skin Color Changes

In lighter skin types, the hemosiderin pigment can be easily seen, giving a peculiar yellowish brown hue to the skin. This pigment may stay on for several months (**Fig. 24.49a, b**). Extended use of energy-based devices like ultrasonic or RF can contribute to this pigmentation. The areas of superficial suction may be hypersensitive to sunlight and may tan very quickly. Local application of bleaching creams like Kojic acid or Hydroquinone may help. Using Q-Switched Nd:YAG 1064-nm laser on this pigment may help to clear it faster.

Dissatisfied Patient

There are patients who, despite objectively satisfactory results, are subjectively dissatisfied. This may be because of the unrealistic expectations. Patients and their relatives must be involved in the decision making. The routine showing of "before and after" photographs of other patients with only perfect results can have negative consequences. If the plastic surgeon is confident of having done a good job and therapeutically having achieved what was planned, he should not succumb to demand for performing another operation.

Secondary Liposuction

One of the most common and important undesired sequelae of liposuction is contour irregularity. Dillerud[44] in a study of more than 3500 procedures found that in no less than 10% of the patients, there were asymmetry, under- or overresection and skin irregularity. The proportion was more in men than in women. The best way to treat a contour

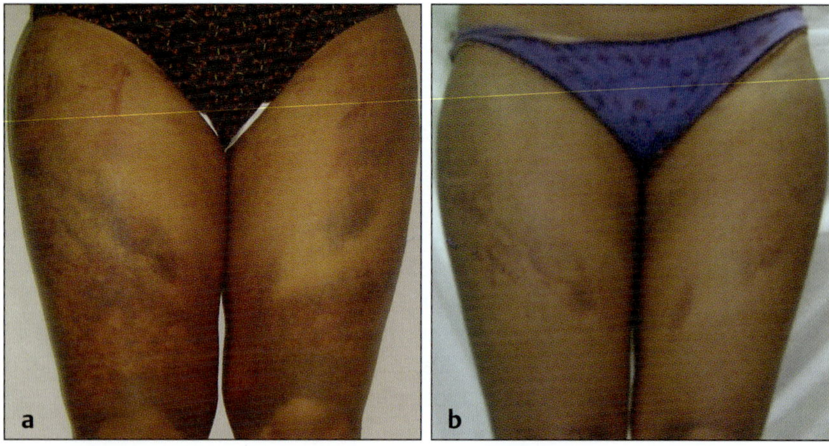

Fig. 24.49 Complication. **(a)** Postliposuction ecchymosis in thigh. **(b)** Ecchymosis clearing with residual hyperpigmentation.

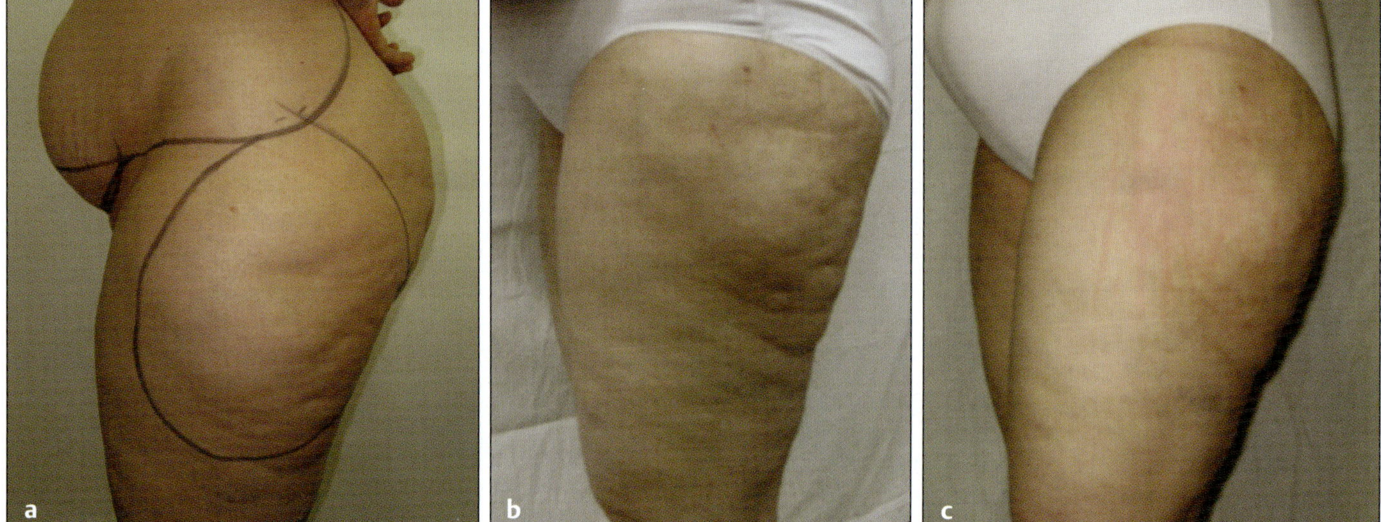

Fig. 24.50 Nonsurgical radiofrequency management of postliposuction irregularities. **(a)** Localized fatty deposit lateral thigh and trochanter with marking for liposuction. **(b)** 3 months after liposuction with residual irregularity. **(c)** After four treatments with nonsurgical radiofrequency to smoothen the subcutaneous residual fat and tightening of the skin.

irregularity is to avoid it. Undercorrection leading to either a residual bulge or step deformity are treated with localized liposuction. There is a very important role to use powered instrument in secondary liposuction as the area to be treated is fibrotic. Overcorrection leading to dimples, grooves, furrows can be treated with touch-up liposuction in the surrounding area and fat transplantation under the depressed area.

Presence of skin fold even after 6 months to 1 year may require a dermolipectomy procedure.

Nonsurgical Energy-Based Devices for Fat Reduction

Energy-based devices have been used for a long time to reduce subcutaneous fat, cellulite treatment, and skin tightening (**Fig. 24.50a–c**). They offer the simplistic nonsurgical treatment with added benefits of no hospitalization and no pain. There is a large group of patients which may benefit from this type of treatments to some extent. Radiofrequency heat, focused ultrasound, and cryofreezing have been used to destroy localized fat in small areas. The fate of the destroyed fat cells and the lipid is still uncertain.

High-focused ultrasound (HIFU) energy can be focused below the skin without causing injury to the skin. The goal is to selectively destroy adipose tissue. The ultrasound waves have frequency of 20 to 20,000 Hz, higher than the audible spectrum and are focused in pulsed mode on a small spot, at a depth of 1.1 to 1.8 cm. Currently, there are two devices ULTRASHAPE using a mechanical effect, and LIPOSONIX using a thermal effect. Clinically, there was no evidence of increased lipid level in the blood after any of these treatments. Both these devices need multiple sessions done at 2 to 4 weeks interval. The second author used ULTRASHAPE for a period of more than 3 years and found it to be not very user friendly. It had a tracking camera and every single area of 6 mm diameter needed to be treated manually. It was found to be labor, time, and cost intensive.

Cryolipolysis causes fat freezing resulting in crystallization of adipose tissue and adipose cell death. An area of skin and subcutaneous fat is kept in firm and continuous contact with the freezing device, for a duration of 30 to 50 minutes with very low suction. The adipose cells undergo "apoptosis" and it is gradually removed through macrophage-mediated phagocytosis over few weeks. The patient feels mild discomfort and has transient erythema with temporary reduced sensation, but no skin necrosis has been reported. But the treated area undergoes fibrosis, making it difficult to do liposuction for the same area at a later date. Some beneficial results have been observed, but long-term benefits are still to be proved.

Injection lipolysis (mesotherapy) chemically reduces the number of fat cells around the injection site. The chemical used is phosphatidylcholine or deoxycholic acid, resulting in adipocyte disruption and death.[45] The use is off-label and there is paucity of evidence-based studies.

The injection is given in a predetermined dose in a marked grid pattern with 1 to 1.5 cm spacing. The dose of 1 to 2 mg (0.1–0.2 mL) is delivered at a depth of 6 to 13 mm for fat reduction and 4 mm depth for cellulite treatment. Patient may experience swelling, redness, bruising, pain, and temporary hardness. The area softens with time and fat reduction takes more than 6 weeks. It needs four to six sessions at 1 to 3 weeks interval for visible result. Soft pinchable fat with tighter skin responds the best. It is effective in treating small areas like submental fat, or as a touch-up procedure for residual fat after liposuction.

In today's body conscious society, liposuction is an extremely popular aesthetic procedure. Even though it may seem like a technically simple procedure for a plastic surgeon, it needs an artistic eye and the skill with an experience to have an aesthetic perspective of the result which can be achieved and an ability to execute the same.

References

1. Wagner BM. Adipose tissue and obesity. Hum Pathol 1985;16(12):1183
2. Coleman WP III. The history of liposuction and fat transplantation in America. Dermatol Clin 1999;17(4):723–727, v
3. Illouz YG. History and current concepts of lipoplasty. Clin Plast Surg 1996;23(4):721–730
4. Flynn TC, Coleman WP II, Field LM, Klein JA, Hanke CW. History of liposuction. Dermatol Surg 2000;26(6):515–520
5. Grazer FM, de Jong RH. Fatal outcomes from liposuction: census survey of cosmetic surgeons. Plast Reconstr Surg 2000;105(1):436–446, discussion 447–448
6. Schrudde J. Lipexeresis as a means of eliminating local adiposity. Aesthetic Plast Surg 1980;4(1):215–226
7. Pitanguy I. Trochanteric lipodystrophy. Plast Reconstr Surg 1964;34:280–286
8. Kesselring UK, Meyer R. A suction curette for removal of excessive local deposits of subcutaneous fat. Plast Reconstr Surg 1978;62(2):305–306
9. Fournier PF, Otteni FM. Lipodissection in body sculpturing: the dry procedure. Plast Reconstr Surg 1983;72(5):598–609
10. Illouz YG. Illouz's technique of body contouring by lipolysis. Clin Plast Surg 1984;11(3):409–417
11. Illouz YG. Body contouring by lipolysis: a 5-year experience with over 3000 cases. Plast Reconstr Surg 1983;72(5):591–597
12. Klein JA. The tumescent technique for liposuction surgery. Am J Cosmet Surg 1987;4:263–267
13. Zocchi M. Ultrasonic-assisted lipoplasty. Adv Plast Reconstr Surg 1998;11:197–221
14. Illouz YG. Principles of liposuction. In: Illouz YG, ed. Liposuction: The Franco-American experience. Beverly Hills: Medical Aesthetics; 1985:21–31
15. Illouz YG, de Villers YJ. Principles of the technique. In: Body LIPO-sculpturing by lipoplasty. Edinburgh: Churchill Livingstone; 1989:63–69
16. Parish TD. A review: the pros and cons of tumescent anesthesia in cosmetic and reconstructive surgery. Am J Cosmet Surg 2000;18:83–93
17. Klein JA. Clinical biostatistics of safety. In: Tumescent technique: tumescent anaesthesia and microcannular liposuction. St. Louis, MO: Mosby, Inc.; 2000:27–31
18. Klein JA. Tumescent technique for regional anesthesia permits lidocaine doses of 35 mg/kg for liposuction. J Dermatol Surg Oncol 1990;16(3):248–263
19. Dhami LD. Liposuction. Indian J Plast Surg 2008;41(Suppl): S27–S40
20. Shiffman Elam MV. Liposuction: principles and practice. Springer. Reduced Negative Pressure Liposuction; 2006; 44:301–304
21. Zocchi M. Ultrasonic liposculpturing. Aesthetic Plast Surg 1992;16(4):287–298
22. Maxwell GP, Gingrass MK. Ultrasound-assisted lipoplasty: a clinical study of 250 consecutive patients. Plast Reconstr Surg 1998;101(1):189–202, discussion 203–204
23. Jewell ML, Fodor PB, de Souza Pinto EB, Al Shammari MA. Clinical application of VASER-assisted lipoplasty: a pilot clinical study. Aesthet Surg J 2002;22(2):131–146
24. Rebelo A. Vibroliposuction: liposuction/liposculpture assisted by compressed air. Int J Cosm Surg 2003;5(1):77–82
25. Flynn TC. Powered liposuction: an evaluation of currently available instrumentation. Dermatol Surg 2002;28(5):376–382
26. Coleman WP III, Katz B, Bruck M, et al. The efficacy of powered liposuction. Dermatol Surg 2001;27(8):735–738
27. Katz BE, Bruck MC, Coleman WP III. The benefits of powered liposuction versus traditional liposuction: a paired comparison analysis. Dermatol Surg 2001;27(10):863–867
28. Blugerman GS. Laser lipolysis for the treatment of localized adiposity and cellulite. World Congress on Liposuction Surgery, Dearborn, MI, October 13–15, 2000
29. Taufig AZ. Hydro-jet-liposuction: a new method for liposuction. Presented at Vereinigung der Deutschen Plastischen Chirurgen meeting, Cologne, Germany; September 2000
30. Paul M, Mulholland RS. A new approach for adipose tissue treatment and body contouring using radiofrequency-assisted liposuction. Aesthetic Plast Surg 2009;33(5):687–694
31. Duncan DI. Helium plasma-driven radiofrequency in body contouring. In: The Art of Body Contouring. March 2019. doi: 10.5772/intechopen.84207

Introduction

Abdominoplasty is one of the commonest aesthetic surgical procedures being performed.[1] Demand for this procedure is growing due to the changing attitudes toward body shape, the influence of social media, and the desire to maintain a youthful figure despite pregnancies. It is not uncommon to see women with minor laxity also seeking surgery. Patients with functional problems due to large pendulous abdomen are the traditional indications for abdominoplasty.[2,3] The procedure has even been reported to improve low back pain in some of these patients.[2] Global increase in bariatric surgery has resulted in patients with extreme tissue redundancy and unique deformities never seen before in human history. The spectrum of cases presenting to a plastic surgeon has thus become diverse and challenging at both ends of the spectrum, as all of them seek a perfect result with low complications. Several publications have, however, reported variably high complication rate for abdominoplasty, especially in obese patients.[4,5] Abdominoplasty has been rated as the aesthetic procedure with the highest complication rates.[6] Several modern advances have enhanced the results and drastically reduced complication rates; however, these changes have not been widely adopted.[7,8] The purpose of this chapter is to describe contemporary abdominoplasty in the context of current knowledge and state of the art, in particular, emphasizing the advantages of the newer lipoabdominoplasty (LABP) and other variants. Abdominal contouring by only liposuction is covered in Chapter 24, "Liposuction and Liposculpture," in Volume VI.

History

Abdominoplasty was described initially as a debulking apronectomy for functional relief.[9,10] Later surgeons reported techniques to save the umbilicus.[11,12] Although Vernon published details of flap undermining and translocation of the umbilicus in 1957, publications in the 1960s by Callia and Pitanguy popularized the operation.[13–15] However, both the concept and technique remained virtually unchanged for three decades.[16,17] Complications like seroma, skin necrosis, and dehiscence as well as aesthetic dissatisfactions were seen in a significant percentage of patients with higher rates in the obese.[18–20] Yet it remained popular and was even combined with other operations.[21,22]

Introduction of liposuction in the 1980s brought a new tool for abdominal contouring; however, it was limited to cases of excess fat without skin redundancy, tissue ptosis, or muscle weakness. Patients having these problems were offered traditional abdominoplasty.[23] Liposuction of the abdominal flap itself was considered risky. The accepted practice was to do the abdominoplasty first and liposuction later or the other way around. But liposuction was found useful in improving the contour in nondissected areas such as the midtrunk, flanks, and back.[24] Alternatively, abdominal liposuction was combined with a simple lower dermolipectomy without flap dissection.[25–27] Tentative guidelines to include liposuction in abdominoplasty were suggested by Matarasso in 1991, along with a classification system for abdominal deformities.[28] In an update in 1995 he advocated adding liposuction to a full abdominoplasty but recommended staying away from the danger zones (Huger zones, **Fig. 25.1**) to preserve flap vascularity.[29]

In 1992, Illouz, the pioneer of liposuction, suggested a different approach. Observing that liposuction caused sufficient "mesh undermining" of the skin flap, he advocated limited undermining and more liposuction, something contrary to the extensive undermining of a full abdominoplasty.[30] In his important publication on high lateral tension closure, Ted Lockwood mentioned liposuction, discontinuous undermining, and perforator preservation but the focus of the paper was on a method of wound closure.[31] It seems that the concept of LABP was ahead of its times. Other significant milestones in the end of last century were: suture obliteration of the dead space described by Baroudi, progressive tension sutures by Pollock, and high superior tension umbilicoplasty by Le Louarn and Pascal.[32–35]

The author started combining full abdominal liposuction and full abdominoplasty with discontinuous undermining in 1995 and observed that liposuction did most of the undermining already, allowing preservation of many perforators.[36] Over time the extent of liposuction was increased and the undermining became limited and discontinuous; superior aesthetic outcomes were noticed and complications were negligible even in the obese patients. This concept and the term "lipoabdominoplasty" was reported by Saldanha et al in 2001 where abdominoplasty was done without undermining[37] and later in 2003 with selective undermining.[38] LABP has now emerged as a safe and powerful method, applicable even in cases of significant abdominal wall obesity.[36] Simultaneous circumferential treatments (liposuction or excisions or both) could now be performed safely due to retention of better vascularity.[39,40]

Aesthetic Concepts

Before attempting abdominoplasty, a surgeon must study and appreciate the features that go to form the "beautiful normal" abdomen and its relationship to adjacent body zones in both sexes. The important landmarks and normal ratios are shown in **Fig. 25.2**. Even significant deviations from these may not be apparent to the patient *before* surgery but are immediately noticed by the patient *after* surgery. Significant anomalies must, therefore, be discussed with the patient preoperatively in front of a mirror. The broad goals of abdominoplasty are summarized in **Box 25.1**.

Box 25.1 Goals of abdominoplasty

- Eliminate tissue redundancy
- Eliminate excess fat in the abdominal wall
- Skin of normal tightness, without folds
- Firm abdominal musculature without diastasis
- Normal mounds and valleys in abdomen
- Normal looking umbilicus in correct location
- A symmetrical fine scar that can be hidden in underwear
- Narrow waist and smooth S curve on the lateral contour
- No distortion of mons pubis

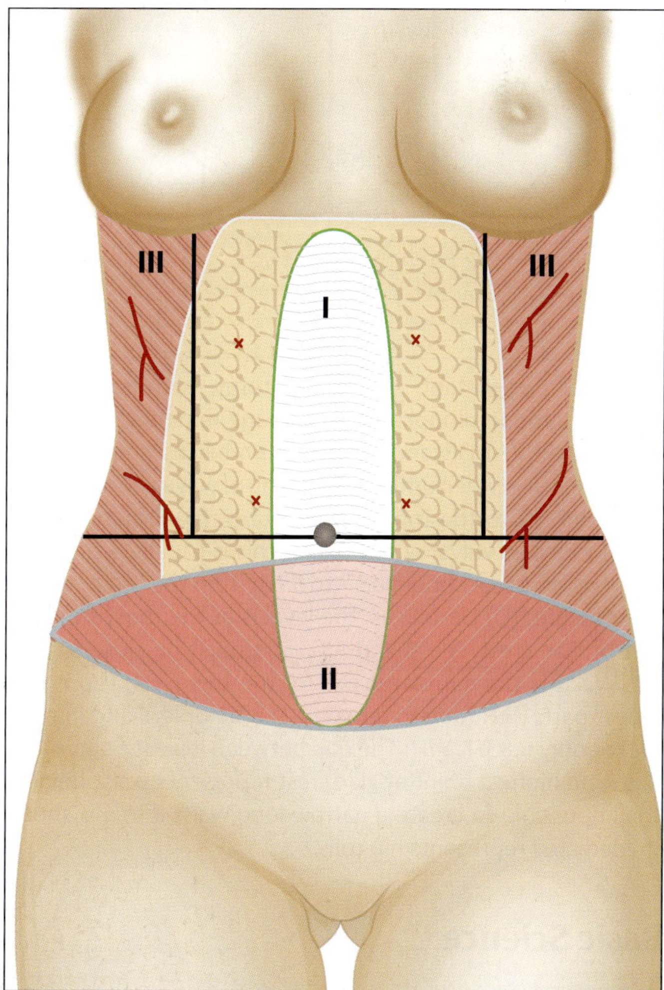

Fig. 25.1 Huger zones. Zone I is central upper zone, mainly supplied by Rectus sheath perforators. Zone II is lower abdomen that is usually removed in abdominoplasty. Zone III is the only remaining source of perfusion in a classical abdominoplasty.

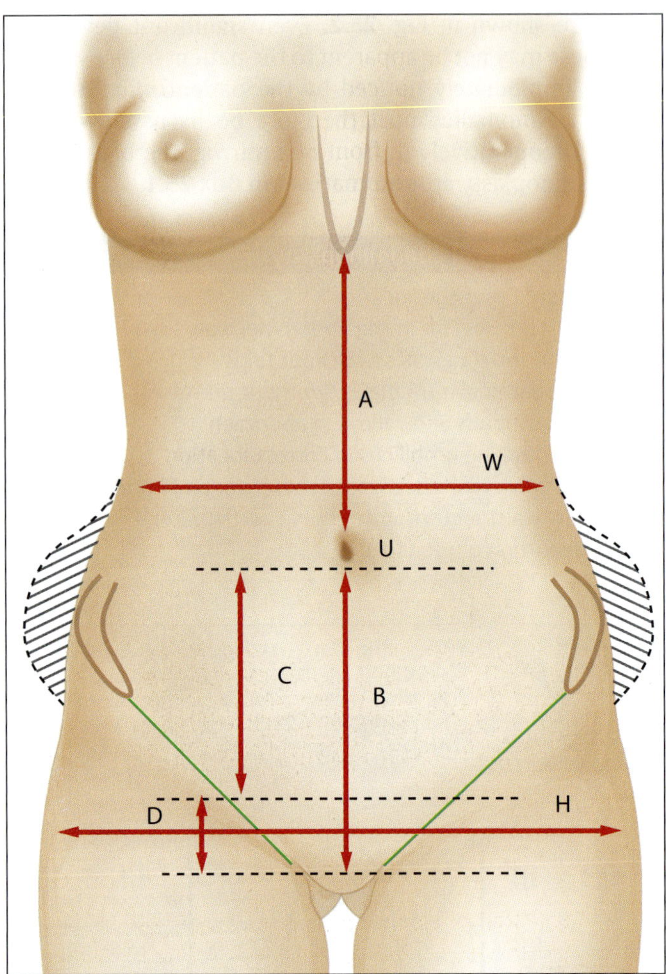

Fig. 25.2 Important surface anatomy and proportions relevant to abdominoplasty. An average female abdomen is represented. (A) Distance between umbilicus and Xiphoid. (B) Distance between umbilicus and top of vulvar commissure. (C) Umbilicus to the top of mons pubis. (D) Distance from top of mons to vulvar commissure; this is usually 5 to 7 cm. The incisional scar should be 7 to 9 cm from the top of vulvar commissure. (U) Umbilicus; the level is at the most superior part of Iliac crest. A = B and A:C ratio must be close to 1.6. (W) Waist is the narrowest part of the torso. (H) Hip is the widest part. W:H ratio in female is 0.72:1 or less and in men it is roughly 0.83:1. WH: The gap between lowest point of rib cage and highest point of Iliac crest represents waist height. It is impossible to create a narrow long waist if WH is short. Shaded area represents hip rolls.

Basic Science

Surgical Anatomy

The standard anatomy of the abdominal wall is well known. Important points of relevance to abdominoplasty are emphasized here.

Layers of Abdomen

It is useful to think of the abdominal wall in layers, starting with the skin. Abdominal **skin** varies from zone to zone especially in the postpartum and postbariatric cases. The skin in the upper half, waist, and flanks is usually thicker and elastic compared to the lower abdomen which may have thin skin and striae. The quality of upper abdominal skin is more relevant since it is relocated to the lower half in abdominoplasty. Poor quality skin in upper segment may compromise the end result, as it is prone to secondary relaxation in the long term. In postbariatric cases, however, there is global thinning and loss of elasticity. Sufficient skin must, therefore, be removed primarily to avoid early return of laxity.

The **fatty layer** may be subdivided into the following layers: true subcutaneous fat, fat of Campers fascia (superficial fat), and deep fat below Scarpa fascia.[41] This trilaminar structure is well defined in all patients in the lower abdomen, irrespective of the degree of obesity.[42] The superficial fat itself is multilayered in the anterior zone due to multiple layers of fibrous tissues in between the fat. The number of layers reduces laterally as the laminae merge and finally fuse along the midaxillary line with the condensed fascia over the external oblique.[43] The deep fat is usually hypovascular, lighter yellow, and arranged as larger globules on the external oblique fascia. The thickness of superficial fat varies in different zones, being several inches thick in some individuals but the deep layer shows less variability.

Scarpa fascia forms the superficial fascia of the abdomen and is surgically important. Its extent and anatomy have been reinvestigated by fresh dissections and computed tomography (CT) scans.[41,43] Lockwood, who developed the concept of high-lateral tension abdominoplasty, described this as a particularly important layer.[44] This layer is strong in lower abdomen and merges with the subcutaneous fibro-fat above the umbilical level in an oblique line.[43] One may raise the abdominal flap either superficial or deep to this fascia (SFS); both variants are described. This fascia is adherent to the skin, muscles, and fascia lata at different places (**Fig. 25.3a–e**). This fact is relevant as it is impossible to pull up the lateral thigh from above this line of fusion (as in belt lipectomy) while it can be used to "hang" the deeper tissues in a lower body lift where the excision goes below this line. It also fuses with the skin and deep fascia below the bra-strap area in some individuals, causing fatty bulges seen so commonly in this area.

The next layer is the **sub-Scarpa fat**, also called deep fat. It is softer; less structured and has larger lobules. It occupies the lower lateral areas and the area of arcus semilunaris reaching up till the level of umbilicus. Reducing this layer is important in achieving a slimmer waistline and creating the lateral valleys. However, leaving a thin intact layer of this fat helps to reduce seroma rates due to prompt adhesion of the flap to this fat. Skin flaps do not adhere well to the shiny surface of aponeurosis, leading to seromas.[8,45,46]

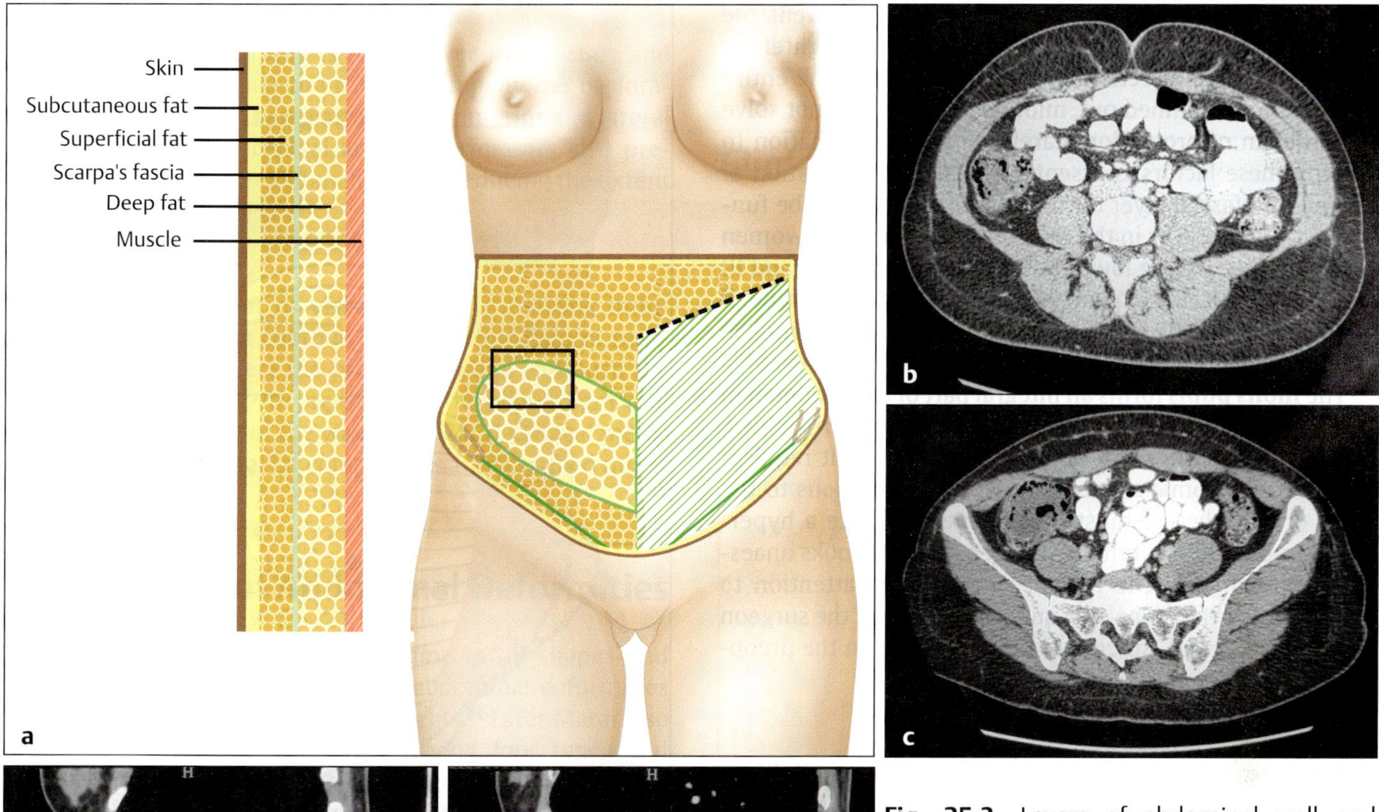

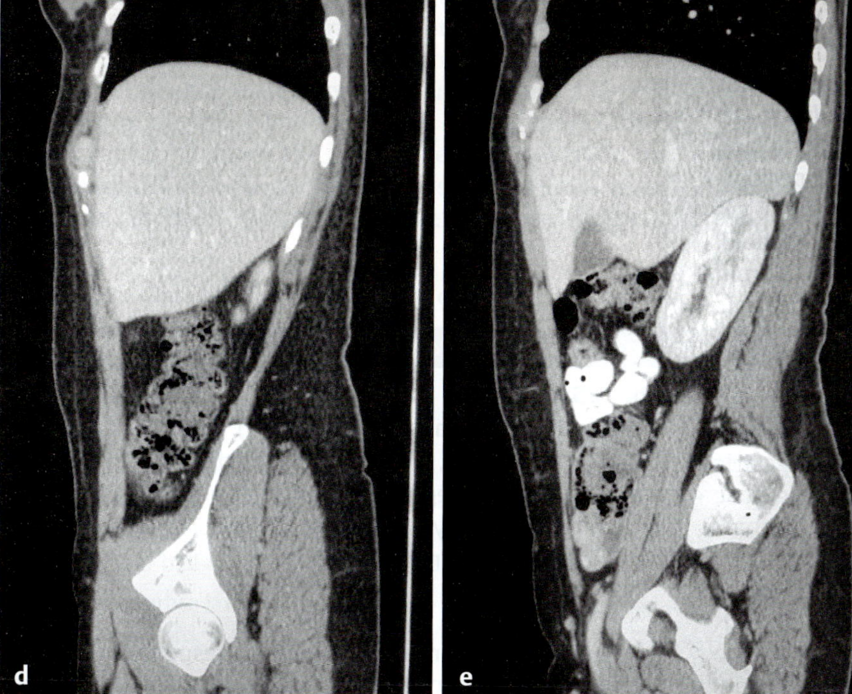

Fig. 25.3 Layers of abdominal wall and arrangement of fascia. **(a)** Schematic diagram: The right side shows superficial fibrofat, window of fat and Scarpa fasica cut out to show deep fat globules. Green shading on left side: usual extent of Scarpa fascia; dotted black line : fusion of Scarpa fascia with superficial fibrofat (eight anatomical variations are described). Dark green line: fusion of Scarpa fascia to fascia lata. Inset shows the layers 1 to 6 at the marked rectangle: skin, true subcutaneous fat, superficial fatty layer, Scarpa fascia, deep fat, and muscular aponeurosis, respectively. **(b, c)** Axial computed tomography (CT) images at umbilicus and lower abdomen: note Scarpa fascia, fusion of fascia at midlateral line, fat compartments, and perforators. **(d, e)** Parasagittal CT sections at mid-clavicular and paramedian lines showing fascia, perforators, and their arborization.

The **musculofascial layers** are well described in anatomy texts; however, the abnormal anatomy of patients coming for abdominoplasty shows wide diversity. There may be several components contributing to myofascial laxity: diastasis or widening of linea alba, an actual gap in linea alba, hernia along the midline, vertical excess of the rectus sheath, laxity of the lateral aspect of rectus sheath, or laxity of fascial parts of the oblique muscles. For these reasons, the extent of abdominal protrusion does not correlate entirely with the extent of diastasis.[47] In some individuals, the rectus muscles have more lateral origins, causing congenital diastasis. It is impossible to approximate such diastasis by standard plication; rectus sheath turnover flaps are needed here (see under “special situations”). Vertical excess of the rectus

Table 25.2 Indications for different techniques of abdominal contouring

	Lipo	Mini	Endo-mini	Limited	Flotation	Inv-T[a]	Std/LABP[b]	Extended or Belt[c]	FDL
Type	0	I	I	II	II	III	IV	V	VI
Upper abdomen	0	0	0	0	0/+	++	+++	+++	++++
Umbilical location	N	N	N	N	High	N/High	Any	Any	Any
Lower abdomen	0	+	0/+	++	++	++	+++	+++	++++
Midline diastasis	0	0	+	++	++	++	Any	Any	Any
Flanks/hips	0/+	+	+	+	+	++	++	+++	+
Back	0/+	0/+	0/+	0/+	0/+	0/+	0/+	++	Any

[a]Inv-T: inverted-T closure is required when the umbilical donor hole remains on the edge of the flap. If the hole is 2 cm above the leading edge, it can be closed separately as a second horizontal scar.
[b]Std, standard abdominoplasty; LABP, lipoabdominoplasty.
[c]Belt, belt lipectomy also called circumferential abdominoplasty; FDL, fleur-de-lis abdominoplasty.

especially antiplatelets and anticoagulants must be checked. History of varicose veins, deep vein thrombosis (DVT), or current varicosity is important. With the proliferation of nonsurgical therapies, it is important to ask specifically about injection lipolysis, laser lipolysis, cryolipolysis, or mesotherapy; patients may not volunteer these facts. These treatments often cause widespread internal fibrosis making further liposuction difficult.[57] A full detailed history must be taken regarding substance abuse especially tobacco. The patient must be informed about the increased risk in smokers and the need to quit completely for 3 weeks before and after surgery.

Examination

Examine the patient as a whole to determine the global shape and obesity before focusing locally. Examination is best done in front of a full-length three-sided mirror. Key points are mentioned in **Box 25.2**. Two special clinical tests are recommended.

Standing Tummy Tuck Maneuver

The patient is asked to tuck in their abdomen and firm up the muscles; the resultant change in lateral profile is noted and shown to the patient. A big change indicates excess visceral fat (which is being pushed inwards by the muscle action). The parietal fat can be pinched against the firm musculature at the same time to assess its thickness. Thus, the relative contribution of parietal and visceral volumes to the overall contour becomes clear (to patient and surgeon). Male patients who have chiefly visceral fat excess can thus be convinced that they will not benefit from abdominoplasty. It is very instructive to ask the patient to grab this external fat roll and remember it. This recall will help to dispel any doubts about fat removal after surgery. The thickness of fat at different locations (upper, mid, and lower) should be measured by pinch meter or ultrasound and documented. A subset of patients will have deep grooves dividing the abdominal fat into two or more rolls. This is due to chronic pressure from a belt, sari, or other garments or due to folding of fat rolls. These grooves need specific attention during surgery but a shadow of the groove may persist. The patient's attention is drawn to this.

Box 25.2 Important points in clinical examination (Done in front of a mirror)

- Standing
  - General shape, waist/hip relations
  - Diffuse upper abdominal fullness (visceral fat)
  - Number of abdominal rolls (parietal fat)
  - Horizontal grooves (may persist after surgery, see text)
  - Upper abdominal skin quality (risk of secondary relaxation if bad)
  - Protrusion of umbilicus (hernia)
  - Lower abdominal panniculus (skin hygiene)
  - Mons pubis (ptosis, bulk, adherence)
  - Hip fat and skin excess (risk of dog-ears, needs specific prevention)
  - Back and bra rolls
  - Shape of buttocks (Fat grafting)
  - "Tummy tuck maneuver" (see text)
    - Big change = excess visceral fat
    - Small change = more parietal fat
- Supine
  - Medical examination for pathology including hernia
  - Scaphoid or convex (convex indicates visceral fat)
  - Head-raising test (measure diastasis)
  - Palpate rectus muscle edges (tone, congenital diastasis)
  - Inspect umbilicus (hygiene, pathology)
  - Perform bimanual simulation test (see text)
  - Assess existing scars

Surgical Simulation Test

In supine position, the back of the patient's couch is flexed 45 degrees and a trial bimanual approximation is done between the supraumbilical skin and suprapubic. If this can be done to within 5 cm of the expected incision level, the patient is suitable for a full abdominoplasty with removal of the umbilical donor hole (type IV). If this is difficult, the patient is warned about possible inverted-T closure (type III).

Scars

Any existing scars including C-section are assessed for quality. The patient is asked to rate her scars as good, acceptable, or bad; this is a subtle way to anticipate her scar tolerance. She is informed that the final scar quality may be worse than her C-section scar; this always elicits surprise. This is a good time to introduce the concepts of factors affecting scar quality, scar permanence, and measures to improve scars.

Diagnosis

It should now be possible to make a comprehensive diagnosis as per **Box 25.3**. The psychological suitability and the likelihood of the patient sticking to a healthy lifestyle are also evaluated and recorded.

Treatment Planning

Choice of Technique

The goals of abdominoplasty are listed in **Box 25.1**. Achieving these goals requires correct treatment planning, which is based on the comprehensive diagnosis and classification type of deformity as guided by **Table 25.2**. **Flowchart 25.1** shows the decision tree in a different way. In types III and above, LABP is the preferred default, unless the abdominal wall has no excess fat (i.e., <1 inch thick). Additional aesthetic procedures may safely be performed concurrently but respecting surgical time and local experience. The suctioned fat can also be used for gluteal or breast augmentation. Addition of nonaesthetic abdominal/pelvic procedures is not encouraged although it has been done safely.[21,58]

Box 25.3 Key questions to be answered as part of comprehensive "diagnosis" in prospective abdominoplasty patients

- What is the classification type of the deformity?
- Is the patient a candidate for abdominoplasty or liposuction?
- Does the patient have realistic expectations?
- Would it be lipoabdominoplasty or modified classical technique?
- Is circumferential treatment (liposuction with or without excision) required?
- What is the likely length of the scar (limited, standard, extended, or circumferential)?
- Is mons lipo/lift required?
- What is the extent of muscle plication/hernia repair and the likely need for a prosthetic mesh? Is plication of external oblique aponeurosis (in global laxity) required?
- Is there need or desire for added procedures (fat graft, buttock contouring, etc.)?
- What is the tendency for bad scars?

Explanatory Note (For Table 25.2)

- Type 0: Use of energy-assisted liposuction has enabled resection procedures to be avoided in select cases (**Fig. 25.6**). Endoscopic techniques even allow myofascial plication in this category, using access from umbilicus and pubis.
- Type I: Such patients with skin laxity restricted to the suprapubic area are corrected by mini abdominoplasty. Formal muscle plication is not part of this operation; however, plication by open or endoscopic techniques can be used if necessary (**Fig. 25.7**).
- Choice between types II and III: Patients of type II with more skin excess in lower abdomen must have the position of umbilicus assessed. If it is low, the abdomen may be reclassified as type III. If umbilicus is normal, it remains as type II and a limited abdominoplasty is indicated without disturbing the umbilicus; however, the umbilicus may end up pointing downwards (**Fig. 25.8**). If the umbilicus is high (umbilicus to pubis >15 cm), it can be shifted to a lower more normal location after internal detachment of its pedicle; this also tightens the upper skin. This is called umbilical flotation (**Fig. 25.9**). The umbilicus is fixed in a Golden proportion of 1.6:1 between supra- and infraumbilical segments.[59]
- Type III: There is upper abdominal skin excess but not enough to stretch all the way to the suprapubic area. Here the skin resection line goes below the umbilicus but upper abdominal flap is raised fully with the umbilical donor hole remaining on the flap. During closure of the wound, if the hole is close to the edge, the intervening skin bridge is excised and the defect is closed vertically (**Fig. 25.10**). If it is away from the edge, it is better to close it as a separate horizontal scar (**Fig. 25.11**).
- Patients with circumferential laxity require extended abdominoplasty or circumferential (belt) abdominoplasty (V). The more advanced cases of truncal ptosis with deformity of buttocks and thighs qualify for a lower body lift, which is a different surgery with different markings.
- Occasionally, one may have to deviate from this algorithm to accommodate the patient's wish especially in the Indian scenario. For example, a nulliparous patient with type III deformity may refuse scars. She will usually not have muscle diastasis. She can get useful improvement with energy-assisted liposuction. However, she must be informed that this is not ideal and is a compromise (**Fig. 25.6**).

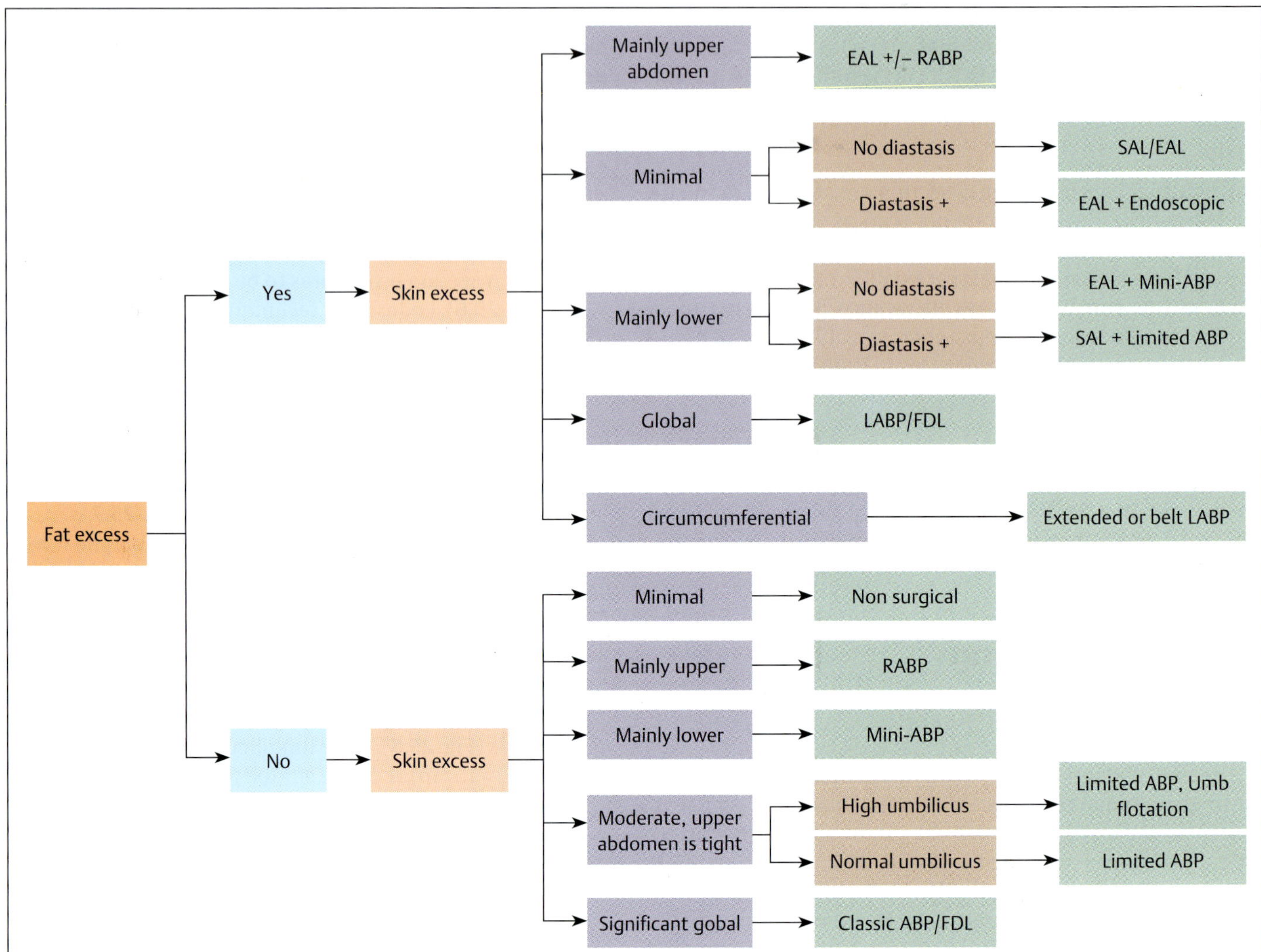

Flowchart 25.1 Algorithm for choice of procedure in abdominoplasty. ABP, abdominoplasty; EAL, energy-assisted liposuction; FDL, fleur-de-lis abdominoplasty; LABP, lipoabdominoplasty; RABP, reverse abdominoplasty; SAL, suction-assisted lipectomy. Excess fat in flanks requires additional flank liposuction. Excess skin and fat in flanks requires extended version of abdominoplasty. Postbariatric cases tend to need circumferential lift. Massive horizontal skin excess will require a vertical component such as fleur-de-lis; in such cases, the dorsal part of a circumferential lift is better done at a later stage.

Managing Expectations and Informed Consent

The success of aesthetic surgery is measured by the satisfaction of the patient; for this, the patient's expectations must match realistic possibilities. Almost all patients expect that they will have a very flat "tummy" and will lose a lot of weight after surgery. The patient must be educated about physiology of weight control; the fat compartments (visceral *vs.* parietal) and the role of muscle tone in achieving the final result. The patient must take responsibility and ownership of visceral fat, body weight, and muscle toning, as clearly these are not changed by abdominoplasty. An illustration like the one in **Fig. 25.5** is very useful during consultation. Written and illustrated leaflets and at least two consultations are recommended to ensure effective retention of all the details. Potential complications are discussed in detail at the second consultation. It has been famously stated that any information given prior to the surgery is part of "*informed consent*," and the same information provided after surgery can be interpreted as an "*excuse*" for a suboptimal result.

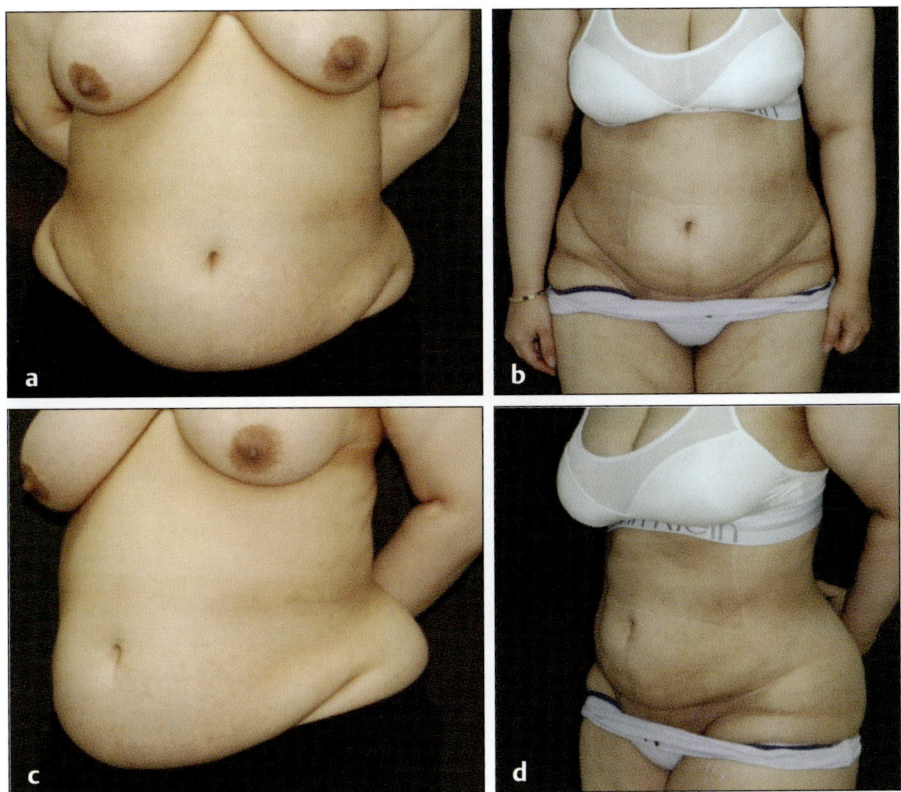

Fig. 25.6 Result of energy-assisted liposuction in a patient who refused abdominoplasty. She had good skin quality and normal muscles. **(a, b)** Pre- and postoperative front views. **(c, d)** Pre- and postoperative oblique views. Early results improve with time.

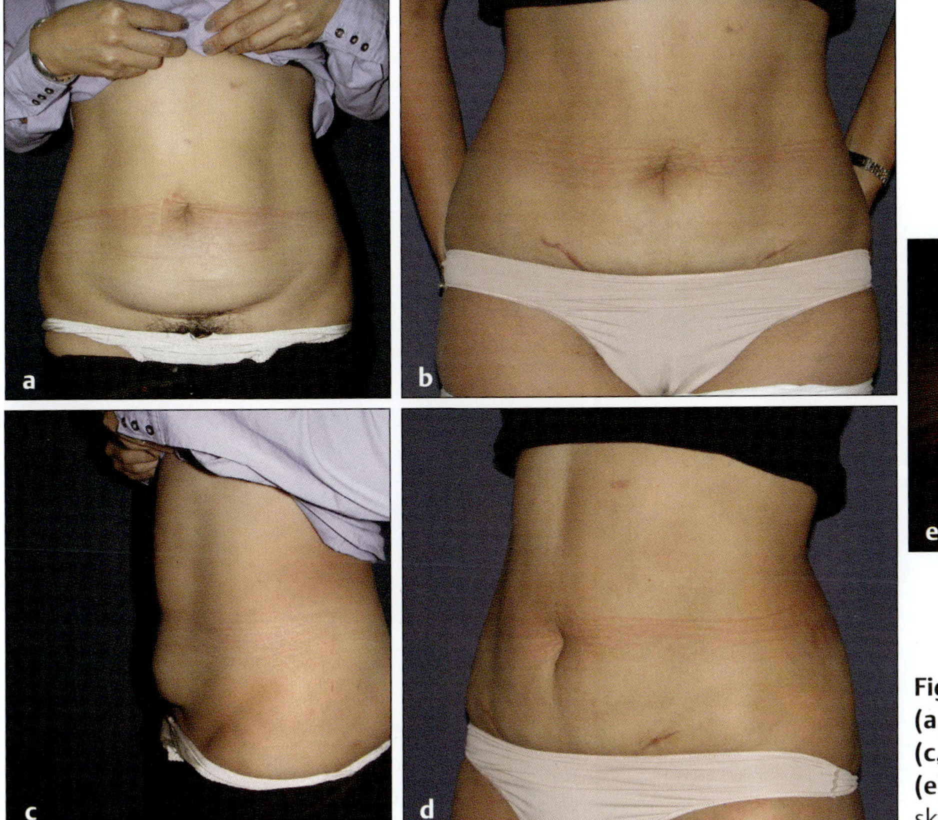

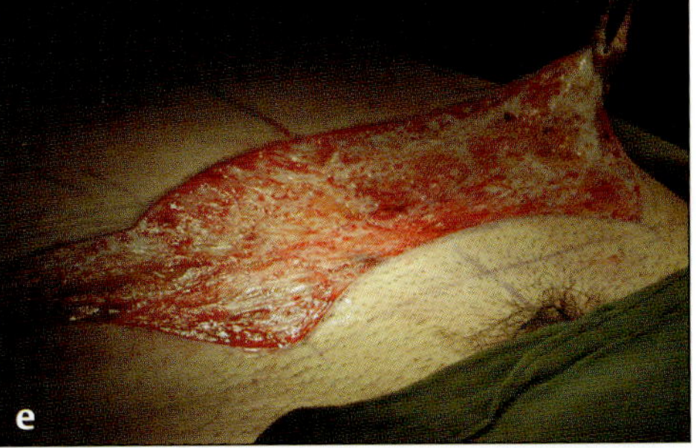

Fig. 25.7 Type I mini abdominoplasty. **(a, b)** Pre- and postoperative front views. **(c, d)** Pre- and postoperative lateral views. **(e)** Intraoperative picture after removal of skin paddle.

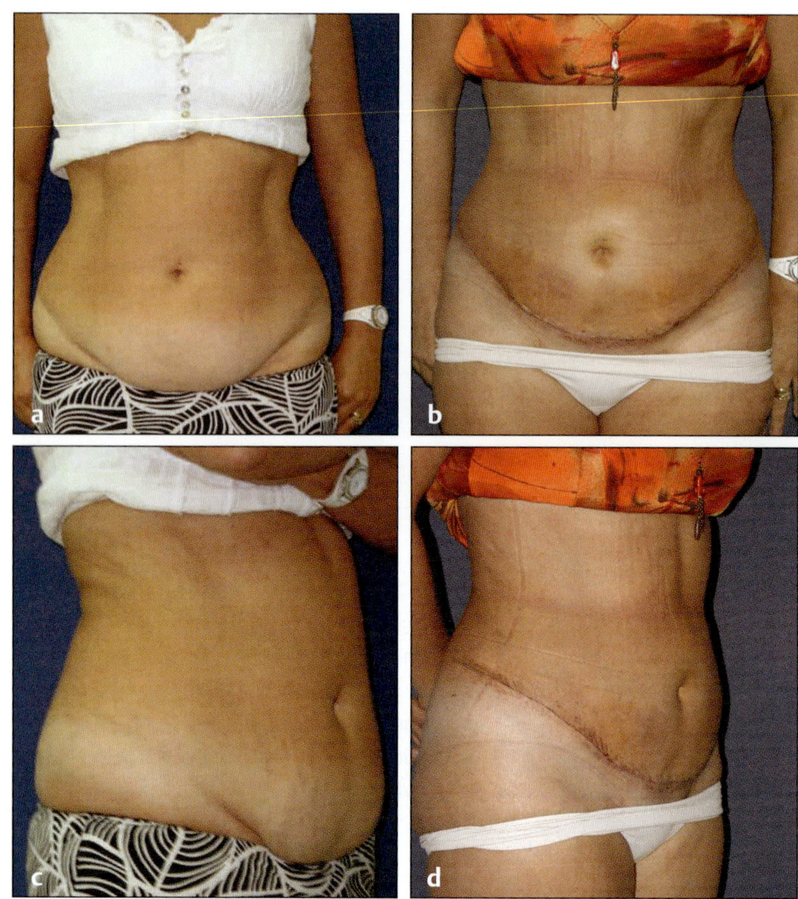

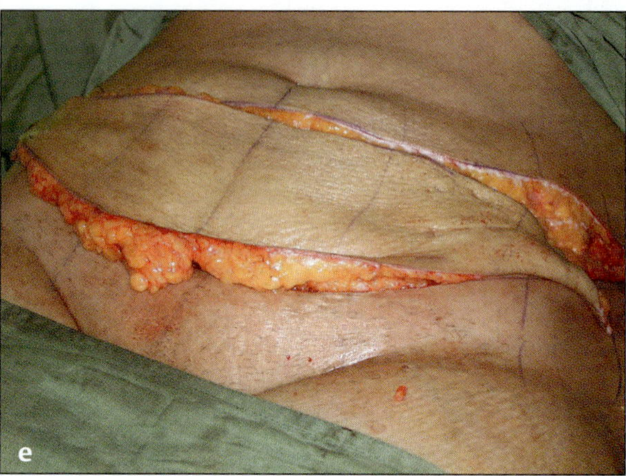

Fig. 25.8 Type II limited abdominoplasty. **(a, b)** Pre- and postoperative front views. **(c, d)** Pre- and postoperative oblique views. **(e)** Intraoperative picture showing extent of dermolipectomy.

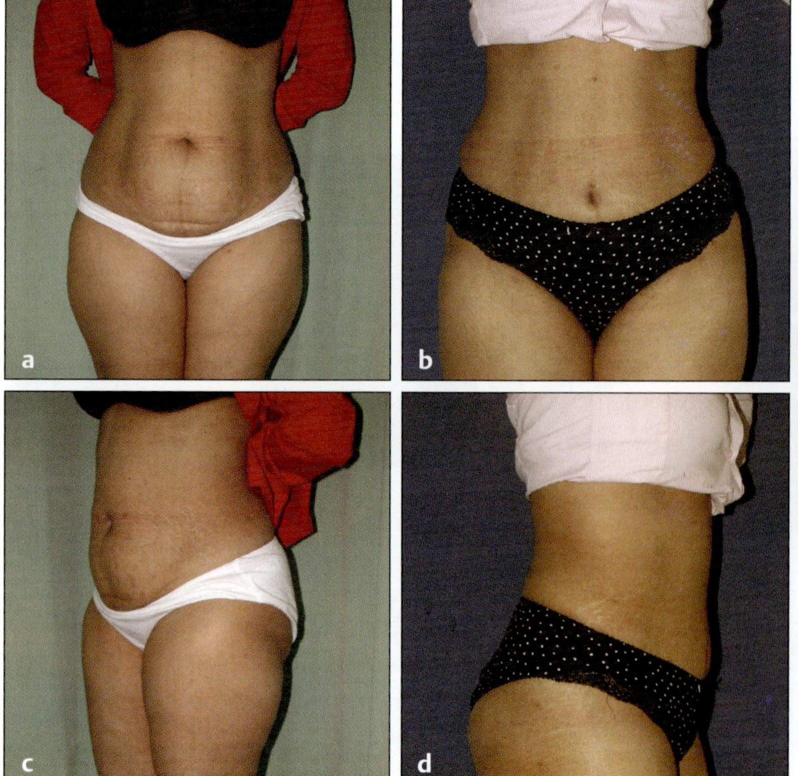

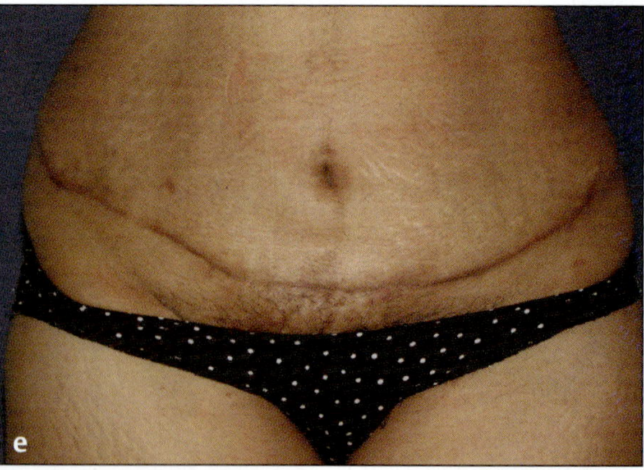

Fig. 25.9 Type IIF limited abdominoplasty plus umbilical flotation. **(a, b)** Pre- and postoperative front views. **(c, d)** Pre- and postoperative oblique-lateral views. **(e)** Close-up of scar and umbilicus. She also underwent liposuction of thighs.

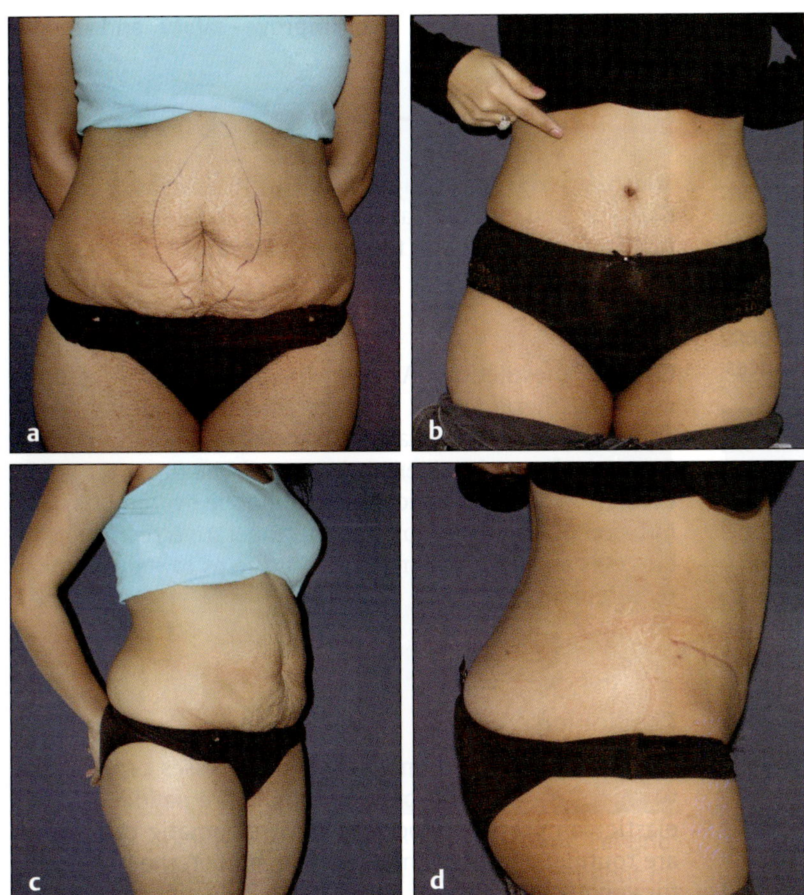

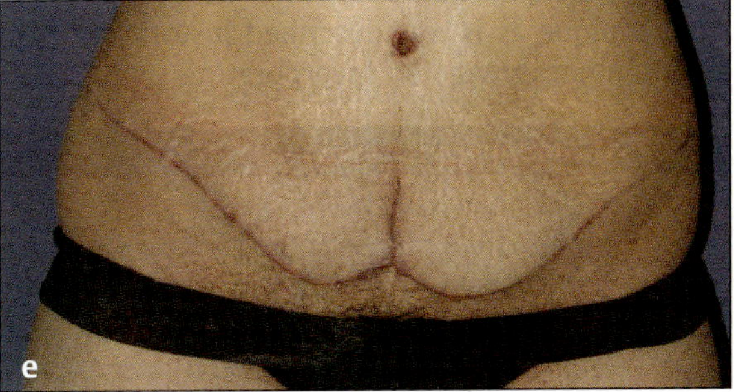

Fig. 25.10 Type III with inverted-T scar. Indicated in a patient with inadequate skin redundancy in upper abdomen. **(a, b)** Pre- and postoperative front views. **(c, d)** Pre- and postoperative oblique-lateral views. **(e)** Close-up of T scar.

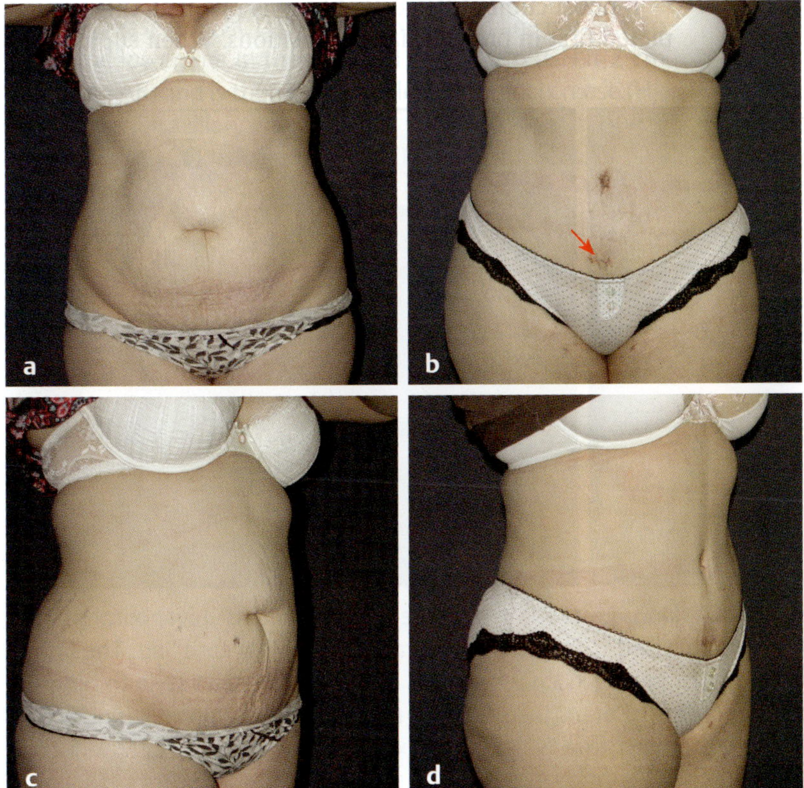

Fig. 25.11 Type III with separate closure of umbilical hole. **(a, b)** Pre- and postoperative front views. **(c, d)** Pre- and postoperative oblique views.

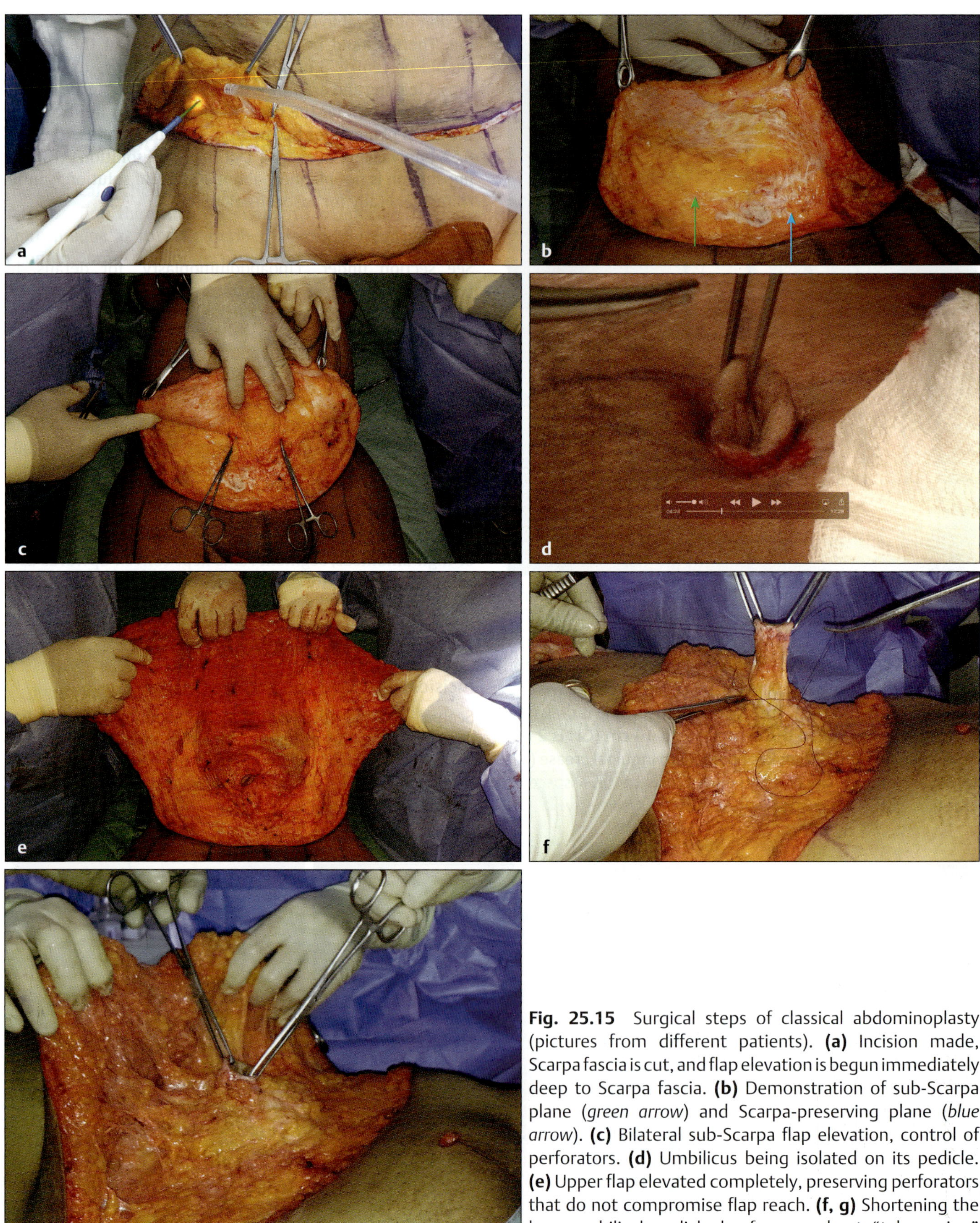

Fig. 25.15 Surgical steps of classical abdominoplasty (pictures from different patients). **(a)** Incision made, Scarpa fascia is cut, and flap elevation is begun immediately deep to Scarpa fascia. **(b)** Demonstration of sub-Scarpa plane (*green arrow*) and Scarpa-preserving plane (*blue arrow*). **(c)** Bilateral sub-Scarpa flap elevation, control of perforators. **(d)** Umbilicus being isolated on its pedicle. **(e)** Upper flap elevated completely, preserving perforators that do not compromise flap reach. **(f, g)** Shortening the long umbilical pedicle by four quadrant "telescoping" sutures to set the skin disc at the level of rectus fascia.

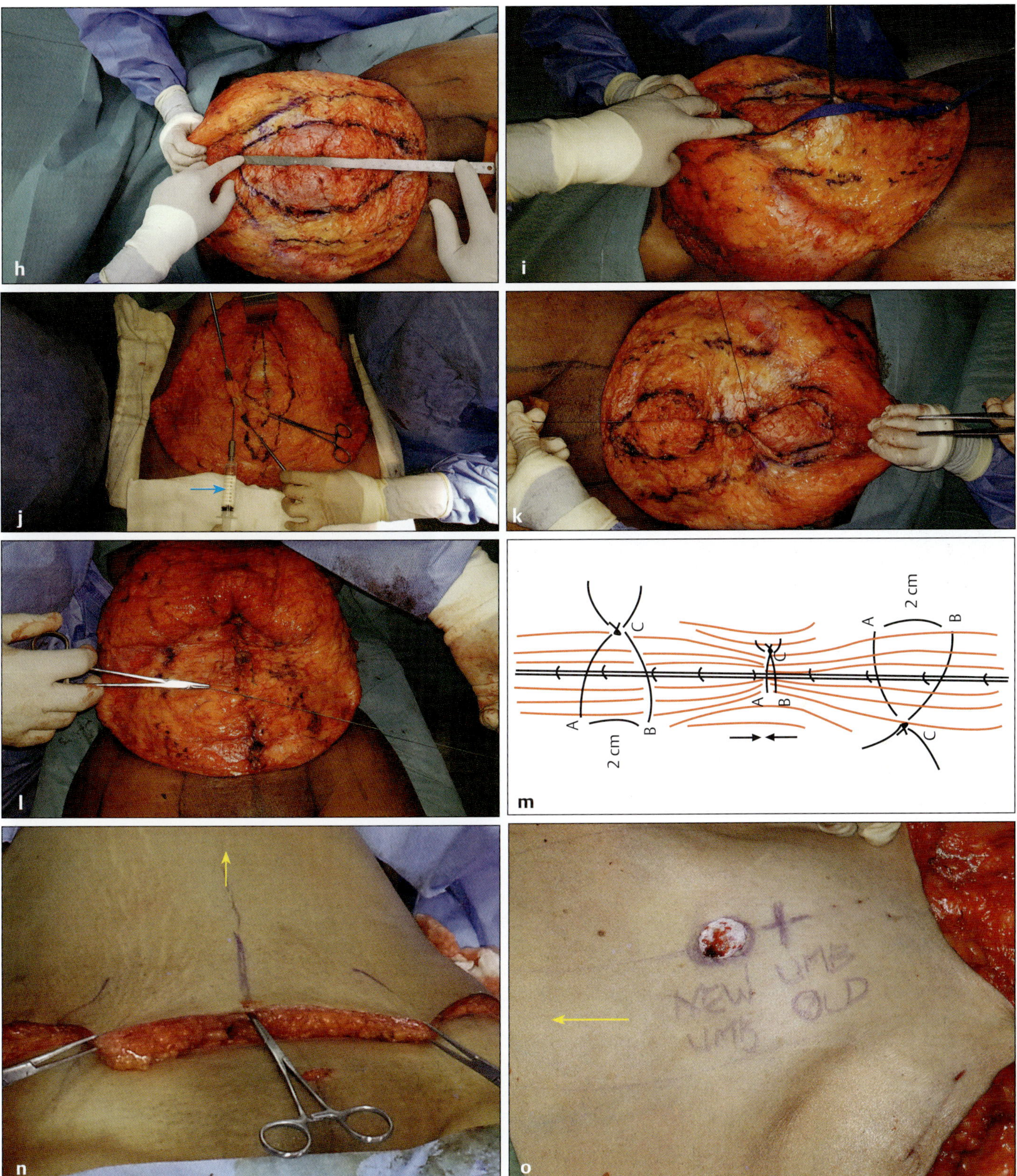

Fig. 25.15 *(Continued)* **(h)** Length of the diastasis in a straight line. **(i)** Measuring the true length of rectus sheath. **(j)** Rectus sheath block by Bupivacaine. **(k)** First layer of rectus sheath repair in progress. **(l)** Completed second layer repair. **(m)** Schema of triangular mattress suture technique to shorten the vertical length of rectus sheath. **(n)** Excess skin flap is resected and trial approximation done, *yellow arrow* points to cranial. **(o)** Position for new umbilicus is marked 1.5 cm cranial to projection point of native umbilicus, skin is de-epithelized.

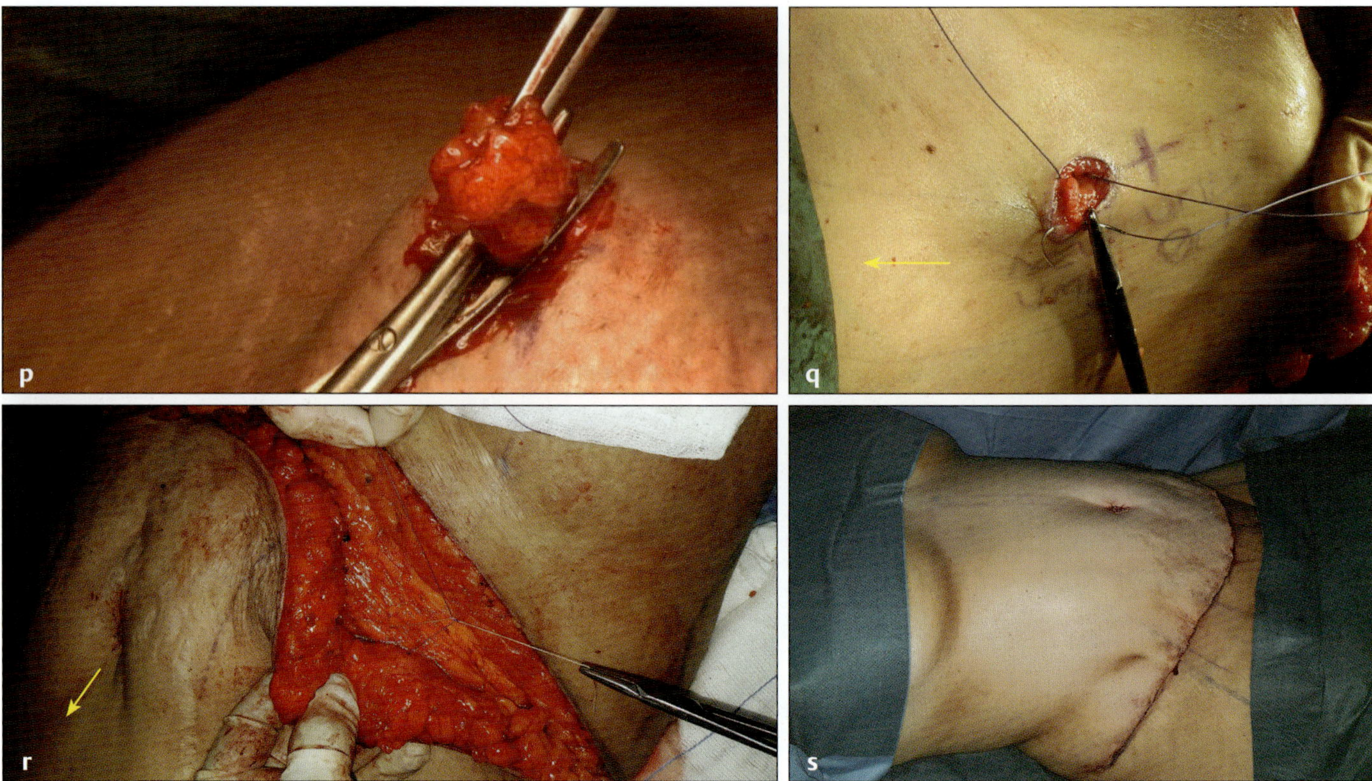

Fig. 25.15 *(Continued)* **(p)** A cone of fat is removed tapering inwards. **(q)** Sutures between dermal fringe and rectus fascia to produce ink-well effect. **(r)** Obliteration of the space under flap by absorbable quilting sutures. **(s)** Final result after layered closure: Scarpa layer, deep dermis, and skin.

The residual infusion fluid acts as a heat sink to minimize collateral damage. Teflon coated nonstick tips remain clean and are recommended. Damaged and burnt tissue is an important promoter of infection, an important concept worth remembering.[66]

Flap Elevation

The white Scarpa fascia is incised and held with Allis forceps. The flap is elevated, with cephalad dissection hugging the undersurface of the Scarpa fascia in an easy avascular plane till the umbilicus. Only the rectus perforators are encountered; these must be tied off.[67] Fat on the external oblique aponeurosis (deep fat) is preserved. Gentle open liposuction can be used to thin this layer. Fat overlying the medial rectus sheath, however, has to be removed to allow plication. (*Variation*: In Scarpa preservation technique the dissection plane is superficial to the fascia but a rectangle of fascia has to be excised in the lower midline to permit plication.) A circular incision is made around the umbilicus keeping the disc about 1 cm in diameter. Incision is deepened and the umbilicus is isolated on its pedicle with a thin layer of fat on it. Flap elevation continues upwards—the plane is now on the anterior rectus sheath and linea alba. Splitting the flap in lower half helps with access. The medial perforators above and below the umbilicus are divided between ligatures—using only diathermy risks them retracting and causing rectus sheath hematoma. Further lateral dissection, which requires cutting the zones of adherence and dealing with more perforators, is best done discontinuously using the surgeon's fingers spread out. Any restraining fibers and vessels are cauterized and cut. Incremental liberation of the flap with frequent checks by pulling it down ensures that we preserve as much vascular supply as possible while ensuring tension-free closure. Complete flap elevation over the costal margins is historical but is still practiced by many. In the author's view this is unnecessary and is the root cause of many complications.[8]

Plication

Full dose of muscle relaxant should be ensured at this stage. Medial borders of rectus muscle and the plication lines 2 cm lateral to them are marked by pen. The medial borders are approximated by continuous over and over sutures, taking 2 cm wide bites with a pitch of 1.5 cm. Separate sutures are used above and below the umbilicus. The lateral lines are then approximated with interrupted horizontal mattress (or figure-of-8) sutures of a soft strong permanent braided suture. Closure should be snug but not tight; the tissues should not become strangulated. *This is an important surgeon-variable feature in postoperative pain.* In patients with marked laxity, additional plication may be done along the linea semilunaris to narrow the waist. Patients with marked protrusion of the abdomen also have increased vertical length of rectus sheath from xiphoid to pubis leading to persistent protrusion after surgery (**Fig. 25.15i**). Transverse plication of the musculature can be done to address this but a simpler triangular mattress technique has been described to reduce this vertical dimension[68,69] (**Fig. 25.15m**).

Different types of sutures have been used for myofascial plication. The author prefers using size 0 or 1 loop polydiaxonone (PDS) or by the barbed variant (Quill or Stratafix) for the first layer and Ethibond No 2 for the second layer. Permanent sutures like polyamide or polypropylene may also be used but the knots must be internalized. Long absorbable suture alone has been shown to be effective in a long-term study.[70]

Rectus Sheath Block

Author prefers rectus sheath block in all the patients. This is done with a 14G, 20 cm long, blunt infiltration cannula inserted into the rectus sheath at the umbilical level via a stab incision (**Fig 25.15j**). Forty milliliters of 0.25% bupivacaine is injected into each sheath by passing the cannula up and down lateral to the line of perforators the access incision is closed. With the new liposomal bupivacaine (Exparel™) the effect of block may last for 96 hours.[71]

Skin Excision

The table is now flexed 30 to 45 degrees and the skin flap is pulled down. Using Allis forceps or d'Assumpcao forceps the lower flap is projected on to the upper flap and markings are made. The excess skin flap is trimmed off after checking repeatedly for tissue tension and symmetry. In the Lockwood's high–lateral tension technique, the midlateral part of resection deviates a bit more cranially, creating greater tension in closure laterally, which also lifts anterior thigh tissues. In most cases, this resection also removes the umbilical donor hole. If the hole is on the border, the lower flap may be mobilized lifting the mons, about an inch can be gained this way and the donor hole can thus be excised. Beyond this, one should not force a tight closure, nor distort the mons pubis but must accept a separate closure of the umbilical hole as a short vertical line or as a separate horizontal closure (type III) (**Figs. 25.10 and 25.11**).

Next, the flap is attached to the lower midline using a single temporary suture. The projection point of the buried umbilicus is marked on the flap but not cut. A new opening is made 1.5 cm cranial to this projection.[35] Making the neoumbilicus higher than the projection point gives immediate flattening of the upper half and relaxes the tension in lower half.[72] A heart-shaped or an inverted triangle is marked and de-epithelized. The dermis is opened via Y-shaped incision and a cone-shaped plug of fat is cored out. This results in a dermal fringe internal to the skin hole. The temporary suture is released and umbilicoplasty is completed (**Fig. 25.15o–q**). The upper part of the flap is now advanced on the abdominal wall by a series of sutures (2–0 rapid Vicryl or equivalent) to perform progressive advancement and obliteration of the dead space. This technique is highly recommended and the extra time is well worth it. Generally, two sutures are used above the umbilicus and six to eight sutures are used per lateral side.

Umbilicoplasty

The beauty of the new umbilicus is still an area for constant improvement. It is especially important in the Indian context, as it may be visible in a *sari*. Important tips for a natural look are: vertically oval shape, superior hooding, all scars being internal, a normal inkwell depression, and avoiding a circular scar which is prone to concentric contracture. There are many variations of this technique; the method described here has been found useful in "skin of color" (**Fig. 25.16**). This technique prevents the formation of a flat superficial umbilicus with visible scars—a deformity seen too often unfortunately.

Closure

Two silicone suction drains are placed and led out through the mons. Alternatively, the lower dead space is obliterated by sutures, and drains are avoided (author's preference). There is no merit in using both measures.[73] Key stitches are placed, guided by premarked grid lines. Layered wound closure is begun by approximating Scarpa fascia on the lower flap to the deep condensed tissue on upper flap. The upper edge is longer than the lower and this needs constant inward adjustment of the upper flap to avoid lateral dog-ears. These fascial stitches relieve tension on skin closure, which is done in two layers. The abdomen is padded and the appropriate garment is applied. Elastic adhesive tapes may cause allergy, blisters or lead to tight bands and are not advised.

Postoperative Regime

The patient is shifted out to her bed directly by using a patient slider in the same Fowler's position. If planned, patient-controlled analgesia can be started. Most patients can be encouraged to walk by evening; they must walk slightly flexed at the hips for 3 to 5 days. Deep breathing exercises, incentive spirometry, and active ankle movements are encouraged. Patients may be routinely discharged home after one to two nights of hospitalization. Straining at defecation must be avoided. A high fiber diet and stool softeners are prescribed.

After Care

Compressive garments are recommended 24×7 for 2 to 3 weeks and only during the day for 3 more weeks. Drains, if used, are removed after daily drainage decreases to 30 mL per day, in any case by seventh day whichever is earlier. Patients begin a program of soft massage using a moisturizer all over the abdomen. This helps rehabilitation, relieves itching and lymph stasis, and restores confidence. The patient can expect feelings of tightness, brief episodes of needle-like

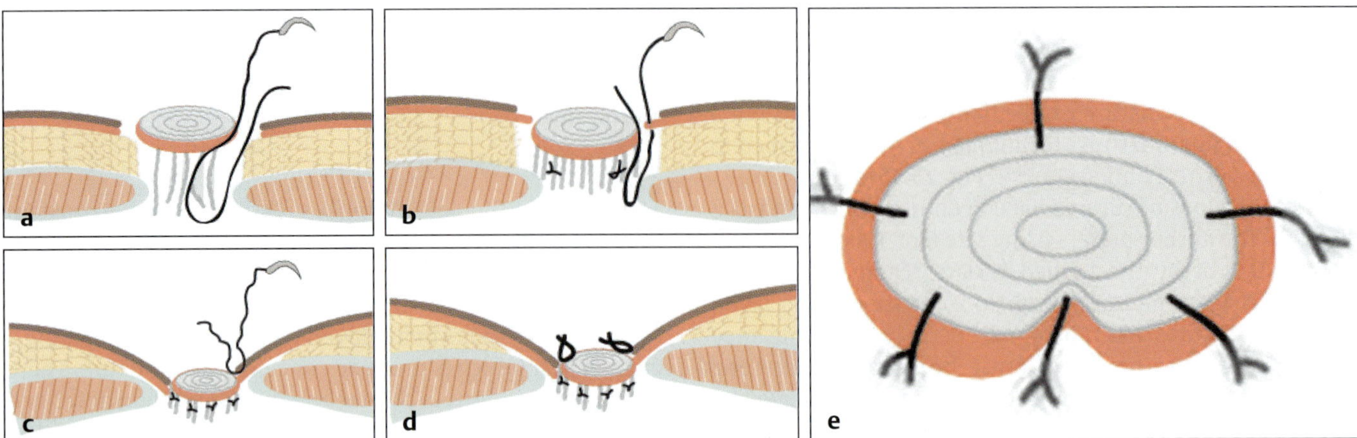

Fig. 25.16 Umbilicoplasty technique. **(a)** Four quadrant sutures are used to telescope the umbilical pedicle and set the skin-disc close to the rectus sheath. **(b)** The dermal fringe on the neoumbilical hole is sutured to the rectus fascia at 3 and 9 o' clock positions. **(c)** The remaining dermal fringe is sutured to the dermis of the skin disc all around. This produces inversion and takes the scar inward. **(d)** Finally, the skin edges are approximated by fast-absorbing fine sutures. The retained periumbilical fat contributes to gentle convexity all around this inkwell. **(e)** V-shaped dart is introduced inferiorly to break the circular scar.

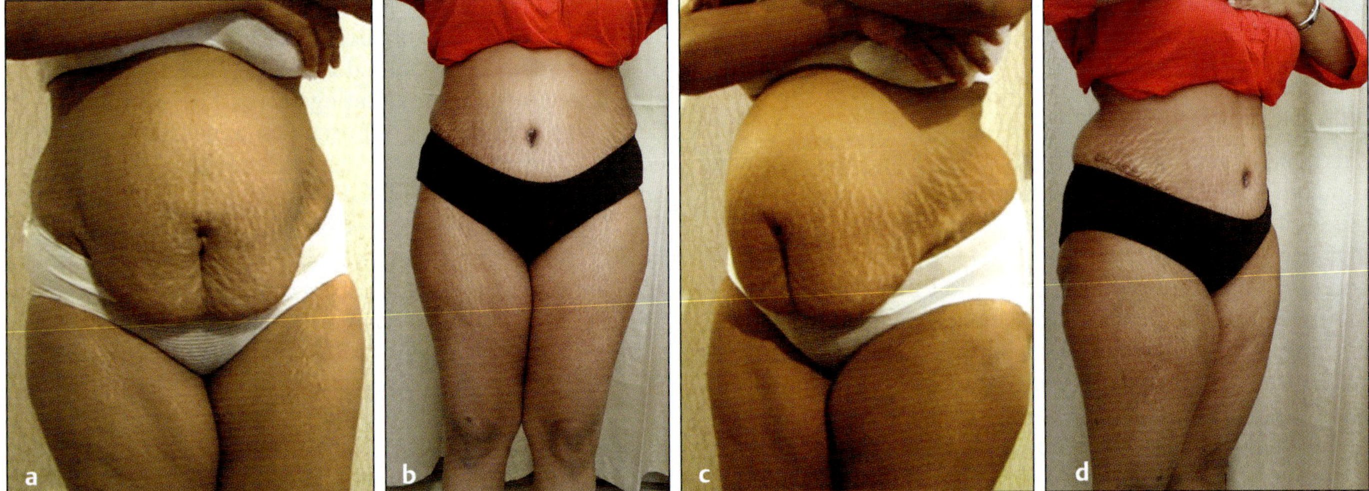

Fig. 25.17 Classical abdominoplasty. Before and after pictures: **(a, b)** front views; **(c, d)** oblique views.

pains, paresthesia, and some numbness in lower central area. Patients can attend office work by the second or third week. Recovery is slower if extensive myofascial plication is done. Result of classical abdominoplasty in a patient of wide diastasis is shown in **Fig. 25.17**.

Technical Variations of Abdominoplasty

Mini Abdominoplasty

It is indicated when there is only limited skin laxity in lower abdomen. Vertical grid lines are drawn and the skin excess is marked as a horizontally long hexagon (rather than ellipse). This ensures freedom from dog-ears. Liposuction is done as indicated. The marked area is de-epithelized (if tissue is very thin) or resected at supra-Scarpa plane. Accurate closure follows (**Fig. 25.7**).

Limited Abdominoplasty

In more advanced cases with skin and myofascial laxity limited to the lower half, a wider paddle of lower abdominal skin is excised together with full repair of lower abdominal muscles. It is possible to work around the umbilicus to continue the midline repair above umbilicus. If the umbilicus is high, it can be detached (floated) to complete the repair, then reinserted at a lower level respecting the golden ratio (**Figs. 25.8 and 25.9**).

Endoscopy-Assisted Abdominoplasty

Individuals having a bulge due to diastasis but without skin excess are candidates for endoscopy-assisted abdominoplasty. It can be combined with a mini abdominoplasty. Men with an epigastric bulge and no skin excess are also ideal.

A short incision in the pubis is used to create an optical space till the umbilicus. Either a second umbilical incision or detachment of the umbilical pedicle affords access to the upper space. Repair can be done by total intracorporeal suturing or by externally introduced sutures retrieved internally. If detached, the umbilical pedicle is reinserted amid the repaired midline.[74,75]

Vest-over Pants Abdominoplasty

Planas described an interesting variation with incision starting at the umbilical level (**Fig. 25.18**). The upper flap is raised and pulled down over the lower skin (vest-over pants) and the lower incision is marked.[76,77] The intervening lower abdominal skin is excised; the remaining steps are the same as in any abdominoplasty. The Planas method has the merit of speed but the surgeon has to be sure of the upper abdominal skin excess before committing to the incision. In a variation of the technique, the author combines this with a type of reverse lift of the lower flap. Thus there will be two flaps, which can then be mutually adjusted for the best contour of upper and lower abdomen. This variant can produce a strong lift of mons and anterior thigh (**Fig. 25.19**). It is a good technique in post-bariatric cases with following advantages: speed, easier access to upper abdomen, flexibility of scar position, bigger resections, and simultaneous mons/anterior thigh lift.[78]

Reverse Abdominoplasty

Excess abdominal tissue has also been tackled in a reverse manner by a submammary incision, lifting the excess in a superolateral vector (**Fig. 25.20**). First described in 1972 with separate resections for upper and lower abdominal excess and two scars, this procedure has also been used as an extended version to correct the entire abdomen in reverse with a single submammary scar.[79–81] Although used rarely, this procedure has been shown to be safe and effective in many reports.[82,83] The indications are:

- Postbariatric patient with significant folds in upper abdomen.
- Patient with greater laxity in upper abdomen and less in lower.
- Existing transverse upper abdominal scar.

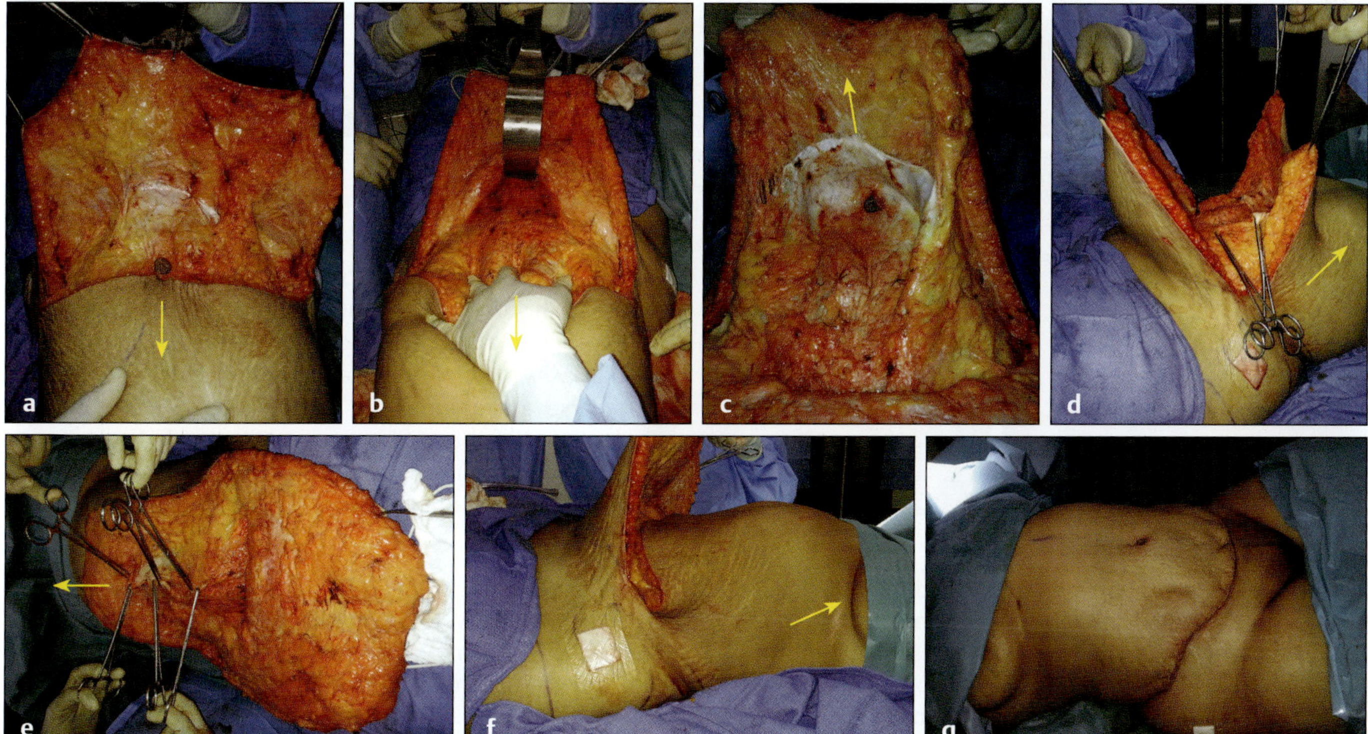

Fig. 25.18 Modified vest-over-pants technique. **(a)** The initial incision is made at the level of umbilicus and lower flap is elevated, *yellow arrow* points to head end. **(b)** Flap elevation reached the pubis to address mons ptosis. **(c)** Upper flap is elevated; white layer is the extremely thinned diastasis. **(d)** The abdominal skin is divided into two flaps. **(e)** Midline plication completed; large lower flap is lying on the thighs. **(f)** The "vest" and "pant" flaps are adjusted, to decide the final level of the lower incision; excess lower flap will be resected. **(g)** Final result.

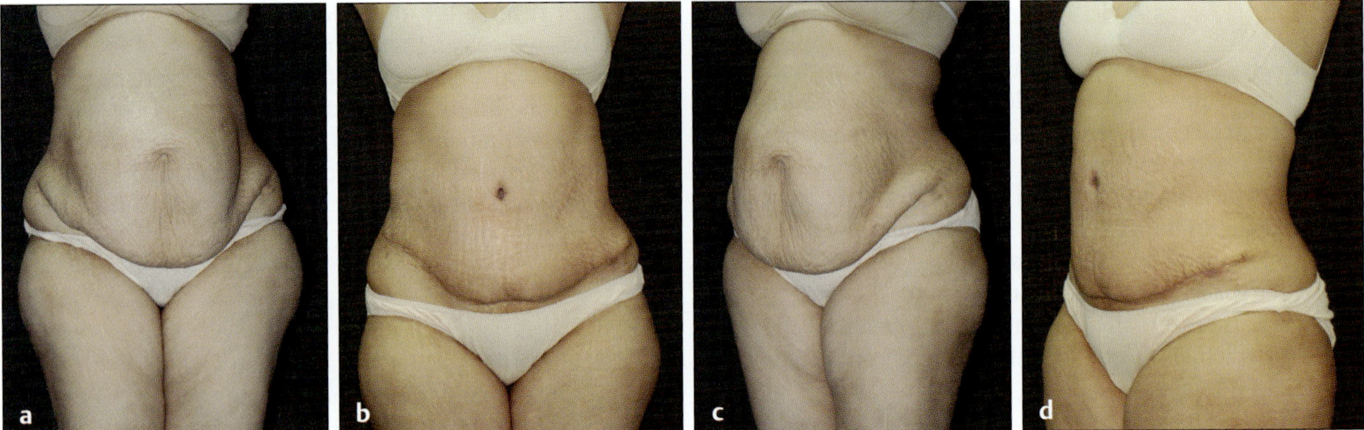

Fig. 25.19 Result of vest-over-pants abdominoplasty. Before and after pictures: **(a, b)** front views; **(c, d)** oblique views.

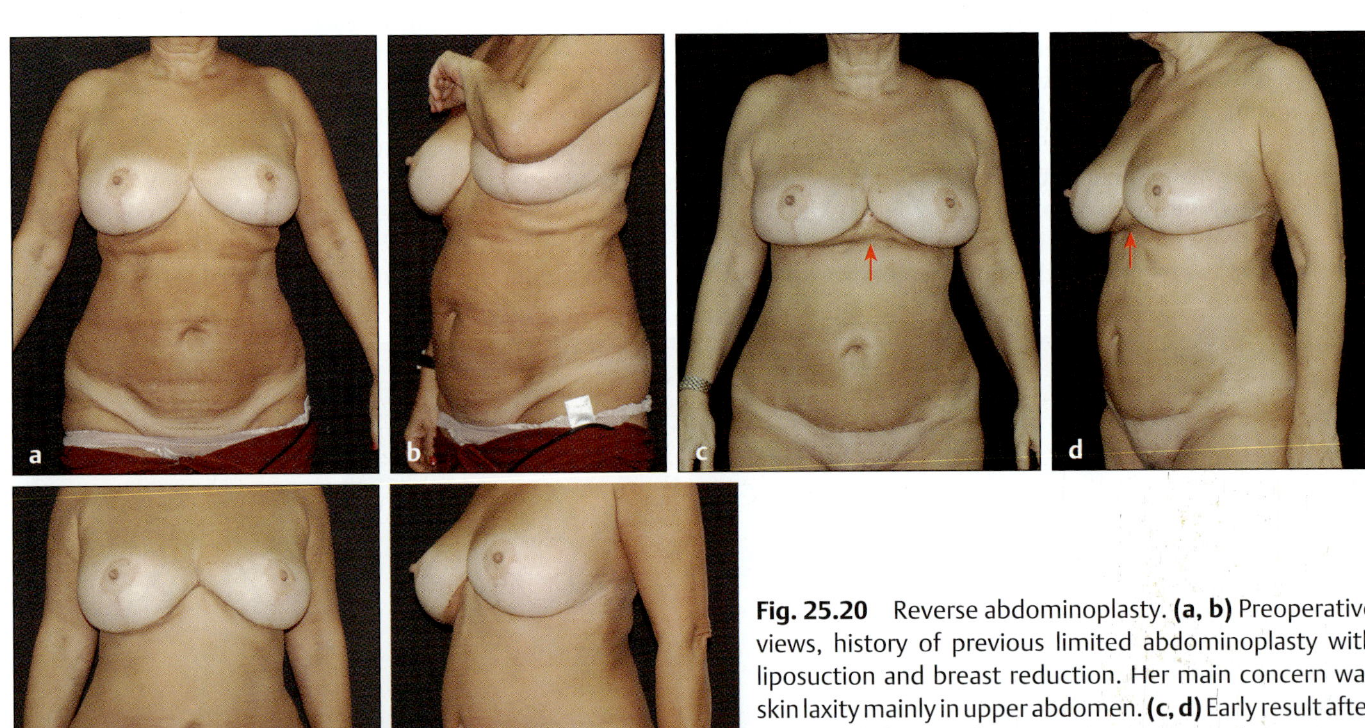

Fig. 25.20 Reverse abdominoplasty. **(a, b)** Preoperative views, history of previous limited abdominoplasty with liposuction and breast reduction. Her main concern was skin laxity mainly in upper abdomen. **(c, d)** Early result after reverse abdominoplasty, using existing inframammary scars and revision of lower scar. Skin excess in substernal area (*red arrow*) was not excised to avoid a scar. **(e, f)** Late result; the skin bulge settles after a few months.

- Simultaneous or previous breast reduction/mastopexy.
- Secondary deformity in upper abdomen.
  - ➢ Tissue laxity due to excess skin/skin and fat.
  - ➢ Uncorrected diastasis in upper part.

In primary cases, starting with submammary incisions connected across midline, the flap dissection is carried down to the pubis after isolating the umbilicus in exactly the reverse of a traditional procedure. Flap vascularity from inferior supply is very robust. Progressive tension sutures or Baroudi-type sutures are used to fix the flap to deep tissues in lower part and to deep fascia in upper part to prevent displacement of IM fold. Umbilicoplasty is done. The excess skin is either trimmed and closure performed at the IM fold or it can even be de-epithelized and used to augment the breast (**Fig. 25.20**).[81]

Employed secondarily, it can be used to correct recurrent or residual problems in the upper abdomen; one may be able to avoid the presternal part of the incision. Combined upper and lower incisions have also been used, keeping the umbilicus and central skin still attached.

Fleur-de-Lis (FDL) Abdominoplasty

Initially described with a midabdominal transverse cut and a vertical lower abdominal component (hence the name meaning lily flower), it now refers to an inverted-T type of resection combining vertical and horizontal skin resections (**Fig. 25.21**). It is indicated in patients with severe global skin laxity such as after multiple pregnancies or massive weight loss. The two main problems with FDL are: unsightly stretched vertical scar (especially in skin of color) and a high incidence of necrosis at the T-junction (**Fig. 25.22e**). Technical tips to avoid these problems: The surgery is conducted in the usual manner till the stage of wound closure. The big disparity between the upper and lower skin is measured in centimeters. An isosceles triangle is marked in the midline of the upper flap with the base equal to this difference reduced by 2 cm; the vertical height is the minimum required for a neat closure. Reducing the base of the triangle by 2 cm ensures that there is absolutely no tension in vertical closure (**Fig. 25.21e**). This triangle is excised including pre-emptive excision of the corners of the T-junction. Layered closure is done taking all the tension on the deep layers so that the skin approximates passively.

En-bloc Resection Technique

This is a variation where the surgeon predetermines the panniculectomy and excises it right in the beginning. The upper flap is then elevated to perform the remaining steps and finish with closure as usual. It has merits of speed and is further explained under "special situations."[84]

Complications

The incidence of complications is variously reported to be from 10 to 20%.[85] It can be reduced drastically by following the above-mentioned principles. Chief culprits leading to complications are: uncontrolled medical conditions, excessive use of cautery at high settings, rough liposuction using

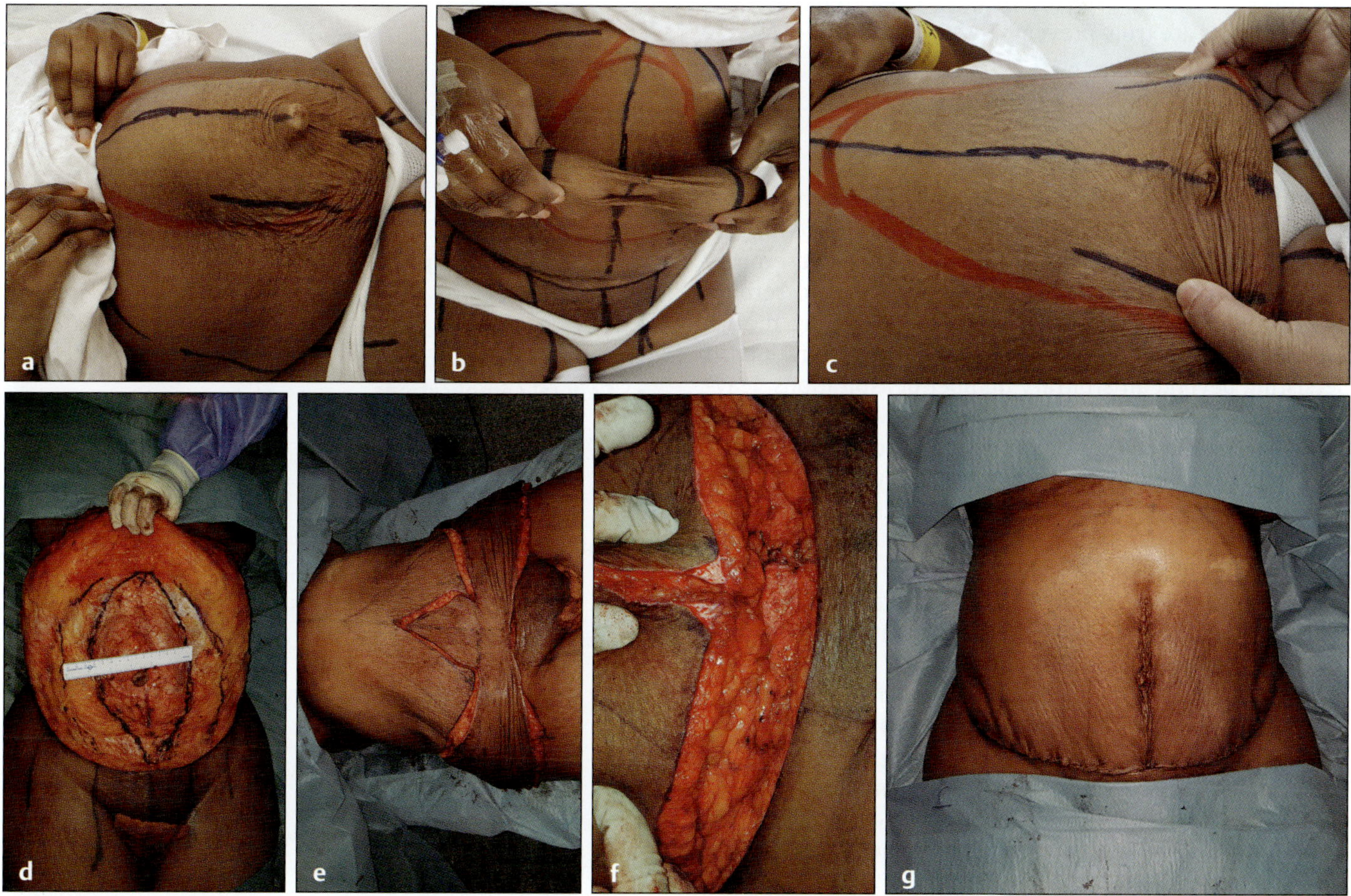

Fig. 25.21 Fleur-de-lis abdominoplasty (FDL). **(a)** Head raising maneuver showing extensive muscle diastasis. **(b)** Skin laxity in horizontal axis needs vertical skin resection. **(c)** Skin laxity in vertical axis needs horizontal skin resection. **(d)** Full display of the diastasis and rectus sheath outlines. **(e)** Fleur-de-lis excision marked. **(f)** Pre-emptive excision of sharp triangles, which are prone for necrosis. **(g)** Completed FDL closure and umbilicoplasty.

large-bore cannulae, widespread mobilization cutting the perforator vessels, leaving the external oblique fascia bare, leaving parasitic fat on flap, leaving large dead spaces (albeit with a drainage), inadequate fascial system repair, wound closure under tension, and concomitant smoking. Obesity is no longer being reported as an independent risk factor especially with LABP, a fact borne out by the author's own experience.[36,86] Infection rates after a clean surgery such as abdominoplasty must be well below 2%. Early infections are usually due to a break in sterile technique or endogenous septic foci. Late infections are usually the sequelae of fat necrosis or seroma.

Classification by Etiopathology

The complications are grouped based on the etiopathology in **Box 25.5**). Such a classification will hopefully bring more clarity and help individual surgeons to pay attention to the etiology and reduce complications. This grouping also guides the management. The dedicated surgeon should never brush off a complication as an unavoidable "fact of life" but must institute serious investigation and soul-searching. Most complications are truly preventable.

Box 25.5 Etiopathologic classification system for postabdominoplasty complications

- **Hemostasis issues**
  - Intraoperative blood loss
  - Hematoma
  - Rectus hematoma
  - Excessive drop in hemoglobin
- **Vascular insufficiency**
  - Fat necrosis
  - Skin necrosis
  - Combined skin and fat necrosis
  - Umbilical necrosis
- **Fluid collection issues**
  - Seroma
  - Leaking seroma
  - Chronic seroma
- **Infective complications**
  - Cellulitis
  - Infected seroma
  - Abscess
  - Necrotizing fasciitis
- **Wound-healing issues**
  - Suture spitting
  - Edge overlap
  - Dehiscence
- **Nerve issues**
  - Hypoesthesia
  - Excessive and prolonged pain
  - Chronic pain
- **Muscle plication issues**
  - Suture/knot problems
  - Recurrence of diastasis
  - Hernia recurrence
- **General complications**
  - Chest complications
  - Venous thromboembolism
  - Myocardial infarction
  - Stroke
- **Potential for malpractice**
  - Peritoneal entry and bowel injury
  - Solid organ injury and bleeding
- **Aesthetic issues**
  - Residual fat
  - Residual skin excess
  - Dog-ears
  - Umbilical issues
  - Abdominal contour
  - Scar problems

Management of Complications

Seroma

Seroma has been assumed to be due to lymphorrhea; this does not seem to be the case. The fluid is more like inflammatory exudate than lymph.[87] Drains do not prevent seromas but the right techniques can. The author has zero seroma rates for over two decades in spite of not using drains. Established seromas may respond to repeated aspirations. If persisting beyond an arbitrary number of aspirations, leaving an indwelling drain or open drainage with a Penrose in situ is better. Chronic seroma is like a pseudobursa with a wall; this needs surgical excision and closure of the space (**Fig. 25.22a**).

Hematoma

Hematoma risk is higher in postbariatric cases, males, and hypertensives (**Fig. 25.22b**). Modest hematomas less than 200 mL may be managed conservatively; larger ones are better evacuated and drained to prevent late seroma and contour deformities. Routine use of Etamsylate, avoiding low-molecular-weight heparins and using pneumatic calf compressions instead, has brought the hematoma rates to zero in the author's practice. Tranexamic acid can also be used routinely and is especially recommended in the high-risk patients.[88]

Ischemia of Flap

The risk of ischemia is higher if there is a transverse scar in the abdominal wall or prior burns. Early signs of ischemia are discoloration and superficial blistering. Releasing a few sutures allows the skin to retract and recover. A portable negative pressure dressing is useful. The skin can be re-advanced later and closed. This strategy may prevent full-scale necrosis. Established full-thickness loss can be allowed to demarcate and heal if small; if larger than 2 cm, it is better

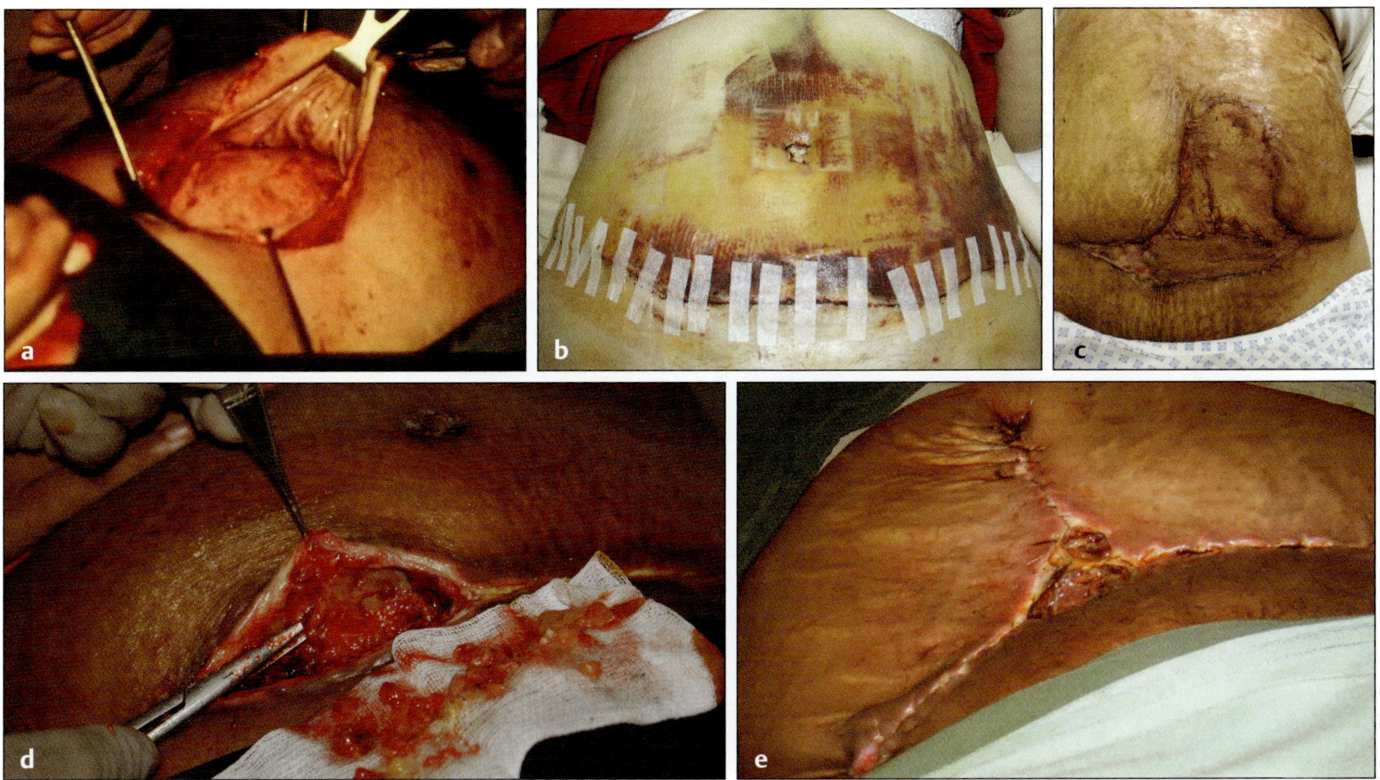

Fig. 25.22 Complications. **(a)** Chronic seroma with a lining looking like pericardium. **(b)** Hematoma in a hypertensive, managed conservatively. **(c)** Triangle-shaped full-thickness necrosis following classical abdominoplasty done elsewhere in a patient with old deep dermal burns. Managed by early debridement, negative pressure wound therapy (NPWT), and skin grafting. **(d)** Fat necrosis, bedside debridement being done. **(e)** Skin-fat necrosis, dehiscence, and sepsis after fleur-de-lis (FDL) abdominoplasty done abroad.

to excise it to prevent infection. Larger raw areas need skin grafting; the graft can often be excised a few months later and skin advanced again (**Fig. 25.22c**).

Fat Necrosis

It presents as hardness with low-grade inflammation, small areas of dehiscence, and chronic serum leakage. The overlying skin shows edema and mild redness. Culture of the fluid is usually sterile and it is futile to use antibiotics. Early debridement of dead fat followed by application of portable negative pressure wound therapy (or dressings) and delayed primary wound closure can solve this rapidly (**Fig. 25.22d**). The author has found ultrasonic therapy to be very useful if there is no open wound. It helps to resolve the edema and induration fast. Sessions are done twice weekly for three weeks.

Dehiscence

Early dehiscence is usually due to excessive tension and poor technique (**Fig. 25.22e**). Prompt resuture in the operating room with use of advancing Baroudi sutures is best. Delayed dehiscence is usually due to fat necrosis and nonadherence of the flaps.

Dog-ears

Dog-ears may become apparent on the sides. Minor issues resolve with time but more significant deformities need a scar revision and touch-up liposuction.

Upper/Lower Abdominal Fullness

Upper fullness is due to either residual fat or not pulling the upper flap sufficiently. This is a difficult problem. Improvements are possible with energy-assisted liposculpture done 6 months later. Lower abdominal fullness needs liposuction, more skin excision, and further muscle tightening.

Lipoabdominoplasty

Definition

LABP refers to the surgical technique of abdominoplasty wherein liposuction is used to mobilize the abdominal flap so that the aims of abdominoplasty can be achieved without performing full surgical undermining of the flap. It is not merely the addition of liposuction to classical abdominoplasty.

The Evolution

Since its invention, liposuction has been applied to contour the abdomen; however, it was mainly used as a standalone procedure. Patients qualifying for abdominoplasty were offered classical abdominoplasty. For over a decade, combining abdominoplasty with liposuction was considered dangerous to the vascularity of the flap and was even specifically contraindicated. Early attempts to combine the two were made in two ways. Either liposuction was selectively applied only to the flanks to improve the bulges there or the skin excision was added to abdominal liposuction in the form of a lower dermolipectomy without mobilization.[25,26,89,90] These surgeries cannot be classified as true lipoabdominoplasties.

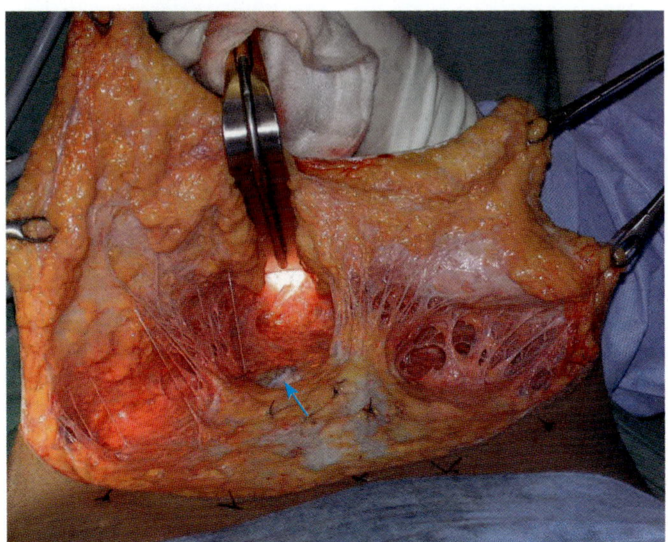

Fig. 25.23 Lipomobilization concept: Honeycomb of spaces created by the liposuction, intact perforators, and their arborization connecting the different perforasomes; the Scarpa fascia is seen on the flap. *Blue arrow* points to umbilical disc.

The author has used liposuction of the abdomen and selective undermining with preservation of perforators from 1995, mainly encouraged by reports that small cannula liposuction spares the blood vessels[50,91] and nerves.[92] The initial cases went without the dreaded complications, leading to progressive increase in the extent of liposuction and decrease in surgical undermining in all patients. The first publication with the name lipoabdominoplasty (LABP) was reported by Saldanha from Brazil in 2001[37] and again in 2003[38] but the concept was already reported in French literature in 1992.[27]

The Concept

LABP is conceptually different—the upper abdominal flap is thinned by liposuction while the neurovascular connections are preserved to a large extent. The flap is now capable of sliding caudally after a bit of discontinuous undermining. This is called "lipomobilization" (**Figs. 25.23 and 25.24**). Neither the extent of skin resection nor the muscle repair is compromised however.

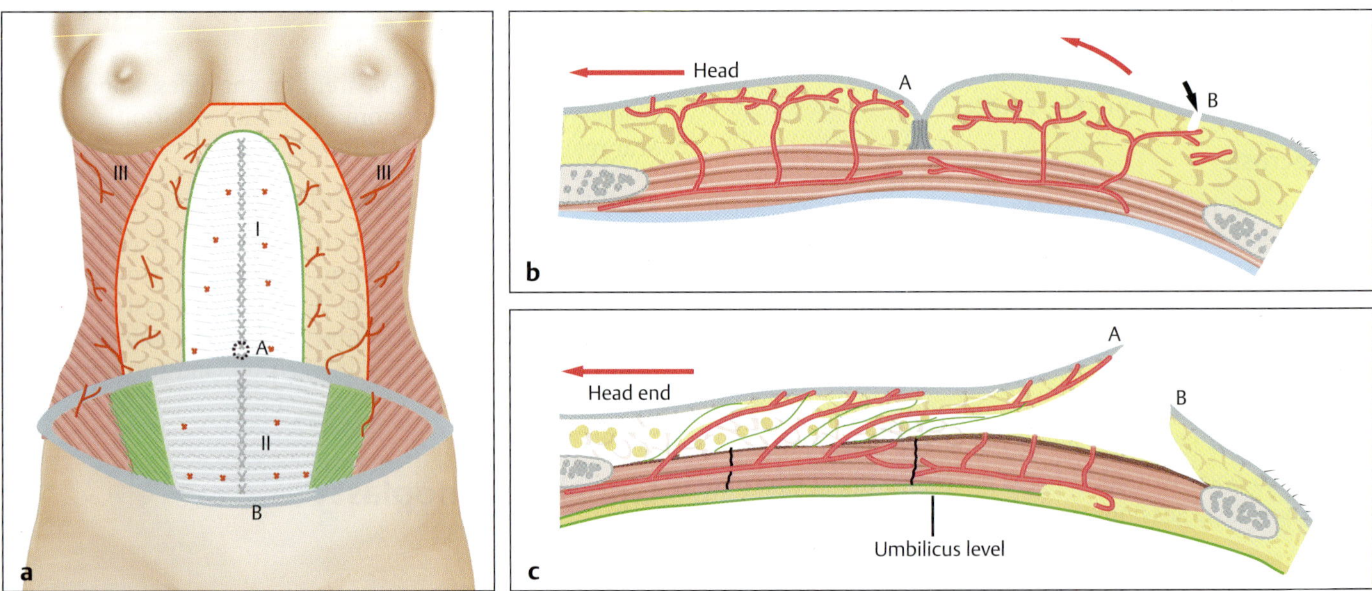

Fig. 25.24 Blood supply of the flap in lipoabdominoplasty. **(a)** The different dissection areas: white central area (I) of tunnel dissection with division of all perforators; *orange shaded* area of selective mobilization with some intact vessels; red striped area (III) of peripheral liposuction with all vessels intact. **(b, c)** Parasagittal view at orange zone: **(b)** Perfusion of intact abdominal skin showing perforators and their arborization in superficial fascia. *Black arrow*: location of incision, point A is at edge of upper flap, point B is at edge of lower incision. **(c)** Showing "tree-top" mobility of the vascular arcades after liposuction; segment AB has been resected, points A and B will be approximated.

Indications and Contraindications

LABP is indicated when the parietal fat is at least 1 inch in pinch thickness. Fat on the flap is considered risky for traditional technique but is an advantage for LABP. The greater the thickness of parietal fat in the upper abdomen, the better the indication and greater the advantages. The concept does not work in very thin abdomens. Excessive visceral fat is a contraindication for any form of abdominoplasty including LABP.

Marking

All the markings are made as in classical technique above. In addition, mark the surface projection of both borders of the rectus sheath, lateral valleys, anterior iliac spines, and lower lateral V shadows in case the patient is very keen on an athletic shape. It is possible to perform high-definition circumferential liposculpture with LABP.[93]

Anesthesia

In the author's practice the initial liposuction (including liposuction of other areas) is completed under local anesthesia with intravenous sedation. This is converted to general anesthesia (GA) before the skin incision, using total intravenous anesthesia (TIVA) technique. This strategy reduces time under GA. TAP blocks may be performed if the skill is available.[61]

Surgical Steps

Patient Position

Surgery begins with the table hyperextended to increase the distance between the xiphoid and pubis which renders tissues taut, facilitating liposuction while drastically reducing the chances of peritoneal entry[94] (**Fig. 25.25**).

Liposuction

Stab incisions are made within the skin to be resected and inside the umbilicus. Klein solution is infiltrated till the tissues become saturated and a bit firm. Peau-d-orange is not created. After waiting 5 minutes for vasoconstriction, liposuction is done in three planes: deep subcutaneous, medium plane, and superficial plane, taking care not to injure the undersurface of skin; this is different from performing a pure liposuction. Movements must be strictly longitudinal without lateral deviations. For every change of direction, the surgeon must come back to the access hole and then change. A 4-mm Mercedes with a bullet nose or a 4-mm Keel cobra is the best for deep and medium levels. A 3-mm Accelerator is used in superficial plane and for midline etching as well as contouring the valleys; it is used with the holes facing deep. Short cannulae are used for contouring the mons pubis and for the costal margins. Liposuction is continued till one of the following end points: skin pinch thickness reaches 1.5 cm or aspirate turns bloody with poor returns.

Energy-assisted and power-assisted techniques can also be used. Ultrasonic, Vaser, infrasonic nutational, and water-jet-assisted liposuctions as well as power-assisted devices are safe and are used by many. However, laser or radiofrequency-assisted liposuctions may be unsafe due to their stated intent to coagulate vessels and produce heat damage.

Incision and Flap Elevation

Incision by scalpel is followed by diathermy blade-tip electrode. Diathermy is set at the minimum effective power setting and "blend" option for efficient smooth cutting. Nonstick Teflon-coated tip with coaxial suction for the smoke is strongly recommended. The superficial inferior epigastric vessels are tied off. The Scarpa fascia is identified and incised bilaterally for an inch. A 3-mm liposuction cannula is inserted and the deep fat suctioned gently. Some fat is left on the external oblique. This step is omitted if the fat pad is thin. The Scarpa fascia is cut all the way and flap elevation begun with diathermy hugging the avascular plane on its undersurface. The flap is elevated till the umbilicus. A honeycomb structure is seen in the upper and lateral abdomen due to the liposuction and here the actual undermining stops (**Figs. 25.23 and 25.25d**). The perforators of DCIA may be cut but can often be saved as well. The umbilicus is circumscribed and isolated on its pedicle. With the help of illuminated retractors and a long-stem diathermy pencil, the upper flap is undermined in a tunnel spanning the divarication and 3 cm lateral to the medial rectus border. A thin parasagittal fascia that extends from the medial rectus border to the skin (normal adhesion line) should be incised carefully since the perforators lie immediately beyond. Hereafter, the surgeon inserts their fingers and mobilizes the flap by lifting and drawing down simultaneously with spread and hooked fingers (**Fig. 25.25g**). This maneuver allows one to identify just the restraining fibers, which are cauterized and divided. Some more perforators (the lateral row) may have to be divided. Progressive and incremental flap mobilization can be seen as this step is repeated. Trial approximation is done with the table flexed 30 degrees to decide on the level of upper incision. In most cases this tallies with the preoperative plan. This is marked for cutting. After repeatedly ensuring correct level, the upper incision is made and the excess tissue excised. The flap is well perfused by branches of intercostals, subcostal, lumbar, and sometimes also the lateral row of rectus perforators and perforating branches of DCIA at the corners (**Fig. 25.24**). The musculature is now exposed to allow a two-layer repair. See under classical abdominoplasty for technique of myofascial repair.

The skin flap is pulled down and temporarily tacked to the lower flap at the midline. Additional mobilization of the lower flap may be needed and mons lift/liposuction may be performed if indicated. Additional contouring and defining liposuction can be done now with thinner cannulae. The umbilical projection point is marked and a new

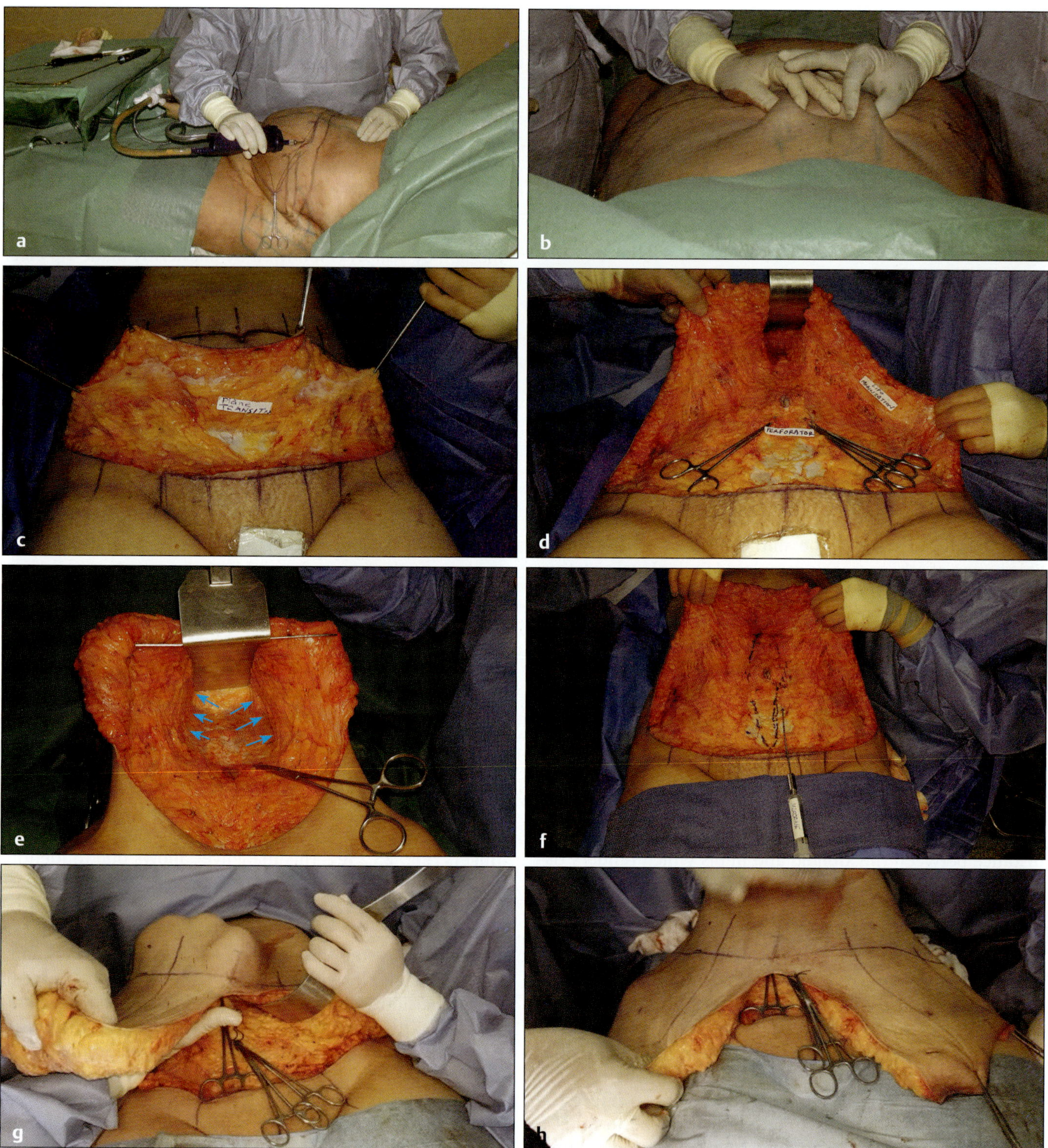

Fig. 25.25 Steps of lipoabdominoplasty (pictures are from different patients). **(a)** Liposuction of entire abdomen, **(b)** to reach fat thickness of 1 to 1.5 cm, taking special care for extra contouring of waists, midline, and lateral valleys. **(c)** Skin flap elevated sub-Scarpa, deep fat layer left intact bilaterally but removed in midline to expose the rectus sheath. **(d)** Flap elevated till umbilicus, lipomobilization seen above this level. **(e)** Broad tunnel dissection of upper abdomen, *blue arrows* show the thin parasagittal fascia connecting medial edge of rectus sheath to the skin (adhesion line). **(f)** Completed flap elevation, note lipomobilization laterally. Rectus sheath block being administered by blunt cannula, **(g)** discontinuous blunt finger dissection in between tethering fibers to improve the reach of flap; fibers may be divided selectively. **(h)** Testing the reach of the flap.

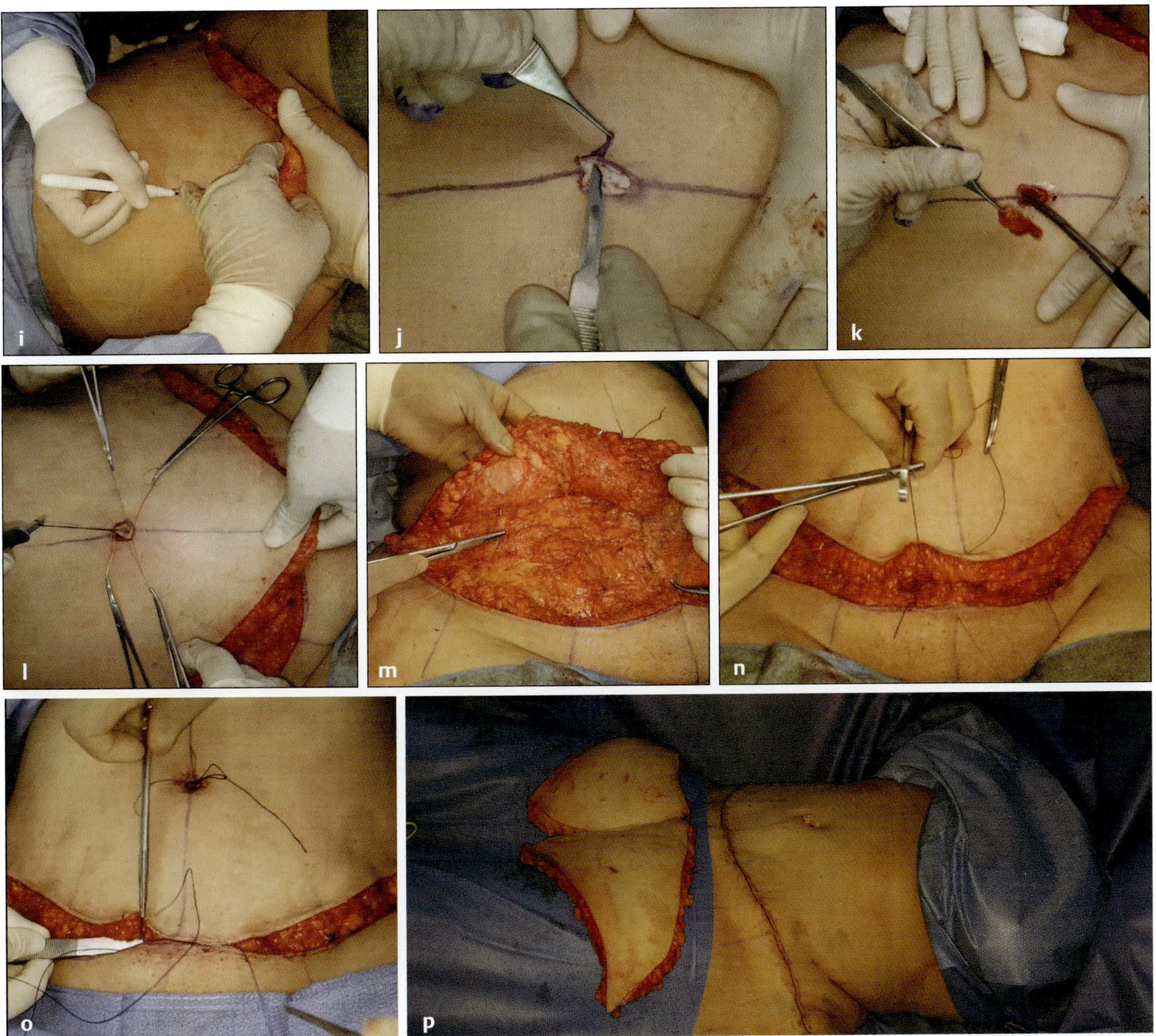

Fig. 25.25 *(Continued)* **(i)** New umbilicus is marked 1.5 cm cranial to projection point of umbilicus. **(j)** Area is de-epithelized and dermis incised. **(k)** Cone of fat removed. **(l)** Dermal edge anchored to rectus sheath to produce ink-welling effect; the umbilical pedicle has already been shortened. **(m)** Quilting sutures applied to close the space under the flap. **(n)** Deep tissues of the flap sutured to Scarpa fascia of lower edge. **(o)** Deep repair completed; skin closure by barbed suture. **(p)** The result: aesthetically perfect abdomen, natural umbilical contours, low symmetric scar and no drains.

umbilical point marked 1.5 cm cranial to this.[35] A new umbilical incision and plasty is made as described under classical abdominoplasty (**Fig. 25.16**). The upper tunnel space is closed by a few quilting-advancing sutures of 2–0 fast-absorbing Polyglactin. The flattening achieved by this is apparent immediately. The deep surface of the lower part of the flap is then fixed to the external oblique aponeurosis by taking quilting stitches of fast-absorbing suture, taking care to stagger the successive rows and to continuously adjust the upper flap medially to correct for length disparity with the lower skin edge. Any excess fat on the skin edges are trimmed preparatory to tension-free closure. Drains are not used; postoperatively a well-fitting garment is applied.

Advantages of Lipoabdominoplasty

The advantages are summarized in **Box 25.6**. This method of abdominoplasty is physiological, comprehensive, and allows

Box 25.6 Advantages of lipoabdominoplasty

- Preserves natural connections
- Better contouring
- Safe in the obese
- Less area of anesthesia
- Less blood loss
- Safe in circumferential surgery
- Safe in presence of horizontal scars
- Versatile
- Less complications
- Suctioned fat available for grafting

complete contouring. Less open spaces are created and tissues seem to adhere and heal rapidly. The technique is trouble free even in diabetics, smokers (provided they stop for 3 weeks), and in presence of upper abdominal scars. In the author's series, there were no seromas or skin necrosis and less than 1% hematomas in over 500 consecutive cases in two decades. Significant wound infections were 2 (0.4%); both were traced to endogenous source in vagina and umbilicus. Several innovations and refinements added to LABP over the past two decades have resulted in an elegant and advanced technique, which is versatile in addressing the entire spectrum of presentations with excellent safety and rapid recovery (**Fig. 25.26**).

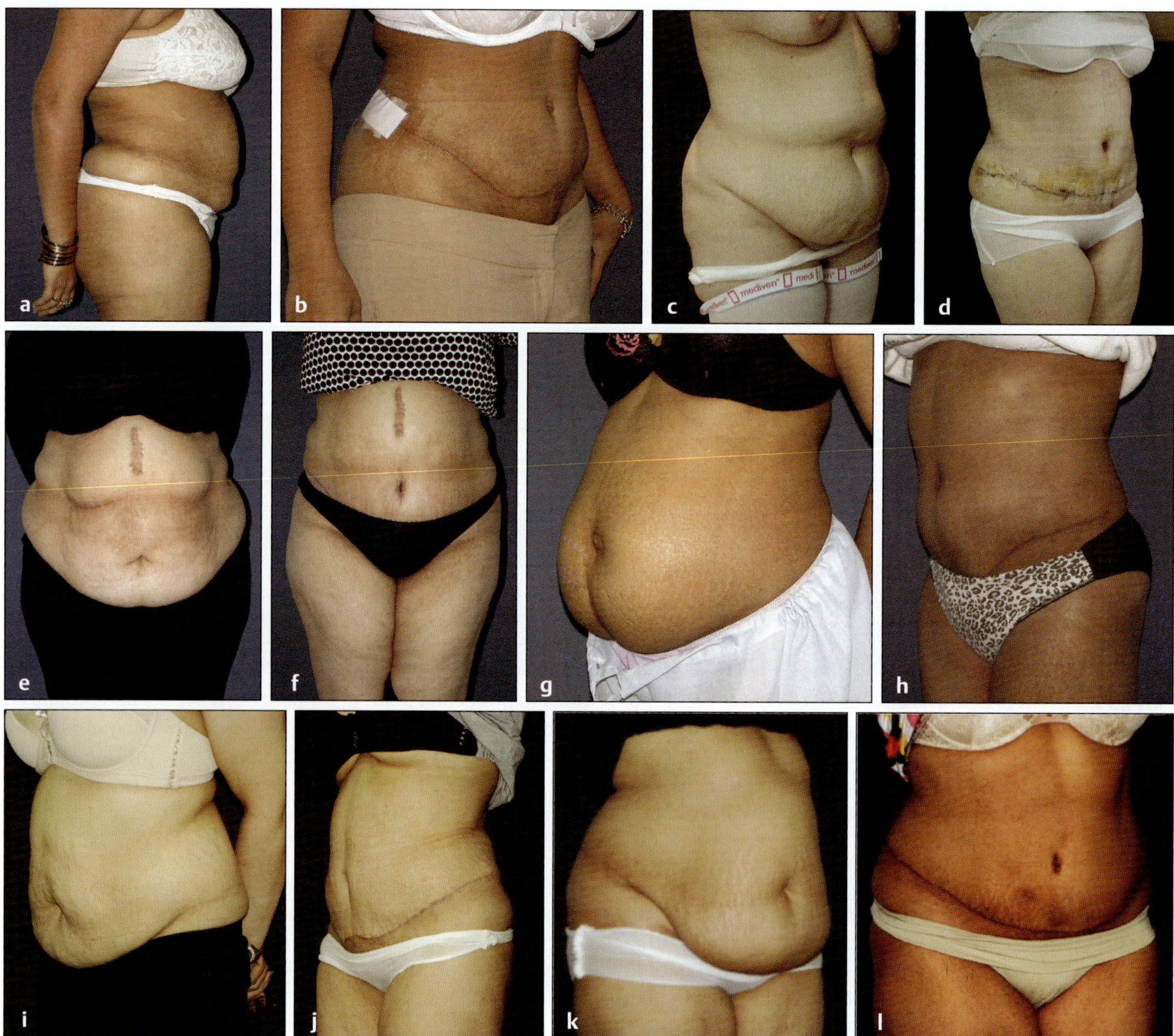

Fig. 25.26 Before and after picture series showing the wide range of patients that can be safely treated by lipoabdominoplasty. **(a–b, c–d, e–f, g–h, i–j, k–l)** The flatness of the abdomen after surgery is mainly determined by visceral fat and residual intrinsic muscle tone.

Special Situations

Some patients present with unique challenges to surgery; strategies to deal with some common situations are given below.

Male Abdominoplasty

A minority of men (without visceral fat excess) are candidates for abdominoplasty. Myofascial plication can be omitted (except when there is congenital diastasis), complete liposuction of the mons pubis, love handles, and muscle contours must be done; the hips rolls must be tackled from front and back. Narrowing of the waist and feminization are to be avoided. The lateral part of scar is kept low and turned down so it can be hidden in male underwear. More care is needed to keep all umbilical scars invisible.

Very Large Panniculus

Patients presenting with massive redundant aprons are challenging; such patients often have comorbidities and limited mobility. Elevating the mega flap in the usual way is tedious, lengthy, and bloody, and complications may be high. A modification of LABP called en-bloc resection is very effective and safe[84] (**Fig. 25.27**).

Technique

A CT scan is obtained to be aware of any hernias. The upper and lower borders of the apron are marked in standing position, going as far laterally and around as needed. Vertical grid lines are marked. In supine position, the upper mark is revised downwards to account for tissue thickness and elastic recoil with gravity eliminated. Surgery starts with infiltration and liposuction of the base of the panniculus. The author performs multiple transfixations at the base to isolate the panniculus; this also helps in hemostasis. Incisions are made and deepened down to but not through Scarpa fascia. Starting at the corners, the entire block of tissue is resected by avulsion in the loose plane created by liposuction. There is surprisingly little bleeding due to avulsion-snapping of small bleeders that shrivel up; any active bleeder must be well controlled. The upper abdomen is then treated by liposuction and LABP proceeds as usual. (Caution! the remaining skin shows elastic recoil after removal of the heavy apron, creating a paradoxical situation of skin tightness during closure. It is advisable to be conservative with the upper resection line and to trim any excess at final closure.) This modification has extended the range of LABP, which can now be safely performed in such "big" cases. The author has used it on several occasions with uniform ease and safety (**Fig. 25.28**).

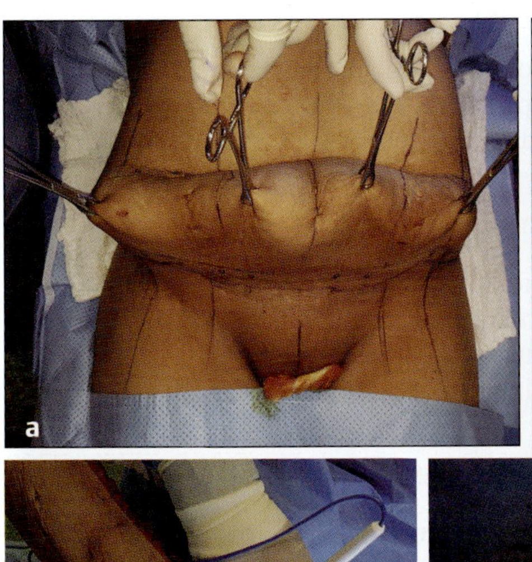

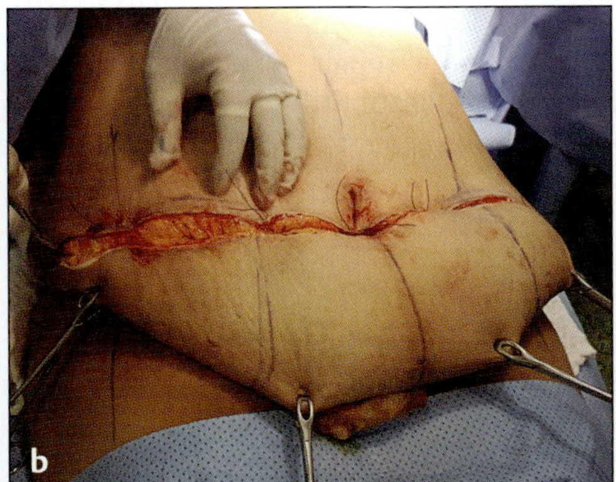

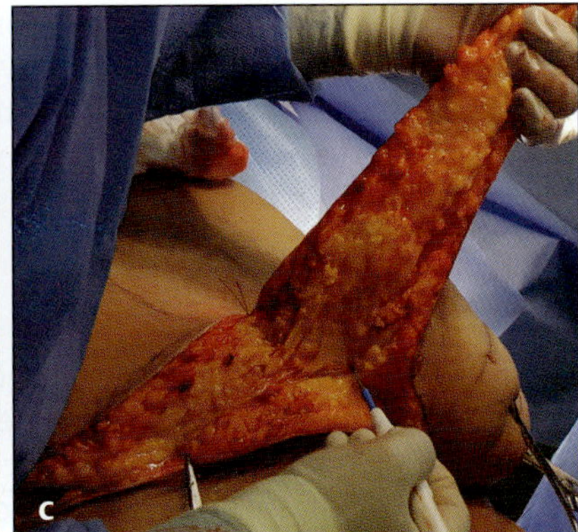

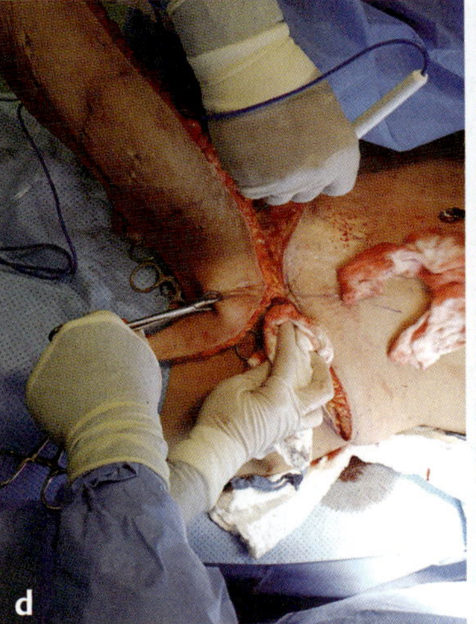

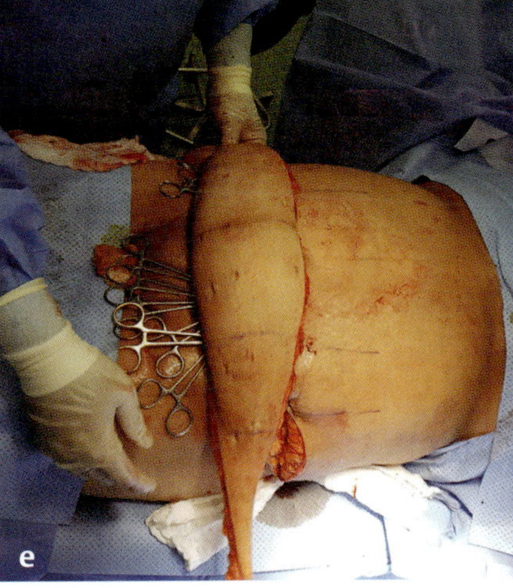

Fig. 25.27 Rapid en-bloc resection of abdominal panniculus. **(a)** Abdominal panniculus is held up; its base is thinned by liposuction and transfixed by several sutures. **(b)** Upper border of the isolated tissue is incised. **(c)** Lower border is incised and the isolated island is being excised by strong avulsion, aided by diathermy. **(d)** Excision from the left side. **(e)** Panniculus excised rapidly.

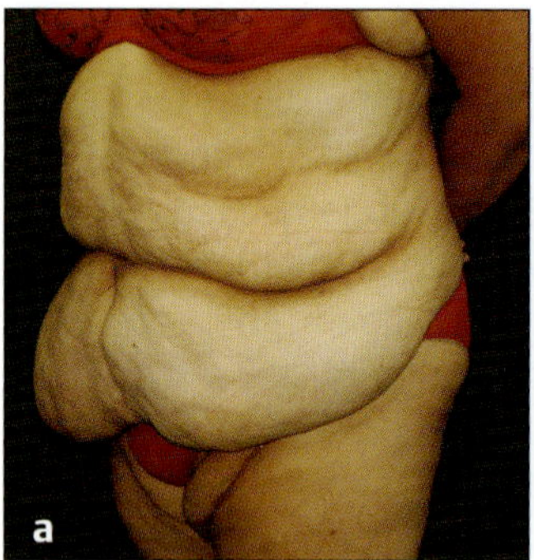

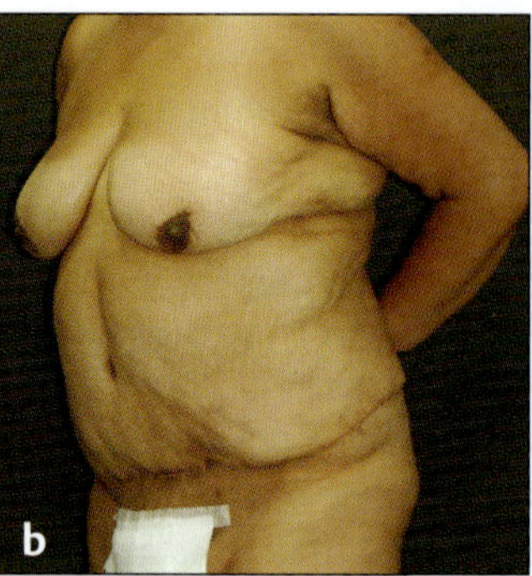

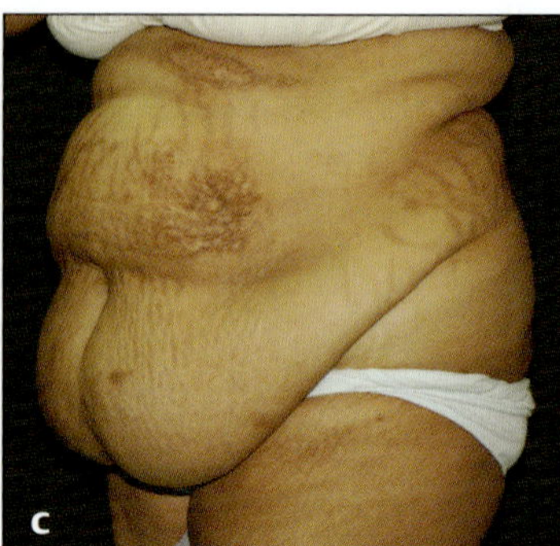

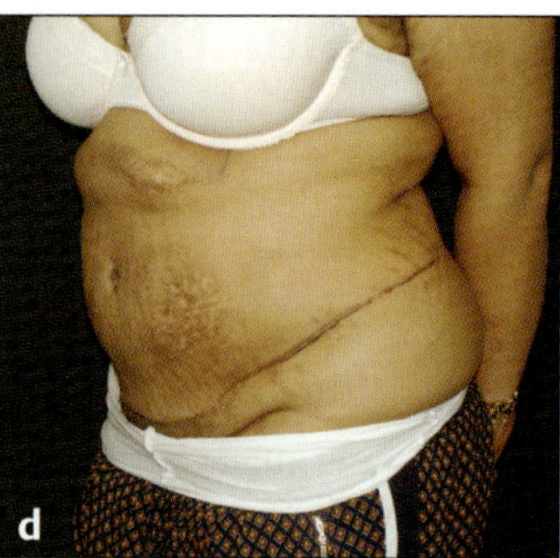

Fig. 25.28 Examples of patients operated by rapid technique. **(a, b)** Before and after photos of a patient with multiple large rolls of redundant tissue. **(c, d)** Before and after photos of a large abdomen with previous deep dermal burns and a large apron of redundancy.

Wide Diastasis

Several options exist to deal with this wide diastasis. One may use bilateral relaxing incisions on the external oblique aponeurosis to reduce the tension on the midline closure.[8,95,96] The resulting composite myofascial flap consisting of the internal oblique and transverses (both more muscular) with the rectus sheath becomes free from the restraint of external oblique aponeurosis and slides medially. There is no risk of hernia in the line of aponeurotomy (**Fig. 25.29**). Anterior rectus sheath turn-over flaps (**Fig. 25.30**) or component separation techniques are other options.[8,97] For larger defects a formal component separation method is used.[98] An inlay mesh may be used additionally.[99,100] Anatomic repair is favored whenever possible to avoid mesh complications. The anesthetist must ensure full relaxation at this stage to ensure that muscle tone does not resist closure.

Congenital Diastasis

This condition is not widely recognized but it exists. It is due to rectus muscles taking origin more laterally. There may also be flaring of the rib margins. Direct plication is difficult and prone to relapse. Bilateral anterior rectus sheath turn-over flaps may be approximated in the midline which in turn brings the muscles closer.[97,101] The exposed tendinous intersections are approximated with strong permanent sutures followed by passive approximation of muscles[8] (**Fig. 25.30**).

Weak Musculature

Such patients need to be prepared well and made to lose visceral fat drastically. Muscle plication is needed in the midline and also along linea semilunaris. A horizontal plication may also be added.[69] A newly described technique of triangular mattress sutures has been shown to shorten the vertical length of the rectus sheath as well (**Fig. 25.15m**).[68] An indwelling urinary catheter can be used to monitor intra-abdominal pressure.[102]

Tight Upper Abdomen

Such patients have insufficient skin laxity for the upper skin to reach all the way to the pubis. There are three possible solutions to this problem: (1) limited lower apronectomy without disturbing the umbilicus, (2) umbilical flotation and lowering the umbilicus, or (3) full abdominoplasty with separate closure of the umbilical donor hole. If umbilical flotation is used, the ratio of upper to lower abdomen should be close to 1.6:1 (Golden ratio).[59]

Previous Liposuction

Manual liposuction may be difficult due to the fibrosis. Ultrasound and power-assisted liposuction works better and has been used in LABP without ill effect.

Distended Umbilicus with Hernia

Dealing with the umbilicus in such cases is a judgment call. If the risk of umbilical necrosis is significant, it is best to excise it altogether and use one of the techniques for creation of a new umbilicus primarily or secondarily.[103,104]

Ventral/Incisional Hernia

Abdominoplasty offers unparalleled access to the entire abdominal musculature and is hence a powerful tool in dealing with ventral hernias, whether primary or recurrent, while also debulking the panniculus. The excellent exposure enables use of advanced reconstructive techniques like fascia turnover, component separation, and inlay mesh to restore normal functional anatomy as well as provide prosthetic reinforcement. A preoperative CT scan is mandatory; LABP can also be used, provided suction is done well away from the hernia as guided by the CT scan. Although laparoscopic hernia repair has become the preferred method, abdominoplasty approach may be a comparable or a better option in selected patients.

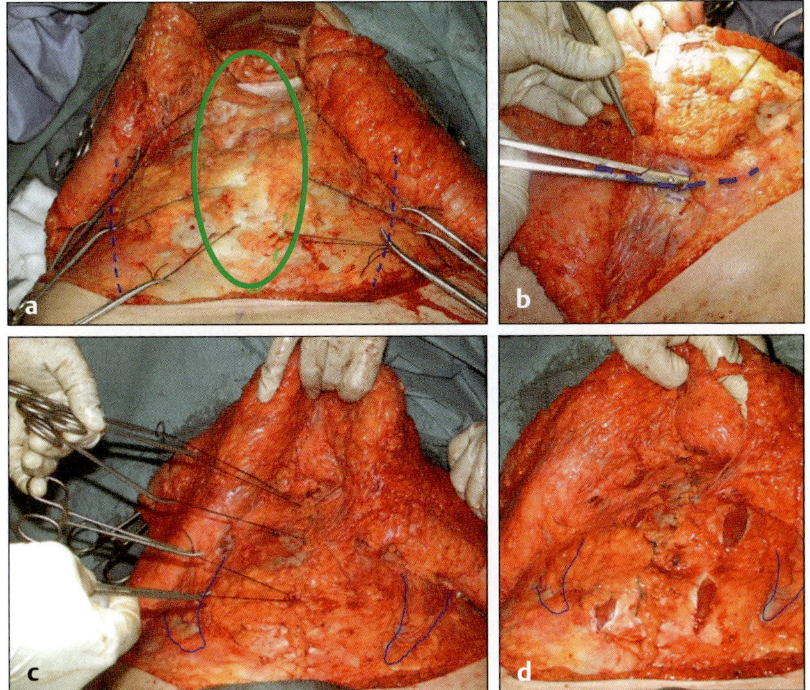

Fig. 25.29 External oblique release technique. **(a)** Anatomy displayed: *green lines*: wide diastasis, *blue broken lines*: outer limits of rectus sheath. **(b)** A small cut is made in the external oblique aponeurosis where it splits to form the anterior sheath. Scissors insert easily in the avascular plane immediately beneath the fascia, which is cut blindly by sliding the scissors. **(c)** Secure midline closure; *solid blue lines* show the widely open edges of aponeurosis **(d)** with the addition of relaxing incisions of anterior rectus sheath as well.

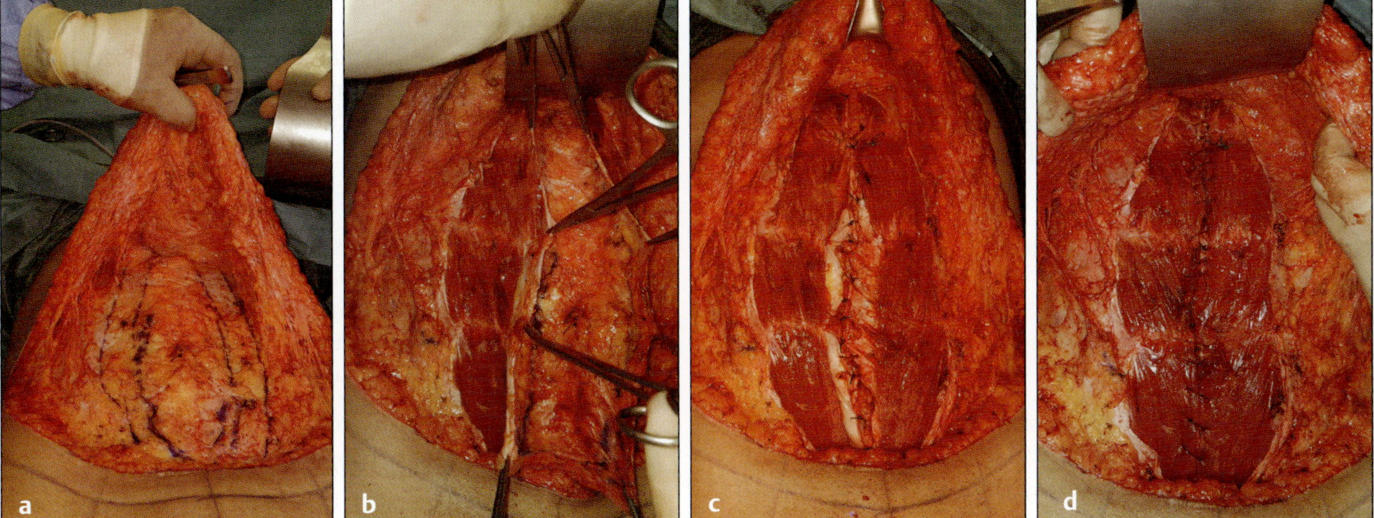

Fig. 25.30 Rectus Sheath turnover technique. **(a)** Inner markings are on medial border of rectus sheath; outer markings show proposed incision on anterior rectus sheath for turnover flap. **(b)** Flaps incised and being dissected off the tendinous intersections. **(c)** Turn-over flaps sutured in midline by permanent sutures. The tendinous intersections will be approximated, the first is done. **(d)** Finally, the muscles are passively joined by absorbable sutures.

Pure Myofascial Laxity without Skin Excess

This is an indication for endoscopic muscle plication with liposuction for contouring.[82]

Circumferential Problems

Increasingly, we get patients whose problems are circumferential. A two-dimensional abdominoplasty is insufficient. It leads to lateral bulges and a dissatisfied patient. Effective options are:

- 3D liposuction and LABP.
- Extended LABP.
- Circumferential LABP or belt abdominoplasty.

3D Liposuction and LABP

This is chosen when there is circumferential fat excess but with good skin elasticity. Surgery starts with liposuction in prone or lateral position under local anesthesia and IV sedation. Grooves below the fat rolls are best treated by subcision and fat grafting using a V-tip dissector-cannula. The patient is then turned supine and LABP proceeds as usual under GA. A majority of patients can be candidates for this as it vastly enhances the "wow" effect of LABP. Concurrent dorsal procedures may not be prudent in FDL type of abdominoplasty.

Extended LABP

In patients with excess tissue over iliac crests (muffin tops), the abdominoplasty marking has to be extended to include these skin rolls (type V). Following liposuction as above, the extensions are excised and closed in two layers using strong sutures to join the Lockwood fascia and superficial fascia of the gluteo-trochanteric complex. The patient is turned and LABP proceeds as usual.

Circumferential Abdominoplasty

This is indicated in patients with circumferential skin laxity. The marking includes a wider paddle in midlateral buttock area for a strong lift but a narrower excision in the dorsal midline to avoid dehiscence. Complete liposuction is followed by an avulsion-type dermolipectomy in the dorsal superficial fascial plane; the fascia is left intact and the subfascial plane is treated only by liposuction; see CT scan images in **Fig. 25.2**. It is important not to expose the shiny fascia on the paraspinal muscles but to stay well superficial; this reduces bleeding, pain, and seromas.

Revisions and Secondary Abdominoplasty

Definitions

Revision refers to small corrections that may be performed in order to improve some aspects of the primary procedure, for example, a partial scar revision or excision of dog-ears. A *secondary procedure* refers to any surgery that is required after an arbitrary long gap such as extensive liposuction or combination of procedures but not a repeat abdominoplasty. A *secondary abdominoplasty* refers to repeating the abdominoplasty in order to address a major issue.

Classification

After examination, these patients may immediately be divided into three groups: (1) convex contour due to visceral fat excess, (2) problems due to errors in the planning or execution of primary surgery or due to complications thereof, and (3) where the benefits of abdominoplasty are waning due to age, subsequent pregnancy, or fat gain in the abdominal wall. The first category needs lifestyle modifications or bariatric surgery if indicated. The second and third groups of patients need careful examination, diagnosis, and planning. Most of them fit into one or more of the following categories:

- Umbilical problems.
- Scar problems:
  - Scar located too high.
  - Hypertrophic scar.
  - Widened scar with contour depressions.
- Residual skin excess in the upper abdomen.
- Residual skin excess in lower abdomen.
- Fat excess in abdominal wall and asymmetries.
- Contour problems in flanks and hip areas.
- Sequelae of previous wound-healing problems/tissue loss.
- Issues with the mons pubis.

Management Strategies

Umbilical Problems

The umbilicus may be too big, too small, dystopic (too high, low, or off-center) or suffer stenosis. Scar hypertrophy and stenosis are treated by intralesional steroid injection, dilatation, and by wearing a silicon rubber stent for 3 months. An abnormal looking big umbilicus can be improved by revision: shortening the stalk, fat grafting to periumbilical area, and breaking the circular scar. Dystopia of umbilicus requires a secondary abdominoplasty; a new additional small scar may result when the umbilicus is restored to its correct position.

Scar Problems

A *scar located too high* is visible above the underwear. If there is secondary laxity of the skin, skin strip excision, progressive advancement, and layered closure solves the issue. If there is no laxity, careful consideration is given to a full-revision abdominoplasty or umbilical flotation. *Scar hypertrophy* is usually addressed by intralesional injections of triamcinolone, 5-fluorouracil, and silicone sheeting/silicone cream therapy. A *wide scar with contour depression* indicates improper closure of the deep tissues and fascia. Appropriate treatment includes liposuction of the upper margin and scar revision with multilayer closure.

Residual Skin Excess in Upper Abdomen

This problem is addressed in the same way as a high scar, (i.e., by a secondary abdominoplasty). Any high diastasis of the recti must also be repaired. Liposuction alone may be enough if the skin quality is good.

Residual Skin Excess in the Lower Abdomen

This problem is due to secondary relaxation of tissues, further weight loss, and inelastic skin. It is easily corrected by further liposuction, excision of the excess skin, and a tension-free closure. This possibility should be discussed preoperatively and included in consent.

Fat Excess and Contour Problems

Usual cause is nonuniform or inadequate liposuction in primary procedure, complications such as seroma/fat necrosis, or further weight gain/pregnancies. Energy-assisted liposuction and fat grafting may be used to break up the divots of fat and internally redistribute the fat.

Tissue Loss

Ischemia of the lower central area results in skin necrosis, infection, and slough. Early debridement and skin grafting can prevent infection, suffering, and severe scarring (**Fig. 25.22c**). After waiting for tissue resolution, the deformity is addressed later using reconstructive principles including the use of tissue expanders. An expert second opinion is very valuable.

Deformities in Mons Pubis

A bulging mons with tissue overhang is easily corrected by liposuction and skin resection. A tight and overresected mons on the other hand is not easy to reverse. If functionally symptomatic, the incision is reopened and the vulva and residual mons are mobilized and refixed at a lower appropriate location using internal stitches. The upper flap is progressively advanced by sutures and anchored to the fascia such that the skin edges approximate without tension. A little fat grafting of the mons pubis may help as well in restoring normalcy.

Summary

Abdominoplasty is one of the most commonly performed aesthetic body contouring procedures. As is true in all surgeries, complete anatomical diagnosis, proper case selection, and comprehensive preoperative counseling are important for a successful outcome. Major improvements of concept and technique in the past two decades have enhanced the safety, range, and scope of abdominoplasty, reduced its complications, and improved the outcome. LABP has now become the default operation. Fat on the abdominal wall is no longer a contraindication while excess visceral fat remains so. Circumferential treatments are shown to be safe. Surgeons aspiring to reach excellence in this field are well advised to study the key historical improvements and incorporate them in their surgical craft.

References

1. Pitanguy I. Evaluation of body contouring surgery today: a 30-year perspective. Plast Reconstr Surg 2000;105(4):1499–1514, discussion 1515–1516
2. Oneal RM, Mulka JP, Shapiro P, Hing D, Cavaliere C. Wide abdominal rectus plication abdominoplasty for the treatment of chronic intractable low back pain. Plast Reconstr Surg 2011;127(1):225–231
3. Staalesen T, Elander A, Strandell A, Bergh C. A systematic review of outcomes of abdominoplasty. J Plast Surg Hand Surg 2012;46(3-4):139–144
4. Swedenhammar E, Stark B, Hållstrand AH, Ehrström M, Gahm J. Surgical training and standardised management guidelines improved the 30-day complication rate after abdominoplasty for massive weight loss. World J Surg 2018;42(6):1647–1654
5. Alderman AK, Collins ED, Streu R, et al. Benchmarking outcomes in plastic surgery: national complication rates for abdominoplasty and breast augmentation. Plast Reconstr Surg 2009;124(6):2127–2133
6. Winocour J, Gupta V, Ramirez JR, Shack RB, Grotting JC, Higdon KK. Abdominoplasty: risk factors, complication rates, and safety of combined procedures. Plast Reconstr Surg 2015;136(5):597e–606e
7. Dutot M-C, Serror K, Al Ameri O, Chaouat M, Mimoun M, Boccara D. Improving safety after abdominoplasty: a retrospective review of 1128 cases. Plast Reconstr Surg 2018; 142(2):355–362
8. Rangaswamy M. Minimising complications in abdominoplasty: an approach based on the root cause analysis and focused preventive steps. Indian J Plast Surg 2013;46(2):365–376
9. Kelly HA. Excision of the fat of the abdominal wall-lipectomy. Surg Gynecol Obstet 1910;10:229–231
10. Thorek M. Reconstructive surgery of the abdominal wall. In: Plastic surgery of the breast and abdominal wall. Springfield, IL: CC Thomas; 1942:245–257
11. Gaudet F, Morestin H. French congress of surgeons, vol. 82. In: French congress of surgeons, Paris; 1905: 125–126
12. Thorek M. Plastic reconstruction of the female breasts and abdomen. Am J Surg 1939;43(2):268–278
13. Vernon S. Umbilical transplantation upward and abdominal contouring in lipectomy. Am J Surg 1957;94(3):490–492
14. Callia WEP Contribuição para o estudo da correção cirúrgica do abdômen em pêndulo e globoso. Técnica original Tese de Doutoramento apresentada a Fac. Méd. USP --São Paulo,1965
15. Pitanguy I. Abdominal lipectomy: an approach to it through an analysis of 300 consecutive cases. Plast Reconstr Surg 1967;40:384–391
16. Regnault, P. The history of abdominal dermolipectomy. Aesth. Plast. Surg.1978; 2:113–123
17. Baroudi R, Moraes M. A "bicycle-handlebar" type of incision for primary and secondary abdominoplasty. Aesthetic Plast Surg [cited 2015 Aug 24] 1995;19(4):307–320
18. Vastine VL, Morgan RF, Williams GS, et al. Wound complications of abdominoplasty in obese patients. Ann Plast Surg 1999;42(1):34–39
19. Rogliani M, Silvi E, Labardi L, Maggiulli F, Cervelli V. Obese and nonobese patients: complications of abdominoplasty. Ann Plast Surg 2006;57(3):336–338
20. Grazer FM, Goldwyn RM. Abdominoplasty assessed by survey, with emphasis on complications. Plast Reconstr Surg 1977;59(4):513–517
21. Hester TR Jr, Baird W, Bostwick J III, Nahai F, Cukic J. Abdominoplasty combined with other major surgical procedures: safe or sorry? Plast Reconstr Surg 1989;83(6): 997–1004
22. Simon S, Thaller SR, Nathan N. Abdominoplasty combined with additional surgery: a safety issue. Aesthet Surg J 2006;26(4): 413–416

23. Matarasso A, Matarasso SL. When does your liposuction patient require an abdominoplasty? Dermatol Surg 1997;23(12): 1151–1160
24. Teimourian B, Gotkin RH. Contouring of the midtrunk in overweight patients. Aesthetic Plast Surg 1989;13(3):145–153
25. Cardoso de Castro C, Cupello AM, Cintra H. Limited incisions in abdominoplasty. Ann Plast Surg 1987;19(5):436–447
26. Dillerud E. Abdominoplasty combined with suction lipoplasty: a study of complications, revisions, and risk factors in 487 cases. Ann Plast Surg 1990;25(5):333–338, discussion 339–343
27. Le Louarn C. Partial subfascial abdominoplasty: our technique apropos of 36 cases. Ann Chir Plast Esthet 1992;37(5):547–552
28. Matarasso A. Abdominolipoplasty: a system of classification and treatment for combined abdominoplasty and suction-assisted lipectomy. Aesthetic Plast Surg 1991;15(2):111–121
29. Matarasso A. Liposuction as an adjunct to a full abdominoplasty. Plast Reconstr Surg 1995;95(5):829–836
30. Illouz YG. A new safe and aesthetic approach to suction abdominoplasty. Aesthetic Plast Surg 1992;16(3):237–245
31. Lockwood T. High-lateral-tension abdominoplasty with superficial fascial system suspension. Plast Reconstr Surg 1995; 96(3):603–615
32. Pollock H, Pollock T. Progressive tension sutures: a technique to reduce local complications in abdominoplasty. Plast Reconstr Surg 2000;105(7):2583–2586, discussion 2587–2588
33. Andrades P, Prado A, Danilla S, et al. Progressive tension sutures in the prevention of postabdominoplasty seroma: a prospective, randomized, double-blind clinical trial. Plast Reconstr Surg 2007;120(4):935–946, discussion 947–951
34. Baroudi R, Ferreira CA. Seroma: how to avoid it and how to treat it. Aesthet Surg J 1998;18(6):439–441
35. Le Louarn C, Pascal JF. High superior tension abdominoplasty. Aesthetic Plast Surg 2000;24(5):375–381
36. Rangaswamy M. Lipoabdominoplasty: a versatile and safe technique for abdominal contouring. Indian J Plast Surg 2008; 41(Suppl):S48–S55
37. Saldanha OR, Pinto EB, Matos WN Jr, Lucon RL, Magalhães F, Bello EM. Lipoabdominoplasty without undermining. Aesthet Surg J 2001;21(6):518–526
38. Saldanha OR, De Souza Pinto EB, Mattos WN Jr, et al. Lipoabdominoplasty with selective and safe undermining. Aesthetic Plast Surg 2003;27(4):322–327
39. Heller JB, Teng E, Knoll BI, Persing J. Outcome analysis of combined lipoabdominoplasty versus conventional abdominoplasty. Plast Reconstr Surg 2008;121(5):1821–1829
40. Brauman D, Capocci J. Liposuction abdominoplasty: an advanced body contouring technique. Plast Reconstr Surg 2009;124(5):1685–1695
41. Chopra J, Rani A, Rani A, Srivastava AK, Sharma PK. Re-evaluation of superficial fascia of anterior abdominal wall: a computed tomographic study. Surg Radiol Anat 2011;33(10):843–849
42. Costa-Ferreira A, Rodrigues-Pereira P, Rebelo M, Vásconez LO, Amarante J. Morphometric study (macroscopic and microscopic) of the lower abdominal wall. Plast Reconstr Surg 2014;134(6):1313–1322
43. Kumar P, Pandey AK, Kumar B, Aithal SK. Anatomical study of superficial fascia and localized fat deposits of abdomen. Indian J Plast Surg 2011;44(3):478–483
44. Lockwood T. Lower body lift with superficial fascial system suspension. Plast Reconstr Surg 1993;92(6):1112–1122, discussion 1123–1125
45. Bhave MA. Can drains be avoided in lipo-abdominoplasty? Indian J Plast Surg 2018;51(1):15–23
46. Friedman T, Coon D, Kanbour-Shakir A, Michaels JV, Rubin JP. Defining the lymphatic system of the anterior abdominal wall: an anatomical study. Plast Reconstr Surg 2015;135(4):1027–1032
47. Brauman D. Diastasis recti: clinical anatomy. Plast Reconstr Surg 2008;122(5):1564–1569
48. Blotta RM, Costa SDS, Trindade EN, Meurer L, Maciel-Trindade MR. Collagen I and III in women with diastasis recti. Clinics (São Paulo) 2018;73:e319
49. Schmidt M, Tinhofer I, Duscher D, Huemer GM. Perforasomes of the upper abdomen: an anatomical study. J Plast Reconstr Aesthet Surg 2014;67(1):42–47
50. Dillerud E, Hedén P. Circulation of blood and viability after blunt suction lipectomy in pig buttock flaps. Scand J Plast Reconstr Surg Hand Surg 1993;27(1):9–14
51. Blondeel PN, Derks D, Roche N, Van Landuyt KH, Monstrey SJ. The effect of ultrasound-assisted liposuction and conventional liposuction on the perforator vessels in the lower abdominal wall. Br J Plast Surg 2003;56(3):266–271
52. Graf R, de Araujo LRR, Rippel R, Neto LG, Pace DT, Cruz GA. Lipoabdominoplasty: liposuction with reduced undermining and traditional abdominal skin flap resection. Aesthetic Plast Surg 2006;30(1):1–8
53. Tourani SS, Taylor GI, Ashton MW. Scarpa fascia preservation in abdominoplasty: does it preserve the lymphatics? Plast Reconstr Surg 2015;136(2):258–262
54. Bozola AR, Psillakis JM. Abdominoplasty: a new concept and classification for treatment. Plast Reconstr Surg 1988;82(6): 983–993
55. Fernandes JW, Damin R, Holzmann MVN, Ribas GGO. Use of an algorithm in choosing abdominoplasty techniques. Rev Col Bras Cir 2018;45(2):e1394 (1–8)
56. Song AY, Jean RD, Hurwitz DJ, Fernstrom MH, Scott JA, Rubin JP. A classification of contour deformities after bariatric weight loss: the Pittsburgh Rating Scale. Plast Reconstr Surg 2005;116(5):1535–1544, discussion 1545–1546
57. Meyer PF, da Silva RMV, Oliveira G, et al. Effects of cryolipolysis on abdominal adiposity. Case Rep Dermatol Med 2016;2016:6052194
58. Sinno S, Shah S, Kenton K, et al. Assessing the safety and efficacy of combined abdominoplasty and gynecologic surgery. Ann Plast Surg 2011;67(3):272–274
59. Abhyankar SV, Rajguru AG, Patil PA. Anatomical localization of the umbilicus: an Indian study. Plast Reconstr Surg 2006; 117(4):1153–1157
60. Ziemann-Gimmel P, Goldfarb AA, Koppman J, Marema RT. Opioid-free total intravenous anaesthesia reduces postoperative nausea and vomiting in bariatric surgery beyond triple prophylaxis. Br J Anaesth 2014;112(5):906–911
61. Araco A, Pooney J, Araco F, Gravante G. Transversus abdominis plane block reduces the analgesic requirements after abdominoplasty with flank liposuction. Ann Plast Surg 2010; 65(4):385–388
62. Klein JA. Tumescent technique for regional anesthesia permits lidocaine doses of 35 mg/kg for liposuction. J Dermatol Surg Oncol 1990;16(3):248–263
63. Davidson SP, Venturi ML, Attinger CE, Baker SB, Spear SL. Prevention of venous thromboembolism in the plastic surgery patient. Plast Reconstr Surg 2004;114: 43e -51e
64. Pannucci CJ, Bailey SH, Dreszer G, et al. Validation of the Caprini risk assessment model in plastic and reconstructive surgery patients. J Am Coll Surg 2011;212(1):105–112
65. Failey CL, Vemula R, Borah GL, Hsia HC. Intraoperative use of bupivacaine for tumescent liposuction: the Robert Wood

Johnson experience. Plast Reconstr Surg 2009;124(4):1304–1311

66. Rubin RH. Surgical wound infection: epidemiology, pathogenesis, diagnosis and management. BMC Infect Dis 2006;6:171–171
67. Skillman JM, Venus MR, Nightingale P, Titley OG, Park A. Ligating perforators in abdominoplasty reduces the risk of seroma. Aesthetic Plast Surg 2014;38(2):446–450
68. Veríssimo P, Nahas FX, Barbosa MVJ, de Carvalho Gomes HF, Ferreira LM. Is it possible to repair diastasis recti and shorten the aponeurosis at the same time? Aesthetic Plast Surg 2014;38(2):379–386
69. Nahai FR. Anatomic considerations in abdominoplasty. Clin Plast Surg 2010;37(3):407–414
70. Nahas FX, Ferreira LM, Ely PB, Ghelfond C. Rectus diastasis corrected with absorbable suture: a long-term evaluation. Aesthetic Plast Surg 2011;35(1):43–48
71. Chahar P, Cummings KC III. Liposomal bupivacaine: a review of a new bupivacaine formulation. J Pain Res 2012;5:257–264
72. Le Louarn C, Pascal JF. The high-superior-tension technique: evolution of lipoabdominoplasty. Aesthetic Plast Surg 2010;34(6):773–781
73. Elbaz JS, Flageul G, Olivier-Masveyraud F. "Classical" abdominoplasty. Ann Chir Plast Esthet 1999;44(4):443–461
74. Zukowski ML, Ash K, Spencer D, Malanoski M, Moore G. Endoscopic intracorporal abdominoplasty: a review of 85 cases. Plast Reconstr Surg 1998;102(2):516–527
75. Eaves FF III, Nahai F, Bostwick J III. Endoscopic abdominoplasty and endoscopically assisted miniabdominoplasty. Clin Plast Surg 1996;23(4):599–616, discussion 617
76. Planas J. The "vest over pants" abdominoplasty. Plast Reconstr Surg 1978;61(5):694–700
77. Planas J, Bisbal J, del Cacho C, Palacin JM. Further advantages of the "vest over pants" abdominoplasty. Aesthetic Plast Surg 1988;12(3):123–127
78. Bracaglia R, D'Ettorre M, Gentileschi S, Tambasco D. "Vest over pants" abdominoplasty in post-bariatric patients. Aesthetic Plast Surg 2012;36(1):23–27
79. Rebello C, Franco T. Abdominoplastia por incisão submamária. Rev Bras Cir 1972;62:249–252
80. Rebello C, Franco T. Abdominoplasty through a submammary incision. Int Surg 1977;62(9):462–463
81. Yacoub C, Baroudi R, Yacoub M. Extended reverse abdominoplasty. Rev Bras Cir Plást 2012;27(2):328–332
82. Matos WN Jr, Ribeiro RC, Marujo RA, da Rocha RP, da Silva Ribeiro SM, Carrillo Jiminez FV. Classification for indications of lipoabdominoplasty and its variations. Aesthet Surg J 2006;26(4):417–431
83. Agha-Mohammadi S, Hurwitz DJ. Management of upper abdominal laxity after massive weight loss: reverse abdominoplasty and inframammary fold reconstruction. Aesthetic Plast Surg 2010;34(2):226–231
84. Pechter EA. Instant identification of redundant tissue in abdominoplasty with a marking grid. Aesthet Surg J 2010; 30(4):571–578
85. Vidal P, Berner JE, Will PA. Managing complications in abdominoplasty: a literature review. Arch Plast Surg 2017; 44(5):457–468
86. Zuelzer HB, Ratliff CR, Drake DB. Complications of abdominal contouring surgery in obese patients: current status. Ann Plast Surg 2010;64(5):598–604
87. Andrades P, Prado A. Composition of postabdominoplasty seroma. Aesthetic Plast Surg 2007;31(5):514–518
88. Rohrich RJ, Cho M-J. The role of tranexamic acid in plastic surgery: review and technical considerations. Plast Reconstr Surg 2018;141(2):507–515
89. Shestak KC. Marriage abdominoplasty expands the mini-abdominoplasty concept. Plast Reconstr Surg 1999;103(3): 1020–1031, discussion 1032–1035
90. Avelar JM. Abdominoplasty without panniculus undermining and resection: analysis and 3-year follow-up of 97 consecutive cases. Aesthet Surg J 2002;22(1):16–25
91. Samdal F, Amland PF, Sandsmark M, Hall C, Aasen AO. Suction-assisted lipectomy does not increase the risk of random flap necrosis in a randomized study in pigs. Aesthetic Plast Surg 1995;19(6):549–553
92. Carpaneda CA. Postliposuction histologic alterations of adipose tissue. Aesthetic Plast Surg 1996;20(3):207–211
93. Hoyos A, Perez ME, Guarin DE, Montenegro A. A report of 736 high-definition lipoabdominoplasties performed in conjunction with circumferential VASER liposuction. Plast Reconstr Surg 2018;142(3):662–675
94. Toledo LS, Mauad R. Complications of body sculpture: prevention and treatment. Clin Plast Surg 2006;33(1):1–11, v
95. Thomas WO III, Parry SW, Rodning CB. Ventral/incisional abdominal herniorhaphy by fascial partition/release. Plast Reconstr Surg 1993;91(6):1080–1086
96. DiBello JN Jr, Moore JH Jr. Sliding myofascial flap of the rectus abdominus muscles for the closure of recurrent ventral hernias. Plast Reconstr Surg 1996;98(3):464–469
97. Kushimoto S, Yamamoto Y, Aiboshi J, et al. Usefulness of the bilateral anterior rectus abdominis sheath turnover flap method for early fascial closure in patients requiring open abdominal management. World J Surg 2007;31(1):2–8, discussion 9–10
98. Ramirez OM, Ruas E, Dellon AL. "Components separation" method for closure of abdominal-wall defects: an anatomic and clinical study. Plast Reconstr Surg 1990;86(3):519–526
99. Heller L, McNichols CH, Ramirez OM. Component separations. Semin Plast Surg 2012;26(1):25–28
100. Heller L, Chike-Obi C, Xue AS. Abdominal wall reconstruction with mesh and components separation. Semin Plast Surg 2012;26(1):29–35
101. Kaya B. Bilateral anterior rectus sheath turnover flaps. J Clin Anal Med 2013;4:506–508
102. Al-Basti HB, El-Khatib HA, Taha A, Sattar HA, Bener A. Intraabdominal pressure after full abdominoplasty in obese multiparous patients. Plast Reconstr Surg 2004;113(7):2145–2150, discussion 2151–2155
103. Bruekers SE, van der Lei B, Tan TL, Luijendijk RW, Stevens HPJD. "Scarless" umbilicoplasty: a new umbilicoplasty technique and a review of the English language literature. Ann Plast Surg 2009;63(1):15–20
104. Ngaage LM, Kokosis G, Kachniarz B, et al. A two-step technique for neo-umbilicoplasty in the abdominal reconstructive population. Plast Reconstr Surg Glob Open 2019;7(7):e2341

Introduction

Obesity leads to a lowered body image. However, a person who has had massive weight loss (MWL) also begins to look very different from what is considered normal. While one may receive accolades for achieving the weight loss, albeit sometimes with help from bariatric surgery, the joy gets somewhat dimmed by the final appearance without ones clothes. Often, skin hangs down in soft, loose folds giving one a sad, dysmorphic look. Add to this the fact that one may benefit from further weight loss if these skin folds are removed. Further, these skin folds make personal hygiene a difficult proposition, leading to fungal and bacterial infections under them, and we have a strong case for removing these.

Massive weight loss is defined as the loss of greater than 100 pounds or 100% above the person's ideal body weight. Some studies[1,2] suggest that bariatric surgery is the only way to produce long-term and stable weight loss. Ghrelin, also known as hunger hormone, stimulates appetite. Cummings et al[3] have shown plasma Ghrelin levels to fall following bariatric surgery, but rise following diet-induced weight loss. Knuth et al[4] compared weight loss in bariatric surgery patients and diet/exercise group. Both groups lost similar amount of weight but the resting metabolic rate was lower in the diet/exercise group. All these studies indicate that diet/exercise group may regain some of the lost weight.

However, a subset of post–bariatric surgery patients, even after massive weight loss do not reach their target weight and may plateau out in the obese or overweight range. In the first instance, a consult with the bariatric surgeon should be arranged. The underlying cause may be anatomical (stretching of gastric pouch, loosening of gastric band, etc.) or behavioral (eating disorder, etc.). Even after ruling out or correcting these issues, patients may still not be able to reach their target weight. They may still have redundant folds of skin which hamper their mobility and personal hygiene. Such patients must not be denied the benefit of body contouring surgery.

Most of the weight loss is in fat. However, the patient is usually left with a large amount of excess skin. The need to remove this excess skin is not only for aesthetic benefit, but also due to health risks. The risk of recurrent skin infections (Intertrigo) and skin breakdown—particularly under the folds of the breasts or abdomen—makes it a problem that is typically covered by insurance companies. The presence of a large pannus prevents patients from losing further weight and having active lifestyles. To address these problems, patients are first evaluated, preferably, when they have reached their plateau of weight loss. Body contouring surgery is planned with patients who are psychologically stable and willing to accept staged operations to achieve the expected goals.

MWL patients have global laxity. Although total body lift in one stage has been described, it is an exception rather than the rule. It is a massive operation that requires a dedicated team, where all team members are well versed with their roles in the surgery. The most common course of action is to do a multistage procedure to correct the global laxity. In this scenario, the area which has to be tackled first becomes an important issue. This decision has to be taken in concert with the patient, depending on the patient's ideal body image.

Body image is defined as a person's feelings of the *aesthetics* or *sexual attractiveness* of their own body, which may be forced onto them by their peers, *social media, or other external sources*. With both ends of the weight spectrum leading to a lowered body image, we need to consider body contouring surgery seriously to help those that might suffer, often quietly, from this malady.

Indications

Surgical management is indicated to get rid of the excessive folds of skin and underlying fat so that the appearance of the patient without clothes resembles the normal morphology, albeit with scars. It is also aimed at preventing repeated skin infections under these folds (**Fig. 26.1**). Most patients of MWL suffer repeated attacks of fungal skin infections under the skin folds. Often, these are compounded by secondary bacterial infection and are resistant to the relevant medications.

It helps further the weight loss already achieved, either by lifestyle changes or bariatric surgery. The redundant skin folds could weigh as much as 8 to 10 kilograms. Their removal, therefore, substantially improves the final weight loss. Sometimes, the surgery is precipitated by physical impediment or issues of personal hygiene caused by the excess skin folds.

It helps improve the patient's body image. These patients have already for years carried around emotional baggage in addition to the excess weight. Even after weight loss, the body still looks quite different from the normal when the clothes are taken off. This deviation from the normal continues to trouble them in spite of the MWL. The patient must be willing to accept staged operations and the resultant scars to achieve the expected goals.

Patient Selection

Patients with MWL often seek remedial measures to get rid of the redundant folds of skin in extremity and truncal areas. However female patients, in addition, are concerned about the deflation and volume loss in areas such as breast and buttock region. Older patients may also experience skin laxity in the facial and neck region. The Pittsburgh Rating Scale[5] (**Table 26.1**) for body contouring after MWL helps to

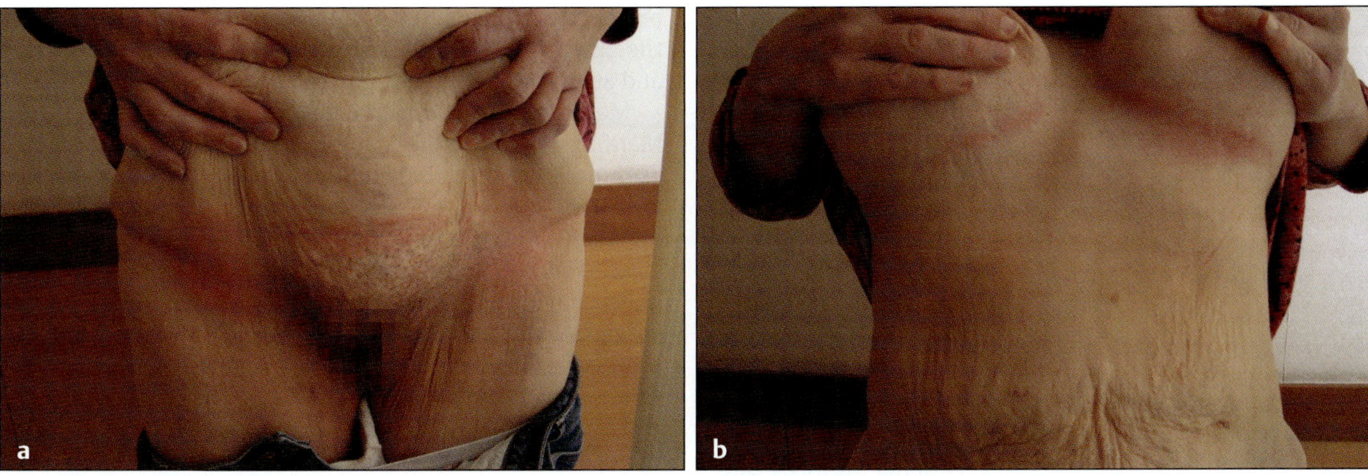

Fig. 26.1 (a, b) Skin infection under skin folds in massive weight loss (MWL) patient.

Table 26.1 Pittsburgh rating scale

Area	Scale	Preferred procedure
Arms	0: Normal	None
	1: Adiposity with good skin tone	UAL and SAL
	2: Loose, hanging skin without sever adiposity	Brachioplasty
	3: Loose, hanging skin with severe adiposity	Brachioplasty+UAL and/or SAL
Breasts	0: Normal	None
	1: Ptosis grade I/II or severe macromastia	Traditional mastopexy, reduction, or augmentation techniques
	2: Ptosis grade III or moderate volume loss or constricted breast	Traditional mastopexy + augmentation
	3: Severe lateral roll and/or severe volume loss with loose skin	Parenchymal reshaping techniques with dermal suspension, consider autoaugmentation
Back	0: Normal	None
	1: Single fat roll or adiposity	UAL and/or SAL
	2: Multiple skin and fat rolls	Excisional lifting procedures
	3: Ptosis of rolls	Excisional lifting procedures

Abbreviations: UAL, ultrasonic-assisted liposuction; SAL, suction-assisted liposuction.
Source: Adapted from Song et al 2006.[5]

classify and grade the degree of deformity and makes suggestions for the possible surgical route to be followed.

The timing of intervention for contouring surgery in MWL patients is critical. Patients often reach their target weight within 2 years of bariatric surgery. Psychological assessment should be part of initial consultation of MWL patients seeking body contouring surgery.[6] They should be asked about the expectations and motivations for body contouring surgery, their body image, and any psychiatric history. Some patients have unrealistic expectations that the body contouring surgery will make their appearance perfect like a person who has had no weight issues before. This difference between expectations and reality should be emphasized and reinforced to the patient so that they understand the result will be far from perfect, in addition to the long scars and need for multistage procedures. Unrealistic motivation (e.g., restoration of relationships) following contouring surgery should be addressed during the initial consultation. Mood swings, feeling of hopelessness, or suicidal thoughts are pointers to underlying psychiatric disorder. In case of doubt, one must take clearance from mental health professionals before embarking on any surgery in patients.

Nutritional deficiencies should be ruled out in these patients. Those achieving MWL through bariatric surgery or by excessive "fad" dieting may have severe vitamin and mineral deficiencies that could compromise wound healing. Intertriginous areas should be inspected for fungal infection and treated with local as well as systemic antifungals and antibiotics before surgery to prevent wound dehiscence.

Contraindications

Medical Comorbidities

Diabetes mellitus, hypertension, heart disease, etc., are contraindications if they are uncontrolled. However, considering that morbidly obese patients often suffer from these conditions, they should not get in the way of body contouring surgery when they are adequately treated and controlled.

Severe Psychological Disorders

Body contouring procedures will always leave the patients with permanent scars, which in our skin types can sometimes be more than just noticeable. Patients MUST be adequately counseled about their extent and location. Failure to do this could set off disillusionment, sometimes with legal implications. Patients who are not willing to accept these scars cannot be taken up for body contouring procedures.

General Counseling Tips

Surgery should be done at a minimum of 1 year after bariatric surgery or 6 months after stabilization of weight loss. The patient should be warned that one may still have residual skin laxity after the surgery. This is because the skin expansion occurs in all directions/vectors of stretch are in all 360 degrees when the patient is obese, whereas most body contouring procedures would trim the laxity only in one dimension.

Choice of surgical procedure is made depending upon the presenting deformity, and no single procedure can be standardized for every patient. The Pittsburgh Weight Loss Deformity Scale[5] provides guidelines as to which procedures may be adopted depending upon the grade of the deformity. However, this is only indicative and cannot be treated as the final word.

Patients should be counseled extensively about the scars that will be left after surgery to prevent disillusionment that could sometimes terminate in litigation. Certain preoperative, intraoperative, and postoperative steps are common for all types of contouring surgery. Where differences exist, they are highlighted in the relevant section.

Preparation of the Patient

Preoperative

Patients' photographs should be taken well in advance of the surgery. Ideally, the patients' photographs should be taken with and without markings. These photographs can be then seen together with the patient. This helps both the surgeon and the patient to see the deformity from a 360-degree perspective. The surgeon can also point out to the patient the amount of excision being planned, the location of scar, and any preexisting asymmetry.

Marking is done with the patient in the upright position. Markings should preferably be made the previous evening as this allows for a final counseling as regard the placement of the scars.

Wash and scrub the operative area twice with antiseptic soapy solution (preferably with povidone-iodine content) on the day prior to surgery and once on the morning of the surgery. Antibiotic cover should be instituted from the day prior to surgery.

Intraoperative

Post-MWL contouring is a lengthy surgery. This necessitates certain precautions to reduce the incidence of adverse events. Hypothermia protocol should be followed to maintain the core body temperature above 35°C. This is done by using a warm prep solution, keeping the ambient temperature at 24°C, using warm intravenous fluid and the use of a body warmer. Hypothermia is known to increase the incidence of complications like cardiac morbidity[7] and surgical site infection.[8]

Positioning of the Patient

Protecting pressure points is paramount in a lengthy surgery. In supine position, a pillow should be kept under the knee to reduce the lumbar lordosis and soft gel pads should be kept under the ankle, elbow, and sacral region. In the lateral decubitus a rolled towel is kept in the dependent axillae to protect the neurovascular structure. The dependent leg is kept flexed and the other leg is kept straight with a pillow in between. In the prone position, with proper pillow placement the abdominal area should be kept free to allow diaphragmatic breathing (**Fig. 26.2**).

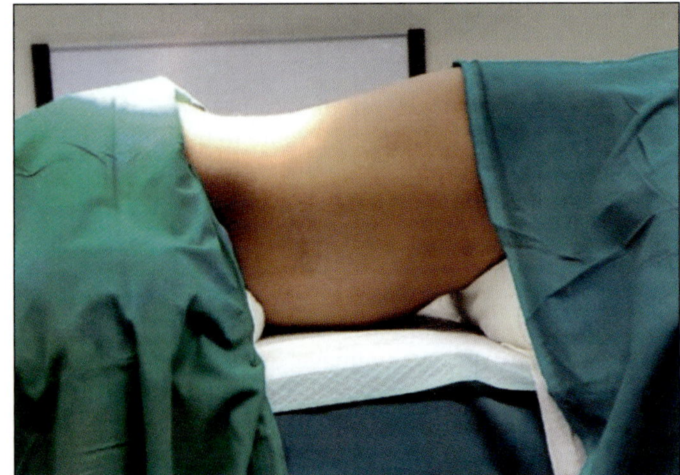

Fig. 26.2 Pillow placement to allow diaphragmatic breathing.

Tailor Tacking

Measure twice and cut once! The final excision is carried out only after confirmation by tailor tacking. This is done for all elliptical excisions like abdominoplasty, thigh plasty, and brachioplasty. Tailor tacking is done by cutting the undermined flap along the reference line drawn preoperatively. Then the undermined flap is approximated to the corresponding point on the opposite flap with the help of a towel clip. This is done at various points along the flap. When applying the towel clip, ensure that it does not produce a constriction band or indentation as this is a sign of excessive tension. It will lead to a scalloped appearance along the closure. Once appropriate tension has been determined then the points along the towel clip are marked to get the final excision margin.

Infiltration

Areas of liposuction and excision are infiltrated as the first step. The composition of infiltration solution is as in **Table 26.2**.

Adrenaline provides profound vasoconstriction, thereby reducing the blood loss and also slowing down the absorption of lidocaine. The safe dose of lidocaine in tumescent infiltration is 35 mg/kg because systemic absorption is slow and occurs over 18 to 36 hours.[9] For this reason, the addition of hyaluronidase is not advisable as it increases the rate of absorption of lidocaine. Lidocaine has an acidic pH which can cause burning paresthesia in the postoperative phase. This is prevented by adding soda bicarbonate in the tumescent solution.

On table, scrub the area with povidone-iodine scrub solution and leave the solution on the patient's skin while the surgeon goes to wash up for surgery. Stockings and a sequential compression device are placed on both the legs for deep vein thrombosis (DVT) prophylaxis. A warming blanket is placed on the upper torso to maintain the core temperature.

Postoperative

There is a uniform similarity in the postoperative management of patients, even though they may have been operated for different body parts. This protocol can safely be followed with minor variations from patient to patient, and body part to body part.

The first dressing change is done at 48 hours, assuming that there is no reason to do it earlier, (e.g., blood soakage).

Table 26.2 Composition of infiltration solution

Normal saline 0.9%	1000 mL
Adrenaline (1:1000)	1 mL (1 mg)
Lidocaine	250 mg
Soda bicarbonate (8.4%)	10 mL

The suture line is swabbed with povidone-iodine and a lighter dressing is re-applied. Wound is inspected again at 48 hours. If there has been no untoward incident, the patient can be allowed to shower over the operated area, and fitted with a corset, which should then be worn continuously (22/24 hours) for a period of 3 to 6 months.

Procedures

The subject of upper body contouring after MWL basically consists of three main areas to be considered:

- The arms, brachioplasty.
- The breasts, in males and in females, as the two present very different problems.
- The posterior upper back, the bra-line back lift.

Brachioplasty

The skin redundancy may be observed only in the proximal ½ of arm, the entire arm extending from axilla to elbow, or the entire arm along with lateral chest wall simulating a bat wing appearance, Any of these can be associated with varying amounts of lipodystrophy.

Patients may be categorized into three subsets: The first group of patients is those with substantial weight loss wherein only a thin layer of skin and underlying fat remains (**Fig. 26.3**). These are the most ideal candidates for the procedure.

The second group of patients presents with a large amount of persistent subcutaneous fat in their arms following MWL (**Fig. 26.4**). These patients should be treated in a staged fashion with aggressive liposuction of the upper arms as the first procedure, followed by an excisional procedure, as a second stage at a later date.

The third group of patients presents with an intermediate amount of subcutaneous tissue (**Fig. 26.5**). These patients may choose between undergoing excisional brachioplasty with a less than ideal result and a staged procedure with liposuction first.

There are conflicting views on whether liposuction should be combined with brachioplasty in cases with moderate lipodystrophy. The author prefers a combined approach as

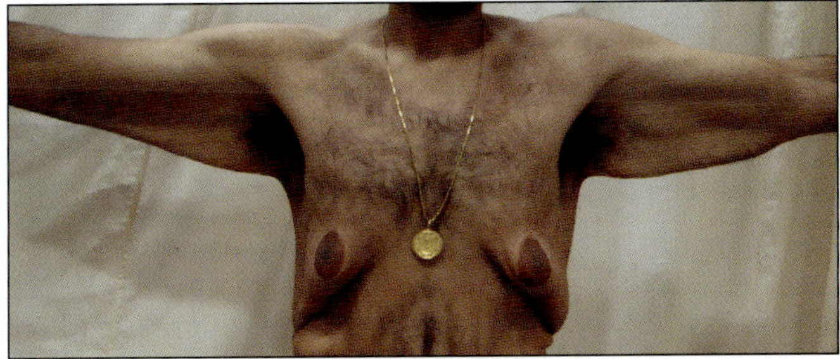

Fig. 26.3 Massive weight loss (MWL) patient displaying thin layer of underlying fat and substantial skin laxity.

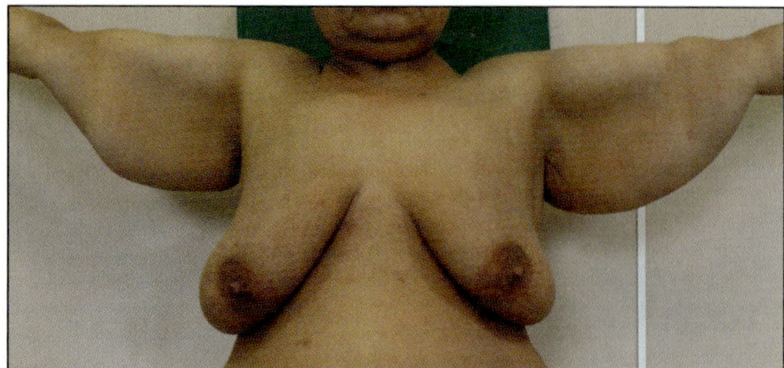

Fig. 26.4 Massive weight loss (MWL) patient displaying skin laxity but with large amount of residual subcutaneous fat.

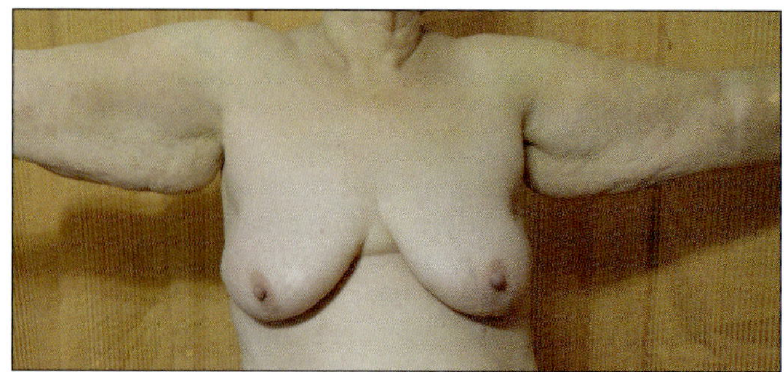

Fig. 26.5 Massive weight loss (MWL) patient displaying intermediate amount of subcutaneous tissue.

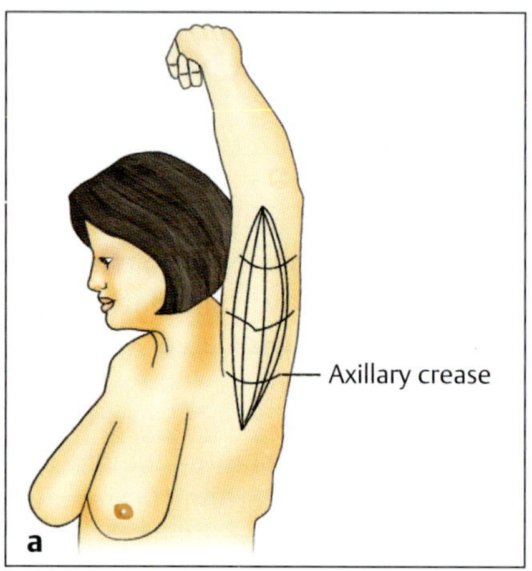

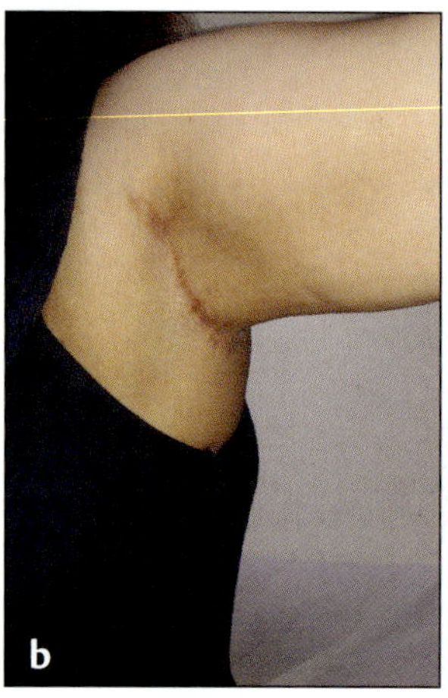

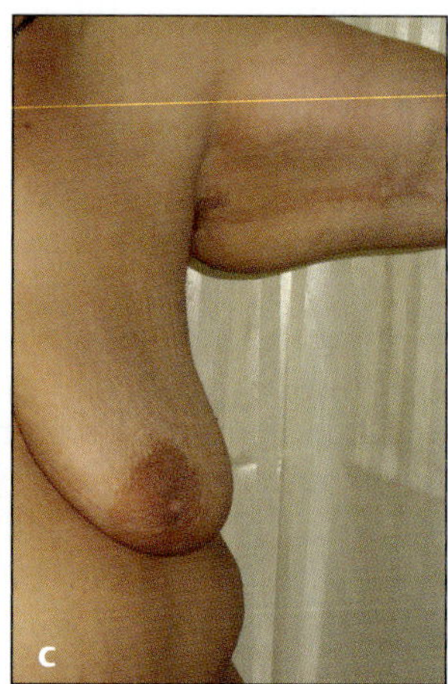

Fig 26.6 **(a)** "Double Ellipse" marking technique (Adapted from Al Aly et al 2016[11]). **(b)** Limited Scar brachioplasty. **(c)** Final scar in bicipital groove.

opposed to a staged protocol, (i.e., a not so aggressive liposuction first, followed by a skin excision at the same sitting). This has the obvious advantage of reducing the cost and recovery time, which is an important consideration among our patients. Furthermore, in a staged protocol, adhesions formed in the subcutaneous tissue following liposuction might impede tissue mobility and the amount of skin excision. Combining liposuction with brachioplasty does not significantly increase the complication or revision rate compared to that of a brachioplasty alone.[10] However, this is in conflict with the author's experience. Aggressive liposuction followed by skin excision at the same sitting does definitely carry a greater risk of wound dehiscence.

Patient selection must be judicious, with enough laxity to justify a scar from elbow to axilla or longer. It is advisable to show them pictures of previously operated patients so that they are aware of the length of the scars, the scar position, and the length of time that it will take the scars to mature.

Procedures Available

Procedures have been described by various authors, who indicate individual preferences for placement of the final scars. Al Aly describes a "Double Ellipse" marking technique[11] (**Fig. 26.6a**) that places the final scar close to the posterior border of the arm. Lawrence Reed describes a "Limited Scar Brachioplasty"[12] which is suitable for minor forms of the deformity. This places the scar in the axillary fold, thus making it invisible when the arms are held by the side (**Fig. 26.6b**). Susan Downey describes a technique that places the scar in the bicipital groove[13] (**Fig. 26.6c**). Each of these techniques has its advantages and disadvantages and can be carefully used in varying forms of the deformity.

- Liposuction—for patients with minimal skin laxity.
- Liposuction + skin excision—for patients with skin laxity and fat excess.
- Skin excision alone—for patients with no fat, only loose skin.

Brachioplasty: Author's Preferred Technique

Method

The patient is asked to hold the arm at 90 degrees to the torso with the elbow also at 90 degrees. The most distal and the most proximal points of the ellipse that form the deformity are marked. Often, the flap will be found to extend onto the lateral chest wall, in which case the incision is extended onto the chest wall, incorporating a Z-plasty at the level of the axilla. A gentle upward curve is marked on the medial aspect of the arm, joining these two points.

The flap of skin forming the excess is folded on itself medially, and a rough assessment is made to ensure that the marked curve does indeed correspond to the folded flap margin. It is safer to err on the side of lesser rather than more skin excision, (i.e., the marked curve is closer to, even hidden by, the margin of the folded flap).

Once this has been ascertained, the marked skin incision is infiltrated with the aforementioned mixture of infiltrate. Having waited sufficiently for the adrenaline to take effect, about 4 to 5 minutes, the skin is incised and the flap is raised at the level of the subcutaneous fat, above the fascia. The author prefers to use blunt dissection interspersed with sharp dissection, but not diathermy dissection as it compromises circulation and increases the incidence of seroma formation.

It is not possible to save all the cutaneous nerves that one encounters, occasionally causing some sensory loss in the medial aspects of the arm and forearm. This is rarely disabling, but should be stressed upon in the preoperative counseling.

Tailor tacking is done before excision to ensure that the arm looks proportionate to the rest of the body and that there are no bands of constriction produced by excessive skin excision at any point along the length of the incision. This is also done to ensure reasonable bilateral symmetry.

The cut margin having been maximally lifted off the deeper tissues is then overlapped on the marked incision and the skin and fat excess is excised. Every effort is made to ensure that no large potential spaces are created due to excessive undermining that could collect hematomas later.

A running stitch of 3–0 absorbable material is used to close the subcutaneous tissue. A running stitch of 4–0 absorbable material is used to make a subdermal closure. A running stitch of the same material is used to make a subcuticular closure of the skin, followed by sterile paper tapes to hold the skin edges together. A soft dressing with cotton rolls is used to lightly compress the operated area (**Fig. 26.7**).

The author believes that it is risky to combine extensive liposuction with skin excision. In addition, it is important that the patient accepts the extent and location of the scar, as well as the possibility of altered sensations on the medial aspect of the arms and forearms. It is better to leave some extra tissue than compromise shape or face serious complications.

Breast Surgery in Males

Skin laxity constitutes the most important component in male breast surgery after MWL. In most cases it is more important than the glandular element. While it is possible for the male patient to “fill” the arm and thigh skin laxity by building up muscles in that area, the chest skin droop is almost impossible to hide.

In addition, the diameter of the nipple-areola complex is often too large for the patient’s newly acquired physique. Evidently, this issue also needs to be addressed to give a pleasing final result. In patients who have had suboptimal weight loss, an additional fold of fat and skin may extend from the anterior chest wall toward the axilla, constituting an additional aspect that requires treatment.

Procedures

Depending upon each individual case, a combination of the following procedures may be required to achieve an optimal final result.

Excision through a conventional lower half areolar incision (Webster)—for minor lipoglandular excess. The author modifies this approach by taking a zigzag incision instead of a linear one.

Circumareolar incision[14] for moderate-to-severe lipoglandular excess, in cases where reduction of the areolar diameter is desirable. A modification of this method is the commonest approach used by the author.

Other options are reduction mammoplasty technique for massive lipoglandular excess and full-thickness grafting of the nipple-areola complex in massive skin ptosis (**Fig. 26.8a, b**).

- “Boomerang” technique for correction of breast deformity after MWL in males (**Fig. 26.8c**).

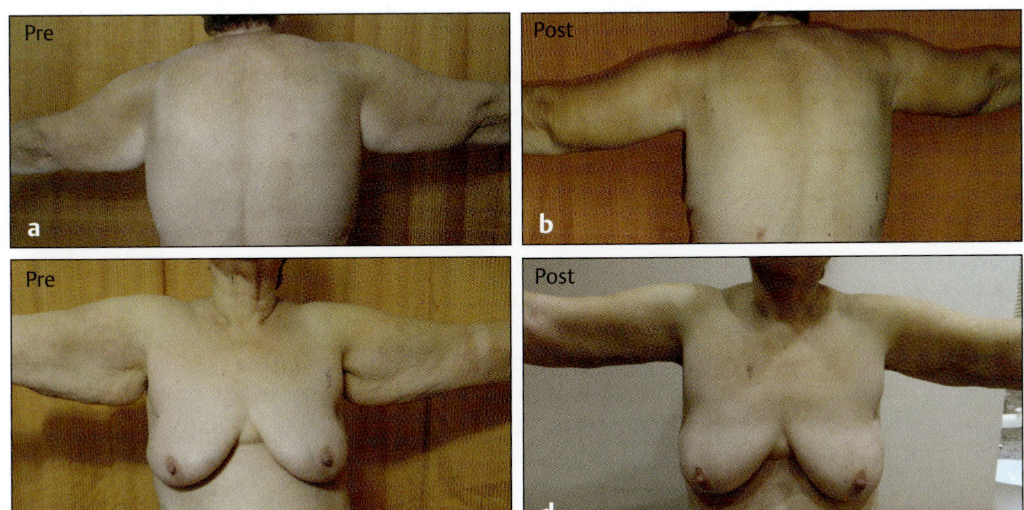

Fig. 26.7 Pre- and postoperative pictures of a brachioplasty patient using the author’s technique. **(a)** Preop posterior view, **(b)** postop posterior view, **(c)** preop anterior view, **(d)** postop anterior view.

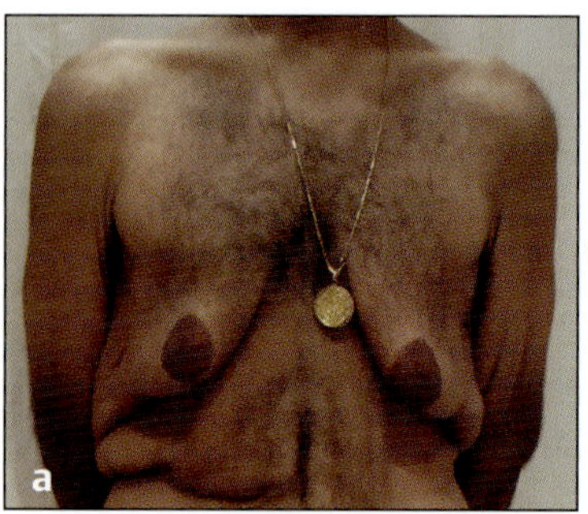

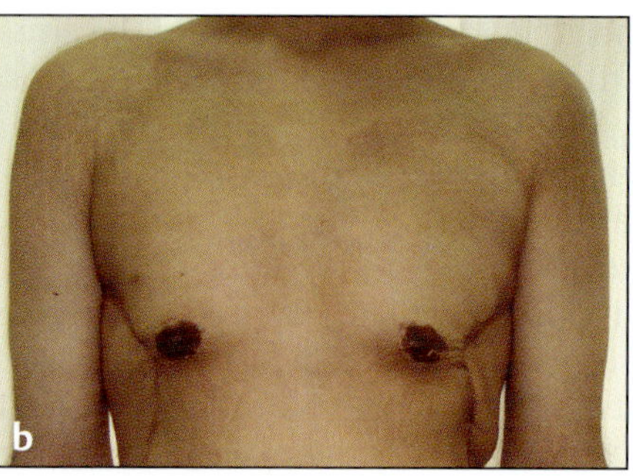

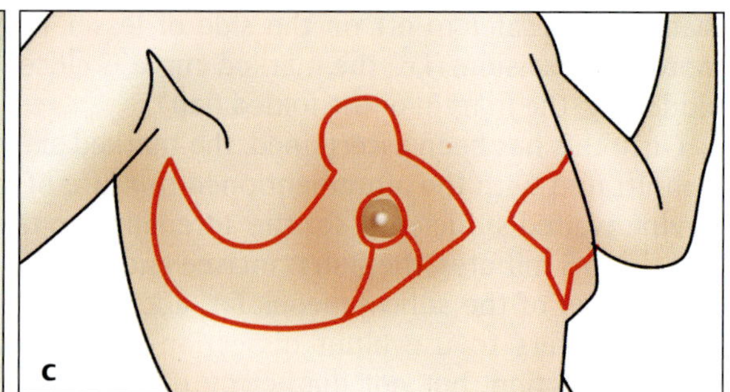

Fig. 26.8 **(a, b)** Pre- and postoperative pictures for patient treated with full-thickness grafting of the nipple-areola complex in massive skin ptosis. **(c)** Markings for "Boomerang" technique of gynecomastia correction. (Source: Mendeley.com.)

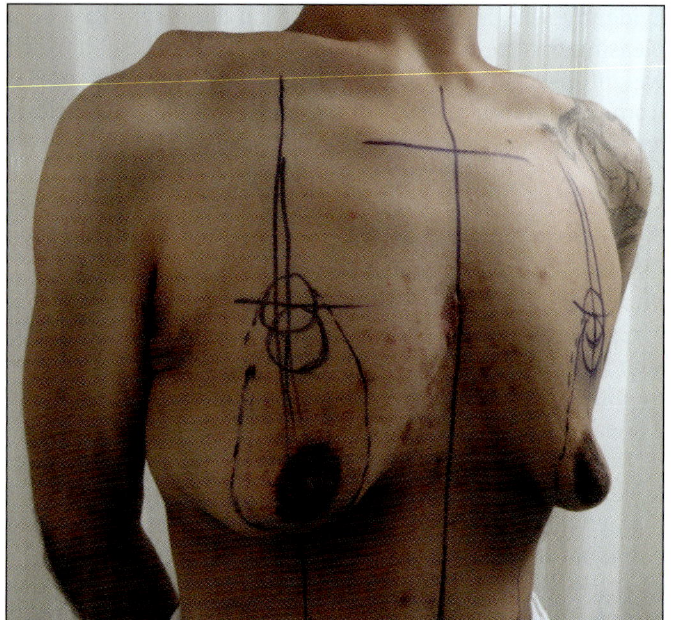

Fig. 26.9 Markings for authors' preferred technique for corrective breast surgery in males following massive weight loss.

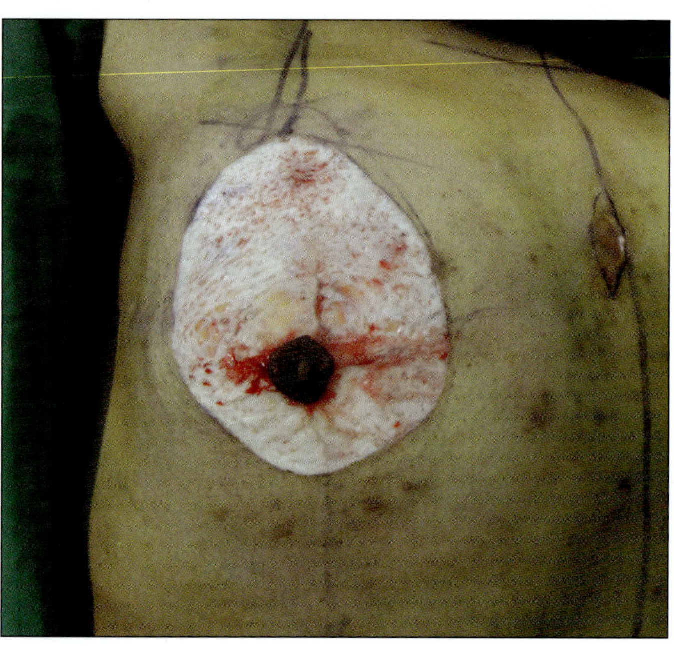

Fig. 26.10 De-epithelialization of ovoid area around the nipple-areolar complex (NAC) to eliminate skin excess.

- Liposuction, generally as an adjunct to reduce fat from the subaxillary region.

Markings are made in the upright position. The mammary meridian is marked. The nipple is marked on the chest meridian on each side in the fourth intercostal space, checking to make sure that this point is approximately at the junction of the upper two-thirds and lower third of the upper arm. A circle of circumference 4 cm is drawn around the nipple to represent the intended areolar position. A similar circle is drawn on the face of the existing nipple-areola complex. An ovoid marking is then made from the top of the upper circle to the bottom of the existing nipple-areola complex, to include all the darker pigmented skin of the native nipple-areola complex (**Fig. 26.9**).

A vertical meridian line is drawn from the lighter skin right across the native nipple-areola complex and extended in the inferior direction to help orientate the nipple-areola complex after de-epithelialization. A similar line is also drawn from lateral to medial for the same purpose.

Without making any incisions, the circle marked on the nipple-areola complex is physically pulled upward to judge whether the skin laxity will allow it to be relocated to its new position. If this is possible, a partial thickness incision is made along the circumference of the ovoid marking, taking care not to make it a full-thickness incision at any point. The entire area within the ovoid is de-epithelized, except the circle of nipple-areola skin on the existing complex (**Fig. 26.10**).

A small segment of the circumference at the lowest part of the incision is then deepened vertically down to the pectoral fascia, and a plane is dissected bluntly to create the submammary space. Another plane is then created in the subcutaneous plane within the glandular tissue, leaving behind at least 1.5 to 2 cm of tissue under the skin. Special care is taken to preserve tissue under the nipple to ensure that it does not become concave on completion of surgery. The entire parenchymal tissue mass between the subcutaneous and subglandular incisions, i.e., the two planes that have been developed, is excised. If required, liposuction is done in the subaxillary area to get rid of fat.

After ensuring hemostasis, and after inserting suction drains, the nipple areolar complex is sutured to its new intended location, starting by fixing it at 3, 6, 9, and 12 o'clock positions first to maintain its orientation. The outer circumference is then sutured to the circumference of the existing nipple-areola complex, "stealing" with every bite to get the minimum amount of wrinkling on the suture line. The author prefers to use a running subcuticular stitch of 4–0 absorbable material. A compressive dressing is placed to prevent hematoma formation. Results in less severe cases using the above technique have been shown in **Fig. 26.11**.

Specific Complications

The greater the laxity of skin that is present, the larger would be the ovoid area that has to be de-epithelized, and hence, the greater would be the wrinkling at the suture line. While this may look alarmingly disfiguring initially, it generally "settles down" over a period of 6 to 12 months if a compression garment has been used (**Fig. 26.12**). The patient, however, must be counseled preoperatively regarding this waiting period.

Another rare possibility is nipple necrosis. To prevent this, the dermal pedicle bearing the native nipple-areola complex should be kept sufficiently thick.

Skin laxity is the most important element that needs to be addressed in male breast surgical correction following MWL. The patient must be warned of the wrinkling that is likely to occur at the circumareolar suture line in cases operated by the de-epithelialization technique that has been described. He should be reassured that in the event of it turning out to be very noticeable, a remedial procedure is possible. In very severe cases, one may be left with no choice but to use the nipple-areolar skin as a full-thickness graft. In these cases, it is necessary to warn the patients about sensory loss on the nipple and areola.

Breast Surgery in Females

Since MWL generally occurs at the expense of body fat, and since the breast consists predominantly of fat, it is evident that the breast will lose shape and size in such patients.

Procedures

The procedure that is most suitable for a given patient depends upon the degree of mammoptosis as well as the surgeon's comfort with the procedure that he normally utilizes.

- Breast augmentation with implants can be done for cases with minor droop, and volume loss.
- Mastopexy with or without implants is preferred in patients with moderate droop, with or without volume loss (**Fig. 26.13**).
- Reduction mammoplasty is reserved for patients with mammoptosis who still retain a substantial breast volume.

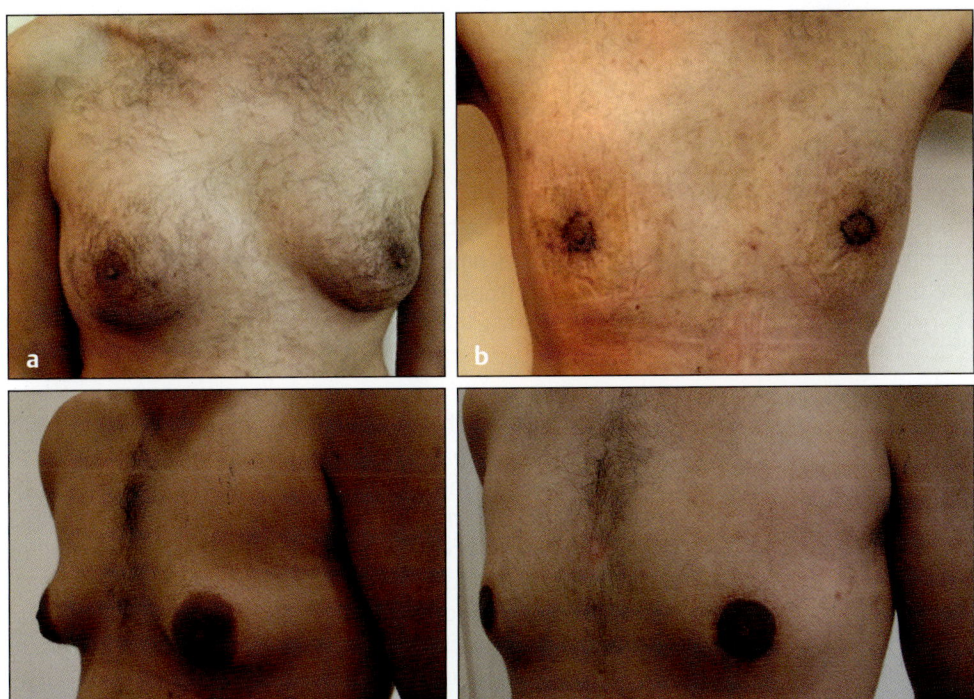

Fig. 26.11 **(a, b)** Pre - and post-operative front-view images of corrective breast surgery in males using circumareolar incision, liposuction and glandular excision. (The images are provided courtesy of Dr Sandip Jain, Mumbai, Maharashtra, India). **(c, d)** Pre- and post-operative lateral view images for corrective breast surgery in males using circumareolar incision for glandular excision.

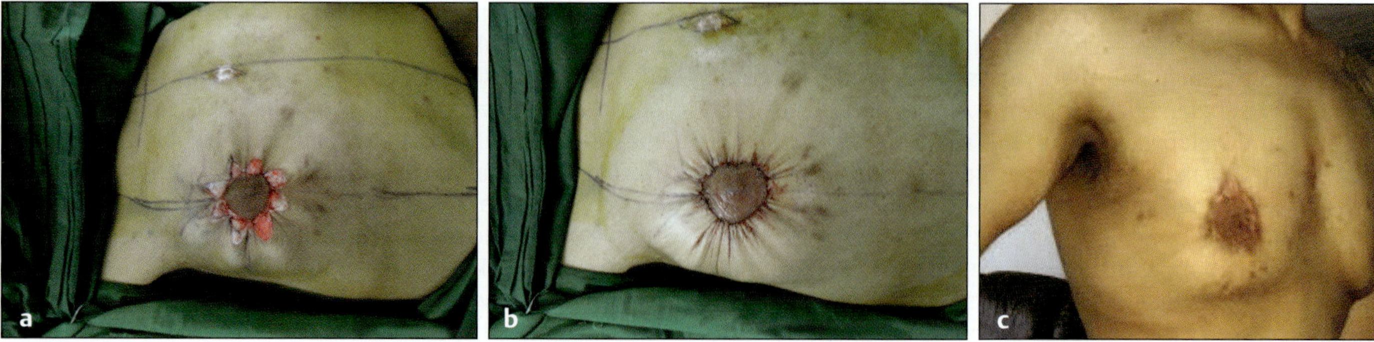

Fig. 26.12 Intraoperative pictures **(a, b)** showing wrinkling of skin at the suture line, and **(c)** showing the final outcome at 6 months (preoperative shown in **Fig. 26.9**).

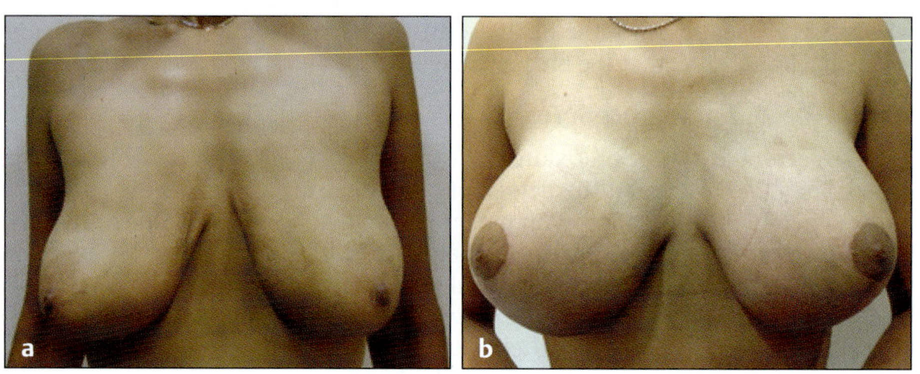

Fig. 26.13 **(a, b)** Pre- and postoperative pictures for mastopexy with implants.

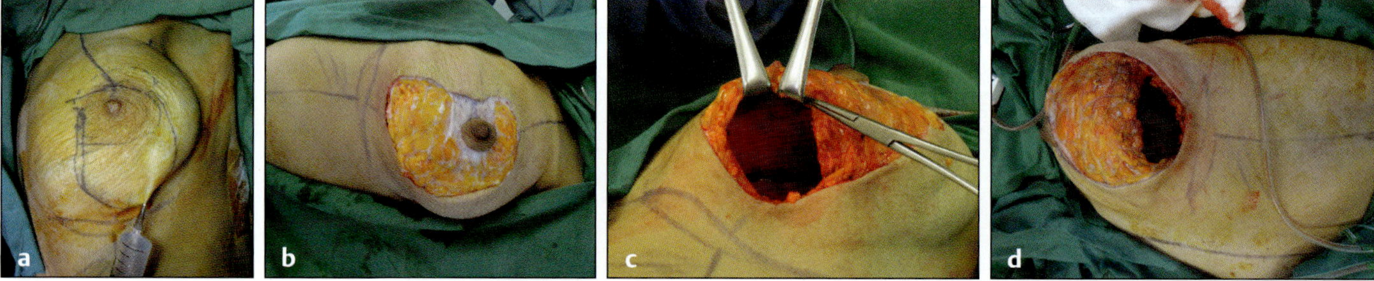

Fig. 26.14 Intraoperative steps for a Hall-Findlay mastopexy with implants. **(a)** Left breast, infiltration along the suture line but not under the pedicle. **(b)** De-epithelialization completed over redundant skin, nipple-areola maintained on dermal pedicle. **(c)** Pocket created in subglandular plane using an inframammary incision. **(d)** Implant in place in the pocket. Drain inserted before implant insertion.

Surgical Technique

For a breast augmentation with implants, the author prefers the submammary approach. If the breast volume is felt to be inadequate, the implant can be placed submuscularly to confer longevity on the procedure. Despite the fact that a massive amount of weight has been shed, there is a significant amount of tissue that can contribute to the overall breast volume. This must be recognized to avoid choosing an implant that is too big.[15]

For mastopexy, the author prefers the technique described by Elizabeth Hall-Findlay using the superomedial pedicle to sustain the nipple-areola complex (**Fig. 26.14**).[16] However, the authors do not encourage implant insertion at the same sitting, since it increases the possibility of complications. If this is found to be essential to provide some shape and volume, the operator is advised to insert the implant submuscularly, to reduce the complication rate (**Fig. 26.15**).

For breast reduction, the author prefers the "vertical dermal pedicle technique" as described by McKissock.[17] Occasionally, the superomedial dermal pedicle technique is used if the volume of tissue in the upper pole is adequate. Results in patients of mammoptosis using the McKissock technique are shown in **Figs. 26.16** and **26.17**.

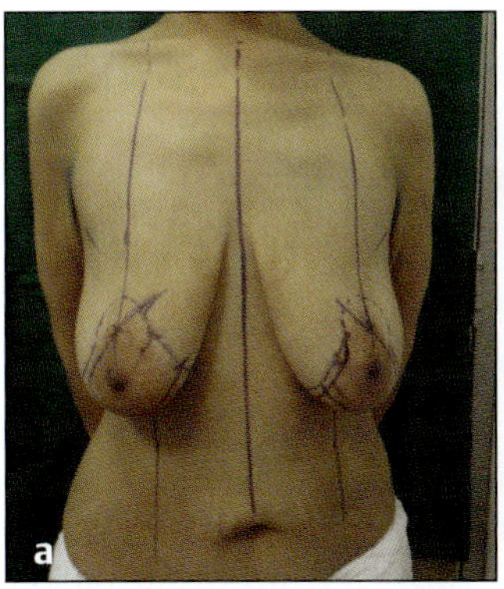
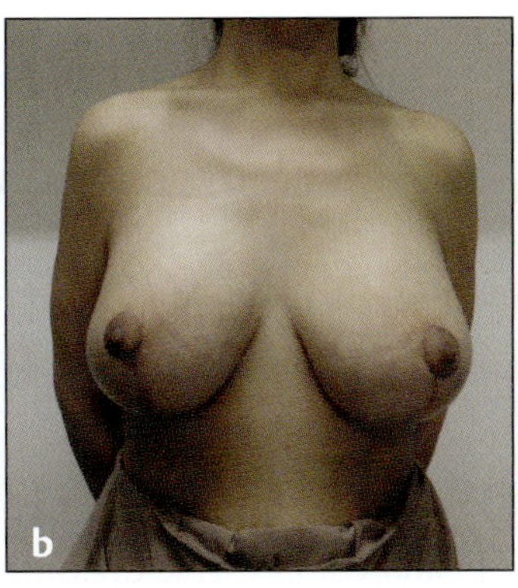
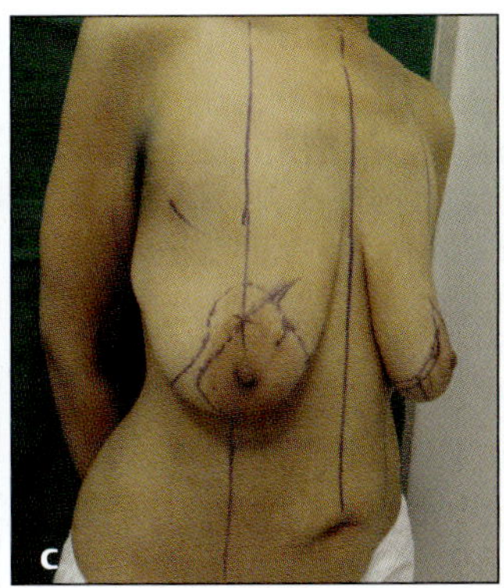
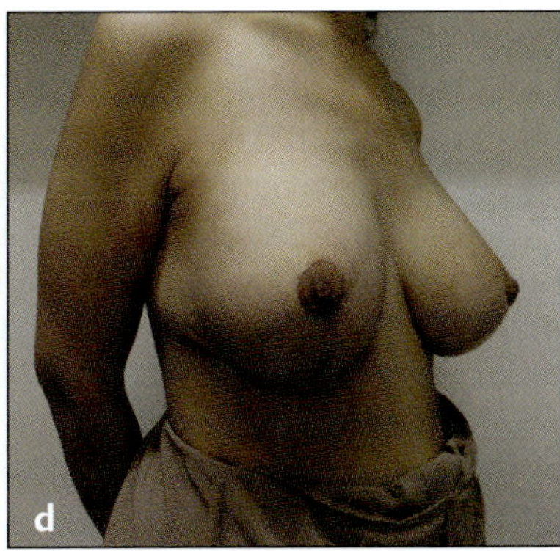

Fig. 26.15 Hall-Findlay mastopexy with implant. **(a, b)** Pre and postoperative front views. **(c, d)** Pre and postoperative oblique views.

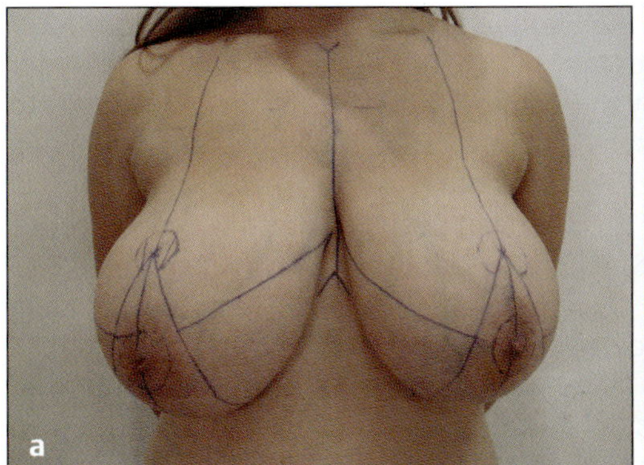
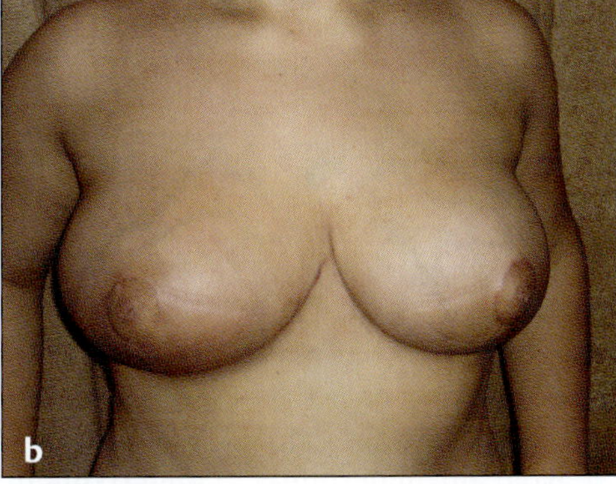

Fig. 26.16 **(a, b)** Pre- and post-operative results of reduction mammoplasty using McKissock technique.

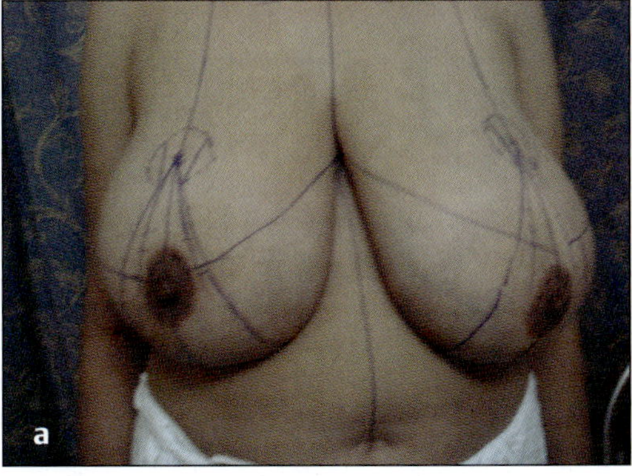
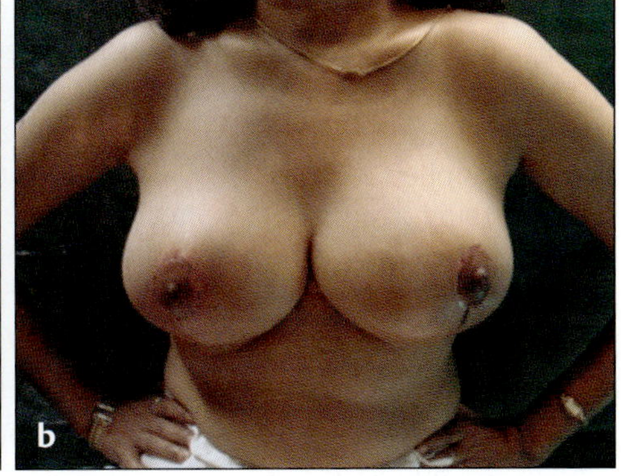

Fig. 26.17 **(a, b)** Pre- and post-operative results of reduction mammoplasty using McKissock technique.

It is extremely important to make a fair judgment of the amount of residual native breast tissue available before choosing any of the above-mentioned procedures. The scarring related to each of the procedures should be clearly explained preoperatively, keeping in mind that Indian skin types are prone to hypertrophic scarring and hyperpigmented scars.

Bra-Line Back Lift

Quite often, the female patient presents with fold of skin and fat just under the bra line. These are caused by adherence of the dermis to the deep fascia of the back, causing the skin to fold over when the patient loses weight. Invariably, the expectation is that a circumferential lower body lift will address the issue by pulling this excess downward. However, this is not the case and a patient should never be misled to think that it would. Excessive skin and fat rolls on the back under the bra can only be successfully attended to by the bra-line back lift, as described by Hunstad.[18]

Procedures Available

This is essentially a stand-alone procedure that does not have too many variations. At best, it could be combined with a breast procedure so as to be able to tackle the troublesome fat rolls that often accompany breast ptosis in the infra-axillary area.

Bra-Line Back Lift: Author's Preferred Technique

The patient is asked to wear her bra and, in the standing position, the outline of the bra is marked with indelible ink on the back, extending the marking to the infra-axillary area if it is part of the surgical plan to address that area. The bra is then taken off and a horizontal line is marked across the middle of the bra marking, extending laterally till the posterior axillary fold on both sides. We now visualize the skin excess on both sides of the midline and two vertical lines are drawn perpendicular to the horizontal line marked in the middle of the outline of the bra, one on each side. An ovoid ellipse is then marked between these two vertical lines in such a way that the margins of the ellipse do not fall outside the bra outlines which were marked at first. Now, the opposing sides of the ellipse are tailor tacked to ensure that we are not excising too much from the skin excess. If at any point along the ellipse it is felt that the skin edges may not be approximate, the margins of the ellipse are pulled toward each other to ensure that the closure does not become very tight.

After infiltrating the standard solution, the incision is made as per the markings. It is deepened down to the fascia overlying the muscle. A full-thickness excision is done of all the tissue contained within the ellipse. Alternatively, the tissue can also be removed by the avulsion method, once the incision is completed. Hemostasis is achieved and the skin edges are brought together. One must avoid any undermining of the skin flaps so that no potential cavity is created that could accumulate a hematoma. If there is more bleeding than expected, a negative suction drain can be placed under the skin. The author prefers the use of 3–0 Monocryl in the subcutaneous layer and a running subcuticular suture of the same material for the skin. Paper tapes are applied to hold the skin edges together. A compressive dressing is applied (**Fig. 26.18**).

Complications

The commonly encountered complications in body contouring surgery for MWL are similar for all body parts and are hence being discussed under a common heading. They can be broadly categorized as early complications, which manifest in the first 2 weeks following surgery, and late complications, which may arise after wound healing.

Early Complications

A **hematoma** should be suspected if the suction drains collect more than 50 to 70 mL in the 6-hour period following surgery (**Fig. 26.19**). The suspicion of active bleeding should be combated with antibleeding measures such as tranexamic acid and compressive dressings. However, strong suspicion should be pursued by re-exploration, preferably, under general anesthesia.

Occasionally, **blistering of the skin** occurs possibly due to a change in the lymphatic flow. Rarely, blisters may form under the paper tape, as a result of the shearing force under them caused by the postoperative swelling or as an allergy to the tape adhesive. The tapes should then be removed along with the blister skin, and the raw area treated as per merit.

Necrosis of the skin flap edges can result in **dehiscence** (**Fig. 26.20**). Small areas of necrosis can be allowed to slough out on their own. As the slough separates, healing progresses underneath. The resultant scar, if unacceptable, can be revised later. Larger areas of necrosis can result from excessive tension during closure, extensive undermining, underlying hematoma or infection, or use of tobacco in the preoperative or postoperative phase. Large areas of necrosis need to be debrided and either resutured, or skin grafted upon the appearance of healthy granulation tissue. This catastrophic adverse event can be prevented by avoiding the risk factors mentioned above.

Extensive undermining, damage to the lymphatics, and shearing forces in the tissue planes contribute to **seroma formation**. In an abdominoplasty, dead space under the superior flap can be obliterated with quilting sutures of 2–0 polyglactin. When raising the flap for excisional contouring, always leave the fat deep to the scarpa fascia behind as the lymphatics travel within it. Undermining should not extend beyond the planned excision. Wearing a corset also immobilizes the flap, reducing the shearing movement, which

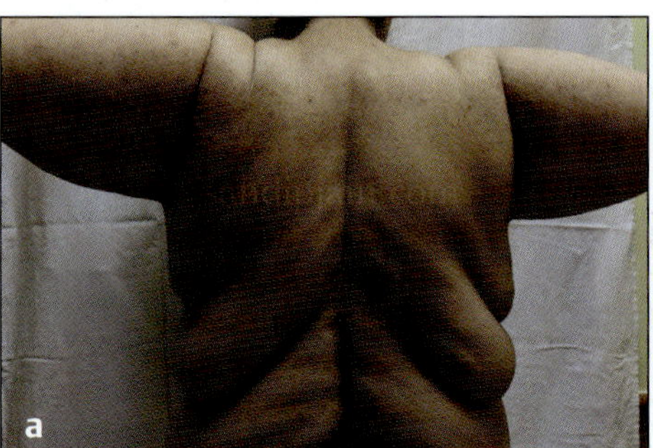

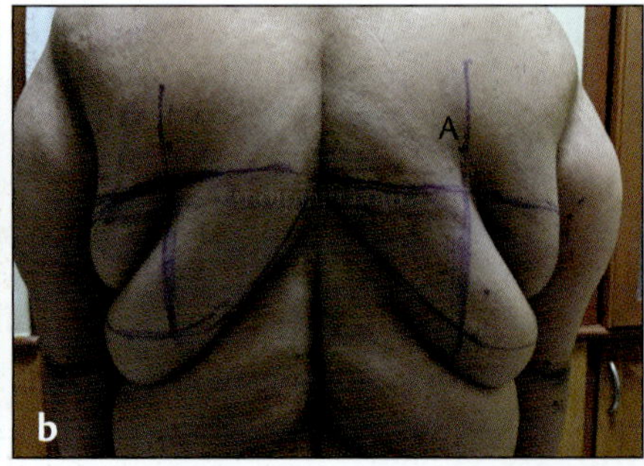

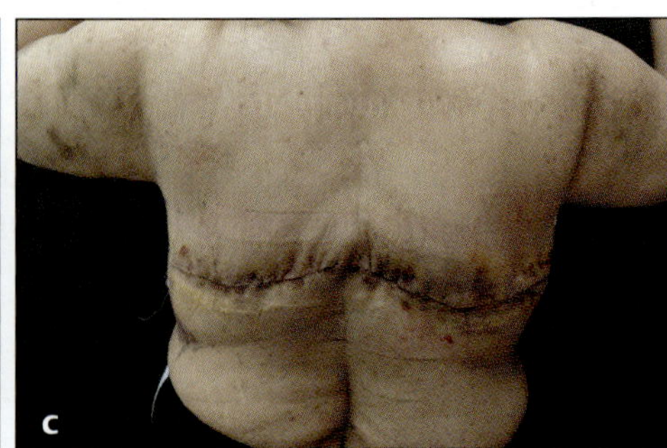

Fig. 26.18 The bra-line back lift: a simple approach to correcting severe back rolls. **(a)** Preop status, **(b)** markings showing Line A, ellipse, lateral extent of incision, and orientation of vertical lines. **(c)** Early postop status. (The images are provided courtesy of Dr Sandip Jain, Mumbai, Maharashtra, India.)

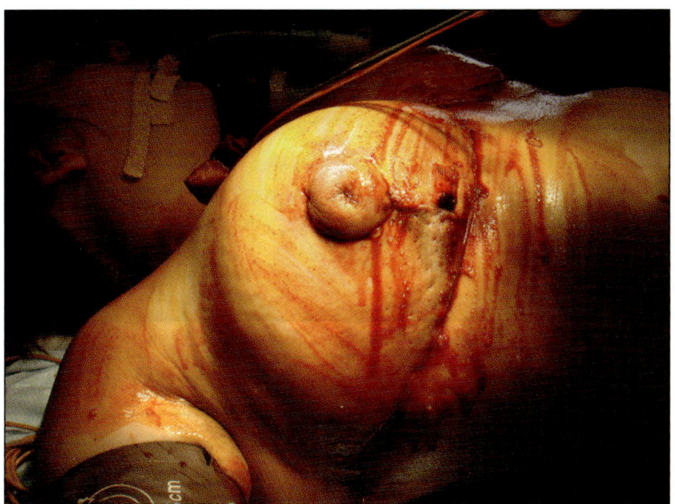

Fig. 26.19 Hematoma in a reduction mammoplasty.

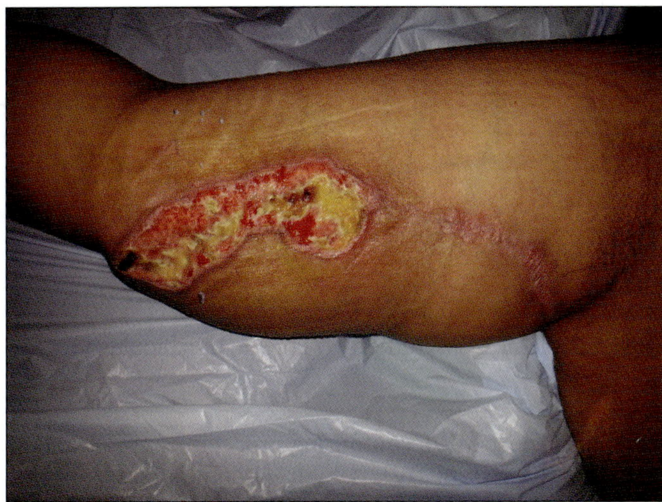

Fig. 26.20 Wound dehiscence in a brachioplasty.

can also help prevent seroma formation. The treatment of an established seroma involves repeated aspiration, percutaneous drain insertion, injecting sclerosing agents[19] in the seroma cavity, or, in extreme cases, excision of the seroma cavity along with its lining. Post-MWL contouring showed a 14% incidence of seroma formation with the highest incidence occurring in circumferential abdominoplasty. A direct correlation was found between the weight of the pannus excised and the incidence of seroma.[20] The authors also believe that using the cautery on cutting mode for flap elevation contributes to a greater incidence of seroma formation.

Late Complications

Fitzpatrick skin types 3 to 6 are more prone to **hypertrophic scarring**. Other risk factors are closure under high tension and delayed healing. Judicious use of silicone gel and corsets in the healing phase can go a long way in preventing hypertrophic scars. Topical silicone gel application twice a day for 6 months is more practicable than whole day silicone gel sheet application as far as patient compliance is concerned.[21]

Fitzpatrick skin types 3 to 6 may show good healing with fine scars in the initial postoperative phase. However 2 to 3 months down the line they may develop **hyperpigmentation or hypertrophy** which can cause dissatisfaction among patients. **Fig. 26.21** shows hyperpigmentation and hypertrophy in a patient 2 years following surgery. The application of topical silicone gel and sunscreen lotion for 6 months can help prevent hyperpigmentation. One study comparing the topical application of silicone gel and Vitamin C for 6 months versus no topical application for scars in Asian skin types showed statistically significant reduction in erythema, hyperpigmentation, and hypertrophy in the former group.[20]

Neurapraxia or division of the cutaneous nerve by cautery, sharp dissection, or retraction can cause **paresthesia** in the territory supplied by the nerve. During brachioplasty, the medial cutaneous nerves of the arm and forearm, which travel alongside the brachial artery and pierce the deep fascia at the midpoint of the arm, are at risk of damage. Keeping the above surface anatomy in mind and leaving a layer of fat on the deep fascia will, in most cases, protect the nerve and avoid the unpleasant side effects of paresthesia. In the event of paresthesia reassure the patient that in the majority of cases, the surrounding cutaneous nerve territory takes over the area of paresthesia in approximately 6 months time.

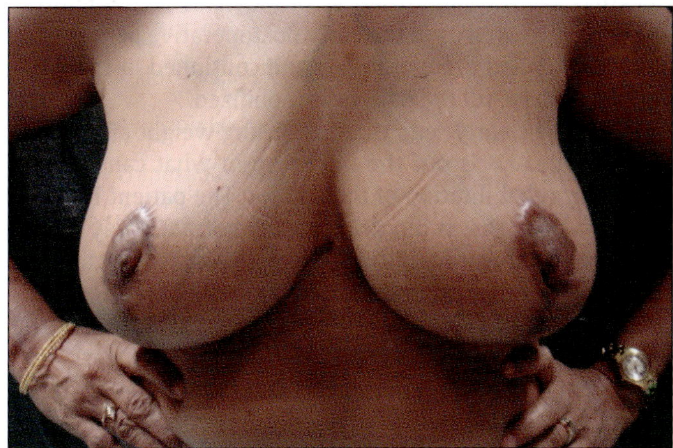

Fig. 26.21 Hyperpigmentation and hypertrophy of scar.

Careful examination and looking at photographs taken at different angles often reveal asymmetry as far as redundancy and residual fat deposits are concerned (**Fig. 26.22**). In some rare cases, asymmetry could be related to the posture of the patient caused by a skeletal deformity. This should be pointed out to the patient during preoperative counseling. After the markings are made, the amount of tissue being left behind should be measured on both sides and adjusted so that equal amounts are left behind, rather than equal amounts being excised. For patients who have undergone MWL, it is advisable to focus on contouring rather than minimum scarring.

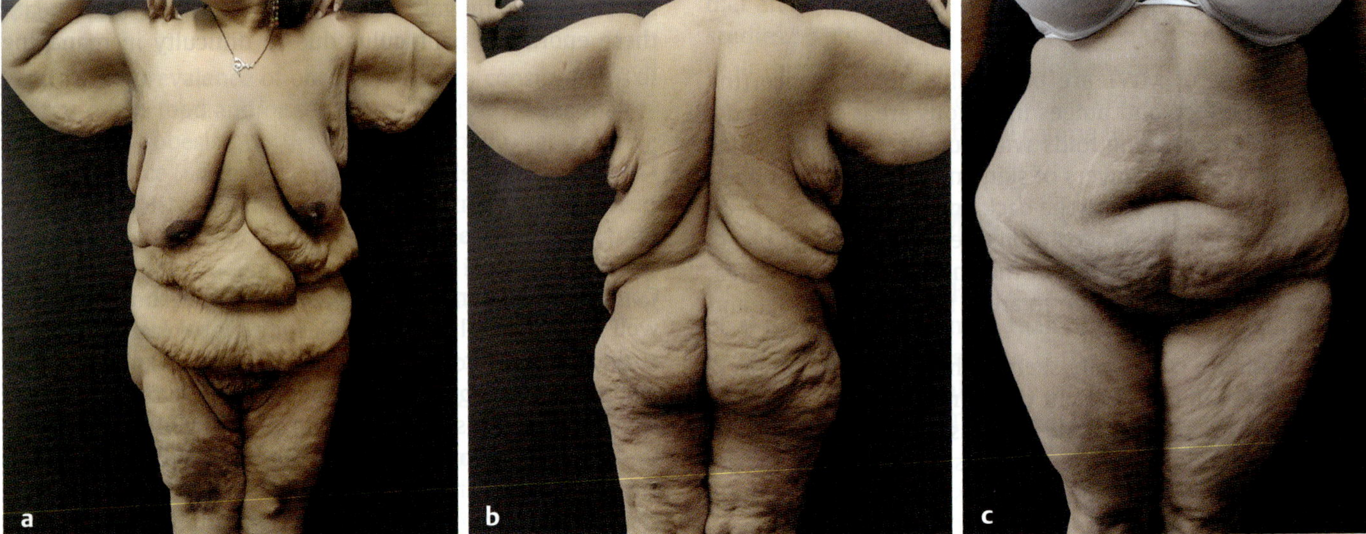

Fig. 27.1 **(a)** Showing mons, hypogastric, umbilical, and epigastric panniculi. Concertina effect can be seen in the thigh, particularly the medial thigh. **(b)** Showing the oblique panniculi in the back and concertina effect in the buttock and thigh and the bulge in the trochanteric area. **(c)** This patient presented with chief complaint of bulges in the flank area and a request for liposuction. However, this bulge is caused by the skin gathering above the zone of adherence in the lateral gluteal area. So it can be corrected by body lifting and not liposuction.

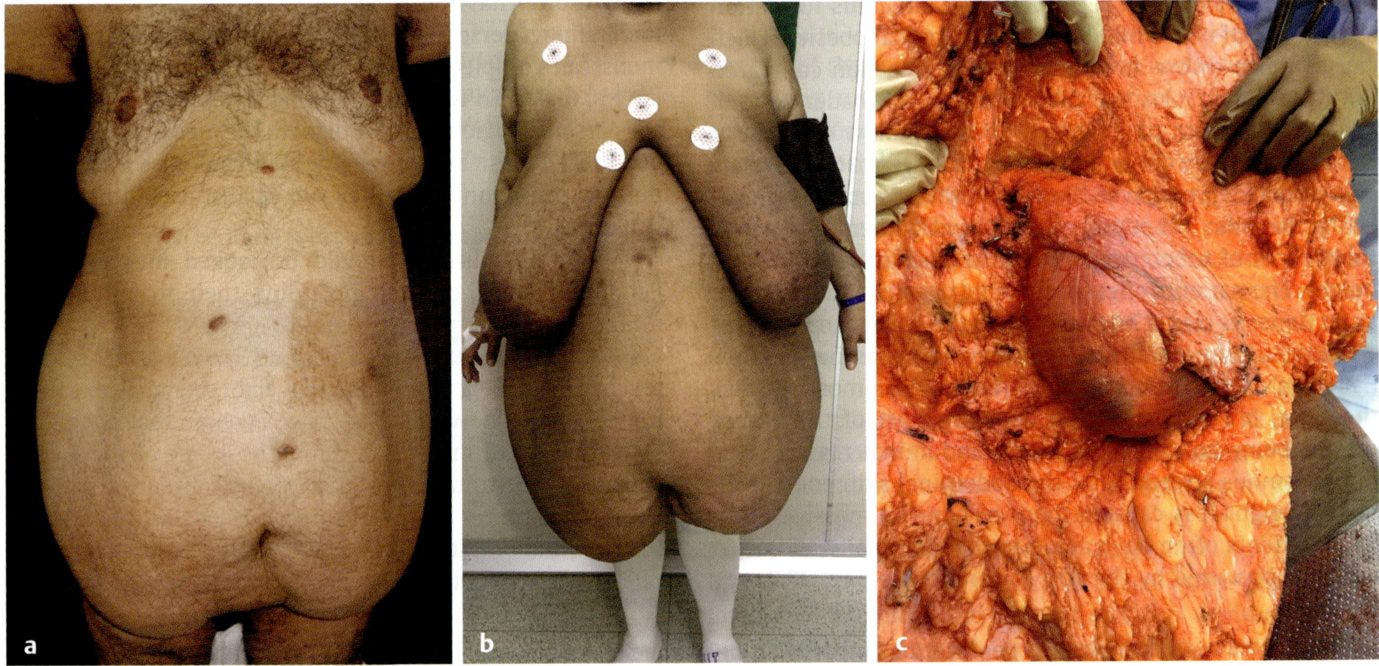

Fig. 27.2 **(a, b)** Panniculus morbidus following massive weight loss. Body mass index (BMI) of (a) and (b) was 39 and 54 kg/m^2, respectively. **(c)** Intraoperative photo of the patient in (b), showing the huge umbilical hernia.

lifestyle with regard to diet and exercise. Promising to do so in the future or after contouring surgery should raise a red flag. This is important to achieve a long-lasting result following contouring surgery.

Detailed information should be sought regarding the type of bariatric surgery, postsurgery recovery, and supplements advised. Malabsorptive bariatric surgery patients are more likely to have their nutritional status compromised.

It is very critical to know a patient's expectations from the body lift surgery. Some patients have modest expectations of just getting rid of folds with the attendant functional benefits from the perspective of improving personal hygiene and/or mobility. On the other end of the spectrum are patients who would expect no less than a bikini body. This may be attainable in patients who have reached their target weight (normal BMI) and have a tall and lean (ectomorph) body frame. However, those with stocky and wide (endomorph) body frames and/or multiple large panniculi should be counseled toward more realistic expectations.

Smoking increases the risk of surgical site infection (SSI), dehiscence, bleeding, and deep vein thrombosis (DVT). It is important to emphasize to the patient that there is no difference in complication rate between heavy and light smoker.[15] So if the patient gives a history of smoking, they should be encouraged to give it up 2 to 4 weeks prior to surgery. Points to be elucidated while taking history of massive weight loss patients are summarised in **Box 27.1**.

Box 27.1 Points to be elucidated while taking history of massive weight loss patients

- Aesthetic concerns
  - Folds
  - Wrinkling of skin
  - Bulges
  - Lack of gap between medial thigh
  - Sagging of buttock
- Functional concerns
  - Inability to exercise due to hanging panniculus
  - Interference with mobility
  - Difficulty in maintaining personal hygiene
  - Bulges in the medial thigh causing friction/burning when walking
- Weight loss history
  - Current weight
  - Maximum weight in the recent past
  - Minimum weight in the recent past
  - How long the weight has been stable
- Any surgery in the past
  - Bariatric surgery: When and what bariatric surgery was done
  - Any other surgery specially abdominal surgery
- Diet: Any particular diet patient is following
- Exercise: What is the exercise routine
- Patient expectations
- Comorbidity, (e.g., hypertension, diabetes, tuberculosis, etc.)
- Smoking history
- Medication
  - Supplements
  - Blood thinner
  - Any other medication
- Any known allergy

Examination

An essential requisite for a comprehensive lower body examination is that the patient be completely disrobed in a warm comfortable environment. The presence of a nurse in the examination room is mandatory. Ideally, one should have a full-length mirror in the room so that surgeon can point out to the patient various deformities and also simulate the surgery being planned. Patients should be examined in multiple positions like standing, sitting, supine, and diving positions. Standing position allows for examination in a circumferential manner with the surgeon sitting at eye level with the lower trunk. The importance of complete exposure with 360-degree examination is amply illustrated by the example in **Fig. 27.3a–f**. Examination points are listed in **Box 27.2**.

Box 27.2 Local examination for lower body contouring

- Body mass index (BMI) (kg/m^2)
- Lower body: Examination of skin
  - Skin folds: Number, location, and orientation
  - Concertina effect
  - Bulges
  - Scar: Location and extent
  - Intertrigo/fungal infection
- Mons ptosis
- Flank ptosis
- Buttock ptosis
- Pinch test
- Localized fat deposit
- Recti divarication
- Abdominal wall hernia
- Per abdomen examination

Body Mass Index

BMI is calculated by a simple formula of kg/m^2 where kg is weight in kilograms and m^2 is height in meters squared. This important information determines the eligibility of the patient to undergo contouring surgery. Generally, the body lift surgery is deferred on any patient with BMI of more than 35 kg/m^2. However, exceptions are made in cases where there is a large heavy panniculus or multiple panniculi. It is obvious that these massive folds of skin will prevent patients from doing proper exercise and so loose further weight. Also surgically removing these folds of skin will by itself cause weight loss in the range of 10 to 15 kg. Therefore, a salvage surgery, such as panniculectomy, can be undertaken in this subset of patients who have less than ideal BMI with the caveat that there is no serious existing comorbidity.

Lower Body Examination

Panniculi, Concertina Effect, and Bulges

The number of folds or panniculi in the abdominal region should be ascertained. Most commonly there is a single panniculus in the hypogastric region (**Fig. 27.4a**). Sometimes hypogastric pannus can be associated with either epigastric

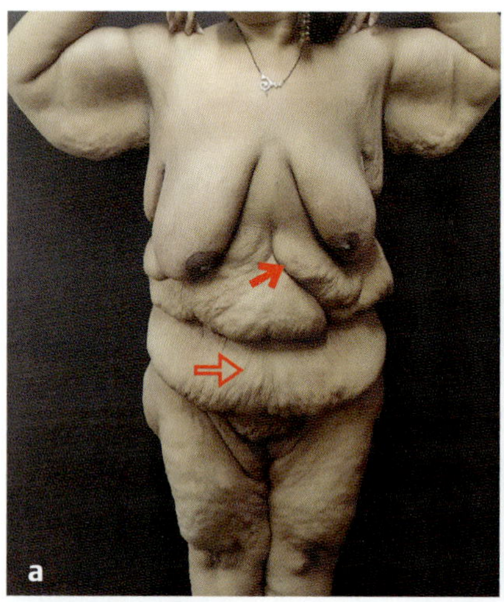
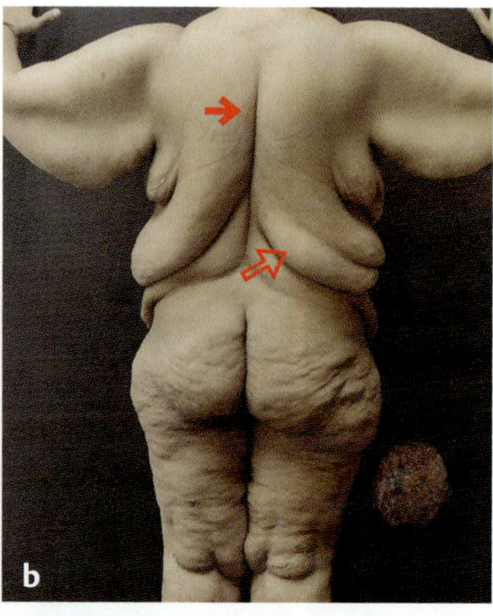

Fig. 27.7 (a) Abdomen showing horizontal folds (*hollow arrow*) and vertical folds (*solid arrow*) signifying vertical and horizontal laxity, respectively. **(b)** Back showing oblique fold (*hollow arrow*) and vertical fold (*solid arrow*) representing oblique and horizontal laxity, respectively.

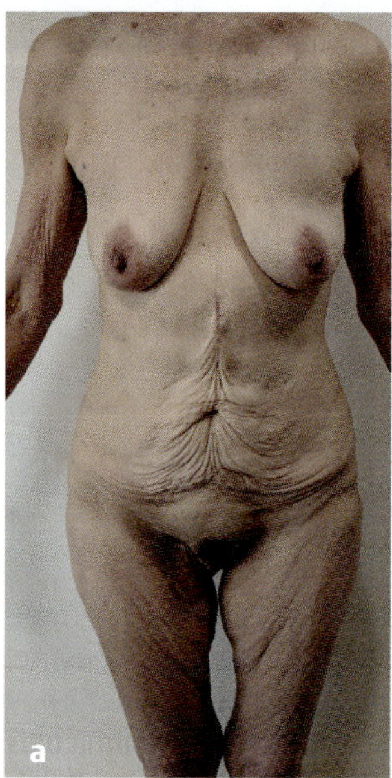
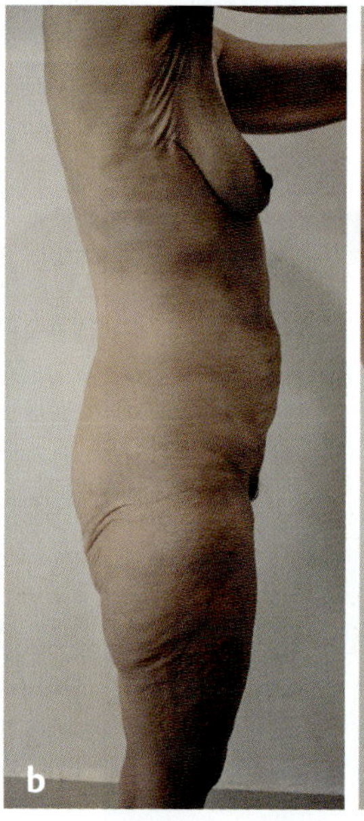
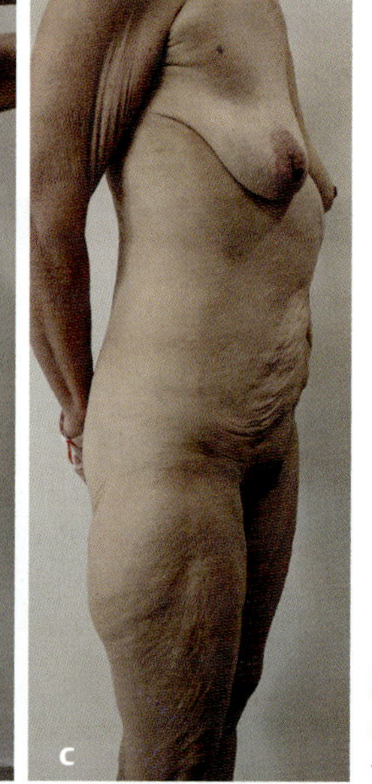

Fig. 27.8 (a–c) More subtle sign of laxity, the concertina or accordion effect, on the abdomen, thigh, and buttock.

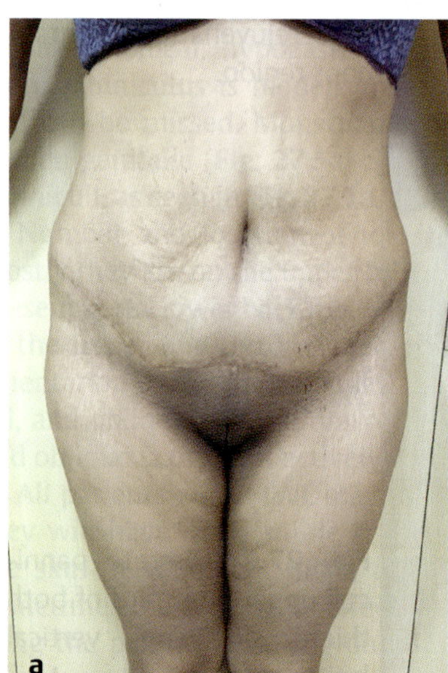
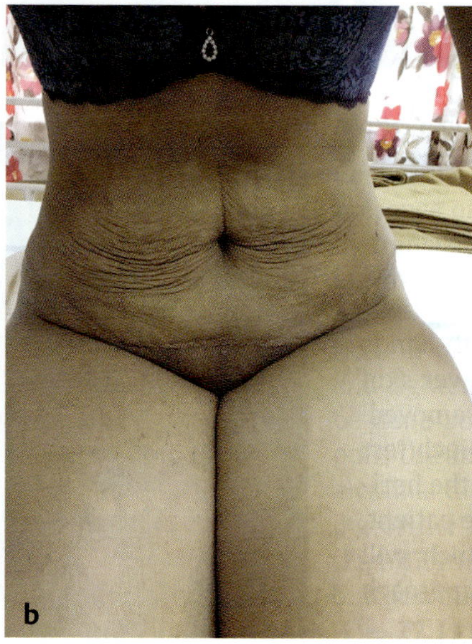

Fig. 27.9 (a) Not so obvious sign of laxity in the abdomen region. **(b)** Same patient in sitting position showing the amplification of concertina effect.

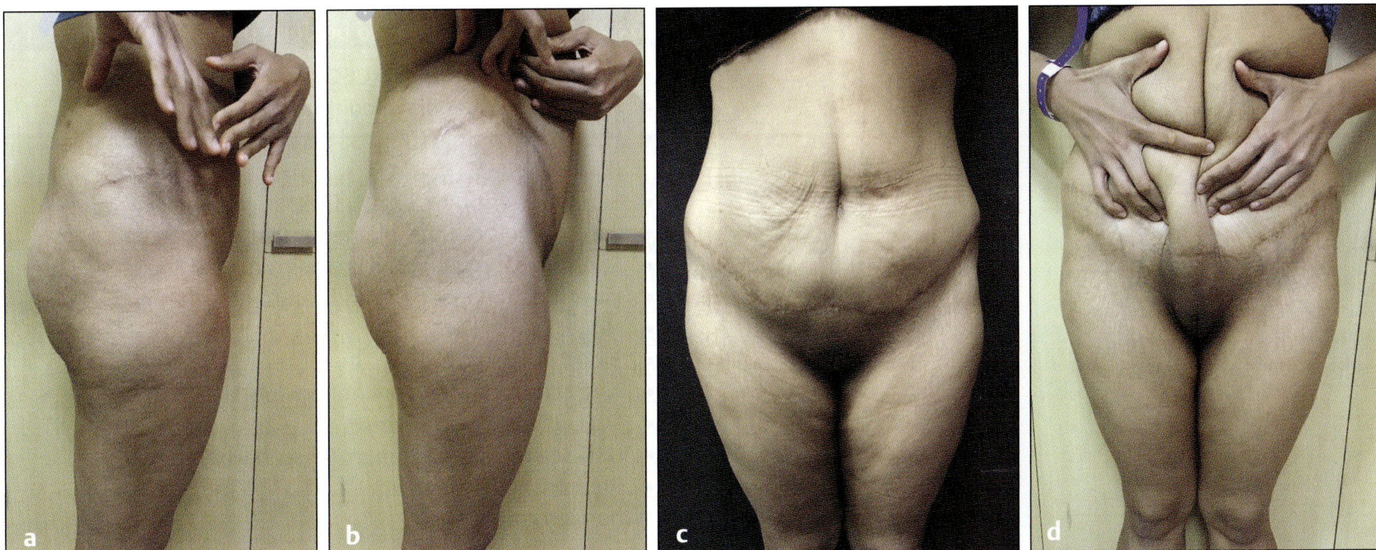

Fig. 27.10 **(a, b)** Translation test done laterally confirms lifting and tightening in lateral thigh. **(c, d)** Translation test done anteriorly lifts and tightens the mons, groin, and anterior thigh.

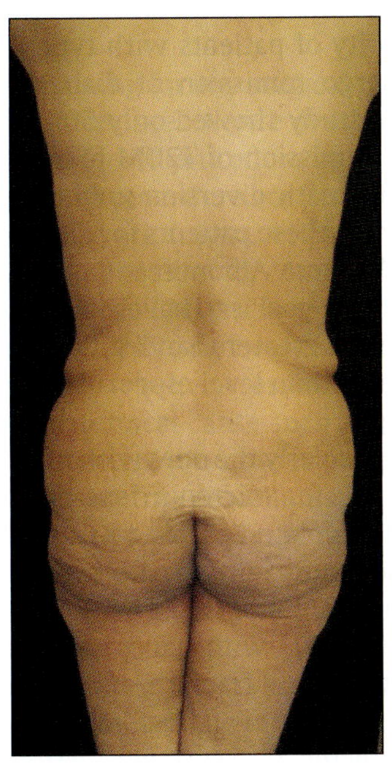

Fig. 27.11 Signs of buttock ptosis: Concertina effect on the buttock. Shortening of natal cleft and elongation of buttock thigh crease.

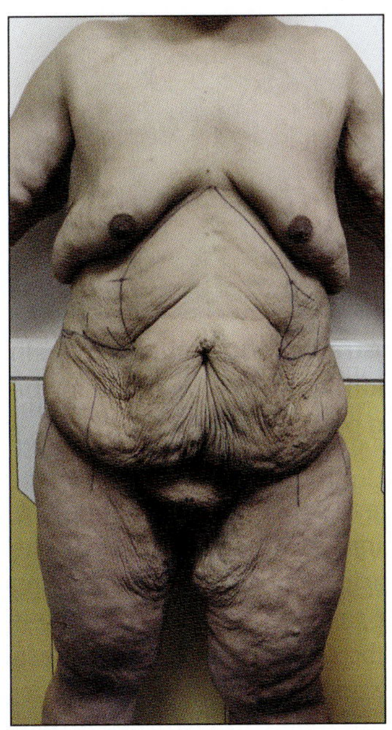

Fig. 27.12 Patient showing vertical and horizontal laxity in abdomen and therefore marked for anchor abdominoplasty along with lower body lift.

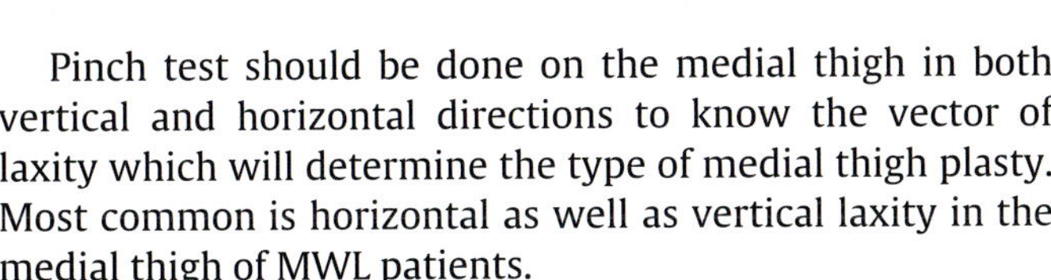

Pinch test should be done on the medial thigh in both vertical and horizontal directions to know the vector of laxity which will determine the type of medial thigh plasty. Most common is horizontal as well as vertical laxity in the medial thigh of MWL patients.

Localized Fat Deposit

Presence of localized fat deposits, which are outside the area of excision, particularly in the epigastric region, anterior thigh, and medial knee, should be noted. This is done by a pinch test which reveals the thickness of subcutaneous fat. Normally pinch thickness over ½ inch suggests the area is amenable to liposuction. However, due to global skin laxity and poor skin tone in post-MWL patients, only areas above 1-inch thickness should be considered for liposuction.

Abdominal Wall Hernia, Recti Divarication

Abdominal wall hernia like umbilical, inguinal hernia or laparoscopic port site hernia can be detected by watching for cough impulse. It is very important to rule these out to avoid inadvertent damage to intra-abdominal organs during liposuction.

In thin patients, diving position gives an estimate of the tone of abdominal muscle (**Fig. 27.13**). Weak tone or recti divarication causes midline bulge in this position. However, obese individuals may show epigastric bulge in the erect

Table 27.4 Elaborates the different vectors of laxity and the corresponding excisional lifts

Types of Excisional lift for MWL patients		
Area—Extent of laxity	**Vector of laxity**	**Type of excisional lift**
Abdomen—circumferential	Vertical	LBL
Abdomen—epigastric	Horizontal	AA
Abdomen—circumferential and epigastric	Vertical + horizontal	LBL + AA
Thigh—circumferential	Vertical	LBL + HMT plasty
Thigh—medial	Vertical	HMT plasty
Thigh—circumferential	Horizontal	VMT plasty
Thigh—circumferential	Vertical + horizontal	LBL + HMT + VMT
Mons	Vertical + horizontal	Mons suspension + horizontal shortening

Abbreviations: AA, anchor abdominoplasty; HMT, horizontal medial thigh; LBL, lower body lift; MWL, massive weight loss; VMT, vertical medial thigh.

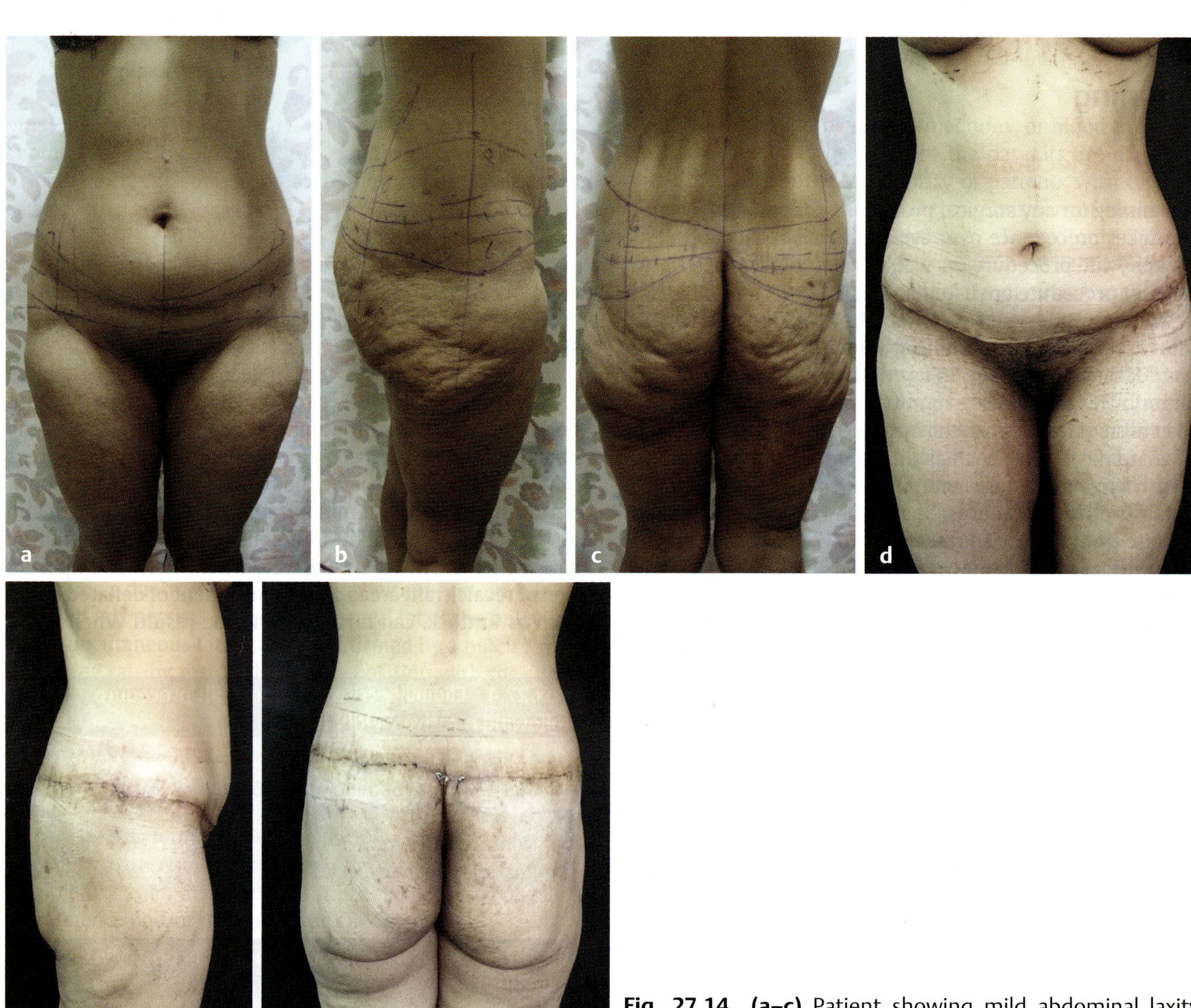

Fig. 27.14 **(a–c)** Patient showing mild abdominal laxity with severe flank and buttock laxity. **(d–f)** After the modified lower body lift where miniabdominoplasty was combined with standard thigh and buttock lift.

liposuction it is important to recall that these patients have global laxity. So the whole body has poor skin tone, compromising the ability of skin to retract post liposuction. Keeping this in mind liposuction when planned should be conservative. Instead of the usual end point of leaving one-fourth inch thickness of fat underneath the skin it should be half-inch thickness instead.

Enhancement of buttock is a contentious issue in lower body contouring surgery for post-MWL patients. The options of buttock enhancement are listed in **Box 27.6**.

In flapless autoaugmentation, following the posterior excision of lower body lift, the inferior flap is rotated up and medially and sutured to the upper flap.[20] So this moves the buttock tissue centrally, where it is deficient. Disadvantage of this technique is elongation of the natal cleft because the longer inferior flap is rotated up and medially to coapt with the shorter upper flap.

Autologous fat transfer (AFT) is another option of enhancing the buttock.[21] The disadvantages of this method are that it cannot be done where donor site is sparse (normal or low normal BMI), unpredictable absorption, risk of fat necrosis, and very rarely fat embolism. However if safety measures are followed then it is one of the simplest options to offer to the patient.[22]

Regarding the flap options, the adipofascial flap is designed by de-epithelializing a medial island of tissue within the posterior excision pattern. The de-epithelialized island of flap, comprising dermis, fat, and fascia, is then mushroomed up by a purse string permanent suture in the fascial layer. The inferior gluteal skin is then undermined and advanced over this island flap giving bulk to the upper buttock.[23] Dirk Richter advocated superior to inferior and lateral to medial plication of adipofascial layer for gluteal augmentation. The inferior gluteal skin is then advanced over this plicated island of adipofascial flap.[24] Colwell described superior gluteal artery perforator flap which was de-epithelialized and shifted into a pocket in the inferomedial aspect of the buttocks.[25] One thing common to all these flap-based gluteal augmentation is the need to undermine the inferior edge of body lift incision. This is done to drape the gluteal skin over the local tissue flap. Most of them also bury a de-epithelialized island of tissue. All these methods, besides increasing the operative time and complexity, increase the risk of wound edge ischemia and dehiscence as well as the risk of seroma, hematoma, and fat necrosis.

Box 27.6 Options of buttock enhancement in post-MWL patients

- Autologous
  - Flapless autoaugmentation
  - Autologous fat transfer
  - Flap based
    - Adipocutaneous
    - Adipofascial
    - Perforator based
- Implant based

Gluteal implants alone have been advocated to fill up and lift up the deflated buttock, thus obviating the need for long incision. However, this was a small series of five patients and a large series of such patients are lacking.[26]

At the other end of the spectrum, there is a school of thought of not doing any buttock augmentation during body lift. This is based on the premise that lower and wider the posterior excision is, the greater the pull on the buttock is. Greater pull translates to more flattening of the buttock. To prevent this Carlos roxo slightly modifies the posterior excision.[27] The post-excision width is narrower medially and wider laterally and also overall the width of excision is conservative. So in addition to less pull on the buttock, on closure the buttock tends to rotate superiorly and medially which in turn leads to desirable medial fullness. In belt lipectomy or central body lift, the posterior excision tends to be more cranial, consequently leading to less pull on the buttock and less flattening.[28] In belt lipectomy, the posterior scar is within 3 cm of the widest part of the pelvic brim, and in lower body lift, it is more than 3 cm caudal to the widest part of pelvic brim. The belt lipectomy targets the tissue around the waist line, so it improves the waist definition and has less lifting effect on the thigh and buttock. Opposite is true for lower body lift. As the incision is lower it has more lifting effect on the thigh and buttocks and less effect on waist definition.

Moreover, a study by Srivastava et al showed no difference in patient satisfaction in lower body lift patients between no augmentation and autoaugmented buttocks.[29] However complications such as wound dehiscence were more common in autoaugmented groups. In the light of above findings, the author uses no buttock augmentation procedure during lower body lift, except on patient request. If possible autologous fat transfer is the only option the author offers (**Fig. 27.15a–f**). As mentioned above, flap-based autoaugmentation violates the sacrosanct principle of no undermining during body lift procedure with its attendant complications. It's trouble not worth taking. Best option is to preserve the deep fat and be conservative with the width of the excision posteriorly so as not to overtly tighten and thereby flatten the buttock. Also in overweight and obese individuals or those with enough subcutaneous fat in the buttock region, the risk of flattening of buttock is not there with lower body lift and no buttock augmentation is required (**Fig. 27.16a–d**). In normal BMI or thin patients a wider excision laterally and very narrow excision centrally will be more appropriate to prevent excessive pull and flattening of the buttock medially and also cause the buttock to rotate up and medially creating desirable medial fullness (**Fig. 27.17a–e**).

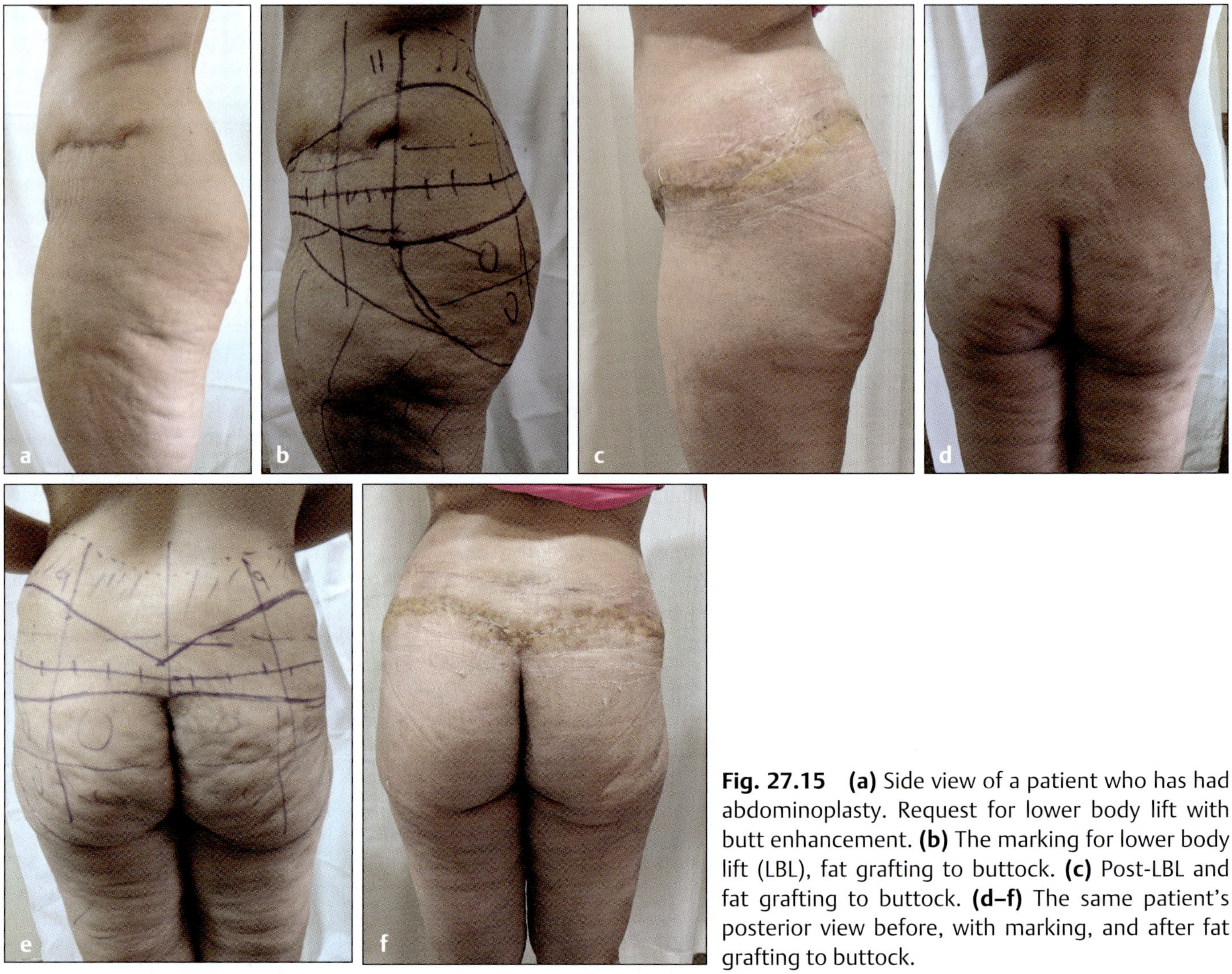

Fig. 27.15 **(a)** Side view of a patient who has had abdominoplasty. Request for lower body lift with butt enhancement. **(b)** The marking for lower body lift (LBL), fat grafting to buttock. **(c)** Post-LBL and fat grafting to buttock. **(d–f)** The same patient's posterior view before, with marking, and after fat grafting to buttock.

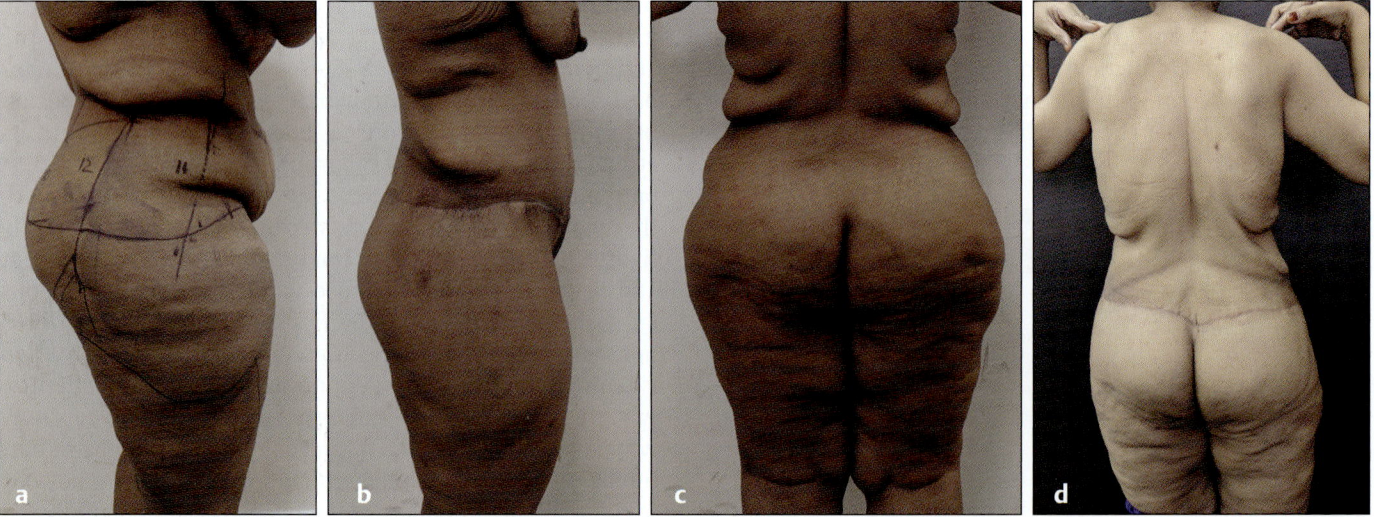

Fig. 27.16 **(a)** Post–massive weight loss (MWL) patient with body mass index (BMI) of 31 and enough subcutaneous fat in the buttock region. **(b)** Following lower body lift with no buttock augmentation. **(c, d)** Same patient's posterior view before and after lower body lift with no buttock augmentation. The buttock projection is maintained.

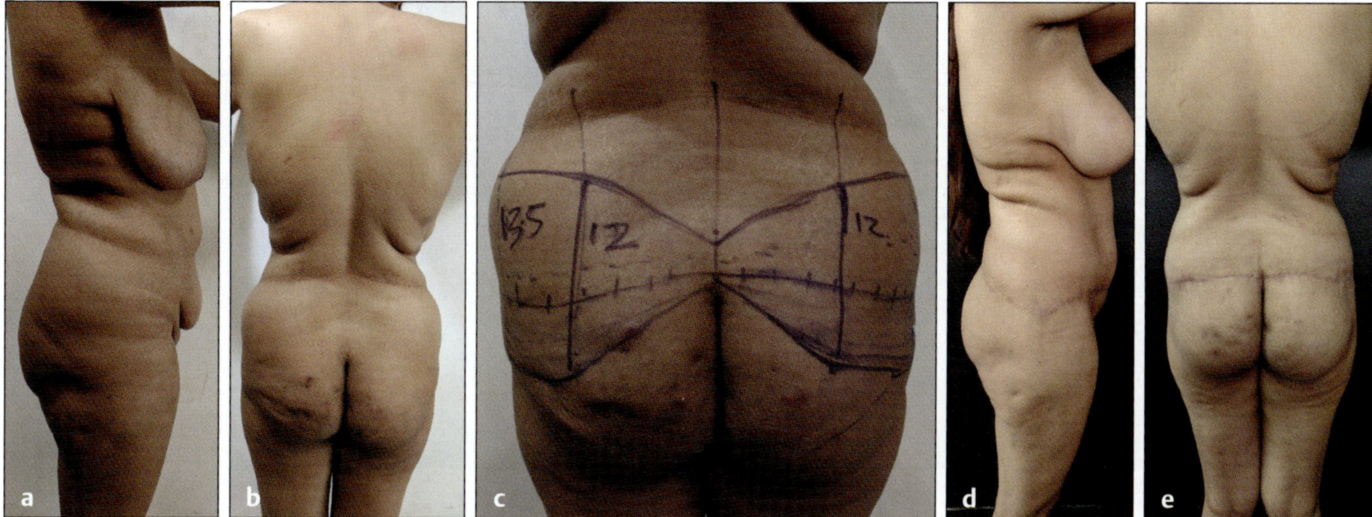

Fig. 27.17 **(a)** Patient post–massive weight loss (MWL) with body mass index (BMI) of 21—side view. **(b)** Post-view. **(c)** Marking of lower body lift showing wider excision laterally and very conservative excision centrally. This causes the buttock to rotate cranially and medially on closure, resulting in medial fullness. **(d, e)** After lower body lift—side and posterior view.

Sequence and Combination of Surgery

Once the type of surgery, excisional lift, liposuction, and buttock enhancement, is decided, the next step would be how to sequence them.

Generally, the lower body is done before the upper body. The reason being the lower body tightening can pull the chest skin and the inframammary crease (IMC) down. So once the lower body lift is done, the final position of the IMC is known. This will allow for more accurate placement of the IMC incision for either breast lift/reduction or augmentation. However some patients may opt for contouring the upper body only and may do the breast only or arms and breast. Such patients must be warned that if they do the lower body contouring later on, it may mar the result of breast contouring surgery done earlier.

Next step in planning would be how to combine the surgeries. Combining surgery is more economical, reduces hospitalization and convalescence time, and is deemed to be as safe as performing the surgery in several stages.[30] The spectrum of combination surgery for lower body contouring can be from only lower body lift to the other extreme of lower body lift + anchor abdominoplasty + vertical and horizontal medial thigh plasty + Mons suspension and horizontal shortening (**Figs. 27.18–27.20**). Any of these combinations can be combined with liposuction and/or buttock enhancement. Preference would be to contour the entire lower body (below the costal margin) in one operation, keeping in mind the Pitanguy principle mentioned earlier. However for a surgeon who has just started doing body lift surgery, it would be advisable to stage the lower body contouring. For instance lower body lift can be done in the first stage and ~3 months later thigh lift can be scheduled.

Regarding upper body lift, one can start off by staging the lower and upper body lifts. In the first stage, lower body lift is done and 3 months later upper body lift (**Fig. 27.21a–i**). As one gains experience one can do the upper and lower body lifts in single admission. On day 1 the lower body lift and on day 4 upper body lift is done with the discharge being on the seventh day (**Fig. 27.22a–f**). This is known as single admission total body lift. However the author has realized that it is better to do this on patients with long and narrow torso as they are better able to tolerate the opposing vector of pull of lower and upper body lifts. Also should be reserved for patients with thin layer of subcutaneous fat as the skin is more pliable (**Fig. 27.22a–f**). This patient had a better result of single admission total body lift as compared with the patient in **Fig. 27.20** where there is still some residual laxity.

The author also prefers to take photographs and print them out and draw the extent of scar on the photograph. This way patients are better able to appreciate the true extent and direction of scar and also serves as a record of having had the discussion with the patient.

Surgical Management

Preoperative Preparation

Presurgery preparations start the evening before surgery. Electrical clippers rather than razor shaving is used to remove all the hair from below the costal margin.[31] Shower is given with chlorhexidine gluconate (CHG) 4% solution the night before and the morning of the surgery. It has been found that preoperative showering with CHG is more effective in reducing the skin staphylococcal colony counts

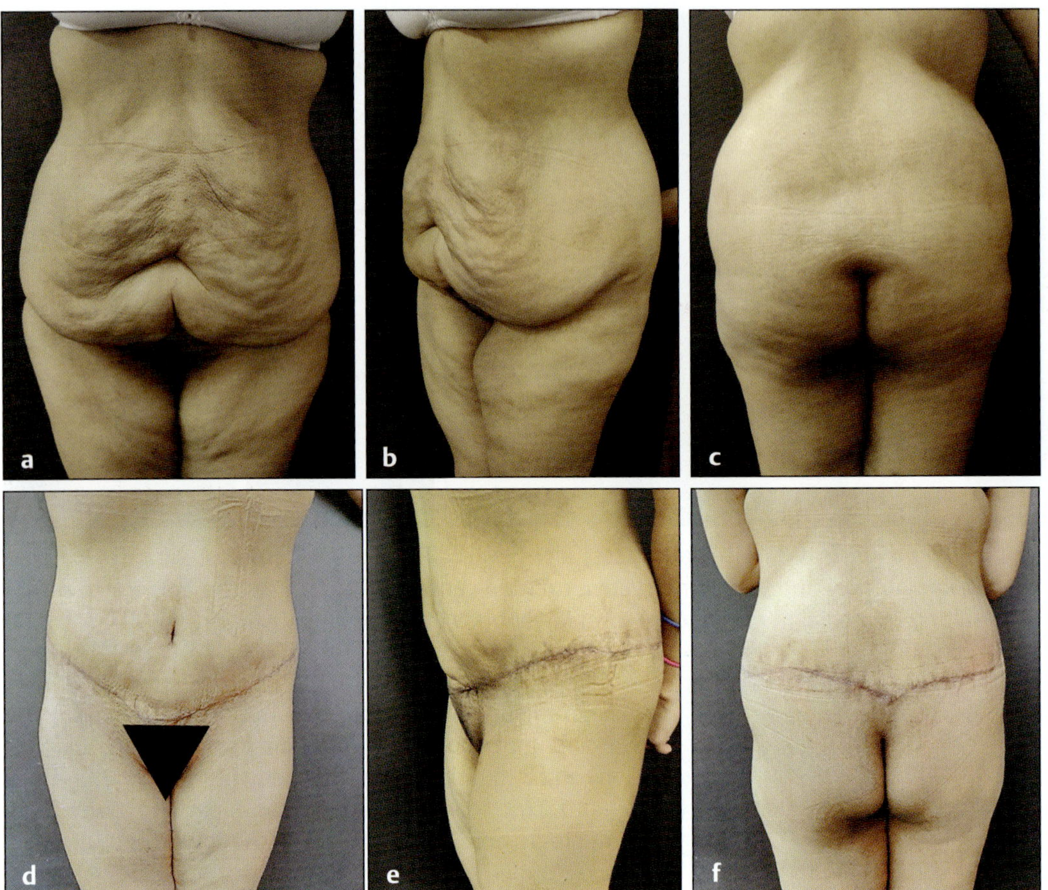

Fig. 27.18 (a–c) Following 41-kg weight loss. **(d–f)** Following lower body lift.

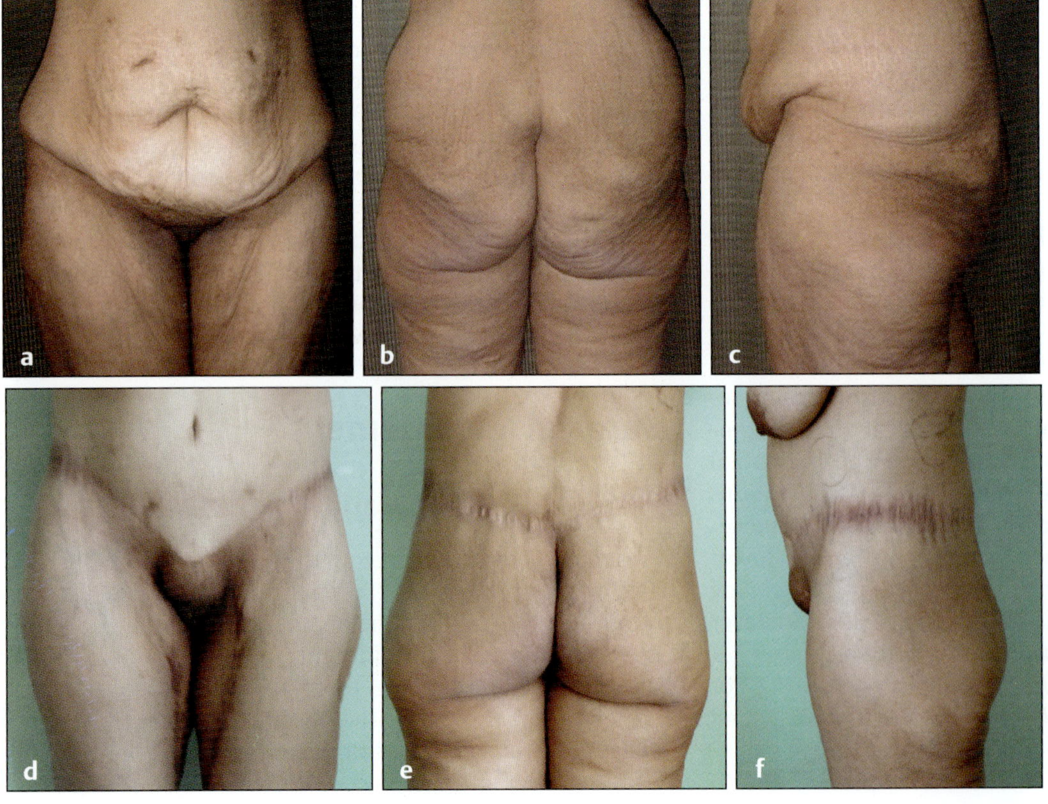

Fig. 27.19 (a–c) Following 55-kg weight loss. **(d–f)** Lower body lift with horizontal and vertical medial thigh plasty and mons suspension and transverse reduction.

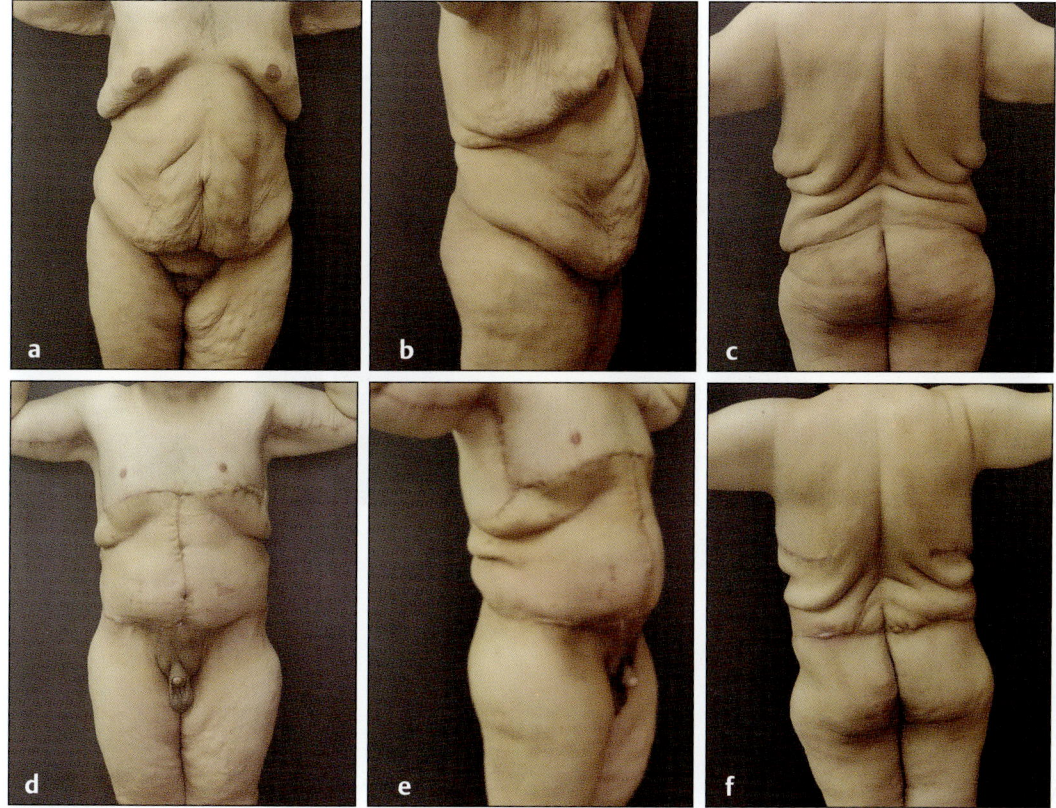

Fig. 27.20 (a–c) Following 114-kg weight **loss. (d–f)** Following lower body lift with anchor abdominoplasty, vertical and horizontal medial thigh plasty, and mons suspension and transverse reduction. This was done on day 1 of admission. On day 4 upper body lift was performed.

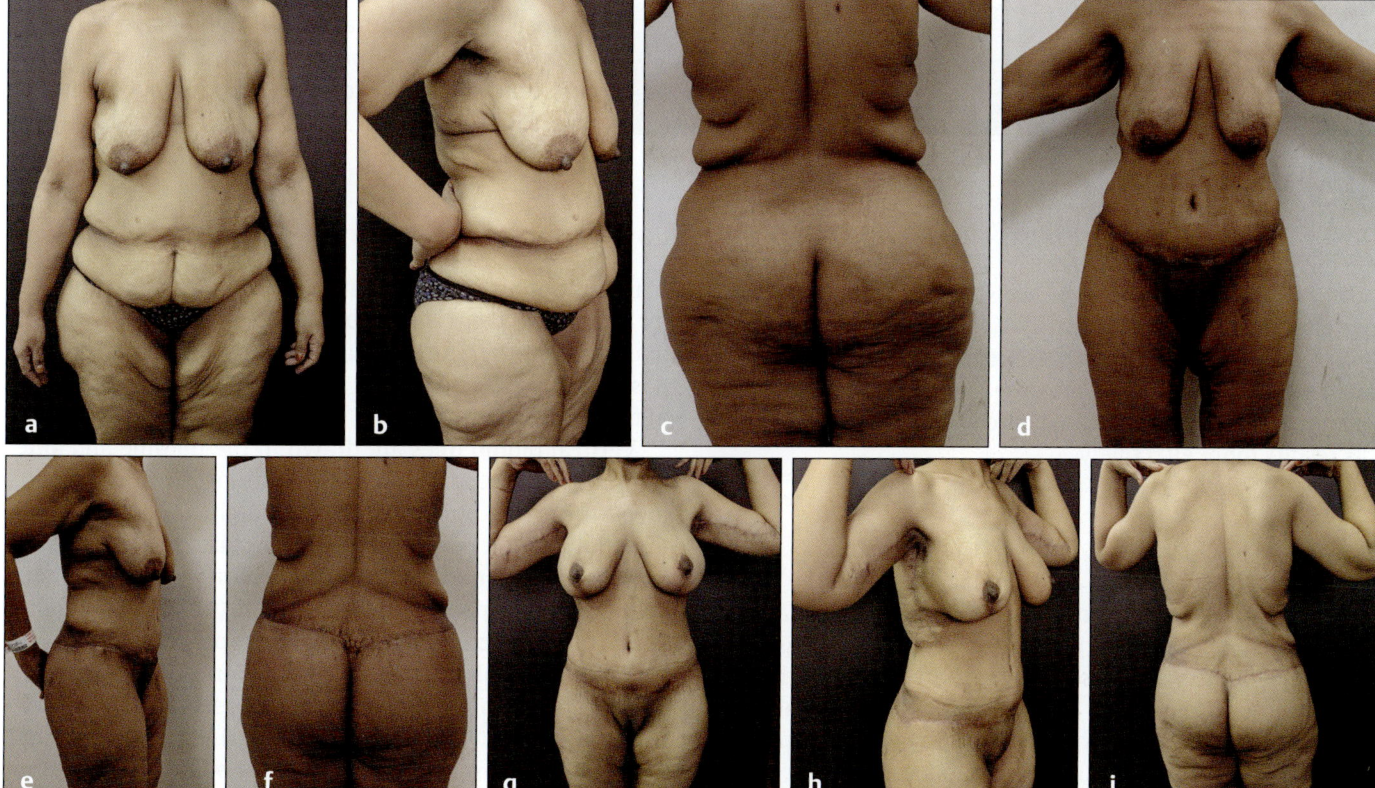

Fig. 27.21 (a–c) Following 50-kg weight loss. **(d–f)** Following first-stage lower body lift + vertical and horizontal medial thigh plasty and mons plasty. **(g–i)** Second-stage upper body lift (brachioplasty + thoracoplasty + augmentation mastopexy).

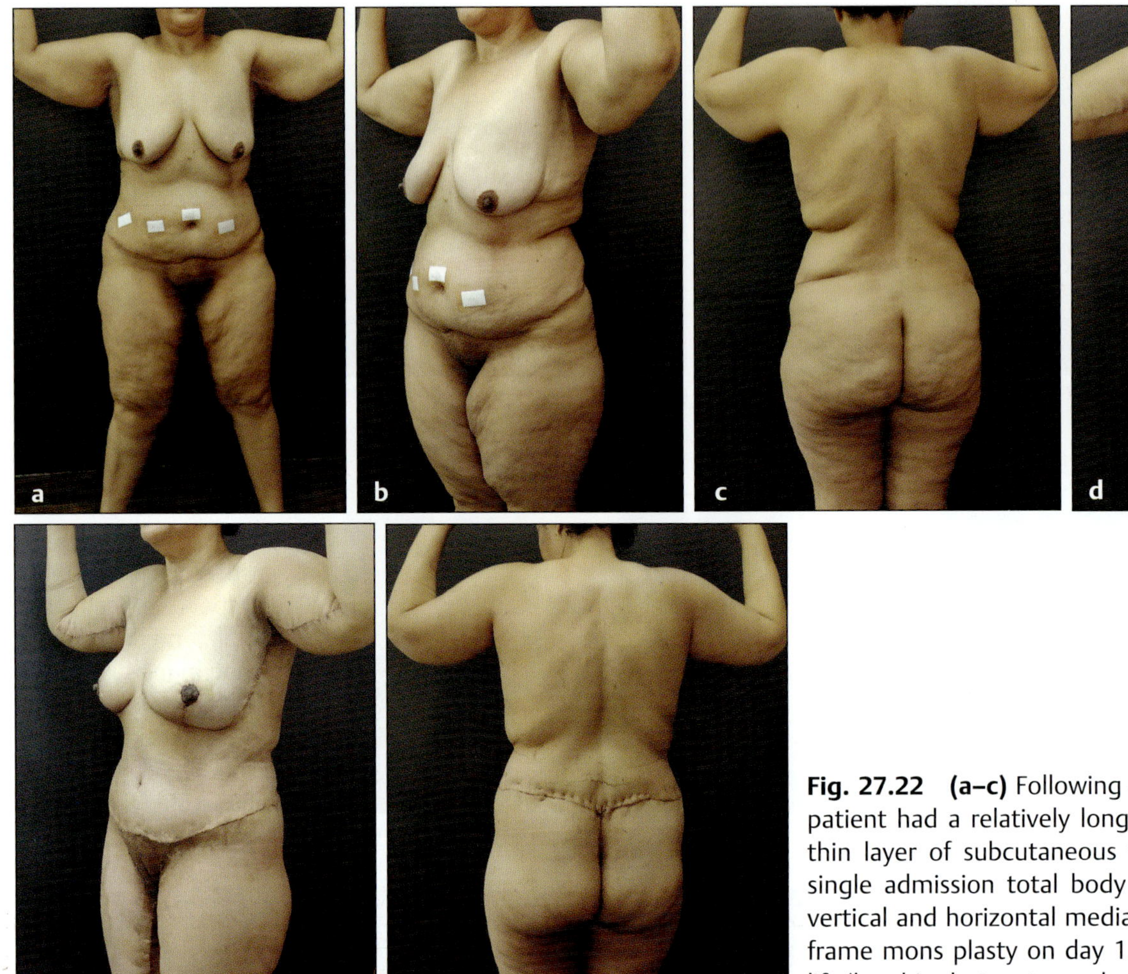

Fig. 27.22 (a–c) Following 40-kg weight loss. This patient had a relatively long and narrow torso and thin layer of subcutaneous tissue. **(d–f)** Following single admission total body lift. Lower body lift + vertical and horizontal medial thigh plasty + picture frame mons plasty on day 1. On day 4 upper body lift (brachioplasty + torsoplasty + autoaugmentation mastopexy).

compared with povidone iodine. Repeated shower is more effective than a single shower.[32]

Photographs are taken in six standard views to completely document the extent of laxity in both upper and lower body **(Fig. 27.23a–f)**. Photographs are taken again after the marking. This allows the surgeon to compare his presurgical plan with the final outcome and therefore critic his results more effectively.

Marking

Marking is done after the above preparation and the evening before surgery. This cannot be overemphasized. Marking the evening before surgery allows the surgeon to leisurely mark the patient and also allows the surgeon to revisit the presurgical plan with the patient. Patients can also be shown the photographs with the markings in place so that they can appreciate the true extent and location of incisions and eventual scars. Two units of packed cells should be cross matched and preserved the evening before surgery.

Lower Body Lift Marking

Marking is done with the patient standing against the wall for support. Patient has to be disrobed completely for the marking and therefore should be made as comfortable as possible and a nurse should be present at all times in case of female patients.

Vertical plumb lines are drawn in the midline and anterior axillary line. Marking of the inferior incision is as follows. The mons pubis is pushed straight up, in a cephalic direction, to the point just before it starts to distort and a mark is made in midline 7 cm from anterior vulvar commissure. Additional points are marked 2 cm (or 2 finger breadth) above the groin crease with the patient pulling the panniculus superomedially. A line is drawn connecting the midline point to the points above the groin crease in a gentle curvilinear fashion (at 45-degree inclination) so that the midline point is the lowest and the lateral most point, at the anterior axillary line, is highest (**Fig. 27.24**). Next the superior incision is marked. In the midline, a point is marked just above

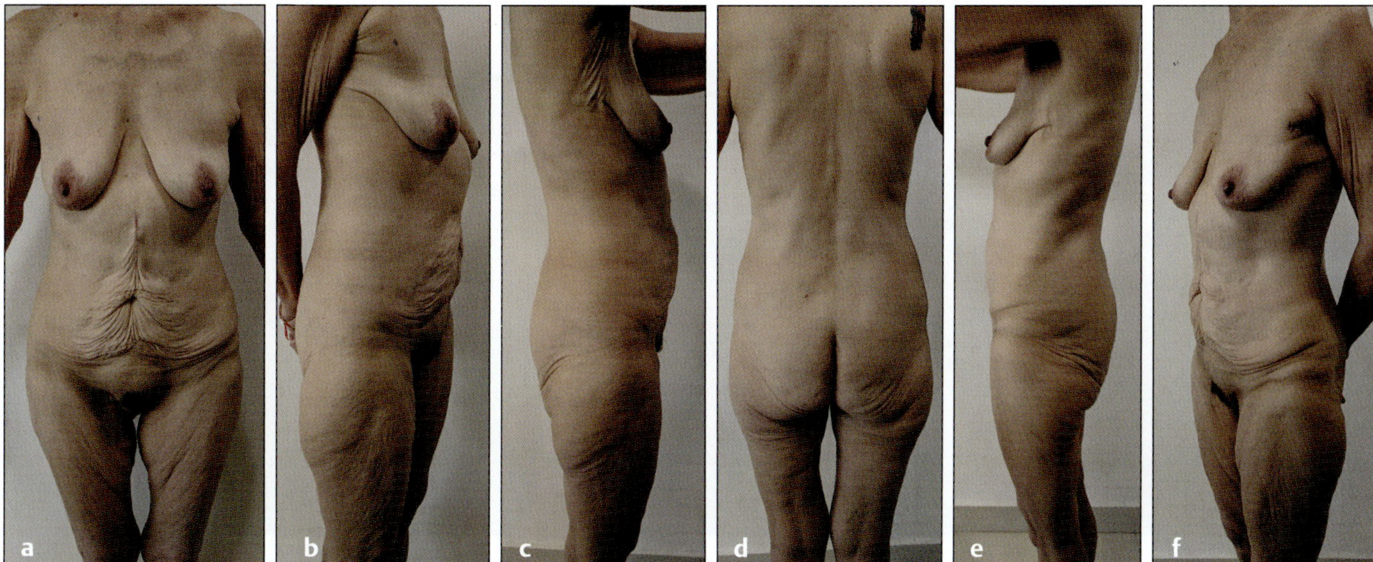

Fig. 27.23 (a–f) Showing the standard six views for lower body contouring.

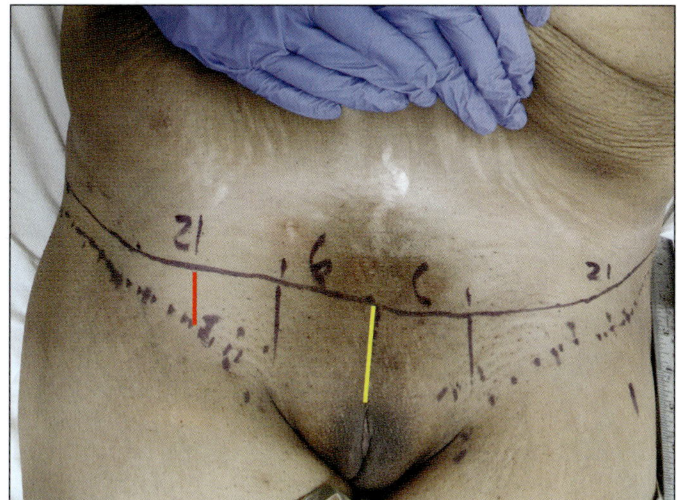

Fig. 27.24 Anterior marking of lower body lift. The midpoint of the inferior marking is 5 to 7 cm from the anterior vulvar commissure (*yellow line*) and the lateral part is 2 to 3 cm from the groin crease (*red line*).

the umbilicus. A pinch test is done to make sure the mons and the superior midline point will come together. Then from this superior midline point, 7 cm lines are marked on either side in a slight caudal direction, corresponding to the width of mons. The superior marking is then extended laterally to the anterior axillary line, and its location is determined again by pinch test.

Next the patient is turned around for the posterior marking. Vertical plumb line is drawn in the midline and posterior axillary line and one in between. These vertical lines are to ensure symmetry of excision and to provide guidance during closure. The inferior incision is marked first. In the midline it starts at the cranial end of the natal cleft. Then it extends laterally in a lazy S fashion. The caudal most point of this line usually corresponds to the posterior axillary line. The superior incision is marked again using the pinch test. The midline pinch test is done with the patient bend down to prevent over excision at this point. The rest of the superior marking extends laterally and in cranial direction, at 45 degree, till the posterior axillary line. The lateral markings are made by simply joining the anterior and posterior markings. Pinch tests are repeated all around, simulating the position in which the patient is going to lie down on the operating room (OR) table, to reconfirm that the superior and inferior markings are going to come together without much tension (**Fig. 27.25**).

Thigh Lift Marking

With the patient standing erect and thighs slightly abducted, a vertical plumb line is drawn from the adductor tubercle down to medial condyle of tibia. This represents the final location of the scar and rest of the marking is done intraoperatively after the lower body lift procedure is complete. The patient is then asked to stand with the thighs adducted together. The vertical line, representing the final scar location, should not be visible from either the anterior or posterior aspect.

Lastly, the area of recalcitrant fat deposits is marked.

Anesthesia and General Care

On the morning of surgery the markings are rechecked and redrawn if necessary. In the OR general anesthesia is given with the patient on the trolley. The anterior markings are then scored with a 24-gauge needle lest they are washed away during surgical prep. Patient is catheterized and below

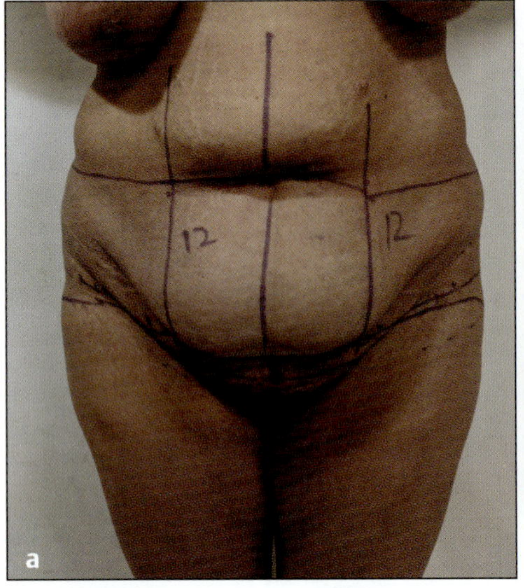

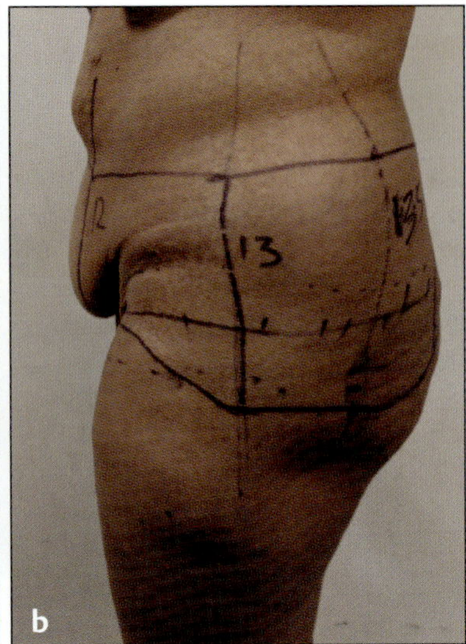

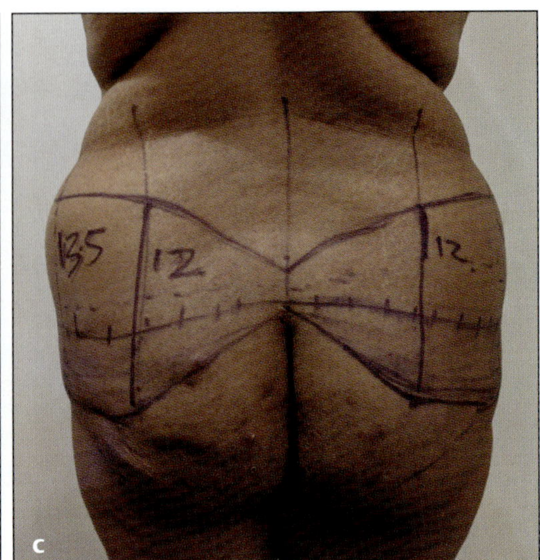

Fig. 27.25 (a–c) Completed marking for lower body lift. The superior marking is estimated by pinch test. To ensure symmetry, width of excision should be measured at predetermined points. (All measurements are in cm.)

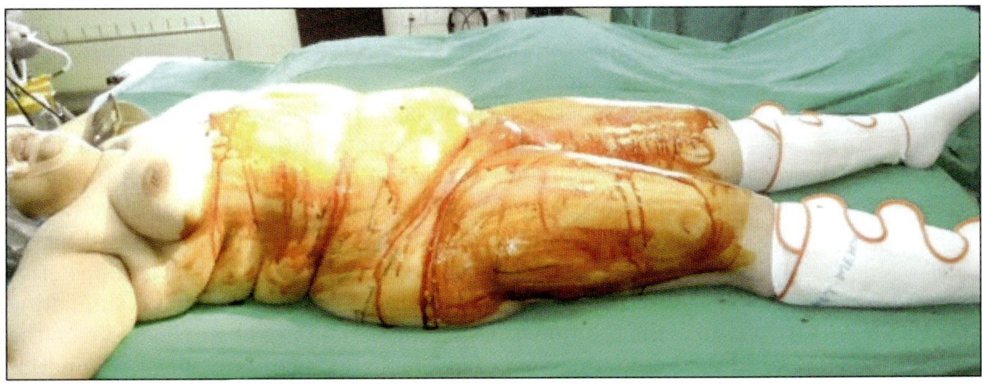

Fig. 27.26 The patient is intubated, marking scored with a hypodermic needle, prepped, and deep vein thrombosis (DVT) stocking and pump applied on the trolley before turning over on to the operating room (OR) table.

the knee DVT stocking and sequential compression devices are applied on both legs (**Fig. 27.26**).

Mild perioperative hypothermia (core temperature <36°C) is common and is attributed to anesthesia-induced loss of thermoregulation.[33] Maintenance of perioperative normothermia (>36°C) is critical in reducing the rate of SSI and the risk of morbid cardiac events. This is especially critical in body contouring surgeries which are of long duration and performed under general anesthesia. One can use forced air warmer (warming blanket), conductive heating mattress, warm IV fluid, and keep the ambient OR temperature at 22°C to maintain perioperative normothermia. Esophageal probe is used in the OR to continuously monitor the core temperature.

Propanol base solution (CUTASEPT, Bode Science Center) is used for the preparation of the skin. Initially, it is applied on the anterior aspect of the lower body. The operating (OR) table is covered with a sterile sheet. Thereafter the patient is rolled on from the trolley to OR table in a prone position. The posterior markings are also scored with 24-gauge needle and then prepped as above.

Pressure points are taken care of by placing gel pads under the knee and anterior iliac spine. It is important that the knee is kept slightly flexed, both in prone and supine position, for the duration of surgery. This is done by placing a folded towel/small pillow under the ankle in prone position or under the knee in supine position. Completely extended knee is known to cause popliteal vein compression which can then lead to DVT.[34]

Surgical Steps

The author applies the following key steps in all his excisional lifts, particularly for lower body, following MWL.

Positioning

Supine/lateral/lateral positioning is preferred by some authors for better lateral resection and more effective liposuction of the hip and trochanteric area.[28] However, this sequence of positioning is easier if the patient is placed on a bean bag on the OR table. The bean bag is inflated to stabilize the patient in lateral positioning.

The author prefers prone-supine positioning. This allows the surgeon to assess the symmetry of both sides following liposuction and excision and also saves time as only one turn is required.

Liposuction

Infiltration is done of the area of recalcitrant fat deposit (marked preoperatively) and also of excision site. The composition of infiltration solution used is given in **Table 27.5**.

Ropivacaine has the same efficacy as bupivacaine but with less potential for cardiotoxicity and neurotoxicity. The amount of lidocaine to be added to the infiltration solution is contentious. One study concluded that decreasing concentration of lidocaine did not alter the intraoperative anesthesia requirement or the postoperative pain control.[35] The lowest concentration used in this study was 100 mg/L of normal saline. Although plasma lidocaine level peaks 8–16 hours after infiltration, its tissue level is subtherapeutic within 4 to 8 hours of infiltration.[36] So lidocaine infiltration may reduce anesthetic requirement intraoperatively, but it cannot be relied upon to provide postoperative analgesia.

Initially the liposuction of the area of recalcitrant fat deposits is done. Most commonly these deposits are found on the trochanteric area, posterior and anterior thigh and upper abdomen.

Liposuction of the upper abdomen helps in two ways. First it discontinuously undermines the superior flap, preserving the vascular perforators, and so it becomes easier to pull it down in caudal direction during closure. Second the thick superior flap is thinned down to the same thickness as the inferior flap, which avoids the superior bulge during closure. If there are no fat deposits in the superior flap then the liposuction cannula, with the vacuum turned off, is used to create the aforementioned discontinuous tunnel. Similarly in the lateral thigh the liposuction cannula is used to create discontinuous channels in the vertical direction. For this the cannula is inserted from the inferior incision of lower body lift.

Next is the excision site liposuction (ESL).[37] This helps in two ways. It debulks the deep fat underneath the SFS. In addition it creates a meshed plane superficial to the SFS which facilitates avulsion excision (to be described later) of the panniculus. This in turn preserves the lymphatic channels, which run deep to the SFS, thereby preventing seroma formation. The author uses no. 6, triport (accelerator tip) cannula for ESL. The end point of ESL is an absolutely thinned out flap of less than half-inch thickness (**Fig. 27.27**).

Table 27.5 Composition of infiltration fluid

Infiltration fluid	Composition
Normal saline (0.9%)	1 L
Lidocaine	300 mg
Adrenaline	1 mg
Sodium bicarbonate (8.4%)	10 mL
Ropivacaine	75 mg

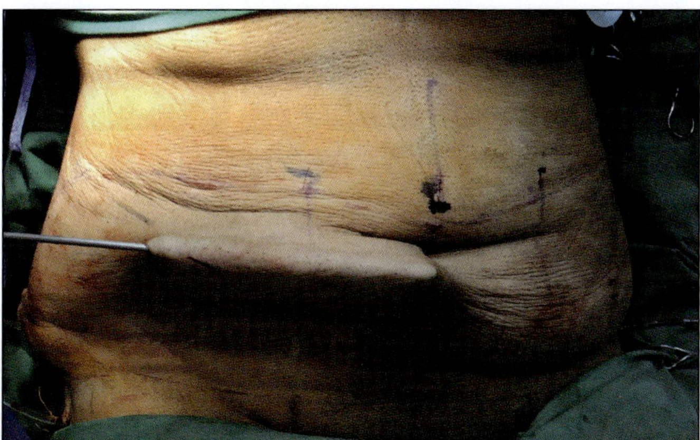

Fig. 27.27 The end point of excision site liposuction showing absolutely thinned-out flap.

Tailor Tacking

Measure twice cut once! This is the underlying principle of tailor tacking. It simulates the closure by approximating the two margins of excision. This is done by either towel clip or skin hooks (**Fig. 28a, b**). The approximation should be done without too much tension.

The marking of thigh lift is done after completion of the lower body lift. In the supine position the thigh to be marked is slightly flexed and abducted. Surgeon with the tip of his digits of one hand presses down on the vertical line on the medial thigh, drawn preoperatively. With the other hand the excess skin is pinched and the assistant applies the towel clip. This is done all along the vertical line. The points of penetration of the towel clip are marked, which gives the anterior and posterior edges of the vertical ellipse of medial thigh plasty (**Fig. 27.29**). Similar tailor tacking is done to mark the vertical excess of the upper medial thigh, if any. This gives a horizontal ellipse, superior edge of which is along the thigh perineal crease. The posterior end of the superior marking ends where the buttock meets the OR table. The anterior end of the superior marking can go up along the lateral border of the mons pubis to join the lower body lift incision (**Fig. 27.30**).

Avulsion Excision

The author uses a scalpel blade to cut the epidermis. Dermal bleeding can quickly add up to a significant blood loss, due to long incisions involved in excisional lift. So it is paramount that diathermy is used throughout once the epidermis is cut with scalpel. The incision is stopped above the SFS and then Kocher clamps are applied to one end of the pannus. The assistant pulls at the Kocher clamp toward him and the surgeon exerts countertraction. The panniculus then smoothly avulses along the meshed plane, superficial to the SFS, created by the ESL (**Fig. 27.31**). For the thigh lift when doing the avulsion excision it is done from proximal to distal to

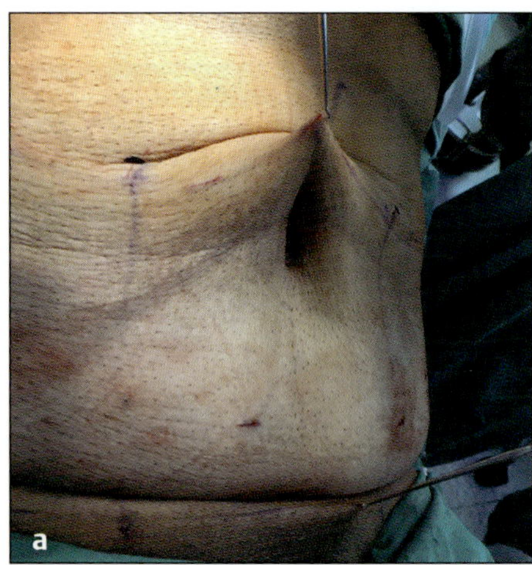

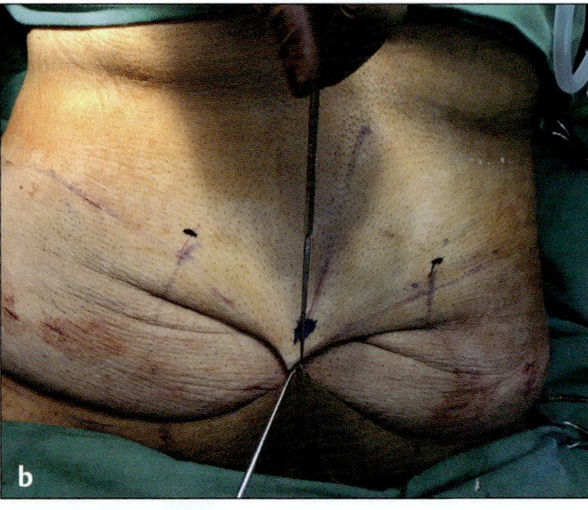

Fig. 27.28 (a, b) Tailor tacking, simulation of closure, being done with skin hooks.

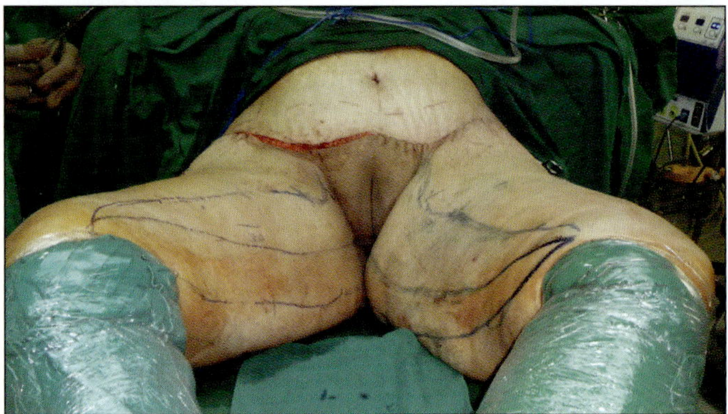

Fig. 27.29 Bilateral vertical medial thigh plasty marking showing the ellipse marked around the proposed line of closure.

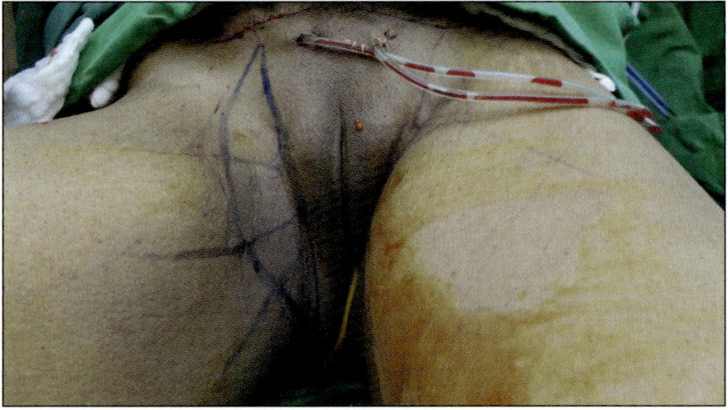

Fig. 27.30 Horizontal medial thigh plasty marking along the thigh perineal crease.

preserve the neurovascular and lymphatic branches. Along the mons thigh junction, the excision should be skin only as lymphatics travel from mons to the inguinal region in a superficial plane. Also the excision should be very superficial near the medial knee as here also lymphatics from the leg congregate and travel in a superficial plane. Hemostasis is done and the area is washed with normal saline to remove any debris.

Tranexamic Acid

This is a plasminogen inhibitor which delays clot degradation. Usually tranexamic acid is given parenterally in doses of 10 to 15 mg/kg repeated three to four times a day. However, parenteral administration carries a small risk of seizures.[38] Therefore, topical application is preferred which is as effective as parenteral administration but without the systemic risk. Usually 3 g of tranexamic acid is mixed with 100 mL of normal saline (3%) and sprayed over the excision site.

Closure

Barbed suture allows for knotless closure which reduces the foreign body load in the wound. This also reduces the closure time as there are no knots to be tied. It also evenly

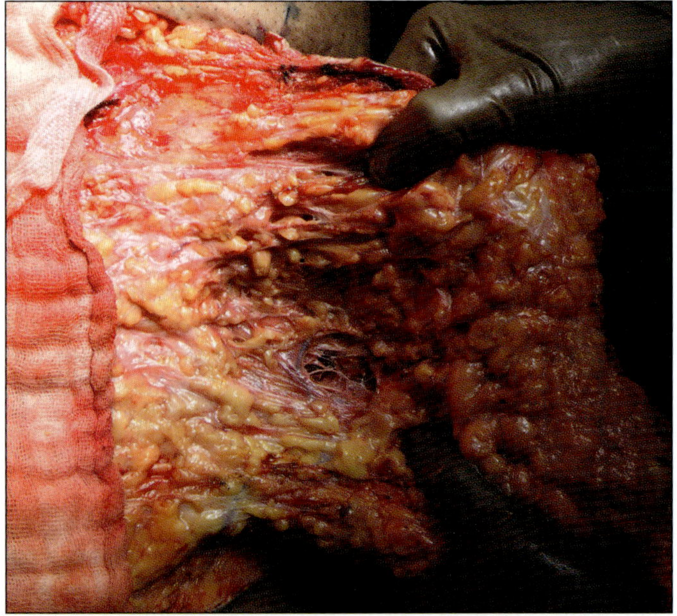

Fig. 27.31 Figure showing avulsion excision along the meshed plane (created by excision site liposuction [ESL]) superficial to superficial fascial system (SFS).

distributes the tension along the closure and is secure.[39] The author uses 2–0 Polydioxanone (Stratafix, Ethicon) bidirectional barbed suture with two 36-cm needles on either end of the suture. The large needle allows a full thickness bite on the thickest of the flap. The first bite is inside out from the subcutaneous fat. It is a bite of deep dermis a cm away from the wound edge, which exits just under the dermis. The second bite on the opposite edge of the wound is outside in. The needle enters under the dermis and takes a bite of deep dermis a cm away from the wound edge and exits from underneath the fat. The needle then takes the third bite, which is of the SFS (3-point suture) (**Fig. 27.32**). Two such passes are made on either side of the first bite and the needles are then pulled in the opposite direction which brings the wound edge together. The assistant continues with closure with one needle and the surgeon with the other. Once the end of the wound is reached a J knot is used to secure the closure. The second layer is 3–0 poliglecaprone (Monocryl, Ethicon) subcuticular suture.

Specific Measures in Relation to Specific Area

Debulking of SFS

Sometimes the SFS is also redundant in the anterior abdomen region. The author has recently started debulking the SFS by removing an ellipse along the superior incision. The SFS is then approximated with 2–0 polyglactin suture. Closed suction drain is placed.

Umbilicoplasty

In the anterior abdomen once the dissection reaches the umbilicus it is cored out in a pyramidal fashion leaving more fat on the stalk as one proceeds toward the base. This is done to preserve the blood supply to the umbilicus. Above the level of umbilicus dissection is performed superiorly in an inverted V fashion right up to the xiphisternum. The lateral limit of this supraumbilical dissection is up to the medial border of rectus abdominis to preserve the perforators. If divarication is present, rectal plication is done with 0-looped nylon, taking bites only at the medial border of rectus abdominis. Rectus muscle plication is strictly avoided in obese patients as it can lead to diaphragmatic splinting and respiratory compromise. The plication is done from xiphisternum to pubes. Cases which do not require plication, the supraumbilical dissection is performed only for few centimeters above the umbilicus. The neo umbilicus opening is made in the form of a cross 2.5 by 1 cm. The dermis of umbilicus and that of neo umbilical opening is then tacked to the external oblique aponeurosis with 3–0 monocryl at 3, 6, and 9 o'clock positions.

Postoperative Care

Patient is directly shifted from the OR table to the patient's bed under surgeon's supervision. The patient is placed in Fowler's position with the knee slightly flexed.

A patient is mobilized within 24 hours of surgery. The drain is removed when it is less than 30 mL/day. Compression garment is placed once the drain is removed. The patient is allowed to wet the area 3 to 4 days after drain removal. This is to allow the drain site to heal. Dressing is required till the healing is complete. Compression garment is to be worn 24/7 for 1 month and thereafter for 12 hours a day for another month. Scar cream for 2 months and sun protection for 6 months are advised once the healing is complete.

Adverse Events

Surgical Site Infection

SSI is an uncommon adverse event. Thigh plasty suture line near the perineum is prone to infection. So the author uses no dressing for the perineal suture line. Instead the patient is instructed to clean the area with antiseptic solution and topical antimicrobial cream application after every visit to the washroom.

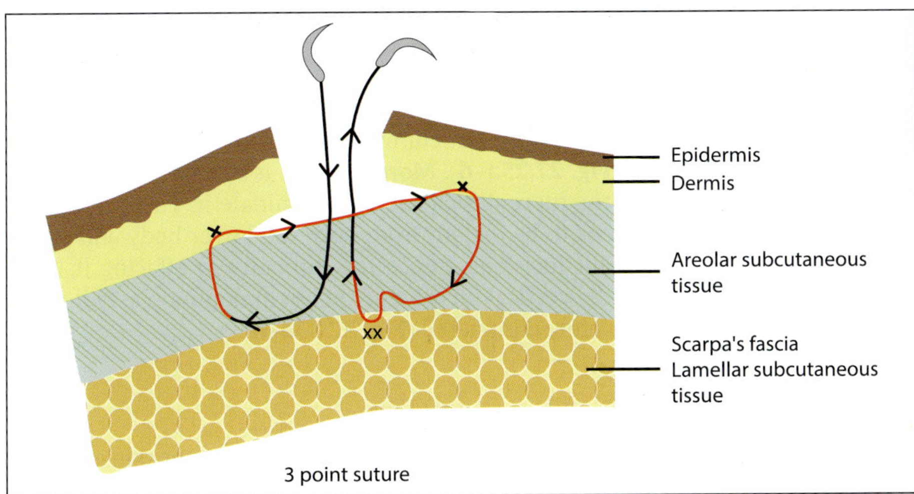

Fig. 27.32 Three-point suture. Full-thickness bite of either wound edge and third bite of SFS (two X). Single X represents bite of deep dermis.

The reduction of SSI is achieved by controlling the systemic and local factors. Systemically comorbid conditions like diabetes mellitus should be well controlled. BMI should be lower than 35 kg/m^2 as obesity increases the propensity to infection.

Micronutrient deficiency particularly of Copper and Zinc and Vit deficiency should be taken care of presurgery as they can increase the susceptibility of infection. Local factors such as clipping rather than shaving of hair, presurgery wash with alcohol-based CHG evening before and morning of surgery, prep with CHG-based solution, maintaining perioperative normothermia, minimizing exposure of tissue by rapidly closing excision site, and proper hemostasis all contribute to reducing the incidence of SSI. SSI can be superficial or deep and the majority of patients are treated by antibiotics covering Gram-positive organisms. Deep SSI can cause wound dehiscence.

Hematoma

Patients with MWL have large perforators which nourish the large panniculus before the weight loss. However, these perforators persist even after the weight loss. At the time of contouring surgery it is prudent to ligate these perforators securely as they can bleed after the blood pressure rises post anesthesia. Besides the above precaution, the author prefers to raise the blood pressure to preinduction level prior to closure, so that bleeders can be detected and ligated or coagulated. Any coagulopathy detected on presurgery tests should be corrected, and diathermy for all incision and excision, avulsion excision, and absolutely no undermining whatsoever are other steps to reduce the incidence of hematoma. The use of tranexamic acid spray lately has also contributed to reduce rebound oozing seen with epinephrine-induced vasoconstriction.

Hematoma if detected should be treated as an emergency and immediately evacuated. A small hematoma can be treated conservatively till it liquifies and then can be aspirated.

Seroma

The most common cause of seroma in excisional contouring surgery is breach of SFS. The importance of SFS in preventing seroma formation was emphasized by Saldanha in his seminal paper.[40] Preserving the SFS layer preserves the lymphatic channels running underneath, and also promotes adhesion of the overlying skin flap. In contrast, the smooth aponeurotic layer facilitates shear movement preventing adhesion of overlying skin flap. The resultant dead space along with disruption of lymphatic channel encourages seroma collection. Obesity and major concomitant liposuction are also risk factors for seroma formation. So in these patients the author prefers to leave the drain for up to 7 to 10 days despite draining less than 30 mL/day. Normally a seroma responds to repeated aspiration and compression. However once the pseudobursa forms it requires surgical excision.

Wound Dehiscence

Common causes of wound dehiscence is hematoma, deep SSI, seroma, excessive tension, compromised blood supply of the wound edges, and poor nutrition. Excessive tension often results at T junction of anchor abdominoplasty and thigh plasty, sometimes leading to dehiscence. Patients should be forewarned about this possibility. Fortunately most of the dehiscence heals with local wound care. Later on scar revision may be required.

Excessive tension can be avoided at the marking stage and during tailor tacking. Especially when excising the anterior abdominal panniculus the patient should not be propped up more than 20 degrees to prevent excessive tension on the wound edges as the patient straightens out in the postoperative phase. Conservative liposuction of the superficial fat compartment and absolutely no undermining will help preserve the blood supply to the wound edges. Poor nutritional status can also impair wound healing. This should be detected and treated prior to surgery.

Minor dehiscence will heal on its own. Almost all dehiscence are treated conservatively with local wound care. Subsequently the scar can be revised. This is a much better option than trying to debride and suture an edematous wound.

Residual Laxity

Patients who have lost upward of 80 to 100 kg generally have multitude of oblique folds in close proximity. This signifies multivector laxity and will be not effaced completely by excising in one or even two directions. In addition to multivector laxity these patients have global laxity, which means the remaining skin, after excising all the folds, is also of poor elasticity. All these combined together predispose to residual laxity/folds despite extensive excisional lifts (**Fig. 27.20e, f**).

The Middle Muddle

The epigastric fold also known as the middle fold is difficult to efface even with combination of upper and lower body lifts (**Fig. 27.25a–d**). More the fold is distant from the incision, the more difficult it is to eliminate it. The middle fold happens to be distant from both the lower body and upper body lift incisions, hence the difficulty in effacing it. Even with the vertical incision of anchor abdominoplasty it is not completely eliminated (**Fig. 27.33a–d**).

Recurrence of Laxity

It is common in patients who have global poor skin elasticity and also weight fluctuation after surgery. Patients should be

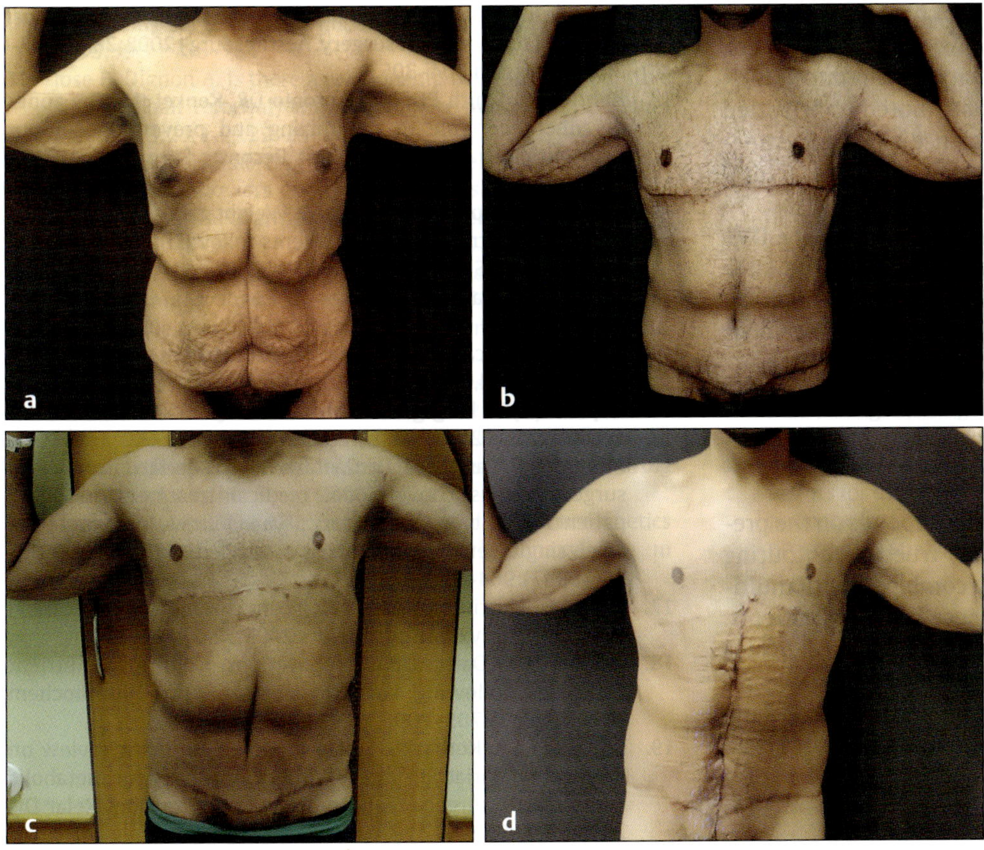

Fig. 27.33 (a) Following 85-kg weight loss. **(b)** Following upper and lower body lift. Patient refused to have anchor abdominoplasty. **(c)** Six months later the middle fold manifests itself again. **(d)** After anchor abdominoplasty some residual middle fold is still seen.

counseled and advised regarding this possibility. They are encouraged to adopt a healthy lifestyle to maintain a stable weight.

Asymmetrical Scars

Asymmetrical scars can mar the final aesthetic result. This can be prevented by taking measurement from a fixed bony point to different parts of the marking and making sure the measurements are symmetrical on the left and right sides.

Hypertrophic/Hyperpigmented Scar

Asian skin has a thicker dermis, with resultant increased collagen density, and higher melanin content compared with Caucasian skin. This encourages vigorous fibroblast response after any insult and combined with presence of higher melanin content results in higher incidence of hypertrophic and hyperpigmented scar in Asian population. The scars also take longer to mature. The patient should be cautioned regarding all the above, during the presurgery counseling.

The more the tension on the closure, the more the risk of hypertrophy and/or keloid formation. All the tension should be borne by the SFS layer. Once the SFS is approximated the skin edges should be kissing each other without sutures.

Other preventive measures for hypertrophic scar are silicone gel application on the scar once the healing is complete. Silicone gel is as effective as silicone sheets with added advantage of higher compliance. Generally, it is used for 2 to 3 months. Author combines silicone gel application along with pressure garment for the same period of time. Pulse dye laser has been found to be effective for treatment of hyperpigmented and hypertrophic scar.[41] Intralesional triamcinolone injection is used for recalcitrant hypertrophic scar or keloid.

Hypovolemia

Patients with restrictive bariatric surgery have limited oral intake and are more prone to postoperative nausea and emesis. This has to be borne in mind in the patients undergoing contouring surgery. The author prefers to give parenteral intravenous fluid for at least 24 to 48 hours postoperatively. Simultaneously, they are encouraged to gradually increase the oral intake of fluids. Otherwise, there is a risk of them going into hypovolemia.

Deep Vein Thromboembolism/Pulmonary Embolism

The incidence of venous thromboembolism (VTE) in western population varies from 33 to 88%. Bagaria et al found the incidence of DVT in Indian population, undergoing major orthopaedic surgery, to be 6.12% with an even lower

Buttock Augmentation

Introduction

> "The most popular image of the female despite the exigencies of the clothing trade is all boobs and buttocks, a hallucinating sequence of parabola and bulges"—Germaine Greer

In recent years, there has been a sudden surge in patients desiring buttock augmentation. This phenomenon can be attributed to the internet/social media effect of showing an hour-glass body shape and fuller derriere. Famous personalities have metamorphosed the concept of beauty by making curvier bodies with prominent buttocks a very enviable trait. Along with this there is a sudden explosion of gyms/fitness and wellness centers where many women wear tights and slacks. Even the normal anatomy of greater trochanteric depression is now called as "hip dips" and many "clients" come asking for their correction. Many times patients also want a fuller buttock projection to improve the shape and make sure their clothes/trousers don't fall flat and achieve a nicer shape. The procedure of buttock augmentation helps in achieving an hour-glass body shape or an "S" curve, a fuller behind and can also correct "hip dips" too!

Buttock augmentation with fat transfer has wrongly been called "Brazilian Butt Lift" for several years, because neither was this surgery described by any Brazilian surgeon nor does it give a lift to the buttocks as no sagging skin is excised.[1] A very important part of this procedure is liposculpting of other adjoining body areas like lower back, thighs, hips, and gluteal region, hence restricting it to just "Butt" doesn't do justice to the term. In recent years it has been advocated to better call it as Safe Subcutaneous Buttock Augmentation.[2] The combination of removal of fat from certain areas of the body and addition to other areas helps in redistribution of fat and changing the body proportions. Only addition of implants cannot achieve the desired results; hence, the popularity of choosing this technique for buttock augmentation. Liposuction of lower back and flanks along with fat transfer to buttocks helps in achieving concavity to convexity, which is aesthetically pleasing.[3]

Controversy

As the case numbers of buttock augmentation with fat increased, it also led to increase in complications, including most dreaded complications of pulmonary fat embolism (PFE), both fatal and nonfatal. A task force under the aegis of Aesthetic Surgery Education & Research Foundation reported 1 in 6214 cases of fatal and 1 in 1931 cases of nonfatal PFE events.[4] Apart from this there are a number of publications reporting such complications.[5–10] The procedure went into so much disrepute that some plastic surgery societies warned their members against performing buttock augmentation procedure.[11,12]

It has been suggested that most of the problems associated with this procedure are due to fat grafting in deeper layers like subfascial and deep muscular layers,[1,4] as there is risk of fat being injected directly into the large gluteal vessels.[13] It is also postulated that fat when injected into deeper subfascial layers raises the compartment pressure. The fat under pressure may be sucked into the deep veins with lower intraluminal pressure.[4,13]

Many surgeons believed that transfer of fat to muscle will help in better survival of adipocytes, based on the principle of muscle having better blood supply as compared to subcutaneous tissue. This thought arises from the knowledge that muscle flaps have better blood supply than fascial flaps.[14] However, the fat survivability depends upon oxygen diffusion and not blood flow. Oxygen tension is same in subcutaneous tissue as well as muscle, and hence, that is the key determinant in fat survival.[13]

Fat transfer to subcutaneous tissue of buttock is safe, but a dilemma arises as to how to inject in sufficient quantity without reaching into deeper layers. Apart from knowledge of anatomy, this procedure demands technical skills and tools to transfer fat aliquots strictly in a subcutaneous plane with enough tissue around to help make this fat survive. There are multiple fascial adhesions between muscular and dermal layers in this region. To make sure that the injected fat remains in subcutaneous space, these fibrous adhesions need to be broken to expand the space using the technique of expansion vibration lipofilling (EVL).[15–18] A power-driven cannula is used to expand the subcutaneous space as well as transfer the fat through pressure system at the same time. Expansion has also shown to improve the survival of grafted fat as pre-expansion and fat transfer have worked for breast augmentation as well.[19,20]

Clinical Anatomy

Clear knowledge of anatomy of the gluteal region is of utmost importance before attempting the buttock augmentation procedure. Muscles of this region are divided into superficial and deep groups. Superficial groups of muscles are large muscles, namely, gluteus maximus, gluteus medius, gluteus minimus, and tensor fascia lata laterally (**Fig. 28.1a**). Smaller deeper muscles are piriformis, obturator internus, gemellus superior, gemellus inferior, and quadratus femoris (**Fig. 28.1b**).[1]

Superior and inferior gluteal arteries (**Fig. 28.2**) are branches of the internal iliac artery. Superior gluteal artery enters this region along with superior gluteal nerve through greater sciatic foramen above the upper border of piriformis muscle and finally divides into superficial and deep branches. The superficial branch enters the deep surface of the gluteus maximus, and supplies the muscle and

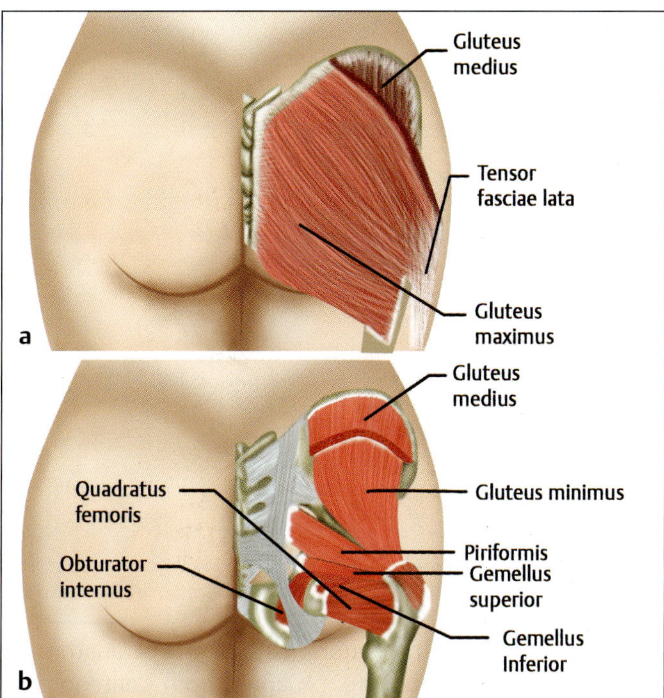

Fig. 28.1 Gluteal muscles. **(a)** Superficial muscles. **(b)** Deep muscles. (Adapted from Villanueva et al 2018.[13])

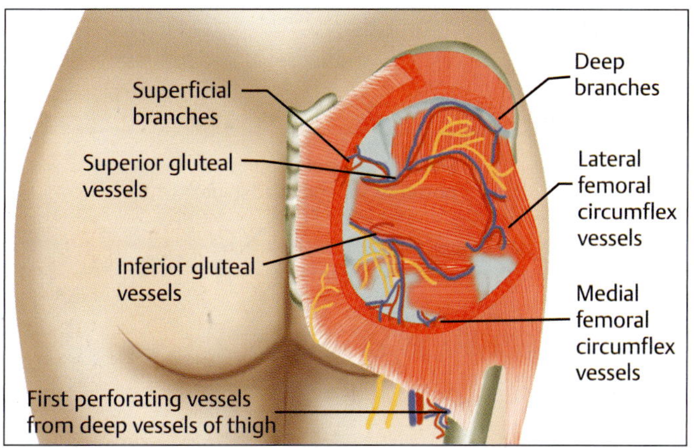

Fig. 28.2 Gluteal vascular anatomy. (Adapted from Villanueva et al 2018.[13])

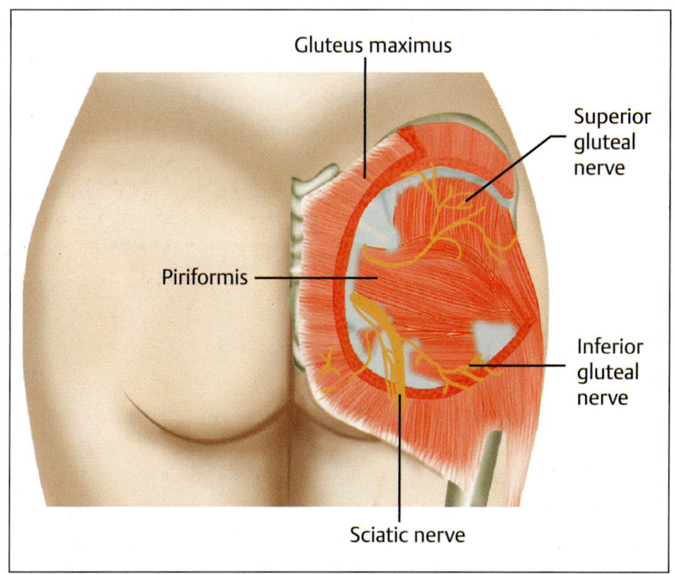

Fig. 28.3 Gluteal nerves. (Adapted from Villanueva et al 2018.[13])

anastomoses with the inferior gluteal artery. A few branches perforate the muscle's tendinous origin, and supply the skin covering the posterior surface of the sacrum, anastomosing with the posterior branches of the lateral sacral arteries. The deep branch lies under the gluteus medius muscle.

Inferior gluteal artery also enters through greater sciatic foramen along with inferior gluteal nerve inferior to piriformis muscle and supplies the lower half buttock region extending into posterior thigh.

Superior and inferior gluteal veins are venae comitantes of their respective arteries and join the pelvic plexus of veins and ultimately drain into the femoral vein. The sciatic nerve enters the gluteal region through the greater sciatic foramen inferior to the piriformis muscle between the superficial and deep group of gluteal muscles (**Fig. 28.3**).[13]

One of the important landmarks (**Fig. 28.4**) in planning buttock augmentation procedure is the posterior-superior iliac spines (PSIS). They define two important aesthetic depressions. The first one being a sacral dimple that forms due to insertion of gluteus maximus at PSIS, along with confluence of lumbosacral aponeurosis and the multifidus muscle. Another depression it forms is sacral triangle with opposite side PSIS and the coccyx being the inferior point. The liposculpting maneuvers should be done to accentuate these two depressions for an aesthetically pleasing result.

Infragluteal fold is formed by thick fascial condensations between the intermuscular fascia and skin. This defines the inferior limit of buttock. Short infragluteal fold limited to the medial half of the total width is desirable, and is often called a "Happy Bottom." Longer fold is formed in aged and deflated buttock with skin excess and gives it a ptotic look, often called a "Sad Bottom."

Lateral depression is formed by greater trochanter and insertions of gluteus mediums, vastus lateralis, quadratus femoris, and gluteus maximus. This depression gives the gluteal region an athletic-toned look, although recently this depression has been defined as hip dips and many patients come for its augmentation to get a fuller and rounder buttock shape.

With this knowledge of muscular and vascular anatomy, one has to be wary of the danger triangle[13] in buttock augmentation. For each buttock, mark a triangle joining PSIS, greater trochanter, and ischial tuberosity (**Fig. 28.5**). This triangle is the zone where all the major vessels and nerves are situated. One should be especially careful in this triangular zone while performing the procedure and always be aware that the tip of the cannula remains superficial.

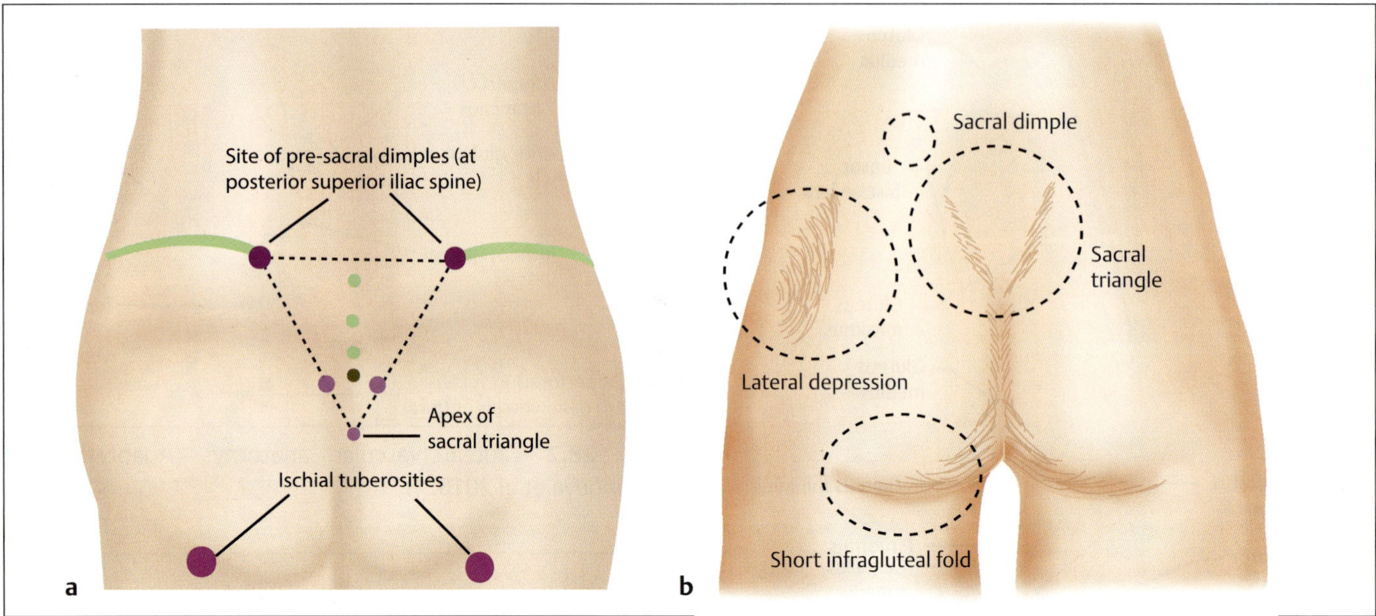

Fig. 28.4 Important anatomical landmarks in planning the buttock augmentation procedure. **(a)** Superficial anatomical landmarks. **(b)** Different features which help in defining aesthetic goals after the procedure. (Adapted from Centeno et al 2018.[21])

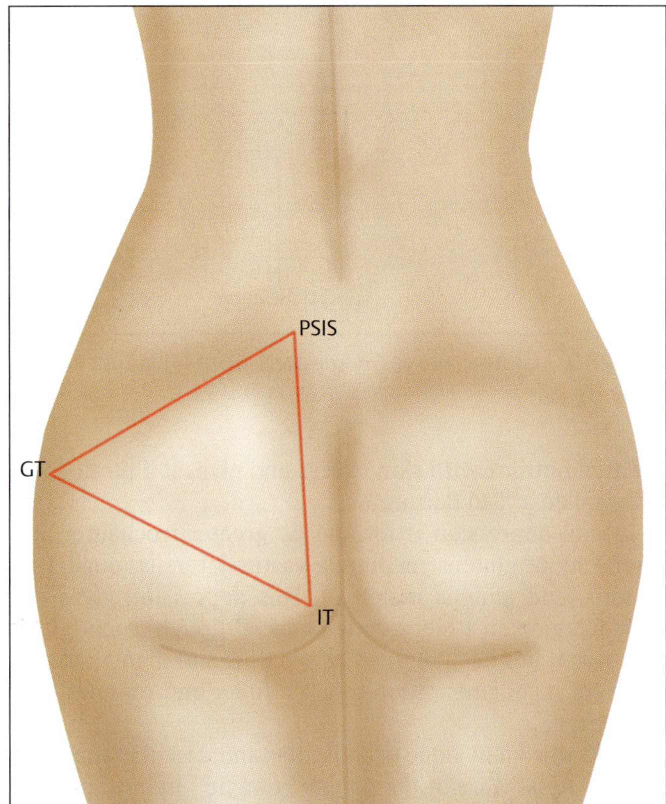

Fig. 28.5 Danger *triangle* in buttock augmentation. PSIS, posterior superior iliac spine; IT, ischial tuberosity; GT, greater trochanter. Deep injection within the area of the triangle increases the risk of vascular or sciatic injury. (Adapted from Villanueva et al 2018.[13])

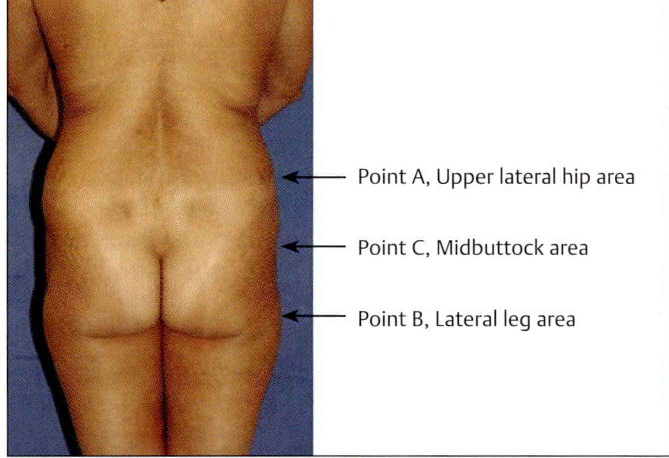

Fig. 28.6 Points which help define different frame types. (Adapted from Mendieta 2006.[22])

Aesthetic Zones and Defining Aesthetic Goals

Buttocks have multiple shapes, and they have been classified into different frames depending upon the pattern of fat distribution.[22] Mendieta has described buttock frame shapes after joining landmark points over the buttock. Point A is the most projecting part in the upper lateral hip, point B is the most projecting part in lateral thigh, and C is the midlateral buttock region which corresponds to greater trochanteric depression (**Fig. 28.6**). Joining points A to B defines the frame shapes of Dr Mendieta (**Fig. 28.7**).

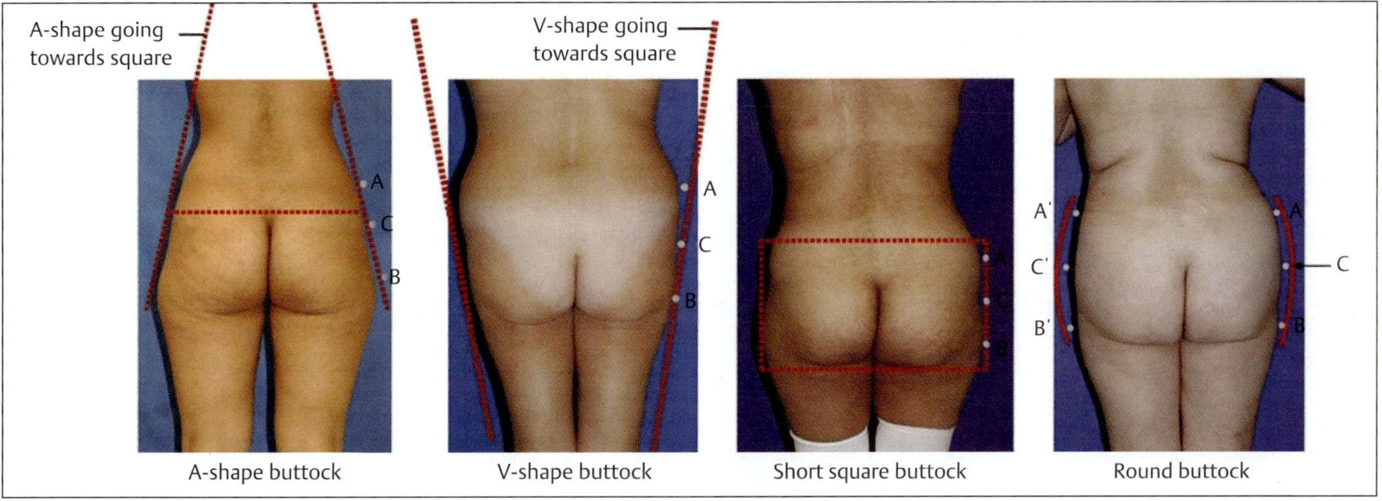

Fig. 28.7 Four different buttock shapes: A, V, square, and round. (Adapted from Mendieta 2006.[22])

Point C helps in differentiating between square and round buttocks. It also aids in grading the trochanteric depression as mild, moderate, or severe. Many times mild depression at point C does not need correction as it improves after liposuction of points A and B.

Square shape being the most common of buttock shapes is also most amenable to treatment by liposuction at points A and B, with point C being fat grafted only when necessary (**Fig. 28.8**). Round-shaped buttocks need improvement of other aesthetic zones around the buttocks to enhance their look. "A" shape buttocks require liposuction at point B and fat grafting of point C if needed (**Fig. 28.9**). "V" shape buttock usually needs liposuction only at point A to achieve well-defined buttocks.

Many times there are intermediate shapes or asymmetry. In such a situation, the surgery is individualized and is executed following the basic principles.

Dr Mendieta has also described ten aesthetic zones of the posterior body which affect gluteal contouring procedure.[23] These zones (**Fig. 28.10**) take into consideration the aesthetics of the back, buttock, and posterior thigh and are important as each of these subunits need to be contorted to achieve a more harmonious and pleasing result. Units 1 to 5 and 8 truly define the gluteal region. Zone 8 corresponds to greater trochanteric depression which needs fat grafting if the patient desires a round shape of buttocks. Zones 3 and 6 are other zones which need fat grafting for gluteal augmentation.

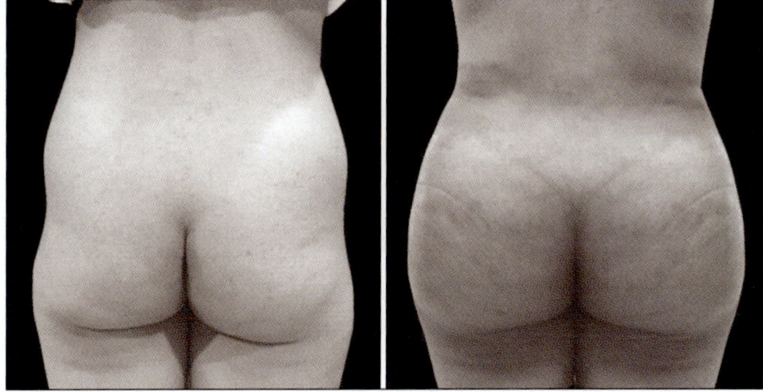

Fig. 28.8 A square-shaped buttock with liposuction of points A and B along with 700 mL of fat grafted to each buttock in two sessions.

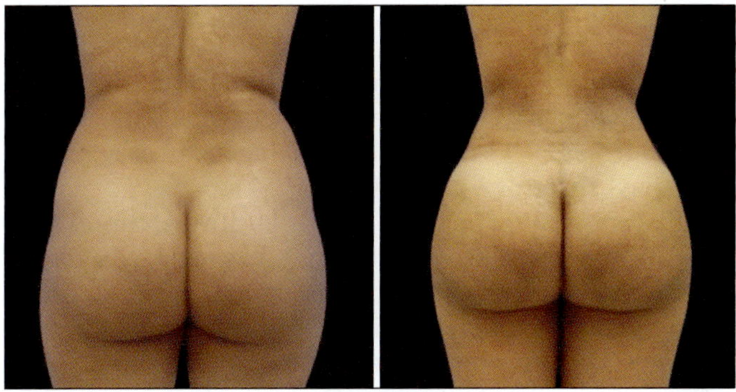

Fig. 28.9 An "A"-shaped buttock with liposuction of point B and 600mL fat grafted to each buttock. Liposuction of flank and upper back has also been performed for further refinement of the results.

Safe Subcutaneous Buttock Augmentation with Fat Transfer

Preoperative Considerations

During preoperative checkup, aesthetic goals need to be defined for each patient. Whether the patient desires projection of buttocks or increase in width or both needs to be ascertained. At the same time, the severity of hip dips (greater trochanteric depressions) should be noted and a discussion carried out with the patient regarding their wish to retain the athletic look or achieve a round buttock shape

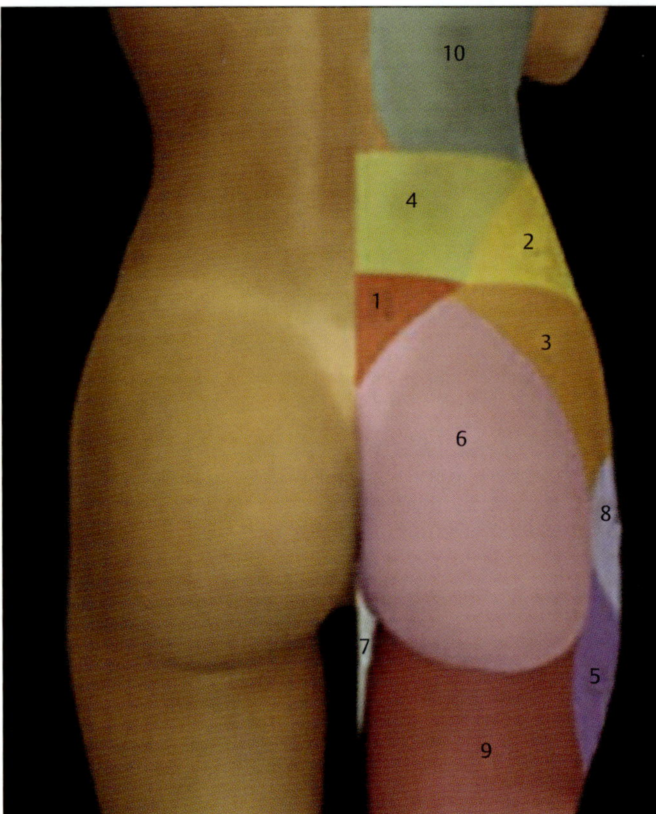

Fig. 28.10 Ten aesthetic units of posterior body as described by Mendieta.[23] 1. Sacrum V-zone; 2. Flank; 3. Upper buttock; 4. Lower back; 5. Outer thigh; 6. Gluteus; 7. Diamond zone: inner gluteal/leg injection; 8. Midlateral buttock point C; 9. Inferior gluteal/posterior thigh junction; 10. Upper back.

by augmentation of the dips. One should always make sure that patient's expectations are kept realistic and in accordance with their anatomical structure. Patient's existing waist:hip ratio should be calculated. The desirable hip:waist ratio for patients wanting a more athletic look with less lateral fullness is >0.7 and for those looking for an exaggerated hour-glass shape or S-curve is <0.7.

Adjacent areas of body fat such as back area, lateral hips, and thigh region along with abdomen also need to be examined, to ascertain the need of liposuction and contouring. The amount of parietal fat, diastasis of recti, or presence of any ventral hernia should be noted. Patients should have sufficient donor site fat to spare. Patients who have very low body fat composition are poor candidates for buttock augmentation with fat transfer; however, they can be asked to gain fat to optimize the yield of fat extraction. Lipoaspirate should be used judiciously in thin individuals. Such patients are therefore asked to prioritize their needs so that fat transfer can be carried out for achieving upper buttock fullness, projection of buttocks, increase in width, or correction of lateral trochanteric depression, according to aesthetic goals.

Thorough medical history is taken and physical examination is performed as for any surgical procedure. History of any hematological disorders, use of anticoagulants, and herbal remedies that increase bleeding risk should be ascertained.[24] Patient should be asked for any personal or family history of pulmonary embolism and in case of doubt, relevant investigations should be done.

Lower extremities are examined to rule out any varicose vein disease as these may increase the chances of venous injury during the surgery. One should record any preexisting sciatic nerve motor or sensory symptoms.

A detailed and informed consent, mentioning the particulars of the procedure, patient's requirements and risks including pulmonary embolism needs to be undertaken after due counseling.

Surgical Technique

Markings

The markings are done in standing position. The zones for liposuction are defined and marked (**Fig. 28.11**). PSIS, greater trochanter, ischial tuberosity, and iliac crest are marked. Iliac crest helps in defining the lower-most region of liposuction and starts off the gluteal region for augmentation inferior to it. It is also a good idea to mark the zones of sacral dimple and sacral triangle so that these areas can also be liposuctioned. Once the buttock area is defined, zones for fat grafting are marked as per plan. Danger triangle (joining PSIS, greater trochanter, and ischial tuberosity) is drawn to ascertain the location of vessels and nerves. Superficial irregularities and cellulites on skin are marked for selective subcision and augmentation as indicated.

Fat Harvest

It is preferable to do this surgery under general anesthesia since large areas like abdomen, upper and lower back, buttock, and thigh region need to be operated. Author prefers to start the surgery with abdominal liposuction. A circumferential or 360-degree liposuction achieves a better contour than selective areas done at different stages. One should consider this as circumferential devolving of the skin from underlying muscle, so that it redrapes and contracts uniformly, which may not occur if performed in multiple stages. Besides, there is no difference in viability of adipocytes irrespective of the donor sites—abdomen, thigh, or flanks.[25–28] With the patient in supine position, the bladder is catheterized. Painting with povidone-iodine solution and surgical draping is done from nipple to infrapatellar region. For liposuction of the lower abdomen two access incisions are given at the lower end of the lateral border of the rectus abdominis. A third incision is placed in the supraumbilical region (**Fig. 28.12a**). For liposuction of the medial thigh two access incisions are taken—one in medial supracondylar region and the other in the medial midthigh. Infiltration of tumescent solution into the abdominal and thigh donor areas is facilitated with power-assisted system and peristaltic pump. Tumescent solution consists of one liter of normal saline with 10 mL of 2% plain lignocaine and one milliliter of 1:1000 adrenaline.

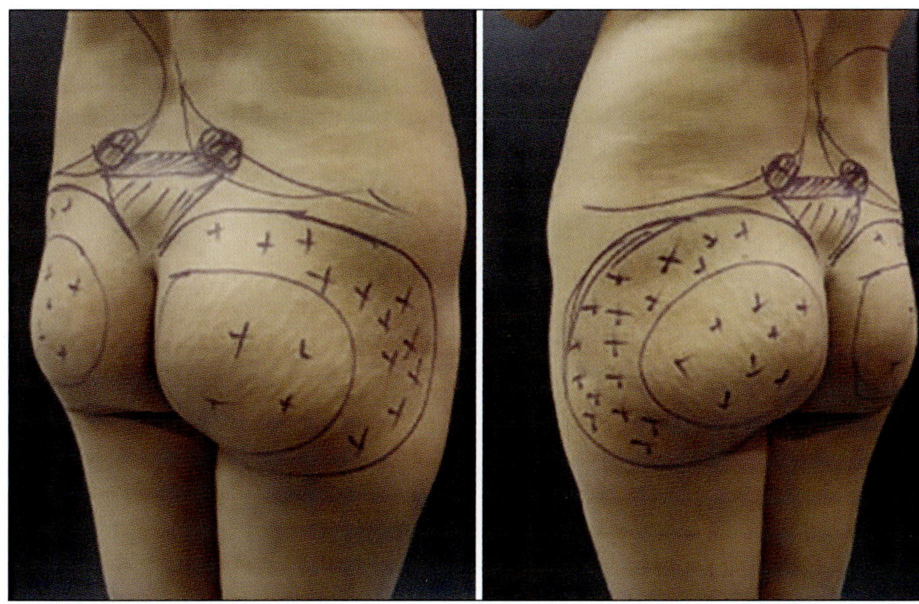

Fig. 28.11 Areas of liposuction are marked in lower back, along with marking of sacral dimples. Buttock outlines are marked with plus signs in the zone where fat grafting needs to be done.

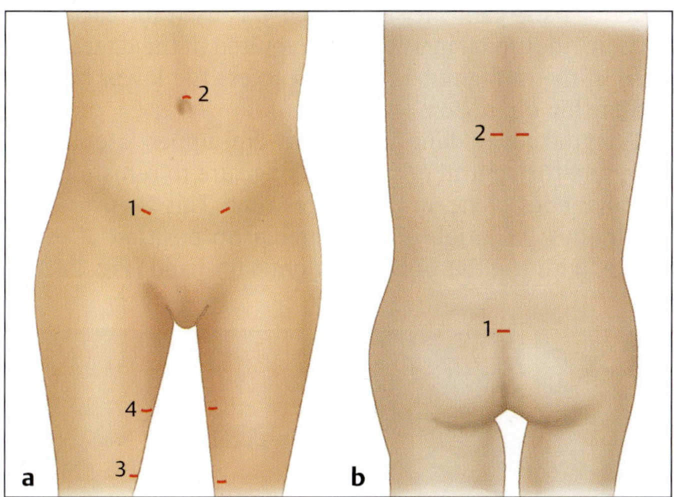

Fig. 28.12 **(a)** Incisions for liposuction of abdomen and thigh. 1. Lower end of the lateral border of rectus abdominis; 2. Supraumbilical; 3. Medial supracondylar; 4. Medial midthigh. **(b)** Incisions for liposuction of back. 1. Superior natal cleft; 2. Paravertebral midback region.

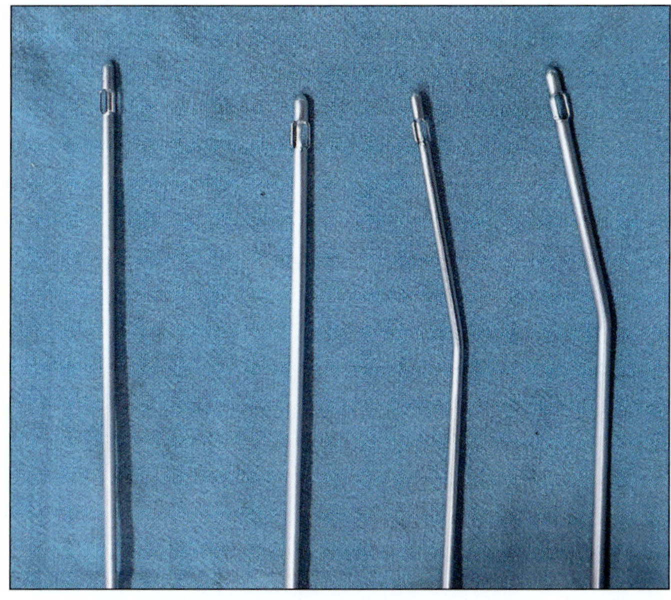

Fig. 28.13 Flared Mercedes cannulas: 4 mm, 5 mm. Angled 4 mm, Angled 5 mm.

Concepts of SAFELipo (Separation, Aspiration, and Fat Equalization) technique[29,30] is preferred using technologies such as ultrasound-assisted lipoplasty (UAL) like VASER (vibration amplification of sound energy at resonance) (Sound Surgical Technologies, Louisville, CO) and power-assisted liposuction (PAL) such as MicroAire (MicroAire Surgical Instruments, LLC, Charlottesville, VA). UAL port is inserted and surrounded by a moist mop. Fat emulsification is done with UAL probe on pulsed mode (V) at 70%. Power-oscillating flared Mercedes cannula (**Fig. 28.13**) without suction is used to release adhesions. Lipoaspiration is performed using 4-mm cannula with flared Mercedes design at a pressure of 500 mm Hg. Using blunt, large-bore cannulas with lower pressure suction for fat harvest has shown to improve viability of adipocytes.[31] The aspirated fat is collected in a calibrated closed sterile canister. Fat equalization is done with MicroAire using 4- or 5-mm cannula with flared Mercedes (basket) tip after disconnecting suction. The access incisions are sutured.

Patient is then turned prone and is placed in a Jack-knife position with silicon blocks placed under the chest and thighs. Cleaning and draping are done from tip of scapula to midthigh region. Access incisions for liposuction are placed in the superior natal cleft and paravertebral region in midback (**Fig. 28.12b**). Liposuction of back is done similarly as was done for abdomen and thighs. Focused liposuction is done in the sacral dimples and sacral triangle zone along with lower back as it enhances the aesthetic appeal by increasing the apparent anteroposterior projection of the buttocks.[32]

Fat Preparation

The collected aspirate is allowed to sediment and all the tumescent fluid is drained. Subsequently, the fat is washed with sterile normal saline to clean the blood and extraneous tissue and allowed to sediment again. The sediment component is then discarded, leaving pure fat behind in the canister. Closed system of fat collection helps in prevention of contamination. In literature, none of the techniques described to process the fat has shown superiority of one over the other.[26] Use of centrifugation in large-volume fat grafting is technically difficult. Total amount of fat left for grafting after two rounds of sedimentation and draining of fluid is nearly 50% of the original aspirate amount. For example, up to 1500 mL of usable fat is collected from a 3000 mL lipoaspirate (**Fig. 28.14**).

Fat Grafting

The most important step in gluteal fat grafting procedure is transfer of fat in the buttock region, which needs to be performed with utmost care using safe surgical tools. ASERF task force recommends the utilization of large blunt injection cannula for fat transfer, using constant motion. Awareness of tip of cannula is to be maintained and it should never be angulated downward. It is also recommended to avoid fat grafting to the muscular layer. Fat transfer is done with the patient in a jack-knife position to make sure that the fat is always transferred in a subcutaneous plane. Lateral decubitus position is not recommended as it is difficult to ensure symmetry between both buttocks.

The separated fat is grafted to designated recipient areas in the buttocks with the subcutaneous-only strategy.[15] Fat is transferred using the EVL technique[18] and the instrument used is a flared Mercedes basket tip 4- or 5-mm cannula attached to power-assisted lipofilling device (**Fig. 28.15**). The cannula is 40 cm in length, either straight or curved. The instrument is powered by a pump with a flow rate of 200 mL per minute. This works on a principle opposite to that of liposuction. Thin cannulas are flexible and may accidentally bend at the interface of syringe and cannula, which can lead to inadvertent deposition of fat at deeper layers,[13] whereas large-bore cannulas are more rigid and ensure precise fat placement and have also shown to increase the survival of adipocytes in large-volume fat grafting.[31,33]

Lipofilling of upper buttock can be done using the same superior natal cleft incision which was used for back liposuction. Additional incisions are required in the lateral one-third of the infragluteal region to access the lower buttock and the hip dip region.

Fat grafting is done in the hip dip, upper lateral buttock, and the central portion, making sure to remain in the subcutaneous plane, in the danger zone. This is ensured by continuous palpation of the cannula tip position at every stroke, with the flat of the nondominant hand (**Fig. 28.16**).

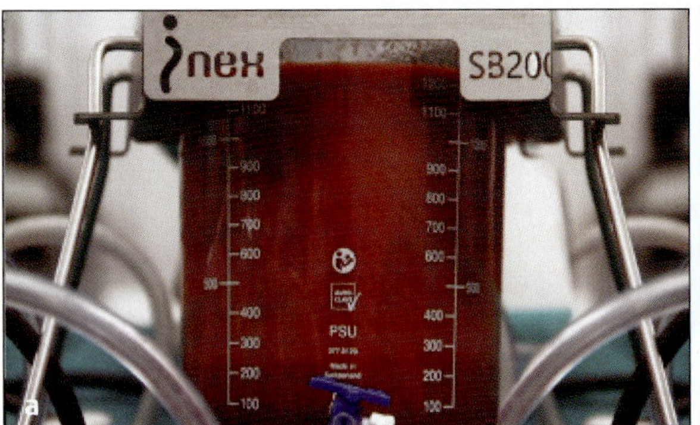

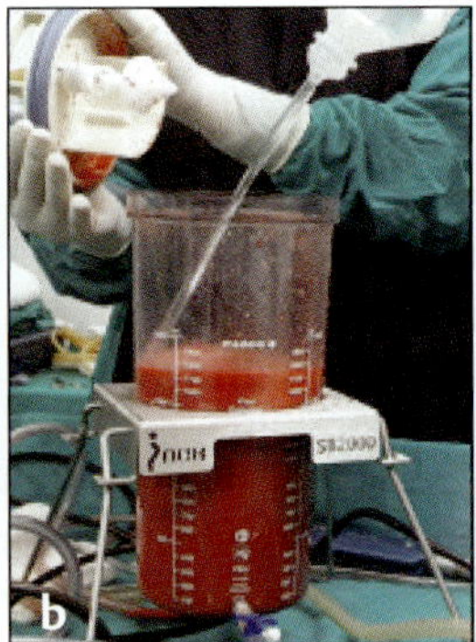

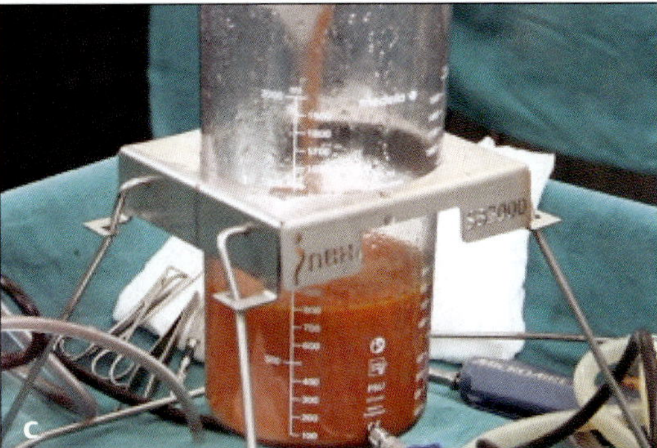

Fig. 28.14 **(a)** Collected fat after liposuction. **(b)** Fat being washed with Normal Saline. **(c)** Pure fat left after washing and decanting.

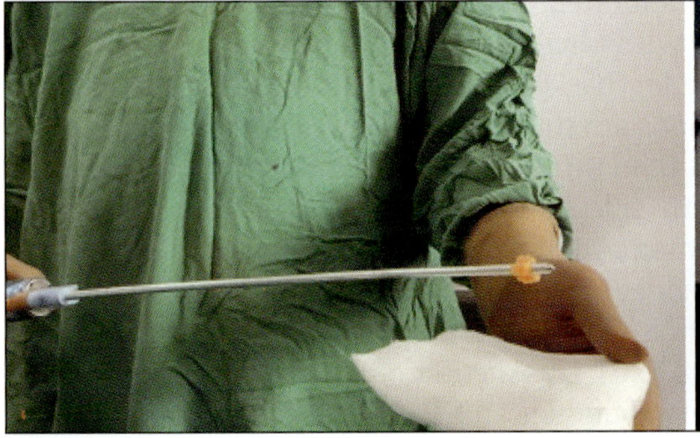

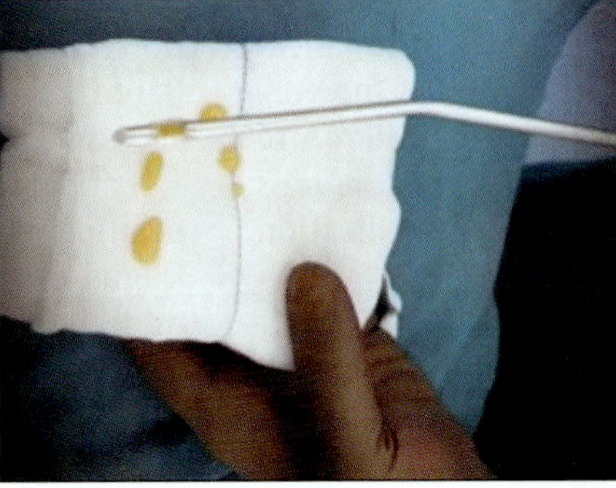

Fig. 28.15 Fat coming out of flared Mercedes cannula.

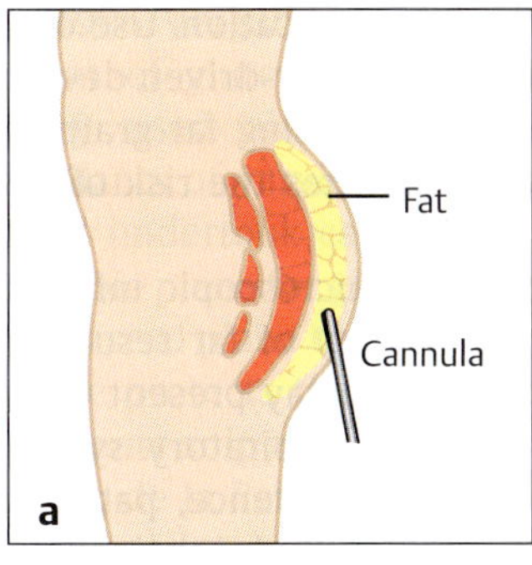

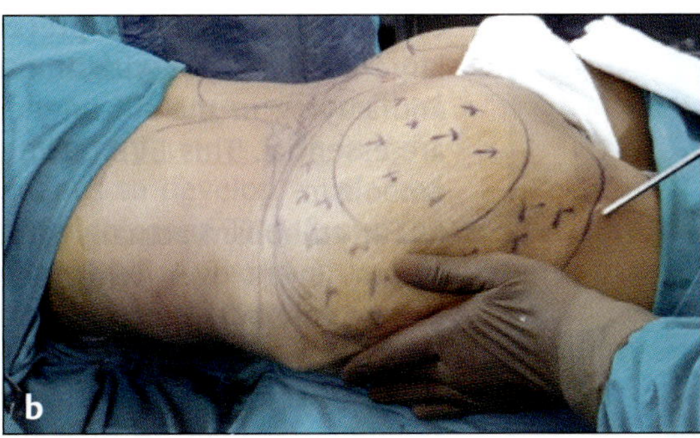

Fig. 28.16 (a) Diagrammatic representation of placement of fat strictly in subcutaneous plane while performing gluteal augmentation. **(b)** Nondominant hand feeling each stroke of cannula and guiding the procedure.

The nondominant hand, thus, plays the most important role in ensuring safety during this procedure. Remaining strictly in the superficial plane especially in the danger zone is of utmost importance to avoid inadvertent injury to vessels and nerves, or direct intravascular injection. There are reports of use of real-time high-frequency ultrasound during the procedure to make sure that transferred fat is restricted to subcutaneous plane.[34] However, intraoperative use of ultrasound probe is cumbersome and adds to the cost as well as operative time.

Continuous motion while lipofilling is of utmost importance. It helps in achieving even distribution of fat cells so that enough amount of well-vascularized tissue surrounds each aliquot of fat. It also prevents continuous fat injection into an injured vessel. Power-assisted oscillating cannula also helps in even distribution of fat by release of adhesions and ligamentous structures. The resultant expansion of the existing subcutaneous space enhances the ease of fat transfer. Multiple passes are made in different directions to ensure homogenous spread of fat. It is also recommended to perform gentle massage in between and at the end of the procedure for even distribution of the fat. Areas of superficial gluteal irregularities and dimple-like depressions are released and fat grafted to even out the skin surface.

It is impossible to accurately know the exact amount of fat required for each patient as it depends upon tissue compliance and skin elasticity. While fat is being transferred, decrease in tissue resistance to cannula movement (as substantial adhesions between muscle and dermis are released) gives an idea of adequate filling. The transferred fat starts getting continuously extruded from the access incision site, which indicates the end point of lipofilling. Also, the skin feels turgid similar to the way it feels after tumescent infiltration. One should avoid overfilling as there is a risk of fat absorption. The high pressure created by overfilling of fat can also, theoretically, increase the chances of pulmonary embolism in cases of venous injury.

Water-tight closure of the access incisions is done to prevent extrusion of the grafted fat. The patient is returned to supine position with pillow placed under thighs to relieve pressure on the buttocks. Emphasis is laid on adequate intraoperative pain management and intravascular fluid balance. A vigilant anesthetist is a quintessential part of the surgical team.

Postoperative Care

Compression dressing is applied at the end of surgery, keeping the buttocks open (**Fig. 28.15**). After a few hours, the dressing is replaced by a compression garment to cover all liposuction areas, keeping the buttock region exposed. Patients are advised to use the pressure garment round the clock for the next 6 weeks except while taking bath. Bathing is encouraged from the next day of surgery.

Early ambulation is recommended, and patients are encouraged to walk 5 to 6 hours after surgery. Mechanical prophylaxis for venous thrombosis by DVT pumps is done in all patients during and immediately after surgery. Chemical prophylaxis is used in high-risk individuals or patients with more than 4 liters of lipoaspirate or surgical duration more than 4 hours, as per the recommendation of American Society of Plastic Surgery Task force on Deep Vein Thrombosis prophylaxis.[35–38]

Offloading or avoiding compression on buttocks is recommended for at least 2 weeks postoperatively. It is recommended that patients sleep in a prone position and sit only on their thighs with special pillows (**Fig. 28.17**) which keep the buttocks off the chair. Cardio and muscle toning exercises are started after 2 weeks of surgery.

Complications

Asymmetry and Contour Irregularities

Subtle asymmetry is not uncommon after the procedure. Many times, asymmetry is present preoperatively which should be pointed out to the patient before surgery. Perfect symmetry between any two body parts is an illusion and should never be chased.

Differential fat absorption between each side is uncommon. Some superficial irregularities may remain due to cellulite, excessive superficial fat transfer, or scar formation. Depending upon each case, correction is planned after 6 months. Excess superficial fat may require liposuction using fine cannula. For small nodular scars, intralesional steroid injections can be tried. Dimpled scars can be corrected by subcision and small fat transfer. Despite meticulous technique, if gross asymmetry happens, one should wait for at least 6 months to ensure complete assessment

Type of Implants

Silicone Gel or Solid Elastomer

Implants with highly cohesive silicone gel with thick shells have a soft and natural feel to them. The projection is more as compared to solid elastomer implants. However, there is an inherent risk of rupture associated with these implants. On the other hand, the solid elastomer implants are rupture-free but have a firm feel to them and provide less projection.[49] At present in the United States, the use of only elastomer implants is permitted for gluteal augmentation. Elsewhere, both cohesive silicone gel type and solid elastomer type are available for use.

Implant Shape

Round implants provide more fullness in the upper and central parts of the buttock, whereas anatomic implants result in more of lower pole fullness (**Fig. 28.19**).

Indications and Preoperative Evaluation

The indications for buttock augmentation with implants are the same as for lipotransfer and include lack of volume, projection, presence of contour irregularity, or gluteal asymmetry. Lean patients with insufficient subcutaneous fat for lipotransfer benefit the most with implant placement in the gluteal region. An ideal patient has lack of projection with little or no ptosis, is of normal weight, has sufficient soft tissue to provide a good cover over the implant, and is free of any comorbidities that might adversely affect wound healing. Obese patients are not good candidates for gluteal implants.[48,52]

Preoperative Preparation

History taking, clinical photography, and patient counseling are done to establish realistic expectations, as described earlier. The buttock shape of an individual is determined by different anatomic components including the underlying bony framework, gluteal musculature, subcutaneous tissue, and the skin. It is essential to evaluate these elements in a patient who is planned for gluteal implant augmentation as the findings influence the choice of pocket for implant placement, type of implant, and the need for adjunctive procedures.[22,48] Assess for:

- Underlying bony framework: Pelvic height and width, spine symmetry, and curvature.
- Gluteus maximus muscle: Height-to-width ratio, muscle base width in relation to distance from midline to midbuttock line, bulk, tone.
- Subcutaneous fat thickness.
- Skin quality, and laxity especially in the infragluteal folds.
- Ptosis: Buttock ptosis is characterized by drooping of skin over the infragluteal fold and presence of skin fold. These can be appreciated on a lateral view of the buttock.

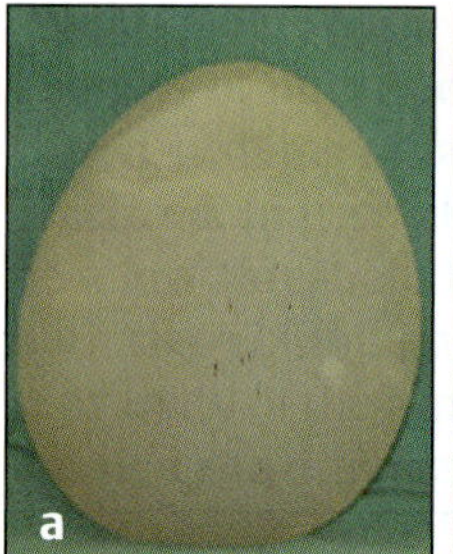
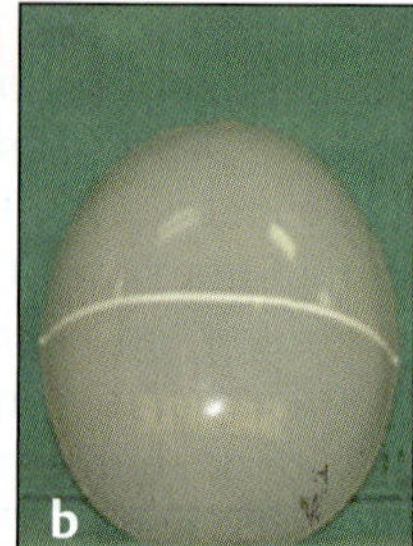
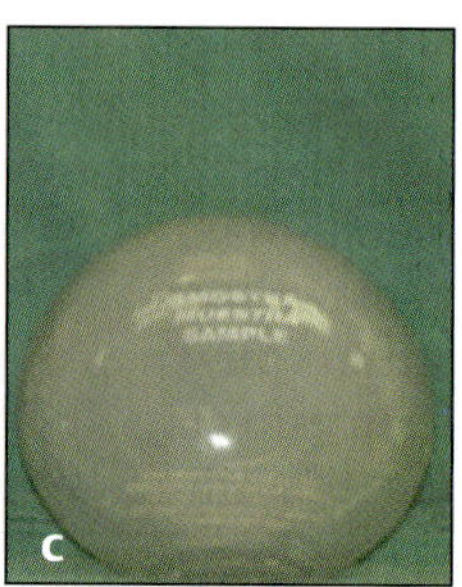

Fig. 28.19 Different shapes of implants available for gluteal augmentation. **(a)** Anatomic. **(b)** Oval: it can have a white line along its equator to facilitate correct placement. **(c)** Round.

Decision-making

Plane of Insertion

Intramuscular and subfascial plane, both can be used in patients with adequate thickness of subcutaneous fat, but in those with strong musculature that might displace the implant, a subfascial pocket is preferred. Patients with thin subcutaneous fat are candidates for intramuscular gluteal augmentation.[48]

Choice of Implant

Those with a short buttock and more lower pole fullness achieve good results with round implants and those with a long buttock are good candidates for oval or anatomic implants.[48] Use of templates preoperatively and sizers intraoperatively helps a great deal in choosing an appropriately sized implant. The base width of the implant should not exceed the base width of the buttocks, as wound healing may be compromised with too wide an implant.[48,52]

Surgical Techniques

Submuscular Implant Placement

Marking

Markings are done in the standing position. The posterior iliac crest and the infragluteal fold are marked, and horizontal lines are drawn from the tip of the coccyx to the greater trochanter on each side. For placing an implant in the submuscular plane, the distance between the iliac crest and the horizontal line should be at least twice the distance from the infragluteal fold to that line, to avoid excessive upper pole fullness (**Fig. 28.20**). The line from tip of the coccyx to greater trochanter corresponds to the inferior border of piriformis muscle and the exit point of the sciatic nerve; therefore, it also marks the inferior limit of the dissection. The implant is placed above this level to prevent any injury or irritation of the sciatic nerve. Above this, a circle of 8 to 10 cm diameter is drawn around 4 to 5 cm lateral to the midline, which represents the implant position and marks the area of subcutaneous undermining and muscle incision.[49,50]

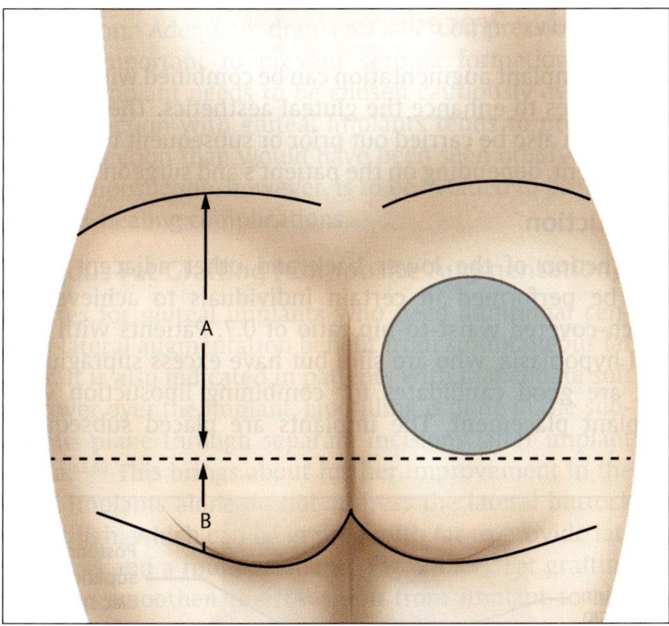

Fig. 28.20 The iliac crest, infragluteal fold, and a line from tip of the coccyx to greater trochanter (*dotted*) is marked on each side. This line corresponds to the inferior border of piriformis muscle and defines the inferior limit of dissection. For placing an implant in a submuscular position, distance A should be at least twice that of B. The blue circle corresponds to the position of the implant. (Adapted from Hidalgo 2006.[49])

Patient Positioning and Anesthesia

The surgery is performed under general or epidural anesthesia. The patient is placed in a prone position with a pillow under the chest and pelvis, with adequate padding of the pressure points.

Incision

A single midline intergluteal or bilateral paramedian incision are commonly employed.[53] The intergluteal incision is 5 to 7 cm long, marked in the midline with its inferior-most point at the tip of the coccyx or 5 cm above the anus (**Fig. 28.21**). The bilateral parasacral incisions are marked 1 cm from the midline in the inferior aspect at the tip of the coccyx and follow the upper gluteal curvature as they reach the upper buttock.

Surgical Technique

The presacral fascia is exposed through the incision, and subcutaneous undermining is done in the region of the previously marked circle (**Fig. 28.19b**). An incision is given in the muscle fascia in the direction of muscle fibers and the fibers are separated till a fine layer of fatty tissue comes into view. This plane lies at least 3 cm deep and is slightly difficult to identify. Once this plane is reached, the pocket is developed. The inferior dissection is limited till the horizontal line

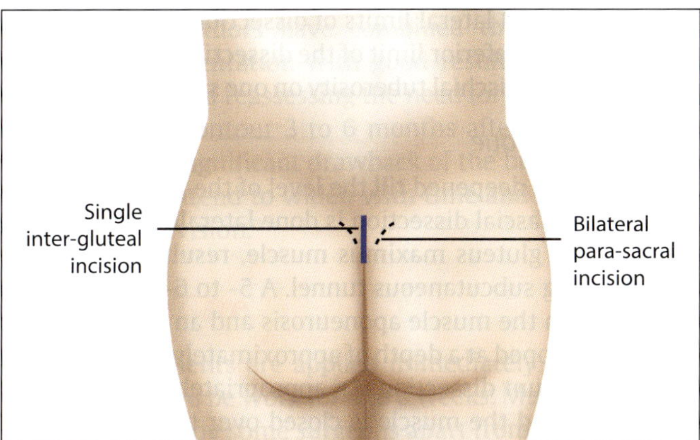

Fig. 28.21 Incision options for gluteal implant placement. Single intergluteal incision and bilateral parasacral incision with minimum 2 cm distance between the two incisions in the inferior aspect. (Adapted from Senderoff 2016.[48])

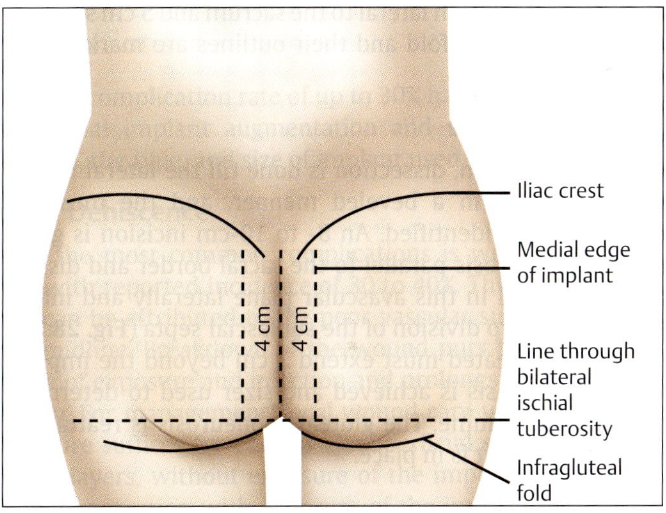

Fig. 28.22 Iliac crests and infragluteal folds are marked. A line is drawn through bilateral ischial tuberosity marking the limit of inferior dissection. Another line 4 cm from the midline on either side determines the site of the medial edge of the implant. (Adapted from Godoy 2018.[56])

as described. Implant size is confirmed with the help of sizers. With the implant in place, the muscle fibers are reapproximated to the overlying fascia and the incision is closed in layers with or without a drain. Similar procedure is carried out on the other buttock.[49,50]

Intramuscular Implant Placement

Marking

Preoperative markings are performed in both standing and seated positions (**Fig. 28.22**). The iliac crest and the infragluteal fold are marked and the area between the two is divided into three equal parts. The implant is to be centered over the middle third around 4 cm lateral to the midline.

Postoperative Care

Mild compression stockings are applied over the dressing on the operating table and continue to be worn for another 6 weeks. Early ambulation is encouraged, and patients are advised to walk with the help of high-heeled shoes for a week, to avoid excessive stretch on the calf muscles. Patients are observed for 24 hours for development of any signs and symptoms of acute compartment syndrome and discharged. Leg exercises are permitted after 2 months and patients are asked to follow up at regular intervals.[67,71]

Complications

Implant augmentation of the calf is a relatively safe surgery with low incidence of complications. Seroma formation, hematoma formation, infection, and wound dehiscence may be encountered with implant insertion. Implant palpability, displacement, rupture, and capsular contracture have also been observed. A unique and serious complication related to implant insertion that deserves a special mention is acute compartment syndrome. Although rare, its development is the most dreaded complication and is usually seen with placement of two implants. Excessive tension in the leg compartments leads to interruption of the blood supply resulting in nerve and muscle ischemia. Early diagnosis and prompt management is crucial for prevention of any long-term disability. Close monitoring of sensations and peripheral pulses should be done for at least 24 hours. Early signs of acute compartment syndrome include pain in excess of what is expected, pain on passive stretch, tense nature of the leg compartment, and presence of numbness or paresthesia. The treatment involves surgical re-exploration and removal of the implants.[67,71]

Conclusion

There is a gradual increase in people desiring aesthetically pleasing buttocks and calves. Buttock augmentation with either fat transfer or implant placement is safe and efficacious. Similarly, calf augmentation with implants is a reliable procedure with good surgical outcomes. Plastic surgeons should be cognizant of these methods to achieve the desired results. A thorough understanding of the anatomy and use of safe techniques aid in reducing complications and enhancing the aesthetic outcomes. With experience, these surgical procedures can be performed efficiently and yield consistent results.

References

1. Del Vecchio DA, Rohrich RJ. A changing paradigm: the Brazilian Butt Lift is neither Brazilian nor a lift—why it needs to be called a safe subcutaneous buttock augmentation. Plast Reconstr Surg 2020;145(1):281–283
2. Del Vecchio D. Common sense for the common good: staying subcutaneous during fat transplantation to the gluteal region. Plast Reconstr Surg 2018;142(1):286–288
3. Ghavami A, Villanueva NL. Gluteal augmentation and contouring with autologous fat transfer: Part I. Clin Plast Surg 2018;45(2):249–259
4. Mofid MM, Teitelbaum S, Suissa D, et al. Report on mortality from gluteal fat grafting: recommendations from the ASERF Task Force. Aesthet Surg J 2017;37(7):796–806
5. Condé-Green A, Kotamarti V, Nini KT, et al. Fat grafting for gluteal augmentation: a systematic review of the literature and meta-analysis. Plast Reconstr Surg 2016;138(3):437e–446e
6. Ali A. Contouring of the gluteal region in women: enhancement and augmentation. Ann Plast Surg 2011;67(3):209–214
7. Cárdenas-Camarena L, Silva-Gavarrete JF, Arenas-Quintana R. Gluteal contour improvement: different surgical alternatives. Aesthetic Plast Surg 2011;35(6):1117–1125
8. Hoyos AE, Perez ME, Castillo L. Dynamic definition mini-lipoabdominoplasty combining multilayer liposculpture, fat grafting, and muscular plication. Aesthet Surg J 2013;33(4): 545–560
9. Marwah M, Kulkarni A, Godse K, Abhyankar S, Patil S, Nadkarni N. Fat fulfillment: a review of autologous fat grafting. J Cutan Aesthet Surg 2013;6(3):132–138
10. Toledo LS. Gluteal augmentation with fat grafting: the Brazilian buttock technique: 30 years' experience. Clin Plast Surg 2015;42(2):253–261
11. American Society of Plastic Surgeons. Plastic surgery societies issue urgent warning about the risks associated with Brazilian butt lifts. https://www.plasticsurgery.org/news/press-releases/plastic-surgery-societies-issue-urgent-warning-about-the-risks-associated-with-brazilian-butt-lifts
12. British Association of Aesthetic Plastic Surgeons. The bottom line: popularity of risky buttock enhancement procedures leading to costliest emergency complications. British surgeons warned not to perform procedures until more data is collected. https://baaps.org.uk/media/press_releases/1630/the_bottom_line
13. Villanueva NL, Del Vecchio DA, Afrooz PN, Carboy JA, Rohrich RJ. Staying safe during gluteal fat transplantation. Plast Reconstr Surg 2018;141(1):79–86
14. McCraw JB, Arnold PG, eds. McCraw and Arnold's atlas of muscle and musculocutaneous flaps. Norfolk, VA: Hampton Press Publishing Company; 1987
15. Del Vecchio D. Common sense for the common good: staying subcutaneous during fat transplantation to the gluteal region. Plast Reconstr Surg 2018;142(1):286–288
16. Del Vecchio DA, Villanueva NL, Mohan R, et al. Clinical implications of gluteal fat graft migration: a dynamic anatomical study. Plast Reconstr Surg 2018;142(5):1180–1192
17. Wall S Jr, Delvecchio D, Teitelbaum S, et al. Subcutaneous migration: a dynamic anatomical study of gluteal fat grafting. Plast Reconstr Surg 2019;143(5):1343–1351
18. Del Vecchio D, Wall S Jr. Expansion vibration lipofilling: a new technique in large volume fat transplantation. Plast Reconstr Surg 2018;141(5):639e–649e
19. Khouri RK Jr, Khouri RK. Current clinical applications of fat grafting. Plast Reconstr Surg 2017;140(3):466e–486e
20. Del Vecchio DA, Bucky LP. Breast augmentation using preexpansion and autologous fat transplantation: a clinical radiographic study. Plast Reconstr Surg 2011;127(6):2441–2450

21. Centeno RF, Sood A, Young VL. Clinical anatomy in aesthetic gluteal contouring. Clin Plast Surg 2018;45(2):145–157
22. Mendieta CG. Classification system for gluteal evaluation. Clin Plast Surg 2006;33(3):333–346
23. Mendieta CG, Sood A. Classification system for gluteal evaluation: revisited. Clin Plast Surg 2018;45(2):159–177
24. Broughton G II, Crosby MA, Coleman J, Rohrich RJ. Use of herbal supplements and vitamins in plastic surgery: a practical review. Plast Reconstr Surg 2007;119(3):48e–66e
25. Rohrich RJ, Sorokin ES, Brown SA. In search of improved fat transfer viability: a quantitative analysis of the role of centrifugation and harvest site. Plast Reconstr Surg 2004;113(1): 391–395, discussion 396–397
26. Del Vecchio D, Rohrich RJ. A classification of clinical fat grafting: different problems, different solutions. Plast Reconstr Surg 2012;130(3):511–522
27. Li K, Gao J, Zhang Z, et al. Selection of donor site for fat grafting and cell isolation. Aesthetic Plast Surg 2013;37(1):153–158
28. Ullmann Y, Shoshani O, Fodor A, et al. Searching for the favorable donor site for fat injection: in vivo study using the nude mice model. Dermatol Surg 2005;31(10):1304–1307
29. Wall S Jr. SAFE circumferential liposuction with abdominoplasty. Clin Plast Surg 2010;37(3):485–501
30. Wall SH Jr, Lee MR. Separation, aspiration, and fat equalization: SAFE liposuction concepts for comprehensive body contouring. Plast Reconstr Surg 2016;138(6):1192–1201
31. Gir P, Brown SA, Oni G, Kashefi N, Mojallal A, Rohrich RJ. Fat grafting: evidence-based review on autologous fat harvesting, processing, reinjection, and storage. Plast Reconstr Surg 2012; 130(1):249–258
32. Mendieta CG. Gluteal reshaping. Aesthet Surg J 2007;27(6): 641–655
33. Wall S Jr, Del Vecchio D. Commentary on: Report on mortality from gluteal fat grafting: recommendations from the ASERF Task Force. Aesthet Surg J 2017;37(7):807–810
34. Cansancao AL, Condé-Green A, Vidigal RA, Rodriguez RL, D'Amico RA. Real-time ultrasound-assisted gluteal fat grafting. Plast Reconstr Surg 2018;142(2):372–376
35. McDevitt NB; American Society of Plastic and Reconstructive Surgeons. Deep vein thrombosis prophylaxis. Plast Reconstr Surg 1999;104(6):1923–1928
36. Iverson RE; ASPS Task Force on Patient Safety in Office-Based Surgery Facilities. Patient safety in office-based surgery facilities: I. Procedures in the office-based surgery setting. Plast Reconstr Surg 2002;110(5):1337–1342, discussion 1343–1346
37. Davison SP, Venturi ML, Attinger CE, Baker SB, Spear SL. Prevention of venous thromboembolism in the plastic surgery patient. Plast Reconstr Surg 2004;114(3):43E–51E
38. Caprini JA, Arcelus JI, Reyna JJ. Effective risk stratification of surgical and nonsurgical patients for venous thromboembolic disease. Semin Hematol 2001; 38(2, Suppl 5):12–19
39. Oranges CM, Tremp M, di Summa PG, et al. Gluteal augmentation techniques: a comprehensive literature review. Aesthet Surg J 2017;37(5):560–569
40. American Society of Plastic Surgeons. Plastic Surgery Statistics Report 2019 [dataset on the internet]. United States: American Society of Plastic Surgeons; 2020. https://www.plasticsurgery.org/documents/News/Statistics/2019/plastic-surgery-statistics-full-report-2019.pdf
41. de la Peña JA, Rubio OV, Cano JP, Cedillo MC, Garcés MT. History of gluteal augmentation. Clin Plast Surg 2006;33(3):307–319
42. Cocke WM, Ricketson G. Gluteal augmentation. Plast Reconstr Surg 1973;52(1):93
43. González-Ulloa M. Gluteoplasty: a ten-year report. Aesthetic Plast Surg 1991;15(1):85–91
44. Robles JM, Tagliapietra JC, Grandi M. Gluteoplastia de aumento: implante submuscular. Cir Plast Iberolatinoamericana 1984;10: 365–369
45. Vergara R, Marcos M. Intramuscular gluteal implants. Aesthetic Plast Surg 1996;20(3):259–262
46. de La Peña JA, Lopez MH, Gamboa LF. Augmentation gluteoplasty: anatomical and clinical considerations. Key Issues Plastic Cosmetic Surg 2000;17:1–12
47. de la Peña JA. Subfascial technique for gluteal augmentation. Aesthet Surg J 2004;24(3):265–273
48. Senderoff DM. Aesthetic surgery of the buttocks using implants: practice-based recommendations. Aesthet Surg J 2016;36(5): 559–576
49. Hidalgo JE. Submuscular gluteal augmentation: 17 years of experience with gel and elastomer silicone implants. Clin Plast Surg 2006;33(3):435–447
50. Hidalgo JE. Submuscular gluteal augmentation. Clin Plast Surg 2018;45(2):197–202
51. Vergara R, Amezcua H. Intramuscular gluteal implants: 15 years' experience. Aesthet Surg J 2003;23(2):86–91
52. de la Peña Salcedo JA, Gallardo GJ, Alvarenga GE. Subfascial gluteal implant augmentation. Clin Plast Surg 2018;45(2): 225–236
53. Mofid MM, Gonzalez R, de la Peña JA, Mendieta CG, Senderoff DM, Jorjani S. Buttock augmentation with silicone implants: a multicenter survey review of 2226 patients. Plast Reconstr Surg 2013;131(4):897–901
54. Cárdenas-Camarena L, Paillet JC. Combined gluteoplasty: liposuction and gluteal implants. Plast Reconstr Surg 2007; 119(3):1067–1074
55. Cárdenas-Camarena L, Trujillo-Méndez R, Díaz-Barriga JC. Tridimensional combined gluteoplasty: liposuction, buttock implants, and fat transfer. Plast Reconstr Surg 2020;146(1): 53–63
56. Godoy PM, Munhoz AM. Intramuscular gluteal augmentation with implants associated with immediate fat grafting. Clin Plast Surg 2018;45(2):203–215
57. Aslani A, Del Vecchio DA. Composite buttock augmentation: the next frontier in gluteal aesthetic surgery. Plast Reconstr Surg 2019;144(6):1312–1321
58. Lee JW, Kang MG, Park SS. Secondary gluteal augmentation: surgical technique and outcomes. Plast Reconstr Surg 2018; 141(6):1371–1382
59. Gonzalez R. Buttocks lifting: how and when to use medial, lateral, lower, and upper lifting techniques. Clin Plast Surg 2006;33(3):467–478
60. de la Peña-Salcedo JA, Soto-Miranda MA, Vaquera-Guevara MO, Lopez-Salguero JF, Lavareda-Santana MA, Ledezma-Rodriguez JC. Gluteal lift with subfascial implants. Aesthetic Plast Surg 2013;37(3):521–528
61. Shah B. Complications in gluteal augmentation. Clin Plast Surg 2018;45(2):179–186
62. Serra F, Aboudib JH, Marques RG. Reducing wound complications in gluteal augmentation surgery. Plast Reconstr Surg 2012;130(5):706e–713e
63. Gonzalez R. Augmentation gluteoplasty: the XYZ method. Aesthetic Plast Surg 2004;28(6):417–425
64. Senderoff DM. Revision buttock implantation: indications, procedures, and recommendations. Plast Reconstr Surg 2017; 139(2):327–335
65. Glitzenstein J. Correction of the amyotrophies of the limb with silicone prosthesis inclusions. Rev Bras Cir 1979;69:117

66. Carlsen LN. Calf augmentation: a preliminary report. Ann Plast Surg 1979;2(6):508–510
67. Andjelkov K, Sforza M, Husein R, Atanasijevic TC, Popovic VM. Safety and efficacy of subfascial calf augmentation. Plast Reconstr Surg 2017;139(3):657e–669e
68. von Szalay L. Calf augmentation: a new calf prosthesis. Plast Reconstr Surg 1985;75(1):83–87
69. Aiache AE. Calf implantation. Plast Reconstr Surg 1989;83(3): 488–493
70. Aiache AE. Calf contour correction with implants. Clin Plast Surg 1991;18(4):857–862
71. Niechajev I, Krag C. Calf augmentation and restoration: long-term results and the review of the reported complications. Aesthetic Plast Surg 2017;41(5):1115–1131
72. de la Peña-Salcedo JA, Soto-Miranda MA, Lopez-Salguero JF. Calf implants: a 25-year experience and an anatomical review. Aesthetic Plast Surg 2012;36(2):261–270
73. Dini M, Innocenti A, Lorenzetti P. Aesthetic calf augmentation with silicone implants. Aesthetic Plast Surg 2002;26(6):490–492
74. Kalixto MA, Vergara R. Submuscular calf implants. Aesthetic Plast Surg 2003;27(2):135–138
75. Nunez GO, Garcia DP. Calf augmentation with supra-preiostic solid prosthesis associated with fasciotomies. Aesthetic Plast Surg 2004;116:295–305
76. Montellano L. Calf augmentation. Ann Plast Surg 1991;27(5): 429–438
77. Cuenca-Guerra R, Daza-Flores JL, Saade-Saade AJ. Calf implants. Aesthetic Plast Surg 2009;33(4):505–513

29

Female Genital Cosmetic Surgery: Rejuvenation and Change of External Appearance

Rakesh Kalra

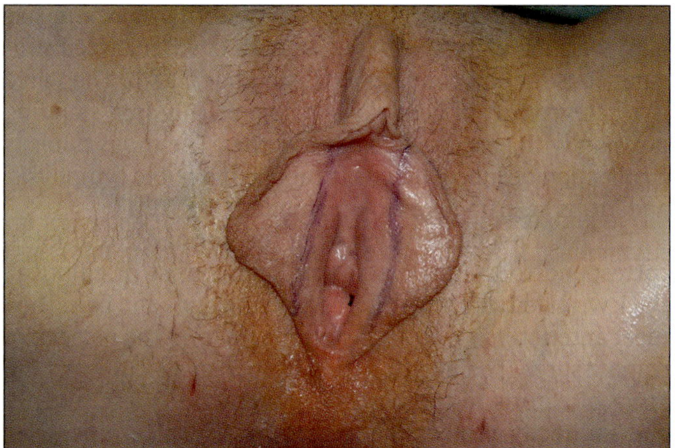

Fig. 29.2 Hart line on labia minora, dividing the mucosal from squamous epithelial surfaces.

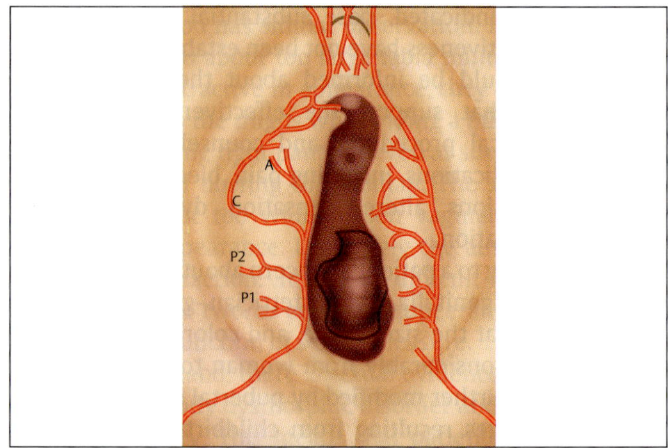

Fig. 29.3 Vascular anatomy of the labia minora. C is central artery, A is anterior branches, P1 and P2 are posterior branches.

narrow, but sometimes can be wide enough to almost form a third fold between the two labia. Its significance is that in some patients, it does disturb the youthful appearance of the genitals, and its trimming or excision produces marked improvement in appearance.

The clitoris consists of erectile glans, body, and crura. It arises from the genital tubercle, and corresponds embryonically to the male penis. Body and glans together are around 2 cm in length and the diameter is less than 1 cm. Prepuce is a protective skin fold and it may leave the glans either partially exposed or hidden completely. Glans is the most innervated and sensitive structure.

Underneath the vulva is the vestibule protected by the hymenal ring, again comprising of an outer tunnel and a deeper tunnel. The outer tunnel consists of the clitoris, the clitoral prepuce, the labia minora, hymen, and the urethral meatus—all structures which are nonhairy and mucosal, lined by secretory glands and having nerve endings. The vestibule is whatever part of genitals that is visible in lithotomy position, except the labia majora and mons pubis.

The blood supply is through the external and internal pudendal artery systems, besides an arborization from the inferior abdominal wall system. The internal, external, and transverse superficial perineal arteries, all branches of the internal pudendal artery, anastomose with the branches of the deep external pudendal artery (**Fig. 29.3**).

The blood supply of the labia minora is rich and extensive. The superficial external pudendal artery anastomoses with the posterior labial artery and further contributions are from the internal circumflex artery. The posterior labial artery runs parallel to the long axis of the labia minora. This initial arch further divides into several other arterial arches, each branch running at right angles to the long axis, and forming a loop under the edge of the minora at its widest dimension, thus providing a rich arterial supply to the labia minora. Such rich vascular supply allows a wide variety of tailoring of the labia minora in a variety of ways (**Fig. 29.3**).

The nerve supply is from the pudendal nerve which is derived from the second to the fourth sacral nerve roots. It enters the pelvis from the lesser sciatic foramen, then through the pudendal canal onward to the ischial spine. The pudendal nerve has three branches: the dorsal nerve of clitoris, the perineal nerve for external genitalia, and the inferior rectal nerve. These, as well as branches of the ilioinguinal, iliofemoral, and posterior genitofemoral cutaneous nerves, supply the sensory nerves to the perineum and external genitalia. Erogenous nerve supply also comes from the pudendal nerve to supply the glans clitoris (**Fig. 29.4**).

Anatomical Changes with Aging

In the young preadolescent females, the strong septa of the superficial system of Scarpa, Colles, and Buck fascia attach the mons and the labia majora to the underlying periosteum. The vestibular clitoris and prepuce are smooth and small in size. This clitoris is surrounded by smooth and pink labia minora hidden within the labia majora from external visibility. The minora envelope the clitoris above as a hood, and they diffuse posteriorly into the perineal body. The labia majora have adequate padding of subcutaneous fat.

Transformations occur in the above normal anatomy at several stages in life. At puberty the labia minora grow and become pigmented. The clitoral prepuce becomes wrinkled and covers the clitoris. Childbirth, pregnancy, and weight gain cause increased fat accumulation and also relaxation of the superficial fascial system. This results in perineal ptosis. The vaginal canal relaxes and the pelvic outlet becomes weaker. Pregnancy causes a larger growth of the labia minora and it starts hanging down externally even more. With additional factors such as redundancy and gravity, the labia minora have increased wrinkling, hypertrophy, pigmentation, nerves, and sebaceous glands.

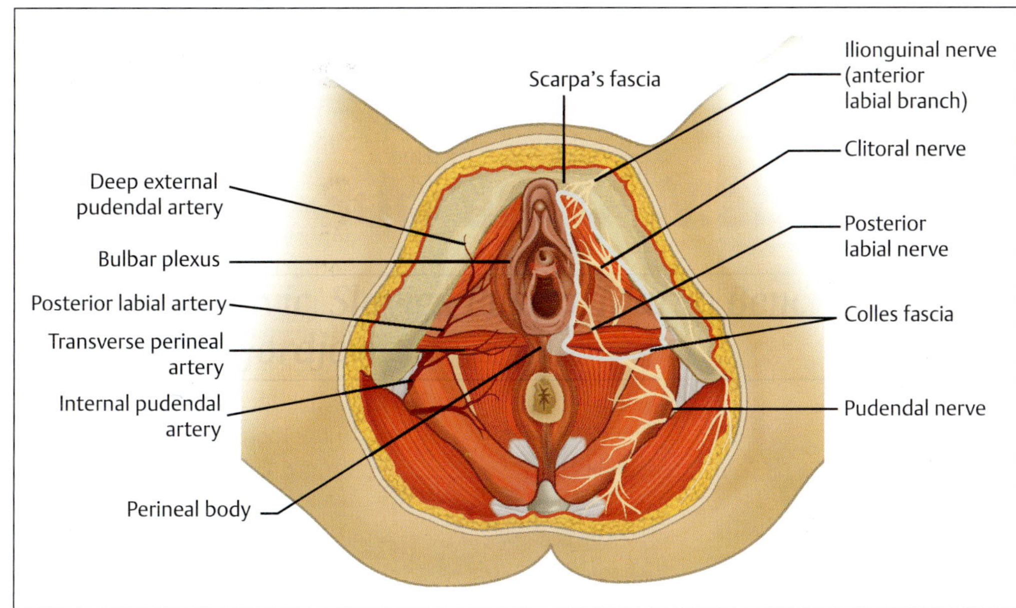

Fig. 29.4 Anatomy of vulva. Blood supply and nerve supply of perineum and vulva.

Excessive weight loss causes reduction of the fat from the labia majora and the mons. As this happens, there is greater wrinkling and ptosis of the labia.

With advancing age, the perineal ptosis goes on increasing, and the external genitalia begin to atrophy. There is an increased loss of subcutaneous fat, increased descent, and reduced secretions from the vaginal mucosal tissues, leading to dryness of the lining of vulva and vestibule, and consequently further mucosal atrophy.

However, these changes do not strictly follow the above events in life. For example, some very thin built women, nullipara, may also have excessive growth of the labia minora, or older women, multipara, may still have a good amount of subcutaneous fat with no hypertrophy of labia minora. Thus, genetic makeup and individual factors also play a role.

The Genital Aesthetics—What Is Normal?

This is a very philosophical question. Beauty has no definition and it is in the beholder's eyes. It has no gauge or measurement to it. For the genitals, there is no criterion for a good or a bad shape that may yet be well defined. The face does have some rules of one-thirds that define good proportions, and the breasts do have some set rules of the size and location of the nipple-areola complex or the kind of fullness and curves that are considered aesthetic. However, when it comes to the genitals, it is still an undefined science of beauty, yet it is possible that not before long, a large number of studies/research works would define standards of beauty. Some workers do mention some criteria, like proposing norms for the length of the labia minora exposed outside at its maximum width, or the fullness of the labia majora, or the amount of exposure of the clitoris from under the preputial hood. But these areas are unlikely to get confined to yardsticks of measurements.

In this chapter we shall be discussing about the shapes of the vulva. The question is, does vulva have a describable shape? We talk of faces being the perfect oval shape, or the square face, or the long or wide face. We speak of shapely legs, a perfect blend of slender thighs rising high into the rounded buttocks. In fact, many descriptive terms have been evolved, for different areas of the face and breasts. Is there anything even as close to the above as far as vaginal shapes are concerned? Not many descriptive terms truly. Actually, the hundreds of shapes of the vulva are all normal. This has been demonstrated by many artists who have taken down the shapes of the vulva either in plaster of Paris casts, or in pictures.

The vulva shapes are compared to a clamshell—open and closed (**Fig. 29.5**). The closed look is the ideal, sought-after appearance, where the two folds of the labia majora fall upon each other, with no exposure of the internal anatomy. The open clam shell appearance is the, as it is called, "not so neat" appearance, where the two labia majora are wide apart, exposing not only large labia minora, but the inner pink vaginal mucosa too at times. This is associated with the aging effects on the genitals.

Clinical Presentation

The aesthetics-related complaints of genitals involve requests for reduction or trimming of the labia minora and reduction of labia majora and mons. The opposite is also often demanded, that is, augmentation of the atrophic, wrinkled labia majora and mons, hymen repairs, vaginal tightening, etc. These are usually surgeries on demand.

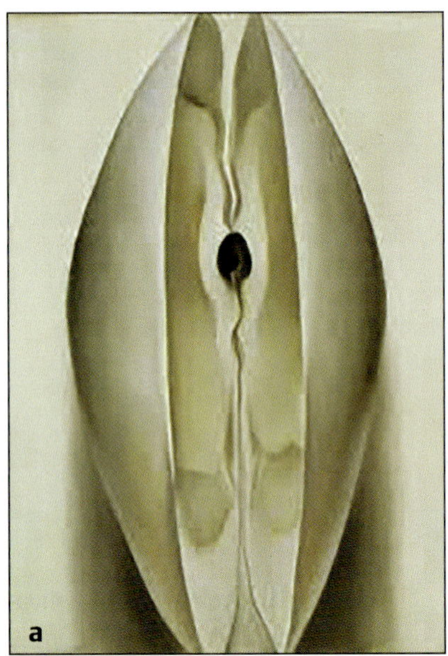
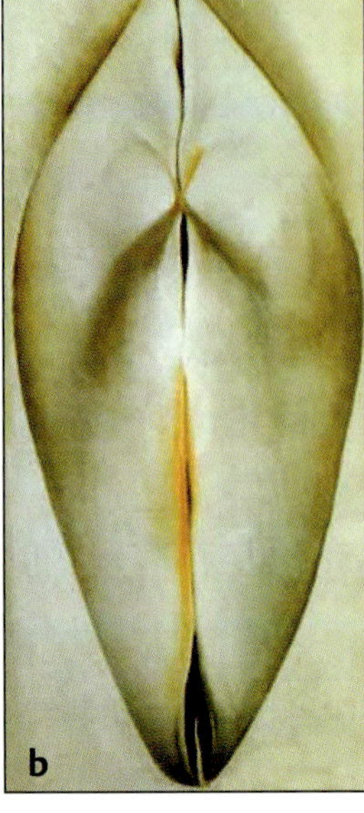

Fig. 29.5 **(a, b)** Open and closed clam-shell appearance of vulva.

Table 29.1 Vaginal rejuvenation procedures

Type of procedures	Procedures
Surgical procedures for external appearance manipulation	• Vertical or triangulated trimming of labia minora • Fat filling for labia majora and the Mount of Venus. Or, for the opposite effect, the mons pubis Liposuction • Excision of the redundant skin intermediate to labia minora and majora
Internal surgical procedures for rejuvenation	• Partial clitoridectomy • Unhooding of the clitoris • Vaginal tightening • Hymenoplasty
Nonsurgical procedures	• Energy-based vaginal tightening-RF and lasers • Fillers and PRP • G-Spot enhancement

Spectrum of Vaginal Rejuvenation Procedures

Different varieties of surgeries are performed in varying combinations depending upon the personal needs and after mutual discussions (**Table 29.1**).

It is observed that if only one of the procedures from among the surgical procedures is done, the external appearance does change, but it is likely to be far from satisfactory. However, when multiple procedures are performed together, then the maximum transformation occurs. Balding or pubic hair-do, tattooing, piercing, etc., all complete the list of decorating the female genitalia, providing a rejuvenated external appearance.

Preop Preparation and Anesthesia

The ideal time for vaginal rejuvenation procedures is immediately after a menstrual period as it gives the patient a time frame of 4 weeks after surgery before the next menstrual flow. This gives enough time for healing of the operated area.

Patients are taken off oral contraceptive pills, blood thinners, and any other medication that could result in abnormal bleeding during surgery for at least 2 weeks. The vulva and the vagina have rich blood supply and one should be careful to avoid excessive bleeding and congestion during surgery. Smokers are instructed to completely stop smoking prior to surgery. Patients may be started on antiseptic vaginal pessaries and broad-spectrum oral antibiotics including coverage for anaerobes 2 to 3 days prior to the surgery.

Most of the surgical procedures for vaginal rejuvenation are done under spinal or general anesthesia with the patient in a lithotomy position. An in-dwelling urinary catheter is passed prior to surgery and kept for 12 to 24 hours following surgery.

Surgical Procedures for External Appearance

Labia Minora Reduction

Labia minora trimming or reduction is the commonest surgery performed, called labiaplasty. Large labia minora, protruding out of the vulva in a standing posture, does become the main reason for women seeking the trimming. Reasons are not purely aesthetic in nature, as there are genuine functional reasons that cause women to seek this procedure.

Motakef classification describes the amount of labia minora protrusion beyond the labia majora.[8]

- Class I: 0 to 2 cm protrusion beyond the edge of the labia majora.
- Class II: 2 to 4 cm beyond the edge of the labia majora.
- Class III: more than 4 cm, beyond the edge of labia majora.

In Felicio classification of labial hypertrophy, there is an additional Class IV to the above classification, with labia minora protruding more than 6 cm.[9]

The minora should be symmetrical, and not protruding beyond the labia majora in the standing position. Banwell classification describes the variations in the area of excess protrusion of the labia minora (**Fig. 29.6**).[10]

- Type I: Upper-third enlargement (winging).

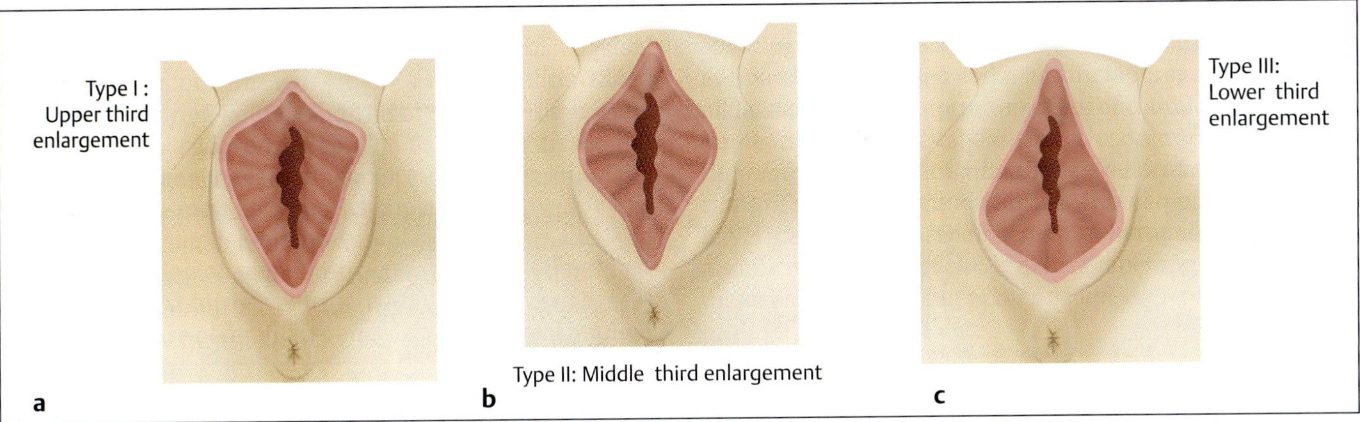

Fig. 29.6 Banwell classification based on site of labia minora enlargement. **(a)** Type I: Upper third enlargement. **(b)** Type II: Middle third enlargement. **(c)** Type III: Lower third enlargement.

- Type II: Middle-third enlargement.
- Type III: Lower-third enlargement.

These two are the most quoted classifications of labia minora hypertrophy. However, these classifications may not be a practical guide at surgery.

There are several techniques described, including de-epithelialization, W-plasty, laser labiaplasty, custom flask, fenestration, and composite reduction.[11] A variety of techniques may be devised or practiced, but these depend upon the surgeon's imagination and innovations.

The Horizontal Technique or "Wedge" Excision

The excess of labia is assessed by pinching between thumb and finger. As the tissue is held in a pinch, the excess labia minora fold looks like a dog ear, and this dog ear is excised with ingenuity. Continuous overrunning suturing produces hemostasis at the edges, and also does away with cut ends of the suture that are usually hurtful to the patient in the postoperative period. Ensure catching the dermis with every suture and eversion of the skin edges. The scar extends in a straight line from the inside, where it gets hidden, but extends to the outside in the hyperpigmented area, where it is likely to get noticed (**Figs. 29.7 and 29.8**).

There are few variations to this technique. The site of excision may vary depending upon the level of tissue excess as per Banwell classification. The wedge excision could be the upper third or lower third. This depends upon the judgment of the surgeon. To avoid notching and scar contracture, a Z-plasty may be incorporated. Alternatively, star excision may be performed (**Fig. 29.9**).[12]

The Vertical or Edge Excision Technique

Direct edge resection was first described by Capraro.[13] This was further refined using lazy "S" incision by Felicio[14] and running "W" incision by Maas and Hage.[15] Alinsod used radio frequency in addition to linear excision for further refinements.[16]

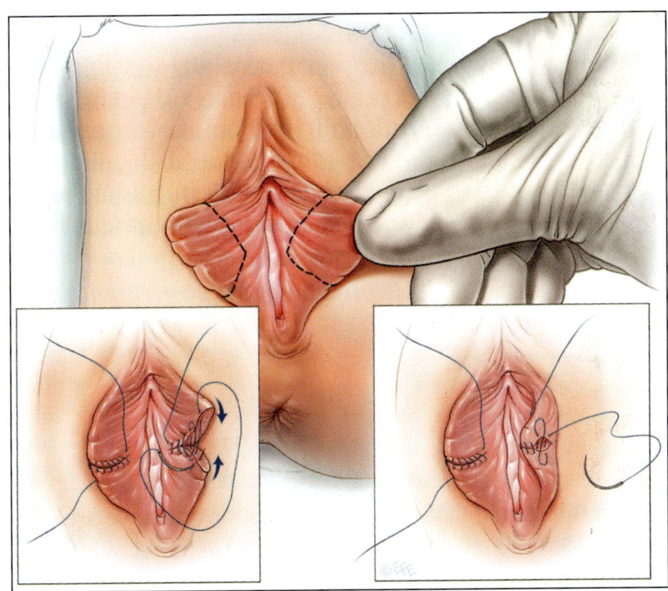

Fig. 29.7 Artist's view of horizontal (wedge) excision.

In this technique, a vertically oriented, curvilinear resection is done, from the take-off point inferiorly, to almost a centimeter of the clitoral hood above. Sufficient extra skin is removed to hide the labia minora from view on normal standing posture. Hence preop marking in this posture is recommended. However, too much should not be removed because this tissue is sensitive and has important role in providing lubrication during sexual intercourse. Thus, an effective balance should be achieved. However, there is a possibility of impaired arousal, lubrication, and inability to achieve orgasm following minora trimming. Suturing of inner and outer layers is done using continuous 5-0 absorbable suture, leaving the two ends long, so that the ends do not prick the sensitive vaginal skin in the postoperative period (**Figs. 29.10 and 29.11**).

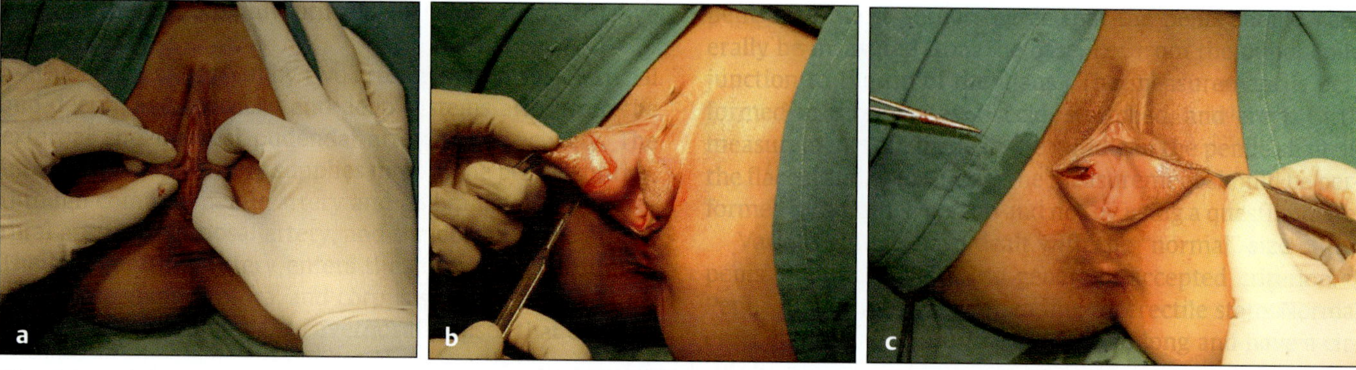

Fig. 29.8 **(a)** Assessing the wedge to be removed by pinching the excess labia minora. **(b)** Incision over the wedge to be excised. **(c)** First suture has been placed on left side, to be followed by suturing both medially and laterally to complete the wedge excision.

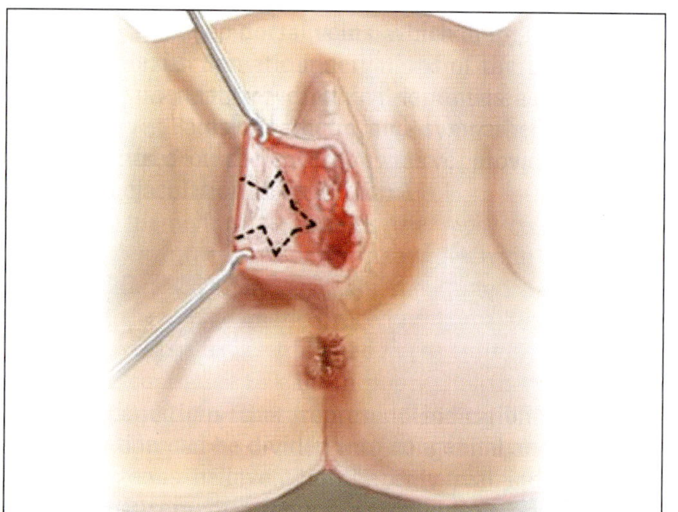

Fig. 29.9 Star labiaplasty is a modification of the wedge excision, utilizing four limbs. (Adapted from Tepper et al 2011[12].)

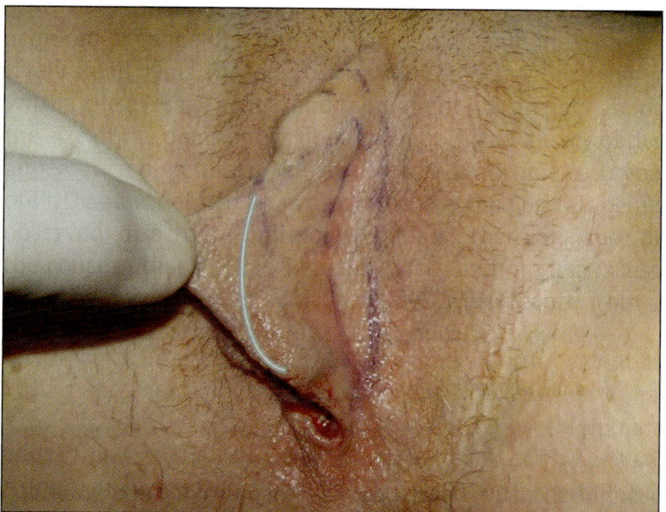

Fig. 29.10 Vertical or the "edge" technique.

There are minor variations of this technique in the form of zigzag excision (**Fig. 29.12a**)[15] and de-epithelialization technique (**Fig. 29.12b**),[17, 18] which are aptly presented in the respective figures

There are several modifications to these two basic techniques of labia minor reduction. Giraldo and González called it "flask" labiaplasty,[19] and inferior and posterior wedge excisions have been described by others.[20–22] Gress described composite reduction labiaplasty, in which the labia minora reduction extends to clitoral hood reduction as well as clitoral protrusion.[23] Ostrzenski described a fenestration labiaplasty.[24]

Complications of Labia Minora Reduction

Hematoma may form within the layers of labia minora. This shall need evacuation and a repeat of deeper sutures to obliterate the dead space. Wound dehiscence occurs following infection, or excessive friction in the postoperative period. Adequate rest, and loose clothings are recommended

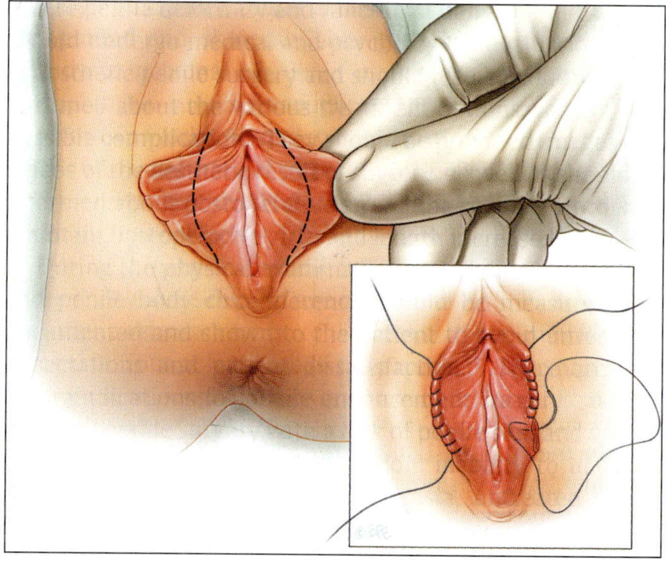

Fig. 29.11 Artist's view of a vertical or edge reduction.

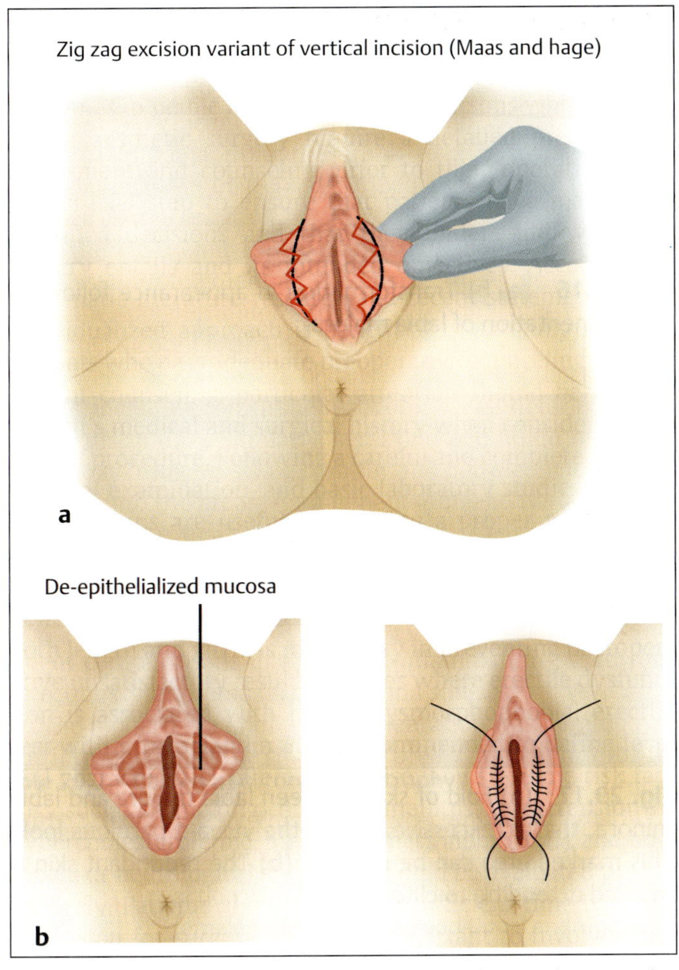

Fig. 29.12 (a) Variation of design of edge technique, by incorporating a series of Z-plasties. **(b)** Variation of design of edge technique, by incorporating a de-epithelialization of the labia both internally as well as externally.

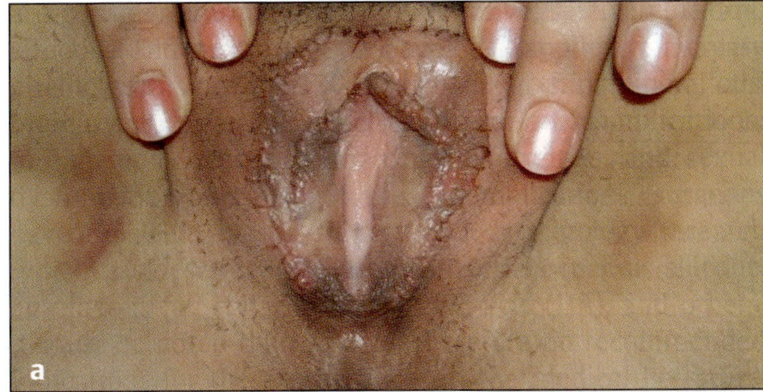

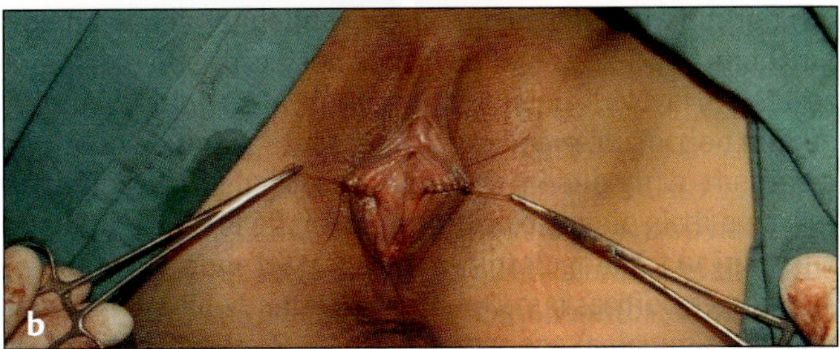

Fig. 29.13 (a, b) Comparing two basic methods of labia minor reduction. **(a)** Serrated edge following the vertical reduction, **(b)** scar extending to exposed surface and risk of notching with horizontal wedge excision.

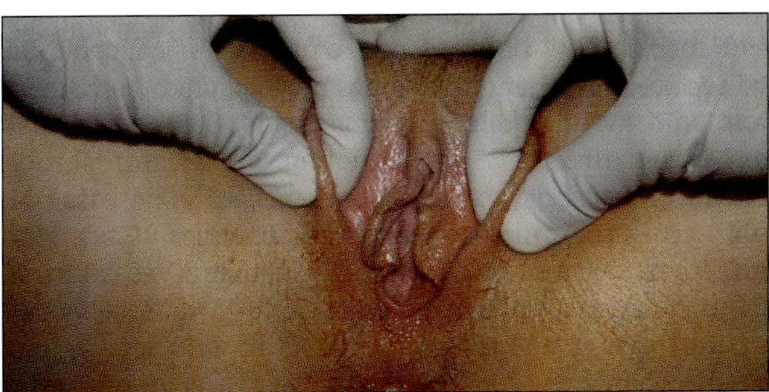

Fig. 29.14 The pinch test preoperatively highlighting the extent of fat depletion from labia majora.

to prevent excessive strain on the operated site. A secondary suturing may be required. Scarring is likely in both procedures, as an edge excision gives an operated look owing to the appearance of a serrated edge, while the wedge excision technique may have visible scar outside the labia minora (**Fig. 29.13**).

Liposculpturing of Female External Genitalia

Fat Filling of Labia Majora and Mount of Venus

Labia majora can have several conditions depending upon simple age-related changes to some pathological processes. For moderate fat loss and atrophic appearance, a pinch test between the thumb and finger suggests the atrophy and is a tool to judge the quantum of atrophy before and during surgery (**Fig. 29.14**).

This atrophic, aged look of the labia majora can be reversed by autologous-fat augmentation. The fat is harvested from any part of the body; however, adjacent inner thigh, and the lower abdomen are preferred with the patient in lithotomy position. The fat is decanted, washed with saline, and injected into the labia majora, with a 1.5- to 2.4-mm cannula using Coleman technique.[25] This is often through the same port used for aspiration, at the posterior commissure area. Relatively more quantity of fat is injected anteriorly and is gradually tapered down in the posterior area (**Fig. 29.15**). Fat is deposited in small aliquots in vertically oriented track lines. Even small pooling of fat has given lasting results in the labia majora. Approximately 15 to 30 mL of fat is injected on each side which is in excess of its requirement allowing for 30 to 40% absorption. A satisfactory result is expected after 3 months (**Fig. 29.16**).

Complications of Fat Augmentation

Absorption and asymmetry: The survival of fat is unpredictable. Thirty to forty percent of fat gets absorbed and may

the corona of the glans, leaving a sleeve of prepuce attached to the glans. The erectile tissues are removed from the corpora cavernosa of the clitoris with preservation of the dorsal neurovascular supply to the glans, within a strip of 1 cm wide soft tissue on the dorsum under the Buck fascia. The corpora are divided proximally where the two roots diverge under the pubic symphysis. The amputation stump is closed with hemostatic sutures.

There are two approaches to this procedure. In dorsolateral approach, the neurovascular bundle is first carefully dissected off the corpora cavernosa. Thereafter, cavernosa are sacrificed (**Fig. 29.21**). In ventral approach, the corpora are first removed without disturbing the dorsal neurovascular structures with expectation of better preservation of sensations of the clitoris.[27]

The glans is reduced by either leaving behind a crescent of corona glandis from 9 to 3 o'clock positions, or else leaving behind a trifoliate, Maple leaf–shaped remnant of the glans, supplied by the dorsal vessels. The three leaves are closed upon themselves, producing a round, small-sized neoglans. Two sutures on either side of the neurovascular bundle, taken with the deeper tissues, anchor the NV bundle deep. Preputial skin is folded upon itself to form a clitoral hood to give a natural appearance. Preservation of the dorsal nerves makes the neoclitoris sensate.

Unhooding of the Clitoris

Clitoral hood is the preputial skin on the dorsum of the clitoris that almost completely hides it. The erogenous clitoris, thus, is usually not amenable to external tactile stimulation, and is one reason why many women are not able to achieve orgasm at intercourse.

Hoodectomy surgically produces partial exposure of the clitoris. The skin hood is lifted at the 12 o'clock position above the clitoris and a probe is passed between the two (**Fig. 29.22a**). The overlying fold of skin is split open, well short of the sulcus (**Fig. 29.22b**). On making a full-thickness dorsal cut, two layers of the hood shall open up. These are sutured to each other (**Fig. 29.22c**) with 5/0 continuous absorbable suture. This effectively exposes the clitoral head, making it more sensitive to sexual stimulation.

There are few variations to hoodectomy. To shorten the hood, two lateral ellipses in the sulcus between the clitoris and the labia minora can be excised. Alternatively, an

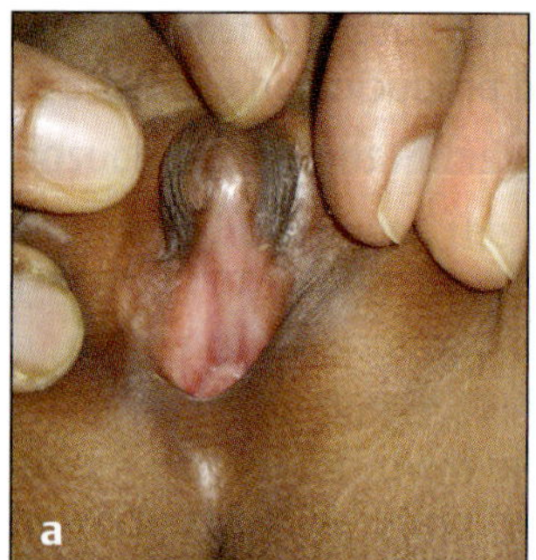
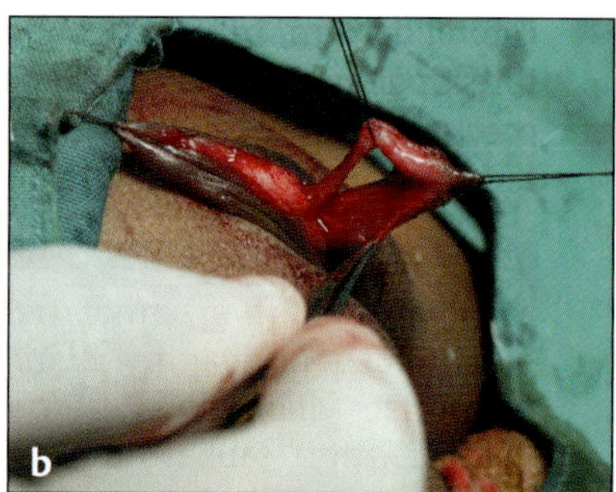
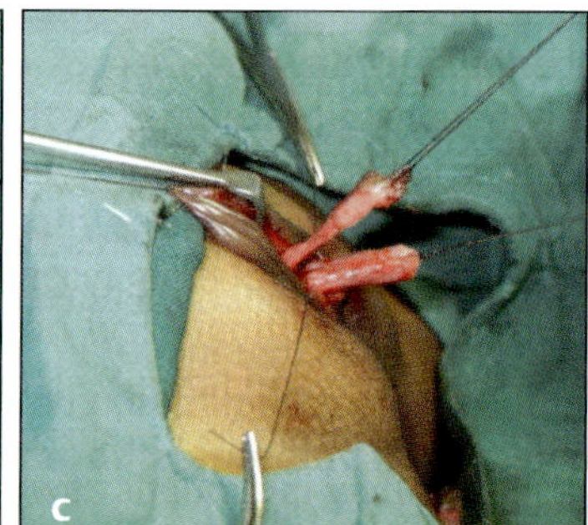
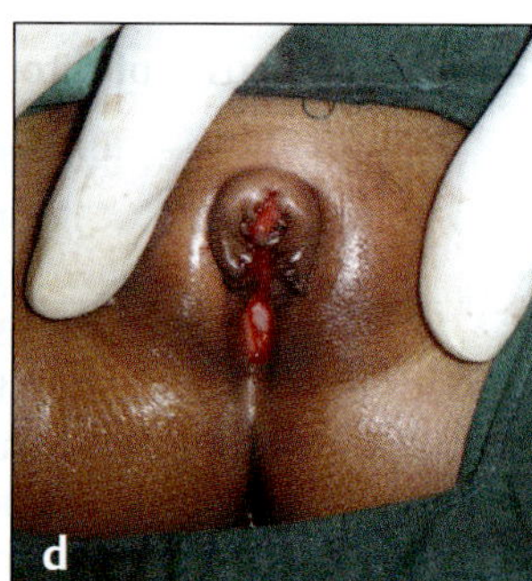

Fig. 29.21 Procedure of a clitoroplasty in a patient with female pseudohermaphroditism. **(a)** Appearance of the external genitalia in a case of female pseudohermaphroditism. The baby has a hypertrophied clitoris/pseudopenis with normal vagina and urethra and preputial hood. **(b)** Dissection of the glans clitoris with the dorsal neurovascular bundle and the corpora cavernosa. **(c)** Separation of the glans from the corpora cavernosa before amputation of the latter at the base. **(d)** Suturing of the glans clitoris into position, with reduction of the preputial hood. (The images are provided courtesy of Dr Milind Wagh, Mumbai, Maharashtra, India.)

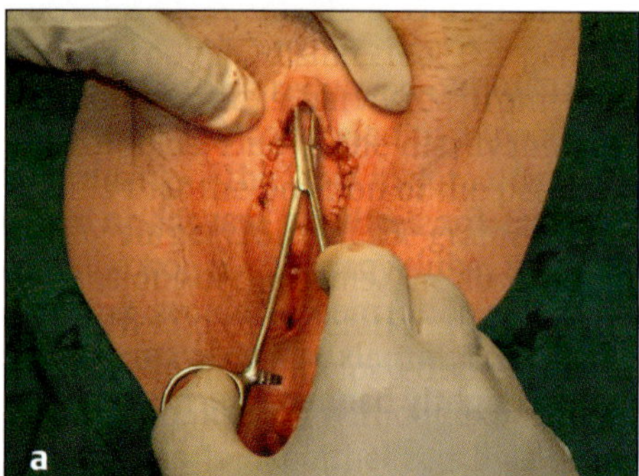
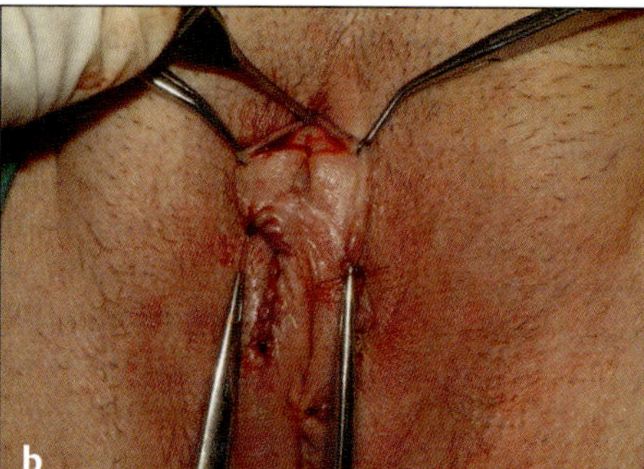
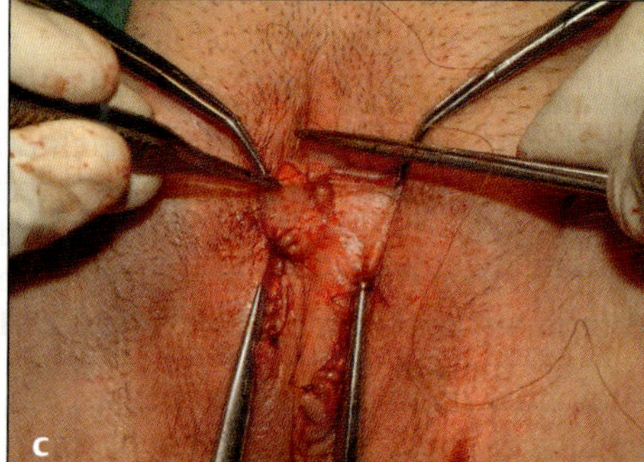

Fig. 29.22 **(a)** The clitoral hood raised at 12 o'clock position over a hemostat. **(b)** The hood divided at the center for about 5 mm, showing the outer and inner layers so displayed. **(c)** The two layers of skin are sutured together using continuous 5/0 round body needle chromic catgut.

inverted U-shaped excision of the skin over the dorsum of the prepuce is done. This should be carefully done as excessive exposure of the clitoris makes it hypersensitive, especially when it comes in contact with the garments.

Vaginal Tightening or Repair of Relaxed Vaginal Outlet

Vaginal tightening is requested by women following one or more vaginal deliveries. They complain of laxity of the vaginal canal, especially the introitus area as compared to predelivery. This is often the result of episiotomies done in difficult vaginal deliveries where the strength of the sphincter ring does not return to normal. This reduces sexual gratification considerably for both the partners.

It is clinically diagnosed by the appearance of a gaping patulous vaginal introitus. On asking the patient to contract the vagina using the pelvic diaphragm, the tightening at the introitus is poor. This is confirmed by a per-vaginal examination. An easy insertion of 3 or more fingers into the introitus and inability of the patient to firmly grip the fingers by contracting her vaginal musculature is indicative of a lax vagina which merits tightening (**Fig. 29.23**).

Examination must rule out urethrocele/cystocele which occurs following the attenuation or rupture of the pubo-vesico-cervical fascia from a loss of support of the anterior vaginal wall resulting in descent of the urethra (urethrocele) or the urinary bladder (cystocele). One should also rule out rectocele which results from the failure of a normal support system after bad obstetric history, resulting in herniation of the posterior vaginal wall and the rectum into the introitus. If any of these conditions are noticed, they should be appropriately managed by the respective specialists.

Surgical Vaginal Tightening

The procedure is performed under spinal or general anesthesia with the patient in the lithotomy position. The surgical procedure entails marking a triangle on the posterior vaginal wall, with the apex in the midline, approximately 12 to 15 cm deep into the introitus, and the two base points placed along the mucocutaneous junction at the introitus.

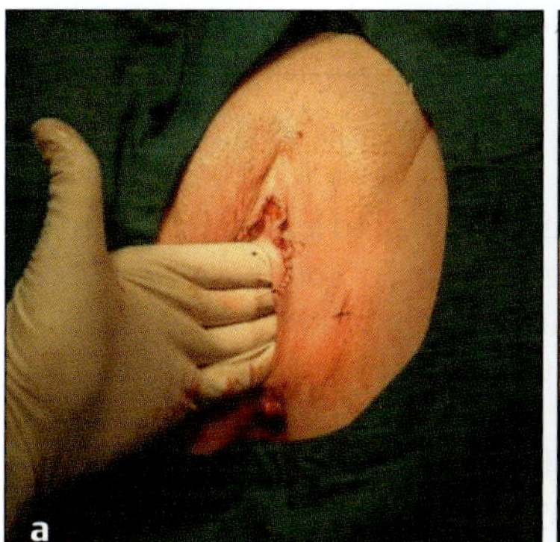

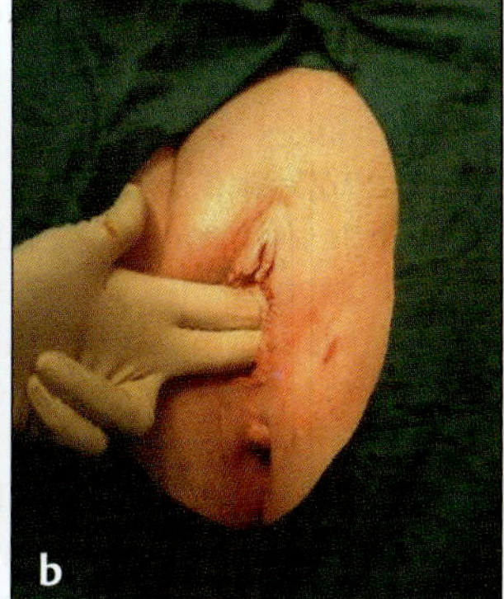

Fig. 29.23 **(a, b)** Loose introitus outlet before surgery, and only two fingers snug after surgery.

When the tightening required is moderate, the base points can be at say, 7 and 5 o'clock positions. If the tightening required is greater, then they can be as high as at 8 and 4 o'clock positions. To assess the position of these base points, a pair of Babcock forceps are placed to hold the mucocutaneous junction and they are pulled together toward the midline (**Fig. 29.24a**). The fingers are then inserted through the introitus to judge the required amount of tightening. Similarly, placement of apex point also varies based on the amount of desired tightening.

The outside skin overlapping the introitus is gently marked as a U pattern of about 2 cm length, so as to expose the ends of the levator muscle and the scar tissue at the introitus (**Fig. 29.24b, c**). Posterior vaginal wall and the marked areas are infiltrated with a hemostatic solution of 1:200, 000 epinephrine.

First the U-flap of skin is raised from the underlying muscles (**Fig. 29.24d**). The careful dissection continues in posterior vaginal wall to elevate the entire triangle of mucosa right up to the apex (**Fig. 29.24e**). The entire skin-mucosal sheet is then excised in one piece. Interrupted buried sutures are placed to approximate the edges of the mucosa. A second layer of continuous 2–0 absorbable suture is used to close the mucosa up to 1.5 to 2 cm from the introitus. The ends of the levator muscle and the covering fascia at the introitus are sutured together with 2–0 Vicryl (**Fig. 29.24f**). The continuous suture of 2–0 Vicryl now completes the opposition of the mucosa right up to the mucocutaneous junction bringing the two base points together (**Fig. 29.24g**). The skin in U-pattern outside the introitus is now sutured with continuous 4–0 Vicryl (**Fig. 29.24h**). At the end of the procedure, two fingers should snugly fit into the introitus (**Fig. 29.24i**).

Postoperatively patient is ambulated as soon as possible. The urinary catheter is removed. Normal attention to personal hygiene is counseled. Antiseptic/Antibiotic vaginal pessaries are used. Patient is advised to abstain from sexual activity for 4 to 6 weeks. Later, it is advised to use lubricant during the sexual activity.

As a result of tightening, especially of the lower one-third to half of the length of the vaginal canal, the Female Sexual Function Index globally improves. At least two-thirds of the operated women report increased satisfaction in sexual life.[3] However, small numbers complained of dyspareunia and low vaginal secretions or lubrication.

Functional vaginal rejuvenation has been tried with elastic silicone threads[28] and by submucosal implantation of Gore-Micromesh in the posterior vaginal wall through two parallel incisions—one at the inner side of the vaginal inlet, and another in the posterior wall.[29] Results are positive only when the mesh is sutured to the fascia and muscles below, and is plicated.

Hymenoplasty

Hymenoplasty or revirgination is requested for a wide variety of reasons. It may be requested by women to avoid a cultural or social backlash for not being a virgin at the time of

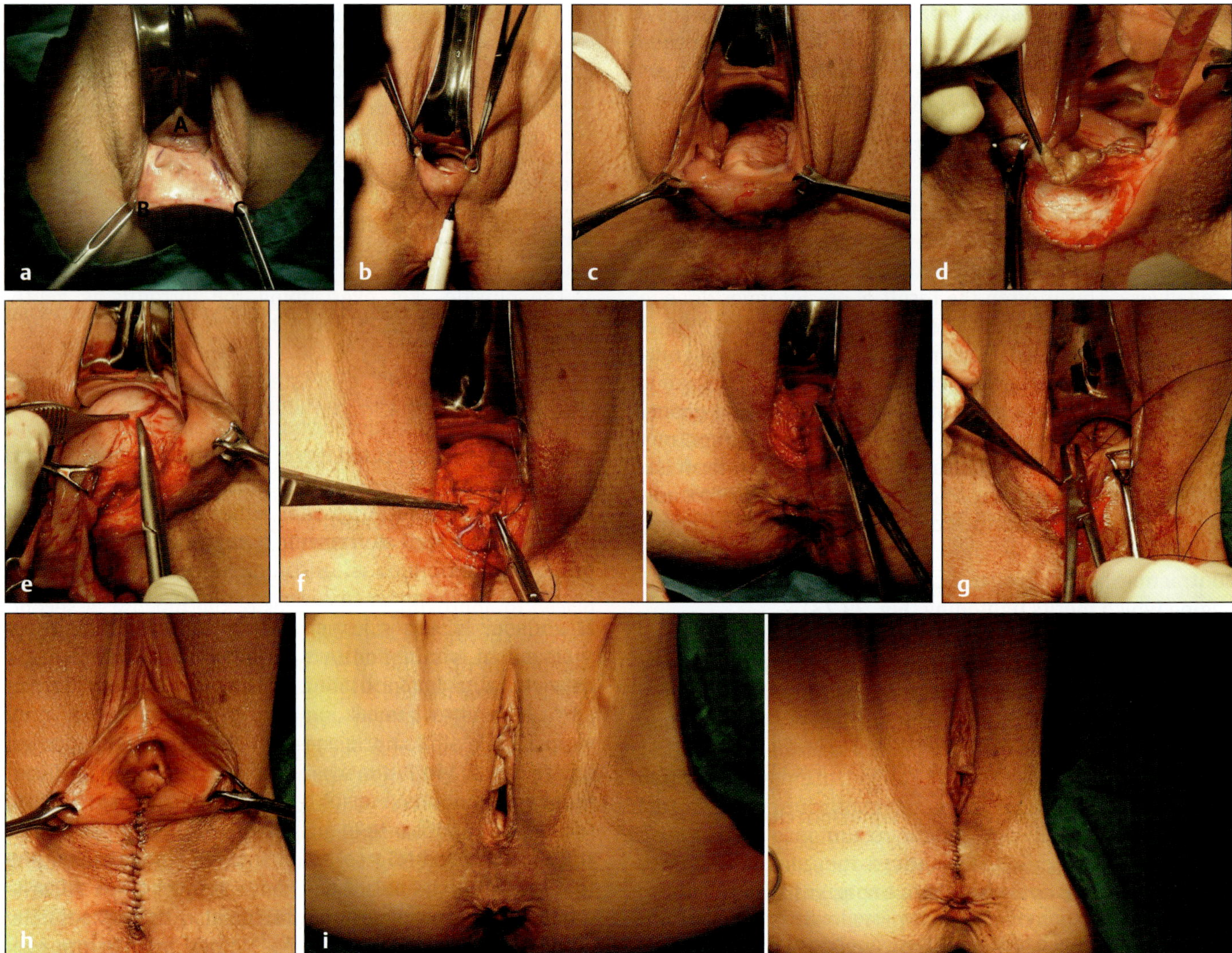

Fig. 29.24 Triangular flap excision on posterior vaginal wall with muscle imbrications. **(a)** Marking of three points over posterior vaginal wall. A is the apex of the triangle. B and C are the variable points over the mucocutaneous junction at the introitus. **(b)** Marking the U pattern on the skin outside the introitus to expose the muscles, **(c)** skin and mucosa marked for dissection and removal for vaginal tightening, **(d)** U pattern of skin outside introitus raised exposing scarred tissue and levator muscle ring underneath, **(e)** excision of posterior vaginal mucosal sheet in one piece. **(f)** Levator muscle repair with interrupted sutures of 2–0 Vicryl, **(g)** closure of mucosa with 2–0 Vicryl, **(h)** final appearance with tightening of vagina and perineum, **(i)** comparison of preop and postop appearance after vaginal and perineal tightening. The length of perineum has significantly increased. (The images are provided courtesy of Dr Milind Wagh, Mumbai, Maharashtra, India.)

marriage. This is requested after penetrative sexual assault or any other personal or social requirement.

The techniques used depend on the status of original hymen. If the hymenal tags are identifiable, they are split using 11 no. surgical blade and adjacent tags are sutured to create the hymen. Several of these adjacent mucosal tags are sutured to one another to create a circular hymenal facsimile with a central aperture. It is also possible to suture together skin tags far from one another across the introitus (**Figs. 29.25 and 29.26**).

In case hymenal tags are absent, two trap door flaps are raised from opposing sides of the vaginal wall. The raw surfaces of flaps are opposed and sutured together (**Figs. 29.27 and 29.28**).

During hymenoplasty, care is taken to leave enough space for the menstrual flow. Healing takes about 3 to 4 weeks. Hence it is ideally done immediately following a menstrual cycle. It is suggested that the hymen should be repaired a few weeks before the expected intercourse, to ensure that it will serve its purpose and would actually tear open. In author's experience, even after many years the reconstructed hymen do not become so fibrosed so as to resist or fail to tear at intercourse. However, postcoital bleeding may be difficult to guarantee in all the cases.

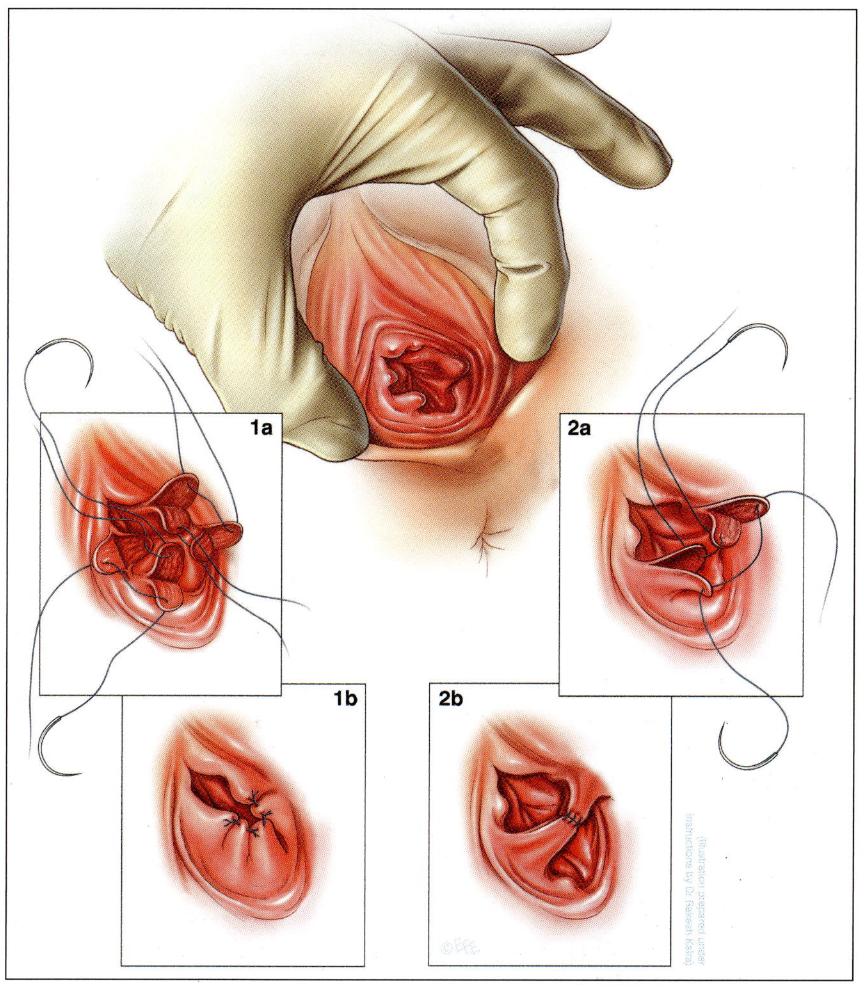

Fig. 29.25 Artist's depiction of suturing of adjacent hymen tags (1a-b) or of tags across the vaginal canal (2a-b).

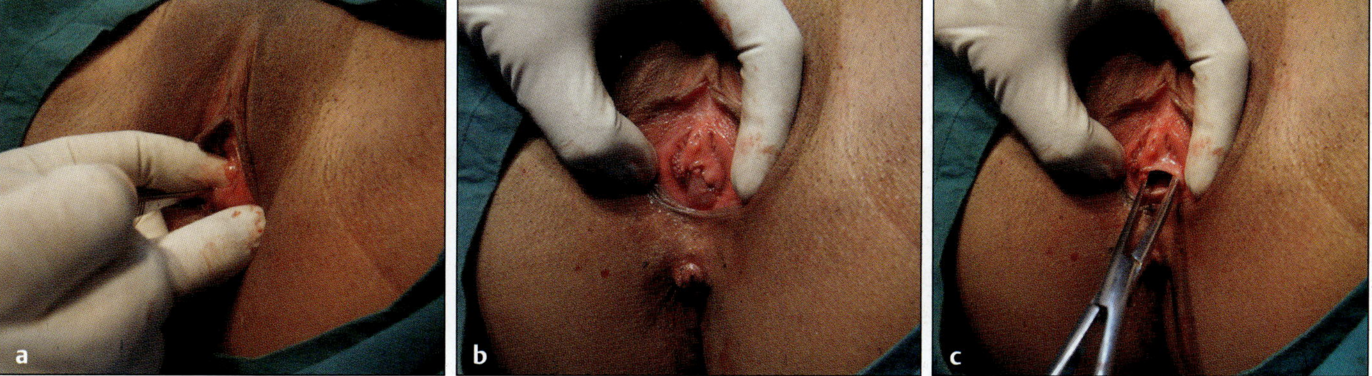

Fig. 29.26 Hymenoplasty using hymenal mucosal tags. **(a)** Tags are demonstrated, **(b)** the tags are sutured around the introitus, **(c)** a central space for menstrual flow is demonstrated.

Combination Procedures of Vaginal Rejuvenation

The rejuvenation surgical techniques have been discussed as independent procedures. However, for achieving the satisfactory result the surgeon should clinically assess the patient, discuss their expectations and possible surgeries. Most of the patients require a combination of procedures for most effective result (**Figs. 29.29–29.32**).

Nonsurgical Vaginal Rejuvenation

Energy-Based Vaginal Tightening—Radiofrequency and Lasers

Vaginal tightening has been tried with radiofrequency and lasers, both attempting to increase submucosal collagen tissue over several sittings. This helps to strengthen and

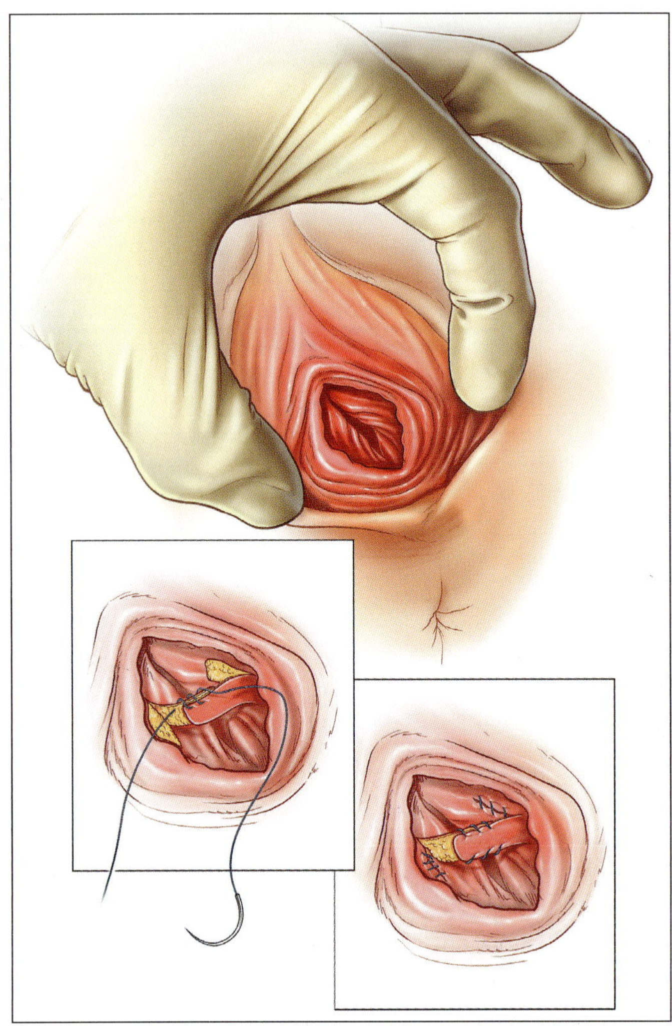

Fig. 29.27 An artist's view of suturing of fresh mucosal flaps raised from adjacent walls of vagina to create a neohymen (3a-b).

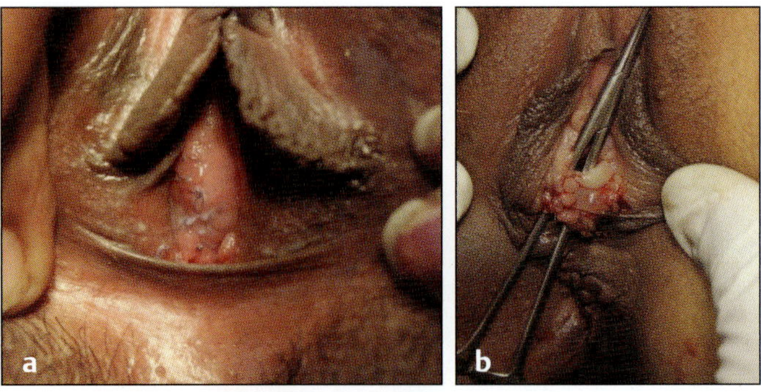

Fig. 29.28 Hymen reconstruction using vaginal mucosal flaps. **(a)** Two flaps have been sutured to reconstruct the hymen; **(b)** a hemostat is inserted to demonstrate the space above and below the hymen to allow menstrual flow.

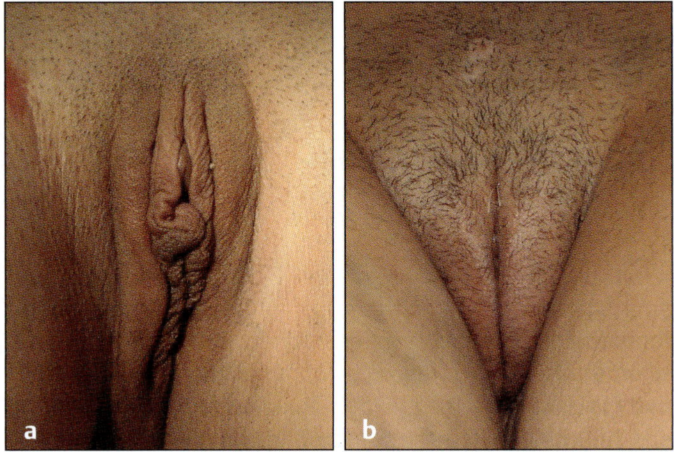

Fig. 29.29 **(a, b)** Atrophic appearance of labia majora augmented by fat, unaesthetic exposure of labia minora trimmed, and redundant intervening fold excised to give a prepubescent appearance.

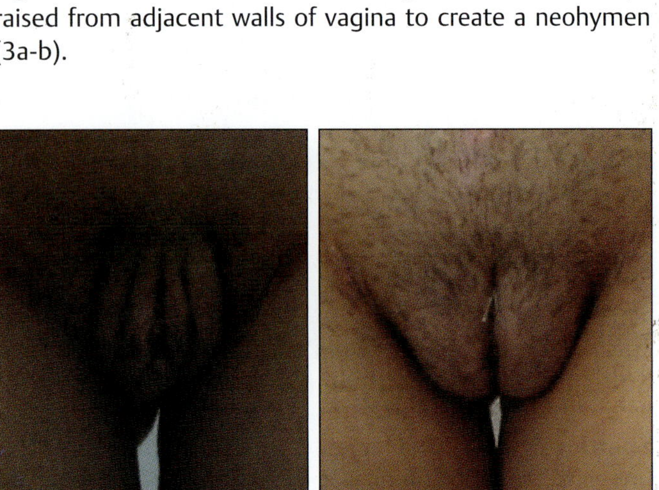

Fig. 29.30 **(a, b)** Atrophic appearance of labia majora augmented by fat, unaesthetic exposure of labia minora trimmed, and redundant intervening fold excised to give a prepubescent appearance.

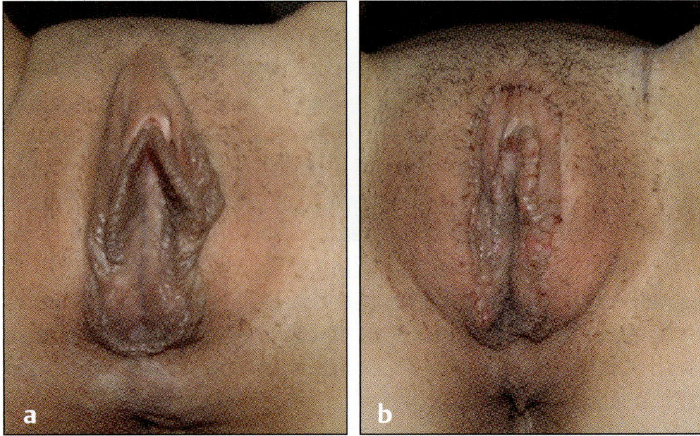

Fig. 29.31 **(a, b)** Atrophic appearance of labia majora augmented by fat, unaesthetic exposure of labia minora trimmed, and redundant intervening fold excised to give a prepubescent appearance.

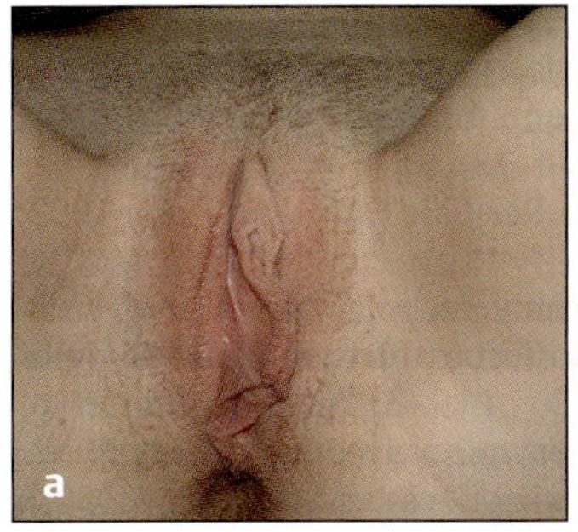

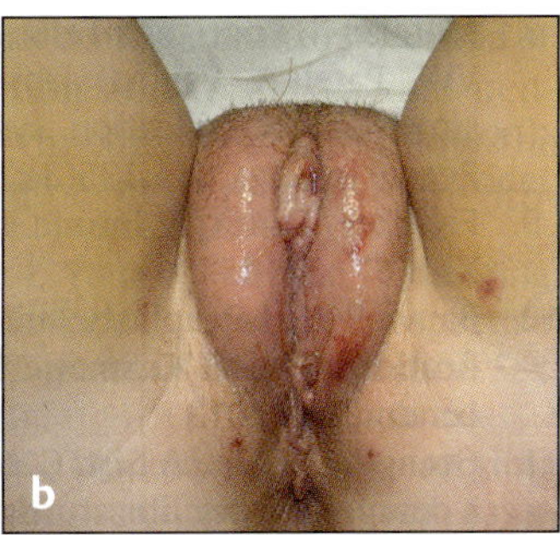

Fig. 29.32 **(a, b)** Reduction of labia minora and fat augmentation of labia majora reduces the patulous vaginal appearance.

thicken the mucosa, thus providing some degree of tightness. This procedure works well in young women, who do not want a surgical scar, and who have just started feeling early loosening of vagina during intercourse. Till date, however, the FDA has not approved any energy-based medical device for vaginal "rejuvenation" or vaginal cosmetic procedures, or for the treatment of vaginal symptoms related to menopause, urinary incontinence, or sexual function.[30]

Fractional CO2 lasers are advertised as conservative, minimally invasive, minimal downtime procedures with no complications and high efficacy. Indications are women with dyspareunia and fibrosis of vaginal mucosae subsequent to episiotomies, and women with altered genital sensation because of vaginal atrophy owing to hormonal changes, menopause, and aging. Histological changes of increased collagen layer have been demonstrated. Other changes brought about by lasers are collagen/elastin contraction, neovascularization, neocollagenases, improved vaginal lubrication, improved elasticity and hydration.[3, 31] It has also been tried to build up mucosal rugosities, especially in women who have, what is called a bald vaginal mucosa, i.e., smooth without any rugosities. The improved rugosities help in achieving better friction during sexual intercourse. For this the CO2 laser is used in continuous mode at 8 to 10 W with defocus. The depth of vaginal columnar rugae vaporization is between 2 and 5 mm width.[32]

The Erbium-YAG laser is nonablative and causes hyperthermia at 65°C. This remodels the vaginal mucosa, causing improved elasticity and tightness. Two treatment sessions are given, at 4 to 6 weeks apart.[33]

Radiofrequency is another device which emits focused electromagnetic waves. This has been classically used for firming up both the face and neck skin. No anesthetic is required for using 75 to 90 J/cm^2 of RF energy.[34]

PRP and Hyaluronic Acid Injections

Vaginal atrophy, dryness, pruritis, irritation, loss of subcutaneous fat, sparse pubic hair, and dyspareunia are the signs of aging. Majority of these conditions that occur postmenopausal are especially because of decreased estrogen levels.

A variety of nonsurgical rejuvenation procedures have been tried alone or in combination. Platelet-rich plasma (PRP) alone, or in combination with fat or hyaluronic acid, has been used with fair results in restoration of labia minora pigmentation along with youthful contour of labia majora.[35, 36] Lipofilling of the posterior vaginal wall, in combination with hyaluronic acid and PRP in the subcutaneous tissue of the surrounding perineum, has been tried, [36] but effectiveness and safety need further studies. Vaginal dryness can be helped with PRP injections which enhance the lubrication.

Many patients suffer from excessive and troublesome lubrication. Ablative lasers can be used on the lateral vaginal walls in a checkboard fashion to reduce the quantum of mucus-secreting glands.

Ablative CO2 and RF can also be used to produce skin lightening, but complications may sometimes produce even further hyperpigmentation.[37] The area is sensitive, and it is better to err on the side of negative, rather than over doing and causing burns with the energy-based devices. Alternatively, perineal skin lightening is possible with local chemical applications. Systemically, vitamin C, pine extract, tranexamic acid, and glutathione have been tried but there is no evidence of their benefits.

G-Spot Injections

Ernst Grafenberg, a German gynecologist, identified a highly erogenous area in the anterior vaginal wall which is supplied by more nerve endings.[38,39] Few years later many authors termed this as the G-spot after the innovator's name. This is on the anterior vaginal wall, about 3.8 to 4.2 cm from the pubic bone about a centimeter below the external urinary meatus. As an anatomic structure it is difficult to identify. Some surgeons enhance this area, by submucosal injection of hyaluronic acid, PRP, or fat.[40] The effect is to protrude the area, and also to increase the surface area, which makes it amenable to greater friction during intercourse. This increases the possibility and duration of orgasm. However, if the vaginal canal is loose, a simple G-spot enhancement may not work unless tightening is done. Hence a proper patient selection and counseling are the keys to success.[41]

Summary and Caution

There has been an increasing demand for the female genital rejuvenation procedures, over the years. In true sense, these fall outside the realm of evidence-based medicosurgical procedures and are truly not medically indicated procedures. Considering the reality of the situation and constant requirement, Canadian Task Force on Preventive Healthcare has enlisted guidelines which caution the specialists before undertaking these procedures.[42]

- The obstetrician and gynecologist should play an important role in helping women to understand their anatomy and to respect individual variations.

30

Aesthetic Surgery of Male Genitalia

Borko Stojanovic, Slavica Pusica, Marko Bencic, Marta Bizic, and Miroslav L. Djordjevic

and are therefore highly utilized in penile reconstructive procedures.[3,4]

The penis is supplied by two arterial systems: superficial and deep. The superficial and deep systems arise from the external and internal pudendal arteries, respectively. The internal pudendal artery supplies most of the penile entities, through common penile artery and its branches: bulbourethral artery, cavernosal artery, and the dorsal penile artery. The bulbourethral artery enters the corpus spongiosum to supply the glans, urethra, and corpus spongiosum. The cavernosal artery supplies the cavernosal sinuses that engorge with erection. The dorsal penile artery travels between the penile crura and the pubis, continuing with the dorsal vein and dorsal penile nerve within the neurovascular bundle. It supplies the dorsal cavernosal bodies and provides redundant blood supply to the glans, urethra, and corpus spongiosum via circumferential branches. Drainage is achieved by superficial and deep dorsal veins, which drain into the preprostatic plexus. Somatic innervations of the penis derive from the pudendal nerve, which continues as the dorsal penile nerve. Parasympathetic and sympathetic innervations are based on the cavernous nerve, providing tumescence and ejaculation[3] **(Fig. 30.1b, c)**.

Aetiopathogenesis

Indications for Penile Enhancement Surgery

Medical conditions that represent indication for penile augmentation can be divided into congenital and acquired. Many surgeons believe that the only real indication for penile enhancement surgery is actually a micropenis, which can be caused by endocrinological disorders or genetic factors. Other congenital anomalies that require aesthetic corrections are hypospadias, epispadias, and intersex disorders, where correction is not only focused on penile size, but also on urethra repair and other aspects of penile appearance. Surgical intervention can also be considered in certain acquired medical conditions that carry the risk of penile shortening, such as penile cancer, various penile injuries, Peyronie disease, and different modalities of prostate cancer treatment (radiation, hormone therapy, radical prostatectomy).

Penile Dysmorphophobia

Some men may be so preoccupied with the size of their penis that they develop a disorder called penile dysmorphic disorder (PDD). PDD is not an actual diagnosis in the DSM (the Diagnostic and Statistical Manual that psychiatrists and psychologists use for diagnosing mental disorders); in most cases it is better considered as a subtype of body dysmorphic disorder (BDD) that focuses exclusively on the penis. These are mostly men with average penis length and circumference. There is no standardized technique for measuring penis size; most authors agree that the penis should generally be measured from the base, i.e., from the pubopenile junction to the tip of the glans.[5] The measurement is performed in three states, flaccid, stretched, and erect. Girth measurements are made in the middle of the penile shaft, in the flaccid and erect states. The measurement should be performed by a trained person and not by using a questionnaire.

Various studies have dealt with the "normal" size of the penis, but there is still no generally accepted criterion.[6–8] Penile dimensions vary depending on erectile state. Normal erect adult penises are 12.7 to 17.7 cm long and have a circumference of 11.3 to 13 cm. In contrast, flaccid penises are 7.6 to 13 cm long with a circumference of 8.5 to 10.5 cm. Knowledge of these normal dimensions is essential for evaluating a request for enhancement surgery.

A patient may be considered to be suffering from some type of penile dysmorphophobia if the patient has no acquired or congenital disease that would result in an objectively small penis, the length or circumference of the penis is within the average range, and the patient has anxiety about the size of the penis or has doubts about the adequacy of the appearance of genitals. The small penis syndrome is a type of PDD and is defined as an anxiety about the genitals being observed, directly or indirectly (when clothed), because of the concern that the flaccid penis length and/or girth is less than the normal for an adult male, despite evidence from a clinical examination to counter this concern.[9]

Preoperative Evaluation

Penile enhancement surgery is associated with the highest reported patient satisfaction and is very effective in cases with penile dysmorphophobia. However, these procedures can lead to numerous intraoperative and postoperative complications that range from mild to difficult, such as severe penile deformity and functional damage. All patients should undergo medical and psychological evaluation prior to aesthetic penile surgery and should also be educated and informed about the various treatment options, results, and possible complications. They should be provided images and videos of the aesthetic result of surgery, as well as should be informed about postoperative stretching regime in order to maintain postoperative girth and length increase.[10,11]

During the physical examination stretched penile length and penile body circumference should be measured and documented and shown to the patient to avoid unrealistic expectations and patient dissatisfaction.[12] There are few contraindications for penile enhancement surgery, such as previous penile surgery with a lack of penile skin and visible scars, confirmed erectile dysfunction, inability to undergo anesthesia, untreatable blood dyscrasia, untreated active infection, or known hypersensitivity or allergy to synthetic materials.

Selection of Patients

Patient selection presents the key to optimizing clinical outcomes in penile aesthetic surgery. Persons who undergo penile aesthetic surgery require a detailed preoperative assessment and counseling prior to their operation. This is a crucial step to ensure that patients have made fully informed decisions and that they understand what the surgery entails and its intended objectives. According to systematic literature research and recent statements, only individualized approach is beneficial in carefully selected patients who pass adequate preoperative counseling. During patient counseling, particular attention should be paid to patient's medical and surgical history when considering the type of procedure. Following a careful and complete history, physical examination, and basic laboratory studies, several examinations are useful in defining a proper method for penile enhancement. Also, additional exams should be done to define penile anatomy and possible associated functional deficits. Preoperative measurement of penile dimensions, both length and girth, is mandatory in preventing postoperative unsatisfactory results. In cases where erectile dysfunction is associated with penile dysmorphophobia, erectile test with prostaglandin E1 is recommended to define level and characteristics of erection. Also, any systemic risk factors such as smoking, diabetes mellitus, hypertension or hypercholesterolemia, high body mass index (BMI), and hormonal or neurological etiologies should be evaluated preoperatively. Patients should be given sufficient time to make a decision for surgery. It is also important to involve their partner, if possible.

Preoperative Care

Penile enhancement surgery is performed under general, spinal, or even local anesthesia according to the patient's condition and surgical team's preference. The patient is placed in a supine position on the operative table. The genitals are shaved and scrubbed with chlorhexidine soap immediately before the incision. Intravenous broad spectrum antibiotics are also administered before the incision and the skin prepped with an alcohol-based solution. There is evidence that alcohol-based chlorhexidine solution is better than povidone-iodine in preventing surgical wound site infection.[13] A surgical incision drape is also placed to decrease undesired skin contact.

Penile Girth Enhancement

Nonsurgical Penile Girth Enhancement: Injection Therapy

The main premise of the use of the injectable materials in penile girth enhancement is that these techniques are considered to be minimally invasive, safe, simple, and effective. Different materials have been applied to increase phallic girth since the 1900s, such as paraffin, mineral oils, mercury, cod liver oil, which led to serious complications: foreign body reactions, scarring, deformities, and sexual dysfunction.[14] Because of these complications, surgeons have relied on plastic surgery and dermatology research which has described the use of materials such as silicone, autologous fat, collagen, hyaluronic acid (HA), and others. It must be noted that, to date, there are no recommended indications for these procedures in the medical literature, nor have any guidelines been suggested.[15] In addition, no injectable filler has been approved by the US Food and Drug Administration (FDA) for use in the penis.[16] Nevertheless, as a growing number of men with penile dissatisfaction pursue esthetic treatment to enhance their penile girth, there is a need for safe and effective procedures. Penile girth enlargement can be done by transferring autologous fat or injecting a soft tissue filler. Soft tissue fillers are classified as nonpermanent (collagen, HA), semipermanent (calcium hydroxylapatite [CaHA] and poly-L-lactic acid [PLA]), and permanent (polymethyl methacrylate microspheres [PMMA], highly purified forms of liquid silicone, and hydrogel polymers) (**Fig. 30.2**).

Autologous Fat Transfer

Autologous fat injections into the dartos fascia are frequently used in phallic image alterations. First described by Panfilov in 2006, augmentative phalloplasty with autologous fat transfer was performed on 88 patients, aged 24 to 54 years. Sixty patients underwent autologous fat transfer only and 28 received additional ligament release. The skin at the base was elongated by V-Y plasty, and the scrotal skin was released by Z-plasty. Initial penis length was 6.5 to 10 cm (average 8.72 cm) and circumference was 8 to 10.1 cm (average 9.18 cm) in flaccid state. At one-year follow-up, 77 patients stated they were highly satisfied, and 8 were fairly satisfied. Three early and late complications were reported.[17]

Preparation

Before surgery, patients should shower and the operative field should be shaved. The donor site is, in most cases, bilaterally from the thighs, but when there is localized adiposity in suprapubic region, liposuction of this area can enhance the final result, as it unveils hidden penis. This type of surgery is usually performed under general anesthesia, but sometimes it can be conducted using intravenous sedation ("twilight anesthesia") combined with a penis root block, which causes an intrasurgical erection. After standard disinfection of the skin, the adipose tissue is harvested.

Through two 0.5- to 0.7-cm subcutaneous incisions in the inguinal region, 200 to 300 mL of the tumescent formula is injected with the infiltration cannula. The tumescent formula (modified Klein solution) consists of 100 mL of regular saline solution containing epinephrine (1:1,000), 20 mL

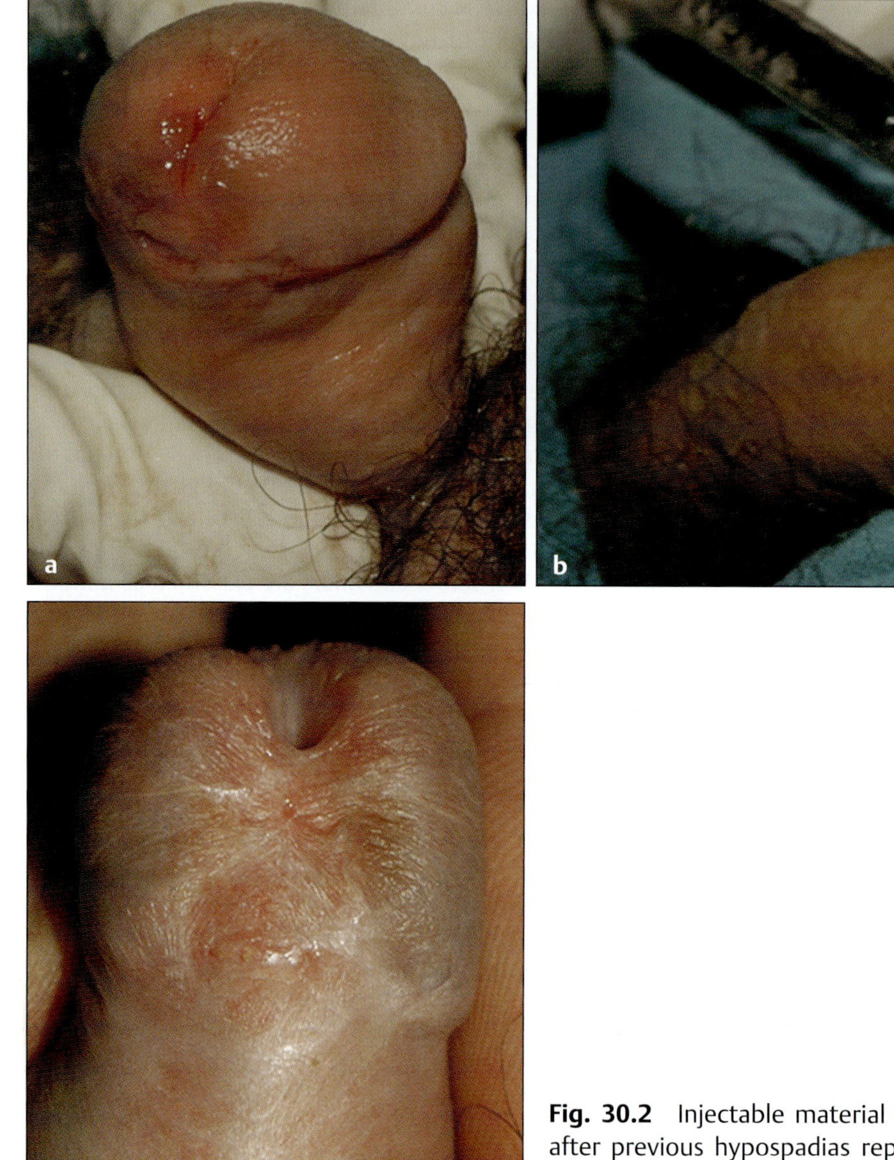

Fig. 30.2 Injectable material for glans augmentation: **(a)** glans deformity after previous hypospadias repair; **(b)** Bio-Alcamid (alkyl-imide polymer) is used for glans contour and deformity correction; **(c)** result after procedure.

of 8.4% sodium bicarbonate and 2% lidocaine. The maximum amount of injected lidocaine should not exceed 35 mg/kg. After additional 15 to 20 minutes, liposuction is performed with a harvesting cannula, using fanlike pattern in the subcutaneous fat layer, going back and forth. About 30 to 60 mL of fat is extracted from the inner side of upper thigh. If more fat is needed, it can be harvested from the front or side of the upper thigh, inner side of the knee, or the lower abdomen.

A fat sieve is used to filter the tumescent solution, blood, and free oil, which are unnecessary fluids during liposuction. Filtered fat is washed in normal saline (500 mL) to remove unnecessary components. The filtered fat tissue is divided into 10-mL syringes using a teaspoon. The capped sampling syringes without the piston are sealed and centrifuged. After centrifugation, the harvested fat separates into three layers. The uppermost layer composed of oil is decanted, and the reddish layer at the bottom composed of blood, water, lidocaine, and fibrous tissue is drained by opening the cap of the syringe. The middle layer predominantly composed of fat is used for the injection.

Penile Autologous Fat Injection

A blunt-tip cannula is typically used for autologous fat transfer into the penis. If we imagine the frenulum on a clock face at 6 o'clock, then the penile skin is punctured at the 11, 1, 3, and 9 o'clock locations around the penis, and the fat is injected into the various layers and directions, with avoidance of the urethral area (5–7 o'clock). Fat is injected throughout the penis, beginning from the distal portion and proceeding to the penile root. When the injections are complete, the penis needs to be moved between two hands and carefully "kneaded." The incisions do not need stitching and they leave no visible scars. Cohesive elastic bandage is necessary to prevent shifting of the fat during change of posture or erections. The patients are advised to abstain from physical activity for 30 days and sexual activity and masturbation for 60 days.

Collagen and Hyaluronic Acid (HA) Injection

Collagen was the first facial filler to be introduced decades ago, and due to its properties like immediate effect and easy administration, it was considered a logical material for penile girth enhancement. Collagen can be sourced and is commercially available from a variety of animal models: human, bovine, and porcine. Bovine collagen derivatives require hypersensitivity testing, as up to 3% of patients receiving these collagens will develop a reaction.[18] Porcine products, due to their manufacturing process, do not require sensitivity testing.[19] While collagen is considered to be relatively safe, it rapidly degrades and has the shortest durability among all of the injectable materials, thus leading to frequent reinjections. Some of the possible side effects are nodules, beading, and granuloma.[20] Although collagen fillers have found their role in aesthetic surgery and are often used as "gold standard" for comparison with other dermal fillers, reports about penile girth enhancement with collagen are anecdotal.

Emerging popularity of HA has revolutionized the use of soft tissue fillers in aesthetic medicine. As an important natural component of human body and a conserved component of all living beings, HA fillers do not possess tissue specificity. Therefore, humoral or cell-mediated immune reactions are extremely rare, and unlike collagen, use of HA does not require allergy testing. The half-life of HA in natural form is within 20 hours, and HA survives only for 1 to 2 days. Crosslinking process is used to stabilize HA, leading to an increased longevity. One of the significant differences between the various HA-based products is the molecular weight of HA used in cross-linking.[21] The most common adverse event is hypersensitivity reactions (~0.02%), while major adverse events include infection, granulomatous reaction, and formation of acneiform and cystic lesions, but they are rare.[22,23] Superficial injection may leave a bluish discoloration (called Tyndall effect). One of the main advantages of HA fillers is that some of the adverse events or migration may be safely reversed with hyaluronidase.

Kwak et al investigated 41 patients who were injected with 20.56-mL HA and followed up for 18 months.[24] HA was injected into the fascial layer of penile body in flaccid state using a 21-gauge cannula with the "Back & Forth Technique" at four locations: 10, 2, 5, and 7 o'clock positions from the base of the penis to the coronal sulcus. They reported that the mean increase in the circumference of girth was 3.9 ± 0.3 cm (3.4–4.4) at 1 month which decreased to 3.8 ± 0.3 cm (3.2–4.2) at 18 months. There was no deformity, inflammation, or any adverse reaction in any of the cases. Another group of 41 patients were injected with HA into their glans penis. They reported increase in glandular circumference of 1.5 cm at 1-year follow-up. There was no sign of inflammation or any serious adverse reaction. The same investigators reported 15% decrease in glandular circumference at 5-year follow-up.[25]

Calcium Hydroxylapatite (CaHA) and Poly-L-Lactic Acid (PLLA)

Calcium hydroxylapatite (CaHA) is an injectable dermal filler that contains uniform CaHA microspheres suspended in an aqueous carboxymethylcellulose gel carrier. It is considered a long-lasting, but nonpermanent, filler, and is highly biocompatible with human tissue. As with all biodegradable dermal fillers, CaHA can be associated with rare incidences of foreign body reactions, but only a handful of case reports have been documented in 10 years of clinical use. CaHA can be associated with local, short-term, injection-related adverse events, which are generally mild and resolve within a few days. Clinical trials that have followed patients for up to 3 years postinjection report no adverse events.[26]

PLLA is a biodegradable, resorbable synthetic polymer which belongs chemically to the alpha-hydroxy-acid group. PLLA has the ability to stimulate fibroblast proliferation and neocollagenesis by foreign body reaction, which stimulates a cellular inflammatory response. Most common adverse effects are formation of papules and nodules (<10%), and if they do not resolve spontaneously, intralesional steroid injection or excision may be needed. Lee and colleagues conducted preliminary study about penile girth enhancement with PLLA injections on 23 patients who were treated with 10 mL of PLGA-based filler and followed up for 6 months. They reported a mean increase of 2.4 cm in the penile circumference. Adverse events were reported in five cases: three cases of injection site induration, one of penile curvature, and one of painful erection. All adverse events were mild, which improved within few months.[17,27,28]

Liquid Injectable Silicone (LIS) and Polymethylmethacrylate (PMMA)

Liquid injectable silicone (LIS), or polydimethylsiloxane, was one of the first materials used for soft tissue augmentation and as sculpturing agent. Use of LIS, since the collagen and other fillers were introduced, is to say at least controversial and highly discussed. Currently, only two LIS products (AdatoSil and Silikon 1000) are approved by the US Food and Drug Administration (FDA). These are only used for treatment of retinal detachment.[29] Proponents of LIS assert that in its highly purified form and with correct application, they are perfectly safe and complications are rare. However, when they occur, due to either large volume of filler or poor techniques, adverse effects can be grave for cosmetic appearance, for instance, granuloma formation, migration to other sites, skin dyschromia, and can only be handled surgically.[23]

Considering that most adverse effects of LIS are in connection to high volume, it is widely accepted that its use in penile augmentation would not be suitable, and most studies regarding this topic point to its unacceptable results. However, Yacobi et al reported the largest series of liquid silicone penile injection in 324 men. The authors performed injections of 5 mL on the dorsal and lateral aspects of the penis, repeated three to six times at intervals of at least 30 days. On average, penile circumference was improved by 2.6 cm (27% increase), and no postoperative complications were noted.[30]

PMMA, which is a synthetic polymer of methylmethacrylate, is a nonabsorbable, biocompatible, and permanent filler material. It consists of 30- to 120-mm-sized microspheres with smooth surface. The most common adverse event is lumpiness, followed by erythema, itching, hypertrophic scarring, and granuloma formation. Yang et al injected 20 patients with 24-mL PMMA for penile enlargement and followed up for 6 months. They reported a mean increase in penile circumference of 3.7 cm at penile base, 4.2 cm at midshaft, and 3.8 cm at distal shaft. The complications were mild asymmetry of penile shape and nodular lesion at the injected site in one patient each. The same investigators also reported results at 1-year follow-up, showing no significant difference between 6 and 12 months.[31]

Surgical Penile Girth Enhancement

Dermal Fat Graft

A dermal fat graft is an epidermis-free graft that comprises all layers of the skin and the underlying subcutaneous tissue after removal of the epidermis.[32] Commonly performed in reconstructive surgery, this procedure transfers high volume of dermis and fat. This has relatively high-graft success rate with low absorption in penile augmentation. The posttransplant survival mechanism of adipose cells is still not known, but there are unproven theories such as the host cell replacement theory and the cell survival theory.

Low fat diet can be recommended 2 to 3 weeks prior to surgery, leading to smaller fat content, thus reducing degenerated adipose cells and improving rate of adipose cells. Both the recipient site and the donor site should be shaved and thoroughly disinfected. For penile girth enhancement, dermofat graft is harvested from the abdomen, flank, or gluteal folds. One of the disadvantages of gluteal dermofat graft is that the position of the patient needs to be changed during surgery. Size of the graft is determined based on the dimensions of the penis. The absorption rate of fat must also be taken into consideration; thus, graft should be 20 to 30% bigger than that anticipated solely on the recipient size. First step is skin incision without exposing the subcutaneous fat. The dermis is deepithelized by peeling off the epidermis using size-appropriate surgical blade. Complete removal of the epidermis is necessary to prevent possible epidermal cysts at graft site. Upon complete deepithelization, dermal incision is extended into subcutaneous tissue and once it reaches adequate depth, dermal fat graft is lifted en bloc. The deep fat layer of the donor site and the subcutaneous tissue are closed by layer-by-layer suturing, which is followed by the skin closure.

The skin below coronary groove of penis should be incised by circular or longitudinal mode, and then sufficient pocket should be created by dissecting up to the Buck fascia as fast as possible, where the harvested dermofat will be placed. For the graft, usually the juxtaposition method to place the fat side of grafted tissue parallel to the base of the recipient site is used. Graft is fixated at several points to penile subcutaneous tissue. In cases where preservation of preputial skin is requested, penoscrotal approach can be used. Longitudinal incision is made at the base of the penis through the scrotal skin and penile body is dissected and separated from the skin. Dermofat is placed around the body and fixed. Inverted penile skin is replaced and penile shaft with graft in place is transposed inside and incision closed (**Fig. 30.3**).

Some authors have reported outcomes for dermal fat grafting in small cohorts. Spyropoulos and colleagues reported a mean increase in penile circumference of 2.3 cm at the base and 2.6 cm at the coronal groove with dermal fat grafting.[33] Xu and colleagues performed dermal fat grafting in 23 patients who simultaneously underwent lengthening with suspensory ligament division. The authors utilized two longitudinal, dermal fat grafts, which were secured proximally to prevent graft migration. At 6 months follow-up, the flaccid girth increased by 1.7 ± 0.5 cm, and patient satisfaction was significantly improved in several domains of the Male Genital Image Score.[34] One of the improvements is the possibility of performing simultaneous dermolipectomy of lower abdominal wall and girth augmentation with dermal fat from the same region (**Fig. 30.4**). Some of the complications that can occur after this procedure are edema, redness, infection, skin necrosis, wound protrusion, penile curvature, epidermal cyst, seromas, and penile deformities.

Allografts

Allograft is an acellular dermal matrix and acquired from donated skin using proprietary processing techniques that are reported to preserve the biochemical and structural components of the extracellular matrix.[35] The main idea behind use of allografts in penile augmentation is that allograft could replace autologous fat and other fillers because of its ability to provide the cosmetic benefit of symmetry and durability without the need for more complex harvesting. Various allografts have been used in penile augmentation such as AlloDerm® (LifeCell Laboratories, USA), MegaDerm® (L&C BIO, Korea), and SureDerm® (Hans Biomed, Korea).[36]

Allograft should be soaked in saline solution with antibiotics 20 minutes prior to graft suturing. Blood is applied on both sides of the allograft and then washed off on only one side. The blood-soaked side should face Buck fascia. The size of the allograft is determined based on the penile

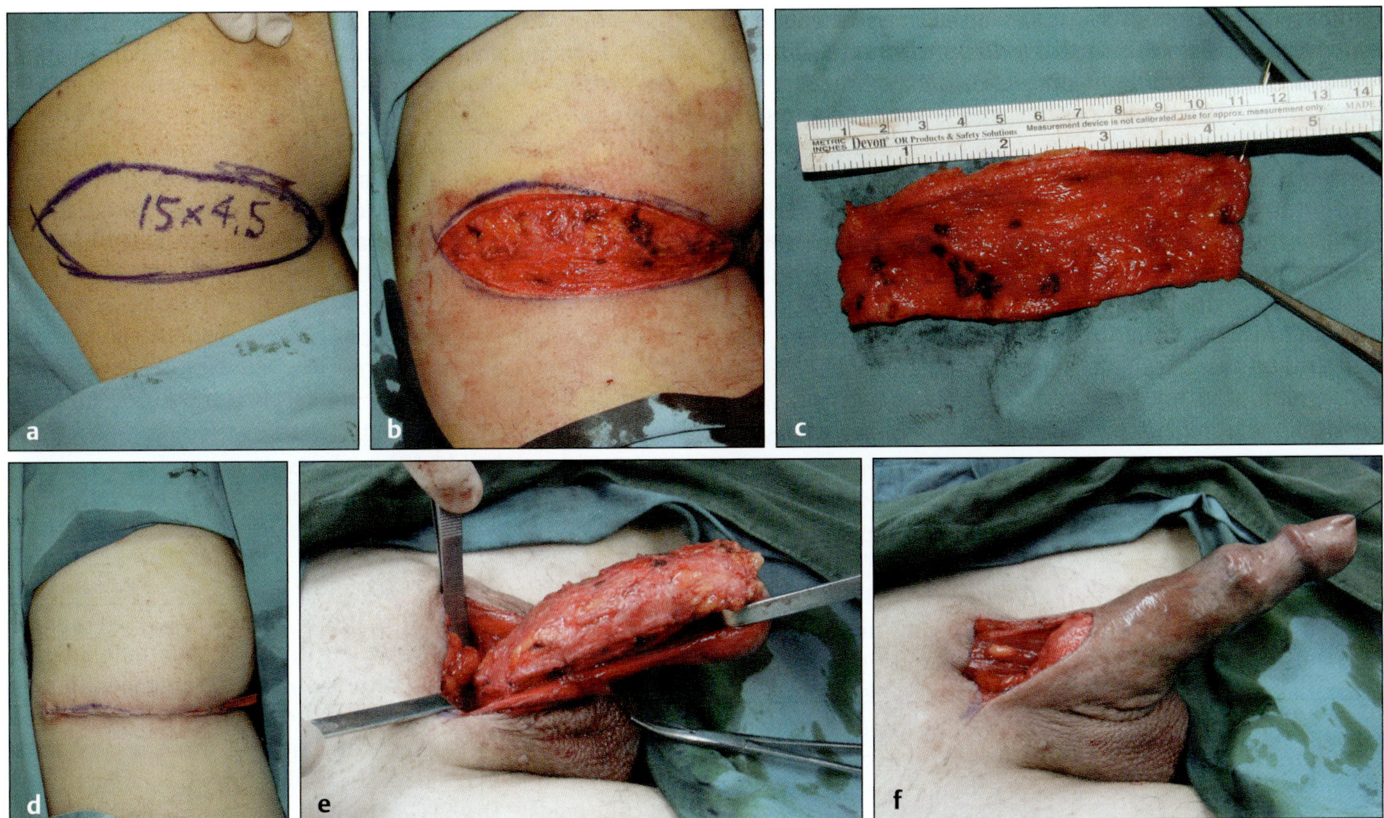

Fig. 30.3 Dermal fat grafting: **(a)** left buttock is marked for harvesting; **(b)** de-epithelialization is done; **(c)** good shape of the harvested graft; **(d)** donor skin closure; **(e)** dermal fat graft is placed around the penile body; **(f)** additional ligamentolysis is done simultaneously before skin closure.

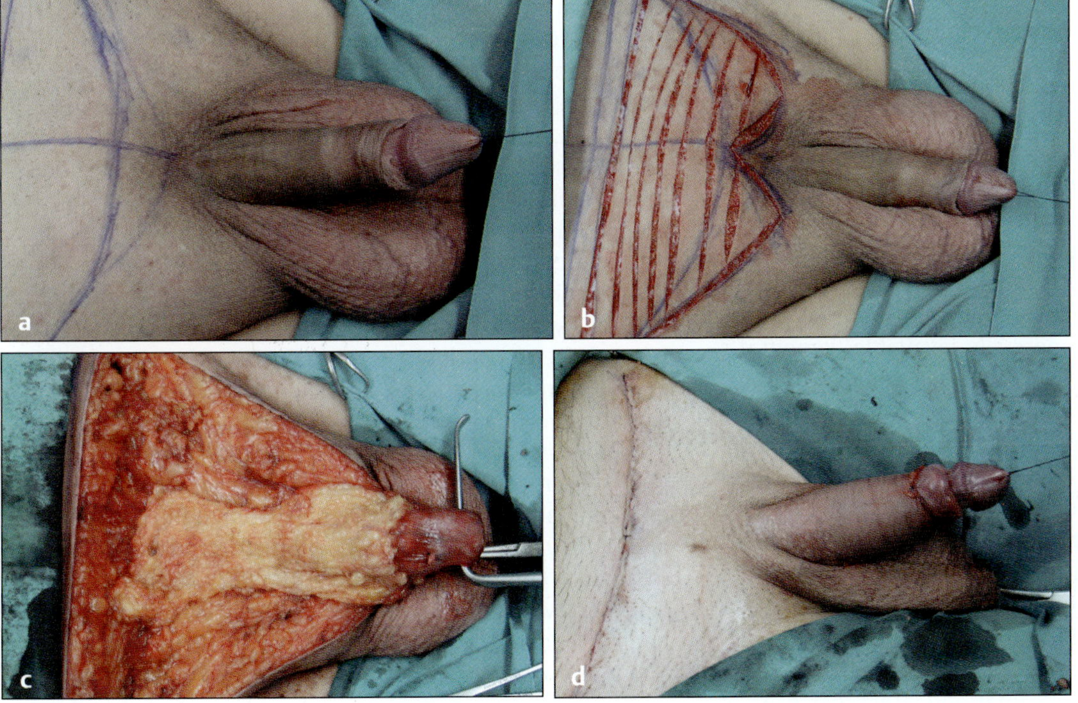

Fig. 30.4 Dermal fat grafting with abdominoplasty: **(a)** lower abdominal wall is marked for removal; **(b)** de-epithelialization is done creating good dermal fat graft; **(c)** dermal fat graft is fixed to the penile body by penile inversion approach; **(d)** appearance at the end of surgery.

dimensions. There are two approaches for graft placement: infrapubic incision and through circumcision incision. In infrapubic approach, transverse incision, Z-plasty, or V-Y plasty can be used. The incision area is spread open until the dartos fascia is found. The index finger is inserted into the incision area to pull out the penis. The allograft is fixated onto the penis at eight points: three on the coronary sulcus, three on the proximal penis, and one on the center of allograft at both corpus spongiosum borders. The penis is placed back into its original position. The dartos fascia, subcutaneous tissue, and skin are sutured. A small drain can be placed in the infrapubic area. For circumcised individuals, incision is made on the entire circumcised portion of the penis. For noncircumcised individuals, incision is made 1 to 1.5 cm below the coronary sulcus, and excess skin may be removed if necessary. Incision is made until the Buck fascia is reached. Then the dartos fascia is separated from the Buck fascia to the root of the penis. Allograft is placed in between the dartos fascia and Buck fascia and fixed in the same manner as in the infrapubic incision method. Then, the penis is placed back into its original position. The dartos fascia, subcutaneous tissue, and skin are closed in layers.

There are several reports regarding postoperative complications. They range from minor to very severe. Bruno et al reported the first two cases of complications following penile augmentation, which led to extensive penile skin necrosis requiring split-thickness skin grafting in both.[37] Solomon et al compared outcomes of girth enhancement with three different acellular dermal matrix materials (AlloDerm®, Belladerm®, Repriza®) placed in a series of 47 patients. Overall, 42% of patients had infectious complications, and 6.4% of cases resulted in total graft loss. There were no differences in complications among the different matrix preparations.[35]

Xenografts

Xenografts are derived from animal tissues (bovine and porcine), and they are subjected to various methods of processing to be suitable for use in humans. Initial rat experiments demonstrated that these grafts promote neovascularization and collagen deposition with decreased inflammatory response as compared to synthetic material. Some of the most popular commercially available xenografts are Permacol—porcine-derived dermal collagen tissue, Lyoplant—collagen implant made from acellular bovine pericardium, SurgiMend—xenogenic acellular dermal matrix derived from fetal bovine dermis tissue, and MegaDerm Ultra derived from porcine dermis.

Size of the graft is determined according to penile dimensions. Multiple transverse and vertical slits are made in the graft. After the surgeon has opted for access, which may also depend on the patient's preferences, blunt and sharp dissection is performed, pocket created, prepared graft is anchored to Buck fascia on the distal, proximal, and lateral parts of the penis using absorbable sutures.

Complications that could occur after surgery are penile edema, wound dehiscence, infection, hematoma, penile skin necrosis, penile curvature, and penile deformity **(Fig. 30.5)**. Alei et al reported the first series of penile girth augmentation with porcine dermal matrix grafts placed through a small penopubic incision. In a cohort of 69 men, the mean increase in flaccid and erect circumferences was 3.1 and 2.4 cm, respectively.[38] All patients experienced self-limited penile edema, and eight patients had either massive ecchymosis or suture dehiscence. In addition, graft fibrosis with reduced penile elasticity occurred in eight patients. Another report from Saudi Arabia revealed high rate of complications after using a porcine xenograft for penile girth augmentation in 18 patients. Postoperative complications occurred in eight (44.4%) patients, two of whom required graft removal. Despite improvement in penile girth, nine (50%) patients were unsatisfied according to a nonvalidated questionnaire.[39]

Biodegradable Scaffolds

In 2006, Perovic et al reported novel technique for penile augmentation by using autologous tissue-engineered, biologically resorbable scaffolds. The technique is based on transplanting autologous cells from dermal tissue onto tube-shaped biodegradable scaffolds (PLGA, poly lactic-co-glycolic acid).[40] Dry PLGA scaffold 50 mm in length, 30 mm in inner diameter, and 3 mm in thickness is first seeded with fibroblasts previously harvested from the patient's serum, and incubated for 24 hours. The surgical procedure starts with a subcoronal incision and penile degloving, followed by placement of two cell-seeded scaffolds around the penile shaft. Shape adjustment is required to keep the urethra and periurethral tissue uncovered and scaffold-free. Careful implantation is necessary to avoid injury to surrounding structures, as well as damage to scaffold, which can result in migration and significant deformation. To prevent possible migration, scaffold is fixed with multiple sutures to fascia. In rare cases of noncompliant skin, they can be placed under lifted neurovascular bundle. Dartos fascia and penile skin are closed in layers **(Fig. 30.6)**.

The preliminary clinical results were encouraging, showing a significantly lower complication rate than reported in previously established procedures, and they included skin necrosis in two patients, seroma in six patients, and wound infection in two patients, all of whom were managed conservatively. Long-term follow-up and possibility of repeated procedure with goal for more girth enhancement has been published recently.[41] One of the main characteristics of the biodegradable scaffolds is their tendency to become almost completely absorbed following implantation. In addition, their study confirmed predisposition of scaffolds to stimulate cell ingrowth, giving a completely new layer to the penile body. Recently, the same group reported histomorphometry and immunohistochemistry studies, based on biopsies of the engineered tissue, and revealed de novo synthesis and accumulation of mechanically stable dartos tissue.[41]

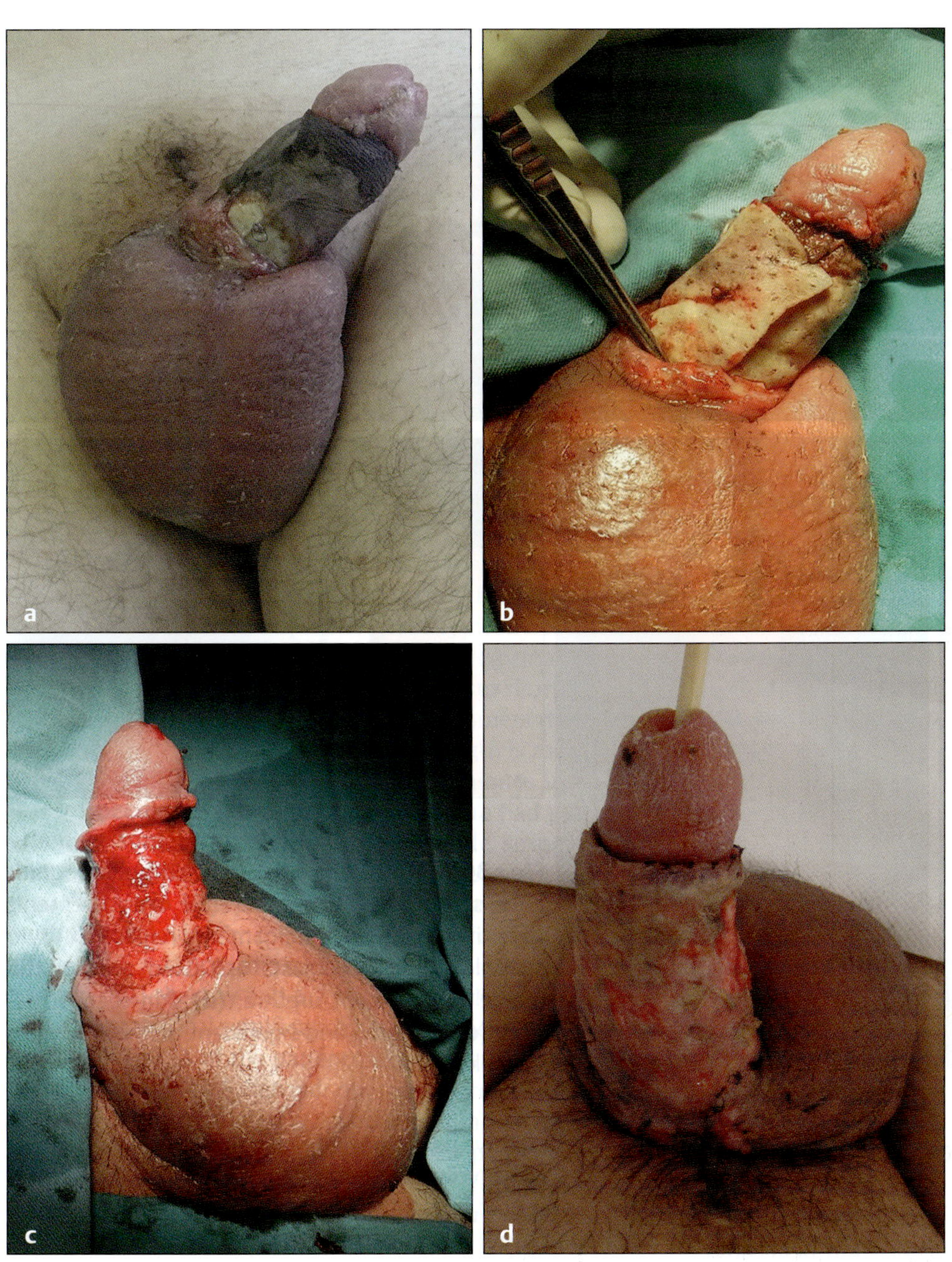

Fig. 30.5 Penile skin necrosis after xenograft insertion: **(a)** appearance after girth enhancement by Permacol; **(b)** removal of necrotic skin (Permacol is visible around the penile body); **(c)** complete removal and refreshment of the penile shaft; **(d)** skin defect is covered with skin grafts.

Venous Grafts

Considering that most of the procedures for penile girth augmentation enlarge penis in flaccid state and not in erectile state, Austoni et al developed a corporoplasty grafting procedure for erectile girth enhancement.[42] After degloving the penis through a combination of circumferential subcoronal and median penoscrotal incisions, bilateral longitudinal incisions are made into the corpora extending from the corporal base to the apex at the glans penis, thereby achieving the corporal expansion. The saphenous vein was then harvested and used as a graft for corporal closure, thereby preserving the girth expansion. In a series of 39 patients, the authors reported a mean erectile girth increase of 1.4 cm. No major postoperative complications were encountered, and there was no change in sexual function postoperatively as measured by nocturnal penile tumescence. Yang et al utilized the same corporoplasty technique, comparing venous and artificial polytetrafluoroethylene (ePTFE) grafts in 20 men with either congenital micropenis or penile dysmorphophobia. The authors reported an increase in erectile girth, ranging from 1.5 to 3.0 cm. All patients had self-limiting penile edema in the immediate postoperative period, but no major complications ensued. Measures of patient satisfaction and erectile function were not reported.[43]

Breast

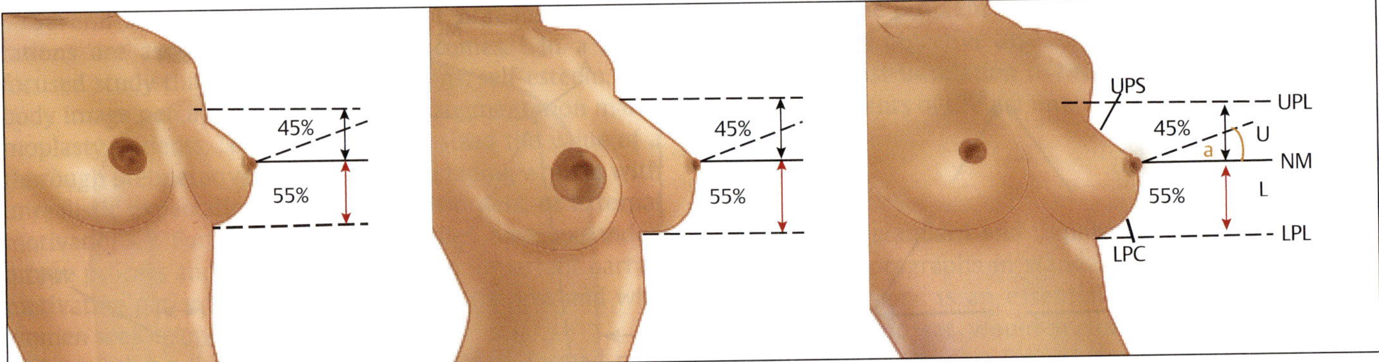

Fig. 31.12 Three-quarter profile view with standard breast parameters. U:L proportion, nipple angulation, contour of upper and lower poles. These images show three different breast sizes: all three models have a U:L ratio of 45:55, straight or concave upper poles, 20-degree upward angle of nipple pointing, and convex lower poles. Abbreviations: U, upper pole; L, lower pole; UPL, upper pole line; LPL, lower pole line; NM, nipple meridian; UPS, upper pole slope; LPC, lower pole convexity; a, nipple angulation. (Adapted from Mallucci and Branford 2012.[20])

While most of their exhaustive work applies mainly to reconstructive surgery, particularly their emphasis on the conus, the footprint, and the envelope of the breast as the three most important entities to be taken into account, the parameters to focus on apply equally well to aesthetic breast surgery.

Hauben et al, in 2003, measuring the anatomic size of the nipple, areola, and breast in 37 normal women aged 20 to 64 years concluded that irrespective of age and bodily habitus the NAC bears a constant 1:3 proportion to the breast.[22]

It is obvious that considerable developmental and morphometric differences exist in the breasts of women from various ethnic groups like the Chinese compared to the European. Several studies have addressed this and have attempted to generate relevant parameters and guidelines.

Qun Qiao, in 1997, carried out a 2-year study to research breast volume and other characteristics in a cohort of 125 young Chinese women, defined standards of breast development among Chinese women and, more specifically, obtained average breast volume and its relation to a variety of parameters.[23] Similarly, Avşar et al, in 2010, published their data on breast anthropometry based on a study of 385 female Turkish undergraduate students and compared it with western women.[24] Such studies have added to the knowledge about the anthropometric data on wide variation in size, shape, and other parameters of the breast.

In addition to such ethnic anthropometric variations, mating-relevant attributes like attractiveness play a huge part in women seeking aesthetic surgery of the breast, and thus it becomes important to be aware of the extent of the role played by them. Studies like those of Dixson et al, in 2015, done in men and women predominantly of European descent tested how variation in breast size and areolar pigmentation affected perceptions of women's sexual attractiveness, reproductive health, sexual maturity, maternal nurturing abilities, and age.[25] Sexual attractiveness ratings increased linearly with breast size, but large breasts were not judged to be significantly more attractive than medium-sized breasts. Small and medium-sized breasts were rated as most attractive if they included light or medium colored areolae, whereas large breasts were deemed more attractive if they had medium or dark areolae.

Lastly, introducing yet another subjective factor, there have been studies looking into variations in preferences between patients and plastic surgeons. In an interesting study, Hsia and Thomson, in 2003, looked into this aspect and demonstrated that plastic surgeons and patients seeking breast augmentation may have drastically different images in mind regarding what constitutes an attractive, natural, and ideal breast shape.[26]

Brody in 2004 asks, in a pertinent editorial aptly titled "The perfect breast: is it attainable? Does it exist?" and goes on to make a few interesting observations. Reviewing anthropology and art literature, he notes that there had never been a scholarly anthropomorphic study or artistic analysis of the breast and nor had there even been a valid statistical evaluation of the range and distribution of breast sizes and shapes.[15] He further observes that the rendition of the nude female breast throughout the history of art reflected how the clothing of the specific time, place, and culture of any given historical era shaped the bosom.

The breast is also the most changeable organ in the body, altering with puberty, weight gain and loss, hormonal balance, pregnancy, lactation, menopause, and plain age. Its shape and relative position also vary with posture. He also pertinently points out that "just in the last hundred years, the idealized breast shape has gone from the Victorian 'monobosom' to the boyish flapper to Jane Russell's full-breasted look to today's Pamela Anderson–like, contractured 'Bay Watch' globules."

As remarked ever so often by so many authors, the final recourse is often the position that "the surgeon's sense of sculptural form must dictate the ultimate decision as to the placement and shape of the breast."

Summary

A comprehensive assessment of the breast in a patient seeking aesthetic enhancement will start with a clear understanding of the normal anatomy both in the conventional sense and in the plastic surgical framework of features such as shape, size, contours, and symmetry. It will further involve appreciation of the subjective and objective measures of the aesthetic standards, accepting the limitations of these measures, being subject to variations across cultures, regions, and periods. Finally, it will also take into consideration the individual patient's expectations both in terms of the breast and the general wellbeing, and the limitations of surgical capabilities.

Thus, a balanced approach to the aesthetic assessment of the breast, applying well-accepted measures coupled with an intrinsic understanding of the aesthetics and a nuanced grasp of the individual patient as a whole, will enable the achievement of a realistic standard of outcome.

References

1. Palmer JH, Taylor GI. The vascular territories of the anterior chest wall. Br J Plast Surg 1986;39(3):287–299
2. Courtiss EH, Goldwyn RM. Breast sensation before and after plastic surgery. Plast Reconstr Surg 1976;58(1):1–13
3. Spear SL, Davison SP. Aesthetic subunits of the breast. Plast Reconstr Surg 2003;112(2):440–447
4. Burget GC, Menick FJ. The subunit principle in nasal reconstruction. Plast Reconstr Surg 1985;76(2):239–247
5. Bailey SH, Saint-Cyr M, Oni G, et al. Aesthetic subunit of the breast: an analysis of women's preference and clinical implications. Ann Plast Surg 2012;68(3):240–245
6. Yalom MA. History of the breast. New York: Ballantine Books; 1998
7. Tebbetts JB, Adams WP. Five critical decisions in breast augmentation using five measurements in 5 minutes: the high five decision support process. Plast Reconstr Surg 2005;116(7): 2005–2016
8. Tebbetts JB. A system for breast implant selection based on patient tissue characteristics and implant-soft tissue dynamics. Plast Reconstr Surg 2002;109(4):1396–1409, discussion 1410–1415
9. Regnault P. Breast ptosis: definition and treatment. Clin Plast Surg 1976;3(2):193–203
10. Penn J. Breast reduction. Br J Plast Surg 1955;7(4):357–371
11. Honigman RJ, Phillips KA, Castle DJ. A review of psychosocial outcomes for patients seeking cosmetic surgery. Plast Reconstr Surg 2004;113(4):1229–1237
12. Nikolić J, Janjić Z, Marinković M, Petrović J, Bozić T. Psychosocial characteristics and motivational factors in woman seeking cosmetic breast augmentation surgery. Vojnosanit Pregl 2013;70(10):940–946
13. Solvi AS, Foss K, von Soest T, Roald HE, Skolleborg KC, Holte A. Motivational factors and psychological processes in cosmetic breast augmentation surgery. J Plast Reconstr Aesthet Surg 2010;63(4):673–680
14. Sarwer DB, Wadden TA, Pertschuk MJ, Whitaker LA. The psychology of cosmetic surgery: a review and reconceptualization. Clin Psychol Rev 1998;18(1):1–22
15. Brody GS. The perfect breast: is it attainable? Does it exist? Plast Reconstr Surg 2004;113(5):1500–1503 Comments 2005; 115(4):1202–1207
16. Tegtmeier RE. A quick, accurate mammometer. Ann Plast Surg 1978;1(6):625–626
17. Galdino GM, Nahabedian M, Chiaramonte M, Geng JZ, Klatsky S, Manson P. Clinical applications of three-dimensional photography in breast surgery. Plast Reconstr Surg. 2002;110(1): 58–70
18. Creasman CN, Mordaunt D, Liolios T, Chiu C, Gabriel A, Maxwell GP. Four-dimensional breast imaging, part I: introduction of a technology-driven, evidence-based approach to breast augmentation planning. Aesthet Surg J 2011;31(8):914–924
19. Westreich M. Anthropomorphic breast measurement: protocol and results in 50 women with aesthetically perfect breasts and clinical application. Plast Reconstr Surg 1997;100(2):468–479
20. Mallucci P, Branford OA. Concepts in aesthetic breast dimensions: analysis of the ideal breast. J Plast Reconstr Aesthet Surg 2012;65(1):8–16
21. Blondeel PN, Hijjawi J, Depypere H, Roche N, Van Landuyt K. Shaping the breast in aesthetic and reconstructive breast surgery: an easy three-step principle. Plast Reconstr Surg 2009;123(2):455–462
22. Hauben DJ, Adler N, Silfen R, Regev D. Breast-areola-nipple proportion. Ann Plast Surg 2003;50(5):510–513
23. Qiao Q, Zhou G, Ling Y. Breast volume measurement in young Chinese women and clinical applications. Aesthetic Plast Surg 1997;21(5):362–368
24. Avşar DK, Aygit AC, Benlier E, Top H, Taşkinalp O. Anthropometric breast measurement: a study of 385 Turkish female students. Aesthet Surg J 2010;30(1):44–50
25. Dixson BJ, Duncan M, Dixson AF. The role of breast size and areolar pigmentation in perceptions of women's sexual attractiveness, reproductive health, sexual maturity, maternal nurturing abilities, and age. Arch Sex Behav 2015;44(6):1685–1695
26. Hsia HC, Thomson JG. Differences in breast shape preferences between plastic surgeons and patients seeking breast augmentation. Plast Reconstr Surg 2003;112(1):312–320, discussion 321–322

Introduction

The ideal breast size and shape vary, depending on anatomic, cultural, social, and personal considerations. Thus, it is very important for the surgeon to understand the patient's desires and expectations and decide whether they can be met. Augmenting the breast can have a very significant positive influence on a woman's self-esteem, perception of body image, relationships, and quality of life.

Breast augmentation remains the most common aesthetic surgery procedure performed worldwide to the tune of 1.8 million cases in 2018.[1] In the United States it has remained the top cosmetic procedure since 2006. In 2019, 0.3 million cases were performed in the United States.[2] This procedure continues to gain in popularity in the developing world, with an increasing middle class with doubling income, easier access to information and service providers via the digital platform. Though numbers in the developing world are nowhere near to those done in the developed world, the goal is the same for all plastic surgeons—happy patients, with good aesthetic results, having minimal complications, and low reoperation rates.

For a procedure that appears so straightforward in theory, to have so many options in terms of techniques and implant designs, makes an astute surgeon alert to equip self with the knowledge to understand the nuances to master this procedure. This is also one of the first major aesthetic surgery procedures freshly graduated plastic surgeons are called upon to independently perform.

First the silicone gel scare in the 1980s and 1990s and now the anaplastic large cell lymphoma (ALCL) issues, breast implants have had more than their fair share of controversies. Thus, it is also pertinent for plastic surgeons to be aware of the historical and current issues relating and relevant to this procedure.

Breast augmentation is a clinical process and not just a procedure. This process starts with a well-informed patient. Thus, it is prudent for us to educate the patient about all the aspects relevant to the procedure. This is often easier said than done, in this information age, where a lot of, both, true and misleading information is posted on the internet, thus confusing the patient. The first step is to explain the process and clear their doubts and allay all concerns adequately, to their satisfaction. This is very important, as their understanding and thus their involvement in the decision-making process is paramount. A well-informed patient with realistic expectations is more likely to be happy with the outcome. The aim of the chapter is to be a compressive guide in this decision-making and execution process.

Breast Augmentation—Indian Perspective

The fascination with large breasted women is as prevalent in India as in other parts of the world. What distinguishes India from the rest of the world is the celebration of the human body, whether it is dancing girls and the exquisitely sensual statues shown in the temples of Khajuraho or our epics and centuries-old books which describe even goddesses and their bodies in detail.[3]

As the aspirational values of the developing world has increased, so too has the popularity of cosmetic breast surgery. A majority of the ladies are from a middle-class background and obviously aiming to improve their social status and personal life. Even so, the reasons why breast augmentation surgery is sought are still very different from the western world. An understanding of these factors helps both doctor and patient in smooth decision making, especially during the consultation process, when often the final decision does not lie with the lady.

Typically, women seeking breast augmentation can be divided into three distinct age groups.

Early twenties resort to improve their matrimonial prospects. Thus at least one of the parents plays a major role in decision making. Another reason is body image issues.

Late twenties to thirties often due to partner demand or because of post-pregnancy body image issues.

Forties to fifties: Usually as a personal wish for a bigger bust or to rectify long overdue post-pregnancy body image issues.

History

The first ever case of successful breast augmentation was reported by Vincent Czerny in 1895, in which he transplanted a lipoma from the trunk to a post-mastectomy breast.[4] Longacre, in 1954, described a local dermal-fat flap for breast augmentation.[5]

In the 1950s and 1960s, many solid alloplastic materials were used for augmenting the breast. These included polyurethane, polytetrafluoroethylene (Teflon), and expanded polyvinyl alcohol formaldehyde (Ivalon sponge). Eventually, they were discontinued because of the significant side-effects, including soft tissue reactions, breast deformity, and breast discomfort. Similarly, semisolid and liquid materials like epoxy resin, beeswax, paraffin, and petroleum jelly were injected into the breast for augmentation and they too were discontinued over a period of time, due to their side effects.[5,6]

Uchida, in 1961, was the first to use silicone for breast augmentation. He injected free liquid silicone into the breast. This was soon discontinued due to the resultant frequent complications like chronic inflammations, recurrent infections, granuloma formation, and sinuses.[6]

The modern era of breast augmentation was heralded by the introduction of the silicone gel breast implant in 1962 by Drs. Cronin and Gerow, manufactured by the Dow Corning Corp., Michigan, USA. This was a two-component prosthetic device with a silicone elastomer shell filled with silicone gel.[7] The shell and the filler have since undergone several modifications.[8]

Evolution of the Mammary Implant

Evolution of the mammary implant is akin to the evolution of silicone and has mirrored the advancements in breast augmentation. There are two main types of mammary implants, silicone filled and saline filled. Both have an outer silicone shell. Silicone is extensively used in our day-to-day life. Silicone is a mixture of semiorganic polymeric molecules composed of chains of monomers. Silicone's utility value is in its viscoelasticity. So, it can be manufactured in a liquid, gel, or rubbery form by modulating the length of the polymer chain and the degree of cross-linking between the chains. As the average length of the polymer chains and the cross-linking between them increases, the viscosity increases, transforming it into a gel state and thus giving it a firmer consistency. *Cohesivity* refers to this viscosity. Modulating the cohesivity alters the gel, making it less elastic and more firm or vice versa. Increased gel cohesivity also gives the implant "form stability," that is, the gel is able to maintain its designated distribution within the implant withstanding extrinsic forces.

Over the years, silicone has proven to be extremely stable and inert when implanted into living tissue, as it is resistant to the action of enzymes—hence its popularity.

The first-generation implants (1962–1970) were smooth surfaced, and had a thick shell with a seam and moderately viscous gel filled in. They had a teardrop shape and had Dacron patches on the posterior surface to prevent rotation. They, however, had a high rate of capsular contracture.[8]

Second-generation implants (1970–1982) had thinner, seamless shells, thinner gel, and a round shape, all to promote a natural feel. However, the thin shells caused a silicone bleed into the fibrous capsule created around the implant.[8]

Third-generation implants (from 1982 onwards) had thicker shells, thicker gel, and a round shape. Thus, the strength and integrity of the implants improved. This led to lesser gel bleeds and lesser implant ruptures.

Fourth-generation implants (from 1986 onwards) were defined by the advances in manufacturing guidelines, which led to strict regulation of implant characteristics of shell thickness and gel viscosity. They had features similar to the third generation, and were in addition available in a textured surface.[8–10]

Fifth-generation implants (from 1993 onwards) have enhanced cohesive, form-stable silicone gel. They have a higher cross-linking of the silicone molecules. They are available in anatomic and round shapes. The teardrop-shaped implants are also called "gummy bear" implants as the highly cohesive, form-stable gel fill maintains the shape of the implant in vivo.[11] Thus in these latest fifth-generation (also called sixth generation) implants, there is a shift in focus from volume to distribution of volume.

Implant Characteristics

There are a multitude of implant parameters which have to be considered to evaluate the advantages of different implant types. Understanding these characteristics helps in deciding the implant best suited for a particular case from the plethora of implant models now available to choose from. The three keys are implant fill, shape, and surface.

Implant Fill

Saline-Filled Implants

These implants are usually inserted empty and once in situ are inflated to the desired volume with sterile saline through a small port. The port is then removed. There is a self-sealing tab at the port insertion site. Arion (France)[12] in 1965 was the first to report his experience with inflatable saline implants. However, Europe soon moved away from saline-filled implants due to the high deflation rates. But its use continued in the United States, as there was a moratorium on gel-filled implants due to the silicone gel controversy.[10] Saline was the only fill material allowed in the United States from 1993 to 2006. Even after the ban has

Summary

In the face of evolving implant technology, all these variables in implant characteristics have brought about a boom in options available to achieve the ideal result. There are now a vast array of implant gels, shells, and fill ratio to choose from. Thus, the plastic surgeon is now better equipped to customize the shape, size, and feel of the breast.

Clinical Considerations

Consultation and Assessment

Every patient turning up for a consultation for a breast augmentation desires the ideal breast. She looks up to the plastic surgeon to fulfill her need. Patient expectations are often driven by social, psychological, and cultural influences. The first step is establishing proper communication with the patient and defining what would be an aesthetically ideal breast in her case.

An ideal breast is one which is attractive, symmetrical, and matches with the size the patient desires, in proportion to her body. The anatomic factors that may limit achieving this ideal should be kept in mind. The patient's build especially the chest shape and size, current breast volume, and skin quantity and quality help decide what is best suited to an individual.

A thorough discussion along with a display of pre- and postoperative photo gallery, and different sized implants, provides a better understanding of the patient's thoughts. This is followed by examination, implant size decision, and explanation of the procedure (**Box 32.1** and **Fig. 32.1**).

Psychological Assessment

Enhancement of a woman's breast size can have a positive impact on her self-confidence, body image, and general approach to life. It can improve a patient's outlook and therefore indirectly affect her relationship with others. Thus, the benefits can far outweigh the physical change achieved.

Box 32.1 Indications for augmentation mammoplasty

- Hypomastia
  - Developmental
    - Primary
    - Secondary: Chest wall deformity
  - Involutional
    - Post-pregnancy
    - Significant weight loss
- Tubular breast
- Cosmetic correction
- Mild ptosis
- Breast asymmetry
- Breast reconstruction

On the flip side, if it is done for reasons other than breast enhancement, it can lead to great disappointment, for patient and surgeon. Toward this, a surgeon should first develop an understanding of the patient's motives for seeking breast enhancement, thus ensuring that her expectations are realistic.

Red flags are women with serious psychological problems who desire breast augmentation. Such patients should be handled with caution as a less than perfect result may even further aggravate her disturbed condition. Similarly, the timing of a request for breast augmentation should be noted. Requests for breast augmentation after personal psychological trauma should also be preferably deferred till her personal situation improves.

Oncological and General Medical Evaluation

Detailed medical history is of paramount importance. All factors that increase the probability of hematoma should be evaluated, bleeding disorders and medicines affecting coagulation, e.g., salicylates, NSAIDS, antiplatelet agents. Family history of breast cancer and breast disease, e.g., fibrocystic disease, should be elicited. One should note the symptoms of breast discomfort and breast pain and patient should be counseled that these problems may not improve by this surgery. Personal history of smoking and any other habits and allergies should be noted. Smokers have higher risk of capsular contracture.[25]

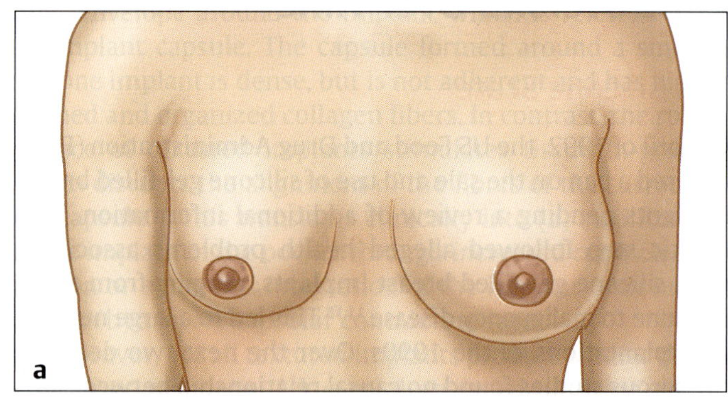

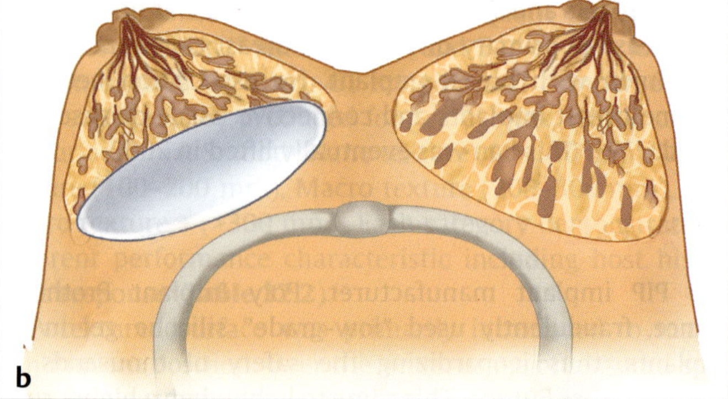

Fig. 32.1 **(a)** Breast asymmetry: cause may be soft tissue or bony. **(b)** Unilateral augmentation mammoplasty for correcting breast asymmetry.

Physical Examination

Physical examination, along with the preceding detailed medical history, helps in deciding the risk factors and appropriateness for breast augmentation (**Table 32.3**).

It is important to note the chest wall shape. A round-shaped chest diverges the breast axes, making the breast appear further apart following augmentation. This shape is made apparent by noting the nipple position and direction, which in this case would be pointing laterally and outwards. Rectangular-shaped chests, on the other hand, make the breast axes parallel, thus making the breast appear closer together postoperatively (**Fig. 32.2**).[25,26]

Operative Planning

Sound preoperative planning and decision making is as important as good surgical technique in achieving desired results. There are five decisions which have to be taken as part of planning. These decisions should be made using quantifiable data and measurements incorporating patient's desires and her physical assessment.

Volume of Augmentation

This is the first step to planning the augmentation. The main stay should be the patients' desire and her idea of a perfect breast. Most women leave it to the surgeon, considering him to be "the expert and thus the best judge." Others express a desire to be normal. Most want a moderate enlargement. Decision making is quicker in a woman who is expressive about her desired size. Showing her photographs of pre- and post-operative results followed by a trial with sizers usually reaches a satisfactory conclusion. It is a bit challenging in a woman who is unsure or not forthright with her thoughts. The brassiere she is wearing, especially the volume of padding and her comments on the same, can be a good starting point.

3D and 4D imaging is now available for measurement and simulation. Such a system can be a good tool to stimulate discussion and help in decision making for the appropriate shape and size of implant or to demonstrate the benefit of a mastopexy on a ptotic breast.[27] It can also be a good marketing tool. Another advantage of using it is that it can reduce operative time for those surgeons who otherwise use sizers intraoperatively to decide optimal fill volume.

Special Situations

Obese Patients

They often have suboptimal aesthetic results as the epigastric bulge camouflages the volume of the augment to some extent. Hence, often higher volume implants may be required for a satisfactory outcome.

Ptotic Breasts

Women with ptotic, moderate-sized breasts and empty upper pole often have a thinned-out skin envelope. Augmentation only, without mastopexy, in these patients

Table 32.3 Points to be noted during physical examination

General examination	• General body shape, chest shape, body posture, body proportions • Symmetry of chest and breast
Chest examination	• Shape, symmetry, anomalies • Assess pectoral muscle
Breast examination	
• Breast position	• Position on chest wall, Ptosis
• Breast size	
• Breast shape	
• Breast width	
• Breast parenchyma	• Consistency, tenderness, lumps/nodularity, amount and distribution
• Breast volume	• vis-à-vis skin envelope
• Breast skin	• Thickness (pinch test), elasticity, stretchmarks, scars
• Breast tightness	• Compliance
• Nipple	• Characteristics, anomalies-inversion/discharge
• Areola	• Position, size/dimensions (diameter/circumference)
Inframammary fold (IMF)	• Crease position in relation to nipple • Distance from nipple in cm (usually <5 cm = short) • Quality—whether distinct IMF delineated
Axilla	• For lymph nodes

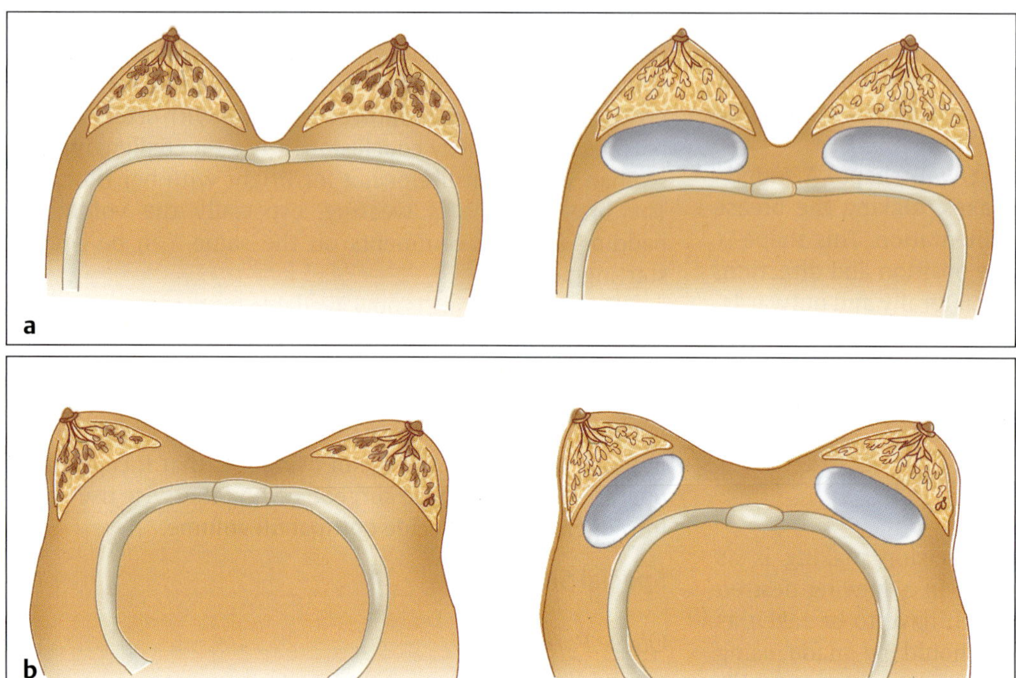

Fig. 32.2 Effect of different chest wall shapes on breast aesthetics. **(a)** Rectangular chest wall makes the breast axes parallel. **(b)** Rounded chest wall makes the breasts appear apart.

can give poor results. The increased breast weight because of the augmentation stretches the lower pole, further accentuating the ptosis.

Implant Selection

Implant Size

The selection process begins at consultation, starting from understanding patients' goals followed by the surgeon's assessment. The dimensions of the implant, that is, the volume, width, and projection of the implant, lead to the desired shape. Breast width of existing breast parenchyma, nipple to inframammary fold (IMF) distance, and maximum anterior pull of the breast skin are important measurements to decide the implant size. These assess the dimensions of the breast and the compliance characteristics of the skin envelope, thus quantifying the ease of accommodating the volume desired. So, for the same chest size, these measurements would vary in virginal, post-weight loss, or post-pregnancy breasts.

To accommodate the variables, for a particular volume, various implant sizes are available in each product range with varying the base width and projection (low, medium, and high profile). As a general rule, the selected implants' base width should be lesser than the existing breast footprint.

Implant Filling

The implant chosen may be silicone gel filled or saline filled. With the advent of cohesive gel and better silicone envelopes, "silicone gel bleed" is no longer an issue. Thus, the need for opting for saline fill as a safer option is eliminated. Gel-filled implants have a softer, more natural feel, as compared to saline-filled implants. Also, the failure of an inflatable saline implant causes an immediate distressing breast asymmetry. However, the final decision should rest with the patient and her concerns about silicone.

Implant Surface Texture

Textured implants have been more popular than smooth implants since the 1990s. They also show a lower incidence of capsular contracture. This incidence is even lesser when they are placed submuscularly or subfacial. The pocket has to be snug in case of textured implants. It should be larger in smooth implants to allow for implant mobility.

This decision on surface texture is only relevant to round implants, as anatomic implants are all textured, so as to prevent rotation. The patient should be informed about the rare but definitive reporting of BIA-ALCL in textured surface implants. For this reason smooth/nano-textured implants are gaining in popularity.

Implant Shape

The round implants are used in the vast majority of patients. However, the proponents of anatomic implant make their point by highlighting the fact that the natural attractive female breast is not hemispherical. The anatomically shaped implant, for a given base width and volume, has less upper pole convexity than a corresponding round implant. However, superior results with anatomic implants remain unproven[25] (**Table 32.4**).

Author feels that surgeons doing higher number of cases should familiarize themselves with the use of anatomic implants too. There is a learning curve to master, to obtain the promised superior results.

Table 32.4 Indications as per implant shape

Round implants	Anatomic implants
• Patient desiring fuller appearance	• Patient who wants a natural appearance and implant that "fits" their breast
• Very small volume augment	• Constricted lower pole breast
• Good breast shape and skin quality	• Thoracic hypoplasia
• Athletic individuals	• Surgeon's preference
• Those desiring very large implants	
• Secondary surgery—to avoid risk of rotating	

Choice of Incision

Of the several surgical approaches described for implant pocket access, the inframammary, periareolar, and transaxillary are the common locations for incision placement. Transumbilical approach is more widely described than used. The choice of incision should be individualized. However, since the gel implants have become standard, the inframammary and periareolar incisions are used in the vast majority of cases (**Fig. 32.3**; **Table 32.4**).

Inframammary Incision

The inframammary incision remains the most popular approach today. This facilitates accurate dissection and implant placement. However, optimal incision placement can be challenging as the position of the inframammary crease changes with surgery. The healed scar is inconspicuous when it lies precisely in the new crease position (**Fig. 32.4a**). It may be more visible, wide, or hypertrophied if it lies above or below the crease.

Periareolar Incision

The periareolar approach was described by Jenny in 1972. Its central location provides the best exposure to the implant pocket. In addition, it facilitates controlled lowering of the IMF under direct vision. In cases with constricted lower pole, the direct access allows easy scoring and release of the lower breast parenchyma (**Table 32.5**).

Periareolar scars are usually inconspicuous if they are precisely placed at the junction of the color change. As there is little tension, the scar quality is usually excellent and hypertrophy is rare (**Fig. 32.4b**). The incision can be lengthened to further ease implant insertion by making it a zigzag (like a series of Ws) (**Fig. 32.4c**). This maneuver also reduces the risk of scar contracture. Periareolar approach is often preferred in secondary cases (with pre-existing inframammary scar) needing capsulotomy or capsulorrhaphy (**Fig. 32.4d**).

Transaxillary Incision

This approach was described by Hochler in 1973. This incision is best suited for saline implants though it can also be used for gel-filled implants. This approach avoids breast scars. Ideal candidates are young patients with good shape and reasonable volume. Dissection is either blunt or endoscope assisted. Blunt dissection is easier but requires experience and expertise. Endoscopic dissection is more complex and has a higher hematoma risk. As the breast pocket is remote from the incision, precise alteration of the IMF is more difficult, as is asymmetry correction. Proper placement of implant is often difficult. Inadequate muscle release with this technique may lead to persistently high riding implants.[22] Given the technical challenges, it is not a technique recommended for the occasional surgeon (**Table 32.5**).

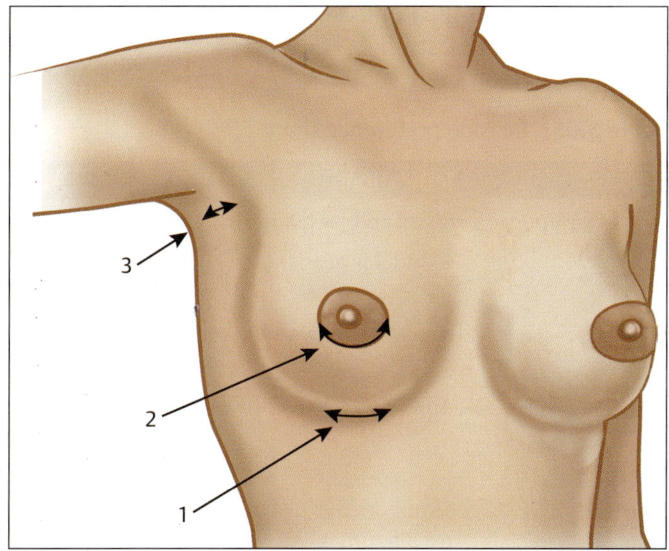

Fig. 32.3 The three popular access incisions for breast augmentation: 1. Inframammary, 2. Periareolar, 3. Transaxillary.

Plane of Implant Placement

Choosing the appropriate plane for implant placement plays an important role in obtaining an excellent outcome in breast augmentation. This in turn depends upon the thickness of tissue cover available and the type of implant selected. The options available are subglandular (submammary/retromammary/prepectoral) and submuscular (subpectoral) (**Fig. 32.5**). Recent options added have been subfascial and dual-plane.

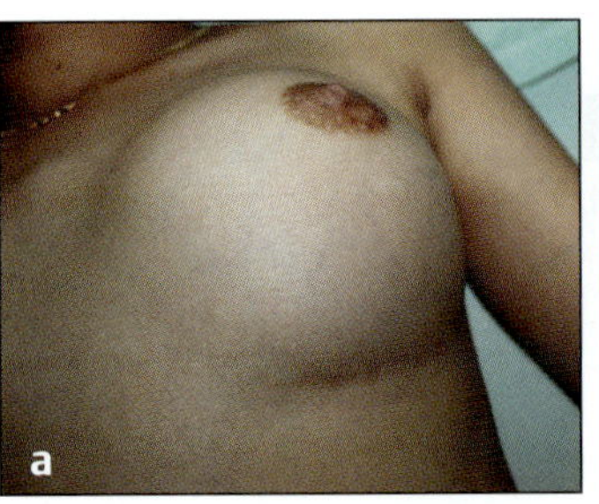
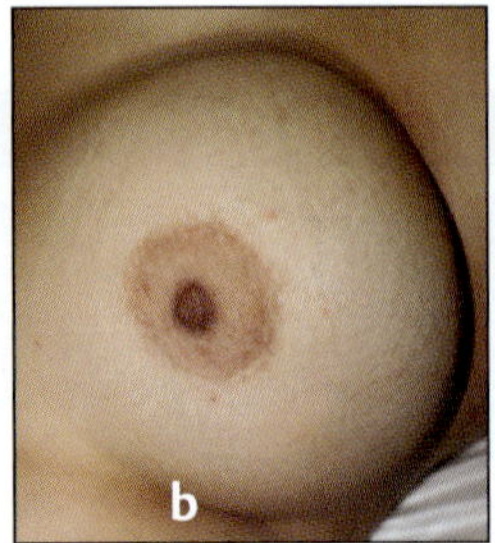
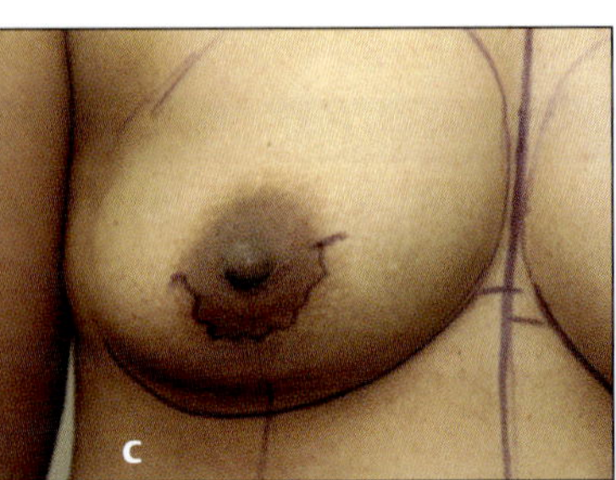
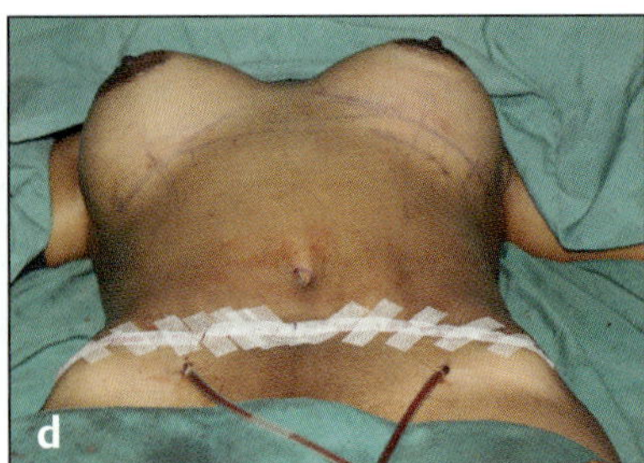

Fig. 32.4 **(a)** Inframammary scar: One year postop—well-healed scar but is perceptible (though barely) even in a fair complexioned patient. **(b)** Periareolar incisions usually heal with inconspicuous scars. **(c)** A useful modification of the periareolar scar—lengthening the scar and breaking the contractile forces. It is the author's preferred incision whenever the areolar diameter is greater than 4 cm. **(d)** Periareolar incisions are ideal for cases where breast augmentation is planned along with an abdominoplasty.

Table 32.5 Incision preference chart

	Indications	Advantages	Disadvantages
Inframammary incision	Small areolar diameter	Immediate access	Optimal scar placement challenging
	Glandular ptosis	Complete pocket visualization	Visible scar • especially in colored skin
	Implant size over 400 mL	Wider access possible (to place larger implants)	Risk of iatrogenic implant rupture during wound closure
	Anatomic-shaped implants	Fold modification	Risk of implant exposure in postop period • if thin soft tissue cover • weight of implant
	Simultaneous placement of pectus excavatum prosthesis	Accurate hemostasis	Scar migration
Periareolar incision	• Adequate areolar diameter (≥4 cm)	• Inconspicuous scar	• Limited exposure of surgical field
	• Concomitant release of constricted lower pole	• Direct access to lower parenchyma	• Parenchyma ducts transected—sterility compromised
	• Considering circumareolar mastopexy	• Best exposure to implant pocket	• Potential risk of increased nipple sensitivity
	• Secondary cases for capsulorrhaphy	• Easy adjustment of inframammary fold (IMF)	• Scar on breast mound
	• Well-defined areolar border		• Higher incidence of capsular contracture
Transaxillary incision	• Request for saline implants	• Avoids breast scar	• Scar visible in sleeveless dresses (common in Asia/India)
	• Special request for this incision		• Inserting gel implants challenging
	• Surgeon who has mastered this technique		• Can't correct tubular breast deformity through same scar
			• Subglandular implant placement difficult
			• Superior implant malposition
			• Revision surgery requires second incision
			• Steeper learning curve

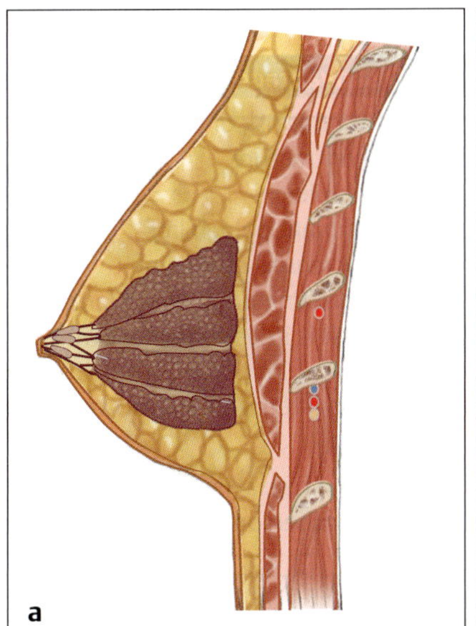

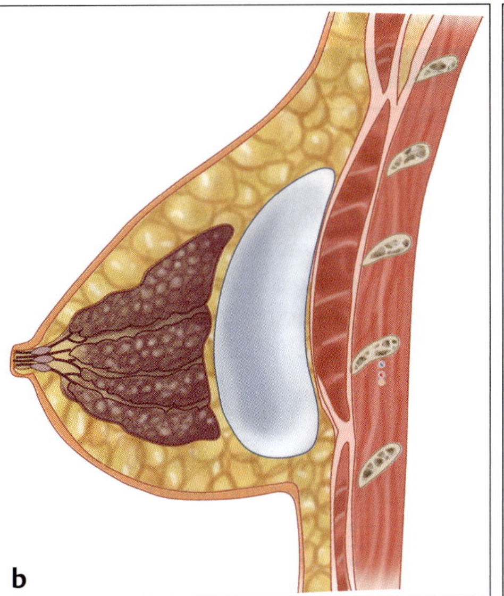

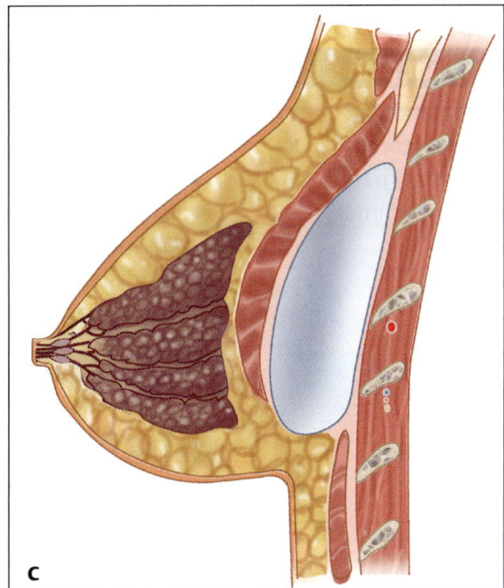

Fig. 32.5 Plane of implant placement: **(a)** preop, **(b)** subglandular, **(c)** submuscular.

Ideally, the best position for a breast implant is in the subglandular plane. This seems to be the anatomically correct plane to give a natural shape and contour to the breast. Earlier, when initial breast augmentations were done, the implants were placed in this plane. However, there was a continued high incidence of capsular contracture around the implants, which led to the preference of the submuscular position. Over time, submuscular plane, for varying reasons, has remained, by far, the more popular choice. The risk of capsular contracture is now shown to be less dependent on the plane of placement, though still reported to be higher in subglandular plane. It can be minimized in either pocket by sound surgical techniques and appropriate postoperative management.

Subglandular Plane

The best candidates for subglandular plane are those with reasonable existing breast tissue volume or mild ptosis. The results show excellent breast projection. Good soft tissue coverage especially in the upper pole is essential to avoid implant palpability (**Table 32.6**).

Subfascial Plane

This plane is created between the pectoralis major muscle and its overlying fascia. The advantages are better support to the overlying breast tissue and an incidence of capsular contracture equivalent to submuscular placement but with better shape and less implant mobility (**Table 32.6**). However, long-term studies are awaited for corroborating the aforementioned benefits, till which time the benefits remain unclear.[28]

Submuscular Plane

This plane is best suited for women with minimal breast tissue and mild or no ptosis. The main benefit of submuscular plane is excellent upper pole aesthetics as the border of the implant is camouflaged by the muscle. However, it is more painful, as it involves division of the pectoralis major muscle (**Table 32.6**).

Dual-Plane Placement

This was first published by John Tebbetts in 2001.[29] The concept is that the implant so placed lies in a dual plane, subpectorally superiorly where the device most needs coverage and subglandular in the lower part to give a natural contour and better projection. Thus it allows the benefits of both techniques (**Table 32.6**).

The muscle is divided at its origin along the IMF, which allows the cut edge of the muscle to glide superiorly and give access to create a large subpectoral pocket. The attachments of the lower part of the muscle to the overlying gland are released, so that the lower cut muscle edge rises, freeing up the lower pole, creating a small subglandular portion. This is referred to as Dual 1 (**Fig. 32.6a, b**). The dissection can be extended, thus raising the muscle edge further superiorly—Dual II (**Fig. 32.6c, d**) and Dual plane III (**Fig. 32.6e, f**).

Complete submuscular implant coverage can be achieved by releasing and dropping the pectoralis major, serratus anterior, and rectus abdominis muscles over the implant. However, this is not popular as it limits lower pole "expansion." Also this causes significant morbidity and pain.

Size of Pocket

Early augmentation procedures involved creating pocket sizes only slightly larger than the implant selected. The pocket size reduced due to the forces of wound contraction in the healing phase. This led to surgeons creating more generous pockets. This dictum still holds true when using

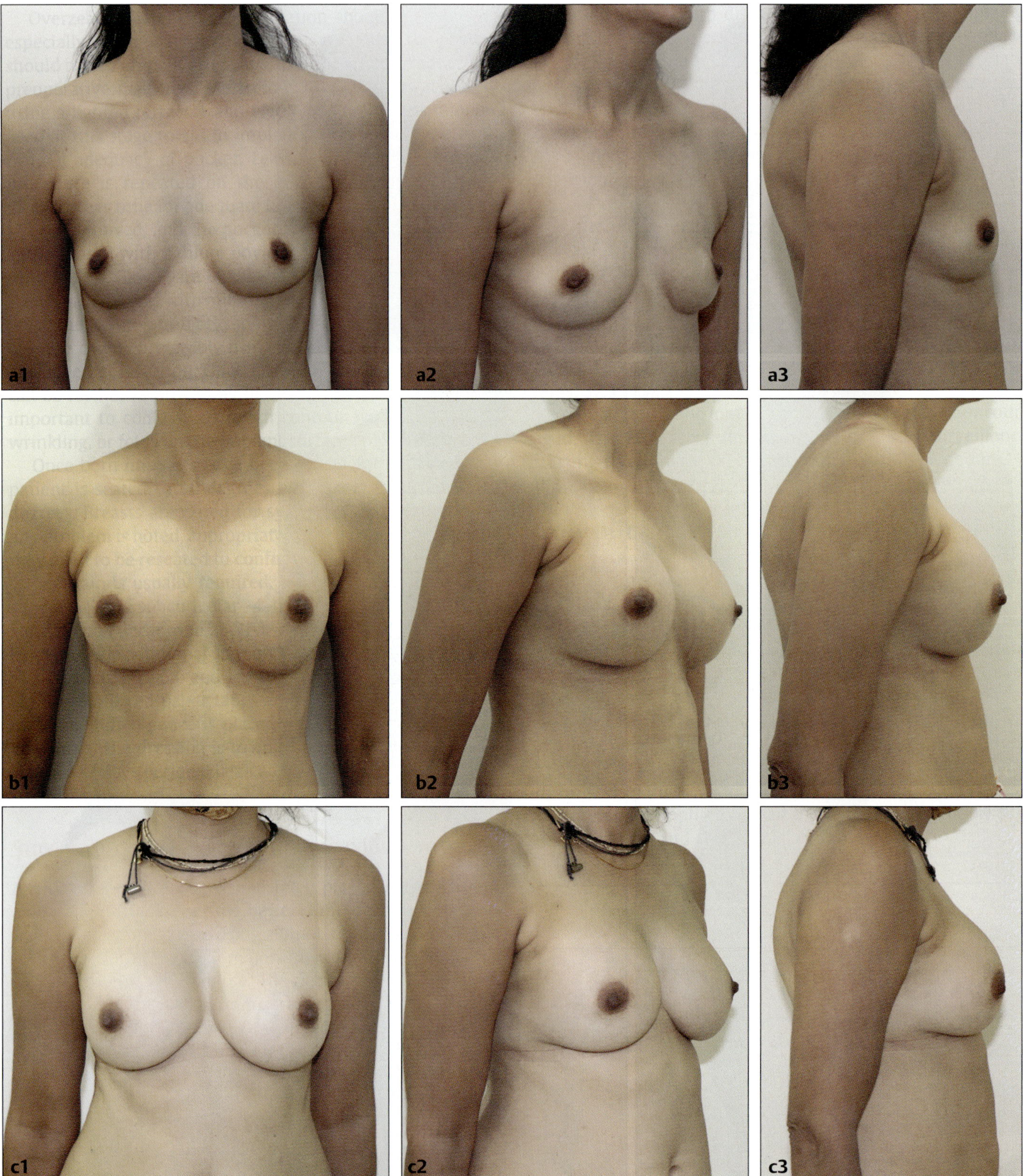

Fig. 32.12 This is a 47-year-old with hypomastia showing postpartum parenchymal atrophy and skin thinning. She desired moderate-sized breasts enough to be a significant change, but not big enough to draw obvious attention. A 275-mL textured surface, round, extra high-profile cohesive gel silicone implant, with a base width of 110 mm and an anterior projection of 45 mm was placed in the submuscular pocket through an inframammary incision. **(a)** Preoperative, **(b)** postoperative, **(c)** long term follow up.

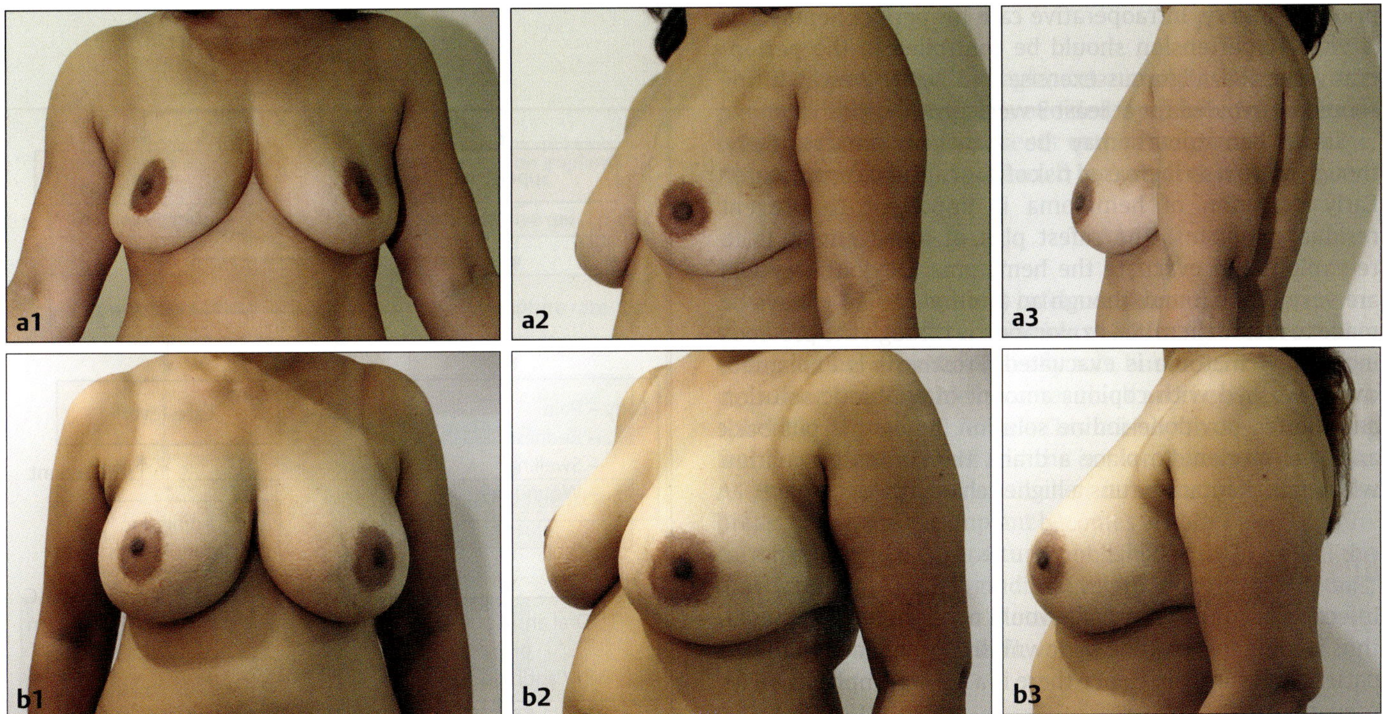

Fig. 32.13 A 46-year-old mother of two with mild ptosis and parenchymal atrophy. **(a)** Breast characteristics of volume vis-a-vis skin envelope, skin elasticity, and laxity led to a decision to choose a 365mL round-shaped textured cohesive gel silicone implant with a base width of 121 mm and an anterior projection of 48 mm. The implant was placed through a periareolar skin incision in the subglandular plane through a transparenchymal route. **(b)** The 5-year postop photographs show good maintenance of volume (indicating minimal glandular atrophy), minimal progress of ptosis (appropriate implants size selection), no implant visibility (good soft tissue cover), and an attractive postoperative breast shape (appropriate plane of implant placement).

Table 32.7 Complications with implant augmentation mammoplasty

Surgical complications	Implant complications	Unsatisfactory aesthetic outcome	Late complications
• Hematoma	• Rippling	• Asymmetry	• Capsular contracture
• Sensory alteration	• Wrinkling	• Muscle animation	• Poor scarring
• Breast pain	• Visibility/palpability	• Double bubble	• Scar hypertrophy
• Seroma	• Implant rotation	• Poor cosmesis	• Keloid
• Infection	• Rupture		• Striae distensae
• Mondor disease	• Extrusion		• Ptosis
• Pneumothorax			• Glandular atrophy
• Galactorrhea			
• Symmastia			BIA-ALCL
• Periprosthetic effusion			
			Reoperation

Abbreviation: BIA-ALCL, breast implant associated–anaplastic large cell lymphoma.

Hematoma

Hematoma occurs most frequently in the immediate postoperative period. However, late presentations are also known. In cases presenting with a delayed hematoma, quite often there is a history of breast trauma. Typically, a postoperative hematoma presents with onset of unilateral pain accompanied by increasing tightness or ecchymosis. Examination shows shape distortion and unilateral enlargement. Investigations reveal a drop in hemoglobin. Presence of a hematoma also increases the risk of infection.

For prevention of a hematoma, medicines including health supplements, herbs, and alternative medications that can affect blood coagulation should be stopped 1 to 3 weeks

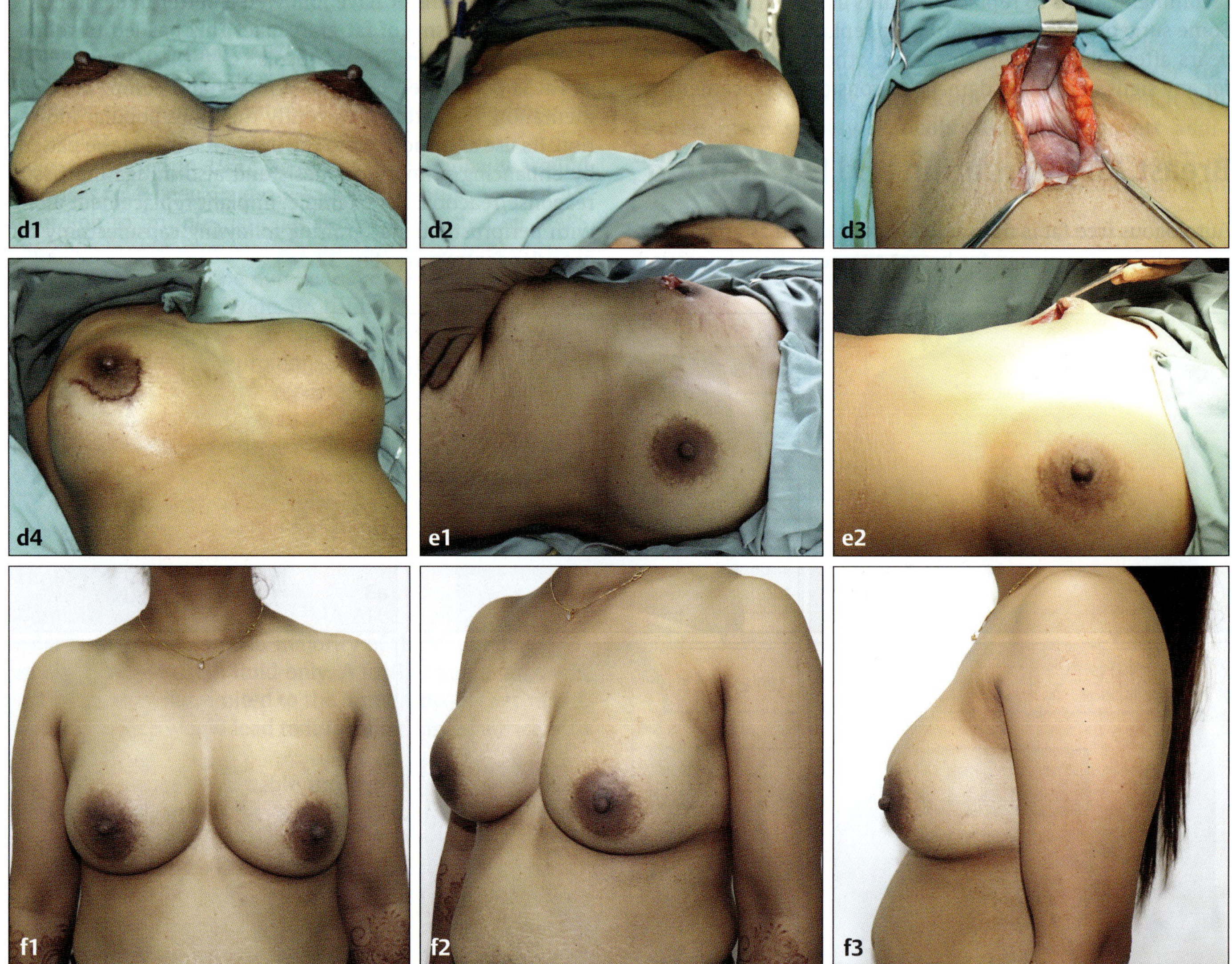

Fig. 32.14 (*Continued*) **(d, e)** Reoperation was done with capsulectomy and implant replacement and fat grafting. **(f)** Five-months postoperative.

At this point in time, fat grafting to the breast remains technique driven. Hence significant variability in outcomes is reported. Nuances of fat grafting to the breast, including outcomes and limitations, are addressed in detail in Chapter 33 on "Role of Fat Grafting in Breast Surgery" in Volume VI.

References

1. ISAPS international survey on aesthetic/cosmetic procedures 2018. https://www.isaps.org/wp-content/uploads/2019/12/ISAPS-Global-Survey-Results-2018-new.pdf. Accessed August 17, 2020
2. Plastic Surgery Statistics Report 2019. https://www.plasticsurgery.org/documents /News/Statistics /2019/ plastic-surgery-statistics-full-report-2019.pdf. Accessed August 17, 2020
3. Mahakavi Kalidas. Kumara-Sambhavam: circa 400 BCE, written in Sanskrit and translated into English by many. Kumara-Sambhavam: the origin of the young god. Trans. Hank Heifetz. Penguin Classic
4. Czerny V. Plastic replacement of the breast with a lipoma. Chir Kong Verhandl 1895;2:216
5. Longacre JJ. Surgical reconstruction of the flat discoid breast. Plast Reconstr Surg (1946) 1956;17(5):358–366
6. Uchida J. Clinical application of crosslinked dimethyl polysiloxane, restoration of breast, cheeks, atropy of infantile paralysis, funnel-shaped chest etc. Jpn J Plast Reconstr Surg 1961;4:303
7. Cronin TD, Gerow FJ. Augmentation mammaplasty: a new "natural feel" prosthesis. In: transactions of the Third International Congress of Plastic and Reconstructive Surgery. Amsterdam: ExcerptaMedica: 1964
8. Maxwell P, Gabriel A. Breast augmentation. In: Neligan P, ed. Plastic Surgery. 3rd ed. USA: Elsevier Inc.; 2013. Vol. 5,Sec. 1: 11.e1–38

9. Ramachandran K. Breast augmentation. Indian J Plast Surg 2008; 41(1, Suppl):S41–S47
10. Adams WP Jr. The process of breast augmentation: four sequential steps for optimizing outcomes for patients. Plast Reconstr Surg 2008;122(6):1892–1900
11. Steinbrech DS, Lerman OZ. Breast implants: background, safety and general consideration. In: Aston SJ, ed. Aesthetic plastic surgery. 1st ed. Saunders Elsevier: 2009:645
12. Arion HG. Retromammary prosthesis. C. R. Soc Fr Gynaco; 1965:5
13. Tebbetts JB. What is adequate fill? Implications in breast implant surgery. Editorial. Plast Reconstr Surg 1996;97(7):1451–1454
14. Gabriel A, Maxwell GP. The science of cohesivity and Elements of form stability. Plast Reconstr Surg 2019; 144(1S Utilizing a Spectrum of Cohesive Implants in Aesthetic and Reconstructive Breast Surgery, 1S):7S–12S
15. Jewell ML, Fickas B, Jewell H. Implant surface options and biofilm mitigation strategies. Plast Reconstr Surg 2019; 144(1S Utilizing a Spectrum of Cohesive Implants in Aesthetic and Reconstructive Breast Surgery, 18S):13S–20S
16. Atlan M, Nuti G, Wang H, Decker S, Perry T. Breast implant surface texture impacts host tissue response. J Mech Behav Biomed Mater 2018;88:377–385
17. Barr S, Hill E, Bayat A. Current implant surface technology: an examination of their nanostructure and their influence on fibroblast alignment and biocompatibility. Eplasty 2009;9:e22
18. Schlenz I, Kuzbari R, Gruber H, Holle J. The sensitivity of the nipple-areola complex: an anatomic study. Plast Reconstr Surg 2000;105(3):905–909
19. Sánchez-Guerrero J, Colditz GA, Karlson EW, Hunter DJ, Speizer FE, Liang MH. Silicone breast implants and the risk of connective-tissue diseases and symptoms. N Engl J Med 1995; 332(25):1666–1670
20. Karlson EW, Hankinson SE, Liang MH, et al. Association of silicone breast implants with immunologic abnormalities: a prospective study. Am J Med 1999;106(1):11–19
21. Duteille F, Perrot P, Bacheley MH, Stewart S. Eight year safety data for round and anatomical silicone gel breast implants. Aesthet Surg J 2018;38(2):151–161
22. Mallucci PL. Ten-year experience using inspira implants: a review with personal anecdote. Plast Reconstr Surg 2019; 144 (1S Utilizing a Spectrum of Cohesive Implants in Aesthetic and Reconstructive Breast Surgery, 1S):37S–42S
23. Tebbetts JB, Adams WP. Five critical decisions in breast augmentation using five measurements in 5 minutes: the high five decision support process. [reprint in PlastReconstr. Surg 2006; 118 (7 suppl): 35S–45S; PMID: 17099482] Plast Reconstr Surg 2005;116(7):2005–2016
24. Hidalgo DA, Spector JA. Breast augmentation. Plast Reconstr Surg 2014;133(4):567e–583e
25. Hirsch EM, Brody GS. Anatomic variation and asymmetry in female anterior thoracic contour: an analysis of 50 consecutive computed tomography scans. Ann Plast Surg 2007;59(1): 73–77
26. Kortesis BG, Bharti G. Maximizing aesthetics and patient selection utilizing natrelle inspire line implants in aesthetic breast surgery. Plast Reconstr Surg 2019; 144 (1S Utilizing a Spectrum of Cohesive Implants in Aesthetic and Reconstructive Breast Surgery, 1S):30S–36S
27. Walden JL. Breast augmentation. In: Aston SJ, ed. Aesthetic plastic surgery, 1st ed. Saunders Elsevier; 2009:661
28. Shen Z, Chen X, Sun J, et al. A comparative assessment of three planes of implant placement in breast augmentation: A Bayesian analysis. J Plast Reconstr Aesthet Surg 2019;72(12):1986–1995
29. Teitelbaum S. The dual plane approach to breast augmentation. In: Aston SJ, ed. Aesthetic plastic surgery. 1st ed. Saunders Elsevier; 2009:675
30. Adams WP Jr, Rios JL, Smith SJ. Enhancing patient outcomes in aesthetic and reconstructive breast surgery using triple antibiotic breast irrigation: six-year prospective clinical study. Plast Reconstr Surg 2006; 118(7, Suppl):46S–52S
31. Wiener TC. The role of betadine irrigation in breast augmentation. Plast Reconstr Surg 2007;119(1):12–15, discussion 16–17
32. Pajkos A, Deva AK, Vickery K, Cope C, Chang L, Cossart YE. Detection of subclinical infection in significant breast implant capsules. Plast Reconstr Surg 2003;111(5):1605–1611
33. Wiener TC. Betadine and breast implants: an update. Aesthet Surg J 2013;33(4):615–617
34. Adams WP Jr, Culbertson EJ, Deva AK, et al. Macrotextured breast implants with defined steps to minimize bacterial contamination around the device: experience in 42,000 implants. Plast Reconstr Surg 2017;140(3):427–431
35. Nahabedian MY, Spear SL. Acellular dermal matrix for secondary procedures following prosthetic breast reconstruction. Aesthet Surg J 2011; 31(7, Suppl):38S–50S
36. Moschetta M, Telegrafo M, Cornacchia I, et al. PIP breast implants: rupture rate and correlation with breast cancer. G Chir 2014;35(11-12):274–278
37. Lindenblatt N, El-Rabadi K, Helbich TH, Czembirek H, Deutinger M, Benditte-Klepetko H. Correlation between MRI results and intraoperative findings in patients with silicone breast implants. Int J Womens Health 2014;6:703–709
38. Shah AT, Jankharia BB. Imaging of common breast implants and implant-related complications: A pictorial essay. Indian J Radiol Imaging 2016;26(2):216–225
39. Basile FV, Basile AV, Basile AR. Striae distensae after breast augmentation. Aesthetic Plast Surg 2012;36(4):894–900
40. Magnusson M, Beath K, Cooter R, et al. The epidemiology of breast implant-associated anaplastic large cell lymphoma in Australia and New Zealand confirms the highest risk for Grade 4 surface breast implants. Plast Reconstr Surg 2019;143(5): 1285–1292
41. Loch-Wilkinson A, Beath KJ, Knight RJW, et al. Breast implant-associated anaplastic large cell lymphoma in Australia and New Zealand: high-surface-area textured implants are associated with increased risk. Plast Reconstr Surg 2017;140(4):645–654
42. U.S. Food & drug administration/FDA takes action to protect patients from risk of certain textured breast implants; 2019. https://www.fda.gov/news-events/press-announcements/fda-takes-action-protect-patients-risk-certain-textured-breast-implants-requests-allergan. Accessed on August 20, 2020

33

Role of Fat Grafting in Breast Surgery

Klaus Ueberreiter

Box 33.4 BEAULI protocol

Preoperatively
- Analgesic sedation or general anesthesia
- Tumescence solution:
  3 L N/S + 150 mL lidocaine 1% + 3 mL adrenaline 1:1000 (+ 37.5 mL sodium bicarbonate 8.4 mVal)
- Warmed to body temperature

Surgery
- Infiltration and suctioning
- Using 3.8-mL rapid harvesting cannula and negative pressure of −500 mm Hg
- Almost constant reinjection of fluid during harvesting
- Collecting the fat and separating it from the liquid and oily debris using the LipoCollector
- Extracting in 50-mL irrigation syringes
- Filling of five 10-mL syringes facilitates counting of grafted volume
- Infiltration with blunt needle of 10 cm length
- Augmentation via one prick incision laterocaudally
- Infiltration of 1 mL per cm^2 in a pearl string pattern
- Maximum volume of fat transfer recommended 300 mL per side

Postoperatively
- Postoperatively compression garment of suctioned region for 4 wk
- Keeping the breasts warm with a spool of wide absorbent cotton
- No cooling, no pressure

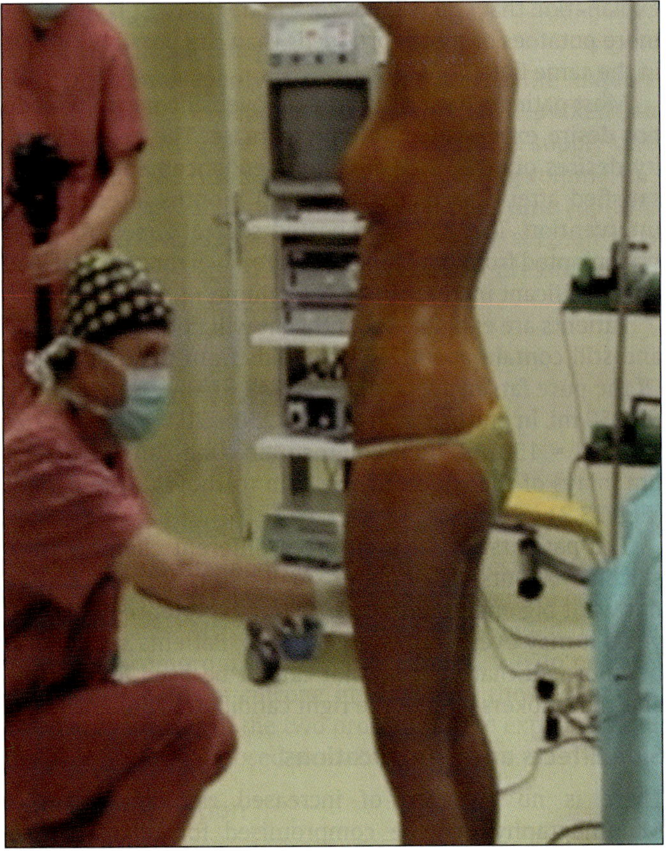

Fig. 33.4 Patient preparation.

Box 33.5 Planning of fat grafting sessions in various indications

- Aesthetic breast augmentation generally requires two fat grafts at an interval of 3 mo; one procedure = ½ cup size
- In case of a capsular fibrosis with implant removal, most patients are satisfied with a single transplant
- Reconstruction after cancer may require up to eight or more fat grafting sessions, especially after radiotherapy

In general, it is planned as per the preference of the patient, and hence this procedure is a typical win-win situation for the patient by getting rid of fat at one site and gaining on the other.

For an ordinary bilateral breast lipofilling you should harvest 600 to 700 mL of fat. We do the markings on the breast only in case of asymmetries.

It is easier to scrub the patient standing in front of the OR table, then making the patient sit back on the table. The legs are draped in sterile cloth by lifting one leg after another. Thus, they are well disinfected all around in a short time. For modesty they come into the theater wearing single-use disposable panty (**Fig. 33.4**). In the last 10 years, problems like fainting have not been observed.

If the procedure becomes more and more routine in one's practice, ready-to-use sterile sets are recommended including the necessary drapes, syringes, sponges, etc. This is cheaper and easier to prepare.

The patient is placed supine on the table. General anesthesia is usually not necessary; we prefer sedation supported by local anesthetics in the tumescence solution. There are always discussions about the harmful effects of local anesthetics. In a study by Keck et al, it was shown that prilocaine has a toxic effect on preadipocytes.[15] Lidocaine in the usual dilution does not seem to have any impact. Another study by Hilkka Peltoniem compared patients with standard tumescence solution under sedation and patients with Ringer solution under high epidural. The magnetic resonance imaging (MRI) volumetric evaluation 6 months postoperatively showed no significant difference in the outcome.[16] Sodium bicarbonate is a buffer solution which lessens the pain during injection of lidocaine. Under sedation it is not necessary and can be excluded.

Infiltration

In the beginning all the marked areas for liposuction are infiltrated in a wet technique. It is not necessary to use a lot of liquid if water-assisted harvesting is being used, as enough fluid is injected during fat harvest. Remember that the tumescence fluid should be at the body temperature.

On each side of the table there is a foot pedal for controlled injection of the fluid. After infiltration of the liposuction areas, the breasts too are infiltrated (about 100–150 mL each) to avoid hematoma and to create more space for infiltration. The suction procedure can be started right away. Only if the procedure is planned entirely under local anesthesia, one should wait for 20 to 30 minutes to have better effect of the local anesthetic. Also, the harvesting takes at least the double time when compared to procedure under additional IV sedation as one needs to work significantly slower.

Typical areas for fat harvest are hips, thighs, abdomen, and flanks. Of course, it can also be harvested from other areas like arms and calves, but this takes more time and the surgical costs could be more.

Fat Harvest

For an ordinary fat graft, you will need 200 to 300 mL per breast. Some fat loss due to destroyed cells of about 10 to 20% should be calculated. That means for an average job of 250 mL per side 600 to 650 mL of fat should be harvested in the LipoCollector for bilateral fat grafting (**Fig. 33.5**). This volume is reached when the lower level of fat comes down to the mark of 400 mL.

Equal portions of fat should be harvested from all the marked sites, (e.g., right thigh in and outside each 150 mL, and left thigh the same amount). In skinny patients it helps if you do a first round, collecting smaller amounts, and then repeat in the same order.

Tip: The harvested fat should be almost bloodless. If the procedure seems too bloody, it might be because of some changes in the adrenaline. Adrenaline should be protected against sunlight, as exposure to sunlight destroys the adrenaline. A new ampoule of adrenaline should be tried or double the amount of adrenaline per liter may be used. There is no harm if higher concentration is used.

Once enough fat is collected, the suction tube is removed from the top and connected to the bottom escape of the lipocollector. The negative pressure must be reduced to −0.3 bar; otherwise, the filter mesh could be damaged. First watery fluid appears in the drain, then it becomes more and more milky. This is due to the emulsified fat. Do not close the drain, because no fat particles will pass the filter and the drained fluid is a waste without any content of valuable tissue like stem cells (**Fig. 33.6**).

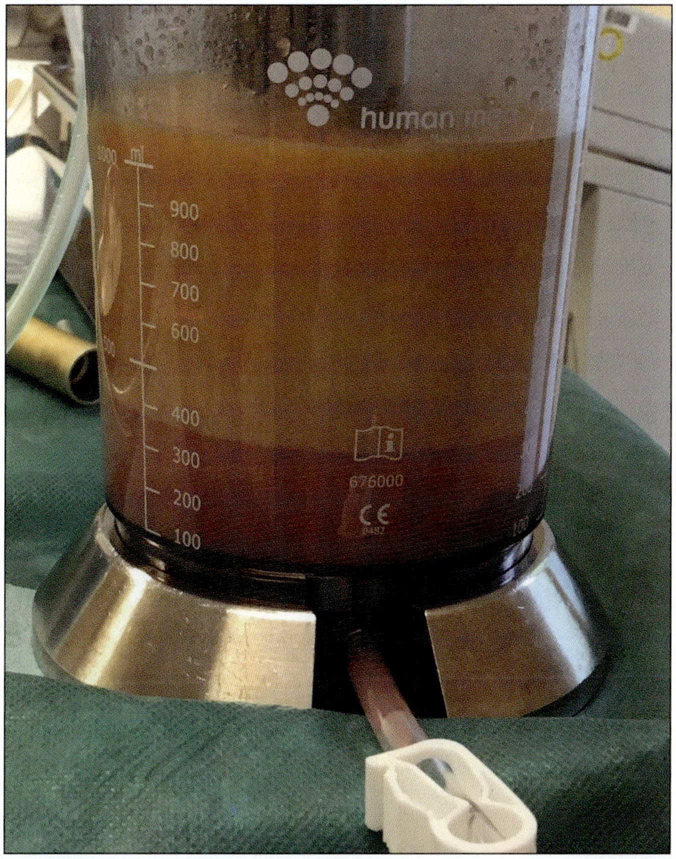

Fig. 33.5 Lipocollector with correct volume for bilateral augmentation.

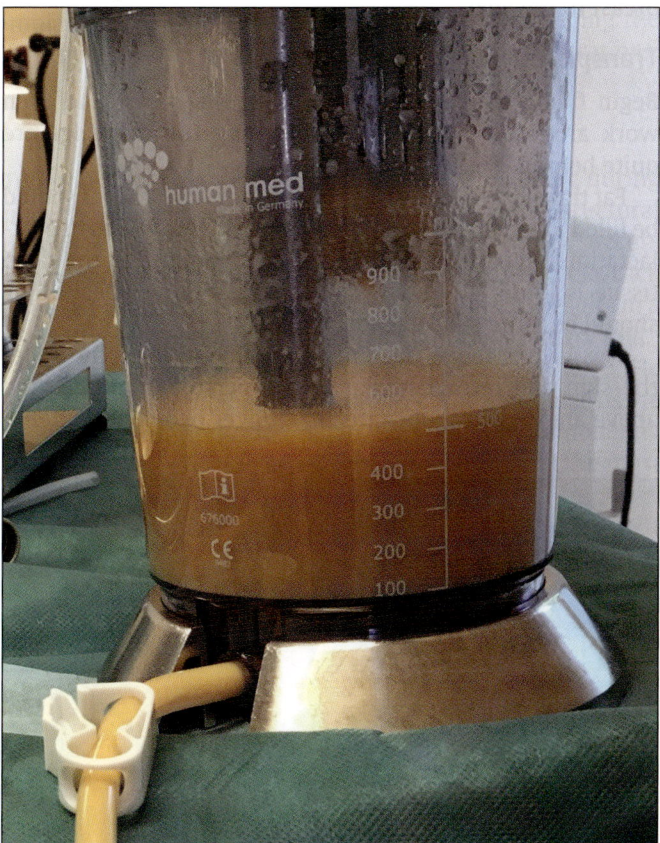

Fig. 33.6 After removing the waste fluid, leave the clip open, even if you observe yellow fat coming out to the waste container. This is only oily emulsion and does not contain any viable cells or stem cells.

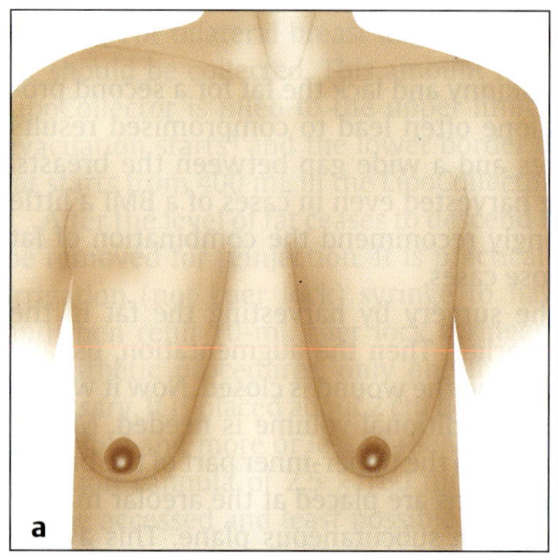

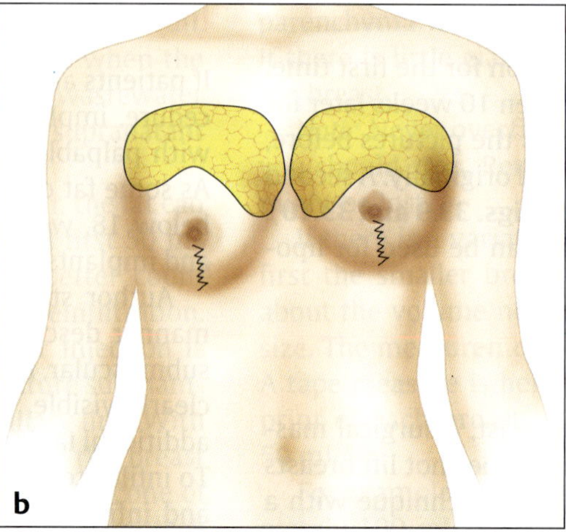

Fig. 33.11 **(a)** Before mastopexy. **(b)** After filling in the cranial area.

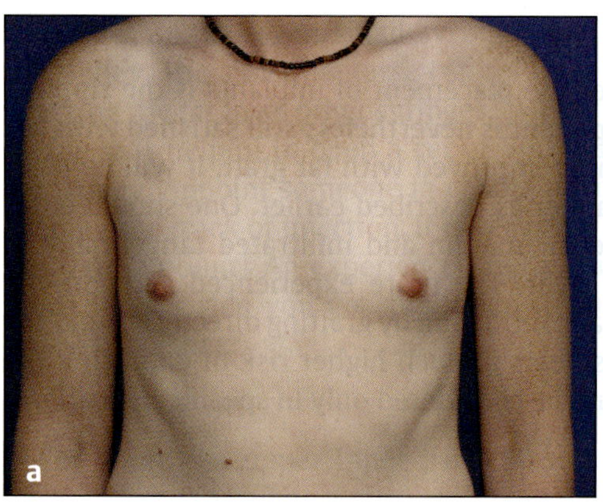

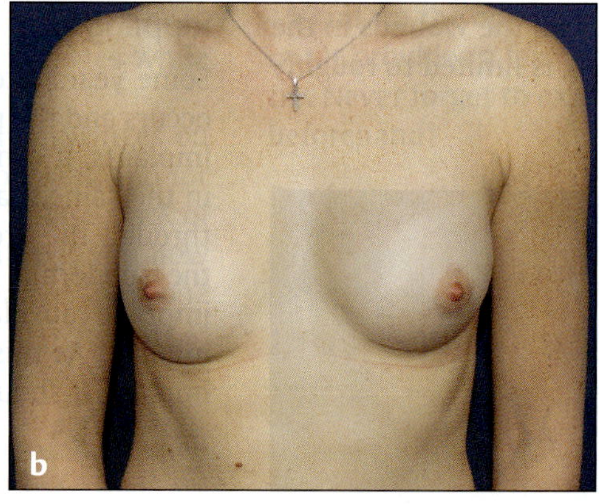

Fig. 33.12 **(a, b)** Combination of small implants and fat graft in one session. (The images are provided courtesy of Dr. Yves Surlemont, France.)

There is a risk of destruction of glandular tissue especially in young patients and large scars are the unfavorable outcomes of corrective surgery of tuberous breasts. It also necessitates multiple implant exchange operations over the lifespan and abnormal submammary fold persists. The author, since 2014, therefore treats tuberous breasts exclusively by fat grafting (**Boxes 33.6** and **33.7**).

The surgery can be done under sedation and takes approximately 60 minutes after little experience. It can be easily done as an outpatient procedure. After 4 days, most patients are able to go back for work.

Marking and Planning

The preoperative markings are done in a standing position as described earlier. Tuberous breasts can appear in a ptotic form, even when the nipple-notch distance is short (below 20 cm). This appearance is caused by a high inframammary fold and not by a ptotic areola complex. Never be tricked into performing a mastopexy in such cases, if the sternal notch-nipple distance is below 20 to 22 cm! Plan to lower the fold!

As a rule of thumb, the new fold should be marked 10 cm below the nipple. The incision for fat injection should be placed below and lateral to the new line. The fat injection will lead to an extension and growth of the skin envelope.

Box 33.6 Ready to use draping set for fat grafting

- Two large table covers
- One anesthesia cloth
- Two leg protectors
- Sponges
- 4 nos 50-mL irrigation syringes
- 6 nos 10-mL Luer lock syringes

Box 33.7 Goals of surgical management in tuberous breast

- New position of the inframammary fold
- Volume enhancement
- Reduction of areola size

Therefore, any reduction in the areola complex will be safer and easier in a second operation.

Fat Injection

The harvesting and infiltration technique of the fat follows Berlin autologous lipotransfer (BEAULI) protocol as discussed earlier (**Box 33.4**). The first step of surgery broadens the breast dimensions and recreates a new inframammary fold (**Fig. 33.13**). The adipose tissue is injected directly subcutaneously according to the preoperative marking. The distribution of the fat graft is subcutaneous and retroglandular. An average of 200 to 250 mL per side can be grafted.

It is important to explain to the patient that immediately after infiltration, the area of the old inframammary fold remains very rigid but after a period of approximately 6 weeks the original fold disappears letting the skin expand itself. The fact that the weight of the transplanted fatty tissue cannot automatically lower the inframammary fold by itself makes this first step surgery decisive.

The second session is performed after an interval of 3 months. The inframammary fold is further filled up with fat in order to stabilize its relocated position. Given the fact that enough tissue layers are established from the previous surgery, the lower quadrants are infiltrated in deep and superficial layers giving a more pleasant round shape to the breast. Hence, usually two sessions are required for the relocation of the inframammary fold (**Figs. 33.14 and 33.15**).

Areolar Reduction

There are a plenty of different ways of areolar reduction. In most cases patients with tuberous breast present with relatively large areolar diameter. About one-fourth of the patients in type I and II, half of the patients in type III, and 75% of patient in type IV are affected. Especially the ratio of the areola size is high considering mostly the small size breast bothers the patients in particular, so the reduction of the nipple-areola complex will be required in most of the cases. The results are better, when the tension is minimal due to the relaxed skin. Usually it is carried out in a second surgery. Preoperatively, we need to figure out if an open or closed areolar reduction is indicated.

Open Areolar Reduction

Double-layer technique: The indication for an open procedure is a relatively big skin excess which cannot be solely reduced by the closed technique without causing a severe protrusion of the areola. Normally, a periareolar incision

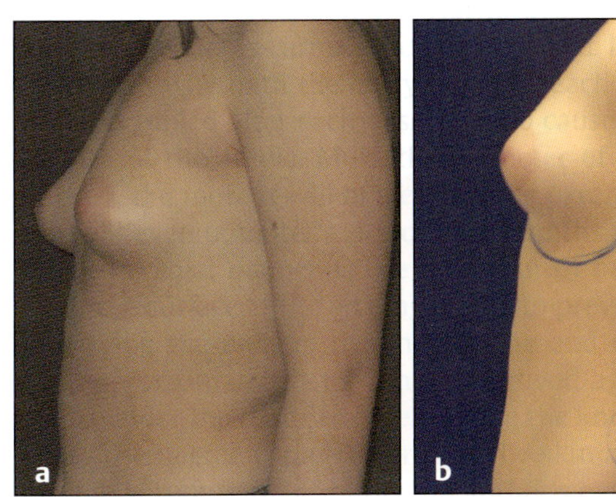
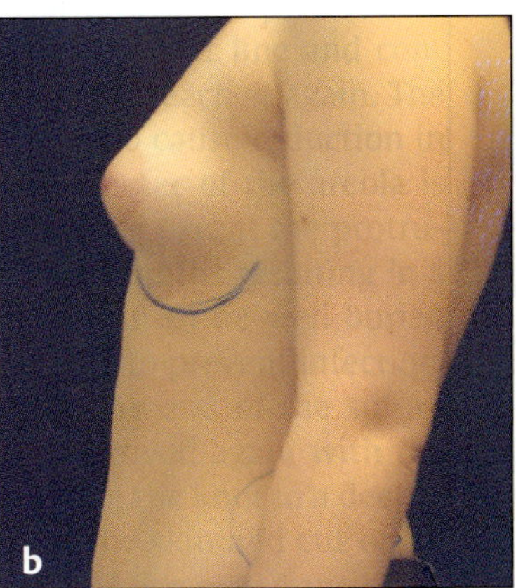
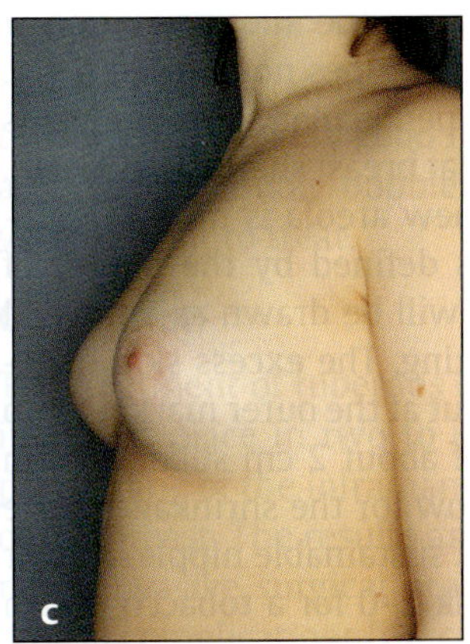

Fig. 33.13 **(a–c)** Goals of surgical management in tuberous breast.

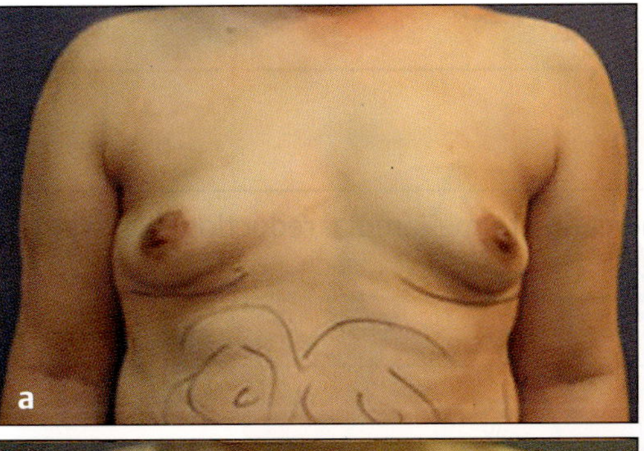
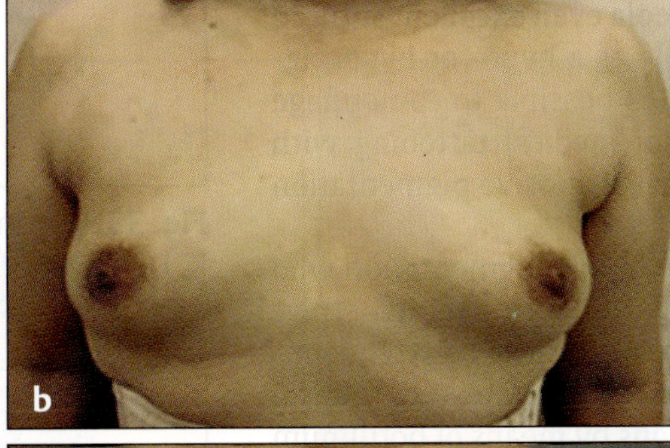
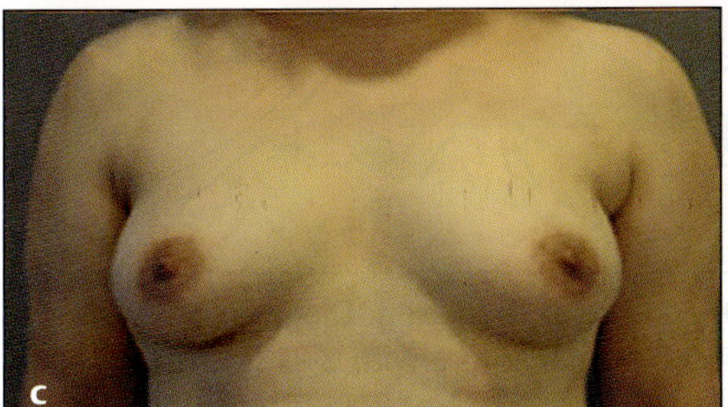
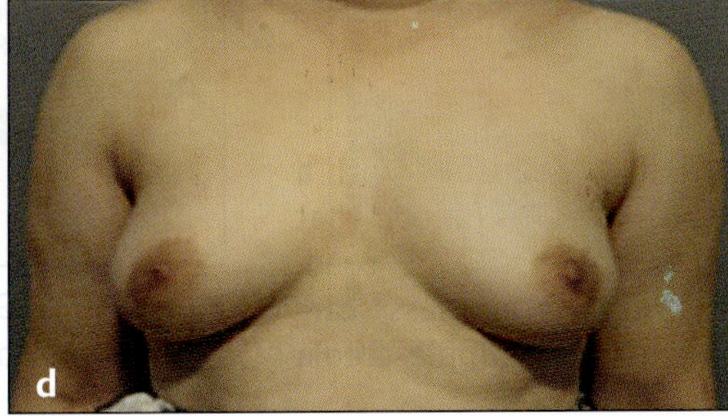

Fig. 33.14 Tuberous breast; **(a)** front view: marking of the inframammary fold and donor site for lipotransfer, **(b)** 17 days after the infiltration of 290 mL of fat on left and 300 mL on right side, **(c)** 6 months postoperatively, **(d)** 9 months postoperatively.

The overall reliable results combined with the less effort, low risks, and minimal complications make this procedure superior to the still widely used treatment with silicone implants. After positive experience with the outcomes, the author performs less and less invasive surgical procedures. Most of the tuberous breast deformities are being treated without exception by autologous fat transfer since 2012.

Box 33.8 Advantages of fat grafting in tuberous breast

- Avoids scars
- No destruction of the glandular tissue
- Very good additional skin growth
- Avoids obligatory follow-up operations

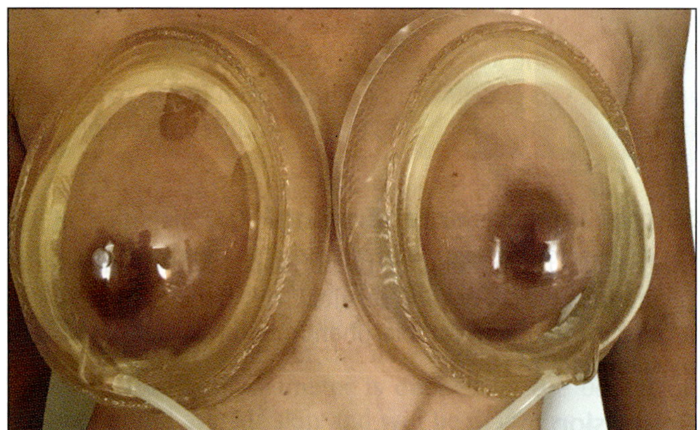

Fig. 33.19 Brava device (presently not available).

Use of External Extension

The idea of external extension devices to enlarge the breast volume is not very new. In the Museum of Hygiene in Dresden, Germany, some suction cups are on display which were sold in the 1950s. In the year 2000 Roger Khouri published his experience with an automated device (**Fig. 33.19**).[21,22] Different sizes of cups are chosen according to the breast size. As the breast volume increases during the application, larger cups will be applied. The original idea was to achieve a moderate breast enlargement without surgery. When fat grafting became a basic treatment in plastic surgery, it was recommended for achieving larger volume augmentation (**Table 33.1**; **Figs. 33.20 and 33.21**).[23,24]

The initial treatment lasts for 4 weeks; the device must be worn 12 hours daily. That is a challenge for the patient, as wearing during daily activities will be compromised due to the increasing size of the cups and at night sleep will be affected by losing the negative pressure which causes alarm and calls for readjustment of the device (**Table 33.1**).

Implant Conversion with Fat Grafting

Introduction

There are multiple reasons for removing implants such as pain, unnatural appearance, infection, capsular contracture, broken implants, general discomfort, and breast implant illness (BII). Ten to 30% of the patients receiving silicone implants have a risk of developing a capsular fibrosis within

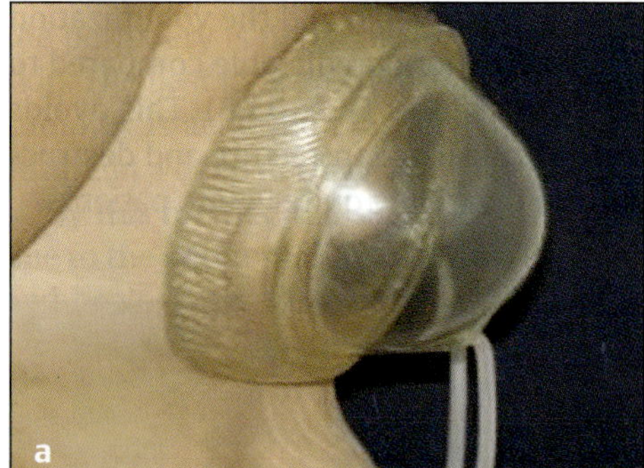

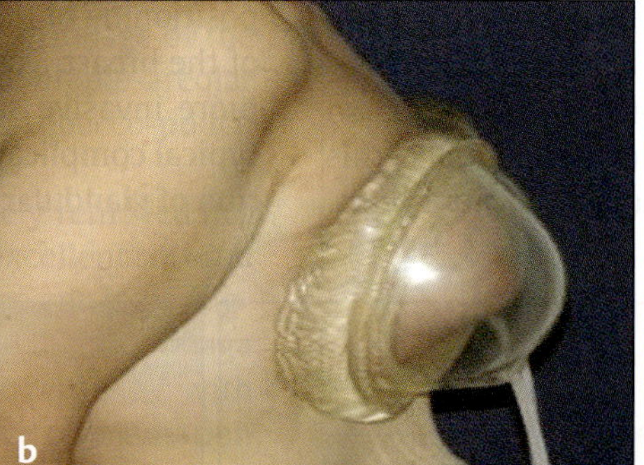

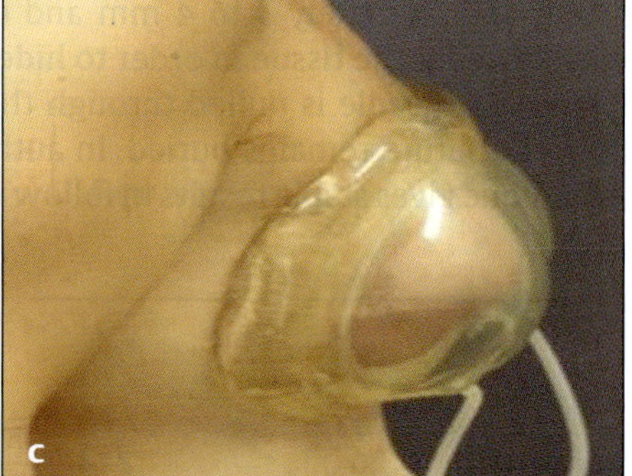

Fig. 33.20 Brava and fat grafting for enlargement of breast. **(a)** Breast before. **(b)** After application of -35mm Hg. **(c)** After 6 weeks of treatment. (The images are provided courtesy of Norbert Heine, Germany.)

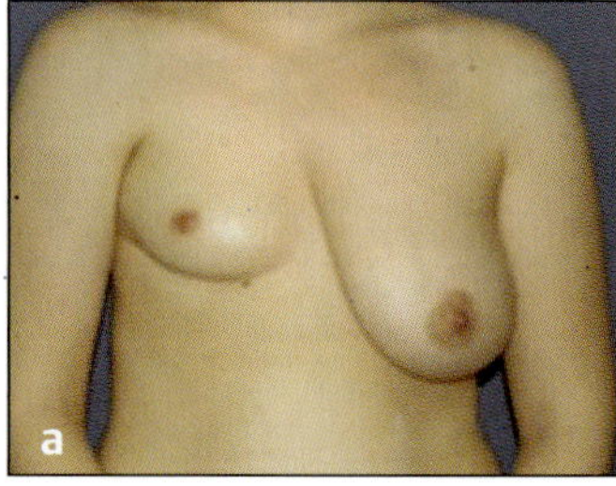

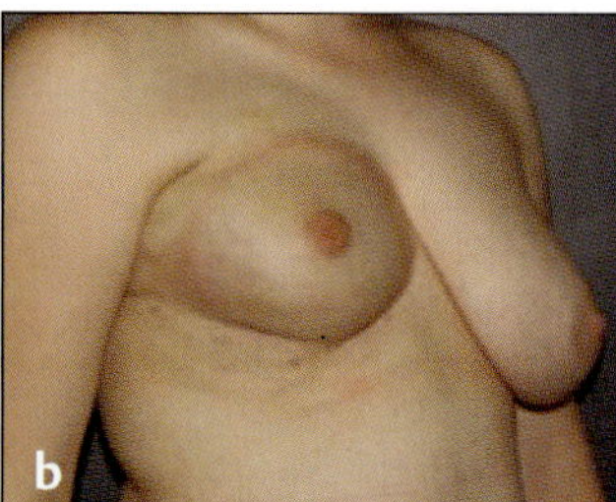

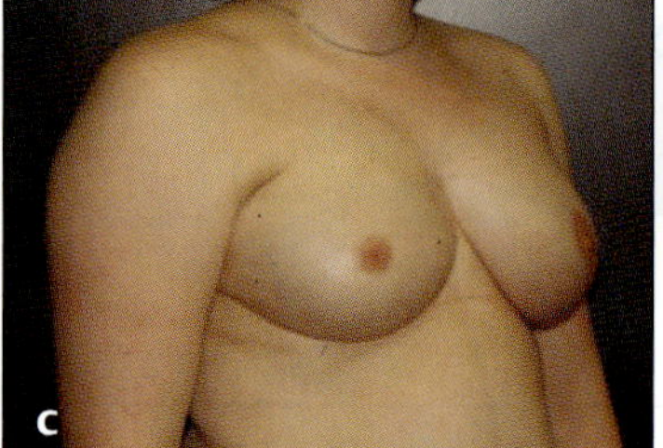

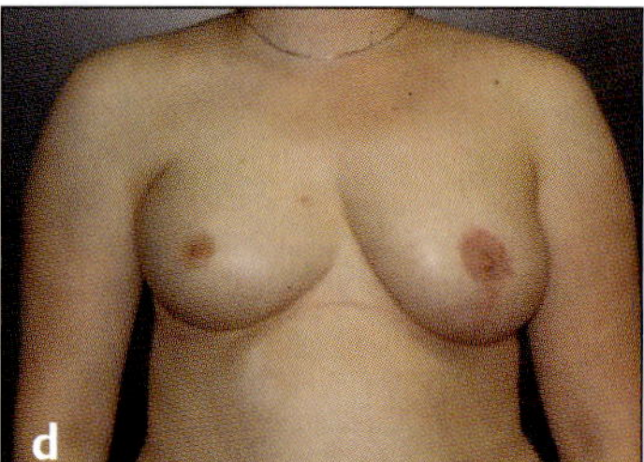

Fig. 33.21 Poland syndrome treated with extension and fat filling. **(a)** Patient with Poland syndrome before. **(b)** After two sessions of extension and filling. **(c, d)** After four sessions of extension and fat graft and reduction of left breast.

Table 33.1 Positive and negative features of Brava

Positive features	Negative features of pre-skin extension
• Reduces tissue pressure, as the pressure kills fat • Enlargement of recipient tissue • Limited skin excess leads to higher tissue pressure • Tight scars adherent to the chest wall can be stretched • Local hyperemia and angioneogenesis shall occur • Immobilization after lipofilling for better vascularization	• Risk of skin lesions • Not always successful in extension of scars • Additional costs • Need of high compliance

a period of 10 years after surgery. In recurrent cases a temporary removal of the implants must be considered.[25–27] Exchanging implants for fat is a procedure with very low complications and high satisfaction rate. During the last years we tried to convince all patients asking for reoperation after implant augmentation to consider this great alternative as a final solution.

Exceptions are heavy smokers and patient without a reasonable amount of available fat tissue. A BMI of 18 has proven to be the lower limit at author's clinic. Occasionally, patients succeed in gaining enough weight to finally undergo a lipofilling procedure. A loss of weight after a lipofilling procedure or fluctuations in weight by 2 to 3 kg has shown only minor impact upon the breast volume later on (**Box 33.9**).

Box 33.9 Ideal patient for exchange of implant to fat grafting

- Nonsmoker
- Tired of reoperations
- Dissatisfied with the form and firmness of breast
- Suffering from BII-associated symptoms
- Afraid of BIA-ALCL
- Desires to take benefit of liposuction

Abbreviations: BIA-ALCL, breast implant-associated anaplastic large-cell lymphoma; BII, breast implant illness.

Technical Approach

The surgery is usually done under general anesthesia and takes approximately 60 to 90 minutes after a period of learning. An inpatient admission for 1 to 2 days is recommended. The patients are being marked preoperatively with the donor sites for fat grafting preferably the tummy/flanks region or upper thighs for logistic reasons if there is no preference from the patient's side. In our clinic we start by harvesting the fat. The procedure of lipotransfer follows the Berlin Autologous Lipotransfer Protocol (BEAULI) as described earlier.

Removing of Implants

In most cases the skin incision of the former implant insertion can be used, specially an incision in the inframammary fold or periareolar incision. The procedure is performed after complete excision of the old scar. Axillary access is not recommended because of the difficulty of accessing the capsule. The dissection goes right onto the capsular surface of the implant. The capsule is incised so that the implant can be mobilized and removed without harming it. Textured Allergan and polyurethane-covered implants are more difficult to extract. In cases of intact implants, the procedure is easier. Nevertheless, after good cleansing of the cavity, inspection of the capsule is done, because in all reported BIA-ALCL cases the tumor was palpable inside the capsule.

If the implant is preoperatively known to be damaged, a radical "en bloc" excision is to be discussed beforehand with the patient. In such situation the disadvantage is the limitation in amount of fat grafting. The author has not encountered any problem after the removal of the damaged implant and a thorough cleaning of the cavity (**Fig. 33.22**). Multiple changes of gloves is paramount, though this may be challenging and time-consuming.

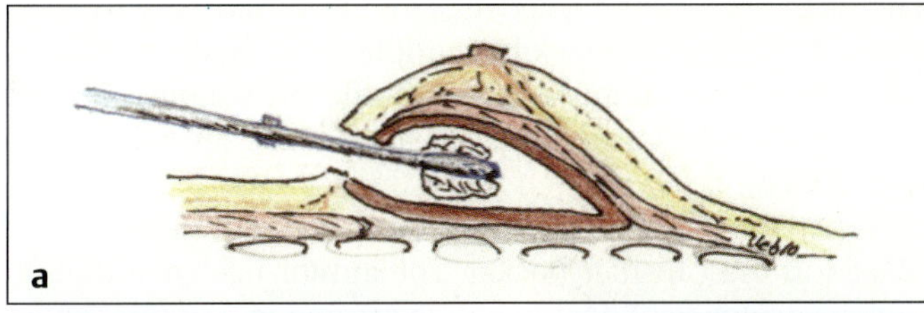

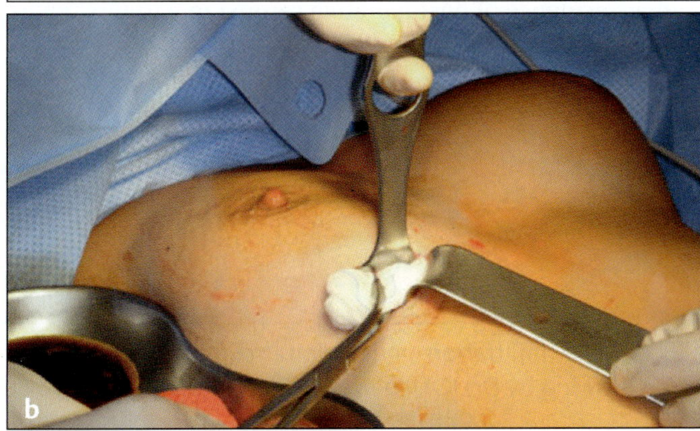

Fig. 33.22 Curette and cleansing of the capsule. **(a)** Diagrammatic representation of capsule cavity after removal of the implant. **(b)** Clinical photograph showing removal of capsule and cleansing of cavity with antiseptic solution. (Prepared as per a drawing by Dr. K. Ueberreiter.)

Fat Injection

In *subglandular implants*, the fat is injected in the pectoralis major muscle. Here approximately 150 mL of fat can be infiltrated without the risk of cyst formation. In *subpectoral implants*, the capsule edge is caught with a Kocher's clamp and pulled slightly for tightening and stretching. The involuntary perforation of the capsule and resulting loss of fat can be thus avoided. The blunt 2 mm diameter, 16 cm length infiltration cannula is inserted right on top of the capsule. The index finger can easily palpate the correct position of the needle from inside of the capsule to prevent perforation. The infiltration is done by performing even pressure on the syringe plunger while withdrawing the cannula tip (**Fig. 33.23**). Each tunnel is infiltrated with about 1 mL so that the fat in a 10-mL syringe is distributed by 10 to 20 fan-shaped movements. If necessary, the position of the clamp is changed.

The subcutaneous infiltration is done almost equivalent to the aesthetic augmentation described in previous section (**Fig. 33.24**).

How Much Fat to Inject?

The amount of transplanted fat should approximately correspond to the former size of the implant but shall not exceed 350 mL. Larger amount is not sufficiently nourished by the surrounding tissue fluid and a lot of the fat may perish (**Box 33.10**).

When the infiltration is almost finished, a drain should be placed in the capsular pocket. The author has encountered higher incidence of postoperative seroma in patients where the capsule is closed without a drain.

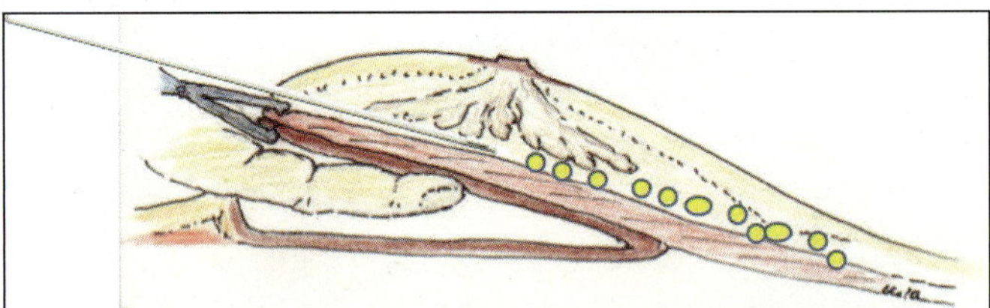

Fig. 33.23 Infiltration under digital control. (Prepared as per a drawing by Dr. K. Ueberreiter.)

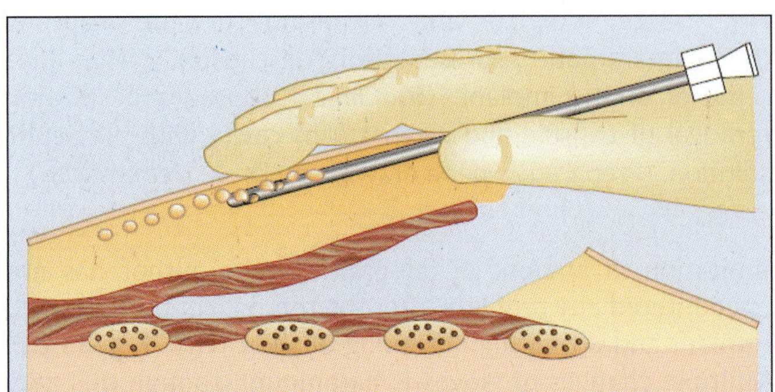

Fig. 33.24 Subcutaneous infiltration. (Prepared as per a drawing by Dr. K. Ueberreiter.)

Seroma

As we are not suturing the capsule anymore, we enable fluids to drain to the subcutaneous layer. If in rare case seroma occurs, it can easily be needle aspirated. At the same time the injection of a corticosteroid helps to avoid a reoccurrence. The subcutaneous layer and the skin are usually closed in two layers of resorbable sutures.

Finally, the area directly above the wound is filled up with fat from an additional prick incision that is commonly done at a lateral point close to the anterior axillary line as it has been explained in the section on aesthetic fat graft (**Fig. 33.25**). The incisions are closed alternatively with adhesive strips (e.g., omnistrips) or sutures. The breasts are wrapped by a cotton dressing. The patient is dressed up with the respective compression garment.

After-care

Compression should be avoided and warmth is maintained to enhance the blood supply. Normal daily activities like walking are allowed, but excessive sports should be avoided. Most patients develop a moderate swelling which increases during the first week and slowly subsides over a period of 4 weeks. The drain is removed the next postoperative day. The adhesive tapes should remain for approximately 4 weeks on the incision scar to prevent keloid formation.

Box 33.10 Key to success in fat grafting

Never try to overfill the tissue planes with fat; higher amount of fat will not increase the survival, rather will cause more complications like higher reabsorption rate and oily cysts

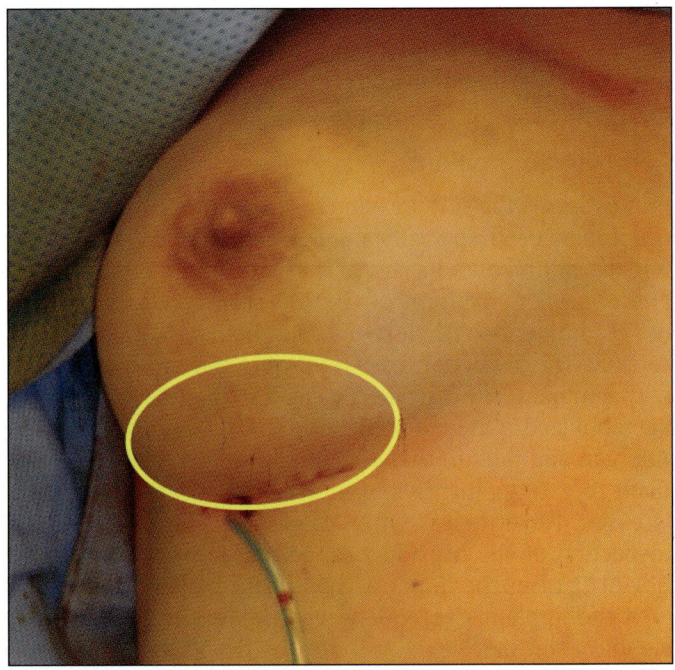

Fig. 33.25 Marking of area for lipofilling from separate incision.

The patient is allowed to take a shower after 2 days of the operation. These patients need to be followed for assessing the long-term outcome (**Figs. 33.26–33.28**).

Removing the Capsule

Within the last few years more and more patients with possible side effects caused by silicone implants reported to our clinic. They are unspecific and comprise among other symptoms fatigue, hair loss, paresthesia, headaches, brain fog, exanthema, depressions, nausea, or palpitations.

Many patients by browsing the internet seem to believe that BII is caused by silicone particles which would be stored in the capsule. Also, the suggestion is made that there are bacteria and fungi accumulated in the fluids surrounding the implants. Others talk of heavy metals being contained in implants and leading to a poisoning of the immune system. All these are not based on scientific evidence. If patients with symptoms of BII are believers of these theories, it is hard to dissuade them out of an "en-bloc" resection. After explanation of pros and cons and detail counseling, the

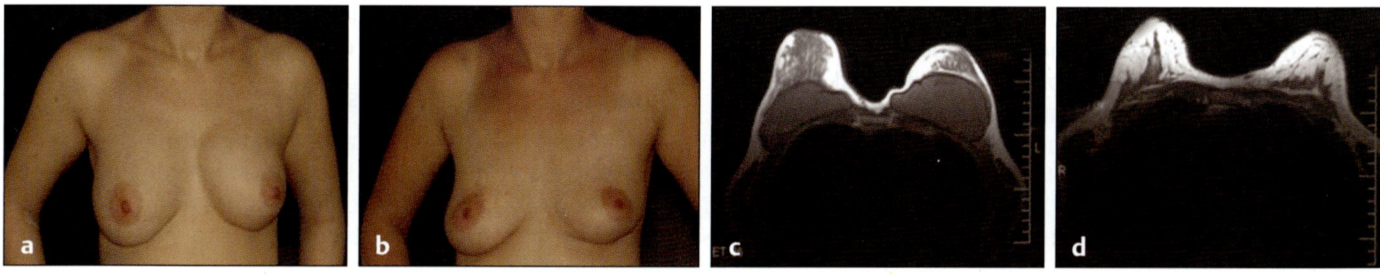

Fig. 33.26 Capsular fibrosis after breast augmentation with silicone implants and after implant conversion with fat grafting. **(a)** Patient's preoperative photograph, **(b)** postoperative photograph after fat grafting. Remaining asymmetry due to removal of left breast tissue at the age of 17 years (now 34). **(c, d)** Magnetic resonance imaging (MRI) before and 1 year after the procedure.

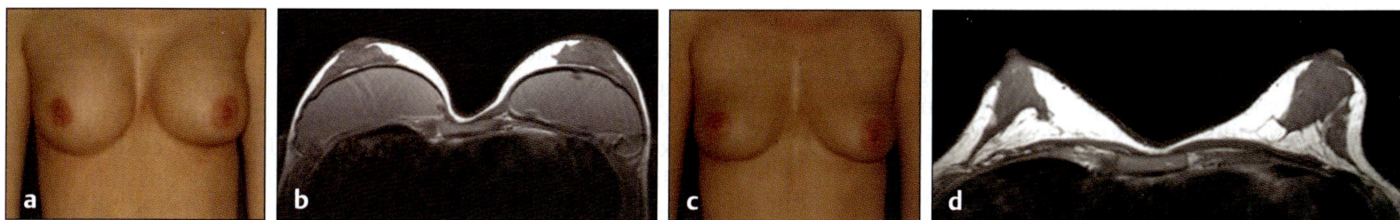

Fig. 33.27 Capsular fibrosis after breast augmentation with silicone implants (right: 305 g; left: 265 g), managed with fat grafting. **(a)** Clinical photograph showing capsular contracture, **(b)** magnetic resonance imaging (MRI) showing implant and contracture **(c)** after implant removal and two sittings of fat grafting (right: 180 mL; left: 160 mL), **(d)** the MRI 8 months later.

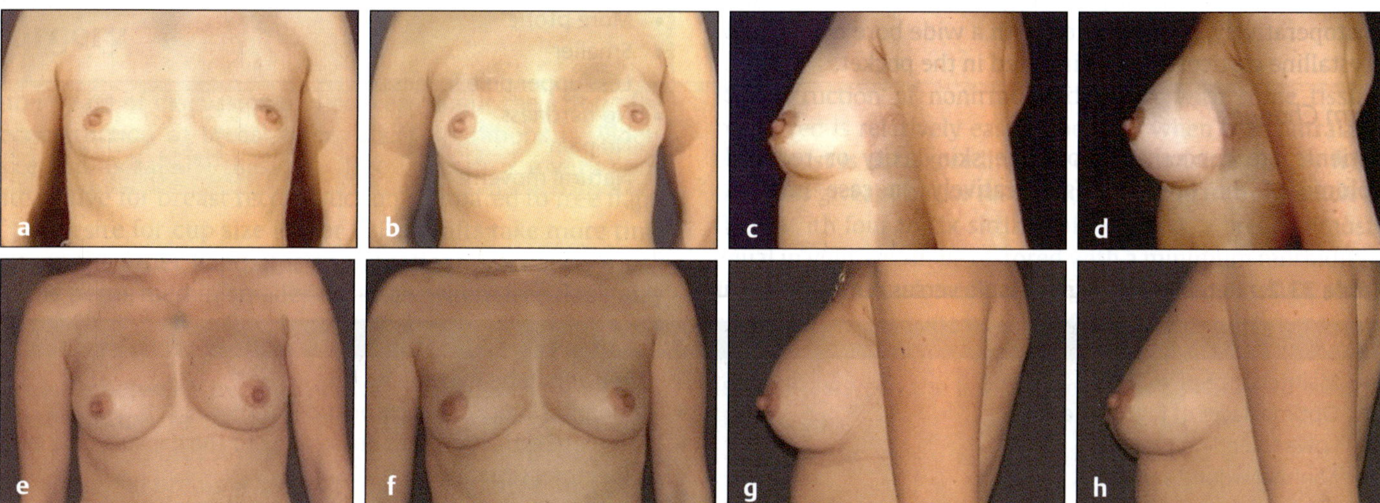

Fig. 33.28 **(a, c)** Patient presenting for breast augmentation. **(b, d)** Bilateral breast augmentation with silicone implants, **(e, g)** same patient 8 years later presenting with capsular fibrosis B III with implants still in place. **(f, h)** Six months after implant conversion with fat grafting.

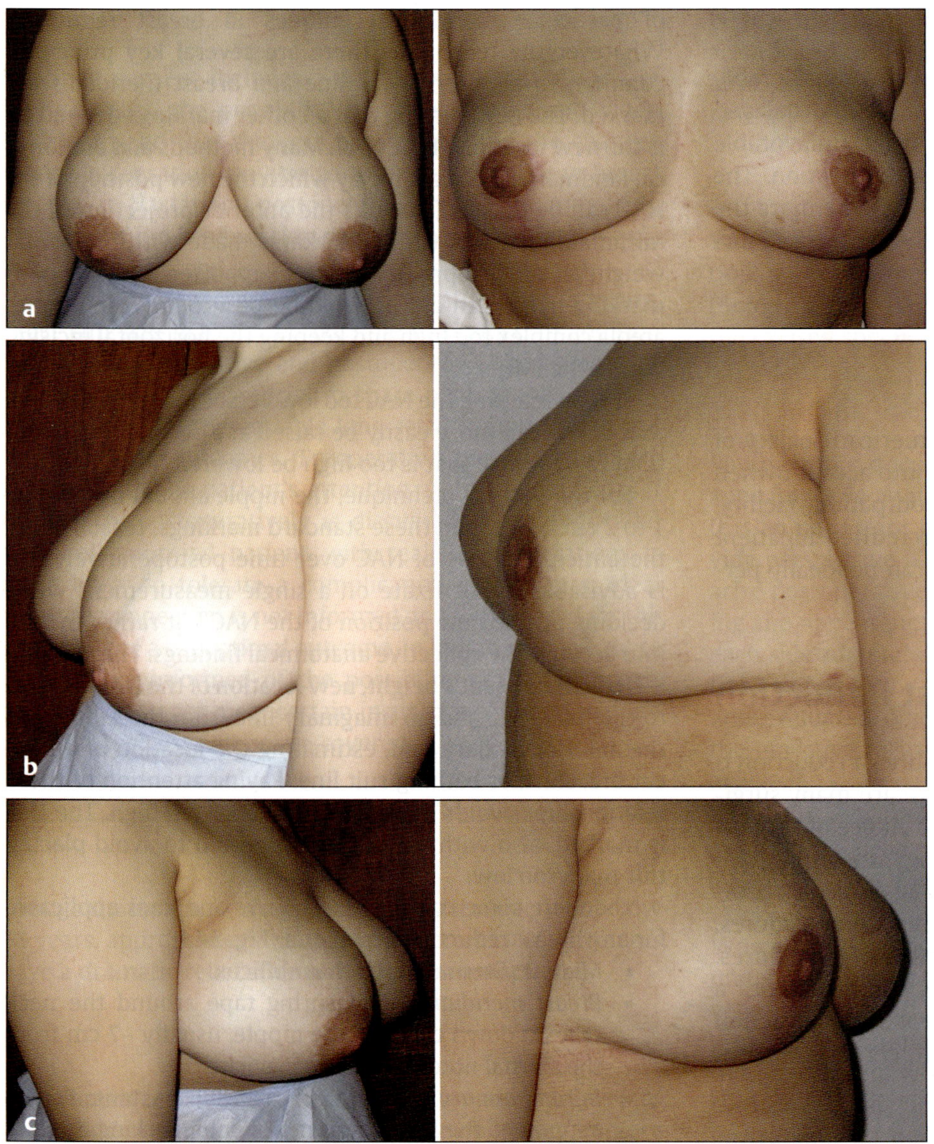

Fig. 34.5 **(a–c)** Before and after pictures of a moderate macromastia. Superomedial flap with Wise closure.

creates adequate projection, and the upper pole contour is round. The nipple should be localized and marked to the highest point of the breast.[29]

- The lateral most point of the inframammary crease when horizontally connected to the breast meridian, it is the point of intersection. This is not a commonly practiced method.

Thus, a rather low-lying new NAC may be marked using any two measures, ~21 to 23 cm level is acceptable. Acceptable NAC width ranges between 38 and 42 mm. Sternal notch to nipple distance should be 21 to 23 cm. Nipple to IMF distance of 6 to 7 cm under maximal stretch gives the ideal projection.

Other measurements that are not commonly practiced but are useful are breast base width, anterior pull skin stretch, soft tissue pinch thickness of the upper pole, and soft tissue pinch thickness at the IMF.[30]

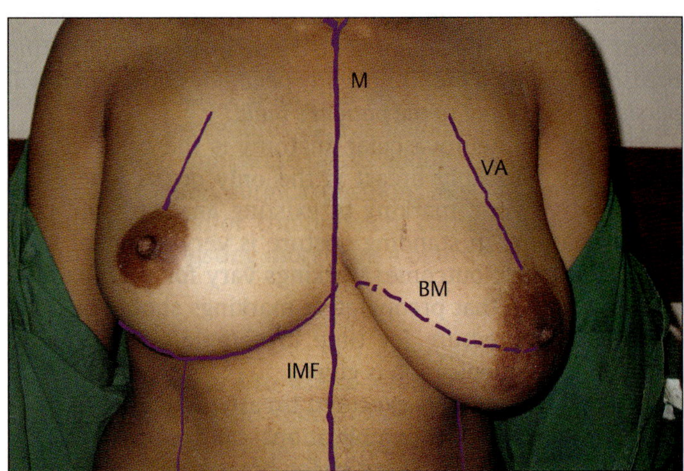

Fig. 34.6 Common landmarks. BM, breast meridian; IMF, inframammary fold; M, midline; VA, vertical axis.

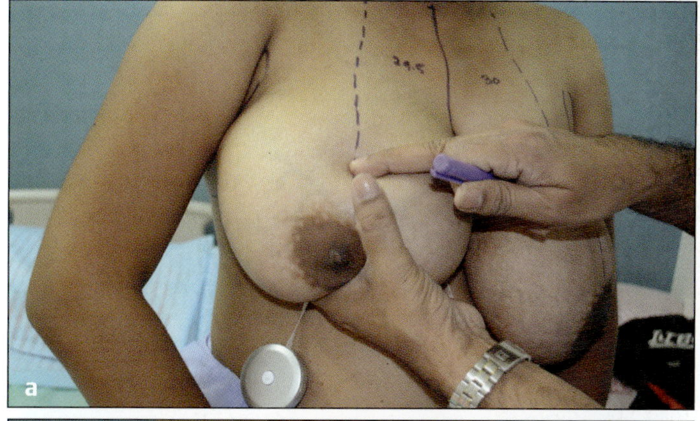

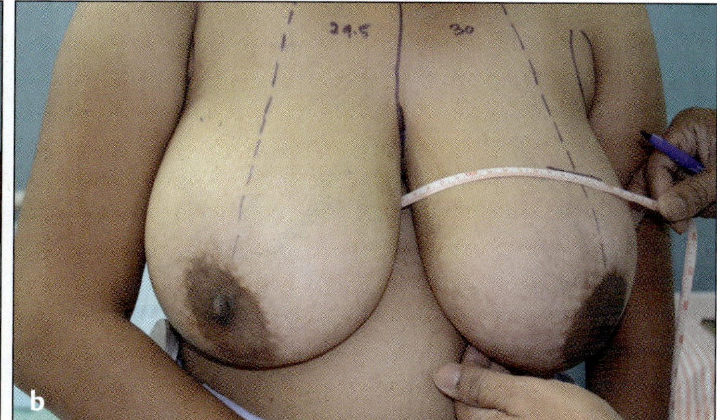

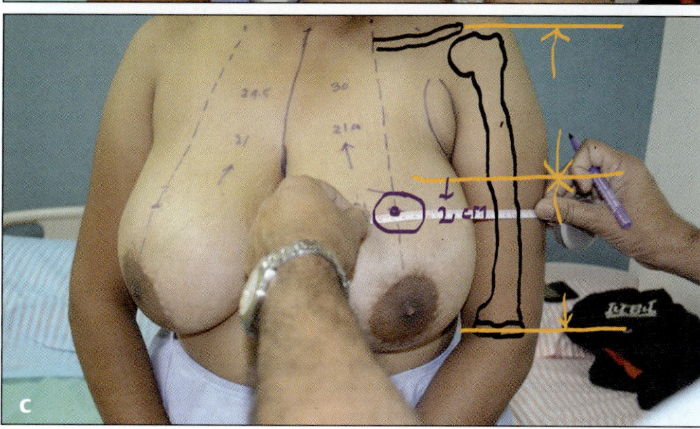

Fig. 34.7 Different ways of marking the future nipple-areolar complex (NAC). **(a)** Anterior projection of inframammary fold (IMF) on to breast meridian. **(b)** Tape measure parallel to IMF on to breast meridian. **(c)** Midhumerus point and 2 cm down.

Markings for Superomedial Pedicle: Hall-Findlay Technique[12]

Once the common landmarks are marked, by gently lifting the breast up and rotating to the left (**Fig. 34.8a**) and to the right (**Fig. 34.8b**), two vertical lines are dropped down from the breast meridian. When major reduction is the plan, more force is used in both directions to include more tissue to be removed. The wider the two lines, the smaller and more projectile is the breast. The lower borders of these lateral markings are joined by a curved line 2 to 4 cm above the IMF. The upper borders are joined by the future periareolar circumference. This line is drawn from a point 2 cm higher than the future nipple and forms a mosque-dome shape instead of the usual open circle (**Fig. 34.8c**). This modification was introduced because it was observed that it leaves a perfect circle areola after suturing and produces less tension on the upper part of the areola and therefore there is less risk of scar widening. The total length of this dome should not exceed 16 cm to prevent later widening. This is a free hand marking. Using silicone template or wire keyhole pattern, the new nipple circumference and the angle can be marked. This helps during the initial learning phase.

The parenchyma to be excised in a small vertical reduction is called "ghost areas" because here the skin is left intact unlike Wise pattern where the skin is also removed en bloc. If the vertical length is unlikely to resolve smoothly by gathering sutures as it happens in moderate to huge reductions, it should be converted to a J, L, or inverted-T closure (**Fig. 34.9a–c**).

Now the superomedial pedicle is marked with a base width of 6 to 8 cm enclosing the NAC of 38 to 42 mm diameter. The upper margin of the flap usually occupies quarter to half of the new nipple circle.

Markings for Inferior Pedicle

Usually it is done with the help of gadgets like wire keyhole pattern. Free hand marking is difficult. Once the future nipple site is marked as mentioned earlier, the vertical limbs of the keyhole pattern is spread 8.5 cm, measured at the 5 cm mark along the wire limbs. The open circle of the keyhole is located with its top 2 cm above the new nipple position. Along the vertical limbs 5 to 6 cm is marked on both the sides[1,5] (**Fig. 34.10**).

The two ends of the IMF are clearly marked. Medially it should stop 3 to 4 cm from the midline. Laterally it should stop along the mammary fold rather than following the lateral fold. The 5 to 6 cm point from the vertical limb should connect to the lateral and medial points of IMF with some adjustments, like a lazy "S," to match the length of both lines.

The inferior pedicle is marked 4 to 6 cm wide and centered on a line from the nipple down to the midpoint of the inframammary incision marking. A cookie cutter of 38 to 42 mm diameter is used to make an impression on the wide NAC.

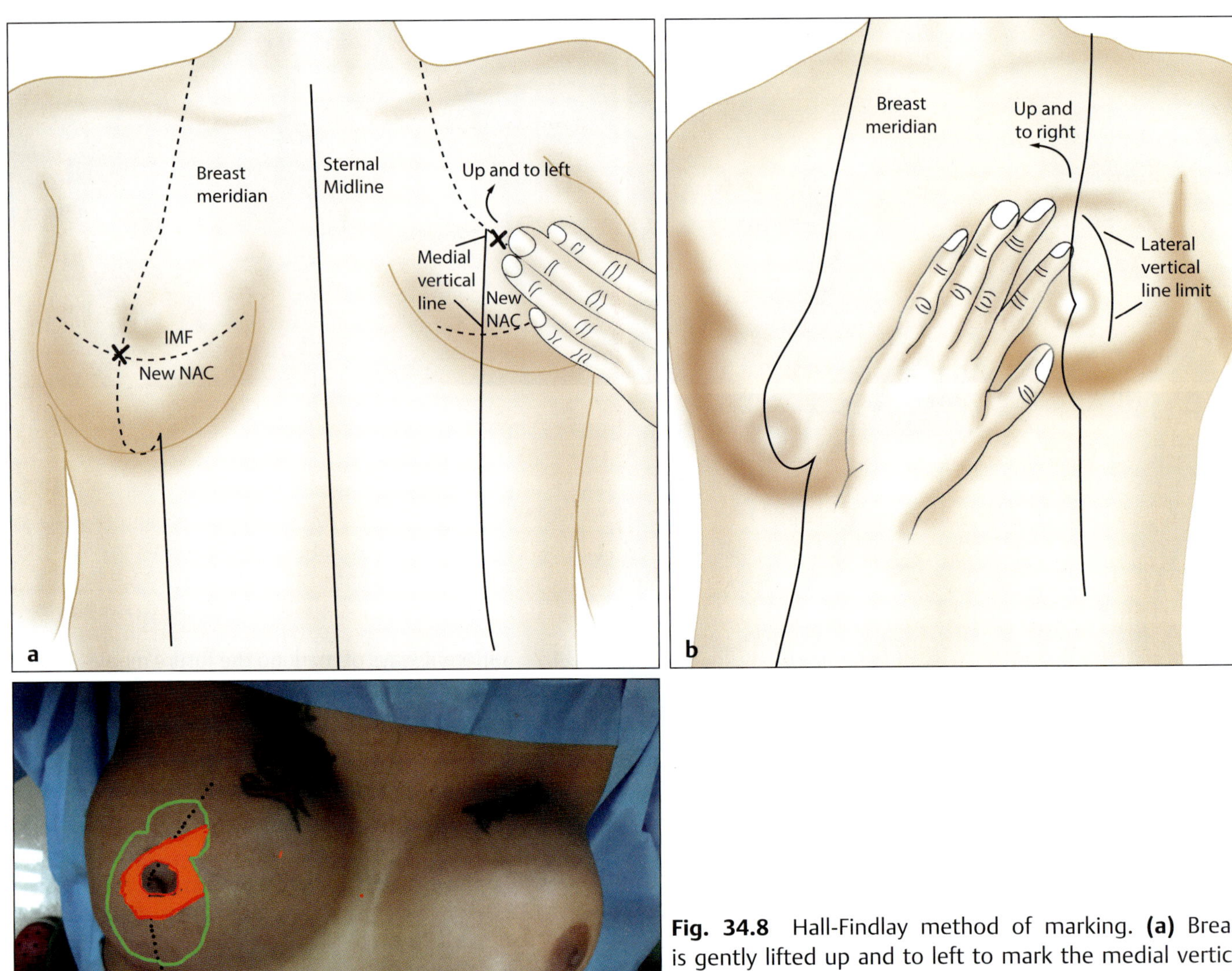

Fig. 34.8 Hall-Findlay method of marking. **(a)** Breast is gently lifted up and to left to mark the medial vertical line. **(b)** Breast is gently lifted up and to right to drop the lateral vertical line. **(c)** Superomedial pedicle sketched on a breast image. IMF, Inframammary fold; NAC, nipple areola complex.

Fig. 34.9 Three options to deal with the lower end of vertical closure when it is longer. **(a)** Box or gathering suture/purse string. **(b)** J-closure. **(c)** Mini inverted-T closure.

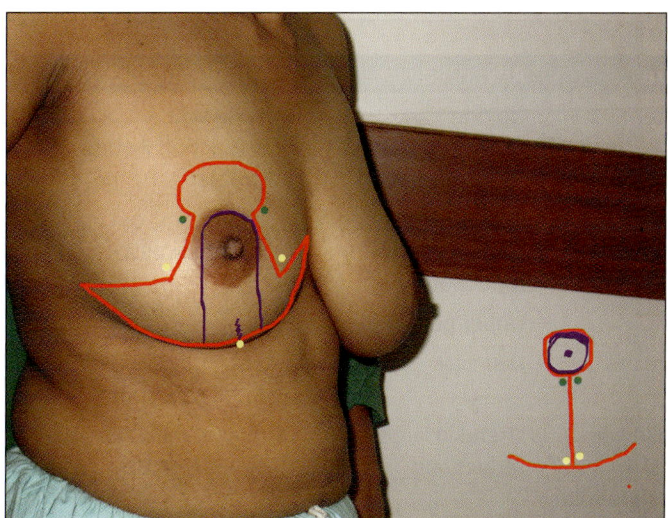

Fig. 34.10 Markings of a Wise-pattern incision with inferior pedicle.

The inferior pedicle is closed as inverted-T. The length of the horizontal limbs is decided by the resection volumes—the more the volume, the longer the limbs. The inferior pedicle with Wise-pattern closure is easy to learn and practice and is safe.

Many breast reduction procedures are mentioned in the literature, but only few are practiced today. The popular techniques are listed in **Table 34.1**.

Surgical Steps of Breast Reduction

Access incisions and creation of pedicle, parenchymal resection, breast shaping, and management of excess skin are four major steps in breast reduction procedures (**Box 34.1**).[40] Preinjection of the breast with epinephrine-containing solution should avoid the planned vascular pedicle to the NAC. The safety and efficacy of epinephrine use and tumescent solution infiltration in reduction mammaplasty have been reported.[41] These methods decrease blood loss and decrease operative times.

Box 34.1 Four key steps in breast reduction

- Access incisions and creation of pedicle
- Parenchymal resection
- Breast shaping
- Management of excess skin

Access Incisions

The most common access incisions are Wise-pattern, vertical, circumareolar, and liposuction.

The Wise-pattern skin incision affords the widest access to the breast parenchyma and can accommodate a variety of pedicles (**Fig. 34.10**). The vertical pattern skin incision affords adequate access to the breast parenchyma (**Fig. 34.11**) but to a lesser degree than the Wise incision. Multiple pedicle options are also possible. The circumareolar, Benelli-type access incision is limited by concentric skin excision around the NAC (**Fig. 34.12**). It offers more limited access to the parenchyma and limited pedicle choice to the NAC. While deciding the incision, one needs to plan the type of pedicle-bearing NAC. There are many pedicles in vogue.

Pedicle Types

Inferior

This is the pedicle popular in north American countries. The blood supply for an inferior pedicle comes from both the deep artery and vein coming up just above the fifth rib and the more superficial arteries from the fifth interspace coursing down around the periphery of the breast and then traveling up in the subcutaneous tissue. In very huge reductions, inferior pedicle is useful. It is usually a pyramidal-shaped flap; its length can be 15 to 20 cm. The pedicle thickness is usually 4 to 5 cm. Wise-pattern closure is usually used. If the NAC becomes avascular over a long pedicle, this is converted to a free nipple graft. Over a period of years the breast bottoms out. Various modifications, such as pedicle-shaping sutures,[42] recruiting more tissues from the central pedicle,[43] have also been used along with this pedicle (**Fig. 34.13**).

Superior

The blood supply for the superior pedicle is from the descending branch of the perforating artery coming from the second interspace of the internal mammary system.

Very short pedicle is used, mainly when there is less ptosis (**Fig. 34.14**). When longer flaps are used, it is likely to kink on itself, and gives good projection. Vertical reduction is the ideal type when superior pedicle is used. The pedicle is plicated to bring the areola up and the undersurface of the fold is sutured to the pectoralis fascia as high as possible.[9]

Superomedial

The descending branches from the second and third perforating branches of the internal mammary system supply this flap. It is one of the robust flaps commonly used in vertical reductions (**Fig. 34.15**). It can be raised with a thickness of 1.5 to 2 cm. Usually 10 to 15 cm long flap is safe. This is ideal for moderate resections and is useful in mastopexies.

Bipedicle

The second, third, descending branches and the deep branches of the fourth perforating branch of the internal mammary system supply this flap. This is useful in very large reduction and revision of breast reduction procedures, where the previous flap was not known. Ideal bipedicle is a vertical bipedicle of McKissock rather than the horizontal bipedicle of Strombeck where the upward movement is restricted (**Fig. 34.16**).

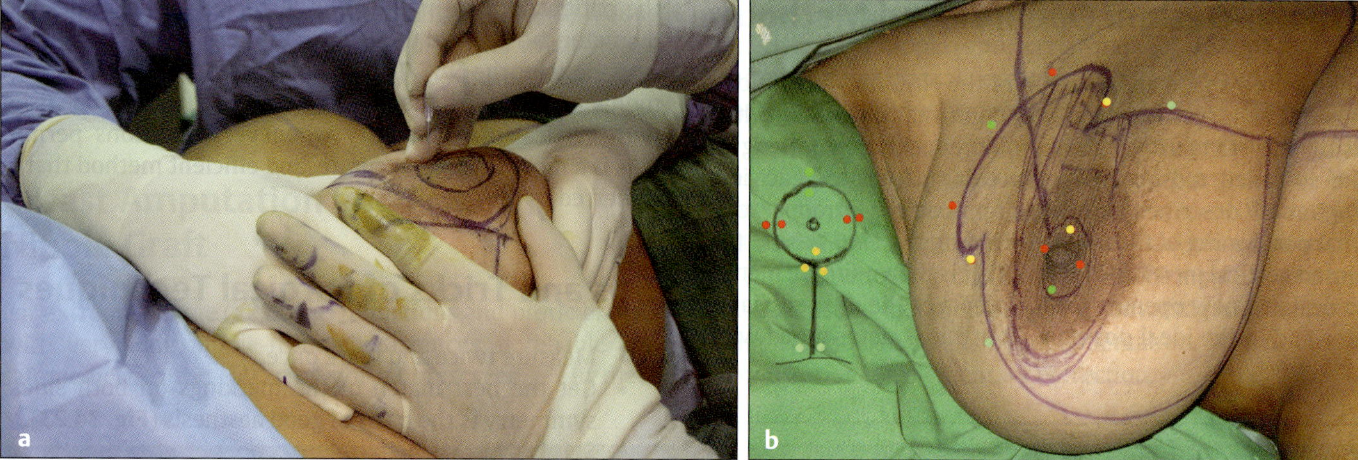

Fig. 34.24 Orientation tattooing using methylene blue. **(a)** Tattoo marking with needle and methylene blue. **(b)** Completed tattoo and the inset showing the final closure.

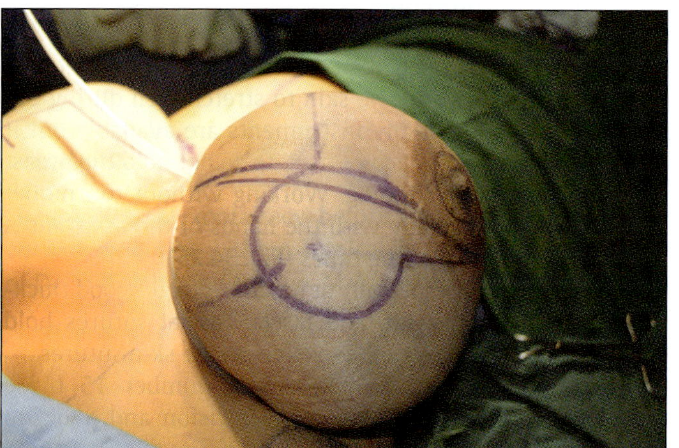

Fig. 34.25 Breast tourniquet—the breast is held taut.

- All the flaps in breast reduction procedures are dermaglandular. There is a very good robust subdermal plexus which supplies the NAC. There are many efficient methods of de-epithelization.[49] There are many ways of doing it, but always make sure the process is away from the nipple so that the NAC is always protected. De-epithelization is done when the flap is taut.
- Flap first (**Fig. 34.27**): The entire procedure depends on the flap carrying the NAC. After de-epithelization, dissect the flap first and protect it from shearing and cutting forces.
- Some inclusion sutures tagging the NAC to the deeper tissue will prevent shearing during movements of the flap and help in moving the flap while dissecting.
- Deep sutures: Try to suture the fat and fascia (SFS) under the dermis together so that there is no tension on the skin closure which is very important for good healing and fine scars. Ted Lockwood has described about the importance of this fascia and these sutures.[50]

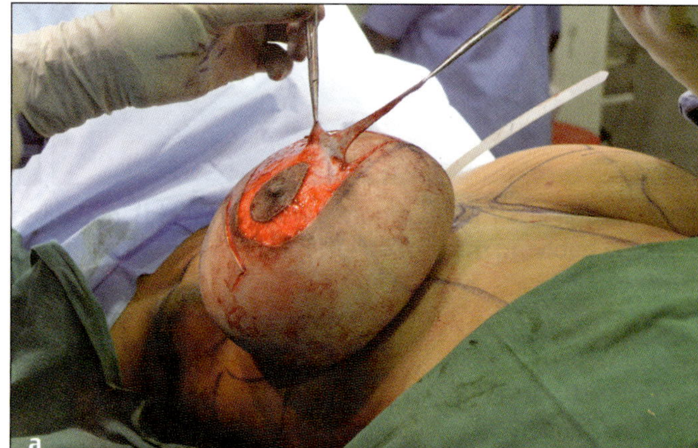

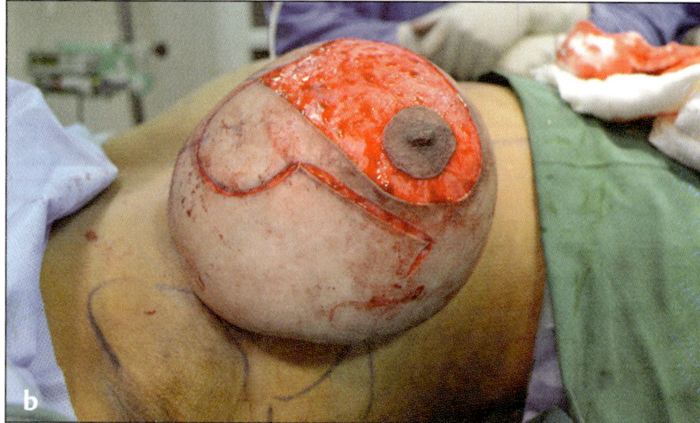

Fig. 34.26 **(a)** The de-epithelization of the pedicle using scalpel. **(b)** After completion of de-epithelization.

- To drain or not: Wrye et al[51] showed no difference in complications between drained and undrained breasts, but when patient satisfaction was evaluated, the patients preferred the early postoperative comfort, early discharge afforded by the absence of a drain.

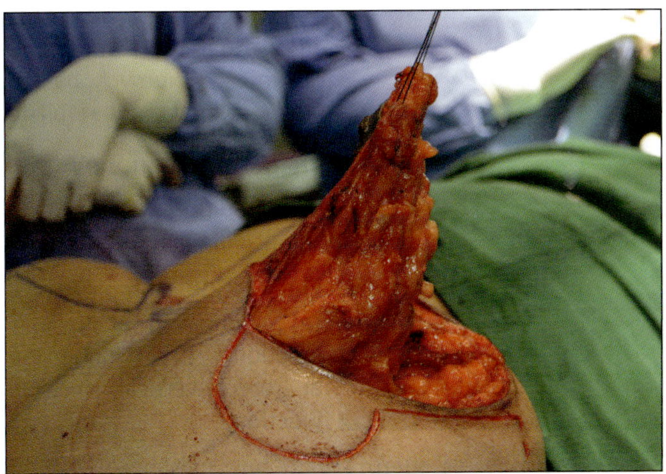

Fig. 34.27 After de-epithelization, the flap is dissected and carefully protected from shearing and cutting forces.

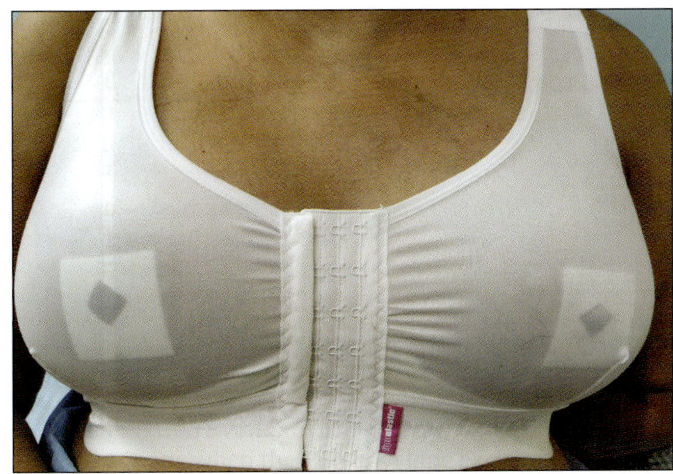

Fig. 34.28 Supportive bra applied immediately after the procedure.

Postoperative Management

Immediate Phase

Dressing and Breast Support

After the subcuticular closure, either skin glue or steristrips are used to reinforce the suture line. A waterproof adhesive dressing followed by on-table application of good supportive bra (**Fig. 34.28**) probably helps in reducing the pain and hematoma. First review and change of dressing after 48 to 72 hours is important to look for hematoma and NAC viability.

If drains are placed, they are typically removed on the first postoperative day. Patients are monitored for nipple viability and hematoma by observing symmetry and firmness. All patients are given instructions to limit physical activity for 2 weeks or more. Activities of daily living are typically resumed on the first postoperative day. An examination confirms the state of the nipple, incisions, skin flaps, and overall breast symmetry. A supportive bra helps to reduce the pain and gives sufficient compression to avoid plastering the breast tightly.

Long-term

A soft elastic nonwire support bra can be worn for the first 2 weeks, and then weaned until the end of the fourth week, when the patient may wear her bra of choice. Follow-up should be arranged at 6 and 12 months to assess final breast shape, symmetry, and NAC sensibility.

Management of Complications

The most common complication, independent of reduction technique, is delayed wound healing. Proper patient selection and surgical planning will help decrease the chances of most of the undesirable outcomes.

Despite all the meticulous care, in the best of the hands and in the optimal patient, complications may occur. Fortunately, most of the complications that occur with reduction mammaplasty can be resolved with favorable outcomes.

Early Complications

Delayed Wound Healing

Delayed wound healing is the most common complication in reduction mammaplasty regardless of technique, and is related to closure with undue tension, underlying pressure from a seroma or hematoma, flap necrosis and ischemia, infection, or comorbidities. Typical locations for wound dehiscence are the T-junction (**Fig. 34.29a, b**). These areas are often managed conservatively. Sometimes, delayed primary closure may be performed.

Poor Nipple Vascularity

Partial or total nipple necrosis can be a devastating complication (**Fig. 34.30**).

Good technique and assistance help prevent the shearing force that depletes the blood supply to the NAC. Timely inclusion sutures where the NAC is sutured to the deeper tissues of the pedicle and on-table orientation tattooing with methylene blue prevent kinking of the pedicles.

Poor Vascularity Detected on the Operating Table

A pale or bluish nipple with limited bleeding on the cut edge warrants very close postoperative observation. Poor or dark blue blood flow from a pin prick is also worrisome. Sometimes, at the end of the procedure, it will turn pink with normal capillary refill. An objective assessment of the blood flow to the nipple is the fluorescein intravenous dye test and a Wood's lamp. Probably the latest intraoperative

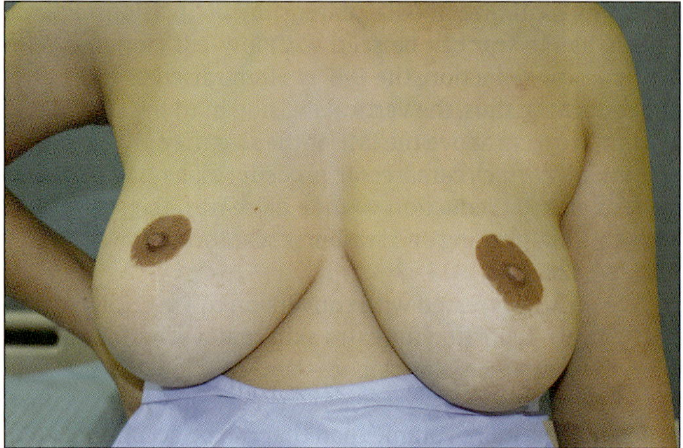

Fig. 34.33 Bottoming-out of the breasts after breast reduction.

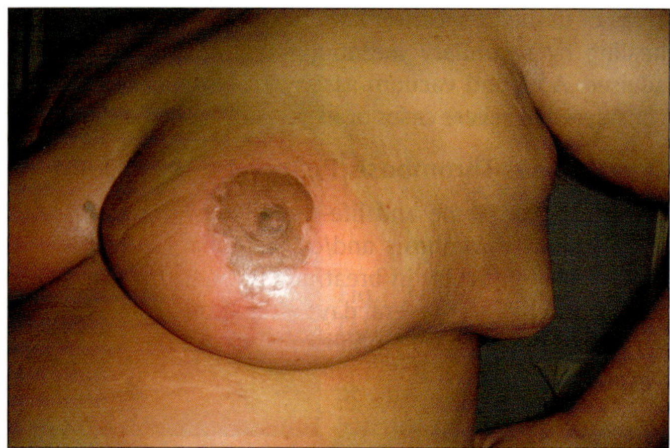

Fig. 34.35 Dog-ear at the lateral end of Wise closure.

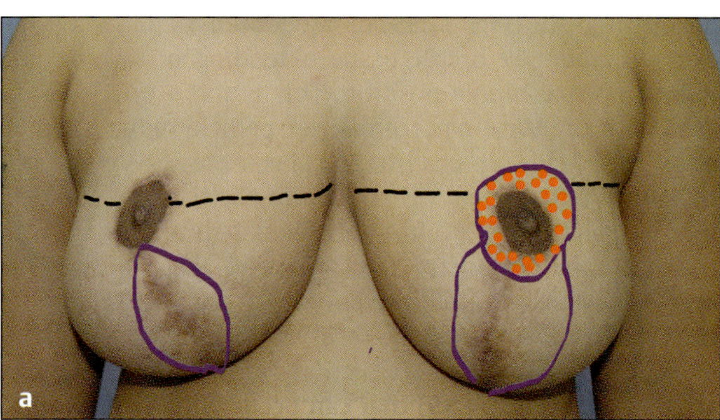

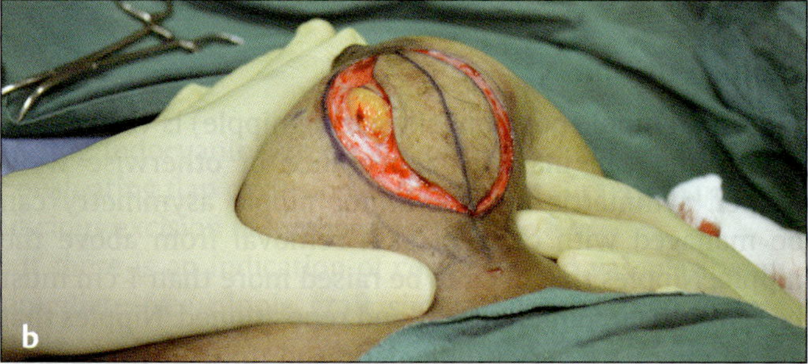

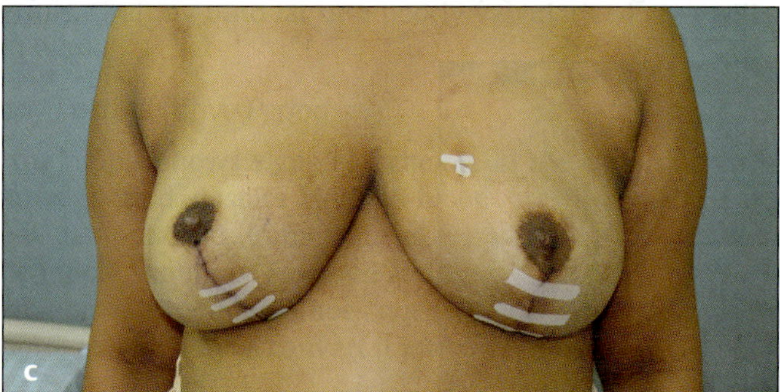

Fig. 34.34 Frank Lista method of correction of bottoming-out. **(a)** If nipple-areolar complex (NAC) is in the ideal position, only inferior wedge excision and closure—right breast. If NAC is in a lower position, a superior pedicle is incorporated—left breast. **(b)** Excision of inferior wedge. **(c)** After correction.

If there is concomitant bottoming-out of the breast, it is best to reshape the breast relative to the nipple. If the nipple is truly too high, it must be repositioned lower on the breast mound, leaving a scar above the nipple.

Asymmetry

Minor asymmetry is inevitable. Significant size asymmetry can be managed with liposuction or further parenchymal resection. Complete revision may be needed if there is gross asymmetry.

Fat Necrosis

Fat necrosis presents as a local area of firm or hard tissue. This is usually noted close to the breast surface, as it is more easily palpated there. Deeper areas of fat necrosis may be diagnosed only by radiography. Should fat necrosis occur, it should be needle aspirated to confirm the diagnosis and to rule out a neoplasm followed by excision or aspiration if symptomatic. Long bulky pedicles are prone for fat necrosis. The calcifications of fat necrosis are macro and the diagnostic differentiation from micro calcifications of malignancy is usually not difficult, provided the operative history is revealed.

Changes in Nipple Sensation

All patients are informed during the consent process that nipple sensation can permanently decrease, increase, or not change after reduction mammaplasty. Early changes in sensation are often temporary and should be managed expectantly until at least 6–12 months after surgery. Multiple reports exist comparing techniques based on sensory outcomes. One demonstrated that no difference exists between medial and inferior dermoglandular pedicles and that resection weight was not a variable in sensory outcomes.[55]

Nipple Retraction

Nipple might lose its projection and appear retracted (**Fig. 34.36a, b**). It can occur following any pedicle technique.

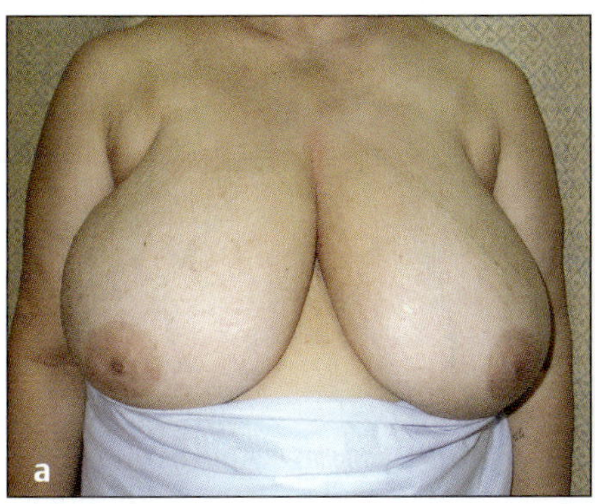
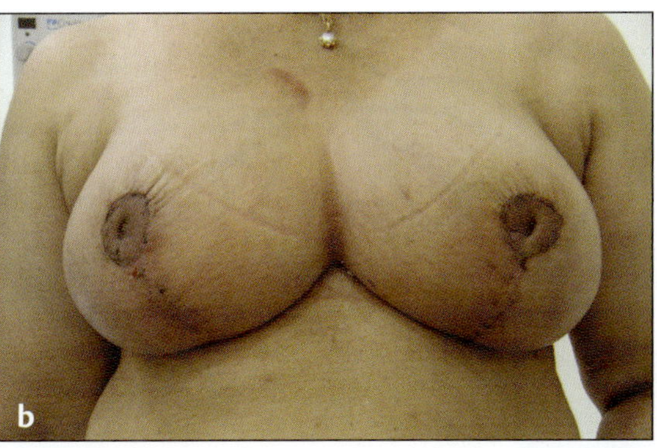

Fig. 34.36 **(a)** Nipple retraction before. **(b)** Nipple retraction after.

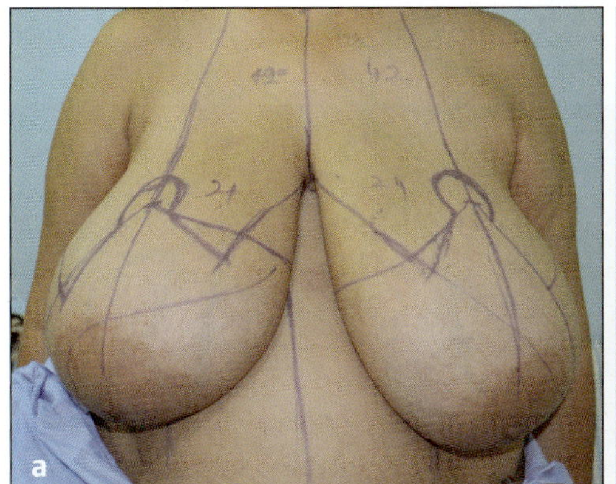
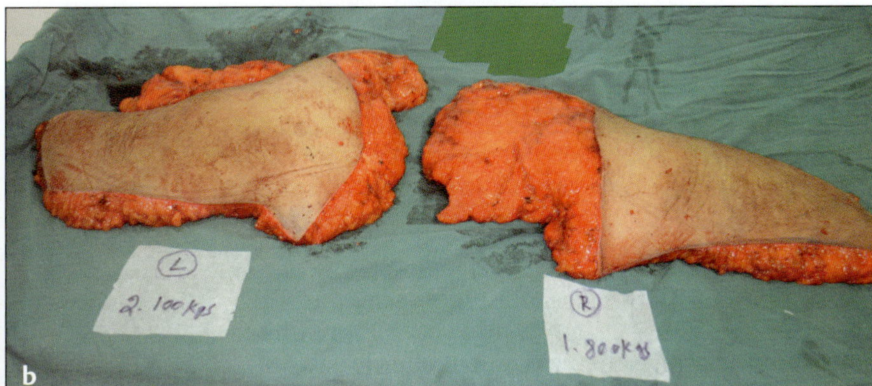

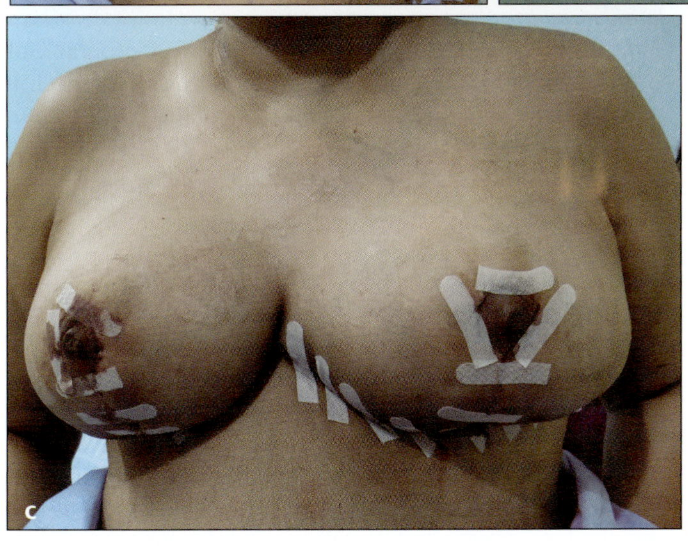

Fig. 34.37 Gigantomastia. **(a)** Before surgery. **(b)** Resected tissues. **(c)** Immediate postoperative image after superomedial pedicle with Wise closure.

Probably it is due to tissue insufficiency at the new nipple position.

Special Situations

Gigantomastia

When more than 2,000 g of tissue is removed, it is preferable to use this term. Superomedial pedicle can be used safely (**Fig. 34.37a–c**). But the risk of complications like nipple loss and later bottoming-out may happen. Amputation and free nipple graft is probably the ideal procedure for gigantomastia.

How to Address the Axillary Fold?

Axillary folds are challenging areas of body contouring, especially when one has to address it along with breast reduction. Young patients with good skin elasticity and firm fat can be suctioned, hoping that skin will redrape in few months. Indian patients have higher incidence of huge fatty folds, which may need excision during the reduction itself to get a good contour (**Fig. 34.38a, b**).

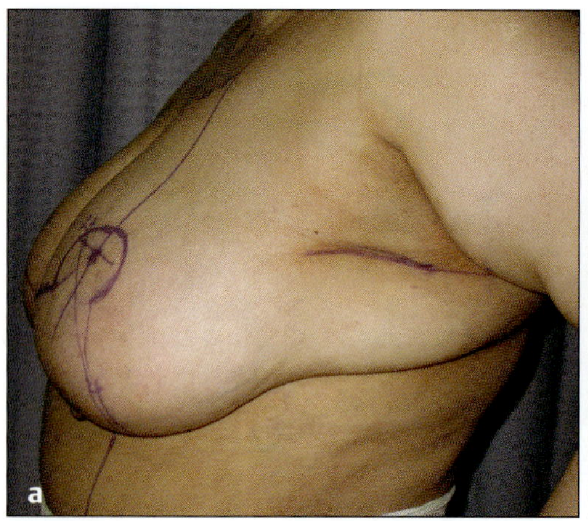

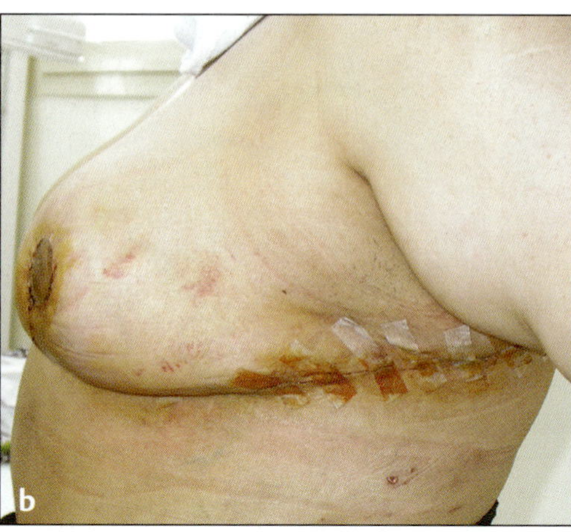

Fig. 34.38 Addressing the axillary fold along with breast reduction. **(a)** Before excision. **(b)** Immediately after excision.

Mastopexy

Introduction

It is customary and logical to include mastopexy along with breast reduction. Both procedures, in principle, appear to be same except that the pexy seems to have less magnitude and minimal scarring. The expectations of the pexy patients are more refined and demanding. The issue is lift along with gain in volume. In most instances, the final results after pexy are critically evaluated and various combinations of augmentation either with silicone or autologous fat are used along with this procedure. At least a mild degree of ptosis is factored into the final result of a well-done reduction mammaplasty, but such residual ptosis may be less acceptable to the small breasted woman with primary aesthetic motivation for undergoing mastopexy.

History of Mastopexy

In 1897, Pousson was the first to describe mastopexy, where large crescents of skin and fat from the superior portion of the breasts were removed and fixed with sutures to the pectoralis major muscle. Other significant stages in history were when Dufourmentel and Mouly[56] in 1961 excised infralateral crescent of skin around the areola and rotated the lateral gland superiorly. In 1971, Goulian described dermal mastopexy,[57] where the concept of skin brassier was fashioned. In 1978, Hinderer and Courtiss[58] further refined the dermal strips to anchor the breast. With the emergence of reliable dermoglandular flaps for NAC in breast reduction procedures, correcting small breasts with ptosis alone became possible. The skin was tailored by the reduction pattern with the glandular tissue retained to provide volume and projection. Gonzalez-Ulloa[59] was the first to recommend concomitant subglandular augmentation of the breast during mastopexy to correct the ptotic hypoplastic gland.

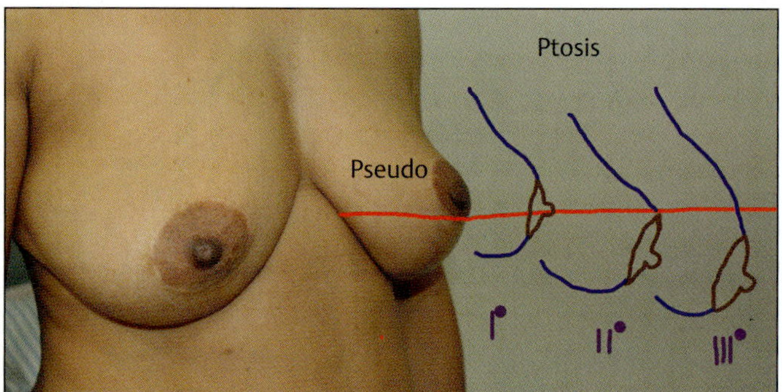

Fig. 34.39 Classification of ptosis. Clinical photograph of pseudo ptosis. Diagrammatic representation of Grade I, II and III ptosis.

Cárdenas-Camarena and Vergara.[60] in 2001 published his experience with one-stage mastopexy augmentation.

Pathophysiology of Ptosis

Breast sags due to various reasons. This natural aging process results in stretching of skin envelope with or without striae and loss of parenchymal volume. The fallen position may be accelerated by constitutional predisposition, in addition to the unfavorable factors in any normal woman like weight loss, pregnancy, lactation, and menopause. Breast after earlier lift will also sag after few years, probably due to the above-mentioned reasons. Ted Lockwood[61] emphasized on suturing the SFS with nonabsorbable sutures to delay this sagging.

Any breast operated for ptosis can and will sag over different time period usually 4 to 10 years and this fact has to be told clearly before surgery and this may need revision.

Regnault[62] in 1976 classified ptosis by degree (**Table 34.3** and **Fig. 34.39**).

Mastopexy can be done alone or in combination with augmentation. For significant ptosis, the same markings of any breast reduction technique, one is familiar with, can be

Table 34.3 Regnault classification of ptosis of breast

Degree of breast ptosis	Description
First degree	Nipple descends to the level of inframammary fold
Second degree	Nipple falls below the fold but remains above the lowest contour of the breast
Third degree	Nipple reaches the lowest contour of the breast
Pseudoptosis	Loose and lax breast sags below IMF but whose nipple remains above the IMF

Abbreviation: IMF, inframammary fold.

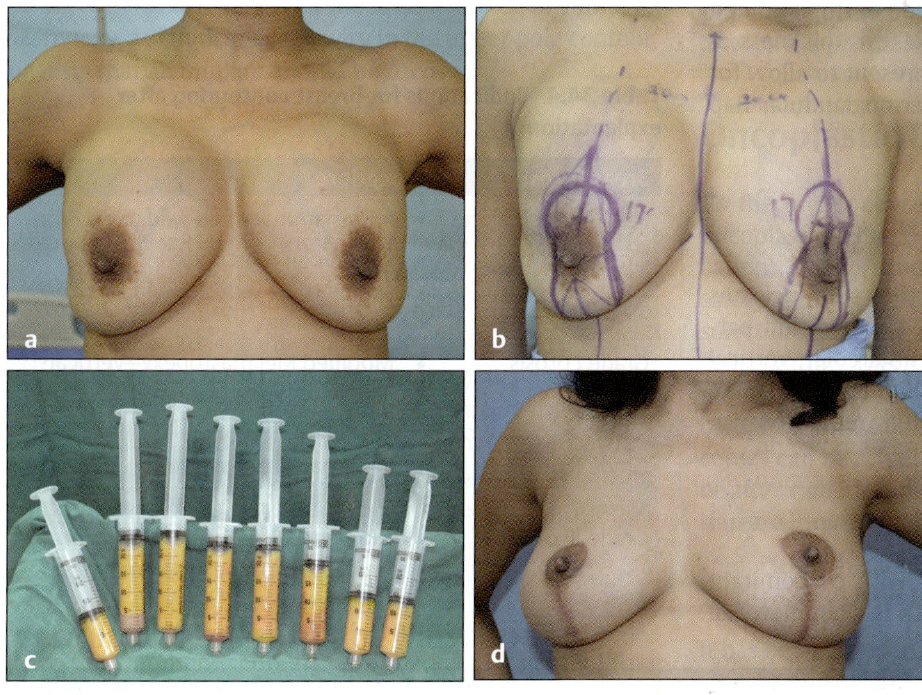

Fig. 34.40 Explantation mastopexy. **(a)** Waterfall deformity. **(b)** Vertical mastopexy plan. **(c)** Fat graft was used to augment after explantation and pexy. **(d)** Three months postoperative image.

used with less of resections. When tissues to be removed are far greater than that to be retained, planning and execution would appear relatively easier than in mastopexy where a surgeon takes some time to learn how little objective elevation is required to bring the nipple to the proper level in a lax small breast where holding and marking itself is very demanding.

In an attempt to rearrange the fallen tissues to add volume and uplift of the nipple complex, the final appearance will show an unnatural flatness to the inferior aspect. These patients must be counseled about this flatness which will correct itself within the first 2 months after surgery. This autocorrection may go beyond the acceptable level to a point of relapse of ptosis which may be cautioned early itself and prepare the patients for possible revision after 6 months.

Combined mastopexy augmentation makes use of a device (implant) that is designed to expand and add volume to the breast with an operation that is structured to lift and tighten the tissue. These opposing forces may end up with difficulties in obtaining expected shape, projection, and volume in addition to the risk of increased complications such as delayed wound healing and exposure of implants, unfavorable scars with capsular contracture.

The recent addition of autologous fat transfer along with mastopexy seems to have a balanced outcome.

Surgical Principles and Procedures

The demand for breast lift and volume augmentation seems to have increased among Indian women.

The upliftment includes the following four options:

1. Mastopexy with modest reduction.
2. Mastopexy alone when tissue volume is adequate.
3. Augmentation combined with mastopexy when there is tissue deficiency.
4. Explantation followed by concomitant mastopexy.

In volume-deficient mastopexy situations, subcutaneous transfer of autologous fat is another useful procedure to augment and rejuvenate the breast (**Fig. 34.40a–d**).

These four different options are sometimes subjective to both patients and surgeons. The end result should balance both to have a satisfied patient.

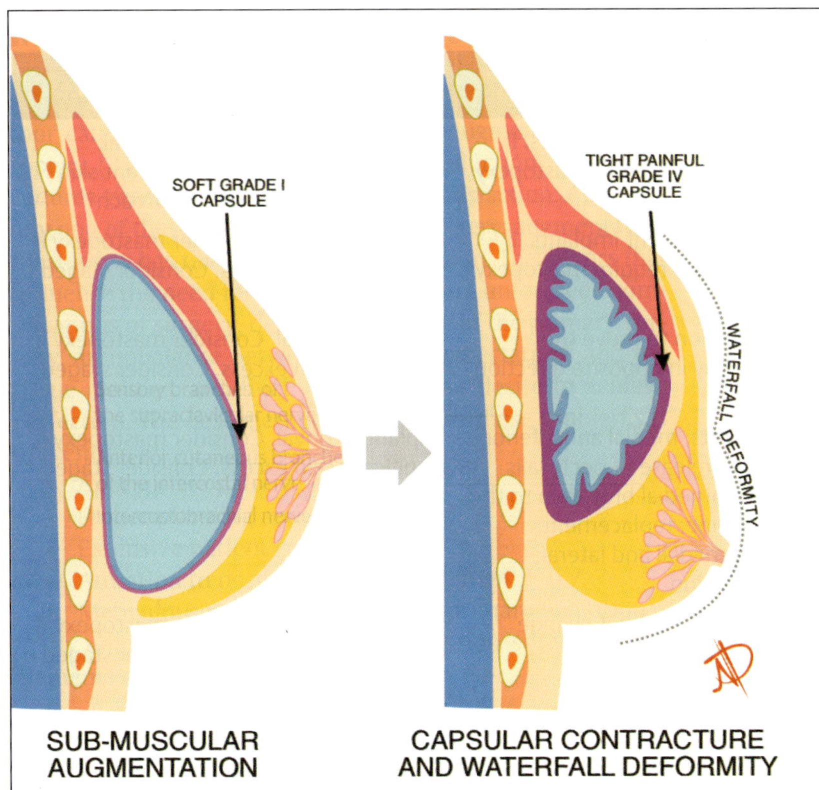

Fig. 35.2 Comparison of the submuscular breast augmentation with Baker grade I capsular contracture versus grade IV and its associated waterfall deformity.

Table 35.2 Original Baker classification of capsular contracture after augmentation mammoplasty[6]

Class I	Breast absolutely natural; no one could tell the breast was augmented
Class II	Minimal contracture; I can tell surgery was performed, but patient has no complaint
Class III	Moderate contracture; patient feels some firmness
Class IV	Severe contracture; obvious just from observation

have been associated with minimal encapsulation.[9] With the awareness of higher incidence of ALCL cases with polyurethane-coated implants, their usage has diminished.[3]

The options available to deal with the capsule are removal of the implant and capsulectomy with or without a replacement with new implants. Access must always be through the inframammary incision, even if the primary augmentation was through another route. This allows for the best access to all parts of the capsule and prevents malposition of the new implant.

The removal is best done in two steps. The implant capsule is opened, and the implant removed first, even in case of a rupture, and the cavity is wiped clean of silicone gel, followed by a total capsulectomy (**Fig. 35.3**). En bloc capsulectomy, which is a misnomer indicating removal of implant with an intact capsule, is not indicated here.[10] The removal of the implant with an intact capsule carries a lot more difficulties and morbidities. This is especially so in a subpectoral augmentation, in a thin patient and a large implant. It would require a much longer incision and has a potential to even cause a pneumothorax, with no advantage to the patient. The indication for an en bloc capsulectomy is limited only to a case of anaplastic large cell carcinoma.[11,12]

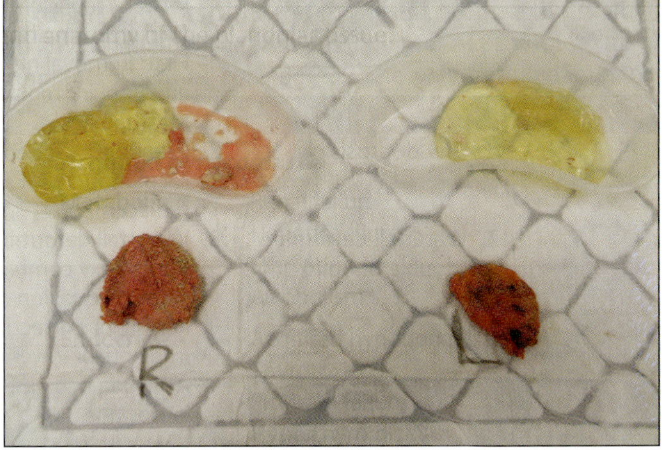

Fig. 35.3 Removal of a ruptured silicone gel implant followed by a total capsulectomy.

In cases with capsular contracture change of the implant pocket from submammary to submuscular is best avoided alongside a capsulectomy. In cases where the breast parenchyma is thinned out and the skin has lost its tone, an exchange of the pocket will allow the denuded anterior surface of the pectoralis to adhere to the undersurface of the skin and will lead to the tethering of the skin/thinned out pectoralis major. This will lead to puckering of the skin with contraction of the pectoralis major muscle.

The footplate of the breast may be violated during a capsulectomy. It is important to assess the footprint, and at times lateral or inferior extensions of the pocket need closure. This is usually done with 2–0 vicryl interrupted sutures.

Meticulous hemostasis of the cavity is essential, as hemorrhage from the denuded pectoralis major muscle or the undersurface of the breast parenchyma is a dreaded complication of this procedure. The serous drainage from the drains for a prolonged period is a common feature of this operation.

Replacement of the implant following capsulectomy is the most preferred option (**Fig. 35.4**). This allows for the skin envelope to be filled and has a better aesthetic outcome. A small number of patients choose not to have a replacement. The aesthetic outcomes in these cases are dependent on the size of the implant removed, amount of the breast parenchyma, and quality of the breast skin envelope. In cases where a large implant is removed, with limited breast parenchyma and stretched skin envelope, there will be significant ptosis (**Fig. 35.5**).

Implant Infection

Infection following primary breast augmentation is around 1.5%. Typically, patients present with symptoms within the first week, although delayed infections up to a few months can occur. Typical symptoms are pain, swelling, erythema, temperature, and occasionally discharge from the incision site. Access to the breast pocket via the inframammary fold (IMF) has the lowest rates of infection. Early antibiotics can be of help, although these patients are likely to develop

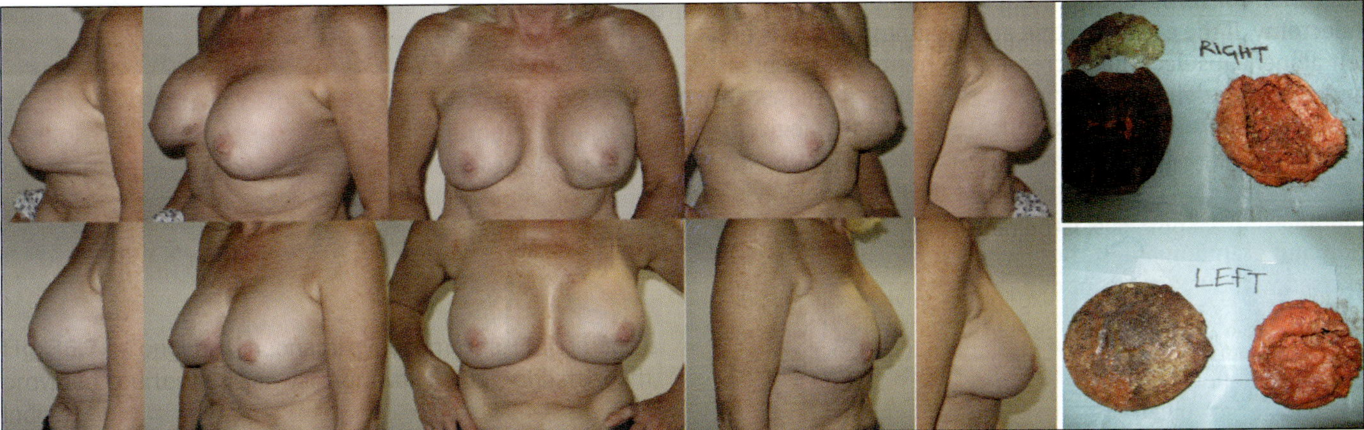

Fig. 35.4 Bilateral submuscular augmentation performed 22 years earlier. She presented with Baker IV capsular contracture and extracapsular rupture of the left breast implant with silicone extravasation in the medial part of the inframammary crease and a "waterfall deformity." The implants were removed, total capsulectomy performed, the inframammary fold was controlled on the left side, with replacement of the implants.

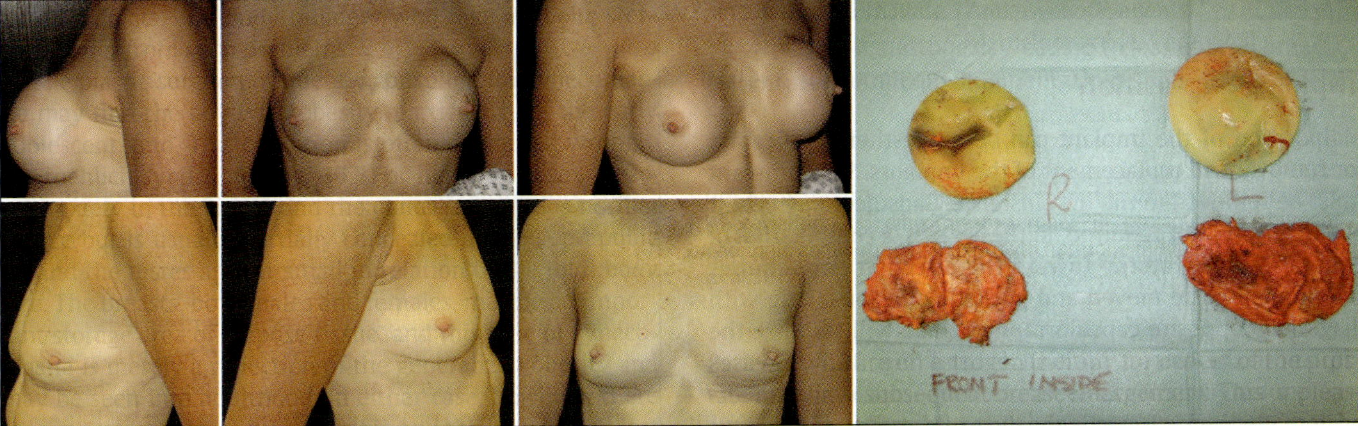

Fig. 35.5 A 30-year-old submammary augmentation with Baker IV capsular contracture, bilateral rupture (magnetic resonance imaging [MRI]), treated with bilateral implant removal and total capsulectomies. The postoperative photos demonstrate loss of volume, ptosis, and skin folds.

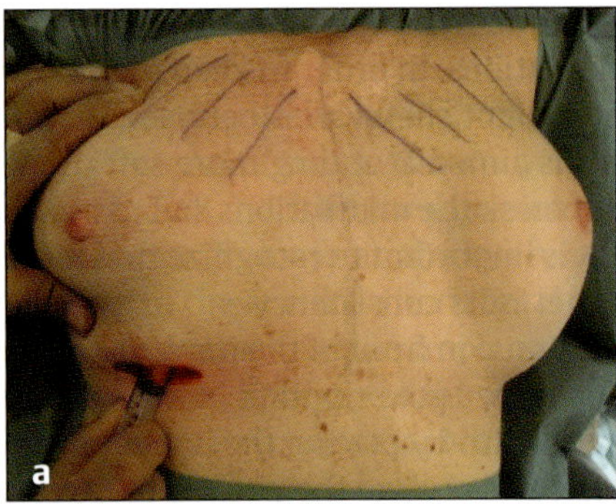

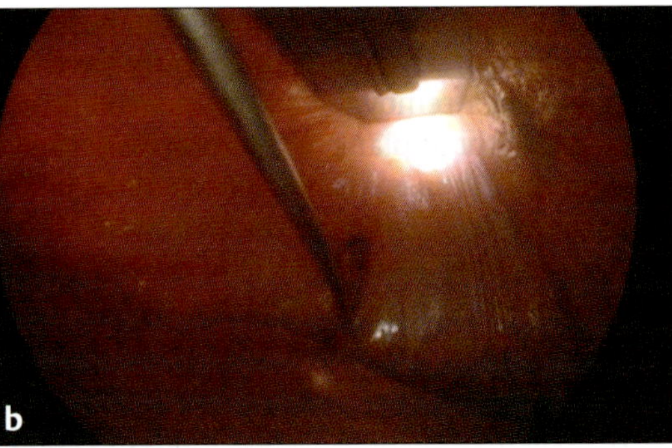

Fig. 35.12 **(a)** Implant removal and lipofilling through the capsule into space between the capsule and the dermis. **(b)** View from within the implant capsule, with retraction of the anterior capsule with a lighted retractor and infiltration of the fat through a puncture in the anterior capsule from within.

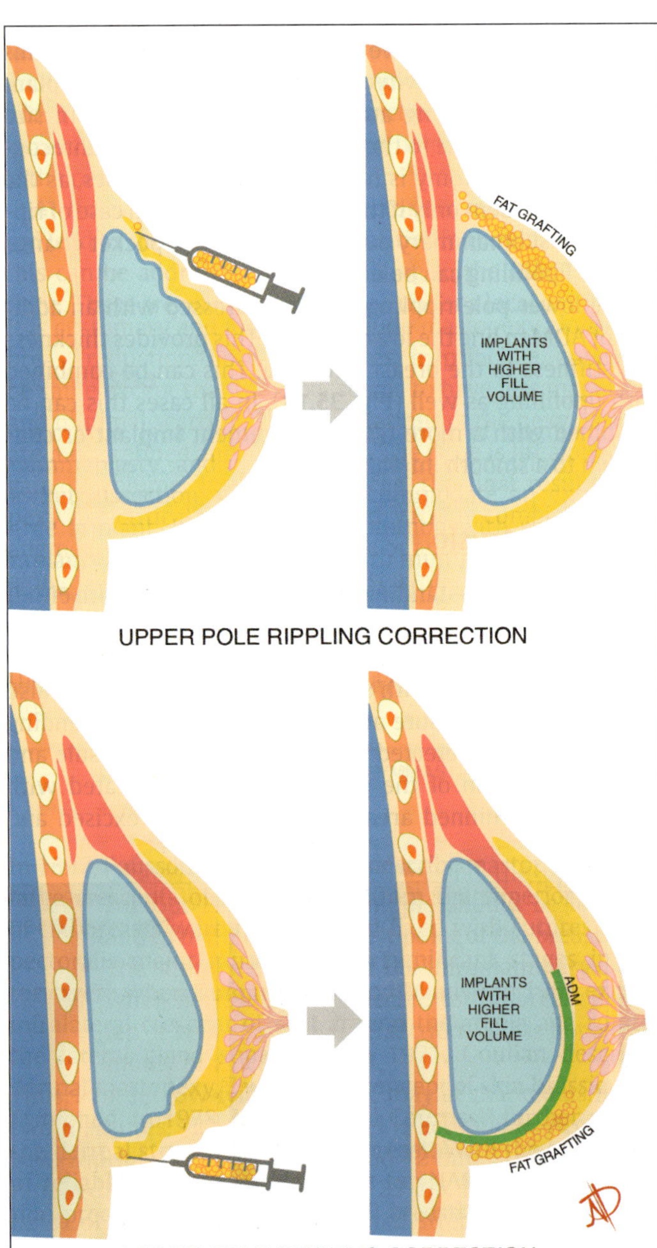

Fig. 35.13 Correction of rippling at the upper and lower poles of the breast with lipofilling and the use of acellular dermal matrix (ADM).

soft tissues sutured over this in layers, which can alter the breast shape. A more robust way would be to excise this and remove the implant to allow the tissues to recover. A new implant can be placed in a submuscular pocket with or without an ADM.

Deflation of Saline Implants

Although not commonly used in our practice, saline implants occasionally do have a role. These implants have the inherent risks of deflation following failure of the implant shell which is more common in textured surfaced implants and those that are underfilled. Treatment involves removing the implant and replacement.

Delayed Sudden Onset Swelling of the Breast

Sudden onset of swelling of the breast many years following the augmentation can be quite disconcerting for both the patient and the surgeon. At times, this is due to a blunt force trauma or unusual exertion of the upper body, such as in sports. But most often this is spontaneous without any particular event. It is essential to aspirate the fluid under ultrasound guidance and send it for cytology. This is to rule out ALCL, albeit extremely rare.[23]

Aspiration of the fluid, resting the arm to avoid excursion of the pectoralis major, and anti-inflammatory drugs are recommended. Majority of patients respond to this. In cases the fluid recurs, removal of the implant, capsulectomy, and replacement are options.

Breast Implant Associated–Anaplastic Large Cell Lymphoma

Breast implant associated–ALCL is a rare but severe complication of breast augmentation.[24] The presentation is acute onset swelling or fluid accumulation in the breast or around an implant, pain, changes in the shape of the breast, and, in some instances, axillary lymphadenitis. Aspiration of the fluid and cytology is mandatory. If proven, the treatment is *en bloc* removal of the implant and the capsule, with or without axillary clearance. Rare cases may require chemotherapy.

Revision Surgery Following Primary Augmentation Mastopexy

This forms a small part of the augmentation practice. Although some centers perform limited periareolar skin resection at the time of an augmentation, in many cases, a full-blown mastopexy with augmentation is limited in numbers. It is by far the most complication-prone aesthetic breast surgery and a leading cause for unsatisfied patients in breast surgery.[25] It has an inherent weakness—by making a pocket for the implant the blood supply to the breast parenchyma and the NAC from the chest wall perforators is lost. This combined with periareolar incision and elevation of the skin reduces the blood supply further. The tightening of the skin over the implant and freed breast tissue further compresses the blood supply, compounded by edema in the postoperative period. Hence, this procedure combines the complications of augmentation, mastopexy, and that of loss of vascularity to the parenchyma and NAC. The first two sets of complications will be discussed under augmentation and mastopexy sections of this chapter.

Nipple-Areolar Compromise

Partial or total loss of NAC, with or without parenchymal loss or fat necrosis, is a devastating sequela of an augmentation mastopexy, albeit it is rare. This is always associated with implant loss. Hence it is essential to appreciate the blood supply to the breast tissues after breast augmentation (**Fig. 35.14**). The wounds must be fully healed, and the scars supple prior to any intervention. A combination of scar revisions, lipofilling, areolar tattooing, and placement of an implant may be considered in stages. Reconstruction of the nipple is usually not possible due to scarring.

Recurrent Ptosis

The inherent loss of skin tone, along with the weight of the implant, contributes to recurrence of the ptosis. Revision mastopexy without capsulectomy, is a safe procedure. If the patient desires a much larger implant to fill the stretched skin envelope or the atrophied breast parenchyma, this can be considered. However, in a patient with recurrent ptosis, increase in the weight of the implant will lead to further ptosis in a short period of time. Further, the ligamentous structures between the dermis and the underlying tissues are severed by the process of elevation of the skin flaps in a mastopexy. Their support to the breast, albeit stretched already, is lost following a mastopexy (**Fig. 35.15**). Hence, recurrence of the ptosis, with or without the weight of the implant, is an understandable consequence.

Poor Scar

Scars which are stretched following an augmentation mastopexy are a common problem. Revision of these can be performed under a local anesthetic. The periareolar scars are

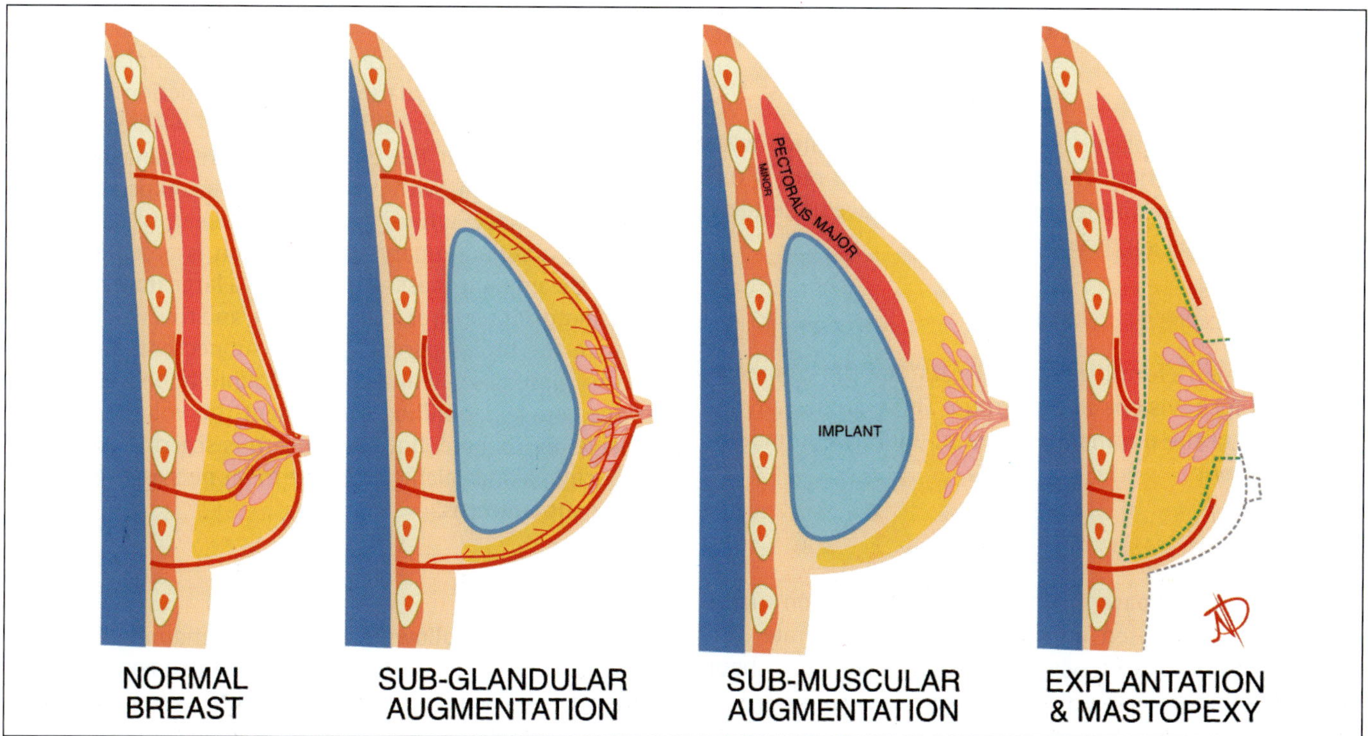

Fig. 35.14 Blood supply of a normal breast, augmented breast, and that in which explantation and mastopexy have been performed.

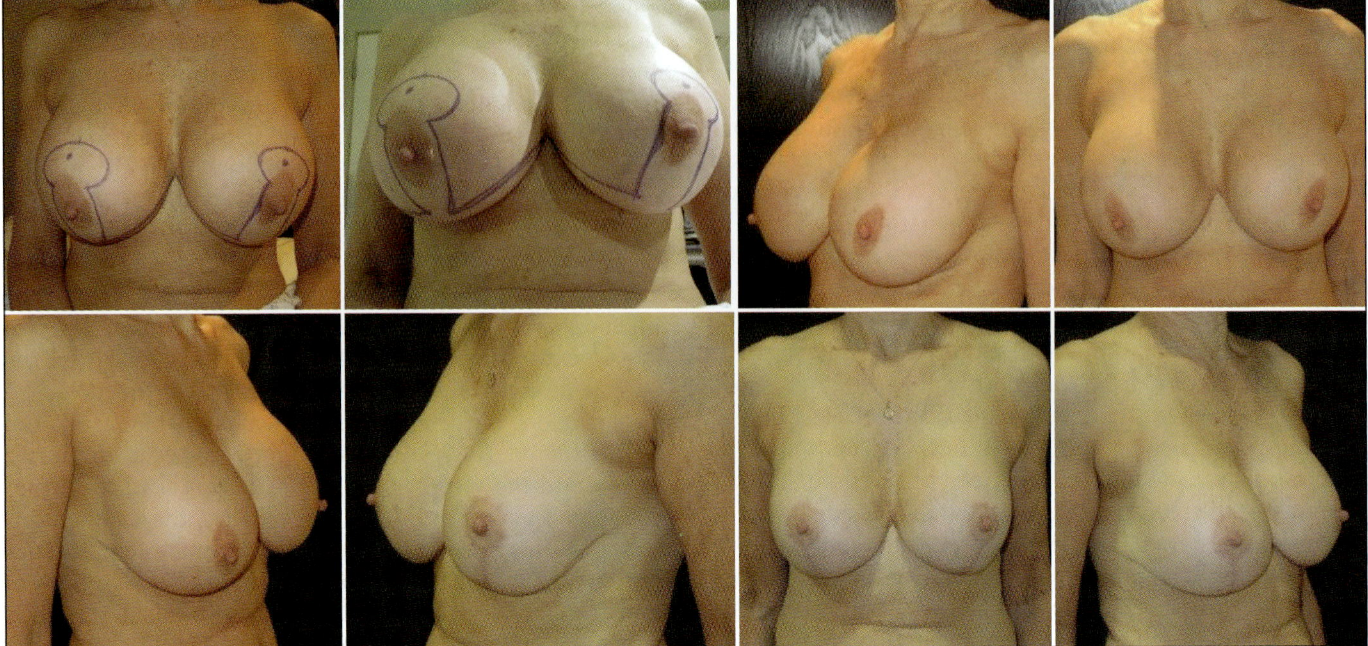

Fig. 35.15 Bilateral subglandular implants performed many years ago. Postpartum ptosis treated with removal of implants, replacement with smaller implants, and mastopexies. Note that capsulectomies were NOT performed in order to maintain the blood supply to the nipple-areolar complex (NAC).

subjected to a centrifugal force constantly and are difficult to prevent from widening. Benelli-type blocking sutures are of minimal benefit in the short term only.

Revision Surgery Following Reduction Mammaplasty

Reduction mammaplasty is an aesthetic procedure with a functional indication. The patient satisfaction rate is the highest of all the aesthetic breast procedures we undertake. However, revision surgeries are common.

Standing Cone Deformities

Standing Cone Deformities or "dog-ears" are the commonest reason for revisions in this group. These are usually on either ends of the inframammary scar, undertaken under a local anesthetic.

Breast Asymmetry

Asymmetry or increase in size, following reduction mammaplasty, is addressed only if significant. Moderate size reduction can be dealt with liposuction with or without skin tightening along the previous scars. A secondary breast reduction is best avoided, due to the risk to the vascularity of the nipple, especially if the details of the primary surgery are not available. In the event this is attempted without the knowledge of the pedicles used in the primary reduction, a free nipple graft technique is preferable.

Excessive Breast Reduction

Excessive reduction in size is an unusual complaint in this group of patients. Estimating the exact reduction amount in the primary surgery is difficult and learnt with experience. It is important that the expectations are managed in the primary operation, with regard to the size expectations. In the rare instance, where the patient is keen to have a size increase, a submammary augmentation is acceptable. The size of the implant must be modest, as a large implant with a large footprint requires a large pocket, and this would devascularize the breast parenchyma. A subpectoral augmentation in these cases will lead to a double bubble deformity in due course. Lipofilling to augment the volume is a reasonable option here, but the concern is scarring within the parenchyma and calcification due to fat necrosis, leading to diagnostic concerns.

Recurrent Ptosis

Recurrent ptosis following a reduction mammaplasty can be addressed by a simple skin-only mastopexy. In these instances, the undermining of the skin flaps has to be minimal. Use of synthetic slings in these cases is best avoided due to the levels of mobilization required.

Nipple-Areolar Loss

Nipple necrosis is a devastating complication of reduction mammaplasty, but fortunately rare. This is usually due to an enthusiastic attempt to elevate the NAC, with a pedicle, in a patient with a very low nipple position to begin with. Intraoperatively, if the nipple perfusion becomes difficult, it must be converted into a free nipple graft technique.

Loss of an NAC is accompanied by surrounding fat necrosis. A resection of the scar and the areas of fat necrosis in the first instance, to achieve primary healing of the wounds, followed by nipple reconstruction, areolar tattooing, lipofilling, or augmentation in multiple stages may be required.

Patients who have already undergone a previous breast reduction with an unknown pedicle or those in which a significant movement of the NAC is required may benefit from a free nipple graft technique (**Fig. 35.16**).

Nipple Malposition

Nipple malposition can occur when the nipple is too high, low, lateral, or medial. The latter three are easier to correct. In these cases, crescentic excision of breast skin in the direction of the new nipple position is required, in addition to refashioning the breast skin flaps around the new nipple-areolar position.

A nipple that is too high is more difficult to correct. If the primary issue is bottoming-out of the breast parenchyma, the nipple can be left in its position, and an elliptical excision of the lower pole of the breast skin and tissues along the IMF will give the appearance of a lower NAC on the breast mound. If this is not possible, then the nipple will require moving by repositioning either using a free nipple graft, with a skin graft above it, or using a V-Y technique. Either of these techniques leaves a scar higher on the breast and can show over brassiere.

Breast Cancer

Malignancy in the breast reduction specimen is again a rare but severe sequela.[26] In these cases, a mastectomy is the only option with or without primary breast reconstruction. We advocate the use of preoperative imaging in those patients close to screening age for breast cancer or those with significant family history, as a proportion of these patients may benefit from therapeutic mammaplasty techniques rather than requiring a mastectomy.

Poor Scars

Scars from a reduction mammaplasty can be hypertrophic or form keloids at times. Patients at greatest risk include young, dark-skinned patients especially Asians and Afro-Caribbeans. Shorter scar techniques such as vertical and L-shaped patterns can be helpful in the smaller breast. Unfortunately, these shorter scar techniques have a higher rate of touch-up surgery as they have a steeper learning curve compared to a standard Wise pattern technique.

In a Wise pattern reduction, it is more common to see thicker scars in the lateral and medial ends of the inframammary scars. Silicone tapes, injections of triamcinolone acetonide, or rarely scar revisions are used to deal with this. Stretching of the scars, especially at the vertical component of the scar, can be dealt with a simple revision.

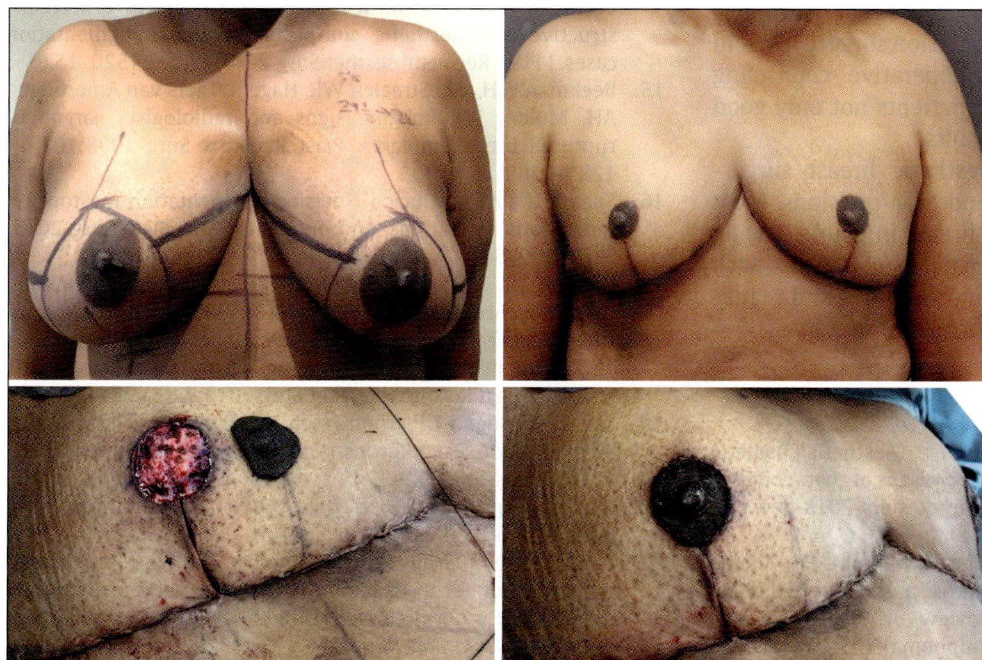

Fig. 35.16 Breast reduction with free nipple graft technique in a patient who had undergone a previous breast reduction with an unknown pedicle 20 years ago.

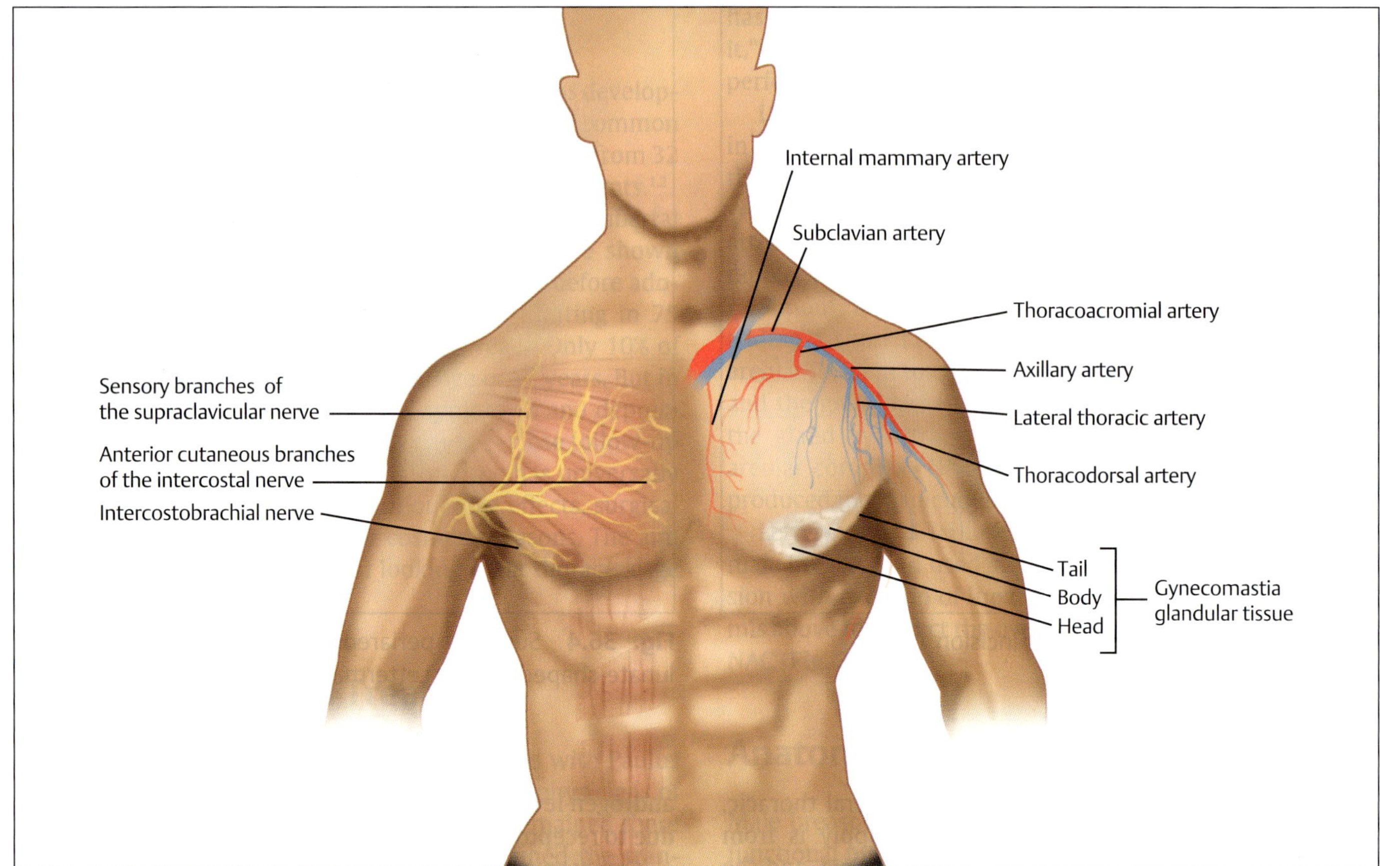

Fig. 36.5 The blood supply and innervation of the male breast and anatomy of the glandular tissue.

Box 36.1 Causes of congenital and acquired gynecomastia

Congenital gynecomastia	
Physiological gynecomastia	
	Neonatal
	Prepubertal
	Elderly
Pathologic factors	
Hypogonadal	Androgen resistance
	Enzymatic deficiency of testosterone synthesis
	Congenital anarchism
	Klinefelter syndrome
Hyperestrogenic	True hermaphroditism
	Congenital adrenal hyperplasia
	Elevated peripheral aromatase

Acquired gynecomastia	
Metabolic	Renal failure
	Hepatic failure
	Starvation
	Alcoholism
Endocrine	Acquired hypogonadism
	Thyrotoxicosis
	Pituitary failure
	Hyperthyroidism
	Anabolic steroids for body building
Neoplastic	Adrenal tumors
	Testicular tumors
	HCG-producing tumors
	Bronchogenic carcinoma
	Pituitary tumors
Miscellaneous	Chest wall trauma
	Spinal cord injury
	Psychological stress
	HIV infection
	Herpes zoster infection

Abbreviations: HCG, human chorionic gonadotropin; HIV, human immunodeficiency virus.
Source: Adapted from Glass.[9]

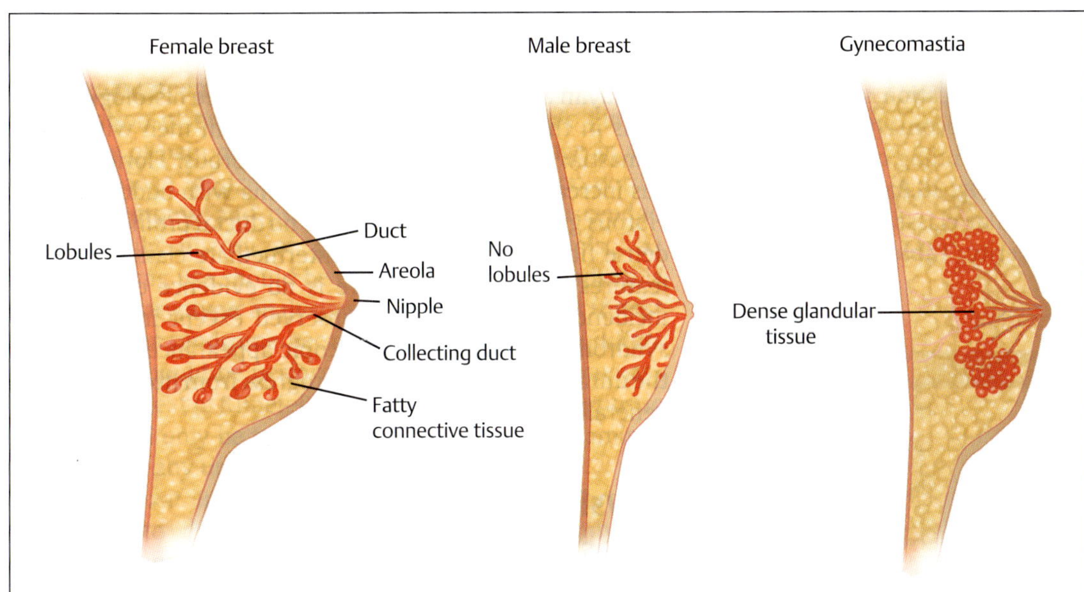

Fig. 36.6 Architecture of the female breast, the normal male breast, and gynecomastia.

Fig. 36.7 Congenital neonatal gynecomastia. (This image is provided courtesy Dr Sanwar Agrawal, Raipur, Chhattisgarh, India.)

Acquired gynecomastia may be pathological or pharmacological. Pathological causes can be primarily endocrine, metabolic, or neoplastic (**Box 36.1**). Gynecomastia may also be caused by numerous drugs which alter the estrogen or testosterone concentrations (**Table 36.1**).[2,13] Marijuana and heroin addicts, and body builders who take anabolic steroids, suffer from such problems.

The plastic surgeon frequently consulted for gynecomastia may find the boy with obesity, particularly of the early adolescent kind. This condition is often diagnosed wrongly as Froehlich syndrome (**Fig. 36.5**) or hypogonadism, creating anxiety in the family and the child. The penis is normal in size but is usually partially concealed in the suprapubic fat and the testes appear small in relation to the total body size. The breasts, both males and females, may be an important storage area of adipose tissue, and this type of gynecomastia is merely a reflection of the generalized obesity and may be seen into adulthood. In either case, however, there is no mammary tissue hypertrophy, and the breast is almost completely composed of adipose tissue.

Gynecomastia also is seen in patients of testicular tumors including chorionepithelioma, seminoma, and teratoma.[14]

Table 36.1 Mechanisms leading to gynecomastia

Mechanism leading to gynecomastia	Drugs causing gynecomastia
Increased serum estrogen	Estrogens, including topical preparations Aromatisable androgens hCG
Estrogen like activity, Decreased serum Testosterone or DHT	Digitoxin, herbal products GnRH agonist or antagonist Leydig cell damage or inhibition Ketoconazole, Metronidazole Spironolactone, Cancer chemotherapy Finasteride or dutasteride
Androgen receptor blockers	Flutamide, bicalutamide Spironolactone Cimetidine, Marijuana
Increased serum PRL	Anti psychotic agents Metoclopramide, Verapamil
Mechanism uncertain	Isoniazid, Amiodarone Antidepressants Human GH, Proton pump inhibitors Highly active retroviral therapy

Abbreviation: DHT, dihydrotestosterone; PRL, prolactin; hCG, human chorionic gonadotropin; GH, growth hormone (Adapted from Sansome et al 2017).[15]

Patients who are on estrogen therapy for cancer of the prostate may have subsequent breast enlargement. This unpleasant and uncomfortable result of necessary treatment may be minimized by the administration of small doses of radiation to the breast but surgical correction is also possible once the condition has stabilized.

Surgical Steps

Surgical steps in gynecomastia through periareolar incision are diagrammatically presented in **Fig. 36.12**.

A small semicircular incision is placed within the areola skin junction (**Figs. 36.10, 36.12a, and 36.13a**). The incision is carried down to the breast capsule.

In nonobese patients, the capsule is well defined. In the fatty or poorly defined enlargement, incision is deepened to 10 to 15 mm. At this point, the skin overlying the breast below the incision is undermined leaving a protective pad of uniform thickness of subcutaneous tissue on the undersurface of the mobilized skin (**Fig. 36.13c**). It must be noted that a thin skin flap over the denuded pectoral fascia will leave a depression as unsightly as the original condition. At the limits of the excision which is usually marked on the surface before the incision, the dissection deepens to bevel or feather the periphery of the disc of breast tissue and/or fat to be removed (**Fig. 36.13d**).

Attention is now turned to freeing the superior half of the superficial fascia of the breast mass. Hooks or Allis forceps or stay sutures are used at the edge of the areola and is pulled toward the operator. The breast mass is incised in a

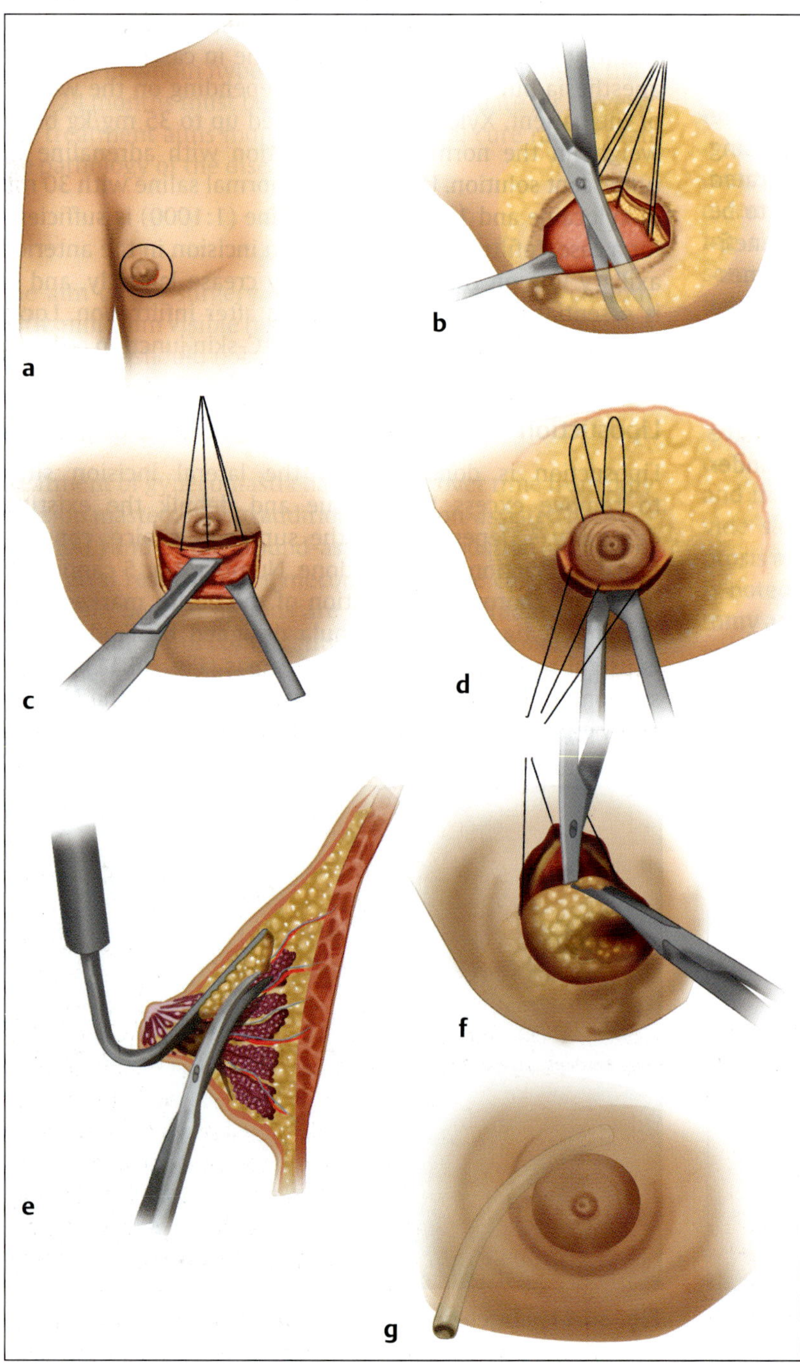

Fig. 36.12 Surgical steps in gynecomastia through periareolar incision. **(a)** Incision in the inferior periareolar margin from 3 to 9 o'clock. **(b)** Separating the skin from the anterior breast in the inferior pole. **(c)** Cutting of nipple and areola, leaving a thick button of tissue below the nipple-areolar complex (NAC). **(d)** Separating the skin from the breast in the superior pole. **(e)** Tapering of the breast in the edges and use of illuminated retractor. **(f)** Separating the breast at the depth from the pectoral fascia. **(g)** Final closure using subcuticular suture with (or without) a drain.

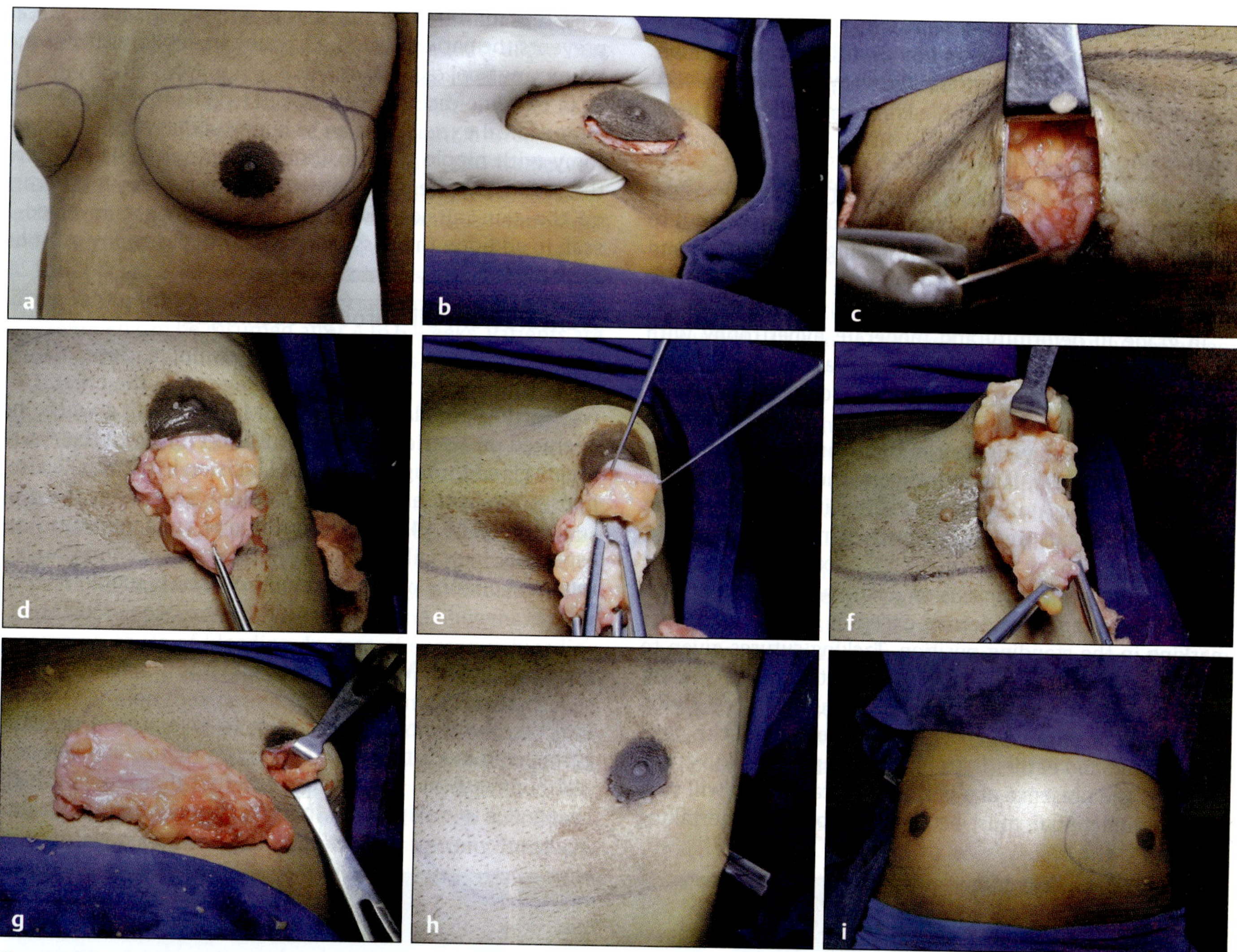

Fig. 36.13 **(a)** Dotted marking at the incision. **(b)** Periareolar incision at the junction of the areola and skin. **(c)** Separating the inferior pole of the gland from the skin. **(d)** Delivery of the inferior pole of the gland through the incision. **(e)** Dissecting through the gland till the upper pole leaving a button of sufficient thickness of gland below the areola. **(f)** The gland freed from all sides delivered through the incision. **(g)** The excised gland with the head, body, and tail. **(h)** Areolar incision meticulously closed with a drain. **(i)** The result at the end of the procedure.

plane parallel to the surface leaving a button or disc of tissue of uniform thickness attached to the nipple. This is usually 10 to 15 mm thick and designed to prevent depression or retraction of nipple (**Fig. 36.13e**). It is wise to leave a somewhat thicker button then one may have thought necessary, as further removal can be done later. The dissection is continued beyond the areola until the anterior face of the breast has been freed (**Fig. 36.13e**).

The gland can be removed in several ways. The gland is grasped and freed from the pectoral fascia using blunt finger dissection or sharp dissection as desired by the operator. When the gland is very large and the edge is difficult to visualize, it may be necessary to split it vertically and remove it into sections. Beveling the edge of the specimen is advisable to secure a more smooth transition at the periphery of the dissection (**Fig. 36.13f**).

After removing the gland the dead space is inspected and irregularities of fatty contours are trimmed carefully (**Fig. 36.13g**). Hemostasis is secured, the cavity is irrigated, and the incision is not closed until the surgery on the second side is completed. Final inspection for symmetry and hemostasis is done and inspection of the contour of the chest may reveal areas where fat removal has been incomplete or irregular or where the contour is not pleasing. This should be corrected. In case of any doubt, drain must be left which could be using a large suction catheter on each side or corrugated drains (**Fig. 36.13h**). The incisions are closed using subcutaneous absorbable sutures, usually of 3–0 Monocryl and subcuticular absorbable suture or skin sutures which need to be cut (**Fig. 36.13i**).

Surgery of gynecomastia requires wide subcutaneous dissection via a disproportionately small incision. Problems

S